Laboratory Diagnosis of Bacterial Infections

INFECTIOUS DISEASE AND THERAPY

Series Editor

Burke A. Cunha

Winthrop-University Hospital
Mineola, and
State University of New York School of Medicine
Stony Brook, New York

1. Parasitic Infections in the Compromised Host, *edited by Peter D. Walzer and Robert M. Genta*
2. Nucleic Acid and Monoclonal Antibody Probes: Applications in Diagnostic Methodology, *edited by Bala Swaminathan and Gyan Prakash*
3. Opportunistic Infections in Patients with the Acquired Immunodeficiency Syndrome, *edited by Gifford Leoung and John Mills*
4. Acyclovir Therapy for Herpesvirus Infections, *edited by David A. Baker*
5. The New Generation of Quinolones, *edited by Clifford Siporin, Carl L. Heifetz, and John M. Domagala*
6. Methicillin-Resistant *Staphylococcus aureus*: Clinical Management and Laboratory Aspects, *edited by Mary T. Cafferkey*
7. Hepatitis B Vaccines in Clinical Practice, *edited by Ronald W. Ellis*
8. The New Macrolides, Azalides, and Streptogramins: Pharmacology and Clinical Applications, *edited by Harold C. Neu, Lowell S. Young, and Stephen H. Zinner*
9. Antimicrobial Therapy in the Elderly Patient, *edited by Thomas T. Yoshikawa and Dean C. Norman*
10. Viral Infections of the Gastrointestinal Tract: Second Edition, Revised and Expanded, *edited by Albert Z. Kapikian*
11. Development and Clinical Uses of Haemophilus b Conjugate Vaccines, *edited by Ronald W. Ellis and Dan M. Granoff*
12. *Pseudomonas aeruginosa* Infections and Treatment, *edited by Aldona L. Baltch and Raymond P. Smith*
13. Herpesvirus Infections, *edited by Ronald Glaser and James F. Jones*
14. Chronic Fatigue Syndrome, *edited by Stephen E. Straus*
15. Immunotherapy of Infections, *edited by K. Noel Masihi*
16. Diagnosis and Management of Bone Infections, *edited by Luis E. Jauregui*
17. Drug Transport in Antimicrobial and Anticancer Chemotherapy, *edited by Nafsika H. Georgopapadakou*
18. New Macrolides, Azalides, and Streptogramins in Clinical Practice, *edited by Harold C. Neu, Lowell S. Young, Stephen H. Zinner, and Jacques F. Acar*
19. Novel Therapeutic Strategies in the Treatment of Sepsis, *edited by David C. Morrison and John L. Ryan*
20. Catheter-Related Infections, *edited by Harald Seifert, Bernd Jansen, and Barry M. Farr*
21. Expanding Indications for the New Macrolides, Azalides, and Strepto-gramins, *edited by Stephen H. Zinner, Lowell S. Young, Jacques F. Acar, and Harold C. Neu*
22. Infectious Diseases in Critical Care Medicine, *edited by Burke A. Cunha*

23. New Considerations for Macrolides, Azalides, Streptogramins, and Ketolides, *edited by Stephen H. Zinner, Lowell S. Young, Jacques F. Acar, and Carmen Ortiz-Neu*

24. Tickborne Infectious Diseases: Diagnosis and Management, *edited by Burke A. Cunha*

25. Protease Inhibitors in AIDS Therapy, *edited by Richard C. Ogden and Charles W. Flexner*

26. Laboratory Diagnosis of Bacterial Infections, *edited by Nevio Cimolai*

Additional Volumes in Production

Antimicrobial Pharmacodynamics in Theory and Clinical Practice, *edited by Charles H. Nightingale, Takeo Murakawa, and Paul G. Ambrose*

Laboratory Diagnosis of
Bacterial Infections

edited by
Nevio Cimolai
Children's and Women's Health Centre
Vancouver, British Columbia, Canada

MARCEL DEKKER, INC.   NEW YORK · BASEL

ISBN: 0-8247-0589-0

This book is printed on acid-free paper.

Headquarters
Marcel Dekker, Inc.
270 Madison Avenue, New York, NY 10016
tel: 212-696-9000; fax: 212-685-4540

Eastern Hemisphere Distribution
Marcel Dekker AG
Hutgasse 4, Postfach 812, CH-4001 Basel, Switzerland
tel: 41-61-261-8482; fax: 41-61-261-8896

World Wide Web
http://www.dekker.com

The publisher offers discounts on this book when ordered in bulk quantities. For more information, write to Special Sales/Professional Marketing at the headquarters address above.

Current printing (last digit):
10 9 8 7 6 5 4 3 2 1

PRINTED IN THE UNITED STATES OF AMERICA

Preface

The science relating to infection has expanded exponentially, and we are all no doubt aware of the difficulties of attempting to assimilate this new knowledge. There are many texts that eloquently describe the clinical aspects of infectious diseases, as well as several that lay out in detail the mechanics of procedure and methodology. Our book makes no pretense of providing voluminous detail on either. Rather, as in the *Laboratory Diagnosis of Viral Infections, Second Edition, Revised and Expanded*, edited by Dr. Edwin E. Lennette (Marcel Dekker, Inc., 1991), we propose that the need is to provide timely and pointed material for the laboratorian and diagnostician to use in selecting and applying diagnostic maneuvers for everyday practice.

Over a decade ago, many predicted that molecular technologies would render most classical diagnostic methods obsolete. Although the trend toward molecular diagnostics increases, there has developed a hybrid of classical and new methods; both equally important no matter how simple or complex. The balance of emphases will no doubt continue to shift in the direction of molecular techniques but perhaps more so due to the increasing number of new pathogens and new disease associations. The chapters by Alex van Belkum and Wil Goessens, David Fredricks, and Marc Struelens highlight this change, its impact, and its future potential. The science, while becoming complex, has nevertheless led to very exciting times for diagnosticians.

New basic science begets new medicine. Within a short period of time, new pathogens have been identified at an unprecedented pace. The revolution in the field of immunocompromised hosts has led to a medical renaissance for bacteria which were in large part deemed innocuous. Old diseases have often been renamed "emerging infections." Given the state of the art, a new pathogen once defined quickly becomes studied to the point where diagnostic tools and genomics are recognized in a few short years. The chapter by Anna Sander on human bartonellosis serves to remind us how quickly progress can be made when scientific minds are so directed.

A primary purpose of diagnostic technologies is to establish certainty, but certainty of diagnosis necessarily evokes interventionist strategies, the most directly influenced being antimicrobial therapy. Antibiotic use, while critical to the beneficial outcome in many circumstances, has become a complex issue, as outlined by John Turnidge and Jan Bell. For many pathogenic bacteria, antimicrobial resistance continues to increase. Molecular techniques have become of value both to determine said resistance and to clarify the epidemiology of change.

The diagnostic laboratory cannot be viewed as a "stand-alone" entity. Its functions are intimately related to patient care and in many respects constitute a form of medical practice. As the applications of diagnostic bacteriology evolve, new diagnostic modes will likely emerge that are in a sense laboratory-based but not necessarily based in the formal microbiology laboratory. For example, John Holton and Dino Vaira illustrate this latter concept thoroughly in their chapter on gastric helicobacters.

Throughout the chapters, we have made use of dendrograms to illustrate the relationship of various bacteria. The intent here was not to provide detailed figures for illustrating DNA homologies but rather to provide a guide for those less acquainted with these relationships in general form.

Our world is as small or as large as we make it; the scientific community is no different. Over the last two decades especially, we have learned much about new diseases and new diagnostic techniques from our international colleagues. Lessons of the past have been rekindled. Globalization has forced us to renew our appreciation of the many communities in which we live in large part because of the various aspects of life that facilitate the transmission of infectious microbes. Accordingly, the input from several international scientists and laboratorians is a reflection of this diversity and of the need to share our knowledge globally. Along this line, I would like to thank Dr. Alasdair MacGowan of Bristol for his comments on Chapter 13. The need to continue sharing our knowledge in this fashion and to view the diverse multinational contributions as being essential to the "big picture" will no doubt remain.

Nevio Cimolai

Contents

Preface   *iii*
Contributors   *vii*

Part I: General Considerations for the Diagnosis of Bacterial Infections

1. A Role for Microscopy Continues   1
    Jochen Gottschalk and Alexander von Graevenitz

2. Applied Systematics   9
    John T. Magee

3. Critical Features of Specimen Collection, Transport, and Processing   33
    Chandar Anand and Nevio Cimolai

4. Serodiagnosis for Bacterial Infections   55
    Nevio Cimolai

5. Molecular Diagnostics: Present and Future   83
    Alex van Belkum and Wil Goessens

6. Searching for the Unknown   117
    David N. Fredricks

7. Molecular Epidemiology   125
    Marc Struelens

8. Determination of Resistance to Antibacterials   147
    John D. Turnidge and Jan M. Bell

9. Blood Culture Systems   189
    W. Michael Dunne, Jr. and Mark LaRocco

10. The Quality Laboratory 211
Nevio Cimolai

Part II: Specific Bacterial Infections

11. Staphylococcal Infections 229
Nevio Cimolai and Frank Espersen

12. Streptococcal and Enterococcal Infections 257
Graziella Orefici, Roberto Nisini, and Christina von Hunolstein

13. Gram Positive Bacilli: *Corynebacterium, Listeria, Bacillus*, and Others 333
Nevio Cimolai and Kathryn Bernard

14. Mycobacteria and Actinomycetes 377
Nevio Cimolai, William A. Black, and Adalbert Laszlo

15. *Enterobacteriaceae* and Enteric Infections 423
Nevio Cimolai, G. Balakrish Nair, Yoshifumi Takeda, and Luiz R. Trabulsi

16. Gram Negative Cocci and Moraxellae 499
Nevio Cimolai and Dominique A. Caugant

17. Gram Negative Infections: Pseudomonads and Other Gram Negative Non-Fermentative Bacteria 527
Kathryn Bernard

18. Gram Negative Infections: *Haemophilus* and Other Clinically Relevant Gram Negative Coccobacilli 557
Jose Campos and Juan A. Saez-Nieto

19. Gram Negative Infections: Gram Negative Zoonoses 581
C. Anthony Hart and Malcolm Bennett

20. Gastric Helicobacters 605
John Holton and Dino Vaira

21. Legionellosis 635
Janet E. Stout and John D. Rihs

22. Bartonellosis 653
Anna Sander

23. Whooping Cough (Pertussis) 687
James C. Paton

24. Anaerobic Infections 705
Nevio Cimolai

Contents

25. Borrelioses   747
   Nevio Cimolai, Jarmo Oksi, and Matti K. Viljanen

26. Treponemal and Other Spirochetoses   777
   Bruno L. Schmidt

27. Chlamydiae   795
   *Lee Ann Campbell, Jeanne M. Marazzo, Walter E. Stamm,
   and Cho-chou Kuo*

28. Rickettsioses (with Q Fever)   823
   Jean-Marc Rolain and Didier Raoult

29. Mycoplasmas   861
   Nevio Cimolai

Index   *893*

Contributors

Chandar Anand   Provincial Laboratory of Public Health for Southern Alberta, Calgary, Alberta, Canada

Jan M. Bell   Department of Microbiology and Infectious Diseases, Women's and Children's Hospital, North Adelaide, South Australia, Australia

Malcolm Bennett   Department of Veterinary Pathology, Centre for Comparative Infectious Diseases, University of Liverpool, Liverpool, England

Kathryn Bernard   Special Bacteriology Laboratory, Canadian Science Centre for Human and Animal Disease, Winnipeg, Manitoba, Canada

William A. Black   Department of Pathology and Laboratory Medicine, University of British Columbia, Vancouver, British Columbia, Canada

Lee Ann Campbell   Department of Pathobiology, University of Washington, Seattle, Washington

José Campos   Reference-Bacteriology Department, Centro Nacional de Microbiologia, Instituto de Salud Carlos III, Madrid, Spain

Dominique A. Caugant   Department of Bacteriology, WHO Collaborating Centre for Reference and Research on Meningococci, National Institute of Public Health, Oslo, Norway

Nevio Cimolai   Department of Pathology and Laboratory Medicine, Children's and Women's Health Centre of British Columbia, Vancouver, British Columbia, Canada

W. Michael Dunne, Jr.   Barnes-Jewish Hospital and Washington University School of Medicine, St. Louis, Missouri

Frank Espersen   Division of Microbiology, Statens Serum Institut, Copenhagen, Denmark

David N. Fredricks   Division of Infectious Diseases, Department of Medicine, Stanford University Medical Center, Stanford, California

Wil Goessens   Department of Medical Microbiology and Infectious Diseases, Erasmus University Medical Center Rotterdam, Rotterdam, The Netherlands

Jochen Gottschalk   Department of Medical Microbiology, University of Zurich, Zurich, Switzerland

C. Anthony Hart   Departments of Medical Microbiology and Genitourinary Medicine, Centre for Comparative Infectious Diseases, University of Liverpool, Liverpool, England

John Holton   Department of Bacteriology, Windeyer Institute of Medical Science, Royal Free and University College London Medical School, London, England

Cho-chou Kuo   Department of Pathobiology, University of Washington, Seattle, Washington

Mark LaRocco   Department of Pathology, St. Luke's Episcopal Health System, Houston, Texas

Adalbert Laszlo   IUATLD/WHO Consultant on Tuberculosis Bacteriology, Nepean, Ontario, Canada

John T. Magee   Department of Medical Microbiology and Public Health Laboratory, University of Wales College of Medicine, Cardiff, Wales

Jeanne M. Marazzo   Division of Allergy and Infectious Diseases, Department of Medicine, University of Washington, Seattle, Washington

G. Balakrish Nair   National Institute of Cholera and Enteric Diseases, Calcutta, India, and Laboratory Sciences Division, International Centre for Diarrhoeal Diseases, Dhaka, Bangladesh

Roberto Nisini   Laboratory of Bacteriology and Medical Mycology, Istituto Superiore di Sanitá, Rome, Italy

Jarmo Oksi   Department of Medicine, Turku University Central Hospital, and Department of Medical Microbiology, Turku University, Turku, Finland

Graziella Orefici   Laboratory of Bacteriology and Medical Mycology, Istituto Superiore di Sanitá, Rome, Italy

James C. Paton   Department of Molecular Biosciences, Adelaide University, Adelaide, South Australia, Australia

Didier Raoult   Unité des Rickettsies, Faculté de Médecine, Université de la Méditerranée, Marseille, France

John D. Rihs   Special Pathogens Laboratory, Department of Laboratory Medicine and Pathology, VA Medical Center, Pittsburgh, Pennsylvania

Jean-Marc Rolain   Unité des Rickettsies, Faculté de Médecine, Université de la Méditerranée, Marseille, France

Juan A. Saez-Nieto Bacteriology Department, Centro Nacional de Microbiología, Instituto de Salud Carlos III, Madrid, Spain

Anna Sander Department of Medical Microbiology and Hygiene, University of Freiburg, Freiburg, Germany

Bruno L. Schmidt Ludwig Boltzmann Institute of Dermato-Venerological Serodiagnostics, Hospital of the City of Vienna-Lainz, Vienna, Austria

Walter E. Stamm Division of Allergy and Infectious Diseases, Department of Medicine, University of Washington, Seattle, Washington

Janet E. Stout Infectious Disease Division, Pittsburgh VA Healthcare System, University of Pittsburgh, Pittsburgh, Pennsylvania

Marc Struelens Department of Microbiology, Hôpital Erasme—Université Libre de Bruxelles, Brussels, Belgium

Yoshifumi Takeda National Institute of Infectious Diseases, Tokyo, Japan

Luiz R. Trabulsi Laboratorio Especial de Microbiologia, Instituto Butantan, São Paulo, Brazil

John D. Turnidge Department of Microbiology and Infectious Diseases, Women's and Children's Hospital, North Adelaide, South Australia, Australia

Dino Vaira First Medical Clinic, University of Bologna, Bologna, Italy

Alex van Belkum Department of Medical Microbiology and Infectious Diseases, Erasmus University Medical Center Rotterdam, Rotterdam, The Netherlands

Matti K. Viljanen Department in Turku, National Public Health Institute, Turku, Finland

Alexander von Graevenitz Department of Medical Microbiology, University of Zurich, Zurich, Switzerland

Christina von Hunolstein Laboratory of Bacteriology and Medical Mycology, Istituto Superiore di Sanitá, Rome, Italy

Andrej Weintraub Department of Microbiology, Pathology, and Immunology, Karolinska Institute, Stockholm, Sweden

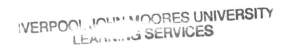

Laboratory Diagnosis of
Bacterial Infections

1

A Role for Microscopy Continues

Jochen Gottschalk and Alexander von Graevenitz
Department of Medical Microbiology, University of Zurich, Zurich, Switzerland

I. INTRODUCTION

This chapter does not describe various types of microscopes, microscopic techniques, and the care of microscopes. Neither does it cover principles and techniques of staining and the use of stains in anatomic pathology. Rather, we try to highlight the continuing importance of microscopy in diagnostic microbiology and the advantages and disadvantages of various techniques and stains. The aim is to help the clinical microbiologist to evaluate a specimen and arrive at a correct bacterial identification.

II. GENERAL FEATURES

Unstained preparations are used in the daily bacteriology routine above all for the determination of motility. It is important that this be done with special slides that allow the drop of the culture to remain undisturbed, and that true motility not be confused with Brownian movement. If "normal" slides are used, the movement of fluid may imitate bacterial motility. The use of darkfield microscopy by now is limited to the search for treponemes; with the decrease of syphilis and the use of fluorescent antibody stains, proficiency in this technique is on the wane.

Stained smears of a specimen allow for the recognition of bacteria and of host tissue cells including morphological features and bacterial-cellular relationships. Thus, they may help decisively in establishing a rapid, though preliminary, diagnosis (e.g., in a sample of spinal fluid). This advantage is lost when large amounts of normal flora that consist of multiple morphotypes are present, e.g., in throat samples. Rough quantitation (from circa 10^5 organisms/mL. on) and determination of the suitability of a specimen for further processing are also possible through stained smears. Smears of cultures may provide additional features that are not recognized in specimens (see below). Correct preparation of the sample for microscopy avoids many pitfalls. Particularly important are the use of clean, defatted glass slides, concentration (e.g., by centrifugation) unless quantification is necessary, a homogeneous distribution of the sample on the slide (e.g., by rolling of a swab), and fixation.

III. INDIVIDUAL STAINS

Most frequently used is the Gram stain which has the advantage of differentiation. Its reliability, however, depends on a number of factors: a) the thickness of the smear versus the time used for decolorization — "thick" areas may not decolorize and "thin" ones may over-decolorize; b) the age of the culture — Gram positive rods, in particular spore-formers, tend to lose Gram positivity with age (1); c) the quality of the staining fluids — precipitation, particularly of crystal violet, may be misinterpreted as Gram positive bacteria; d) non-microbial features of a sample — mucous may be misinterpreted as long Gram negative rods, and high protein levels may coat bacteria and interfere with decolorization (2); and e) "non-textbook" staining — several Gram negative genera are able to partially retain the Gram complex, such as *Moraxella* and *Acinetobacter* spp. (3). Others stain weakly only [e.g., *Legionella* and some anaerobes (4)]. Still others do not stain at all or stain poorly such as *Treponema pallidum*, most mycobacteria, mycoplasmas, chlamydiae, and rickettsiae.

Recognition of bacteria in stained smears is largely a matter of experience. Regular outlines and sharp corners in the case of rods are in favor of bacteria but bacterial shapes may be distorted by heat fixation (in our experience, this does not happen often), or may change from the effect of antimicrobial treatment. Beta-lactam antibiotics, as an example, may cause filamentous forms or oval cells (5).

Some of the problems mentioned are amenable to solutions. These are: i) filtration of staining fluids; ii) use of a small sample regularly distributed over a marked area of the slide; iii) use of young (preferably ≤ 24 hrs.) cultures for staining; iv) use of prolonged (2 min.) staining with the counterstain, or use of carbol fuchsin instead of safranin (4); v) fixation with methanol instead of heat (4); vi) staining of anaerobes in an anaerobic chamber (6); vii) daily quality control using Gram positive and Gram negative organisms; and viii) additional use of tests that correlate well with "textbook" Gram stain coloration.

These include:

• KOH test: 3% KOH disrupts Gram negative cell walls and releases viscous DNA which forms a string when a colony suspension on a slide is raised with a loop. Errors may occur with *Bacillus*, *Listeria*, and anaerobic Gram positive rods (which may be KOH-positive) as well with fastidious nonfermentative Gram negative rods such as *Acinetobacter*, *Moraxella*, *Agrobacterium*, *Brucella*, *Kingella*, *Sphingomonas*, and *Ochrobactrum* which may be KOH-negative (7).

• LANA test: 4% L-alanine-4-nitro-anilide is split by Gram negatives into alanine and a yellow compound, 4-nitroanilide. Errors are less frequent than with the KOH test and may occur with '*Corynebacterium aquaticum*', *Gardnerella*, and a few other Gram positive rods (LANA-positive) as well as *Moraxella*, and some anaerobic Gram negative rods (which may be LANA-negative) (8,9).

The use of non-specific or special stains may be of additional help in the clinical laboratory. As compared to the Gram stain, methylene blue improves staining of *Neisseria*, some Gram negative rods, and of *Treponema vincentii*; it stains eukaryotic cells less strongly (4). The Wayson modification also stains bacteria - dark blue, protein (e.g., mucous) - light blue, and inflammatory cells - light blue to purple. It also stains *Yersinia pestis* and *Francisella tularensis* better and seems to be more sensitive than the Gram stain (4). Acridine orange separates bacterial and fungal from mammalian cells by orange versus yellow to green fluorescence, has a higher clinical sensitivity and, of course, a higher analytical sensitivity when cytospin perparations are used. Its main application is for body fluids. If excessive host cells are present, interpretation may become difficult (4).

The Giemsa stain is rarely used presently since staining of *Chlamydia trachomatis* is, if ever, done by immunofluorescent techniques. Its main application is in rickettsial and ehrlichial bacteriology.

Stains that are aimed at specific structures, i.e., capsules, spores, flagella, and granules, are also used less today than in decades past. Typing of pneumococci by capsular swelling is not done in most routine laboratories, particularly since DNA fingerprinting can be used for typing (10). Spore stains seem unnecessary in view of the fact that spores show up as unstained structures (one per bacterial cell) which could, at best, be confused with vacuoles which, however, are irregular in outline and often multiple. Flagellar stains are not favored by most bacteriologists because of the numerous difficulties associated with their use. If flagella need to be shown at all, e.g., for some non-fermentative Gram negative rods (3), electron microscopy may be a better method for presentation. Important structural staining techniques are the Neisser or Albert stains which highlight metachromatic granules of corynebacteria with blue coloration. While these granules are not specific for *C. diphtheriae* and are generally found only if the bacterium has been cultured on Loeffler or Pai slants, the presence of blue stain on both ends of the rod and characteristic Y and V positioning of the organisms are very suggestive of *C. diphtheriae*.

Immunofluorescence stains with fluorescein-conjugated monoclonal antibodies are routinely performed for a few bacteria, e.g., *Legionella pneumophila*, *Chlamydia trachomatis*, *Treponema pallidum*, *Bordetella pertussis*, and *Francisella tularensis*. The sensitivity of direct stains is suboptimal, however, and specificity may also be a problem particularly if polyclonal antibodies are used (*Legionella* versus *Pseudomonas* spp., *Bacteroides fragilis*, *B. pertussis*, and *Stenotrophomonas maltophilia*).

Of the mycobacterial stains, those that include the fluorescent dye auramine O (with or without rhodamine B) are used extensively today since screening is easier than with the traditional hot (Ziehl-Neelsen) or cold (Kinyoun) acid-fast stains. Auramine stains are less specific, however, and must therefore be confirmed if positive (11). Acridine orange also stains mycobacteria. It is to be kept in mind that: a) "rapid growers" (e.g., *M. fortuitum*, *M. chelonae*, *M. abscessus*) may stain poorly, but may stain alternatively with the Gram procedure, b) certain species have microscopically significant features, e.g., "barred" forms for *M. kansasii* or very short forms for *M. avium*. Complete acid-fastness occurs only in mycobacteria while other aerobic actinomycetes such as *Nocardia*, *Gordona*, *Tsukamurella*, and sometimes *Rhodococcus* are only partially acid-fast, i.e., they stain only with a modified Kinyoun stain (11).

IV. DEPENDENCE OF MICROSCOPIC FEATURES ON SPECIAL CIRCUMSTANCES

Bacterial identification from a stained smear is fraught with difficulties but is often necessary in emergency situations. It is, of course, impossible to mention all bacterial morphologies as exhibited under certain conditions. A few examples should suffice.

S. pneumoniae usually shows diplococcoid forms in human samples but is able to form short chains in liquid (e.g., blood) cultures. Lancet shapes are not found in all cells, some are ovoid. Chains of streptococci are poorly recognizable in smears that are taken from solid media but are more easily seen in those from liquid media (13). Short chains and pairs are not specific for *S. pneumoniae* but may also be observed among other streptococci [e.g., *S. milleri*, *Lactococcus*, *Enterococcus*, *Leuconostoc*, *Facklamia*, *Globicatella*, and *Vagococcus* (12)]. Some streptococci may be difficult to recognize as such because they may form rod-like forms [e.g., *S. mutans* and *S. sanguis* (13)], particularly in aging cultures.

Neisseriae show diplococcal forms in smears from direct material but in cultures, single organisms are more frequent; polychromasia is the rule. On some occasions, tetrads are observed. *N. elongata* and *N. weaveri* have rod shapes (14). *Acinetobacter* spp. tend to have diplococcoid forms in older cultures from solid media while early growth in liquid media and growth in the presence of beta-lactams yields rod forms (3).

The accuracy of classifying Gram negative rods from microscopy of direct smears has been examined (15). When three morphotypes were defined (*Enterobacteriaceae* as plump rods; *Pseudomonas* spp. as elongated rods; and *Bacteroides*/*Haemophilus* spp. as narrow short rods) the overall accuracy was 76%. Recognition of these morphotypes, however, appeared to provide little benefit in suggesting antimicrobial treatment.

V. SAMPLE MICROSCOPY

Direct microscopic examination of clinical specimens is still a valuable source of information in bacterial infections. Three different areas will be covered: i) microscopic localization and morphology in prokaryotic and eukaryotic cells; ii) some general parameters that determine the clinical significance of microscopic results for patient material under scrutiny; and iii) special samples and rejection criteria.

A. Cells

Besides bacterial cell morphology, which is described in detail elsewhere (16), the presence and kind of eukaryotic cells and the localization microorganisms in relationship to host cells provides some basic information about a clinical sample. Principally, two kinds of eukaryotic cells can be found in clinical specimens: blood and epithelial cells. White blood cells in large numbers are indicative of inflammatory processes but not exclusively of bacterial infections. At the onset of bacterial infections and sometimes during the active infectious process itself, white blood cells may be missing. Some grading systems for the evaluation of clinical specimens use the numbers of white blood cells as rejection criteria (17,18). The presence of epithelial cells in a clinical specimen may suggest two possibilities: the material is actually derived from an area that is covered by epithelial cells, or the material is derived from an area not covered by epithelial cells but contaminated subsequently by material containing epithelial cells. For these reasons, some grading systems for smear evaluation also use the number of epithelial cells as important criteria (17,18,19).

B. Parameters

Sensitivity and specificity of microscopy of a clinical specimen depend on different factors. For example, less than 10^5 bacteria/mL cannot be seen in a Gram stained clinical specimen. Therefore, the value for analytical sensitivity never reaches 100%. The same is true for specificity. With some exceptions there are no microscopic differences between infectious bacteria and indigenous flora. Due to better specificity, microscopic examination of materials obtained from usually sterile body sites generally is of much greater value than evaluation of bacteria in material with contaminating indigenous flora (e.g., cerebrospinal fluid versus sputum). In order to circumvent this difficulty, rejection criteria were established for clinical specimens with contaminating indigenous flora.

C. Special samples and rejection criteria

1. Cerebrospinal fluid

A Gram stain of centrifuged cerebrospinal fluid in episodes of suspected bacterial meningitis remains a quick and specific method for diagnosing bacterial meningitis. With adequately trained staff, sensitivity for *Haemophilus influenzae, Neisseria meningitidis*, or *Streptococcus pneumoniae* is about 75 to 90% as compared to culture (20). Overall specificity, i.e., recognition of any bacteria as such in a Gram stain from cerebrospinal fluid, is probably near 100%. After pretreatment with antibiotics, there may be a substantial loss of overall sensitivity to 40 - 60% (20).

2. Other materials from usual sterile body sites

Gram stain may be helpful from all materials of sterile body sites with few exceptions: bile, blood (uncultivated), and solid material such as bone.

3. Lower respiratory tract

Sputum

Routine Gram stained smears of sputum are required by almost all clinicians. Gram stained smears are necessary for quality control, but there is some doubt about the clinical value of information that is obtained from Gram stained smears of sputum. The number of squamous epithelial cells (SEC) per low power field (100x) serves as a quality control parameter. If the number of SEC exceeds 25 per low power field, rejection of this sputum is recommended (21). In this case, there is a high probability that so-called sputum is in fact mainly saliva.

Endotracheal suction aspirates (ETSA)

The number of SEC per low power field (100x) serves in ETSA assessment as a quality control parameter as well (19). If more than 10 SEC per low power field are present or if no organisms are seen in the Gram stain, rejection of the ETSA has been recommended (19). Subsequent growth of Gram negative rods in culture in the absence of microorganisms in a Gram stain may be considered mere colonization from the oropharynx.

Bronchoalveolar lavage (BAL)

In patients with suspected ventilator-associated pneumonia, microscopic examination of cells from BAL also yields criteria for the clinical relevance of bacterial findings. When more than 5% of PMNs from BAL contain bacteria, pneumonia can be suspected with sensitivities up to 91% and specificities of 78 to 79% (22,23). The presence of SEC in large numbers suggests contamination with oropharyngeal material.

4. Genital tract

Gram stain of cervical, urethral, and/or rectal swabs in suspected gonorrhea may be helpful. Gram negative diplococci are highly suggestive of *N. gonorrhoeae* (24-26). Since species of *Neisseria* cannot be differentiated morphologically, a definitive diagnosis can only be made by culture (14,27).

Routine culture for *G. vaginalis* from a vaginal swab is often required from clinicians. Gram stain of a vaginal swab can serve as a quality control measure. If more than 25 lactobacilli per low power field (10x10) are visible, the specimen may prove to be unreliable for culture (28).

VI. AGAR MICROSCOPY

This technique has been in decline but some believe that the use of a light microscope with transillumination or incident light can be of considerable help for identifying cultures. Examples for the value of this approach include: a) aerial and/or vegetative mycelium in *Nocardia*, b) α- and β- hemolysis which is considerably facilitated by observation of red blood cells through transillumination, and c) colony features, e.g., "molar tooth" apperance among *Actinomyces* spp. or the "crossed cigar" phenomenon in *Actinobacillus actinomycetemcomitans* (16).

VII. CELL CULTURE MICROSCOPY

Cytotoxicity assays for bacterial toxins are still the gold standard for detection of *Clostridium difficile* toxin or some toxins from diarrheagenic *Escherichia coli*. Cytotoxicity assays benefit from some experience with cell cultures as well as special technical equipment, e.g., microscopes for cell cultures, which are often not available in microbiological laboratories (see Chapters 15 and 24).

REFERENCES

1. Carlone GM, Valadez MJ, Pickett MJ. Methods for distinguishing Gram-positive from Gram-negative bacteria. J Clin Microbiol 1983; 16:1157-1159.
2. Alter D, Josephson S. Gram-positive *Neisseria* meningitis. Arch Pathol Lab Med 1999; 123:444.
3. Schreckenberger PC, von Graevenitz A. *Acinetobacter, Achromobacter, Alcaligenes, Moraxella, Methylobacterium*, and other nonfermentative Gram-negative rods. In: Murray PR, Baron EJ, Pfaller MA, Tenover FC, Yolken RH, eds. Manual of Clinical Microbiology. Washington DC:American Society for Microbiology, 1999:539-560.
4. Woods GL, Walker DH. Detection of infection or infectious agents by use of cytologic and histologic stains. Clin Microbiol Rev 1996; 9:382-404.
5. Lorian V, Sabath LD. Penicillins and cephalosporins: differences in morphologic effects on *Proteus mirabilis*. J Infect Dis 1972; 125:560-564.
6. Johnson MJ, Thatcher E, Cox ME. Techniques for controlling variability in Gram staining of obligate anaerobes. J Clin Microbiol 1995; 33: 755-758.
7. von Graevenitz A, Bucher C. Accuracy of the KOH and vancomycin tests in determining the Gram reaction of non-enterobacterial rods. J Clin Microbiol 1983; 18:983-985.
8. Leonard RB, Ohlson S, Newcomb-Gayman PL, Carroll KC. Comparison of "Gram-sure" with vancomycin disks in distinguishing between Gram-negative and Gram-positive rods. Am J Clin Pathol 1995; 104:69-71.
9. Bamarouf A, Eley A, Winstanley T. Evaluation of methods for distinguishing Gram-positive from Gram-negative anaerobic bacteria. Anaerobe 1996; 2:163-168.
10. Lefevre JC, Faucon G, Sicard AM, Gasc AM. DNA fingerprinting of *Streptococcus pneumoniae* strains by pulsed-field gel electrophoresis. J Clin Microbiol 1993; 31:2724-2728.
11. Gruft H. Evaluation of mycobacteriology laboratories: the acid fast smear. Health Lab Sci 1978; 15:215-220.
12. Facklam R, Elliott JA. Identification, classification, and clinical relevance of catalase-negative, Gram-positive cocci, excluding the streptococci and enterococci. Clin Microbiol Rev 1995; 8:479-495.
13. Hardie JM. Genus *Streptococcus*. In: Sneath PHA, Mair NS, Sharpe ME, Holt JG, eds. Bergey's Manual of Systematic Bacteriology. Baltimore:Williams & Wilkins, 1996:1043-1071.
14. Knapp JS, Koumans EH. *Neisseria* and *Branhamella*. In: Murray PR, Baron EJ, Pfaller MA, Tenover FC, Yolken RH, eds. Manual of Clinical Microbiology. Washington DC:American Society for Microbiology, 1999:586-603
15. Bartlett RC, Mazens-Sullivan MF, Lerer TJ. Differentiation of *Enterobacteriaceae, Pseudomonas aeruginosa*, and *Bacteroides* and *Haemophilus* species in Gram-stained direct smears. Diagn Microbiol Infect Dis 1991; 14:195-201.
16. Murray PR, Baron EJ, Pfaller MA, Tenover FC, Yolken RH. Manual of Clinical Microbiology. 7th ed. Washington DC:American Society for Microbiology, 1999.
17. Murray PR, Washington JA III. Microscopic and bacteriologic analysis of expectorated sputum. Mayo Clin Proc 1975; 50:339-344.
18. Sharp SE. Algorithms for wound specimens. Clinical Microbiology Newsletter 1999; 21:118-120.
19. Morris AJ, Tanner DC, Reller LB. Rejection criteria for endotracheal aspirates from adults. J Clin Microbiol 1993; 31:1027-1029.
20. Greenlee JE. Approach to diagnosis of meningitis. Infect Dis Clin North Am 1990; 4:583-598.
21. Geckler RW, Gremillion DH, McAllister CK, Ellenbogen C. Microscopic and bacteriological comparison of paired sputa and transtracheal aspirates. J Clin Microbiol 1977; 6:396-399.
22. Chastre J, Fagon JY, Bornet-Lecso M, Calvat S, Dombret MC, al Khani R, Basset F, Gibret C. Evaluation of bronchoscopic techniques for the diagnosis of nosocomial pneumonia. Am J Respir Crit Care Med 1995; 152:231-240.
23. Jourdain B, Joly-Guillou ML, Dombret MC, Calvat S, Trouillet JL, Gibert C, Chastre J. Usefulness of quantitative cultures of BAL fluid diagnosing nosocomial pneumonia in ventilated patients. Chest 1997; 111:411-418.
24. Goodhart ME, Ogden J, Zaidi AA, Kraus SJ. Factors affecting the performance of smear and culture tests for the detection of *Neisseria gonorrhoeae*. Sex Transm Dis 1982; 9:63-69.
25. Janda WM, Bohnhoff M, Morello JA, Lerner SA. Prevalence and site-pathogen studies of *Neisseria meningitidis* and *Neisseria gonorrhoeae* in homosexual men. JAMA 1980; 244:2060-2064.

26. Rothenberg RB, Simon R, Chipperfield E, Catterall RD. Efficacy of selected diagnostic tests for sexually transmitted diseases. JAMA 1976; 235:49-51.

27. Koumans EH, Johnson RE, Knapp JS, St. Louis ME. Laboratory testing for *Neisseria gonorrhoeae* by recently introduced nonculture tests: a performance review with clinical and public health considerations. Clin Infect Dis 1998; 27:1171-1180.

28. Spiegel CA. Bacterial vaginosis. Clin Microbiol Rev 1991; 4:485-502.

2

Applied Systematics

John T. Magee
Department of Medical Microbiology and Public Health Laboratory, University of Wales College of Medicine, Cardiff, Wales

I. INTRODUCTION

A striking characteristic of living things is their enormous diversity of form. In size alone, there is variation from the blue whale and the sequoia tree to the smallest bacteria and on into the area where the living and non-living intermingle amongst the viruses and prions. These creatures combine to form the complex, dynamic equilibrium that is the ecology of Earth's biosphere, which shows constant slow variation as new creatures evolve and others become extinct. Life's variation in form and ecological function is well beyond the capacity of an individual to comprehend in any detail. Biologists have been driven to divide its diversity into comprehensible groups, and to learn how to distinguish these groups.

This process of division, description, naming, and identification of groups has evolved into a branch of science in its own right termed systematics. At first sight, the process appears simple particularly to the modern biologist who has an established classification system and who may not have had the inclination or time to understand its origins or to comprehend the huge scientific effort that is involved in its construction. In fact, the process involves a subtle and fascinating blend of intuition, philosophy, mathematics, statistics, and computation that finds applications in subjects as diverse as biology, the social sciences, archaeology, and research on artificial intelligence.

This chapter will give only a brief introduction to the underlying science of systematics. The main thrust will be on areas that are encountered by applied microbiologists, particularly medical bacteriologists. For those who seek a deeper understanding of the science and its controversies, Cowan's publications provide stimulating and humorous insights (1-4), and there are several introductory texts (5,6). The works of Sneath and Sokal provide a definitive guide to the basis of numerical taxonomy (7,8), also reviewed in a monograph from a viewpoint that includes non-biological applications (9). Several volumes include comprehensive reviews of the theory, technology, and practice of bacterial systematics (10,11,12). In general biology, the definition of the species concept still arouses regular and vigorous discussion, and a recent symposium covers these arguments (13).

II. THE DISTINCTION BETWEEN CLASSIFICATION AND IDENTIFICATION

A fundamental and frequently misunderstood concept of systematics is the distinction between classification and identification. Classification is a discovery process in which a set of objects is studied to determine a group structure that takes into account their differences and similarities. Cowan (2) gave the example of classifying hardware fixing products. A collector might present a variety of products to a taxonomist as a jumbled heap. Screws, bolts, nails, and glues form obviously distinct groups – the 'kingdoms' of fixing apparatus – and detailed analysis of screws might divide them into cross or straight slot, countersink, or round head, and then by size. The result of the study would be a set of drawers, each containing a relatively indistinguishable group of objects – the species. Each drawer would have a distinct name in some agreed system of nomenclature, e.g., half-inch straight head #6 wood screw, and the name and a description or photograph could be attached to the drawer. At this stage, the classification is complete, and the system would be handed on to an applied practitioner of fixings.

The carpenter might like this classification, and decide to adopt it. Henceforth, he will take new fixings, compare them to the descriptions on the drawers, and, having identified them, place them in the appropriately named drawer. The carpenter's task of identification does not involve producing new drawers, names, or descriptions; it centres on sorting new objects into a pre-existing system. The system is useful in many practical contexts; the name is a short-hand description, readily communicated to suppliers and other carpenters, and the fixings are classified into distinct kingdoms and species that reflect their properties and use.

The example may appear artificial in these days of mass production, but there was a stage of hand-made production when screws and nails, like bacteria, did not come with a standardized manufacturer's label. Organisms in general, and bacteria in particular, exist in a system where the ability to diversify and adapt to continuous change is essential to survival. The task of classifying bacteria into species is not simple. Those who regard labels like *Staphylococcus aureus* and *Escherichia coli* as godgiven names that are indelibly stamped on every cell would do well to revise their opinion in light of the enormous efforts that are required to create a classification of the bacteria and in light of the continuing uncertainties of the subject.

III. NOMENCLATURE

A. Formal nomenclature

A formal species name comprises a generic and specific epithet that is published in italic type. This unique label refers to the formal description of the species that is current at the time of publication. Where there is controversy, or an earlier description better fits the group of organisms and identification procedures involved, an author may specify the intended formal description, e.g., *Listeria monocytogenes* (Pirie, 1940). After first usage in a document, the genus epithet is usually abbreviated. There are no agreed lists for genus abbreviations; previous usage and considerations of clarity must guide authors. Reference to other formally defined groups in the hierarchy can also be made, e.g., the *Archaebacteria*, the *Enterobacteriaceae*, *Pseudomonas* sp. (a single species of the genus *Pseudomonas*) or *Pseudomonas* spp. (several species of the genus). Formal group names at these higher levels may be printed in 'trivial' form, e.g., pseudomonads for *Pseudomonas*. This may avoid the inconvenience and ugliness of excessive italic text, or reflect an author's disdain of the classification at these higher levels, but note that trivial names do not carry the precision of the formal nomenclature.

These formal names have precise meanings and allow for concise unequivocal communication of the properties of an organism in a universally-accepted technical language. The publication of formal descriptions prevents them from being debased by any misuse. It is indefensible practice to publish a formal italicized name in a sense other than that of the implied description, or to italicize a trivial name that carries no formal description.

The formal nomenclature is supervised by the International Committee for Systematic Bacteriology (ICSB), under the rules of the current Bacteriological Code (14) and is defined by various publications of the ICSB. The Approved Lists (15,16) define those historical species names that were accepted as being validly published during a major nomenclature revision. More recent changes appear in two forms: papers proposing new nomenclature in the *International Journal of Systematic Bacteriology* (*IJSB*), and proposals published in other journals but also submitted for citation in the lists of validly published proposals that appear in each issue of the *IJSB*. Numerous subcommittees of the ICSB aid the core committee with recommendations and advice on specific areas of the nomenclature or more general systematic problems. The ICSB and the subcommittees meet regularly, usually at conferences that are organized by the International Union of Microbiological Societies, and minutes are published in the *IJSB*. Most of the meetings are open to participation by all interested parties. A list of names with standing in the nomenclature can be found at http://www-sv.cict.fr/bacterio/.

The current status of bacterial classification is reviewed in the editions of Bergey's Manual of Determinative Bacteriology (17) as published in each decade. Some regard Bergey's Manual as defining the current formal nomenclature, although changes occur more rapidly than the publication cycle, and it has no formal link with the ICSB. Both, however, draw on the same pool of expertise.

The current Bacteriological Code (14) is essential reading for those intending to propose new formal names. Minimal acceptable standards for species descriptions are being formulated for specific groups of bacteria by the various ICSB subcommittees (18-20), and these should also be consulted. New nomenclature may be proposed in either the *IJSB*, or in other journals. If the latter course is taken, a copy of the published paper should be sent to the *IJSB* so that a citation can be included in the lists of validly published proposals. Where new species of culturable bacteria are proposed, a type strain must be designated, and a culture of this strain must be deposited with a recognized service culture collection. Guidance on names for new species is available in the Bacteriological Code (14) and in articles by Bousefield (21) and MacAdoo (22). Those who propose new nomenclature would do well to consider difficulties in pronunciation or excessive length of names that might inconvenience their colleagues world-wide. Provisions for the designation of (currently) non-culturable species have been published (23,24).

B. Trivial names

Trivial names are not supported by a formal code of rules. Group names like 'the enterobacteria' and 'fecal streptococci' are not published in italic type, and may be intended to convey quite different concepts from apparently synonymous formal names like 'the *Enterobacteriaceae*'. Their use involves the concept that organisms can be classified in many distinct ways, some of which are useful in applied branches of biology, but involve groupings that differ from those of the formal classification. Taking Cowan's example again, a scrap metal dealer might group fixings quite differently in his business affairs and in fixing a broken chair at home. Humans routinely use overlapping and contrasting classifications that are appropriate to different contexts, and microbiologists are no exception.

These terms form an essential part of the technical language of bacteriology and allow complex concepts to be communicated efficiently. The difficulty lies in their lack of formal description. Their misuse can lead to misunderstanding and debasement to the point where the original concept can no longer be conveyed. The 'enterobacteria', for example, may be intended as a synonym for the *Enterobacteriaceae*, or to cover those *Enterobacteriaceae* that are found as commensals or pathogens in human enteric flora, or may include these and other Gram negative enteric bacteria, e.g., *Pseudomonas aeruginosa*. Authors who introduce such new terminology are advised to provide a full and carefully worded definition that can be cited readily.

These terms are often self-explanatory, however, and they define groups of clear practical significance. They often ignore formal divisions, e.g., respiratory pathogens delineates a widely varied group of species with no conceivable connection in the formal hierarchy. Equally, subsets of species within a genus can be defined, e.g., the coagulase-negative staphylococci (CNS). Even these varied terms do not fully account for the conceptual groupings that one uses at the bench. Looking at a mid-stream urine culture, *Staphylococcus saprophyticus* is clearly included in the pathogen group, but not other CNS; for a catheter urine, any CNS in large numbers may be significant; for a skin swab, CNS are commensals; for a CNS-positive blood culture, one examines the request form for mention of indwelling devices before judging significance. These shifting judgements reflect the many distinct ways of grouping bacteria that are required for work in the applied science. Away from the bench, however, this deft and subtle juggling of concepts can readily lead to errors in logic or communication; in research and papers, it is wise to stay with the tight clear definitions of the formal classification.

IV. ORGANISMS

A. Pure culture

Without organisms, there would be little point in classification or identification. The first step in either process is to obtain a pure culture. Failure of technique at this stage will inevitably lead to erroneous results in characterization tests. A single, well-separated colony should be taken from growth on non-selective solid medium and checked for uniform colony morphology on a non-selective purity plate. There are no valid short-cuts for this process, and it may yet fail, even for the most expert practitioner, due to the inclusion of micro-colonies of a cryptic contaminant. Where unusual reaction patterns are encountered, it is wise to culture the organism on a broad range of rich, non-selective media with prolonged incubation under a wide variety of conditions, and to examine the plates under a stereo microscope for contaminants. In large studies, the author has found it wise to prepare blood agar purity plates for all cultures at each stage in characterization, to examine these after standard incubation, and then to incubate for a further 72 hrs. at room temperature for re-examination with a plate microscope. This is a minimal, economic method of screening for contamination problems which may occur in cultures from the most reputable of sources.

At this stage, the culture is termed an 'isolate' in medical laboratories. The same clone of organisms may figure as re-isolates from the same patient, or as multiple isolates from several patients in an outbreak. Given reasonable proof of close similarity in typing tests, an investigator may call a set of isolates a strain, to indicate his/her belief that all of these isolates share a recent common clonal origin. Description of a set of organisms as strains indicates a belief that these are distinct isolates which are taken from varied unconnected sources and with little possibility that any of the isolates have been recently derived from the same clone. These terms have clearly defined and distinct meanings, and they should be used with care to prevent debasement of critically important terminology.

B. Preservation of cultures

The next stage is to preserve the strain in long term storage. This must be performed soon after initial isolation since cultures undergo selective adaptation to laboratory conditions. In earlier times, subculture was termed re-isolation, rightly emphasizing the possibility of the gradual evolution of strains that is inherent in 'storage' by serial subculture. Early microbiologists were limited to this option, and they consequently appreciated the adaptive pliability of bacteria at first hand. Modern microbiologists no longer see variation as an everyday occurrence and are less alert, but the bacteria have not lost their ability to change. Once in pure culture, a strain should be sub-cultured from a sweep rather than a single colony in order to minimize the possibility of selecting an altered sub-clone. Freeze-dried storage is normally employed for large culture collections. Storage on beads in glycerol broth at -40°C or -80°C is a more convenient and less laborious method that is adopted widely for interim storage and smaller collections.

C. Reference cultures

Cultures of reference organisms can be obtained from the various national culture collections. These are essential for quality control of characterization tests, and are indispensable reference points for classification studies. They should be obtained directly from the culture collection, cultured, and stored immediately. Quality control cultures can be revived and propagated by serial subculture for a limited time before renewal from storage. It is tempting to maintain strains in frequent use solely by long term serial sub-culture, but this is unacceptable practice. Economic stringencies have encouraged a tendency to obtain collection strains at second hand, but this is also bad practice; there have been incidents where mislabeled reference strains have been exchanged between laboratories thus causing considerable confusion (25).

V. CHARACTERIZATION TESTS

These tests generate the data that is used in classification and identification. Detailed methods for conventional tests can be found in Cowan and Steel's Manual for the Identification of Medical Bacteria (4). It is important to understand their nature, limitations, advantages, and disadvantages in both contexts before moving on to the methods that are used to analyze the data for either purpose. At another level, one must also understand the nature of the data that tests yield.

A. The nature of characterization data

1. Bi-state variables

Results from many conventional tests are viewed as bi-state variables; that is, the results may be either positive or negative. Most established data analysis systems for identification and classification are based on bi-state variables, and so there is a strong tendency to re-code other types of test results into this format.

2. Non-interpretable results

In fact, most 'bi-state tests' may occasionally yield a non-interpretable result for a variety of reasons. Most commonly, indeterminate results occur because an organism brings the test to the borderline between a true positive or negative reaction. Underlying reasons for this are discussed below. Another reason is that the organism fails to grow because of an unsuitable basal medium. If the test system is unsuited to the metabolism of the organism, e.g., when carbohydrate fermentation tests are applied to highly oxidative organisms, the result may appear valid, but should really be termed non-applicable. There are difficulties in coping with these non-interpretable results in most analysis packages.

3. Multi-state variables

Some tests yield multi-state results. These may be ordered, e.g., colony size small, medium, or large; or non-ordered multi-state variables, e.g., colony color. Taking these examples for ordered variables, the difference between the small and large colony strains is greater than the difference between small and medium forms. For non-ordered multi-state tests, the difference between red-, yellow-, or white- colony strains is considered equal. These tests can often (and, sometimes, better) be fitted into bi-state schemes by considering them as multiple variables each with a bi-state result, e.g., colony size < 1 mm., colony size 1 to 2 mm., colony size > 2 mm., colony red, colony yellow (but not colony white, as this is assumed for non-pigmented strains). The danger of over-enthusiastic translation to bi-state variables is that a single character with many observable states may assume an unwarranted importance in the results.

4. Continuous variables

Other tests may yield continuous variables – numeric measurements that may take any value in a range. It may be possible to convert these into bi-state variables after consideration of the distribution of results. Taking terminal pH in glucose broth as an example, Figure 1 shows a clear partition of isolates into four groups: strong and weak acid-producers, non-acid producers, and alkali producers. By 'thresholding' at minimal in the distribution, one can readily convert this into four bi-state variables: terminal pH <5.8; terminal pH 5.8-6.9; terminal pH 7.0-7.6; and terminal pH >7.6. Most test results reflect some underlying continuous variable that has been truncated to a bi-state variable by 'thresholding' as discussed below in the context of fermentation tests. For continuous variables that show less well-differentiated distributions, a good statistical approach is to measure test reproducibility and to 'standardize' the results by dividing the actual result by the mean within-strain standard deviation.

5. Pattern data

Pattern data that are obtained from fingerprinting techniques comprise many interdependent continuous variables. These data may be analyzed with multivariate statistics (26) or neural network approaches (27). Many microbiologists find this level of mathematics intimidating, but the analyses can be processed through 'black-box' programs given sufficient development effort.

B. Phenotypic tests

1. Microscopic morphology

Conveniently observed micro-morphology characters are limited by the resolution of the light microscope, may be highly dependent on culture conditions, and usually vary widely between cells in a film.

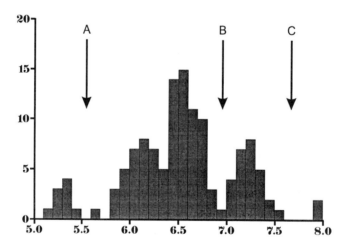

Figure 1 Histogram indicating terminal pH in sugar-containing medium for strains of Gram negative anaerobic bacilli. The markers indicate alternative thresholds for discrimination of strong acid production (A), weak acid production (B), or alkali production (C). (Unpublished data contributed by Professor BI Duerden, Cardiff, Wales)

Cells may be coccoid, cocco-bacillary, rods, spirals (flexible or rigid), or pleomorphic. Subtleties of shape can be telling clues in identification; the 'typical' lanceolate (spearhead-shaped) pneumococcus and the bean-shaped diplococci of the pathogenic neisseriae are well known. Club-shaped cells are often seen in the corynebacteria. Pseudomonads sometimes show gradually tapering cells with sharply rounded ends. Length-to-width ratio varies among bacilli, from the thin flexing rods of some mycobacteria, to the broad rigid boxcar-shaped cells of some *Bacillus* or *Clostridium* species.

Cell arrangement can also be characteristic and may indicate the preferred order of division planes during reproduction and any propensity for cells to remain attached post-division. This is particularly so among the cocci. Diplococci are considered typical in films of pneumococci and neisseriae, chains in the streptococci, square and cubical arrangements in the micrococci, and irregular clusters in the staphylococci. Chains, or sometimes bundled chains, are seen in *Bacillus* spp., and snapping division of club-shaped cells yields the characteristic 'Chinese letter' appearance that is seen for some strains of corynebacteria. For the experienced eye, the shape, size, and arrangement of a few 'typical' cells which are scattered throughout a film is as characteristic as a signature; to the inexperienced, the same film can be an uninterpretable jumble of cells of varying morphology and in random arrangements.

Staining characteristics also vary from the straightforward to the subtle. Positive (purple) or negative (red) cell staining in Gram's method is a major character in identification, and delineates groups with distinct cell wall composition. Gram positive organisms may show variable staining, with patchy staining of the cytoplasm (often associated with storage granules, spores, or pre-spores) or cell wall, or they may only show a positive reaction in the early exponential growth phase. Some strains, however, particularly among the clostridia and *Bacillus* spp., fail to produce a frankly positive Gram reaction. Inexperienced microbiologists readily fall into this trap with disastrous results, collecting say, environmental pseudomonad isolates that later prove to be mostly strains of *Bacillus* spp. Unequivocal identification of asporogenous, frankly Gram negative *Bacillus* or *Clostridium* strains can be taxing even for the most expert microbiologist. Similarly, the methods that are derived from the original Ziehl-Neelsen stain vary somewhat in specificity, and it is wise to familiarize oneself with the range of acid-fast, or acid and alcohol-fast organisms that yield a positive result in the local method.

Stains for organelles are rarely performed in routine medical bacteriology. Spores, capsules, flagellae, nuclei, and some types of storage granules can be visualized in light microscopy by specific staining. Fimbriae and other small organelles can be visualized in electron microscopy, and fimbriae may be detected indirectly by their hemagglutination or other agglutinin activity. Spore frequency, shape, size, position within the cell, and their distortion of cell shape are all important observations in the identification of *Bacillus* and *Clostridium* spp.

2. *Macro-morphology of cultures*

Features of surface colonies that are commonly recorded include: size, color, opacity, surface appearance, cross-sectional profile, and edge structure. These are highly dependent on the medium, growth conditions, and length of incubation. For an expert microbiologist working with familiar and well-standardized media and incubation conditions, however, these characters are often sufficient for presumptive identification to the genus or species level.

Hemolysis arises from many distinct mechanisms, and is assayed on several media. In the United Kingdom, blood agar is commonly made with 5% horse blood, but practice varies between countries. This can lead to differences in observed reactions as some mechanisms of hemolysis require red-cell species-specific receptors. A specialized identification test, the CAMP test, involves synergistic hemolysis of sheep red cells that are pre-treated with staphylococcal delta-toxin and by a toxin that is produced by *Streptococcus agalactiae*.

The importance of close examination of plate cultures cannot be over-rated. This is the mainstay of identification in the routine laboratory. For the taxonomist, sorting by colony morphology will frequently show presumptive species groupings that closely predict the results of prolonged formal classification studies. In all microbiological work, detailed examination of purity plates is essential to prevent errors due to contaminated cultures. Pure culture is the basis of bacteriology. It may be unfashionable to emphasize this basic skill, but the author's experience is that it is essential. No matter how esoteric or sophisticated the methodology, at some stage an undetected contaminated culture can make nonsense of results.

Features of growth in liquid or semi-solid media provide less discrimination. As with colony morphology, the medium, growth conditions, and incubation time are often critical variables. The pattern of growth may depend on oxygen requirements, motility, piliation, hydrophobicity of the cell surface, and ability to flocculate. At the extremes, strains may grow as a thin surface pellicle (often most pronounced for highly piliated and strictly aerobic organisms), as a deposit at the bottom of the broth, as a band midway in the depth of a semi-solid medium (microaerophiles), or give uniform turbidity.

3.   Growth requirements

Gaseous requirements for growth

Strict aerobes grow only in the presence of oxygen (or in the presence of a suitable oxidizing substrate such as nitrate, e.g., *Pseudomonas aeruginosa*), strict anaerobes grow only in the absence of oxygen, and facultative aerobes grow under aerobic or anaerobic conditions. Microaerophiles prefer oxygen concentrations that are lower than those which are obtained in room air. Capnophilic organisms prefer (and may require) carbon dioxide-enriched air. Facultative aerobes that are obligate capnophiles can be readily mistaken for obligate anaerobes since they grow in carbon dioxide-enriched anaerobic gas mixtures but not unenriched air. Some laboratories rely on this for the isolation of capnophiles, but the expense of a CO_2-enriched incubator is well redressed by increased isolation rates from cerebrospinal fluids and sputa. An inexpensive alternative is the classic candle jar. *Campylobacter* spp. are microaerophiles that prefer (or sometimes require) some hydrogen in addition to reduced oxygen concentrations.

There are variable degrees of anaerobiosis, measured in redox potential or E_h, and some 'anaerobes' will grow at quite high E_h, while others are extremely sensitive to trace amounts of oxygen. Note that highly oxygen-sensitive organisms die rapidly in surface spread plates which are left unincubated on the bench. Delays before plates are placed in an oxygen-free environment can markedly reduce the yield of anaerobic organisms. One solution to this problem, widely practised in the 1980s, was to place plates for anaerobic incubation in a holding jar that is gassed with oxygen-free nitrogen. When sufficient plates had accumulated, the jar was taken to full anaerobiosis and incubated. This has fallen from favour, but constitutes a reasonable, economical alternative to purchasing an anaerobe cabinet for poorly financed laboratories.

Temperature requirements

Psychrophilic organisms can grow at low temperatures (2-5°C) and have a growth optimum between 20-30°C. Mesophiles may grow in the range of 10-40°C and have a growth optimum between 30-40°C. Thermophiles may grow in the range 40 to 100°C and have a growth optimum above 40°C. Medical microbiologists rarely encounter organisms with a growth maximum that is less than 37°C for obvious reasons (with the exception of superficial infections with *Mycobacterium marinum*, *M. ulcerans*, or *M. haemophilum*). Little is lost, however, by incubating primary plates at 35-36 °C, and the occasional isolate that would struggle to grow at 37 °C is more likely to be detected. Temperature growth range can play a critical role in the epidemiology of organisms, e.g., *Listeria monocytogenes* which can grow in food products that are stored in a refrigerator.

Osmotic and salt requirements

Most organisms of medical importance grow well at physiological osmolarity and NaCl concentrations. Some, particularly the vibrios and organisms of marine origin, prefer or require raised NaCl concentrations. L-forms, mycoplasmas, and spheroplasts are often osmotically labile. Extreme halophiles or osmophiles require raised NaCl concentrations or media with high osmotic pressure. Many Gram positive cocci will withstand high salt concentrations.

Adaptability is the key to bacterial survival. Wherever there is a niche with available energy and water, bacteria will be found. The various species have adapted to an enormous range of physical and chemical growth conditions. Examples of extreme environments in which bacteria grow include: rock interstices on the Antarctic plateau; deep sea volcanic vents; mine effluent water that is contaminated with heavy metals at pH 2.0; alkaline lakes at pH 12-14; and hot, high salinity pools. So far as the bacteria are concerned, humans are merely another ecological niche that has evolved for their occupation.

Chemical requirements for growth and growth tolerances

Bacteria vary widely in their chemical growth requirements. Some can grow with only nitrogen, phosphate, carbon (and energy) sources, and trace elements. Others have a host of requirements as they are unable to synthesize key co-factors, purines, pyrimidines, amino acids, or porphyrins. At the extreme, obligate intracellular parasites have such broad requirements that they can grow only with the support of the biochemical synthetic capacity of the parasitized cell. Medical bacteria often have a broad range of chemical requirements, possibly as a result of the evolutionary loss of biochemical pathways whose products can be obtained from the host.

Minimal media contain only a nitrogen, phosphate, and carbon source, and trace elements may be carried over from the major constituents and water. The growth requirements of organisms may be explored by the addition of pure vitamins, amino acids, etc., to such a medium. More complete media, such as nutrient agar, contain a source of vitamins and co-factors (e.g. yeast extract) and a mixed amino acid source (e.g. peptone), and supply adequate growth factors for many species. The addition of 5% blood further enlarges the range of species that grow. Beyond this, lysed blood agar, chocolate (heated blood) agar, and addition of hemin, lecithovitellin, or other specialized supplements may allow species with broad requirements to grow.

Reliable and reproducible rich growth media are the heart of diagnostic microbiology. Economizing on media constituents may drastically affect isolation rates. Equally, good medium constituents can yield poor media if preparation is poor; diligent staff, good preparation apparati, and strict quality control of every batch of medium is essential for a fully functional diagnostic laboratory. The preparation and control of identification media is a particularly specialized branch of media preparation where expertise has largely been lost with the introduction of identification kits. For those who wish to prepare their own identification media, the author's advice is that meticulous and accurate preparation technique and quality control are absolute requirements for success.

Those bacteria that are pathogenic for humans tend to show limited tolerance to extreme conditions. The exceptions to this rule have been exploited to give a range of useful selective and enrichment media, and some fairly specific tests for identification. For example, tolerance of selenite, tellurite, and azide are a basis for the selection of salmonellae, *Corynebacterium diphtheriae*, and *Listeria* respectively. Tolerance of bile salts is exploited in selection and identification of enterobacteria and enterococci. Dyes, such as brilliant green, are often tolerated by only a few species. It should be noted that the concentrations of these agents are critical to success. Some, particularly dyes, are not manufactured to high purity, some interact chemically with other medium constituents, and many are toxic for man. Good quality control and appropriate safety procedures are essential in the preparation of such media. Those who attempt to devise dye tolerance-based tests or selective media are advised to assess several batches of the dye from a variety of commercial sources before publication.

Chemical growth requirements figure in several identification tests. These include the classic tests to show requirements for porphyrin precursors (X factor) and NAD (V factor) in *Haemophilus*. V factor is common in nature, and media are readily contaminated thus giving false-negative V requirement tests. Growth factor requirements form the basis of auxotyping for *Neisseria gonorrhoeae*.

4.   *Tests for oxidative metabolic pathways*

Three basic tests for the mode of energy metabolism in bacteria are the oxidase, catalase, and Hugh and Leifson O/F tests. They reflect the presence of components of a functional electron transport system, and clear results for these three tests along with microscopic morphology, staining, and motility will generally guide an investigator to a reliable identification at the genus level. Oxidase and catalase reactions can be assessed rapidly on primary cultures, but the O/F test is slower, is not amenable to commercial identification formats, and so has fallen from favour. It should not be forgotten if other initial identification tests are not informative. Further tests which reflect oxidative metabolism are those for growth in the presence of cyanide and azide, reduction of nitrate (to nitrite or beyond), reduction of nitrite, production of gas (nitrogen) from nitrate, utilization of citrate or malonate, and production of hydrogen peroxide.

5.   Tests for sugar metabolism

Many 'biochemical' identification tests are based on the metabolism of 'sugars'. Table 1 systematically lists the sugars and related substances that are commonly examined. Most of these tests examine for production of acid, but the format varies between bacterial groups in both the basal medium and the pH indicator that is employed. The concept of 'thresholding' is an important key to understanding the diversity of test format and to designing new tests.

Examination of a large number of isolates in lactose peptone water acidification, for example, might yield the distribution of pH measurements as illustrated in Figure 2a. The figure shows two populations, each with a clearly distinct terminal pH. The ideal point to place a threshold which separates the two populations is at A where the two distributions fuse at a minimum frequency. This would minimize the proportion of uninterpretable results. A threshold at B would give a large proportion of uninterpretable tests, and would falsely divide one population. The best indicator system would have a narrow range of color change at A, or failing this, the medium buffering or substrate concentration might be adjusted to bring the threshold pH to that of a suitable indicator. Figure 2b illustrates the population frequencies for a test that is unlikely to yield clear and reproducible results. Figure 2c illustrates distinct populations, but with a narrow minimum in the distribution, and an indicator system that fails to adequately discriminate between them. 'Thresholding' is rarely mentioned in papers, but it is a concept that might well be considered more in design to prevent the introduction of poorly reproducible tests that yield a high proportion of uninterpretable results.

Table 1   Sugars and related substances that are commonly used in the investigation of fermentation, utilization, and chromogenic enzyme tests.

Three carbon polyols:	glycerol
Tetrose sugars:	D (-) erythrose, D (-) threose
Tetrose sugar alcohols:	erythritol
Pentose sugars:	L (+) arabinose, D (-) ribose, D (+) xylose
Deoxy-hexose sugars:	L (+) fucose, L (-) rhamnose (isodulcitol)
Hexose sugars:	fructose (levulose), galactose, glucose (dextrose), mannose, sorbose
Hexose sugar alcohols:	D sorbitol, D mannitol, dulcitol (D galactitol), adonitol
Hexose sugar acids:	gluconate
Amino hexose sugars:	D glucosamine, D galactosamine
Disaccharides:	cellobiose, lactose, maltose, melibiose, sucrose (saccharose), trehalose, turanose
Trisaccharides:	melezitose, raffinose
Polysaccharides:	glycogen, inulin, starch, chitin
Glycosides:	esculin, amygdalin, arbutin, salicin
Six-membered ring polyol:	inositol

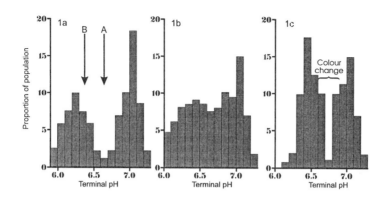

Figure 2 Problems of test 'thresholding'. In 1a, a threshold at A is optimal, separating clearly distinct populations, but a threshold at B includes a proportion of acid-producing strains as negative, and gives equivocal results for 7% of isolates. In 1b, there is no inherent division into two populations, and no possibility of obtaining meaningful and non-equivocal results. In 1c, there are clearly distinct and well separated populations, but the indicator system has a broad pH range in which equivocal results would be obtained thus enclosing ca. 21% of the strains.

Common end-products of carbohydrate metabolism include CO_2, acetate, lactate, formate, and acetyl methyl carbinol. CO_2 production (or CO_2 and hydrogen from formic hydrogen lyase activity) can be detected with an inverted Durham's tube in glucose peptone water, and acetyl methyl carbinol can be detected by the Voges-Proskauer test. The methyl red test reflects the acidity of the end product mix.

Detection of sugar metabolism often depends on acid production. More direct tests for individual enzymes (e.g., glucosidase, galactosidase, amylase, fucosidase, glucuronidase, and sialidase) have been introduced, starting with chromogenic substrates such as ortho-nitro phenyl D-galactoside (ONPG) and esculin, and progressing to the highly sensitive methyl umbelliferone-tagged fluorogenic substrates.

Bacteria rarely fit into the rigid and simple systems that we desire, and their behaviour in identification tests for carbohydrate metabolism is no exception. Species of several genera (notably the aerobic spore-forming bacilli and the pseudomonads) fail to produce acid from sugars in the classic fermentation formats because they metabolize the sugars to CO_2 (and the peptone base to ammonia) rather than to incompletely oxidized acidic products. For strongly oxidative organisms with less fastidious requirements, an ammonium salt base will reveal utilization of the sugars. Other problems include: bleaching of indicator systems under anaerobic conditions; and non-specific enzyme systems that metabolize many sugars and so reflect a single character in a range of tests, e.g., for *Acinetobacter* (28). There are also several groups of asaccharolytic bacteria, and these are poorly identified in identification systems which are largely based on saccharolytic activity. It is best to review the substrates that these organisms are likely to encounter in nature and to utilize tests that are likely to reflect their metabolism. A notable success of this approach is the clear discrimination of species of anaerobic Gram positive cocci as determined with tests for enzymes that are involved in proteolysis and amino acid metabolism (29).

6. Tests for protein and amino acid metabolism

Assays for production of indole and H_2S were amongst the earliest of identification tests, reflecting the importance that microbiologists once placed on the olfactory sense, but which are now largely ignored for safety considerations. Tests for digestion of gelatin and casein, and the 'mixed' test for saccharolytic and proteolytic activity in litmus milk soon followed. The pattern of digestion of meat granules in broth by clostridia is an important test. Nitrogen metabolism is revealed by tests for lysine, ornithine, and arginine decarboxylase, arginine dihydrolase, phenylalanine deaminase, and urease. The tests for specific arylamidase activities represent a breakthrough in characterization by greatly improving the identification of asaccharolytic organisms. Other assorted tests for metabolism of amino acids are those for decomposition of tyrosine and for hydrolysis of hippurate (benzoyl glycine). The tube and slide tests for staphylococcal coagulase are amongst the most rapid species-specific identification tests that are employed in diagnostic bacteriology, and they offer an excellent example of familiarity by breeding a host of variant methodologies.

7.   Tests for lipid metabolism

The classic test is for lipase and lecithinase on egg yolk agar. Tests for digestion of Tweens 20, 40, and 80, and of tributyrin have also been introduced.

8.   Tests for nucleic acid and purine/pyrimidine base metabolism

The test for DNAase is the most frequently encountered, but there are also tests for phosphatase and decomposition of xanthine. The metabolism of heterocyclic nitrogen compounds is often neglected in identification and characterization tests.

9.   Tests based on cell wall receptors

Cell surface structures, i.e., the wall and cell membrane, are the interface between the bacterial cell and its environment. They govern much of the host-parasite interaction in bacterial disease, and research into pathogenesis often centers on cell surface receptors. Many important sub-species (epidemiological typing) systems are ultimately derived from this work, e.g., O, H, and K serotyping, phage typing, M and T serotyping, etc. Fewer tests have emerged from this work for the differentiation of species, but several are important in the differentiation of the Gram positive cocci, e.g., optochin, lysostaphin, and lysozyme susceptibility, bile solubility, and the Lancefield antigens.

C.   Chemical analysis of cell components

Formal chemical analysis of cell components has thrown considerable light on the classification of bacteria. Polypeptide bridging sequences in cell wall peptidoglycan, wall and membrane long chain fatty acid composition, and isoprenoid quinones and other carriers in the electron transport chain have all contributed to the nomenclature. Chemical analysis at this level, however, is beyond the resources of most diagnostic laboratories. With one notable exception, these analyses have remained the province of biological chemists.

   The work of Moss and his colleagues (30) has produced a system for identification which is based on long chain fatty acid composition. These lipids are found in the cell membrane and cell wall, and their quantitative and qualitative composition is highly species-specific, but depends also on growth medium and incubation temperature. The acids are extracted into a suitable organic solvent from cells that are grown under standardized conditions. They are methylated, and the volatile methyl esters are then analyzed by gas-liquid chromatography. The resulting profile can then be compared with those of standard reference organisms, grown under the same conditions, to yield an identification. The whole process has been packaged as the semi-automated Sherlock Microbial Identification System (MIDI Inc., Newark, New Jersey) that is in routine use at many major reference centres and commercial laboratories.

D.   Fingerprinting methods

There are a wide variety of instrument-based techniques that are applied in taxonomic studies, but none have yet found their way to routine identification. Microbiologists seem to prefer to work with tube and pipette-based technology, rather than the instrument-based technology fingerprinting methods, and their potential has been largely ignored except by a few enthusiasts and specialized units.

Briefly, pyrolysis gas-liquid chromatography and pyrolysis mass spectrometry (31) yield pattern data that reflect whole-cell composition. They operate by rapid thermal degradation of cell samples in the absence of oxygen which is then followed by separation and quantitation of the products. Matrix-assisted laser desorption and ionization time of flight mass spectrometry, commonly termed MALDI-TOF-MS, has recently been applied to whole-cell bacterial specimens with promising results (32). This is a rapid method in which cell material is decomposed in a laser beam and the molecular fragments are separated and quantified by time of flight spectrometry. Unlike pyrolysis techniques, cells are dried in a quinone-derivative matrix, which distributes the energy input and ionizes the fragments. The cell polymer fragments so obtained are much larger than the 20 to 500 Dalton fragments that are obtained in pyrolysis, and the results are more amenable to chemical interpretation.

Infra-red spectrometry and its more modern derivative, Fourier-transform infra-red spectrometry (33,34), again yield pattern data that reflect whole-cell composition, but by quantitative analysis of the infra-red spectrum of cells. In Raman spectrometry and UV excitation Raman spectrometry (35), absorption lines that are normally part of the infrared spectrum are revealed as modulations of monochromatic visible or ultra-violet light respectively. UV excitation has the advantage that the contribution of specific polymers, DNA, RNA, or proteins, to the spectrum can be overwhelmingly enhanced by tuning the excitation light to a frequency that is specifically absorbed by the polymer.

Sodium dodecyl sulphate polyacrylamide gel electrophoresis (SDS-PAGE) of whole cell proteins or outer membrane proteins also yield pattern data, but in this case for the protein constituents of the cell. Cell proteins are liberated by lysis, the peptides are separated by boiling in the presence of mercapto-ethanol, and they are linearized and charged by the addition of the SDS anionic detergent. The peptides can then be separated according to molecular weight in electrophoresis, and the band pattern visualized by staining (36).

All of these methods have been applied in taxonomic studies of bacteria, and, with the exception of the electrophoretic techniques, can be applied to the analysis of single cells. By and large they are rapid, have non-species-specific methodology with simple specimen preparation, are automated or are capable of automation, and can cope with large numbers of specimens. All require careful standardization of growth conditions. The pattern data that they yield often requires quite heroic mathematical analysis, but this can be handled readily by modern computers, and the results, which are well worth the effort, yield highly discriminatory data at all levels from genus through species and down to sub-species typing.

E. Molecular methods

The discovery that DNA was the basis of heredity, like many subsequent major advances in molecular biology, originated from work with bacteria. The first of the molecular characterization techniques was the assay for the ratio of guanine and cytosine to adenine and thymine base pairs in chromosomal DNA (G+C ratio, usually expressed as a percentage). This proved highly informative in taxonomic studies at the genus level, but was too prolonged and complex for routine identification. DNA-DNA hybridization followed and, although this is even more demanding and time consuming than base ratio estimation, it has been accepted as the gold standard for designation of bacterial species (37). Strains of the same species show 70% to 100% hybridization (with a difference of 5°C or less in thermal stability) when standardized against a same-strain control. This has been calculated as reflecting 96% to 100% sequence identity of the genome (38).

1. Conserved genes

As molecular techniques advanced, it was realized that some genes show a high degree of sequence conservation. Presumably, these genes code for RNA or protein molecules whose functional expression is essential to metabolism. A large portion of the RNA or amino-acid sequence is critical to this functionality. An example is the small sub-unit ribosomal RNA gene where the gene product has a complex three-dimensional structure. This structure is dictated by internal folding about complementary intramolecular base sequences and binding to ribosomal protein components, and is essential for protein synthesis. Presumably, most mutations within the gene yield products that are non-functional, or have such poor functionality that mutated clones fail to compete. These genes evolve slowly, and show a high level of sequence homology across wide taxonomic divisions. The best documented examples of conserved genes are those that code for the 16S and 23S ribosomal RNA components, heat shock proteins, and RNA and DNA polymerase components. The most useful are those that have highly conserved unique sequences that are suitable for universal primers at both the 5' and 3' ends, thus allowing for amplification by PCR or other similar techniques.

These conserved genes have become an important tool for taxonomists. Initial work on the direct sequencing of 16S rRNA showed strong intra-species conservation and inter-species variation. With the introduction of rapid and automated sequencing, and by exploiting the polymerase chain reaction to amplify specific sequences and then the cycle reaction to sequence them, a large bank of sequence data became available. Comparison of these sequences has revolutionized our ideas on the evolution of life and has markedly affected views on the evolutionary inter-relationships of bacterial species. These conserved genes have also become targets for molecular characterization and identification, and techniques have evolved to exploit their unique taxonomic properties.

2.   Probe-based detection and identification of species

This relies on documentation of a target DNA sequence that is present in all members of a species (or genus) and that is absent from all other organisms. An example is the mycobacterial insertion sequence, IS6110, which is present in most strains of the tuberculosis group (*M. tuberculosis*, BCG and *M. bovis*), but that is not found in other bacteria. For specimens showing acid-fast bacilli, rapid identification to this group would be a strong indication of disease and thus pre-empt prolonged confirmation by conventional culture. Furthermore, highly sensitive and specific sequence detection might be a substitute for microscopy particularly for specimens other than sputa when microscopy is difficult and where organisms tend to be sparse. Several probe-based identification techniques have been introduced on this basis.

Briefly, a target-specific oligonucleotide is synthesized and labeled, often with a fluorescent or enzyme marker. This is then hybridized with test DNA, and binding of the label indicates the presence of the target sequence, and so, the target organism. Methodological formats vary widely: from in situ hybridization with detection of hybridization in single cells to extraction of DNA from specimens or cultures with or without amplification which is followed by solid or liquid phase hybridization and detection of bound label (39). The methods tend to be costly, but are rapid and specific. Each individual probe method tests for a single group, species, or genus with a unique probe, and often with unique detailed methodology. These are in reality specific detection, rather than identification methods, but they could be developed to embrace a wider role (see below).

3.   Sequencing-based identification

The large database of 16S rRNA gene sequences and the increasing availability of automated sequencers has prompted several reference laboratories to take up this approach. The 16S rRNA gene is amplified from a DNA extract of the strain with universal primers, the products are purified and cycle-sequenced, and the sequence is compared with those in the ribosomal RNA database. Often, the variations in the first 300 to 500 bases of the 16S rRNA gene are sufficient to allow for identification thus avoiding the necessity for tedious full sequencing of the gene with intermediate lead primers. This is only a little slower than phenotypic identification for rapidly growing organisms provided that full sequencing is not required. It is too costly and inconvenient for routine use, but it is becoming the method of choice at larger centres for those isolates that prove difficult to identify by normal methods. A proportion of these difficult strains are likely to be of previously unrecognized species, and there would be considerable advantages if some international system was instigated to record the 16S rRNA sequence, conventional test reaction patterns, and clinical details for these strains. A full 16S rRNA sequence will probably become part of the minimal requirements for the description of new species within the next decade.

4. Restriction digest-based identification

Again, this depends on documentation of a sequence that shows intra-species variation and within-species conservation, and exists between two highly conserved and unique sequences that can be exploited as PCR primers. DNA is extracted from the organism (or specimen, if the method has a sufficiently robust amplification step), and the target sequence is amplified in conventional PCR. Amplification is confirmed by electrophoresis which should reveal a product of the expected molecular size. The product is digested with a restriction endonuclease, and the restriction products are separated by electrophoresis. Sequence variations at the sites of endonuclease cleavage cause variation in the pattern of products (Figure 3) and so, with the suitable choice of the restriction enzyme (experimentally-based or deduced from known sequence data), each species yields a distinct and characteristic digest pattern that can be stored in a library for comparative identification. Normally, two digests are analyzed from two restriction enzymes with distinct cutting sites in order to obtain discrimination over a range of species and to confirm the identification.

Essentially, this approach detects sequence differences in the target gene but avoids the necessity for full sequencing. It is an inexpensive alternative with costs that are closely comparable to conventional phenotypic identification kits. With two electrophoresis steps and an enzyme digestion, however, identification requires 24-30 hours, and is no more rapid than conventional kits for most organisms. The advantages are evident for slow growing or fastidious organisms or for species that are difficult to identify by conventional methods because they are asaccharolytic or give irreproducible results in conventional tests. The potential for identification by gene amplification directly from the specimen is also

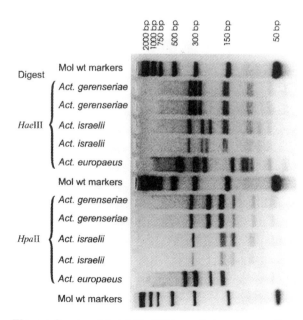

Figure 3 Amplified 16S rDNA restriction enzyme digests for medical isolates of actinomycetes. The figure illustrates clear species-specific banding patterns. (Unpublished data, courtesy of V. Hall)

attractive particularly for slower growing genera. This approach has been exploited for the identification of mycobacteria (40), actinomycetes (41), and the *Clostridia* (42). Although this approach is primarily an identification tool, it may also be useful in screening for previously unrecognized species amongst routine isolates of less well-documented genera.

5. DNA arrays, microelectronics and the future

Microbiologists have resisted automation for a considerable time, but there are new developments that hold promise for a clear path to automated diagnosis of infectious diseases. DNA hybridization methods have been miniaturized to the point that nearly a million distinct oligomer probes can be attached to a space that is smaller than a conventional microscope slide (43). There are less than 1000 bacterial pathogens, perhaps 1000 viral pathogens, and less than 500 fungal and protozoan pathogens of man. Clearly, even if as many as 10 oligomer probes were required for unequivocal detection and identification of each of these species, there would be massive excess capacity on these high-density arrays. There are two problems with the current state of this technology. The hybridization results are read by fluorescence from tagged bases that are introduced during amplification of the specimen's nucleic acid, and so the readers are bulky and costly. Also, the DNA arrays are still made in comparatively small runs for quite limited research applications, and thus are costly.

Neither of these problems is insuperable, and several methods for direct electronic detection of hybridization results are being developed (44). Equally, the costs of micro-electronic devices now lie mainly in their development. A high-density oligomer array with electronic detection would probably be less complex than a 10 megabyte memory chip which currently retails at about $10. All that is required to bring costs to this level is the development process and a massive market, and this will certainly come once the potential of these devices in bedside diagnosis is recognized.

Two other technologies are required to achieve a hand-held instrument that is capable of automated diagnosis. One is a miniaturized clean-up processor that will take the specimen (urine, CSF, blood, liquefied sputum, or sample liquid that is expressed from a damp swab) extract, concentrate the bacteria and/or mammalian cells, and then lyse them to produce free nucleic acids. The other is a miniaturized nucleic acid amplification processor that will replicate the required range of species-specific target sequences from this specimen-derived nucleic acid mixture.

The first of the above technologies is at a very early stage of development, but mixtures of *E. coli* and mammalian red cells have been separated: the bacteria are then lysed by a current pulse in a micro-miniaturized device (45). Target sequences in the recoverable bacterial DNA were then amplified and detected. The most promising line of research in this area is in electrodiaphoresis where suspended particles can be manipulated in electric fields and then differentiated and separated according to their electrostatic properties. Complex micro-miniaturized devices have been produced that are capable of separating red and white blood cells, or mixtures of several bacterial species (46).

The second technology is at a more advanced stage. Micro-miniaturized processors have been devised for almost every known nucleic acid amplification procedure (e.g., 47). An example of the latter is of a continuous flow PCR processor with amplification in two to twenty minutes and with re-use after a flush cycle (47). Several broad range nucleic acid amplification processes are in current use, and these could well be adapted to the requirements for diagnosis in infectious diseases given sufficient impetus.

If these three technologies can be developed to the point where each of the required devices can be manufactured and coupled to one another in a functional bedside diagnostic instrument, there will certainly be a revolution in medicine and in microbiology.

VI. BACTERIAL CLASSIFICATION – A HISTORY

A. An overview of the history in the context of general biology

Several themes in bacterial classification are linked to advances on fundamental research in biology. One of these is the influence of characterization technology. While plants and animals exhibit a host of readily-observed morphological and developmental features, the size and simple unicellular organization of bacteria limits the number of morphological characters that can be observed. The search for adequate numbers of characterization tests drove bacteriologists towards an ever increasingly biochemical approach at a time when other biologists found morphological characters to be adequate. Consequently, bacteriology has played a leading role in many important advances in biochemistry and, later, molecular genetics.

Another theme has been the search to position bacteria in the classification and evolution of life. In 1838, they were first named bacteria and grouped with other microscopic organisms by Ehrenberg. They were then claimed, unsuccessfully by Haekel in 1866, to lie with the Protista or Monera. The latter group included the fungi, algae, and protozoa. They were then placed with the plants by Cohn (48). Bacteria then played a leading role in Pasteur's disposal of the commonly held theory of spontaneous generation of life. After being cast into a taxonomic wilderness, with the most vague of botanical connections as the *Schizomycetes*, it was finally realized that bacteria, blue green algae, and archaebacteria shared a common and unique cellular organization (49,50). The split of cellular organisms into the prokaryotes (bacteria, blue green algae, and archaebacteria) and eukaryotes provided an ironic inversion of prior arguments that bacteria belonged to the plant or animal kingdoms which are now subgroups of the eukaryotic organisms. This story may well continue: molecular techniques show that several groups of eukaryotic micro-organisms represent evolutionary lines whose divergence preceded the division of plants and animals (51).

The above theme intertwines with arguments on phylogeny – the study of evolutionary pathways of life forms. Botanists and zoologists have struggled to fix an evolutionary tree of life from fossil evidence for nearly 200 years. Bacteriologists opted out of this struggle because clearly there was no fossil evidence for the evolution of such microscopic organisms. Having turned their back on evolutionary approaches for a century, bacteriologists then originated the techniques of molecular phylogeny in the 1970s. The evolutionary tree was derived from sequences of conserved genes, particularly the small ribosomal sub-unit RNA, and provided several surprises. It also prompted a successful search for the microfossils of prokaryotes. Currently, controversy rages on the evidence for fossilized bacteria in meteorites and their extraterrestrial origins. Techniques, which unequivocally identify and characterize fossilized prokaryotes, may well provide further surprises in regards to the evolution of life on Earth and, perhaps, elsewhere.

These views are consistent with the recognition that eukaryotic mitochondria and chloroplasts are symbiotic prokaryotic organisms. Evidence from mitochondrial 16S rRNA sequencing studies is consistent with the evolutionary descent of mitochondria from bacteria, and this work has aided in establishing lines of descent amongst the eukaryotes. The breadth of the symbiotic association between prokaryotes and eukaryotes is only beginning to be appreciated. Other intracellular structures of eukaryotes, such as hydrogenosomes and some 'organelles' of motility, are also clearly bacterial symbionts. Some single-celled eukaryotes contain so many distinct symbiotic prokaryotic 'organelles' that they might be regarded better as ecosystems that co-operate within a eukaryotic cell (52).

Medical microbiologists should remember that bacteriology deals with an enormous diversity of organisms which is far larger than the few hundred species that cause human disease. The interactions of bacteria with man are not limited to pathogenesis, but include functions in the ecology that is essential to all life, such as the nitrogen cycle, and include symbioses that are basic to the existence of eukaryotic organisms. Bacteria are the most simple of single-celled organisms, and this simplicity has been a key in the resolution of many fundamental questions on the workings of life.

B. A brief overview of the history

Linnaeus recognized the need for an internationally-recognized system of nomenclature for living organisms. He suggested a system of 'Latinized' binomials with the leading epithet (e.g., *Escherichia*) denoting a broad group of organisms or genus, and the trailing epithet (e.g., *coli*) denoting the specific group within the genus, i.e., species. Linked with a formal description for each species, this system provides a concise and precise technical vocabulary that bridges speciality and nationality.

Microbes had already been observed by van Leeuwenhoek, and these were entered into Linnaeus' earliest classification as six species of the genus *Chaos*. The next true advance came in the late 19th century with sterilization and aseptic handling techniques, liquid and solid media, and pure culture. Characterization technology advanced rapidly. Strains could be isolated in pure culture, and their colonial morphology and growth features in liquid and semi-solid media could be observed. The staining techniques of Gram and Ziehl-Neelsen completed a set of characterization methods that are still the mainstay of identification in the routine diagnostic laboratory.

Experimentation with media soon gave the fermentation, utilization, and physiological tests that have evolved into the panel of conventional 'biochemical' tests that are still employed by diagnostic laboratories. This explosion of information resulted in a tattered beginning to bacterial classification. Pragmatism was the order of the day in medical microbiology, with the purpose of distinguishing newly discovered pathogens, rather than placing them in ordered groups. Equally, scientists in each of the applied disciplines named and described species without reference to work in other branches. For about forty years, a host of concurrent bacterial classifications were generated, each specific to a particular branch of microbiology, or even a particular department.

Ferdinand Cohn (48) made the first attempt to bring some order to this chaos by classifying bacteria with a botanical bias of hierarchical identification keys and with the assumption of within-species invariance of characters that remained ruling features of bacterial classifications for more than eighty years. This attempt at academic classification, and the contrasting attitude of the pragmatists, colored subsequent events with factions and attitudes that are recognizably derived from events of over a century ago.

The diversity of classifications began to coalesce in 1923 with the publication of the first edition of Bergey's Manual. The efforts of Buchanan were particularly important during this phase. This represented the beginning of the formal classification with a system for naming new species and with a limit to further proliferation of descriptions and names for the same organism. The influence of Cohn is clearly marked in the hierarchical keys that were adopted in Bergey's Manual and most of the early classifications.

These keys are based on two assumptions. The first is that there is an inherent hierarchy of 'importance' in the characters that are used to distinguish between bacteria. For example, the Gram staining reaction was often regarded as a principal test and applied initially in the key to separate a group of Gram negative organisms from the Gram positive ones. The covert assumptions were that these two groups represented lines that had diverged early in evolution, and that the Gram reaction was highly conserved. Based on this, one could reasonably assume that this division also reflected fundamental differences in organization thus dictating many observable differences between the groups. In contrast, production of gluconate, for example, would be regarded as a character of low precedence and would be relegated to the deeper levels of the key where genera were being split into species.

The problems with hierarchies of importance for characters lay in these covert assumptions. There was no evidence for evolutionary precedence of any characters at that time, and their priority was a matter of opinion. Shuffling these priorities could produce many distinct keys and hierarchies, and this potential was fully realized in subsequent editions of Bergey's Manual to the continuing annoyance of pragmatist factions who cared little for the hierarchy but found the changes in generic epithets inconvenient. Microscopic morphology and staining characters were regarded as primary tests and were possibly influenced by the primacy of morphology in more general biology. Equally, the assumption that these 'important' characters were conserved was unproven. We know now, from 16S rRNA sequencing, that the Gram negative bacteria probably represent multiple distinct evolutionary lineages, while the Gram positive group originated later as a single evolutionary line rather than being a 'primitive form'.

This discussion highlights a rift in systematic opinion that is important to microbiologists. The pragmatists and purists have had a shifting balance of support that has been reflected in the varying shape of formal bacterial systematics through the century. The extreme pragmatists follow Locke in seeing species as a man-made concept that is imposed on a continuous spectrum of biological diversity. For them, a classification is only justified in its utility for applied microbiology; divisions above species have neither reality nor use. The extreme purists see the species designation as an Aristotelian archetype, i.e., the lowest layer in the hierarchy of real biological divisions (species, genus, family, order, class, phylum, and kingdom) that accurately reflect a linear branching tree of evolution.

The hierarchy thus changed with each new edition of Bergey's Manual, and, in retrospect, each was wrong in some ways and correct in others. The next major advance came with numerical taxonomy where the heritage of botanical assumptions of test invariance and the hierarchical importance of characters was discarded in a single step.

Sneath, working on bacteria, and Sokal, working concurrently on insects, both discarded these assumptions as invalid, and they produced a revolutionary alternative approach to classification. In their scheme of numerical taxonomy, all characters have equal weight, there is no assumption of test invariance, and subjective judgement is largely limited to choosing the levels of similarity at which species, genera, etc. are named.

This major change in the methods of formulating classifications was quickly followed by parallel changes in the approach to identification. Identification keys could be designed to cope with intraspecies character variation but their complexity increases exponentially with increasing numbers of variable characters. A new format for identification was evolved, and it became the mainstay of routine identification with the successive editions of Cowan and Steel's Manual for the Identification of Medical Bacteria (4). This was followed by numerical identification (53) which remains the most rigorous method of identification from 'biochemical' test results.

The concept of polyphasic taxonomy was introduced by Colwell (54), and it has been applied widely by experienced taxonomists. This was a further break from the idea that classification should be based on a hierarchy of importance of characters. Colwell suggested that classifications which are based on the widest possible range of distinct characterization systems would give a nomenclature with prolonged stability. This was a refreshing change in philosophy for a subject that was destabilized throughout its history by ephemeral changes as tests fell in and out of fashion.

Considerable in-roads were made in classifying the diversity of bacteria during subsequent years. In 1980, the publication of the Approved Lists of Bacterial Names (15,16) marked a major consolidation and rationalization of species nomenclature. It facilitated the elimination of early errors, synonymous names, and descriptions, and it also simplified access to the nomenclature. About 2,300 species names were validated in the 1980 Approved Lists, and the number of formally recognized species names doubled in the following two decades.

Bacterial taxonomists had also begun to explore a much wider range of characterization techniques. The morphological, 'biochemical', and serological tests were supplemented with gas liquid chromatography, chemical analysis of cell wall polymers and electron transport chain components, protein electrophoresis, and a wide range of physico-chemical fingerprinting techniques. Only a few of these approaches were sufficiently simple, rapid, and inexpensive to find routine applications in identification, but their contribution to advances in classification was enormous.

The use of nucleic acid analysis began with base ratio analysis, and proceeded to DNA-DNA hybridization. The capability of this approach for distinguishing species was well recognized from the 1970s, and it is now the final arbitrator of species status among bacteria (37). Bacteriology is the only area of biology where there is general acceptance of a single and unequivocal definition of species status. It is ironic that this unique consensus has been achieved in a subject where the underlying species concept is more elusive than in any other area of biology.

From the 1980s, molecular biology has had a progressively greater influence on bacterial systematics. DNA-DNA hybridization and 16S rRNA sequencing played a major role in untangling the complex taxonomy of the pseudomonads and many other groups. This increasing predominance has brought some problems. Classifications which are based on conventional tests, hybridization, and 16S rRNA sequencing do not show invariable agreement, and the areas of disagreement bring considerable practical and conceptual difficulties. The sequencing techniques, however, have brought some scientific basis for a phylogenetic classification of bacteria (55).

VII. IDENTIFICATION

Consideration of specimen microscopy results and colony morphology from a range of media usually divides new medical isolates into three categories: commensals or contaminants of no significance, possible pathogens, and probable pathogens. This triage is mainly based on colonial morphology, and is an art rather than a science. As with all pattern recognition processes, it is difficult to document or teach in a formal setting. The expertise that is required to sort isolates into these categories with confidence and accuracy only comes with long periods of one-to-one training at the bench which is a costly but essential process that can be difficult to justify to paymasters. Without this triage, laboratories would be faced with an unsupportable identification workload.

Many of the probable and possible pathogens can be identified further with simple rapid tests – coagulase, Gram stain, oxidase, catalase, or serological tests for surface antigens, e.g., Lancefield grouping, or poly-O and poly-H *Salmonella* sera. Some isolates are adequately identified by these or other simple overnight tests. A residual number, however, require formal identification, and this is now largely performed with commercial kits. The first stage is to select an appropriate test panel that is based on the preliminary tests. A common error is to select a panel that is suited to the identification of fermentative Gram negative bacilli for an isolate with oxidative metabolism; this can often be avoided with an oxidase test and an observation of the pattern of growth on aerobic and anaerobic isolation media.

A. Numerical identification

This approach, like numerical taxonomic analysis, allows for character variation and also allows for equal weighting of characters. It is based on a matrix of known character frequencies for the taxa, and it assumes that: a) the isolate to be identified cannot be a member of more than one taxon, and b) the isolate is a member of one of the taxa in the matrix. An example of a numerical identification is shown in Figure 4, and the approach has been almost universally adopted in commercial kits where printed lists of identifications for common result profiles are supplied or where the full analysis is performed by a program package. It is important to note that there are two quite distinct sets of indices that should be examined to verify an identification result. One set describes the equivocal nature of the result – an uncertainty of choice between the best-fitting taxon and other taxa. The other set describes the 'strangeness' of the isolate – the extent of difference between the reaction pattern of the isolate and the mean reaction pattern of the first-choice taxon. Low similarities to the first choice taxon may indicate that the isolate does not belong to any of the taxa that are listed in the matrix.

Common sources of erroneous identifications include mixed cultures, poor inoculation, incubation in sub-optimal conditions, inaccurate reading of results, submission of isolates to an unsuitable test panel, and poor species resolution of the matrix.

The accuracy of identification systems is difficult to assess because 'gold standard' methods of identification have shifted markedly over the years, and are always time-consuming, difficult, and costly. Estimates of error rates vary from <10% for systems with twenty or more tests, when working with well-described groups such as the *Enterobacteriaceae*, to >25% for small numbers of tests and poorly documented groups. The author's experience is that those systems with larger test panels, clear reactions, and large well-documented identification matrices give greater confidence in results.

Identification Matrix:

| | Known proportion of isolates of the species giving a positive reaction in tests: | | | | | | | | | | Maximum |
Species	1	2	3	4	5	6	7	8	9	10	likelihood*
A	.90	.01	.05	.99	.99	.50	.99	.95	.99	.99	.38
B	.99	.90	.05	.75	.01	.99	.99	.05	.01	.99	.58
C	.90	.99	.01	.95	.95	.10	.01	.01	.01	.99	.69
D	.95	.50	.02	.95	.90	.01	.01	.10	.01	.99	.34
E	.01	.99	.01	.20	.01	.01	.99	.01	.95	.01	.70
F	.05	.99	.90	.99	.01	.99	.05	.01	.75	.01	.57
G	.95	.05	.90	.99	.99	.05	.90	.99	.01	.10	.60

* - The maximum likelihood is the likelihood of identification for an isolate with the best possible fit to the species. It is calculated by multiplying the proportion of positive reactions together across the row, substituting (1-proportion) if the proportion is less than 0.5 (i.e. the best fit result is negative). For species A, this is .90 x (1-.01) x (1-.05) x .99 x .99 x .50 x .99 x .95 x .99 x .99 (i.e. .38). The isolate reaction pattern in tests 1 to 10 is: + + - + + - - - - +. Calculate the likelihood of obtaining the isolate reaction pattern for each species by multiplying the expected proportions giving the isolate reaction together for each species. If the isolate reaction is negative, substitute (1-proportion) for that test. For species A, likelihood is: .90 x .01 x (1-.05) x .99 x .99 x (1-.50) x (1-.99) x (1-.95) x (1-.99) x .99 = 2.07x10^8.

Now calculate the further identification parameters for each species [examples given for species A].

Log probability = Log$_{10}$(likelihood) [= Log$_{10}$(2.07x10^8) = -7.68]

Modal likelihood = likelihood/maximum likelihood [= 2.07x10^8/.38 = 5.4x10^8]

Identification score = likelihood/sum of likelihoods for all species [= 2.07x10^8/1.03 = 2.0x10^8]

Relative likelihood = likelihood/highest likelihood value [= 2.07x10^8/.69 = 3.0x10^8]

Log probability and modal likelihood are measures of the 'strangeness' of the isolate – how unlikely it is that the pattern of reactions of the isolate would be produced by an isolate of that species. Identification score and relative likelihood are measures of 'equivocality' – how much doubt there is between the first and second choice species.

Identification Indices:

| | Known proportion of isolates of the species that give a positive reaction in tests: | | | | |
Species	Likelihood	Log probability	Modal likelihood	Identification score	Relative likelihood
A	2.07x10^8	-7.6819	5.4x10^8	2.0x10^8	3.0x10^8
B	5.91x10^7	-6.22834	1.0x10^6	5.7x10^7	8.6x10^7
C	0.69	-0.16226	1.0	0.67	0.99
D	0.34	-0.46333	1.0	0.33	0.50
E	9.61x10^{11}	-10.0175	1.4x10^{10}	9.3x10^{11}	1.4x10^{10}
F	1.15x10^9	-8.93846	2.0x10^9	1.1x10^9	1.7x10^9
G	4.38x10^7	-6.35868	7.3x10^7	4.2x10^7	6.4x10^7

The parameters indicate an equivocal identification and there is doubt whether the identity is species C or D. Further tests would be required for a firm identification.

Figure 4 Numerical identification: a worked example.

Identifications that show poor equivocality or 'strangeness' indices are not uncommon, however, and should be examined further by an expert eye. In the routine laboratory, the concern is mainly for the mistaken identification of more rare, but highly pathogenic, isolates as common low-grade pathogens. Such errors have been documented (56).

A species name brings with it a host of information and covert assumptions, and it should be ascribed to an isolate with due caution. There is an unavoidable tendency to assume that new isolates are typical of a species in all features, both in vitro and in vivo, and it may be prudent to moderate this view in some cases. A note that an isolate was atypical in laboratory tests, and may thus show atypical features in vivo may be appropriate in some cases. A frank admission that no species name could be ascribed with any certainty may be appropriate in others. This is an admission that bacteria do not always fit into well-defined species groups, or that we have only begun to catalogue the enormous diversity of bacterial species; this is not an admission of incompetence.

REFERENCES

1. Cowan ST. Taxonomic rank of the *Enterobacteriaceae* 'groups'. J Gen Microbiol 1956; 15: 345-349.
2. Cowan ST. The microbial species – a macromyth? In: Ainsworth GC, Sneath PHA, eds. Microbial Classification. Cambridge:Cambridge University Press, 1962:433-455.
3. Cowan ST. A Dictionary of Microbial Taxonomy. Cambridge:Cambridge University Press, 1978.
4. Barrow GI, Feltham RKA. Cowan and Steel's Manual for the Identification of Medical Bacteria, 3rd edition. Cambridge:Cambridge University Press, 1993.
5. Logan NA. Bacterial Systematics. Oxford:Blackwell Science, 1995.
6. Priest FG, Austin B. Modern Bacterial Taxonomy. London:Chapman & Hall, 1994.
7. Sokal RR, Sneath PHA. Principles of Numerical Taxonomy. San Francisco:Freeman, 1963.
8. Sneath PHA, Sokal RR. Numerical Taxonomy: The Principles and Practice of Numerical Classification. San Francisco:Freeman, 1973.
9. Dunn G, Everitt BS. An Introduction to Mathematical Taxonomy. Cambridge:Cambridge University Press, 1982.
10. Goodfellow M, Minnikin DE, eds. Chemical Methods in Bacterial Systematics. London:Academic Press, 1985.
11. Goodfellow M, O'Donnell AG, eds. Handbook of New Bacterial Systematics. London:Academic Press, 1993.
12. Stackebrandt E, Goodfellow M, eds. Nucleic Acid Techniques in Bacterial Systematics. Chichester:John Wiley and Sons, 1991.
13. Claridge MF, Dawah HA, Wilson MR, eds. Species: The Units of Biodiversity. London:Chapman & Hall, 1997.
14. Sneath PHA. International Code of Nomenclature of Bacteria, 1990 Revision. Washington DC:American Society for Microbiology, 1992.
15. Skerman VBD, McGowan V, Sneath PHA. Approved lists of bacterial names. Int J Syst Bacteriol 1980; 30:225-420.
16. Skerman VBD, McGowan V, Sneath PHA. Approved Lists of Bacterial Names (Amended Edition). Washington DC:American Society for Microbiology, 1989.
17. Holt JG - ed. Bergey's Manual of Systematic Bacteriology. Baltimore:Williams & Wilkins, 1984.
18. Levy-Frebault VB, Portaels F. Proposed minimal standards for the genus *Mycobacterium* and for description of new slowly growing *Mycobacterium* species. Int J Syst Bacteriol 1992; 42:315-323.
19. Ursing JB, Lior H, Owen RJ. Proposal for minimal standards for describing new species of the family *Campylobacteriaceae*. Int J Syst Bacteriol 1994; 44:42-45.
20. ICSB Subcommittee on Taxonomy of the Mollicutes. Revised minimal standards for description of new species of the class Mollicutes. Int J Syst Bacteriol 1995; 45:605-612.
21. Bousefield IJ. Bacterial nomenclature and its role in systematics. In: Goodfellow M, O'Donnell AG, eds. Handbook of New Bacterial Sytematics. London:Academic Press, 1993:318-338.
22. MacAdoo TO. Nomenclatural literacy. In: Goodfellow M, O'Donnell AG, eds. Handbook of New Bacterial Sytematics. London:Academic Press, 1993:339-358.
23. Murray RGE, Schleifer KH. Taxonomic note: a proposal for recording the properties of putative taxa of procaryotes. Int J Syst Bacteriol 1994; 44:174-176.
24. Murray RGE, Stackebrandt E. Taxonomic note: implementation of the provisional status *Candidatus* for incompletely described prokaryotes. Int J Syst Bacteriol 1995; 45:186.
25. Mackenzie DWR, Odds FC. Non-identity and authentication of two major reference strains of *Candida albicans*. J Med Vet Microbiol 1991; 29:225-261.
26. Magee JT. Whole organism fingerprinting. In: Goodfellow M, O'Donnell AG, eds. Handbook of New Bacterial Systematics. London: Academic Press, 1993:383-427.
27. Goodacre R, Timmins EM, Burton R, Kaderbhai N, Woodward AM, Kell DB, Rooney PJ. Rapid identification of urinary tract infection bacteria using hyperspectral, whole organism fingerprinting and artificial neural networks. Microbiology 1998; 144:1157-1170.

28. Hauge JG. Kinetics and specificity of glucose dehydrogenase from *Bacterium anitratum*. Biochem Biophys Acta 1960; 45:263-269.
29. Murdoch DA. Gram-positive anaerobic cocci. Clin Microbiol Rev 1998; 11:81-122.
30. Moss CW, Dees SB. Identification of micro-organisms by gas chromatography-mass spectrometric analysis of cellular fatty acids. J Chromatogr 1975; 112:595-604.
31. Magee JT. Analytical fingerprinting methods. In: Goodfellow M, O'Donnell AG, eds. Chemical Methods in the Classification of Prokaryotes. Chichester:John Wiley and Sons, 1994:523-553.
32. Claydon MA, Davey SN, Edwards-Jones V, Gordon DB. The rapid identification of intact microorganisms using mass spectrometry. Nature Biotechnol 1996; 14:1584-1586.
33. Naumann D, Helm D, Labischinski H, Giesbrecht P. The characterisation of microorganisms by Fourier-transform infrared spectroscopy (FT-IR). In: Nelson WH, ed. Modern Techniques for Rapid Microbiological Analysis. New York:VCH Publishers. 1991:43-96.
34. Goodacre R, Timmins EM, Rooney PJ, Rowland JJ, Kell DB. Rapid identification of *Streptococcus* and *Enterococcus* species using diffuse reflectance-absorbance Fourier Transform infrared spectroscopy and artificial neural networks. FEMS Microbiol Lett 1996; 140:233-239.
35. Nelson WH, Sperry JF. UV resonance Raman spectroscopic detection and identification of bacteria and other microorganisms. In: Nelson WH, ed. Modern Techniques for Rapid Microbiological Analysis. New York:VCH Publishers, 1991:97-143.
36. Vauterin L, Swings J, Kersters K. Protein electrophoresis and classification. In: Goodfellow M, O'Donnell AG, eds. Handbook of New Bacterial Systematics. London: Academic Press, 1993:251-280.
37 Wayne LG, Brenner DJ, Colwell RR, Grimont PAD, Kandler P, Krichevsky MI, Moore LH, Moore WEC, Murray RGE, Stackebrandt E, Starr MP, Truper HG. Report of the *ad hoc* committee on reconciliation of approaches to bacterial systematics. Int J Syst Bacteriol 1987; 37:463-464.
38. Stackebrandt E, Goebel BM. Taxonomic note: a place for DNA-DNA reassociation and 16S rRNA sequence analysis in the present species definition in bacteriology. Int J Syst Bacteriol 1994; 44:846-849.
39. Persing D, Smith TF, Tenover FC, White TJ. Diagnostic Molecular Microbiology. Washington DC:American Society for Microbiology, 1993.
40. Rocha AD, Leite CD, Torres HM, deMiranda AB, Lopes MQP, Degrave WM, Suffys PN. Use of PCR-restriction fragment length polymorphisms analysis of the hp65 gene for rapid identification of mycobacteria in Brazil. J Microbiol Methods 1999; 37:223-229.
41. Hall V, O'Neill G, Magee JT, Duerden BI. Amplified ribosomal DNA restriction analysis for identification of *Actinomyces* species. J Clin Microbiol 1999; 37:2255-2261.
42. Vaneechoutte M, Cartwright CP, Williams EC, Jäger B, Tichy H-V, De Baere T, De Rouck A, Verschraegen G. Evaluation of 16S rRNA gene restriction analysis for the identification of cultured organisms of clinically important *Clostridium* species. Anaerobe 1996; 2:249-256.
43. Johnston M. Gene chips: array of hope for understanding gene regulation. Curr Biol 1998; 8:R171-R174
44. Lamture JB, Beattie KL, Burke BE, Eggers MD, Ehrlich DJ, Fowler R, Hollis MA, Kosicki BB, Reich RK, Smith SR, Varma RS, Hogan ME. Direct detection of nucleic acid hybridization on the surface of a charge coupled device. Nucleic Acids Res 1994; 22:2121-2125.
45. Cheng J, Sheldon EL, Wu L, Uribe A, Gerrue LO, Carrino J, Heller MJ, O'Connell JP. Preparation and hybridization analysis of DNA/RNA from *E. coli* on microfabricated bioelectronic chips. Nature Biotechnol 1998;16:541-546
46. Pethig R. Electrokinetic manipulation of bioparticles. In: Coombs RRH, Robinson DW, eds. Nanotechnology in Medicine and the Biosciences. Amsterdam:Gordon & Breach, 1996:153-168.
47. Kopp MU, Mello AJ, Manz A. Chemical amplification: continuous-flow PCR on a chip. Science 1998; 280:1046-1048.
48. Cohn F. Untersuchungen über bacterien. Beitr Biol Pfl I heft 1872; 2:127.
49. Murray RGE. Fine structure and taxonomy of bacteria. In: Ainsworth GC, Sneath PHA, eds. Microbial Classification. Cambridge:Cambridge University Press, 1962.
50. Gibbons NE, Murray RGE. Proposals concerning the higher taxa of bacteria. Int J Syst Bacteriol 1978; 28:1-6.
51. Sogin ML, Silberman JD, Hinkel G, Morrison HG. Problems with molecular diversity in the *Eukarya*. In: Roberts DMcL, Sharp P, Alderson G, Collins M, eds. Evolution of Microbial Life. Cambridge:Cambridge University Press, 1996:167-184.
52. Fenchel T. Eukaryotic life: anaerobic physiology. In: Roberts DMcL, Sharp P, Alderson G, Collins M, eds. Evolution of Microbial Life. Cambridge:Cambridge University Press, 1996:185-203.

53. Willcox WR, LaPage SP, Holmes B. A review of numerical methods in bacterial identification. Antonie van Leeuwenhoek 1980; 46:233-299.
54. Colwell RR. Polyphasic taxonomy of bacteria. In: Iizuka H, Hasegawa T, eds. Culture Collections of Microorganisms. Tokyo:University of Tokyo Press, 1970:421-436.
55. Woese CR. Bacterial evolution. Microbiol Rev 1987; 51:221-271.
56. Batchelor BI, Brindle RJ, Gilks GF, Selkon JB. Biochemical misidentification of *Brucella melitensis* and subsequent laboratory-acquired infections. J Hosp Infect 1992; 22:159-162.

3

Critical Features of Specimen Collection, Transport, and Processing

Chandar Anand
Provincial Laboratory of Public Health for Southern Alberta, Calgary, Alberta, Canada

Nevio Cimolai
Children's and Women's Health Centre of British Columbia, Vancouver, British Columbia, Canada

The process of establishing a laboratory diagnosis of a putative infectious process involves a series of critical steps in order to facilitate a rapid and accurate detection of the etiological agent or agents involved. All of these must be understood and optimized in order to achieve the best outcome for the patient (1). These include pre-analytic steps of specimen selection, collection, transport and, if necessary, storage (2); analysis of the specimen in the laboratory; and post-analytic steps of reporting and interpretation, and timely delivery of the report to the physician for possible therapeutic intervention. From the laboratory perspective, the quality of microbiological specimens is perhaps the single most crucial factor influencing the value of results obtained, and consequently the pre-analytical stage is perhaps the most critical step. Most microbiological specimens are highly perishable, and poorly collected and transported samples may not only result in failure to recover important pathogens, but may also misdirect therapy towards a contaminating commensal organism with potential adverse effects.

In this chapter we consider the pre-analytic stage of selection and collection of optimum samples, their transport to the laboratory in a safe manner and in a manner that does not compromise the specimen integrity and viability of the etiological agents, and conditions of storage of the samples which cannot be processed immediately upon receipt in the laboratory. As well, we provide an overview of critical features that are relevant to the processing of these samples.

I. SPECIMEN COLLECTION AND TRANSPORT

A. The specimen must be clinically relevant

Specimens should be collected from the site where the infecting organism is most likely to be found and with as little external contamination as possible (3). In some cases, a single sample may be appropriate, whereas in others, samples from multiple sites may improve recovery of the etiological agent. For example, in the case of pneumococcal pneumonia, in addition to the expected presence of bacterium in respiratory specimens, blood cultures are frequently positive, and often provide a definitive diagnosis. For wounds, the more relevant specimen may be a swab which is taken from the advancing margin of the lesion or the abscess wall, and not simply pus or exudate where organisms may be non-viable. For a surface lesion, and depending on the circumstance, swabbing superficially can be inadequate. Specimen collection may benefit if the lesion is opened; purulent material from the advancing edge can be expressed onto a swab or aspirated using syringe and needle. The specimen of choice for a decubitus ulcer is a tissue biopsy; the bacteriology from swabs often represents surface colonization and a needle aspirate may not always sample the pathogens adequately to achieve a diagnosis. Sample for culture of lower respiratory secretions must be sputum that is raised by deep cough and not only saliva. For the diagnosis of *Streptococcus pyogenes* pharyngitis, swabbing of the peritonsillar area should avoid contact with the oral cavity. A nasopharyngeal (but not throat) swab is the preferred specimen for the diagnosis of pertussis. In acute otitis media, a swab of the external ear canal does not sample the causative organisms in the presence of an intact tympanic membrane, and tympanocentesis may be necessary to obtain a suitable sample. For the diagnosis of gonococcal infection in females, an endocervical (but not vaginal) specimen is most relevant.

B. Clear and explicit step-wise instructions for specimen collection and transport should be provided

Collection of specimens is frequently delegated to individuals who do not understand the requirements and consequences of such procedures. Most specimens for microbiology tend to be collected by non-laboratory personnel including physicians and nurses, by patients themselves, and only in a few cases by trained laboratory staff (phlebotomists). Therefore, laboratories need to provide clear and simple-to-understand instructions for the collection of each type of specimen. These can be in the form of a collection manual or instruction cards that are made available at nursing stations, physician offices, and collection stations; alternatively in hospital settings, the instructions can be incorporated in ward manuals. In settings where order entry is electronic, instructions can form part of the menu for ease of reference.

Components of these instructions should include safe collection, optimal specimen collection procedures, use of transport media, specimen transport information, and instructions on completing requisitions and for the labeling of specimens. Importantly, criteria that are used by the laboratory to reject improperly selected, collected, or transported specimens should be made clear. Exact reasons for any exceptions to these rules should be detailed to the laboratory on submission of the specimen.

For specimens to be collected predominantly by a patient, e.g., sputum, mid-stream urine, or stool, easy-to-follow written instructions should be handed to the patient. These should be supported by concise verbal instructions from the nurse/physician. In an era of globalization and mobile populations, it is of value to consider the need for alternate communication strategies when English or other local language is not the patient's own.

Periodic in-service for nursing, medical staff, and allied health professionals in the collection of good quality samples is helpful to reinforce the laboratory's requirements as is a regular laboratory newsletter or similar communication. On-going interaction between pathologists/microbiologists and the primary physicians in communities and hospitals needs to be cultivated and maintained to assist the physicians in the selection of optimum samples.

It is critical to provide updates to the instructions before the laboratory introduces any changes of consequence. Regular revisions of the collection manuals are essential.

C. Patient identification, and relevant clinical and epidemiological information must be provided

Unlike other clinical pathology sub-specialties, in medical microbiology the processing of a specimen is commonly individualized and is dependent on a number of different factors, e.g., the type of sample, site from which it is collected, the anticipated pathogen, and above all, the clinical features. The laboratory selects the most appropriate approach for confirming a suspected diagnosis based on the information provided by the physician on the requisition that accompanies the specimen. Additionally, there are often no fixed values in medical microbiology, and the information provided becomes crucial in the accurate interpretation of clinical relevance of the organisms so isolated. The value of relevant clinical and epidemiological information for quality of service cannot be understated, and ongoing efforts need to be made in order to encourage the clinicians to provide the same.

The minimum information required includes full name, care (or hospital) number, age or date of birth, sex, address, ordering physician's name and address for return of reports and contact if necessary, specific anatomic site, and type of specimen. Physicians should also provide the laboratory with a clinical impression or suspicion of particular and perhaps unusual organisms, current or contemplated antibiotic therapy, immune status if relevant, as well as any pertinent travel and epidemiological history.

In practice, a laboratory's request for information is very often not complied with. Physicians may be encouraged to provide maximum information by requisitions that are designed in whole or in part specifically for medical microbiology and for ease of use. Such a requisition may include the use of check boxes with elements of illness history, significant past history, immune status, intended antibiotic treatment, and exact nature and source of specimen. Finally, the most critical is the date and time of actual collection, since this will help in establishing the transit time to the laboratory, which is critical to the interpretation of the results and for quality assurance purposes.

Ongoing interaction between the physician and the laboratory need to be encouraged since this places the laboratory in a position of being able to advise on the selection and collection of the best possible specimen. The value of such dialogue cannot be underestimated (4).

D. The specimen container must be adequately labeled

In a busy hospital unit where more than one specimen is collected at a time, there exists the possibility that the requisition may become separated from the specimen.

Sufficient information, legibly written, must be provided on a firmly attached specimen label so that the specimen can be matched with the requisition when it is received in the laboratory (5). This is particularly important in a setting when an electronic request generates an on-line printed requisition in the laboratory and the specimen arrives unaccompanied by a hard copy requisition (6).

For adequate identification, the minimal information that is required includes the patient's first and last names, hospital or clinic number which serve as a valuable cross-reference on the name, the anatomical site from which the specimen was taken, name of the physician, and the date and time of collection.

Although the microbiology laboratory treats every specimen as being potentially infectious in the era of Standard or Universal Precautions (7), specimens that are from patients who are particularly known or suspected to have a dangerous and high risk pathogen should be so labeled for the benefit of the portering and the laboratory staff, e.g., suspect brucellosis. Similarly, a clear indication on the label, that the specimen requires emergency handling (STAT testing), serves as a flag to minimize the chance of it being missed as such.

E. The timing of specimen collection must be optimum

For the best opportunity to recover the causative micro-organisms, an optimum time for collection of specimens has to be established on the basis of current knowledge of the natural history and pathophysiology of the infectious process (8).

1. Phase of the disease

The causative agents of an infectious process are more likely to be detected during the acute phase of an illness; certain sampling sites may be better than others. For example, in typhoid fever, *Salmonella typhi* is often recovered in blood culture during the first week of illness, and in culture of feces and urine in second and third weeks respectively. The detection of *Escherichia coli* O157:H7 from stool samples is maximal during the first three days after the onset but decreases progressively (9); a week after the disease process was initiated, the likelihood of recovery will be minimal in most circumstances. For serological diagnosis, optimally-timed serum samples that are collected in the acute and convalescent stages of the disease process are required.

2. Time of day

There are no particular time restrictions for the collection of a single sample. First morning urine or sputum specimens which are collected on three consecutive days are useful for the diagnosis of renal and pulmonary mycobacterial infections since the organism is concentrated in such samples. Samples that are collected at other times of the day may be satisfactory as well. Gastric aspirates for mycobacteria are optimally collected as the early morning sample since the overnight ingestion of sputum improves the sensitivity of isolation.

Twenty-four hour collection of urine and sputum should be rejected since there is a high risk of contamination and overgrowth with more rapidly growing commensal organisms. This practice is unnecessary in view of the sensitivity of current culture techniques.

The optimum timing of blood culture is dependent on the clinical state of the patient. In conditions such as endocarditis, brucellosis, typhoid fever, and other uncontrolled infections, bacteremia is continuous and timing of sample collection is not influenced. In most other infections which result in bacteremia, the presence of bacteria is intermittent and the optimum timing of blood culture is influenced by several considerations (see Chapter 9).

3. Relationship to administration of antimicrobials

As a rule, specimens should be collected before antimicrobial agents have been administered. Some organisms are rapidly killed by appropriate therapy and may not be recovered altogether; others are only suppressed and may re-grow after cessation of treatment. If a culture sample has been taken after initiation of antibacterial therapy, the laboratory should be informed (through a properly completed requisition) so that counteractive measures, e.g., addition of penicillinase or specimen dilution, may be considered.

The collection of samples for antimicrobial drug levels (peak and trough levels) need to be correlated with the administration of the antibiotic.

F. Repeat samples should be limited

Processing of more than one properly collected sample from an anatomical site within a twenty-four hour period does not improve the chance of establishing the etiology of infection, but the duplication does add to unnecessary laboratory cost. Well-defined limits for the collection of specimens from the same anatomic site need to be established and rigidly applied. Once a definitive diagnosis has been established, subsequent cultures generally are governed by the patient's clinical state or as a test of cure. In the latter situation, the cultures are collected ideally after the effects of antibiotics have disappeared. In other situations, mainly involving the gastrointestinal tract, the number of infecting organisms may be small or excretion may be intermittent, e.g., salmonella carriage in a food handler. For evaluation of such cases, examination of three specimens that are collected on alternate days may be warranted.

In general, the following specimens need only be examined:

Once in 24 hours:

Upper respiratory [throat, nose (rarely indicated), oral cavity, ear, sinus], urine, stool, rectal, male genital, female genital - aerobe (endocervix, vaginal, urethra, placenta, vulva, lochia, perineum), female genital - anaerobe (placenta, Caesarean section, endometrium, uterus, culdocentesis, Fallopian tube, cervical aspirate, ovary, Bartholin's gland), lower respiratory (tracheal, bronchial, sputum), surface (burn, cyst, decubitus ulcer, exudate, laceration, lesion, paronychia, skin, stoma, suture, ulcer, vesicle), surgical (abscess, aspirate, hematoma, drain, exudate, fistula, intravenous catheter, purulent exudate, wound).

Up to three specimens in 24 hours:

Blood culture.

Specimens with no restrictions: (limitations may be due to accessibility)

Body fluids (amniotic, pericardial, joint, peritoneal, ascitic), bile, bone marrow, cerebrospinal fluid, lower respiratory tract (transtracheal aspirate, lung biopsy), surgical specimen (biopsy, bone, tissue).

There is growing evidence that the yield of routine enteric bacterial pathogens from stools of patients in hospital who develop diarrhea after three days of admission is extremely low (10). Patient variables must be considered which may increase the risk for these pathogens, e.g., food brought into hospital, e.g., food ingested during day pass, e.g., hospital's record for food-borne or water-borne pathogens. It has been suggested that bacteriological examination of such specimens may, therefore, be limited, e.g., detection of toxin of *Clostridium difficile*. Careful consideration again should be paid to the underlying clinical illness.

G. Contamination with normal (indigenous) flora during collection processes must be minimized

The skin and all mucosal surfaces are populated with indigenous flora and often may also acquire a transient flora or even become colonized for extended periods with potential pathogens. This is particularly true of patients in the hospital environment who are quite ill, immunocompromised, receiving antimicrobial therapy, intubated, catheterized, or who are in high intensity areas such as intensive care units. The collection of specimens from such patients or from sites, which are normally colonized, without precautions to minimize external contamination, could lead to erroneous results and may result in inappropriate treatment. Special care must be taken to minimize contamination during collection process. Special procedures are required to distinguish organisms which are the cause of an infective process from those which are part of the normal flora or those that constitute abnormal colonization.

The approach to the collection and management of specimens can be considered according to whether a site is normally sterile or is colonized with normal flora:

a) specimens from sites which are normally sterile (e.g., joint, pleural, CSF, blood culture): these specimens are collected by percutaneous aspiration after surgical preparation of the overlying skin. The recommended procedure involves cleaning with a germicide (2% iodine, povidone-iodine) application or 70% alcohol, with a contact time of at least two minutes in most cases. These specimens can often be cultured without selective media unless an initial Gram stain of the smear suggests contamination during collection.

b) specimens from sites that have normal flora or specimens that are collected through sites with normal flora: for infections that are caused by pathogenic micro-organisms that are not normally part of the indigenous micro-flora, it may suffice to examine only for known pathogens, e.g., *Streptococcus pyogenes* in pharyngeal specimens, enteric pathogens such as *Salmonella* spp. or *Shigella* spp. in stool specimens, *Neisseria gonorrhoeae* in genital specimens.

Organisms which are part of normal flora, either as indigenous or as transient colonizers, may be responsible for the infectious process at the same or contiguous sites, and determination of their pathogenic role may become difficult. In the case of urinary tract infections, adequate cleaning of the periurethral area and the perineum followed by a mid-stream specimen suffices routinely. Also, use of techniques such semi-quantitative cultures will also aid in differentiating commensal organisms from those that are involved in the disease process.

In other situations, however, such as a lower respiratory tract infection with anaerobic organisms or a complicated urinary tract infection, these measures may not be helpful. It may be possible to entirely or relatively bypass the area that contribute the commensals, and thereby sample directly from the site of infection. Respiratory secretions can be collected by bronchial aspiration or by protected brush, and urine specimens may be collected by suprapubic aspiration. Such invasive procedures, however, are necessary only in exceptional circumstances.

Other techniques that are used during the laboratory processing of the specimen, such as scoring for sputum samples (11) and presence of epithelial cells in smears of wound swabs, allow for some degree of assessment of contamination.

H. Sufficient quantity to complete all examinations that are requested must be collected

Routine processing of a microbiological specimen usually involves multiple procedures such as stained smears and inoculation to several different media. Sufficient material is necessary for each step. Culture of a specimen containing less than sufficient material to complete all required procedures has the potential to yield false negative or misleading results. To avoid this, the laboratory needs to establish the minimum quantity of material that it requires in order to adequately process a specimen, especially when multiple cultures are requested on the same specimen. It is usually easier to obtain an adequate sample during the stage of active infection when purulent material is plentiful. In mild or chronic infections, the amount of exudate or purulent material may be small and it may be difficult to obtain sufficient material especially if a swab specimen is obtained.

Generally, the amount of sample collected on a swab is limited even when much purulent material is present. During the process of inoculation to multiple solid and liquid media, the material on a swab progressively decreases with each successive medium inoculated, and the number of organisms available to be deposited on the last media is smaller as compared to the first. As such, a swab specimen is not considered to be the specimen of choice. Swab specimens, however, are easier to collect and are often the most common type of specimen received in a clinical laboratory.

If multiple requests are made on a single specimen, e.g., broncho-alveolar lavage for routine, mycobacterial, fungal, *Legionella* and viral cultures, sufficient quantity must be collected to permit all examinations. If sufficient quantity is not submitted, cultures should be limited to those that can be inoculated without compromising the completeness after allowing the physician to assign priority.

Rectal swabs are most often inadequate to diagnose gastrointestinal infections and must not be accepted as a substitute for diarrheal stool sample except in children or in acutely ill patients where acquisition is a significant problem. The sensitivity of blood cultures for detecting bacteremia/septicemia has improved significantly with the collection of large volume blood draws.

I. Optimum recovery of pathogens is ensured by the collection of a good quality specimen

Specimen for culture may be submitted in different forms. Swabs are often used for procuring many common types of specimen for culture, but their value is variable and limited. Other than samples of blood and body fluids, tissue samples constitute the most ideal specimens.

Tissue specimens should be placed into a sterile container and transported to the laboratory immediately. A large piece of tissue can be transported as is, but a few drops of non-bacteristatic sterile saline may be added to a smaller sample to help prevent dehydration during transportation.

Frankly purulent drainage or material such as pus that is aspirated with syringe and needle are also very good samples.

The amount of material that is collected on a swab is usually small. Also, swabs have a tendency to dry out and need to be submitted in transport media. Two swabs may be needed if antigen detection is also required in addition to Gram stain and culture. Swabs are made of different materials which may in themselves have limitations; these deserve consideration. Swabs are most often made of materials such as cotton, calcium alginate, dacron, or rayon, and have wooden, plastic, or wire handles. Each material, individually and in combination, may have disadvantages. Cotton swabs may contain residual fatty acid, which can inhibit certain fastidious organisms such as *N. gonorrhoeae*. This toxicity can be remedied by treating the swab with Sorensen's buffer (pH 6.7). Calcium alginate swabs on flexible wire are used to collect urethral and nasopharyngeal specimens, but can release toxic products which can inhibit certain organisms (12) (e.g., herpes simplex virus) and interfere with tests for direct detection of bacterial antigens. Dacron (polyester) or rayon swabs offer an alternative. PCR reactions may also be influenced by varied constituents of swabs and transport media. Swabs tend to dry out rapidly particularly when they contain only scant clinical material. As such, it is necessary to use swabs in conjunction with transport media as described below. The majority of laboratories use commercially-prepared swabs in conjunction with in-house or commercially-prepared transport media.

Other types of specimens include body fluids, some of which, such as joint fluids, blood, CSF, and urine, are normally sterile and are submitted to the laboratory without the use of transport media. It is essential that the laboratory receive the entire specimen and not a swab sampling of it.

J. Suitable specimen containers must be used

Specimens must be collected in sterile containers which are best purchased and provided by the laboratory. If purchased by a third party, the laboratory should approve each individual type of specimen container for its suitability. The size of the containers should ensure ease of collection, especially when the specimen is obtained by patients themselves. Wide-mouthed containers reduce the potential for contamination of the outside surface during the collection process, especially for samples such as sputum and urine. The containers must have tight-fitting lids which render them leak-proof during transport to the laboratory. Leaky specimens pose a hazard both to non-laboratory staff, who often do not have adequate training in biosafety, and also to the laboratory staff who do.

A wide variety of containers with commercially-prepared transport media, or as swab-transport systems, are available and widely used.

The collection of specimens for the isolation of anaerobic organisms requires a special anaerobic transport container. A number of these are available from commercial sources.

K. The specimen must be collected and transported in a safe manner

Universal or Standard Precautions (13) must be maintained when collecting and transporting clinical specimens. These precautions assume that all patients are potentially infectious for blood-borne pathogens, and blood and body fluids from every patient are to be treated as potentially infectious. Basic precautions in obtaining specimens require the use of appropriate barrier precautions in order to prevent skin and mucous membrane exposure: a) use of gloves and lab coat or gown, and the addition of mask and goggles if there is potential risk, b) needles, lancet, etc., to be handled carefully, c) sharps discarded in an approved puncture proof container, d) needles not to be re-capped by hand, and e) hands to be washed thoroughly after gloves are removed or immediately if contamination takes place.

The specimen should be placed in a leak proof container to ensure that there is no contamination externally. This in turn should be placed in a sealable plastic bag that is labeled with an appropriate biohazard symbol and which has an external pouch for the requisition. Leaking samples should preferably not be transported; another sample should be collected if possible.

The requisition must not be placed in the bag with the specimen nor wrapped around the specimen as the requisition will be contaminated if the specimen develops a leak. Instead, it should be kept outside of the bag.

Syringes should not be sent to the laboratory with attached needles. The material should be inoculated into an appropriate transport container if feasible. If the specimen is particularly minute and may be lost during the transfer, the needle may be removed with a safety device and with the syringe capped.

Transport from a distant site to the laboratory falls under regulations which pertain to the transport of dangerous goods, these are legislated in most countries and also governed by the International Air Travel Association (IATA) for shipment by air as discussed below.

L. Transport

The primary objective for performing bacteriological analysis of a specimen is to accurately identify the causative organism of the infectious process, and as such, it is imperative that the bacterial content of specimen is maintained as close as possible to the original state at the time of collection with minimum alteration. The bacteria originally sampled may multiply if the specimen is allowed to stand for prolonged periods on the hospital ward. This may also result in overgrowth by relatively faster growing commensal organisms that are present in some specimens. Such overgrowth could interfere with the isolation of pathogenic micro-organisms especially if the latter were initially present in small numbers. The number of pathogens may decrease if the specimen is maintained under adverse environmental conditions, e.g., prolonged refrigeration in the laboratory prior to processing. Such alteration is relevant when quantitation of bacteria is a critical component of the analysis. Many microorganisms are susceptible to adverse environmental conditions such as changes in temperature (*Neisseria meningitidis*), oxygen (anaerobic bacteria), changes in pH (shigellae), or excessive drying (a relative exception is *S. pyogenes*). Specimens that are likely to contain these and other organisms such as *Bordetella pertussis* or *Neisseria gonorrhoeae* often benefit from immediate application to appropriate media at the "bedside" (14). It is, therefore, essential for the specimen to be delivered promptly to the laboratory - ideally, within the same hour of collection for the results to be most valid.

It is not always possible for the laboratory to achieve these parameters. If prompt transport to the laboratory is not possible, special preservatives or holding media (transport media) must be used. These ensure viability of the pathogens, maintain their original numbers and suppress overgrowth by commensal organisms in specimens that are to be in transit for longer than one hour.

Specimens such as urine and body fluids constitute good culture media and are capable of supporting rapid growth of pathogenic and commensal organisms if held for more than thirty minutes at room temperature. Since the determination of a urinary tract infection is in large part based on the quantitation of bacteria in the urine specimen, it needs to be processed within thirty minutes of collection unless it is immediately refrigerated and transported to the laboratory in a cold state to arrive within two hours of collection. If this is not possible, a convenient mechanism for bedside inoculation is the use of Dipslides or equivalent (15). Alternatively, preservatives such as boric acid or commercially available urine transport kits containing boric acid and sodium formate preservative may be used (15,16).

Most other specimens that cannot be transported to the laboratory within a few hours of collection require the use of a transport medium to maintain them in their original state. Many different transport media have been described and these are available commercially either as separate media or as part of a swab–transport medium system. These systems keep bacteria viable while at the same time relatively discourage their growth. They also protect bacteria against dessication, oxidation, and adverse pH changes. In general, the main constituents of a transport medium are buffers which maintain pH, thioglycollate (a reducing substance to prevent oxidation), and semi-solid non-nutritive agar which is unfavorable to overgrowth of rapidly growing organisms. Charcoal may be added to absorb fatty acids and non-specific toxic components that are present in the specimen and that may potentially damage fastidious organisms such as *N. gonorrhoeae* and *B. pertussis*.

Salmonellae and shigellae can be recovered from fecal samples for up to a week, *Vibrio cholerae* for up to three weeks, and *Yersinia enterocolitica* for over a month in refrigeration, in appropriate transport media. *Streptococcus pyogenes* survives well on pharyngeal swabs transported in a dry state and the use of silica gel in the transport containers prolongs its survival for up to three days.

Specimens for chlamydia and mycoplasma culture can be transported and stored in mycoplasma growth medium, nutrient broth which is enriched with serum, or ideally in sucrose-phosphate transport medium (2-SP) which is specifically formulated to maintain viability of these organisms (17). 2-SP medium, which has antibiotics added to it, is also used for the isolation of chlamydia and genital mycoplasmas (see also Chapters 27 and 29).

Most transport media maintain bacteria in a steady state for up to twenty-four hours after which there is a steady decline in the number of viable organisms, and as such the specimen must be transported to the laboratory as quickly as possible despite the use of a transport medium.

Stuart's medium (modified), Amies' medium (modified), Cary-Blair medium, varied specific anaerobe transport media, and 2-SP medium for chlamydia and mycoplasmas are examples of some transport media. The most commonly used transport medium is the modified Stuart's transport medium. Commercially, these are often incorporated into a combined swab-transport medium system. Often these media can be stored at room temperature for as long as one year without deterioration.

M. The time limit between collection of the specimen and its receipt in the laboratory should be defined

Specimens which are not preserved or not sent in transport media need to be delivered to the laboratory promptly. In a hospital setting, the recommended limit between collection of most specimens and their delivery to the laboratory is within two hours. If this timing cannot be complied with, transport media should be used. It is desirable to have the following specimens transported to the laboratory within a shorter period of time (i.e., 15-30 minutes): cerebrospinal fluid, other sterile body fluids or aspirates, small amounts of tissue samples (larger biopsy tissue can be maintained for twenty-four hours in transport systems), intravenous catheter tips, specimens that are collected by syringe and needle (e.g., from cellulitis), eye specimens (e.g., corneal scrapings) and gastric aspirates. Such time limits obviously would be difficult to achieve in transporting specimens from remote sites, e.g., physician offices. In these settings, the use of appropriate transport media should be mandated.

Although organisms can survive for prolonged periods in transport media, there is a time-related decline in their numbers after twenty-four hours. Failure to isolate pathogenic organisms from specimens received in the laboratory after a delay of more than twenty-four hours does not imply their initial absence. As such, if the laboratory chooses to process such specimens, a qualifying statement may be made which associates the delay in transit with the possibility of a false negative outcome. Transport times of twenty-four hours for blood or bone marrow aspirate which are collected and inoculated directly into broth for culture and held to at least room temperature are relatively acceptable.

N. The temperature limit for transport must be defined

The temperature at which a specimen is transported, be it in its original form or in transport media, affects the quality of the specimen. Transport at room temperature may result in the viability of some pathogenic organisms in specimens becoming compromised and in overgrowth of rapidly growing organisms. This becomes a critical issue for specimens such as urine, whose bacteriology is dependent on quantitation of pathogenic organisms. Most specimens can be transported to the laboratory at room temperature. *Hemophilus influenzae* and pathogenic *Neisseria* spp. are sensitive to cold temperatures and as such, specimens from sites which are likely to harbour these, such as those of cerebrospinal fluid, eye, middle ear, and genital must not be refrigerated. Other specimens such as stool (for *Campylobacter* spp., *Shigella* spp., *Vibrio* spp., *Yersinia* spp.), intravenous catheter tips, gastric lavage, bronchial lavage and sputum, catheter and mid-stream urine are compromised at room temperature and need to be transported at 4°C if transport time exceeds two hours.

Specimens that cannot be processed promptly upon receipt in the laboratory will need to be stored pending inoculation. The conditions under which they are stored and the duration of storage may compromise their quality.

Optimum storage temperatures of specimens which cannot be processed immediately on receipt in the laboratory are as stated above for transport of specimens.

O. Mailing and shipping of specimens from a location distant to the laboratory must conform to regulations

The type of specimen and the proximity to the laboratory of the location of its origin, determines the mode of packaging and shipping for transportation to the laboratory.

The specimens originating from locations that are in close proximity to the laboratory, such as within a hospital, can be transported by hand as previously detailed.

Specimens which originate from locations that are remote from the laboratory, either within the community or from another town, require ground or air transportation by couriers, mail, or airlines. In most countries, such transportation falls under statutory regulations that govern the transport of dangerous goods which include infectious substances and diagnostic specimens. Packaging and shipping needs to conform to local statutes for ground and air transportation and also International Air Transport Association (IATA) regulations for air transportation.

Regulations with respect to the transport of infectious substances and diagnostic specimens have been developed and are regularly updated by the United Nations Committee of Experts in the form of the United Nations Recommendations on the Transport of Dangerous Goods. These have been adopted by most western countries in their entirety or in major part, as a basis for their own statutes. The regulations and the stringency with which they are applied, however, vary from country to country, and as such, it is beyond the scope of this chapter to consider these individually. It is recommended that readers become familiar with the regulations in their own jurisdiction in addition to the requirements of bodies such as IATA and International Civil Aviation Organization (ICAO). The requirements applicable to packaging, documentation, and shipping of infectious substances and diagnostic specimens are complex and require specific training. Most national and also IATA requirements mandate formal training and certification for individuals undertaking transport of dangerous goods.

A key component of the regulations is proper packaging and documentation for transportation which in turn is based on the category of regulated material, i.e., whether it is a diagnostic specimen or an infectious substance. It is important to understand the distinction between these two groups.

Infectious substances are those substances known or reasonably expected to contain pathogens which are known or reasonably expected to cause infectious disease in animals or humans. These include etiological agents and some diagnostic specimens [i) below] that are submitted for initial diagnostic work-up. Such substances are classified in Division 6.2 of IATA regulations under UN #2814. Shipment of specimens and etiological agents which fall within Division 6.2 require documentation and packaging which conform to IATA/ICAO packing instructions (PI) 602 as intended for the transport of infectious substances.

Diagnostic specimens are divided into three groups:

i) those known or reasonably expected to contain pathogens in risk group 2, 3, or 4. Specimens transported for the purpose of initial or confirmatory testing for the presence of pathogens fall within this group and their packaging, documentation, and shipping has to conform to those for infectious substances as above.

ii) those for which a relatively low probability exists that pathogens of risk group 2 or 3 are present. Specimens that are transported for the purpose of initial diagnosis for other than the presence of pathogens, or specimens that are transported for routine screening, fall within this group. Documentation and packaging is required to conform to IATA/ICAO PI 650 which is intended for diagnostic specimens.

iii) those known not to contain pathogens. There are no special regulations applicable to these other than Universal or Standard Precautions.

Some countries such as the United States have an additional special infectious substances category for agents which can cause serious illness or death. These include multi-resistant organisms and organisms that potentially can be used as biological weapons. Special regulations apply to these over and above those for transport of dangerous goods.

Basic steps for packaging of infectious substances are as follows: the sample is contained in a primary container that has a positive seal, is wrapped with enough absorbent material to absorb all liquid in the event of breakage, and is placed in a closed leak-proof secondary container. If there are multiple primary receptacles included in a secondary container, each must be individually wrapped. The secondary container is placed in a UN-approved outer container. An itemized list of contents should be inserted between the secondary and the outer container. Labeling of the outer container should include labels with the name, address, and phone number of the consignor and consignee, the UN number, and an infectious substance class 6.2 biohazard label to confirm the contents. A properly completed shipper's declaration for dangerous goods must accompany the weigh bill.

Diagnostic specimens should be packaged according to IATA/ICAO PI 650. These are similar to those above except that the requirements for packaging are not as rigid and an outer box is only required to be of adequate strength for its capacity, mass, and intended use. Labels indicate the content to be clinical specimens, and a shipper's declaration is not needed.

For the shipping of samples with coolants such as dry ice, special requirements of the packaging to allow for adequate ventilation for CO_2 to escape from the package, and appropriate labeling and documentation are needed.

Numerous approved shipping containers are available commercially. If in doubt as to the classification of the clinical specimen, it is safer to follow the most stringent packaging instructions.

P. A special case for anaerobes

A variety of anaerobic bacteria (see also Chapter 24) colonize skin, the oral cavity, the upper respiratory tract, the gastrointestinal tract, and the female genitourinary tract in large numbers. These sites are colonized with a variety of aerobic bacteria as well, although the anaerobes usually outnumber the aerobes by several fold. As such, the examination of specimens for anaerobes from these sites may provide misleading information, and their examination is generally discouraged. As well, the potential for contamination with anaerobes of specimens that are collected through these sites is considerable. Therefore, it is essential to collect specimens from the actual site of infection by by-passing the site of normal flora (18).

Specimens which are appropriate for the isolation of anaerobic organisms include: pus which is aspirated with syringe and needle from an abscess (swabs are much less desirable), tissue biopsy material, protected brush bronchoscopy specimens, supra-pubic aspirations of urine, and blood or body fluid which is collected aseptically.

Specimens which are inappropriate for culture of anaerobic organisms include: superficial skin swabs, urine other than suprapubic aspiration, sputum, throat swab, nasopharyngeal swab, bronchial washing, vaginal, cervical or urethral swab, and stool or rectal swab.

The properties of an optimum specimen, as previously described for the isolation of aerobic pathogens, equally apply to specimens for anaerobic culture. An ideal specimen is the tissue sample that is collected aseptically. Purulent material which is collected by syringe and needle without contamination by commensal flora from adjacent sites constitutes the next best specimen.

Methods as described above for collection and transport of aerobic organisms are generally inadequate for successfully culturing anaerobic organisms. The lethal effect of atmospheric O_2 must be neutralized from the time the specimen is collected until it is appropriately cultured in the laboratory. Transport of clinical specimens, therefore, becomes one of the most critical factors in the isolation of anaerobic organisms. A number of satisfactory and commercially-prepared collection/transport systems are available for this purpose. Instructions that accompanying the commercial collection kits must be followed.

Transport medium for anaerobes is best pre-reduced and anaerobically sterilized, and is generally composed of modified Cary-Blair or Amies medium, an indicator of anaerobiosis such as rezasurin (colorless under anaerobic conditions but turns pink in the presence of O_2), and reducing substances which maintain adequate oxidation-reduction potential. Inoculated media should be transported at room temperature and arrive in the laboratory within two to three hours.

If only a swab specimen can be collected, it should be maintained in an anaerobic tube that contains pre-reduced anaerobically-sterilized transport media. Specimens thus collected and transported enable the survival of most non-anaerobic organisms, and as such, can be cultured for aerobic organisms as well as for the intended anaerobic organisms.

II. PROCESSING

A. Developing a "culture"

As for the appropriate collection and transport, the processing of clinical specimens in the laboratory benefits from value-added knowledge that is contributed by the individual(s) who submit(s) the material and by the laboratory staff who must carry out the tasks of analysis and review. Whereas it may be difficult to have the primary care-giver detail considerable information outside of the few points that may be possible on most laboratory requisitions, it is equally the responsibility of the laboratory staff to understand their clients (see Chapter 10) and hence the likely needs of their patients. These needs, for example, will differ whether the patient is from the community and non-compromised or whether the patient is from a hospital where various mitigating circumstances may bias the approach to medical care. The needs will also vary given the complexity of the underlying patient morbidity and the degree of diagnostic information that a physician, general or specialist, wishes to acquire. The laboratory therefore needs to weigh the given information in many circumstances after the specimen is received and before it is initially processed by preliminary set-up. In addition, the laboratory also needs to re-evaluate such information during the process of analysis and subsequent reporting. It is the responsibility of the laboratory to interact with its clients in order to gain the most relevant information when it is required above and beyond that which is received in the standard format from requisitions; the service which provides this form of consultation must be dynamic, timely, and knowledgeable. Essentially, there must develop a "culture" among user and provider that recognizes, and then benefits, from the work that is performed in the bacteriology laboratory.

B. The predictive value of results

The pre-analytic phase of specimen collection must take into consideration the likelihood that a given specimen will yield relevant diagnostic information. Likewise, the use of diagnostic information must be tempered with an understanding of how probable it will be that a given result will indicate that an etiological agent is found. For example, *S. pyogenes* is the most common bacterial cause of pharyngitis that will be sought by the clinical laboratory. The frequencies for positive throat swabs often range from 5-30% depending on the patient population. Of concern, however, is the fact that many individuals in the community are carriers for this bacterium and the carriage frequency in itself may be as high as 5-

15% depending on the population (19). It is inevitable, therefore, that "positive" specimens will be obtained from a symptomatic patient when in fact the putative pathogen was not the etiological agent. The latter concept is even more critical when one examines the relevancy of other particular bacteria from respiratory specimens. Both *S. pneumoniae* and *H. influenzae* are common causes of respiratory tract illness, e.g., otitis, sinusitis, and pneumonia. Yet, they are also found as normal commensals in the upper respiratory tract and indeed may be relatively present in overabundance as an overgrowth phenomenon during times of active viral upper respiratory infections. The finding of these bacteria from samples of the oropharynx and nasopharynx have meagre predictive value for the presence of the same in the aforementioned sites of infection (20). In contrast, the finding of *P. aeruginosa* in the respiratory specimen of a child with underlying cystic fibrosis may be associated with a good predictive value for the actual presence in the lower respiratory tract (21). In relevance to reports from Gram staining, it is even more critical that the finding of a particular morphotype be understood in the context of how likely it is to reflect the presence of a pathogen.

C. Maintenance of specimens

Although clinical specimens should be obtained and thereafter transported on a timely basis, there are many circumstances where a return to the original specimen may be desirable. In the worst case scenario, specimens may not have been processed accurately. Whereas proportionately few such mistakes are likely to occur, the high numbers of bacteriology specimens that are submitted makes it probable that such errors will happen. In many circumstances, it will be possible to re-collect, but it is also possible that the circumstances prohibit the latter, e.g., privileged site for collection (such as a surgical specimen or a spinal fluid), e.g., initiation of antimicrobial agents. In addition, the potential to return to the original specimen may prove useful when isolates are lost, when further analyses may be required on a retrospective basis (for those micro-organisms that may be sufficiently preserved by refrigeration), or when Gram or other staining requires a repeat. Refrigeration at 4°C is the most practical method for the short term maintenance of specimens, and freezing at –70°C is optimal for longer term preservation. The practicality of specimen maintenance at 4°C must obviously be assessed on an individual basis but the following serves as a rough guide for common specimens: urine, stool – 3 days; respiratory, wound, CSF, body fluids, gynecological – 7 days. Common sense must prevail for how these may be used. For example, a sample should be recollected if possible if the search was intended to include *N. gonorrhoeae* which is considerably labile. In contrast, a stored sputum may still be useful for tuberculosis work several days later. It is incumbent upon the laboratory to realize and then notify (even in the report) if such delays in processing are likely to impede the search for a relevant pathogen.

D. Maintenance of records

The maintenance of reports is often mandated by accreditation bodies and is officially part of the patient record of care. In addition, however, it may prove of value to have access to working documents for varied reasons. Historically, the work in progress was often recorded by the bacteriology laboratory on back copies of the original requisition if not on a laboratory-generated worksheet. This record establishes continuity for the day-to-day work that is required, but also provides for material that may be of value in retrospective review. The extent of work-up as well as any errors may be seen. Nevertheless, there is a current trend to establish a paperless laboratory. The latter may prove workable but must fundamentally acknowledge the value of having a reasonable work record. Overall, the work record should be held for an acceptable period of time, e.g., 6-12 months minimum.

E. Enrichment culture

Enrichment culture essentially consists of liquid medium, and the major need that enrichment fulfills is the desire to ensure that any quantity of a possible pathogen is found from a specimen especially when it is possible that the determination by swab/solid medium culture may be limited in some circumstances. The type of enrichment is determined by the specific need. In addition to the actual finding of a pathogen (all-or-none) or the simple increase of numbers, enrichment may also serve to facilitate the resuscitation of a pathogen that has already been subjected to an antibiotic; this dilutional effect on the specimen may also serve to help decrease the concentration of other non-specific inhibitors. The enrichment broth may serve as a better format for the resuscitation of bacteria that have been subjected to extremes of the environment, e.g., dessication. The broth is also a medium that will remain hydrated for many days in contrast to the solid medium which is subject to pressures of drying after 2-3 days even within humidified incubators. Atmospheric gradient in a broth can be achieved with the presence of a reducing agent and hence serve as an important adjunct for anaerobic cultures. As well, enrichment culture may allow for more specimen volume to be sampled in contrast to traditional agar media and may thus be of value if not only because it allows for more specimen to assessed. The standard blood culture (see Chapter 9) serves as the best example of the latter.

By way of either chemical or antibiotic constituents, enrichment broths may provide for selection, i.e., the pathogen of choice is promoted while the other potential bacteria from the source may be suppressed. Such selective enrichment is used in many different settings, e.g., enteric enrichment media (see Chapter 15), e.g., mycobacterial enrichment (see Chapter 14) (see Table 1). This approach serves as a mechanism to ensure that the pathogen is not overgrown by either other more hardy bacteria or those which are originally present in larger numbers. In addition, there may be other mechanisms for enrichment that are a function of temperature or growth substrate restriction, e.g., both *Yersinia enterocolitica* and *Listeria monocytogenes* can be enriched during prolonged incubation at 4°C over several weeks in conventional broths (22,23), e.g., *Nocardia* enrichment may occur with the restriction of carbon sources for other bacteria.

In the current era where blood culture media are highly sophisticated and are indeed performing essentially to the limit, it has been of value to use these for the purposes of non-selective enrichment for a variety of specimens, but these should include especially those specimens that arise from otherwise sterile sites, e.g., joint fluid, e.g., paracentesis fluid.

Regardless of enrichment broth, however, the overuse of this strategy may have its limitations. Every manipulation of the clinical specimen carries with it a risk for extraneous contamination. Although the latter contaminants are usually readily acknowledged, there may be circumstances where

Table 1   Examples of common use enrichment in clinical bacteriology.

type	selective	basis
thioglycollate broth	no	facilitates growth of a wide variety of aerobic and anaerobic bacteria
brain-heart infusion	no	supportive of many fastidious bacteria; with or without supplements, e.g., hemin, vitamin K
CNA broth	yes	colistin/nalidixic acid antibiotic supplementation; enrichment of Group B streptococci from female genital specimens as a screening technique
enteric media (e.g., GN broth, e.g., selenite broth)	yes	suppression of normal enteric flora; enrichment of enteric pathogens; subculture times may be critical
mycobacterial enrichment (e.g., Middlebrook 7H9, e.g., Dubos Tween, e.g., BACTEC)	yes	generally inhibit most bacteria except mycobacteria; automated format speeds detection

even likely contaminants may have a higher probability for being true pathogens. The latter is particularly an issue with coagulase-negative staphylococci. Enrichment, when used alone, also limits the observer from understanding the yield of bacteria on a quantitative basis. Whereas some pathogens may be significant on an all-or-none basis, the amount of growth in some circumstances may reflect the likelihood that an isolate is a contaminant or not. The amount of growth and its timing to recognition may also have implications relating to the efficacy of antimicrobial therapy. Therefore, it is usually most appropriate to combine liquid and solid media where possible. In so doing, the laboratorian must develop a rational scheme for inoculation of media and this should take place in the order of non-selective to selective.

F.   Selection versus differentiation

As detailed above, selection of pathogens from a milieu of non-pathogens, or for the determination of complex mixtures, is commonly required. Apart from achieving selection with broth enrichments, it is much more common to achieve selection through a variety of solid media. The selection is accomplished by the addition of varied antibiotics, dyes, or chemicals otherwise (e.g., bile salts, sodium chloride). In most circumstances, selection is relative; it may be highly efficient (e.g., TCBS medium for *V. cholerae*) or much less specific (e.g., MacConkey medium with crystal violet – generally non-specific for members of *Enterobacteriaceae*). Although the intention is to select for a given pathogen, it must be remembered that some forms of a particular pathogen, however infrequent, may be susceptible to the selective process, e.g., some campylobacters may be inhibited by the antibiotics that are routinely used in varied campylobacter selective media.

Differentiation simply implies that a medium has the ability to impart variable phenotypic qualities to bacterial growth, either of the growing colony or of the surrounding medium, and thus one may be able to highlight heterogeneity of microbes from a specimen or at least strongly denote the suspect pathogen. Almost all media have some ability to facilitate differentiation but particular media are so designated due to the pre-determined effort to provide such discrimination, e.g., MacConkey medium for *Enterobacteriaceae*, e.g., egg yolk agar for anaerobes.

Obviously, then, it is possible to fashion media which are selective and differential whether or not they provide for enrichment.

G.   Specimen concentration

In contrast to enrichment per se, where a small volume of specimen may be incubated with a larger volume of broth, specimen concentration essentially compacts the larger specimen so that it may be processed in a smaller volume of medium. Such concentration can be achieved with centrifugational forces of 1500-2000 g. Specimen concentration is generally applicable to specimens with larger volumes and especially those that come from otherwise sterile sites. Such specimens, for example, include cerebrospinal fluid, pleural and pericardial fluid, joint aspirates, and paracenteses. There will obviously be a practical limit to the volume that may be concentrated, and maximal volumes of 50 ml. suffice in most circumstances. Concentration of large volumes will also, however, increase the probability of finding contaminants. The example of peritoneal returns from continuous ambulatory peritoneal dialysis serves to illustrate these issues. When samples of dialysis fluid were cultured for determining the presence of bacterial pathogens in the scenario of peritonitis, early studies often examined a small portion. Thereafter, it became recognized that the centrifugation of greater amounts led to an increased number of positive dialysates. Recommended volumes increased from 5 to 10 to 50 ml.; indeed some even recommended that entire bags of dialysis fluid be cultured (up to several litres) (24). Whereas there was no doubt that the largest volumes yielded greater numbers of positive specimens, the increment achieved after >50 ml. was used was often simply contaminant, e.g., coagulase-negative staphylococci. One must therefore accept that a practical limitation should exist.

Concentration for the purpose of finding at least some pathogens is a time- honoured approach for tuberculosis (see Chapter 14).

H. Tissue processing

In addition to swabs and fluids, tissue may be submitted for bacteriology. It is often useful to have the Gram stain performed on a tissue imprint if this is feasible. The tissue should first be inspected for obvious areas of disease if it is large and heterogeneous. A representative sample of the diseased area should be selected and this should include the area corresponding to the infection core as well as the leading edge if possible. Thereafter, homogeneity prior to processing for routine bacteriology can be achieved in a number of ways. The tissue can be ground with a mortar and pestle; this is often needed for samples that prove difficult to disrupt. Alternatively, soft tissue can be simply chopped or minced with a scalpel in a smaller vessel.

I.   Quantitative culture

The combination of usual solid and liquid media that are utilized for routine cultures generally provides for a measure of semi-quantitation which is often useful for estimating the burden of microbes and perhaps even for determining whether the putative pathogen is likely causing disease or is present as a component of the commensals. Nevertheless, a more strict quantitation process has been recommended for several individual specimens. Regardless of the example, though, it is critical that specimens for the latter be transported and then processed in a timely fashion so that bacterial growth does not occur in the interim.

Quantitation for urine cultures has been time-honoured and a significance criterion of $\geq 10^8$/L. of a pure pathogen was often rigorously followed. It is apparent that lesser quantities of a pure pathogen may be important, and thus a strict observation of the latter limit may be inappropriate (25). Furthermore, such quantitative criteria may not necessarily apply to non-typical urinary pathogens and for patients who have complex underlying morbidity. Quantitative culture of peripheral intravenous catheter tips has been promoted as a mechanism to define catheter infection and there is a reasonable correlation with colony counts ≥ 15 from an agar roll-tip technique (26). It is important to recognize, however, that the latter is not necessarily applicable to catheter lines that have been obtained from other sites, e.g., central venous lines. Quantitation of sputum bacteriology has been used for the purposes of follow-up during the treatment of patients with underlying cystic fibrosis who have an acute-on-chronic respiratory decompensation. These patients commonly have high counts of pseudomonads (often 10^5-10^8/ml. of sputum) during active infection (27). One must first though have a patient who can reliably cough a deep sputum specimen; many of the younger CF patients are unable to produce such a sample. The comparison of quantitations before and after treatment may be susceptible to collection error, and hence this approach is not commonly used. As an extension of the latter concept, quantitation may be useful in confirming bacterial pneumonia among other patients when high quantitations of bacteria are obtained from protected brush specimens as acquired via bronchoscopy ($\geq 10^4$/ml.) (28); the latter may be useful for documenting aspiration pneumonias but often does not provide additional information to that which has been acquired from routine semi-quantitative methods. Bacterial quantitation of burn biopsies has some predictive value in burn wound sepsis, but has relatively limited application (29).

J.   Scoring schemata

Routine bacteriology is graded with semi-quantitative techniques as mentioned above. Spreading of the specimen in three to four quadrants of the agar medium can thus be translated respectively into a 1+, 2+, 3+ or 1+, 2+, 3+, 4+ semi-quantitative descriptions of growth as it occurs in these areas. The semi-quantitation is obviously subject to the variability which is inherent among technologists. Alternatively, the latter numbers may be translated into the descriptions: scant (very light or very little), light, moderate, or heavy growth.

Microscopy is one area that has lent itself to standardized scoring schemata in order to more precisely provide for reproducibility among the observer. In the most time-honoured of these, Gram-stained sputa are scored for contamination by the observation for numbers of epithelial cells (11); as well, the suitability of the specimen is partially assessed by the enumeration of white blood cells (30,31). Overall, the intent is to provide some assurance that quality specimens are being delivered. In the second best and more contemporary example, Gram-stained smears of vaginal swabs are assessed for their compatibility with an appearance that is indicative of bacterial vaginosis (32,33). Studies have shown that interobserver variability can be improved when a well-defined set of objective criteria are used for such scoring methods.

K. When is the Gram stain of value?

The Gram stain has been routinely applied to most specimens that enter the laboratory almost as an automatism when the specimen is initially set-up. On a practical basis, however, there are a limited number of specimens that the Gram stain will be of value for. Furthermore, even among the latter, the actual use of the Gram stain result by the physician is applicable to only a small proportion for most specimens, and the report is often not seen. The latter dilemma, although disappointing, is nevertheless a reality, and the primary physician obviously balances the relevancy of such information with patient care and other needs. The laboratory must therefore decide what is relevant in the given context.

Gram stains are generally not indicated for upper respiratory specimens, urine, stool, and screening samples for antimicrobial resistance. Gram stains are advocated for lower respiratory specimens, tissue, sterile body fluids, most female genital specimens, male genital specimens, wounds, eye, middle ear, and abscesses. The value of Gram staining for superficial wound specimens, which have a high probability for containing coagulase-negative staphylococci and other skin commensals, remains dubious.

One must not forget the relevance of the Gram stain to the benchtop. Although the primary physician may not make frequent use of Gram stain results, the information should be viewed by the technologist when bacterial growth is initially observed on routine media; discrepancies should be accounted for.

L. Correlation with pathology

Most bacteriological specimens are obtained without any associated sampling of the diseased site for histopathological purposes. The availability of tissue, however, offers a unique opportunity to further assess the importance of bacterial cultures. Preferentially, the tissue for histopathological examination should be obtained from a site that is contiguous to that which is being sampled for bacteriology. The latter in essence serves to confirm that an isolate is directly associated with a disease process, and may explain why there is a discordance between expectations and actual bacteriology. Like the Gram stain, the histopathological examination is a direct measure of specimen quality. Given that an infectious process may not necessarily affect a tissue consistently throughout, the proximal collections for histopathology are important. A more common example of error in this regard is the collection of separate biopsies from bone during a suspect osteomyelitis; separate biopsies may be processed for each of two purposes rather than using a common area for both. In addition to processing in the bacteriology laboratory, Gram stains are also likely to be performed on tissue sections directly (34).

M. Post-mortem microbiology

The examination of tissue from the post-mortem state for the purpose of establishing infection is fraught with many difficulties, and indeed there continues to be some controversy with respect to the approaches which are most appropriate (35,36). Most of the published work in this area comes from the autopsies of adults, but recommendations for the processing of pediatric, fetal, and placental material have been discussed. The occurrence of agonal spread and transvisceral contamination serve to disseminate potential pathogens from sites that have commensal flora. Despite the latter, it is critical to approach the autopsy as if it were a sterile procedure if one is to minimize contamination. Sites which have been apparently contaminated may be seared superficially in order to minimize the contamination of the deeper tissue.

Cultures should be acquired from tissue that is proximal to that which is examined histopathologically. The autopsy should be performed as soon after death as is convenient. The process should ideally be one where the pathologist works from normally sterile tissue towards normally contaminated organs later. The specimens so acquired should be stored and transported appropriately in order to minimize overgrowth. Like clinical specimens from patients, each specific transport requirement should be considered when multiple pathogens are of concern. When multiple sites yield the same bacterium, the probability of identifying a pathogen increases. In the end, the contribution of post-mortem microbiology must be assessed in close proximity to the gross and microscopic findings.

N. Specimens for nucleic acid analyses

The era of molecular diagnostics has brought with it a new dimension in the needs for transport and processing. The bacterial substance for direct detection is genomic material, and thus viable bacterium is not required. Although it may initially seem that the ability to detect inactive bacterium thus implies that much less stringent precautions are required for specimen transport, this is not necessarily the case since both DNA and RNA (the much lesser common target in bacteriology) are susceptible to degradation from either autolytic or exogenous enzymes. Thus, refrigeration, as for typical bacteriology specimens, is preferred. Repetitive freeze-thawing of specimens may, however, be associated with a relative loss in quantitation. The impact of the latter will depend on the initial quantity of bacterium.

The pre-treatment of specimens prior to genetic amplification is considerably variable and has often been a function of the best possible process that is compatible with maximal amplification. Considerations need to be given to buffers, whole cell digests, lytic agents, and specimen concentration (see Chapter 5). There are a considerable number of variations for the latter with almost every bacterial amplification method that has yet been described.

The need for separate facilities has been touted in order to reduce contamination from laboratory sources of genome (37). As well, treatment of the amplification reaction with varied reagents has been recognized to further prevent this problem (38,39). Although much of the current pre-treatment for genetic amplification is still largely manual, there is great prospect that automation and robotics will simplify the laboratory work.

O. Antigen detection

There are many examples where bacterial antigen is detected by immunofluorescence or enzyme immunoassay as detailed throughout this text, but there are few common examples where the detection of bacterial antigen (carbohydrate) directly from clinical specimens is accomplished with agglutination. Examples of the latter include the detection of Group B streptococci, *S. pneumoniae*, *H. influenzae* type b, and varied meningococcal serogroups. Specimens for the latter should be refrigerated even though in general the carbohydrate nature of the antigen is quite stable. As liquid specimens are often used for the latter (e.g., CSF, pleural fluid, urine), antigen detection is performed on supernatants which have been heat-treated.

Cross-reactions with other bacteria must be considered. For example, it is not uncommon to have pneumococcal-like polysaccharide expressed by varied viridans streptococci. Cross-reactions with *Haemophilus* and meningococcal antigens can occur for urine specimens when significant fecal contamination has occurred. In the case of Group B streptococcal antigen detection from urine, it is not uncommon to have the same organism on the skin surface due to stool contamination; thus, the detection of the Group B antigen in urine does not necessarily confirm that a systemic infection has occurred in a neonate. Furthermore, whereas there is plenty of experience in applying some of these antigen detection agglutination methods to the aforementioned specimens, they should not be applied to unusual specimens for which little experience has been gained, e.g., application of *H. influenzae* type b antigen detection to brain tissue.

P.   Standing protocols

Documentation of processing practices in procedural manuals is an accepted component of standard laboratory practice. In addition, however, it may be desirable to design standing protocols for the bacteriological processing of specific clinical specimens; these may include non-bacterial processing as well, e.g., virology, mycology, parasitology. Such standing protocols may apply to very privileged specimens, e.g., brain biopsy, lung biopsy, liver biopsy, and lymph node. The need for such protocols is driven by the concern that only a limited access to tissue will be had, and that the tissue availability for any retrospective testing will be limited. In addition, it may be prudent at times to over-examine a tissue when the clinical information is not easily obtained. The maintenance of excess tissue will also be of some future benefit if the needs subsequently prove to exceed the standing protocol.

The need for standing protocols will depend on the pattern of medical practice in a given context. For example, if a large proportion of bronchoscopies in a given institution are performed for the purposes of diagnosing acute pneumonia in adults, such a protocol may be useful. If, however, the vast majority of such investigations have historically had very little to do with infection, e.g., more to do with structural and physiological concerns, it may be better to leave the processing to the specific requests as made by the attending physician.

Q.   Specimen rejection and re-collection

For a variety of reasons, specimens may be unsuitable for processing. Concerns may include inappropriate sampling for the diagnosis of a given pathogen or infection, inappropriate transport, excessive delay between collection and processing, excessive contamination of the transport vessel, and lack of appropriate labelling for either of the specimen or requisition. For specimens that are easily accessible, re-collection should be promoted, e.g., sputa (failed Q score), e.g., urine. If the specimen is unique, the problem should be documented and the dilemma discussed with the attending physician in order to understand how important it may be to process whatever has been received. Exceptions which are accepted should be documented and a record of the deficiency should be noted on the final report.

Random and rare problems in this regard are expected when the laboratory processes voluminous numbers of specimens; the common occurrence of such problems should be taken as material for resolution in quality assurance loops. For the purposes of specimen rejection and re-collection, it is better to view remediation as a positive feedback and with the desire to be educational rather than punitive.

Out-right rejection of specimens may be clearly applicable in some circumstances. Obvious duplicate specimens constitute one such example. The routine culture of vomitus or neonatal gastric aspirates is generally not indicated. Urine catheters should not be sent in replacement of urine. Anaerobic cultures of the nasopharynx, oropharynx, stool, and vaginal swabs do not have much if any value.

R. Standard processing

Experience, personal (institutional) preferences, and the particular context for the specimen all influence the choice of bacteriological media that will be chosen for processing of specimens. The Gram stain, for example, may modify standard processing given that extra-ordinary expectations arise. For sputa from patients with cystic fibrosis, the presence of pseudomonads creates a need for selective and differential media that might otherwise not be used for a routine sputum. Urine specimens from catheterized elderly or from patients with atonic bladders may carry a greater mixture of coliforms. Figure 1 illustrates the general spectrum of bacteriological media that are usually selected.

The numerous chapters in this text, which cover specific bacteriology, detail the various exceptions which must be considered for special specimens or samples, and these include at least: *Actinomyces* spp., actinomycetes, *Bartonella* spp., blood culture, *Brucella* spp., chlamydiae, *C. diphtheriae*, enteric pathogens, *F. tularensis*, *H. ducreyi*, *H. pylori*, *Legionella* spp., mycobacteria, mycoplasmas, *N. gonorrhoeae*, rickettsiae, and vibrios.

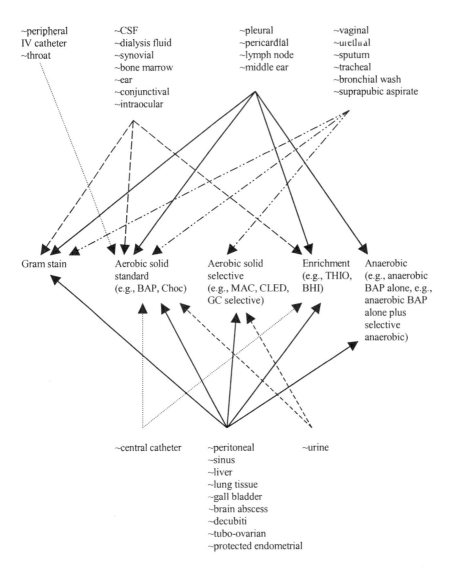

Figure 1 Standard processing selections for varied clinical specimens. BAP = blood agar plate; CHOC = chocolate agar; THIO = thioglycollate broth; BHI = brain heart infusion broth. Not all media examples will necessarily be chosen; the specific chosen examples depend on the nature of the specimen.

REFERENCES

1. Morgan MS. Perceptions of a medical microbiology service: a survey of laboratory users. J Clin Pathol 1995; 48:915-918.
2. Wilson ML. General principles of specimen collection and transport. Clin Infect Dis 1996; 22:766-777.
3. Washington JA. Effective use of the clinical microbiology laboratory. J Antimicrob Chemother 1988; 22:S101-S112.
4. Bartlett RC, Mazens-Sullivan M, Tetreault JZ, Lobel S, Nivard J. Evolving approaches to management of quality in clinical microbiology. Clin Microbiol Rev 1994; 7:55-88.
5. Cook JH, Pezzlo M. Specimen receipt and accessioning. In: Isenberg HD, ed. Clinical Microbiology Procedures Handbook. Washington, DC:American Society for Microbiology, 1992:1.2.1-1.2.4.
6. Valenstein PN, Howanitz PJ. Ordering accuracy: a College of American Pathologists Q-Probes study of 577 institutions. Arch Path Lab Med 1995; 119:117-122.
7. National Committee for Clinical Laboratory Standards. Protection of Laboratory Workers from Infectious Disease Transmitted by Blood, Body Fluid, and Tissue. Wayne, PA:National Committee for Clinical Laboratory Standards, 1991.
8. Shea YR. Specimen collection and transport. In: Isenberg HD, ed. Clinical Microbiology Procedures Handbook. Washington, DC:American Society for Microbiology, 1992:1.1.1-1.1.30.
9. Tarr PI, Neill MA, Clausen CR, Watkins SL, Christie DL, Hickman RO. *Escherichia coli* O157:H7 and the hemolytic uremic syndrome: importance of early cultures in establishing the etiology. J Infect Dis 1990; 162:553-556.
10. Rohner P, Pittet D, Pepey B, Nije-Kinge T, Auckenthaler R. Etiological agents of infectious diarrhea: implications for requests for microbial culture. J Clin Microbiol 1997; 35:1427-1432.
11. Heineman HS, Radano RR. Acceptability and cost savings of selective sputum microbiology in a community teaching hospital. J Clin Microbiol 1979; 10:567-573.
12. Lauer BA, Masters HB. Toxic effect of calcium alginate swabs on *Neisseria gonorrhoeae*. J Clin Microbiol 1988; 26:54-56.
13. Committee on Infectious Diseases. 1997 Red Book: Report of the Committee on Infectious Diseases. Elk Grove Village, IL:American Academy of Pediatrics, 1997.
14. Dowda H, Nelson CF. Evaluation of two transport systems for gonorrhea cultures. J Clin Microbiol 1979; 9:441-443.
15. Jewkes FE, McMaster DJ, Napier WA, Houston IB, Postlewaite RJ. Home collection of urine specimens – boric acid bottles or Dipslides? Arch Dis Child 1990; 65:286-289.
16. Lum KT, Meers PD. Boric acid converts urine into an effective bacteriostatic transport medium. J Infect 1989; 18:51-58.
17. Dubuis O, Gorgievski-Hrisoho M, Germann D, Matter L. Evaluation of 2-SP transport medium for detection of *Chlamydia trachomatis* and *Neisseria gonorrhoeae* by two automated amplification systems and culture for chlamydia. J Clin Pathol 1997; 50:947-950.
18. Holden J. Collection and transport of clinical specimens for anaerobic culture. In: Isenberg HD, ed. Clinical Microbiology Procedures Handbook. Washington, DC:American Society for Microbiology, 1992:2.2.1-2.2.6.
19. Pichichero ME. Group A streptococcal tonsillopharyngitis: cost-effective diagnosis and treatment. Ann Emerg Med 1995; 25:390-403.
20. Cimolai N. Bacteriology of the upper respiratory tract: what is important? Can Fam Phys 1988; 34:2155-2159.
21. Ramsey BW, Wentz KR, Amith AL, Richardson M, Willims-Warren J, Hedges DL, Gibson R, Redding GJ, Lent K, Harris K. Predictive value of oropharyngeal cultures for identifying lower airway bacteria in cystic fibrosis patients. Am Rev Resp Dis 1991; 144:331-337.
22. Embil JA, Ewan EP, MacDonald SW. Surveillance of *Listeria monocytogenes* in human and environmental specimens in Nova Scotia, 1974 to 1981. Clin Invest Med 1984; 7:325-327.
23. Van Noyen R, Vandepitte J, Wauters G, Selderslaghs R. *Yersinia enterocolitica*: its isolation by cold enrichment from patients and healthy subjects. J Clin Pathol 1981; 34:1052-1056.
24. Dawson MS, Harford AM, Garner BK, Sica DA, Landwehr DM, Dalton HP. Total volume culture technique for the isolation of micro-organisms from continuous ambulatory peritoneal dialysis patients with peritonitis. J Clin Microbiol 1985; 22:391-394.
25. Stamm WE, Counts GW, Running KR, Fihn S, Turck M, Holmes KK. Diagnosis of coliform infection in acutely dysuric women. N Engl J Med 1982; 307:463-468.

26. Maki DG, Weise CE, Sarafin HW. A semiquantitative culture method for identifying intravenous catheter-related infection. N Engl J Med 1977; 296:1305-1309.

27. Kilbourn JP, Campbell RA, Grach JL, Willis MD. Quantitative bacteriology of sputum. Amer Rev Resp Dis 1968; 98:810-818.

28. Pollock HM, Hawkins EL, Bonner JR, Sparkman T, Bass JB Jr. Diagnosis of bacterial pulmonary infections with quantitative protected catheter cultures obtained during bronchoscopy. J Clin Microbiol 1983; 17:255-259.

29. McManus AT, Kim SH, McManus WF, Mason AD, Pruitt BA. Comparison of quantitative microbiology and histopathology in divided burn-wound biopsy specimens. Arch Surg 1987; 122:74-76.

30. Murray PR, Washington JA II. Microscopic and bacteriologic analysis of expectorated sputum. Mayo Clin Proc 1975; 50:339-344.

31. Bartlett JG, Brewer NS, Ryan JJ. Laboratory Diagnosis of Lower Respiratory Tract Infections, Cumitech 7. Washington, DC:American Society for Microbiology, 1978.

32. Spiegel CA. Diagnosis of bacterial vaginosis by direct Gram stain of vaginal fluid. J Clin Microbiol 1983; 18:170-177.

33. Nugent RP, Krohn MA, Hillier SL. Reliability of diagnosing bacterial vaginosis is improved by a standardized method of Gram stain interpretation. J Clin Microbiol 1991; 29:297-301.

34. Brewer NS, Weed LA. Diagnostic tissue microbiology methods. Human Pathol 1976; 7:141-149.

35. Koneman EW, Minckler TM. Postmortem microbiology. Crit Rev Clin Lab Sci 1970; 1:5-23.

36. Du Moulin GC, Paterson DG. Clinical relevance of postmortem microbiologic examination: a review. Hum Pathol 1985; 16:539-548.

37. McCreedy BJ, Callaway TH. Laboratory design and work flow. In: Persing DH, Smith TF, Tenover FC, White TJ, eds. Diagnostic Molecular Microbiology: Principles and Applications. Washington, DC:American Society for Microbiology, 1993:149-159.

38. Isaacs ST, Tessman JW, Metchette KC, Hearst JE, Cimino GD. Post-PCR sterilization: development and application to an HIV-1 diagnostic assay. Nucleic Acid Res 1991; 19:109-116.

39. Longo MC, Berninger MS, Hartley JL. Use of uracil DNA glycosylase to control carry-over contamination in polymerase chain reaction. Gene 1990; 93:125-128.

4

Serodiagnosis for Bacterial Infections

Nevio Cimolai
Children's and Women's Health Centre of British Columbia, Vancouver, British Columbia, Canada

I. WHY SERODIAGNOSIS ?

Serodiagnosis is essentially a function of the humoral antibody response to infection. For both historic and practical considerations, it has taken precedence over the measurement of cell-mediated immune responses for infection. Serodiagnosis has been a time-honoured application of considerable benefit, and it continues to be a broadly-applicable major tool despite the advances that have been made in molecular and ancillary diagnostics. From a historical perspective, serodiagnosis has played a large role in laboratory diagnostics at times when culture methods were especially fallible and when pathogens were emerging or not truly defined. Indeed, for some fastidious pathogens, serodiagnosis has often been the first diagnostic method that was available. For some non-cultivable pathogens, the potential to clone organism-specific genome and then express antigens, especially proteins, in vitro has provided even further justification to invoke serodiagnosis.

There are several reasons why serodiagnosis may be desirable as a primary or ancillary diagnostic mode for a given infection:

- the bacterium may not be practically cultivable, e.g., syphilis,
- the bacterium is cultivable, but culture is delayed or technically difficult, e.g. bartonellosis,
- it may be difficult to obtain sufficient quantity of the bacterium for either culture (i.e., needs to be viable) or genetic methods, e.g., advanced Lyme disease,
- the site of infection may be difficult to sample for other methods,
- the pathogen is new but fastidious, and serodiagnosis is among the easiest methods to newly create,
- the serological response is unique to the given pathogen, and endemic seroprevalence is exceedingly low,
- the serological response is consistently strong and, when sought, is highly diagnostic of the infection,
- the serological assay may be commonly reactive at the time that the patient presents with an illness,

> ➤ serodiagnosis may continue to serve as the single standard by which other methods are judged, perhaps even as the reference method,
> ➤ the applicable form of serodiagnosis may be easy to perform and may lend itself to automation which can facilitate the assessment of large volumes,
> ➤ the serological test may simply be more cost-effective than other methods, especially if it can be reasonably implemented in a point-of-care fashion,
> ➤ the serological method is a necessary adjunct to culture, genetic detection, or other methods in order to raise the sensitivity of overall diagnosis for the patient cohort,
> ➤ screening may be better accomplished serologically, and,
> ➤ serology may be needed not for diagnosis per se, but rather to establish the state of immunity which by its presence will necessarily rule out the likelihood of an illness.

The decision to choose serological methods realistically is often a function of several of these reasons rather than any one in particular. Table 1 details examples of bacterial infections for which serodiagnosis is likely to be of some value.

II. WHY NOT SERODIAGNOSIS ?

Equally to the reasons for the use of a serodiagnostic method, there may be several arguments for the use of another diagnostic modality if not any. These include:

> ❖ the onset of the infection is rapid (e.g., measured in hours to a few days), and there is insufficient time for a humoral immune response to develop (which may require 5-10 days at least),
> ❖ the serological response may be delayed for some patients and may extend well into the second or third week after onset,
> ❖ there may be a high endemic seroprevalence in the population, thus leading to a problem of non-specificity (such pre-existing antibody may be a function of the bacterium being a component of usual normal flora),
> ❖ culture or genetic detection or other diagnostic methods may provide a more timely or accurate answer,
> ❖ the infection may repeat (e.g., relapse or reinfection), and an anamnestic response rather than predominantly IgM response may be found, thus posing problems to IgM detection,
> ❖ excessive delay in the performance of a serological test may occur if forwarding to a reference or regional centre is involved,
> ❖ specimen acquisition may have to be repeated for the purposes of comparing a convalescent sample to an acute sample in order to determine that a response to infection has occurred,
> ❖ there may be age-related differences in the ability to develop a humoral response,
> ❖ non-specificity may arise as a consequence of cross-reactivity to other bacterial or non-bacterial antigens,
> ❖ the immune response may be variable and activated to different antigens for different patients (e.g., variable response to ASOT or anti-DNAase during streptococcal infections),
> ❖ the antibody response as measured conventionally in serum may not accurately reflect the response to an infection at a mucosal or other site,
> ❖ the infection may be so common that high antibody titres, including IgM, may be found as a consequence of an infection from months past rather than a recent one,
> ❖ empiric therapy with an antibiotic may be commonly used despite the availability of a serological test,
> ❖ the illness that is anticipated is generally mild, and a diagnostic test may have no major impact,
> ❖ the test is only rarely performed,
> ❖ the adjunctive role of serology in addition to the other diagnostics modes is excessively minor,

❖ cost may be a concern in underdeveloped regions,

❖ the use of the serological test may simply be temporary as new technology has evolved another and more useful test,

❖ there may be an obvious contraindication for the specific test format (e.g., anticomplementarity in the complement fixation (CF) test, e.g., anti-red blood cell antibody in indirect hemagglutination, e.g., non-specific agglutination in particle agglutination tests),

❖ there may be excessive interobserver variation for the test to be consistent on a run-to-run basis,

❖ the response may not be specific when heterophil antibodies are assessed,

❖ the test may not lend itself to point-of-care (i.e., it may not be portable), and,

❖ assessment of a newborn's response may be hindered by the presence of maternal antibody that has crossed the placenta.

The use of serodiagnosis may then be a function of the competing pros and cons as detailed above.

Table 1 Role for serology in bacterial infections. Abbreviations: EIA – enzyme immunoassay; IFA – indirect immunofluorescence; WB – Western Blot; IHA – indirect hemagglutination; CF – complement fixation; MIF – microimmunofluorescence; ASOT – antistreptolysin O; CT – cholera toxin; MHA-TP – micro-hemagglutination assay for *T. pallidum*. See respective chapters for full details.

Bacterial species or genus	Proposed, not commonly used, or historical importance	Established use
Bacillus anthracis	EIA (protective antigen)	
Bartonella spp.	EIA	IFA
Bordetella pertussis		EIA
Borrelia spp.		IFA, EIA, WB
Brucella spp.		agglutination
Burkholderia pseudomallei	IHA	
Campylobacter jejuni	EIA	
Chlamydia spp.	EIA	CF, MIF
Clostridium tetani		(protective antibody)
Corynebacterium diphtheriae		(protective antibody)
Coxiella burnetii	EIA	MIF, CF
Ehrlichia spp.		MIF
Escherichia coli O157:H7	O157 LPS	
Francisella tularensis		EIA, agglutination
Helicobacter pylori	LA, WB	EIA
Legionella spp.	EIA	IFA
Leptospira spp.		agglutination, IHA, EIA
Mycobacterium leprae	EIA	
Mycobacterium tuberculosis	EIA	
Mycoplasma pneumoniae	IHA	CF, EIA, IFA, WB
Nocardia spp.	EIA	
Rickettsia spp.	IHA, CF, Weil-Felix test	MIF, EIA
Salmonella typhi	Widal test	
Staphylococcus aureus	teichoic acid antibodies	
Streptococcus pyogenes	antihyaluronidase	ASOT, antiDNAase
Treponema pallidum	WB	non-treponemal, MHA-TP, IFA, EIA
Vibrio cholerae	vibriocidal antibody, anti-CT	
Yersinia enterocolitica	agglutination, EIA (limited serogroups)	
Yersinia pestis	IHA, EIA	

III. CONVENTIONAL APPROACHES TO SERODIAGNOSIS

There are several considerations which are integral to a serodiagnostic method regardless of whether it is being used for bacterial or other infections. These points are otherwise recognized as conventional approaches in the serodiagnosis of infection.

If a measurable humoral response occurs within 7-10 days of the onset of infection, many patients will not have been ill for a sufficient period of time in order for such a response to have taken place. A single sample which has sufficient titre will not be apparent in less than 5-7 days. Paired sera may therefore be desirable in order to compare titres; the initial sample will often be non-diagnostic in itself, but the acquisition of a convalescent serum will allow for a comparison as a consequence of the change. A change in antibody titre between these two samples will often require 5-7 days, although two weeks will usually ensure the same if the initial serum has a low titre. If the patient is seen late in the illness, both titres may be nearly equivalent, but high. Alternatively, a patient who is seen several weeks late into the illness may have evidence of declining titres. A change between the early and late samples, regardless of increment or decline, should be at least $\geq$four-fold. Two-fold variation is not uncommon as a matter of the error that is inherent in such breakpoints; however, it must also be understood that a small percentage (usually <5% and depending on the method used) may also have four-fold changes as a matter of such error. As an exception, changes in the ASOT for *Streptococcus pyogenes* infection may be considered significant for lesser than four-fold changes (1).

The use of a single serum titre will depend on the normal distribution of the serology results in the unaffected population. The specific titre of significance will balance the sensitivity of detection versus the non-specificity relating to the normal distribution (see VII.C.1. and Figure 7).

Early infection is most often best determined by an IgM response if it reliably occurs. Commonly, IgM will be detected by 7-10 days depending on the nature of the pathogen. For example, IgM responses are frequently observed in such a time frame during the course of *Mycoplasma pneumoniae* respiratory infection among otherwise normal individuals (2). In contrast, it is not uncommon to see a delay in the IgM response to *Treponema pallidum* during primary syphilis (3). Although EIA, IFA, radioimmunoassays, and immunoblotting can be specifically designed to detect IgM responses, several other assays measure the combination of IgG and IgM inadvertently, e.g, agglutination and CF. IHA is mainly a measure of IgM (4), and neutralization assays are especially a measure of IgG outside of the immediate period of infection (5).

Humoral responses have typically been assessed by the use of patient sera rather than other body fluids or samples. The use of sera necessitates that a sufficient systemic response be achieved whether by way of the pathogen entering deep tissue or by mobilization of the immune response (i.e., antibody-producing B cells) from distal sites of infection to the immune cell pool. Sera provide for reasonably consistent samples such that specimen sampling variation or error is minimized. For some infections, however, the major response may be mucosal rather than systemic.

It is desirable to have a unique immune response with little opportunity for either prior recognition of the antigen or previous infection. Since several pathogens are derived from the pool of normal flora, and since others may infect on a recurrent basis, it is possible for the immune response to be anamnestic rather than primary. IgM responses may or may not be lesser, or indeed absent, in such a secondary response, and IgG may predominate.

IV. ANTIGENS AND ANTIGENIC RELATIONSHIPS

A. Antigens

1. Antigen type

Antigens for serodiagnostic assays come in various forms which range from whole bacterium to synthetic peptide. Whole bacteria are often chosen as the initial form for consideration so that processing may be kept to a minimum. Components of bacteria such as capsular carbohydrates, outer membranes or their individual proteins, lipopolysaccharides, exoenzymes, and toxins can also potentially be used as antigens after purification. Some such purifications may consist simply of crude extractions. The use of purified bacterial components may reduce non-specificity and may indeed be a conclusion of the prior recognition that some antigens are more immunostimulatory than others.

Complex antigens are more difficult to standardize given the multitude of epitopes than may exist. Highly purified antigens, such as polypeptides, however, may yet possess several antigen recognition sites. All of these sites may compete for an antibody response, and some may maintain dominance in this respect over others (6). The foci for antibody recognition may or may not be the sites of the antigen that are critical to pathogenesis (7). Nevertheless, virulence factors tend to be recognized more often than not.

2. Antigen modification

Although antibody recognition sites may consist of small carbohydrate or polypeptide regions, more complex conformations that are dependent on secondary or tertiary folding patterns of the structure may also serve to stimulate a response. The latter appearance to the immune system may be subject to change when antigens are prepared in different ways. For example, antigen in the form of whole cell bacterium is often inactivated onto glass slide supports where the sequence of labeling takes place for immunofluorescence studies; the variations of either heat, acetone, formalin, and ethanol fixation have the potential to change the accessibility of antigens (8). In addition, the purification or fixation method may also actively change the antigen through chemical processes. For IFA, acetone fixation is often preferred.

3. Antigen carriers

Agglutination methods often use whole bacterial cells, whereas some may have the antigen bound to solid phase supports such as latex particles or red blood cells. Antigens may have preference in their avidity to some supports and not others. For example, some bacterial lipopolysaccharides (LPSs) may have greater affinity for red blood cell receptors in the form of passive adherence (9) whereas other LPSs will bind to red blood cells only after 'tanning' (surface modification) (10,11), and yet others will not bind well at all.

Plastic, nitrocellulose, nylon, and glass are variably suited for the binding of different antigens. Solid supports for antigen-antibody reactions must be assessed in an experimental fashion in order to determine the optimal format.

4. Variable antigenic factors

Not all antigens that induce humoral responses are necessarily accessible to the antibody response as assessed by a particular technology. Antigenic processing within macrophage and other immune cells exposes the antibody generating system to a large repertoire.

Virulence factors are often targets of the immune response during active infection, although this is not always true. For example, B. pertussis reinfection is very uncommon after a community-acquired whooping cough illness in the absence of immunization (12). Antibodies are directed to a number of virulence factors in the latter circumstance. In borrelioses, strong antibody responses are generated towards the variable outer surface membrane proteins. Yet in several toxin-related illnesses, e.g., due to verotoxigenic *E. coli* or diphtheria or tetanus (13), a strong antibody response to the specific virulence factor does not necessarily arise during the course of an active infection (14). A strong anti-diphtheria toxin response develops much more likely after immunization with diphtheria toxoid than it does after natural infection.

Although the substrate for the antibody interaction may be seemingly an inactive molecule, several serodiagnostic assays are based on the ability of the antibody to entirely block or mitigate an enzymatic process, e.g., ASOT for *S. pyogenes* infections (a form of neutralization).

Some antigen forms inherently have an inability to stimulate the immune system. For carbohydrates, such an inability is best exemplified by the poor response to pneumococcal capsules, meningococcal capsules, and *H. influenzae* type b capsule among children under the age of two years (15-17). The linkage of such antigen to an antigenic carrier may enhance the response markedly, e.g. conjugate vaccine of *H. influenzae* type b (18).

The method of serodiagnosis in itself may significantly bias the spectrum of immune response that is measured since particular antigens may not become available. For example, chloroform-methanol extraction of *Mycoplasma pneumoniae* is used to partially purify a glycolipid extract (19); the latter is used in the traditional CF test and does not include a measure of the anti-polypeptide responses to the bacterium which are considerable. To the contrary, the resolution of *M. pneumoniae* polypeptides by SDS-PAGE prior to immunoblotting ensures that glycolipid antigens are essentially absent from the immunological assessment.

5. 'Retro-fitting' antigens

Molecular technologies offer a way of providing antigen. In the past, the antigen was often initally assessed in a random fashion for its ability to induce an immune response even before it was known whether the antigen was likely to be an important structure. Genetic methods now often provide some indication of whether a virulence factor of some type is being produced. Hence, it is now possible to determine gene sequences and then construct short peptides for the purposes of determining immune response (20). The latter approach has the potential benefit of allowing for the creation of antigens that are of greatest use for serodiagnosis while also providing for a mechanism to delete either cross-reactive or non-reactive sites. Such a method has already been applicable to the design of serodiagnostic tests for viruses that not as yet cultivable although their genomes are well studied (21), i.e., there is potential application to infections that are caused by non-cultivable bacteria.

B. Antigenic relationships

1. Cross-reactivity

Antigenic cross-reactivity may serve as a problem in the application of serodiagnostic assays. Such cross-reactivity may be relevant to antigens that are common intragenera, intergenera, and between bacterium and non-microbial antigens. The cross-reactivity may relate to large complex structures or to single small epitopes.

Among Gram positive bacteria, for example, teichoic acids are somewhat homologous for different species; they may even cross-react with mammalian cell surface antigens such as those on red blood cells (22). For Gram negative bacteria, there is often cross-reactivity among LPSs (23). Bacteria not uncommonly share some similarity of the occasional carbohydrate structure and those of animal or plant tissue, e.g., the glycolipid antigen of *M. pneumoniae* that is used in the CF test (24).

Cross-reactivity, though, does not always imply that the assay will not be valuable. If the antigens are partially similar or induce low-affinity antibodies to the other antigen, it is possible that they will be problematic when low serum dilutions are evaluated but absent at the higher diagnostic titres. Also, such cross-reactivity may be minor compared to the more prominent responses that are obtained against other antigens of the same bacterium.

2. Strain variation

It is desirable to choose antigens for serodiagnostic assays that are least susceptible to variation from isolate to isolate and to the pressures of selection or random change after passage through the host. The antigenic variation that is inherent to the realization of serotyping or serogrouping demonstrates the potential problems in this regard. For example, the numerous capsular polysaccharides of *S. pneumoniae* pose a problem both for serodiagnosis and immunization even though they are key virulence factors (25). Apart from actual change in the laboratory, it may be a predetermined fact that existing and circulating strains are heterogeneous from one region to another. The latter concern was realized in the different responses that are measured in some European patients with Lyme disease versus those in North America (26; see also Chapter 25).

Frequent passage in the laboratory of a strain that is used as the antigenic substrate may lead to an attenuation in virulence but also to a significant change in the antigenic make-up of the bacterium. The in vivo expression of some antigens is not necessarily mimicked in laboratory systems. The use of a near 'wild-type' isolate in contrast to a frequently-passaged or registered strain may be preferable. The latter may not prevent the realization of the immune response on an all-or-none basis, but it may blunt the appreciable response considerably.

3. Do laboratory responses always mimic human responses?

Infection in animal models or vaccination in the same context are often used early to predict the major antigens that may be relevant to human infection. In many circumstances, such studies do indeed determine the major antigens that are shared, but this is not always the case. Some antigens may not necessarily be expressed in the same fashion or at all in human versus experimental animal infections. This should not be surprising since there are several relatively unique infections that primarily infect humans and not other mammals, and vice-versa.

The development of monoclonal antibodies is not spared from such restrictions since they are most often of murine origin and since there may be a great difference in the responses of mouse and human.

It is critical to realize therefore that laboratory studies of immune responses in animals are only a platform on which to realize the complexity of the area if not to gain some partial insight into the anticipated reactivities.

4. The diversity of the immune response

Various bacterial antigens may serve to drive the development of immune responses after natural infection or vaccination such that subsequent disease is prevented. These 'protective' antigens are potential substrates for serodiagnostic assays. Yet, the response to protective antigens does not always equate with the maximal humoral response that may be the most suitable target for serodiagnosis. In fact, it may be the difficulty in achieving a response to protective antigens that allow the pathogen to be a recurrent offender.

The determination of a 'positive' antibody status, if specific, is primarily an indicator of exposure and immune response to a bacterium. The organism may have caused an invasive infection, a superficial infection, or simply existed in a commensal state. The functions of such antibody can be variable. The antibody may simply recognize an antigenic component, but the actual antigen-antibody binding may have no subsequent consequence. Indeed, some of the recognized antigens may be internal and may have been exposed only after the ruptured cell has been exposed to the immune system during the course of infection or phagocytosis. Alternatively, antibody may activate other components of host defences to the extent that antibody-mediated killing results as occurs with complement fixation and activation. As well, the opsonization of bacteria after antibody binding will facilitate some activities of phagocytic cells. The method for antibody measurement may therefore be inclusive or not inclusive of the potential for such antibody interactions. Antibody that is measured by EIA will likely include both forms of active and inactive antibody, whereas neutralization assays select for antibody that is active by its antibacterial action. It cannot be assumed therefore that 'positive' status means protection in full or in part. In fact, many infections may recur despite previous infection and despite the presence of copious amounts of circulating antibody. Furthermore, whereas circulating neutralizing antibody may have the ability to inhibit bacteria in the bloodstream completely or in part, there is no guarantee that such a measure in the blood has much to do with protection at a privileged site, e.g., mucosal or intracerebral. Thus, correlations for serodiagnosis and for protection must be established separately.

V. THE NON-SPECIFICITY OF THE HUMORAL IMMUNE RESPONSE

A. Non-specific responses

The immune system has a repertoire of antibody-producing cells which have the capability of producing antibody to antigens of various types. This innate potential exists even before an individual is exposed to these particular antigens. Given this inherent potential, it is possible therefore that a non-specific stimulation of B cells, which are previously committed to an antibody response of one sort or another, may give rise to an antibody response that is specific to an antigen. The actual affinity of this antibody to the antigen may be weak or strong, and the titre of such antibody is most often low. Nevertheless, it is conceivable that some form of event, perhaps inflammatory and associated with cytokine activation or direct B cell stimulation, may be capable of inciting an antibody response to a bacterial antigen even though the particular bacterium has not actually caused infection. Furthermore, it is possible that an infection may stimulate a non-specific response via polyclonal activation (27). Such an event was proposed by Biberfeld with respect to *Mycoplasma pneumoniae* infection (28).

The development of various autoantibodies, or at least increments of, during infection is a good example of how a pre-disposed antibody response may be stimulated non-specifically (29). For example, rheumatoid factor production (an IgM anti-IgG) is not uncommonly induced during *M. pneumoniae* infections (30). Among those individuals who develop such a response, the titre will be elevated within 2-4 weeks of the acute illness and will then subside in the next several months. Therefore, it is possible that non-specific responses will arise and dissipate during the same time that bacterium-specific responses are also occurring.

B. Heterophil antibody response

Heterophil antibodies are those which arise during the context of an infection, but which react with antigens that are not those of the primary infectious agent. The heterophil antibody may be directed to host tissue or another microbe. The mechanism for heterophil antibody development may be that as detailed above via non-specific polyclonal stimulation. It is possible, however, that the infection itself is intimately responsible for the exposure of the antigen. The bacterium may have some antigen that binds to a receptor, perhaps changing the form of that receptor to make it more enticing to the immune response (31). It may also be that the immune response reacts primarily to the bacterial adhesin but secondarily to the attached hosts receptor. Furthermore, there is the potential that the bacterium or the host are responsible for modifying an antigen as a consequence of the infection itself, e.g., proteolytic mechanism or other.

Cold agglutinins that develop during *M. pneumoniae* infection are good examples of heterophil antibodies that arise during the course of bacterial infections (32). They are IgM antibodies that are directed to the I antigen of some eukaryotic cells, and it is believed that I-like antigens in the respiratory tract serve as principal receptors for *M. pneumoniae* adhesins. Although cold agglutinins are not used much in current mycoplasma diagnostics, this example was nevertheless exploited for such purposes in the past for certain patients (see Chapter 29). Another heterophil antibody response appears to occur during active syphilis, and it is the basis for the non-treponemal tests known as VDRL and RPR (33; see also Chapter 26). The antigen in the latter example is lipoidal, and it is made up of cardiolipin, cholesterol, and lecithin. There is still some uncertainty about what role each of either eukaryotic antigens or of bacterial lipoproteins have in the induction of the latter, but yet such an immune response has been highly useful for diagnostic purposes and continues to enjoy considerable use as a marker of active infection.

VI. A SYNOPSIS OF DIAGNOSTIC METHODS

There has been a natural progression of both simplicity and complexity among serodiagnostic assays which has depended on the evolution of scientific endeavour. It is clear that experience begets the pattern of approach that has been then used for the serodiagnosis of the next pathogen. There has been considerable influence from the development of viral serodiagnostics as this field was naturally of priority given the inherent difficulties that existed with virus detection. The trends and problems have been exemplified by a detailed review of serodiagnosis for *Mycoplasma pneumoniae* which serves as a template for the progress in other areas of diagnostic bacteriology (34).

There have been many comparisons of the serological techniques that are detailed in this chapter. The relevant particulars are highlighted in individual chapters. Perhaps it is best to acknowledge that generalizations can be made, but that the implementation of any technique is very much dependent on the particular pathogen and its pattern of disease causation. Overall, there have been trends toward standardization (and hence transportability), automation for large specimen numbers, and point-of-care testing.

A. Bacterial agglutination

This method was among the earliest available due to the simplicity of the approach. Whole bacterial suspensions are inactivated and standardized to a density such that a visual agglutination will be viewed after reactivity with serial dilutions of patient sera. The assessment of agglutination can take place in tests tubes or in a microtitre format (35). Coloration of the bacterial suspension may enhance the visualization of the reaction. The agglutination will mainly be a function of the interaction between antibody and the antigens which are accessible on the bacterial surface. The antigen-antibody complexes are quite large since the whole bacterium is involved.

This method is applicable to bacteria that grow extracellularly and that are of sufficient size to be seen in a turbid suspension. The method is insensitive when compared to most if not all current methods. Nevertheless, a well-standardized of assay of this sort can be produced with a minimum of resources (36).

B. Diffusion assays (immunodiffusion)

This approach in essence is a form of agglutination assay that is facilitated by the stability of a solid medium (such as agarose) for visualization of the reaction. The antigen must diffuse from the point of source (e.g., well), and so it will necessarily differ from typical bacterial agglutination because the antigen must be smaller in order to migrate through the solid support. The antigens are potentially several bacterial products which may range from cell wall products to intracellular products. The interaction of antigen and antibody is then apparent as a precipitin band in the agarose between the source of antigen and the source of antibody. The diffusion of antibody and antigen are passive, and thus migration occurs in all directions from the source well. The latter will then allow for antibody to migrate and bind antigen, but much of the antigen and antibody are not part of this interaction given their centrifugal migration. This effect diminishes the sensitivity of the assay, and it is uncommonly used in diagnostic bacteriology. The nature of the reaction also prevents there being opportunity for quantitation of the antibody-antigen reaction, although on a cursorial basis, the intensity of banding is a function of the amount of this interaction. These assays would typically require up to 18-24 hrs., and the reactive band(s) could be viewed with the assistance of a stain.

The interaction of antigen and antibody can be focused with the use of a mild electric current which will send these particles in an opposing direction (counterimmunoelectrophoresis; CIE) (37). This will necessarily speed the reaction as well as ensure that the antigen-antibody contact is maximized. Nevertheless, CIE is still overly insensitive compared to contemporary methods (38), and it was only temporarily used for antigen detection rather than antibody detection.

C. Carrier particle agglutination

The above methods depend on the direct visualization of antigen-antibody interactions which may not be prominent, and thus there was an obvious inclination to create some format that would enhance the appreciation of such a reaction. The attachment of antigen to a larger, more visual support, was thus favoured.

There have been many solid supports for this purpose, and these have included latex beads, gelatin particles, red blood cells (3-5% suspensions), and others (39-41). Usually, the antigen is bound to the support passively although in the case of red blood cells, the binding can be passive if it is possible or active via a modification of the red blood cell surface, e.g., tanning from tannic acid exposure. Latex particles for this purpose are <10 μm. All of these supports and their binding to antibody are relatively stable so that reagents may be maintained for months. Assays may be performed on a slide or similar solid support, or in a tube or well. The nature of these reactions lends itself to rapid tests which may require only the dilution of the serum prior to testing.

Reactions are a function of both IgG and IgM, although it appears from the research in indirect hemagglutination (IHA) that IgM is more commonly detected. The IHA titres are essentially patterned according to the maximal IgM response, and the human response tends to be better among young patients, i.e., children and young adults, rather than older adults who may have less of an IgM response. The latter thus allows for potential use in rapid diagnostics. The sensitivity of IHA approaches that of other methods such as enzyme immunoassay.

Non-specific reactions can occur, however, due to the agglutination of the carrier particle rather than bacterial antigen, and this may occur for up to 5-10% of all assays (42). For example, antibody may recognize various surface antigens of the red blood cells. Controls for the latter must therefore be included. In addition, the agglutination reaction in itself may be problematic to read for some serum dilutions, especially those that are at the break-point of the antigen-antibody interaction (so-called equivocal reactions). When a single serum dilution is used, such equivocal results may occur in up to 1-5% of tests depending on the carrier particle and antigen.

A variation of this approach is the red blood cell-IgM capture assay. In this format, antibody to the μ chain of IgM is bound to the red blood cell (Figure 1). The tagged red blood cell thus acts as the visual carrier. Serial dilutions of serum are admixed with the carrier particles which bind IgM, and a standardized antigen is added last (43).

D. Growth inhibition or neutralization

Antibody inhibition of bacterial enzymatic activity or bacterial growth can both be exploited for the purposes of serodiagnosis. For the former, a bacterial enzyme or exotoxin can be neutralized by serial dilutions of serum prior to performing a biological assay which detects the activity. Anti-streptolysin O and antiDNAase testing of sera in the context of *Streptococcus pyogenes* infections are the most

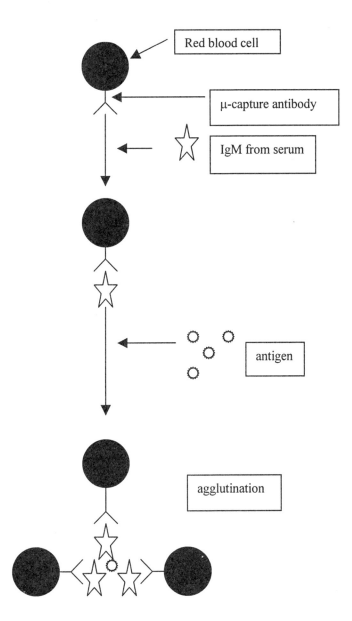

Figure 1   RBC-IgM capture serology.

common current applications of this method (6,44). This variation requires that the bacterial product be partially or fully purified. This method is evidently dependent on the fact that all isolates of a given bacterium that causes the infection be capable of producing the product and that there be a common antibody response normally to that product which is likely to be a virulence factor.

Neutralization of an infectious agent is synonymous with growth inhibition. Serial dilutions of sera are reacted with the infectious agent, and the agent is then cultivated in vitro. Such an approach was commonly used for diagnostic virology, but also served as a measure of protective antibody for some purposes (45). Antibody may be inhibitory in the presence or absence of complement depending on the micro-organism. The measure of inhibition can occur by monitoring growthdirectly or by monitoring the lack of production of a bacterial product or effect, e.g., metabolic inhibition and colour change from pH indicators (46). This approach is a better detector of IgG rather than IgM, although IgG, IgM ,and IgA are all participants in inhibition, and thus the antibody peak is usually later in onset than for those methods that detect mainly IgM. These assays usually require one or more days to complete because of the inhibition end-point. Low titres may appear due to cross-reacting antibodies which have formed as a result of responses to other bacteria. If patients have received antibacterial agents, these may falsely give the impression of high titres due to the metabolic inhibition or bacterial cell death that occurs. The likelihood of prior antibiotic use will depend on the specific infection.

E. Complement fixation

From an historical perspective, it was desirable to enhance the sensitivity of serodiagnostic assays, and this was in part most likely to be achieved by enhancing the quality of the detector systems for antigen-antibody reactions. Again, trends in the virology serodiagnostics served to provide initiatives in these regards. In the CF method, the complement fixation of the antigen-antibody reaction is exploited (47). When the amount of antibody as a result of infection increases, there is more potential to fix complement in the presence of a fixed amount of antigen. The fixation of complement is determined by a detector system which will utilize complement to achieve a biological effect. In the traditional CF assay, a sensitized red blood cell is used as the indicator mechanism so that unfixed complement (implying the presence of less antibody) is bound to the antibody lysin that has been reacted with the red blood cell and will result in red blood cell lysis. If complement is bound to the antigen-antibody complex, it will not be available for red blood cell lysis, and thus the red cells will remain intact. The visualization of intact versus lysed red blood cells in reaction wells will then serve as the end-point for the antibody dilution (Figure 2).

The CF test requires rigorous control and standardization, but quality reagents are available through commercial vendors (48). Critical variables in the performance of the assays particularly include the source of complement, the quality and source of hemolysin, suitability of indicator red blood cells, and the antigen. The preparation of the components as well as the run of the test proper necessitates more than one day for completion. Nevertheless, the CF test may be configured to assess reactivity with more than one antigen in the form of a testing panel and with the use of the same detector system. The CF test is usually performed in a reference laboratory setting.

Traditionally, the CF test has often been used as a standard for which to compare other serological assays. Antibody detection is particularly a function of IgM in acute infections although both IgM and IgG are complement-fixing (48). High standing titres above a particular threshold or four-fold increments between acute and convalescent sera are used for diagnosis. The sensitivity of CF approaches that of current enzyme immunoassays, but the latter are favoured due to simplicity. For some infections, sensitivity may be suboptimal, e.g., CF for chlamydiae.

Some sera may have anticomplementary activity that can interfere with the assay, and this will be detected by appropriate controls. Anticomplementarity of sera can be a marker for Q fever on occasion (49).

F. Immunofluorescence

Indirect immunofluorescence has found many uses in diagnostic bacteriology, and it continues to be used for several examples. The bacterial substrate is usually either agar- or broth-cultivated bacterium, or it may be bacterium that is grown in eukaryotic cells [e.g., chlamydiae or rickettsiae (50,51)] or that is cell-associated [e.g., sometimes used for *Bartonella henselae* serology (52)]. The bacterium, with or without its eukaryotic cell associate, is fixed onto glass. The substrate is then exposed to serial dilutions

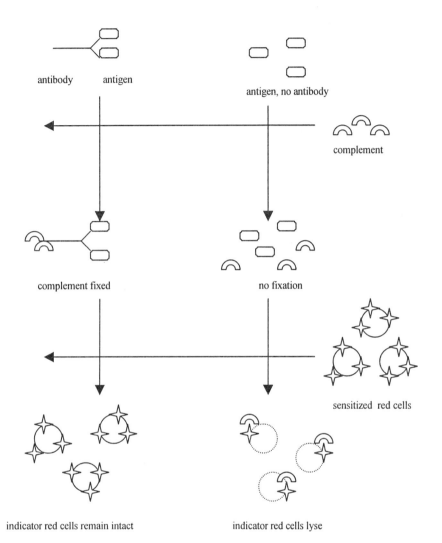

antibody   antigen

antigen, no antibody

complement

complement fixed

no fixation

sensitized red cells

indicator red cells remain intact

indicator red cells lyse

Figure 2 Complement fixation serology.

of serum in different slide wells, and a fluorescence-tagged antibody is then used to detect the human antibody (Figure 3). The signal must be read with an appropriately filtered fluorescence microscope The detector antibody may be specific for either IgG or IgM. Historically, the availability of consistent fluo-rescein-tagged conjugates was a problem, but this problem has been diminished considerably. In addi-tion to fluorescein, there are a number of other fluorochromes that may be used to label antibodies. Both the fixation method and the nature of the bacterial isolate may affect the quality of fluorescence. The most important variable is the observer who must judge gradations of fluorescence intensity despite whatever scoring method or criteria are used to determine a fluorescence end-point. For this reason alone, there may site-to-site variation in the determination of IFA titres. The assessment is best carried out by those who have considerable experience with fluorescence microscopy rather than in centres where specimens are not commonly acquired.

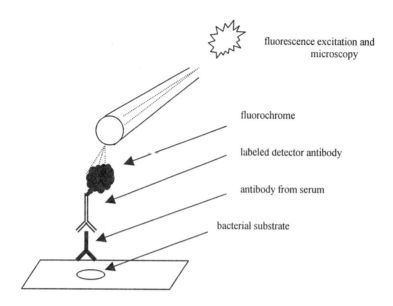

fluorescence excitation and
microscopy

fluorochrome

labeled detector antibody

antibody from serum

bacterial substrate

Figure 3   Indirect immunofluorescence assay.

The ability to detect IgM facilitates the use of IFA for rapid diagnosis, and an IFA can be completed in the course of several hours. IgM titres of significance in IFA tend to be relatively low and certainly in comparison to IgG titres. Changes in IgG-IFA of four-fold or greater will also be deemed significant as they are for CF serology. Many IgM-IFA assays have been commercialized in the past, and some continue to enjoy use. There is generally a good correlation with other IgM methods. IgM-IFA may be susceptible to non-specificity from rheumatoid factor.

The above conventional IFA uses a solid support on which the interpretation of identity is based on a direct visualization through microscopy, but solid phase fluorescence assays may also be assessed through automated readers. This is the basis for the FIAX system (53). Furthermore, fluorescence markers can be used in liquid phase assays whereby the antibody-antigen interaction is occurring in a liquid phase rather than on a solid support.

G. Radioimmunoassay

The use of a radioisotope label was a natural progression from fluorescein and other labels, and the method of measurement had the potential to enhance signal detection and sensitivity. Overall, the use of radioimmunoassay with solid supports is relatively obsolete in bacterial serodiagnosis and has generally been replaced by enzyme immunoassay over the last 15 years. Although radioisotopes do provide for greater sensitivity in comparison to other methods, this gain may be compromised by issues relating to background signal. The difficulty in appreciating 'signal-to-noise' has always been of primary importance in the development of a useful assay, and interpretive 'grey' zones necessarily arise. The use of radioisotopes and the special circumstances surrounding their use has been the major strike against this technology.

Radioimmunoprecipitation (54) with radiolabeled bacterial antigens has served mainly as a research tool to understand the humoral immune response much like contemporary immunoblotting, but it has not surfaced as a major serodiagnostic mode despite having the potential to be used as a confirmatory test.

H. Solid phase immunoassays

The advent of solid phase immunoassays with enzyme-labeled antibodies (enzyme immunoassays; EIA) has proven to be one of the most important advances in contemporary serodiagnostics, and such assays have been widely used for all areas of microbiology diagnostics as well as for many other medical (non-microbial) diagnostics (55-57). The variations of EIA are many, but the more commonly-used approaches have included indirect EIA, antibody-capture EIA, and antibody-capture double sandwich EIA of varied sorts (Figures 4-6).

A variety of enzymes have been used for EIA, but the most common ones are peroxidase and alkaline phosphatase. Essentially it is desirable to label antigen or antibody with an enzyme so that the binding does not interfere with the enzymatic activity which will then be available to convert an enzyme substrate; the change in substrate will be an indicator of the amount of antibody that is present in the serum. As is evident from the Figure below, the indirect EIA is simple, and it has been favoured for most serodiagnostic assays. This format is susceptible however to false-positive results since the binding of test serum antibody can occur more readily to the solid support or to components of the antigen preparation that are bound to the solid surface but that are not true bacterium-specific antigens. As well, in a direct competitive fashion, the indirect EIA will also be susceptible to false-positive assays due to high concentrations of the generic antibody in the serum specimen which non-specifically bind to the solid support. For these reasons, antibody-capture assays have been promoted by some. The latter may use labeled antigen as the detector system or a complex sandwich system in which labeled antibody is used as the detector.

Whether of the indirect or antibody-capture variations, EIA can be configured to selectively assay for IgM or IgG or IgA antibody; again, the IgM systems will be of value for timely diagnoses potentially with the use of single sera. EIAs are amenable to accurate standardization, automation for rapid turn-around, and high volume capacity. Assays can be completed over 3-5 hrs., and some rapid methods have decreased the overall reaction time to ½ to 1 hr.

The type of antigen that is used can vary from whole bacterium to sonicates or extracts to components whether purified or synthetic (direct synthesis of peptides or recombinant). These antigens may be proteins, lipids, or carbohydrates, or combinations of the same. They can be absorbed passively onto the

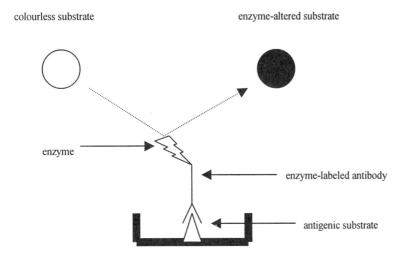

Figure 4   Indirect enzyme immunoassay.

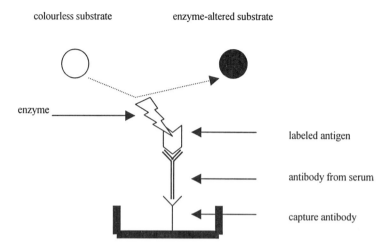

Figure 5   Antibody-capture enzyme immunoassay.

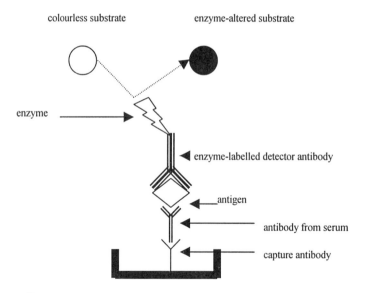

Figure 6   Antibody-capture double sandwich enzyme immunoassay.

solid support or actively fixed. Alkaline carbonate (pH~9.0-9.5) buffers enhance the binding of many antigens to the common solid supports. Plastic and variations thereof are most commonly used as the solid supports, and the configuration of wells which can bewashed suits the system the most. The use of beads for the binding surface area or the use of other supports such as glass, nitrocellulose, and nylon have also received attention. Once the antigen is absorbed onto the solid support, there remains the capacity for the same support to bind antibody from the serum sample in the same fashion, and thus the remaining binding sites require blocking with some other substance(s). Suitable blocking solutions have included buffers with albumin, gelatin, and skim milk, although there are many other possibilities. There have been several attempts to enhance the enzymatic activity through a variety of mechanisms (e.g., avidin-biotin signal amplification), but most of these advances have yielded only marginal gains in sensitivity and often at the expense of other problems that arise usually in regard to specificity. Nevertheless, the quality of conjugates has tremendously improved over the last two decades, and affinity-purified antibodies are readily available. The use of monoclonal antibodies rather than polyclonal monospecific antibodies has also been of value. In some systems, non-enzymatic labels may be used; chemiluminescence has made use of the oxidation of compounds to chemiluminescent end-products. The use of automated readers has simplified the task of interpretation and adds a measure of quantitation that is reproducible.

Although the standard solid phase immunoassays involve the layering of antigens and antibodies, there are many commercial serodiagnostic products which are emerging and which make use of the same immunoassay principle but in a rapid assay format and with a simple one-step membrane assay. Some of these are quickly finding their way into practical use, e.g., *Helicobacter pylori* serology (58). Both traditional solid phase immunoassays and rapid membrane assay variations are potentially useful for screening purposes since high volumes may be handled or simply due to the simplicity of the methods respectively.

Disease-specific IgM is detected as early as 5-7 days after onset of some infections although 7-10 days is more typical. IgG determinations can be made for acute and convalescent sera, although the desired minimal variation in EIA readings for a positive diagnosis may be the subject of debate. Interpretive criteria usually include a 'grey zone' of equivocal readings given that the enzyme activity takes place on a continuous spectrum. The choice of a specific diagnostic threshold continues to be the major problem with these immunoassays. Blocking assays, where competition for antibody is achieved by the use of another antigen-specific antibody, may be used for confirmatory purposes, although such an approach is usually used in the context of assuring positive results when solid phase immunoassays are used for antigen detection. Antibody avidity can also be assessed by these immunoassays, although this has not practically been of much value for serodiagnosis.

The nature of these immunoassays is such that a maximization of sensitivity may allow for antibody to be detected for several months to a year after the acute infection, even for IgM assessments. The latter may be problematic if the pathogen of concern has the potential to infect on a recurrent basis.

Rheumatoid factor may interfere with the accurate interpretation of IgM results. Excessive antigen-specific IgG may also interfere with IgM determinations. For either of these problems, the interference may be eliminated by a preaborption of test sera for IgG prior to the IgM assessment.

I.   Liquid phase immunoassays

Rather than use a solid support to facilitate antigen-antibody interactions as detailed above, a liquid phase will nevertheless be suitable for many such determinations (59). Essentially, changes in enzyme activity or fluorescence can be appreciated as the binding of antigen and antibody modifies the activity of the label. The assays can be configured in a one-step format, and automated readers may be used to standardize the interpretation on a quantitative basis. Since the reaction must remain in the fluid phase, the nature of the antigen must allow for the immune complex to remain suspended, and thus this format is usually of benefit for smaller antigens, e.g., components, enzymes, or toxins, rather than whole bacteria or large complexes. Such a method, for example, is amenable to the determination of antibiotic levels, e.g., aminoglycosides. Liquid phase immunoassays are also known as homogeneous assays.

J.   Immunoblotting

In essence, conventional immunoblotting (commonly referred to as Western blotting) for serodiagnosis is but a variant of solid phase EIA (60-62). The major difference is that microtitre well solid phase EIAs usually have a colorimetric indicator that is indirectly indicative of the presence of antibody, whereas the reactivity of antibody to specific antigens can be visualized in an immunoblot of segregated bacterial antigens.

Most antigens for immunoblotting are resolved in a linear fashion with reducing sodium dodecyl sulphate polyacrylamide gel electrophoresis (SDS-PAGE) (63). They are arranged in a gradation of molecular weights from highest to lowest over the migration path. Although some antigens may appear to have a particular migration rate as correlated with molecular weight standards, they may truly have a different molecular weight due to the conditions of the electrophoresis and the structure of the antigen. The resolved pattern of antigens are transferred to a solid support which will then allow for the exposure to serum antibody and the enzymatic labelling for antibody detection. Solid supports can include nylon, nitrocellulose (most commonly), and other charged cellulose derivatives. Most of the structures that resolve in conventional SDS-PAGE are wholly or partially polypeptides. Nevertheless, it is possible to resolve patterns of glycolipids using other techniques and to follow the latter with immunoblotting, but such an approach is rarely investigated. It must therefore be acknowledged that the antigens which are recognized from immunoblotting have been preselected by the process that has been chosen for resolution and that the size or nature of the antigens may appear different than the native structure due to pre-reduction.

Immunoblotting can be made selective for IgM, IgG, or IgA antibodies by the use of appropriate conjugated-detector antibodies. The nature of the test will potentially provide a confirmatory method of serology over other methods which use indirect indicators of antigen-antibody interaction. This is best exemplified by the use of immunoblotting for Lyme disease (see Chapter 25). The pattern of visualized response that corresponds to diagnostic confirmation may include one or several antigens.

There is considerable variation in the humoral response to most bacteria and such heterogeneity is likely to be seen with immunoblotting where many antigen reactivities are being assessed at one time. Whereas there may be some very dominant antigens that are commonly recognized, many other antigens may be the subject of inconsistent recognition. Furthermore, such recognition is not absolute in a positive or negative sense since gradations of positivity can be seen for any given antigen (64). Indeed, the methodolocrical details of the procedure can greatly affect the outcome of immunoblotting. As well, it is possible to see some run-to-run variation in antibody response patterns. Some antigens may be common to several bacteria and must therefore be viewed cautiously as serodiagnostic indicators, e.g., flagellar proteins of borreliae and treponemes (65). Although immunodominant antigens can be present, the specificity of a reaction pattern is likely to be greater if more than one such antigen is used in the positive assessment criteria.

In the 1980s, standardization of immunoblots was a major dilemma (66), but there has been much improvement in this general area such that commercial immunoblots have become trustworthy. The translation of positive immunoblot patterns to diagnoses for all regions of the world must be viewed also with caution since it may be assumed that the antigen reactivity should be similar when a common antigen substrate is used. With the example of Lyme disease (see Chapter 25), it has become apparent that North American and European isolates do potentially have some significant structural variations.

The modest complexity of immunoblotting, even when the substrates are entirely commercialized, will necessitate that the method be used for small numbers of specimens and usually for a confirmatory purpose rather than for the testing of larger batches of samples.

The production of whole cell polypeptide profiles, which may be tainted by other proteins from growth media, does raise the theoretical concern of increasing the opportunity for being inclusive of non-specific antigens, i.e., the more, the greater the chance for non-specificity. In this regard, the future holds promise for devising recombinant and purified antigens which may circumvent this dilemma (67).

Immunoblotting can be a very sensitive technique and essentially comparable to EIA methods. As the total antibody to a given bacterium extinguishes months after the infection, the change in immunoblot pattern may vary such that reactivities to lesser common antigens disappear first (68).

VII. GENERAL ASPECTS OF UTILIZATION

A. Specimen collection

Serum is generally the specimen of choice for most assays. It will be available after the removal of clotted blood. Some assays require the heat inactivation of sera in order to remove complement. For immunoblotting, plasma may also suffice since the essential antibody remains; the centrifugation of whole blood that has been anticoagulated with various anticoagulants may suffice. The needs for each serodiagnostic method should be considered.

The transport of sera from distant sites or though mail has led to the consideration of dried sera (69). These may be hydrated in the recipient laboratory prior to use. Such transport has been assessed and it is generally favourable especially for IgG studies and especially for screening purposes where there is likely to be a large quantity of antibody. IgM, however, is somewhat susceptible to such manipulation if it is considerable, but not on an all-or-none basis.

The assessment of mucosal antibody as a marker for infection has received comparatively little attention. The acquisition of consistent mucosal samples is much more likely to be fraught with difficulty. As an example, the detection of salivary antibody is becoming popular in *Helicobacter pylori* serodiagnosis (70, 71; see also Chapter 20).

B. Screening versus confirmatory assays

The processing of large volumes of sera for any test can be a challenge for even the largest laboratories. Nevertheless, automation of commercially-available and well-standardized tests has allowed the diagnostic laboratory to at least overcome some of these challenges. Although some assays are not entirely specific, e.g., EIAs, they may be designed to ensure that the vast majority of possible positive diagnoses are not missed. That is, the diagnostic threshold is adjusted to enhance sensitivity. Such an assay is then tailored to function as a good screening test since it is relatively assured that positive diagnoses will not be missed. This elevation in threshold, however, will likely lead to overdiagnosis, and so the presumptive positive assays from initially screening may benefit from the corroboration of positivity from another assay. The latter assay may then be referred to as the 'confirmatory' test.

Immunoblotting has been used as a confirmatory test for screening EIAs in virology diagnostics, e.g, hepatitis C and HIV, and a similar approach has been used for Lyme disease serology. Although the nature of immunoblotting with its identification of bacterial specific antigens seems suited to a confirmatory test, it is the specificity of the assay rather than the actual format that matters. In this sense, it is possible to have confirmation with the use of any serodiagnostic method as long as the assay has been proven to be of high specificity. For example, for syphilis serology, screening non-treponemal tests are most commonly used, and these assays are very sensitive for active disease. Due to the potential for biological false-positives, however, a positive screening test will be followed by a confirmatory treponemal test such as the MHTP or FTA (see Chapter 26). Confirmatory tests may be single or multiple.

Overall, a lesser expensive, more easily performed, and automated test will serve best as a screening procedure. Confirmatory tests usually are more cumbersome and costly. Otherwise, there are many circumstances where a single serological assay may be used for both screening and confirmation.

C. Assessment criteria

1. Threshold criteria

The definition of thresholds for positive and negative assays merits careful consideration. In general, there are very few if any serodiagnostic assays which function perfectly well with the use of strictly positive and negative results. The extent of the 'grey-zone' is dependent on several variables. The determination of cut-off values is initially dependent on the comparison of serological values for the sera of individuals who are asymptomatic and well, and for the sera of those who are truly infected as determined by other definitive means. The serological values that are between these poles represent the 'indeterminate' zone. If the distributions between diseased and non-diseased are far apart, then it is likely that few positives will be false-positive and few negatives will be false-negatives. If the distribution of serological values for these populations overlap, the issue of non-specificity will be more of a concern. The overlapping values may then be considered the zone of 'equivocal' results. If the positive threshold is moved closer to the higher values of the diseased group over a curved distribution, the assay will be enhanced in specificity but compromised in sensitivity. In contrast, the biasing of the threshold towards lower values that are more common for the non-diseased group will lead to improved sensitivity but lesser specificity (Figure 7). The specific choices here must be determined with the knowledge of what missed diagnoses or overdiagnosis means in any given context, and hence they are dependent on experience that must be acquired with application in the field.

2. Measures of utility

The performance utilization of serodiagnostics tests are commonly described in terms that often serve as numeric comparators. Four main terms are initially of common use:

- *Sensitivity*: ratio of true positives to true positives and false negatives. It indicates the probability that all infections are being determined.
- *Specificity*: ratio of true negatives to true negatives and false positives. It indicates the probability that an uninfected individual is truly uninfected.
- *Positive predictive value*: ratio of true positives to true positives and false positives. It indicates the probability that the positive test is truly indicative of infection.
- *Negative predictive value*: ratio of true negatives to true negatives and false negatives. It indicates the probability that the negative test is truly indicative of no infection.

Each of the above ratios is commonly expressed as percentages. Whereas these terms are commonly used for initial assessments and then for test-test comparisons, it is not uncommonly forgotten that the predictive values of the test are very much dependent on the pre-test likelihood that the particular infection exists among the given population. Therefore, if an infection is likely to be common among a patient population, the predictive value of a positive test will likely be better given that many positives will truly be acquired from patients who are ill with that infection. To the contrary, if the infection is extremely uncommon, even a very sensitive and specific test may be problematic to apply since the positive tests may more likely occur among those who are truly not diseased. Furthermore, the nature of endemic seroprevalence and disease commonality also affect these values. If the infection is very common and may repeat itself for a given patient over a short period of time, the presence of pre-existing antibody may confound the results. Even if the disease is uncommon but yet may have been experienced, and the antibodies so developed persist, again the appreciation of the test may falter. The assessment of serodiagnostic assays in field conditions must be emphasized.

D. Quality standards

Most commercial serodiagnostic assays offer control positive and negative sera for simultaneous assessment with unknown patient specimens. In assays such as EIA and CF, these sera are important to ensure that the assay has performed within the expected standards, and yet they may also be important to the calibration of the assay itself.

Use of proficiency testing for serodiagnostic methods is valuable and should be routinely considered (72-75).

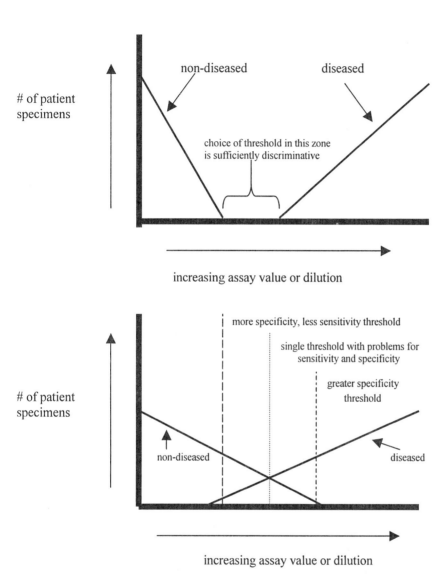

non-diseased   diseased

# of patient
specimens

choice of threshold in this zone
is sufficiently discriminative

increasing assay value or dilution

more specificity, less sensitivity threshold

single threshold with problems for
sensitivity and specificity

greater specificity
threshold

# of patient
specimens

non-diseased   diseased

increasing assay value or dilution

Figure 7   Impact of threshold decisions for determining cut-off criteria in serodiagnostic assays.

E. Automation and robotics

The configuration of several methods lend themselves to automation, and this may facilitate rapid throughput and conserve on cost. The natural evolution in this field is to automate more and to be more inclusive of a greater array of diagnostic tests. Some serodiagnostic assays are uncommonly used, however, and it may be preferable to use manual techniques.

Whereas the performance of these diagnostic assays in a highly automated scenario may be standardized, they are all too often seen as simple input-output maneuvers whereby specimens are rapidly processed and results are rapidly disseminated, much like the performance of routine blood counts or blood chemistries. Such a view of operations will necessarily place less emphasis on important consid-erations such as appropriate utilization and valid application. In the field of diagnostic virology, it is apparent that many if not the majority of serological requests are either not appropriate or have little value in patient management. The same is likely to be true of bacterial serodiagnostic tests. The ramifi-cations of inappropriately chosen tests can be just as important as those for the lack of investigation.

F. Point-of-care testing

As in all of medicine, it would be desirable to have most answers available at the earliest possible con-venience and within the shortest time possible. Naturally then, there has been an interest in bringing some of the serodiagnostic assays to the bedside, clinic, or otherwise very closeby (76,77). This would be most applicable to tests which facilitate rapid diagnosis and which have some immediate impact on patient care. Much effort has already been directed to such assays for the purposes of infectious diseases whether for serological purposes or direct bacterial detection. In this regard, there have been several successes and with the promise of more to come as innovative technologies emerge.

Several point-of-care tests, however, have been commercialized and utilized, but with the subse-quent experience that they are less sensitive (and considerably so for some) than the standards which previously existed. It then requires testing in field conditions to determine what impact this compromise may have on clinical care. There are truly few comprehensive studies of cost-effectiveness in the appli-cation of serodiagnostics tests in general. Furthermore, point-of-care tests are often designed with the hope of accessibility for those who may be lesser skilled than laboratory staff proper. As simple tests may be placed in the hands of lesser skilled individuals, a new version of performance problems arise. For example, the simple appreciation of latex agglutination may be sufficiently mistaken to cause sig-nificant misdiagnosis in unexperienced hands. It may be prudent at times to consider comparing such bedside rapid tests to the existing standard, and to ensure that the test provider is sufficiently informed in order to carry out the procedure accurately.

VIII. COMPLICATING FEATURES

A. Natural variation of the immune response

The factors that effect an immune response are many and go much beyond the details of the bacterium in itself. Given the genetic variation in humanity and given that this translates into variability in the im-mune system, it is not surprising that hetereogeneity in the humoral responses to infection should exist. This is often evident at least among age groups where the very young and perhaps very old have less of a response, and for different reasons, to certain antigens. For example, children under the age of two may respond less to bacterial polysaccharides than other children (15-17). Yet other closed populations or even smaller genetic groups, e.g., families, may response very poorly to select or several antigens.

Immunodeficiency of some sort may lead to no responses, poor responses, or delayed responses. The application of serodiagnostic assays must assure that such limitations are acknowledged.

B. Rheumatoid factor

Rheumatoid factor is a description of an antibody form in vivo which is directed to other antibody of the same host (78,79). For example, the most common form of rheumatoid factor is IgM anti-IgG. An IgG anti-IgG may also be found. In serodiagnostic assays, especially of the indirect type, e.g., indirect EIA, rheumatoid factor may interfere with the accurate determination of true antibody that is directed to the bacterial antigen of interest. In an IgM test, IgM rheumatoid factor may bind to IgG that is directed to the bacterium. Since the IgG will likely remain bound to the antigen (and hence the rheumatoid factor), a subsequent assessment for IgM with the use of an anti-IgM secondary antibody may detect the rheumatoid factor rather than true antibacterial IgM.

Rheumatoid factor is much more prevalent in human sera than would be indicated by the number of individuals that are afflicted by rheumatoid arthritis alone. In many infections, rheumatoid factor is generated by some unknown mechanism during active inflammation.

In at least IgM assays, rheumatoid factor can be removed with an IgG absorbent prior to the assay.

C. Confirming specificity

As previously indicated, immunoblots have served in the capacity of confirmatory serology for some infections. Another method to examine specificity of the immune response may include active absorption of sera with the target antigen. That is, specificity can be inferred if the antibody can be removed after reaction with and then precipitation with the bacterial substrate, usually whole cell. These can be more easily conducted with whole cells that have surfaced exposed antigens rather than component antigens such as toxins which are excreted with the bacterium. There must be a standard, however, for the amount of antibody reduction that should be anticipated given that even cross-reactive antibodies can be reduced by such a process of absorption. There have been few examples where such a confirmatory approach has been adopted outside of the research arena.

D. Maternal-fetal transfer

The maturing placenta begins to allow for IgG to cross its maternal-fetal barrier during the mid-second trimester. Maternal IgG will be more plentiful in the fetal circulation towards the end of a full gestation. IgM is sufficiently complex a molecule that it is not found in fetal circulation unless produced by the fetus itself. Thus, the presence of organism-specific IgM at birth or thereafter is an indication of fetal or newborn infection. Maternal IgG may persist in the newborn for up to six months (range usually 4-12 months), and this may confound serological assays if IgG is the main target for detection. Thus, serological tests for syphilis will often be positive in the newborn when the mother is infected. Infection of the newborn may then require a serial follow-up of newborn titres. A comparison of newborn to maternal titres may also be of some value. At the present time, there is no practical method to differentiate maternal and newborn IgG antibody.

E. Antibiotic effects

An immune response will typically occur during an invasive disease from most bacterial pathogens regardless of whether its measurement is diagnostic or not. Antibiotic therapy has the potential to reduce the amount of an immune response given that antibacterials will prevent bacterial replication and may then abruptly terminate an infection at the time immunity is to be induced. For many infections, the disease is so advanced by the time treatment and diagnosis are had such that antibiotics will have little impact to abrogate antibody development. There are some examples, however, where it is believed that early treatment can both reduce the disease course and hinder antibiotic development. In streptococcal pharyngitis, the ASOT may be affected by antibiotic use. As well, early use of an appropriate antibiotic may diminish the serological response to *Mycoplasma pneumoniae* infection.

F. Humoral versus cell-mediated immunity

The use of an antibody measurement to indicate past or active infection is time-honoured. Likewise, the use of skin testing for the purposes of demonstrating cell-mediated immune responses and hence current or previous infection has also withstood the test of time for some purposes. Nevertheless, the use of in vitro cell-mediated immunity assessments have not been explored to their fullest for diagnostic purposes (80,81). There is the possibility that a complete understanding of immunodiagnostic strategies which are potentially available is biased due to the conventional approaches that most investigators choose to follow. Perhaps even combinations of 'immunodiagnostics' may be the best approach for some infections.

REFERENCES

1. Gray GC, Struewing JP, Hyams KC, Escamilla J, Tupponse AK, Kaplan EL. Interpreting a single antistreptolysin O test: a comparison of the "upper limit of normal" and likelihood ratio methods. J Clin Epidemiol 1993; 46:1181-1185.
2. Hirschberg L, Krook A, Pettersson CA, Vikerfors T. Enzyme-linked immunosorbent assay for detection of *Mycoplasma pneumoniae* specific immunoglobulin M. Eur J Clin Microbiol Infect Dis 1988; 7:420-423.
3. Young H. Syphilis: serology. Dermatol Clin 1998; 16:691-698.
4. Fernald GW, Clyde WA, Denny FW. Nature of the immune response to *Mycoplasma pneumoniae*. J Immunol 1967; 98:1028-1038.
5. Okazaki N, Akema R, Takizawa K. A sensitive method for detecting the fermentation-inhibition antibody to *Mycoplasma pneumoniae*. Microbiol Immunol 1991; 35:871-878.
6. Neurath AR, Strick N, Lee ES. B cell epitope mapping of human immunodeficiency virus envelope glycoproteins with long (19- to 36- residue) synthetic peptides. J Gen Virol 1990; 71:85-95.
7. Relf WA, Cooper J, Brandt ER, Hayman WA, Anders RF, Pruksakorn S, Currie B, Saul A, Good MF. Mapping a conserved conformational epitope from the M protein of group A streptococci. Pept Res 1996; 9:12-20.
8. Wilkinson HW, Brake BJ. Formalin-killed versus heat-killed *Legionella pneumophila* serogroup 1 antigen in the indirect immunofluorescence assay for legionellosis. J Clin Microbiol 1982; 16:979-981.
9. Morooka T, Matano H, Umeda A, Oda T, Amako K, Karmali MA. Indirect hemagglutination assay for antibodies to *Escherichia coli* lipopolysaccharides O157, O111 and O26 in patients with hemolytic uremic syndrome. Acta Paediatr Jpn 1995; 37:469-473.
10. Cabau N, Crainic R, Duros C, Deonyel G, Gaspar A, Bronnert C, Boue A, Horodniceanu F. Freeze-dried erythrocytes for an indirect hemagglutination test for detection of cytomegalovirus antibodies. J Clin Microbiol 1981; 13:1026-1030.
11. Sawada T, Rimler RB, Rhoades KR. Indirect hemagglutination test that uses glutaraldehyde-fixed sheep erythrocytes sensitized with extract antigens for detection of *Pasteurella* antibody. J Clin Microbiol 1982; 15:752-756.
12. He Q, Mertsola J. Epidemiology and prevention of pertussis. Curr Opin Pediatr 1997; 9:14-18.
13. Schneerson R. Similarities between the pathogenesis of and immunity to diphtheria and pertussis: the complex nature of serum antitoxin-induced immunity to these two diseases. Clin Infect Dis 1999; 28:S136-S139.
14. Greatorex JS, Thorne GM. Humoral immune responses to Shiga-like toxins and *Escherichia coli* O157 lipopolysaccharide in hemolytic-uremic syndrome. J Clin Microbiol 1994; 32:1171-1178.
15. Greenberg DP, Ward JI, Burkart K, Christenson PD, Guravitz L, Mracy SM. Factors influencing immunogenicity and safety of two *Haemophilus influenzae* type b polysaccharide vaccines in children 18 and 24 months of age. Pediatr Infect Dis 1987; 6:660-665.
16. Lee CJ, Banks SD, Li JP. Virulence, immunity, and vaccine related to *Streptococcus pneumoniae*. Crit Rev Microbiol 1991; 18:89-114.
17. Gotschlich EC, Rey M, Triau R, Sparks KJ. Quantitative determination of the human immune response to immunization with meningococcal vaccines. J Clin Invest 1972; 51:89-96.
18. Force RW, Lugo RA, Nahata MC. *Haemophilus influenzae* b conjugate vaccines. Ann Pharmacother 1992; 26:1429-1940.
19. Marmion BP, Plackett P, Lemcke RM . Immunological analysis of *Mycoplasma pneumoniae*. 1. Methods of extraction and reaction of fractions from *Mycoplasma pneumoniae* and from *Mycoplasma mycoides* with homologous antisera and with antisera against *Streptococcous* MG. Aust J Exp Biol Med Sci 1967; 45:163-187.
20. Poisson F, Baillou F, Dubois F, Janvier B, Roingeard P, Goudeau A. Immune response to synthetic peptides of hepatitis delta antigen. J Clin Microbiol 1993; 31:2343-2349.
21. Wang JT, Wang TH, Lin JT, Sheu JC, Lee CZ, Chen DS. Improved serodiagnosis of post-transfusion hepatitis C virus infection by a second-generation immunoassay based on multiple recombinant antigens. Vox Sang 1992; 62:21-24.
22. Knox KW, Wicken AJ. Immunological properties of teichoic acids. Bacteriol Rev 1973; 37:215-257.

23. Perez-Perez GI, Hopkins JA, Blaser MJ. Lipopolysaccharide structures in *Enterobacteriaceae, Pseudomonas aeruginosa,* and *Vibrio cholerae* are immunologically related to *Campylobacter* spp. Infect Immun 1986; 51:204-208.

24. Plackett P, Marmion BP, Shaw EJ, Lemcke RM. Immunochemical analysis of *Mycoplasma pneumoniae.* 3. Separation and chemical idenification of serologically active lipids. Aust J Exp Biol Med Sci 1969; 47:171-195.

25. Zielen S, Buhring I, Strnad N, Reichenbach J, Hofmann D. Immunogenicity and tolerance of a 7-valent pneumococcal vaccine in nonresponders to the 23-valent pneumococcal vaccine. Infect Immun 2000; 68:1435-1440.

26. Hauser U, Krahl H, Peters H, Fingerle V, Wilske B. Impact of strain heterogeneity on Lyme disease serology in Europe: comparison of enzyme-linked immunosorbent assays using different species of *Borrelia burgdorferi* sensu lato. J Clin Microbiol 1998; 36:427-436.

27. Braun MG, Gross WL, Muller-Hermelink HK. Morphological differentiation of human lymphocyte subpopulations following polyclonal stimulation with bacteria and lectin. Immunobiology 1988; 177:220-232.

28. Biberfeld G. Antibodies to brain and other tissues in cases of *Mycoplasma pneumoniae* infection. Clin Exp Immunol 1971; 8:319-333.

29. Horn MP, Gerster T, Ochensberger B, Derer T, Kricek T, Jouvin MH, Kinet JP, Tschernig T, Vogel M, Stadler BM, Miescher SM. Human anti-F-epsilon-RI-alpha autoantibodies isolated from healthy donors cross-react with tetanus toxoid. Eur J Immunol 1999; 29:1139-1148.

30. Mizutani H, Mizutani H. Immunologic responses in patients with *Mycoplasma pneumoniae* infections. Am Rev Resp Dis 1983; 127:175-179.

31. Feizi T, Loveless RW. Carbohydrate recognition by *Mycoplasma pneumoniae* and pathologic consequences. Am J Resp Crit Care Med 1996; 154:S133-S136.

32. Petz LD. Autoimmune and drug-induced hemolytic anemia. In: Rose NR, De Macario EC, Fahey JL, Friedman H, Penn GM, eds. Manual of Clinical Laboratory Immunology, 4th Ed. Washington, DC:American Society for Microbiology, 1992:325-343.

33. Creighton ET. Rapid plasma reagin (RPR) 18 mm circle card test. In: Larsen SA, Hunter EF, Kraus SJ – eds. Manual of Tests for Syphilis. Washington, DC:American Public Health Association, 1990:103-112.

34. Cimolai N. Serodiagnosis of the Infectious Diseases: *Mycoplasma pneumoniae.* Norwell, MA: Kluwer Academic Publishers, 1999.

35. Arimitsu Y, Kmety E, Ananyina Y, Baranton G, Ferguson IR, Smythe L, Terpstra WJ. Evaluation of the one-point microcapsule agglutination test for diagnosis of leptospirosis. Bull World Health Organ 1994; 72:395-399.

36. Brandao AP, Camargo ED, da Silva ED, Silva MV, Abrao RV. Macroscopic agglutination test for rapid diagnosis of human leptospirosis. J Clin Microbiol 1998; 36:3138-3142.

37. Holliday MG. The diagnosis of Legionnaire's disease by counterimmunoelectrophoresis. J Clin Pathol 1980; 33:1174-1178.

38. Sharma M, Datta U, Roy P, Verma S, Sehgal S. Low sensitivity of counter-current immuno-electrophoresis for serodiagnosis of typhoid fever. J Med Microbiol 1997; 46:1039-1042.

39. Lieberman D, Lieberman D, Horowitz S, Horovitz O, Schlaeffer F, Porath A. Microparticle agglutination versus antibody-capture enzyme immunoassay for diagnosis of community-acquired *Mycoplasma pneumoniae* pneumonia. Eur J Clin Microbiol Infect Dis 1995; 14:577-584.

40. Cimolai N. Particle agglutination. In: Cimolai N, ed. Serodiagnosis of the Infectious Diseases: *Mycoplasma pneumoniae.* Norwell, MA, USA:Kluwer Academic Publishers, 1999:57-63.

41. Holliman RE, Johnson J, Duffy K, New L. Discrepant toxoplasma latex agglutination test results. J Clin Pathol 1989; 42:200-203.

42. Taylor P. Evaluation of an indirect haemagglutination kit for the rapid serological diagnosis of *Mycoplasma pneumoniae* infections. J Clin Pathol 1979; 32:280-283.

43. Coombs RR, Easter G, Matejtschuk P, Wreghitt TG. Red-cell IgM antibody capture assay for the detection of *Mycoplasma pneumoniae*-specific IgM. Epidemiol Infect 1988; 100:101-109.

44. Nelson J, Ayoub EM, Wannamaker LW. Streptococcal antidesoxyribonuclease B: microtechnique determination. J Lab Clin Med 1968; 71:867-873.

45. Simhon A, Lifshitz A, Abed Y, Lasch EE, Schoub B, Morag A. How to predict the immune status of poliovirus vaccinees? A comparison of virus neutralization at a very low serum dilution versus ELISA in a cohort of infants. Int J Epidemiol 1990; 19:164-168.

46. Senterfit LB, Jensen KE. Antimetabolic antibodies to *Mycoplasma pneumoniae* measured by tetrazolium reduction inhibition. Proc Soc Exp Biol Med 1966; 122:786-790.

47. Palmer DF. Complement fixation test. In: Rose NR, Friedman H – eds. Manual of Clinical Immunology, 2nd Edn. Washington, DC:American Society for Microbiology, 1980:35-47.

48. Cimolai N. Complement fixation. In: Cimolai N – ed. Serodiagnosis of the Infectious Diseases: *Mycoplasma pneumoniae*. Norwell, MA:Kluwer Academic Publishers, 1999:39-51.

49. Cowley R, Fernandez F, Freemantle W, Rutter D. Enzyme immunoassay for Q fever: comparison with complement fixation and immunofluorescence tests and dot immunoblotting. J Clin Microbiol 1992; 30:2451-2455.

50. Teysseire N, Raoult D. Comparison of Western immunoblotting and microimmunofluorescence for diagnosis of Mediterranean spotted fever. J Clin Microbiol 1992; 30:455-460.

51. Wong YK, Sueur JM, Fall CH, Orfila J, Ward ME. The species specificity of the microimmunofluorescence antibody test and comparisons with a time resolved fluoroscopic immunoassay for measuring IgG antibodies against *Chlamydia pneumoniae*. J Clin Pathol 1999; 52:99-102.

52. Sander A, Posselt M, Oberle K, Bredt W. Seroprevalence of antibodies to *Bartonella henselae* in patients with cat scratch disease and in healthy controls: evaluation and comparison of two commercial serological tests. Clin Diagn Lab Immunol 1998; 5:486-490.

53. Thompson TA, Wilkinson HW. Evaluation of a solid-phase immunofluorescence assay for detection of antibodies to *Legionella pneumophila*. J Clin Microbiol 1982; 16:202-204.

54. Huisman JG, Winkel IN, Lelie PN, Tersmetter M, Goudsmit J, Miedema F. Detection of early anti-p24 HIV responses in EIA- and immunoblot-negative individuals: implications for confirmatory testing. Vox Sang 1987; 53:31-36.

55. Wreghitt TG, Morgan-Capner P. ELISA in the Clinical Microbiology Laboratory. London, UK:Public Health Laboratory Service, 1990.

56. Crowther JR. Enzyme Linked Immunosorbent Assay. Totowa, NJ, USA:Humana Press, 1995.

57. Deshpande SS. Enzyme Immunoassays: From Concept to Product Development. New York, NY:Chapman and Hall, 1996.

58. Vaira D, Holton J, Menegatti M, Ricci C, Landi F, Ali A, Gatta L, Acciardi C, Farinelli S, Crosatti M, Berardi S, Miglioli M. New immunological assays for the diagnosis of *Helicobacter pylori* infection. Gut 1999; 45:S23-S27.

59. Gibbons I, Hanlon TM, Skold CN, Russell ME, Ullman EF. Enzyme-enhancement immunoassay: a homogeneous assay for polyvalent ligands and antibodies. Clin Chem 1981; 27:1602-1608.

60. Bjerrum OJ, Heegaard NHH. CRC Handbook of Immunoblotting of Proteins. Boca Raton, LA, USA:CRC Press, 1988.

61. Baldo BA, Tovey ER. Protein Blotting: Methodology, Research, and Diagnostic Applications. New York, NY:Karger, 1989.

62. Dunbar BS. Protein Blotting: A Practical Approach. Oxford, UK:Oxford University Press, 1994.

63. Laemmle UK. Cleavage of structural proteins during the assembly of the head of bacteriophage T4. Nature 1970; 227:680-685.

64. Kowal K, Weinstein A. Western blot band intensity analysis: application to the diagnosis of Lyme arthritis. Arthritis Rheum 1994; 37:1206-1211.

65. Cooke WD, Bartenhagen NH. Seroreactivity to *Borrelia burgdorferi* antigens in the absence of Lyme disease. J Rheumatol 1994; 21:126-131.

66. Anonymous. Interpretive criteria used to report Western blot results for HIV-1 antibody testing – United States. MMWR 1991; 40:692-695.

67. Burkert S, Rossler D, Munchhoff P, Wilske B. Development of enzyme-linked immunosorbent assays using recombinant borrelial antigens for serodiagnosis of *Borrelia burgdorferi* infection. Med Microbiol Immunol 1996; 185:49-57.

68. Hammers-Berggren S, Lebech AM, Karlsson M, Andersson U, Hansen K, Stiernstedt G. Serological follow-up after treatment of *Borrelia* arthritis and acrodermatitis chronica atrophicans. Scand J Infect Dis 1994; 26:339-347.

69. Fenollar F, Raoult D. Diagnosis of rickettsial diseases using samples dried on blotting paper. Clin Diagn Lab Immunol 1999; 6:483-488.

70. Christie JM, McNulty CA, Shepherd NA, Valori RM. Is saliva serology useful for the diagnosis of *Helicobacter pylori*? Gut 1996; 39:27-30.

71. Reilly TG, Poxon V, Sanders DS, Elliott TS, Walt RP. Comparison of serum, salivary, and rapid whole cell blood diagnostic tests for *Helicobacter pylori* and their validation against endoscopy based tests. Gut 1997; 40:454-458.

72. Bakken LL, Callister SM, Wand PJ, Schell RF. Interlaboratory comparison of test results for detection of Lyme disease by 516 participants in the Wisconsin State Laboratory of Hygiene/College of Pathologists Proficiency Testing Program. J Clin Microbiol 1997; 35:537-543.

73. Guy EC, Robertson JN, Cimmino M, Gern L, Moosmann Y, Rijpkema SG, Sambri V, Stanek G. European interlaboratory comparison of Lyme borreliosis serology. Zentralbl Bakteriol 1998; 287:241-247.

74. Bakken LL, Case KL, Callister SM, Bourdeau NJ, Schell RF. Performance of 45 laboratories participating in a proficiency testing program for Lyme disease serology. JAMA 1992; 268:891-895.

75. Magnarelli LA. Quality of Lyme disease tests. JAMA 1989; 262:3464-3465.

76. Halpern NA, Brentjens T. Point of care testing informatics: the critical care-hospital interface. Crit Care Clin 1999; 15:577-591.

77. Kost GJ, Hague C. The current and future status of critical care testing and patient monitoring. Am J Clin Pathol 1995; 104:S2-S17.

78. Milgrom F. Development of rheumatoid factor research through 50 years. Scand J Rheumatol 1988; 75:S2-S12.

79. Chen PP, Fong S, Carson DA. Rheumatoid factor. Rheum Dis Clin North Am 1987; 13:545-568.

80. Kammer GM. T-lymphocyte activation. In: Rose NR, De Macario EC, Fahey JL, Friedman H, Penn GM, eds. Manual of Clinical Laboratory Immunology, 4th Ed. Washington, DC:American Society for Microbiology, 1992:207-212.

81. Fletcher MA, Klimas N, Morgan R, Gjerset G. Lymphocyte proliferation. In: Rose NR, De Macario EC, Fahey JL, Friedman H, Penn GM, eds. Manual of Clinical Laboratory Immunology, 4th Ed. Washington, DC:American Society for Microbiology, 1992:213-219.

5

Molecular Diagnostics: Present and Future

Alex van Belkum and Wil Goessens
Department of Medical Microbiology and Infectious Diseases, Erasmus University Medical Center Rotterdam, Rotterdam, The Netherlands

I. INTRODUCTION OF CONVENTIONAL MICROBIOLOGY

Since the era of Koch and Pasteur, medical microbiology has matured into a multi-disciplinary, increasingly high-tech science. Based on microscopic observations and culture of microorganisms, infectious diseases could initially be diagnosed and treated, whereas ultimately preventative strategies could be designed as well. Determination of the presence of microbial agents remains the key issue in medical microbiology. The optimal way of identifying pathogens in the laboratory has evolved from primitive strategies which were used by its pioneers into an ever-increasing number of elegant antigen-detecting assays. Recently, separate microbial antigens could be identified by means of immunological assays, and the use of poly- and mono- clonal antibodies allowed for the development of a large array of primarily protein-based diagnostic procedures and instruments. Laboratory expertise in biotyping, definition of susceptibility to antimicrobial agents, production of bacteriocins, protein and phage analyses, and the use of several chromatographic procedures was acquired and is available to many microbiology laboratories. During the past two decades, however, another major shift has occurred in the development of diagnostic tests: nucleic acids were discovered to be the identification targets of choice for the detection of a large number of different microbial pathogens. DNA, with its mere four building blocks and its relative chemical stability, proved to be an excellent template for a wide variety of diagnostic applications. Obviously, nucleic acids are the core substances that are found in all forms of microbial life. For this and other reasons to be discussed below, molecular diagnostics has grown in importance for the detection of many, if not most, agents of infectious diseases. The major principles, fields of application, today's trends, and future developments will be the topics for discussion herein.

II. NUCLEIC ACID STRUCTURE AND ITS RELEVANCE TO MICROBIAL IDENTIFICATION

Nucleic acid molecules are relatively simple with respect to the complexity of their building blocks: both RNA and DNA are constructed each with the use of only four nucleotide triphosphates. In the double helical conformation, not only is the chemical structure straightforward, but also the physical conformation is relatively homogeneous. This makes DNA an especially stable and homogeneous compound that is quite easy to purify. Moreover, the linear nature of the molecules facilitates in vitro reproduction by either enzymatic or chemical syntheses. As a useful laboratory consequence, DNA synthesis can be performed using fully automated, pre-programmable equipment. Although there are limitations in the size of the molecules that can be synthesized, fabrication of DNA and RNA oligonucleotides is common practice in the molecular microbiology laboratory. Naturally occurring nucleic acid molecules come in a variety of shapes and may specify a diverse array of functions, many of which go beyond the scope of this review. It is important to realize, however, that structures such as plasmids, transposons, insertion elements, gene cassettes and operons, bacteriophage genomes, repeat motifs and microbial chromosomes all have their own unique potential value for use in molecular diagnostics.

A. Conventional staining and labeling technologies

Most of the conventional stains for nucleic acids intercalate into the double helical molecule and induce fluorescence after transillumination by ultraviolet light. Ethidium bromide is likely the most often used compound in this respect. DNA and RNA can also be labeled by the incorporation of radioactive isotopes, either in the format of nucleotide precursors or by the action of phosphorylating agents. Direct chemical modification, e.g., with the help of alkylating agents, provides another labeling possibility. Alternatively, DNA can be labelled, chemically or enzymatically, with various small haptens, such as fluorescein, digoxigenin, and rhodamine among others. The availability of antibodies that are specific for these small molecules has enabled the development of a wide spectrum of immunological procedures for visualizing nucleic acids in general. Finally, DNA molecules can be equipped with complete enzymes, thus making enzymatic detection of the molecules straightforward and easy. The current technological possibilities allow for the multi-color painting of specific chromosomal regions, for instance. The application of a certain staining procedure is guided by many practical criteria. Sensitivity and specificity issues, technical expertise that is required, cost, nature of the diagnostic target, and the number of tests to be done on a daily basis are all important in the final decision making process. Many of the above issues have been recently reviewed in more detail (1).

B. Hybridization characteristics

The interaction between two complementary DNA or RNA molecules, which gives rise to the generation of a (partial) double helical segment as stabilized by specific hydrogen bridges between the base moieties in the pairing strands, is called hybridization. Hybridization truly is the fundamental core of modern DNA diagnostics. It determines both the sensitivity and the specificity of all nucleic acid detection and identification assays. The opposite of hybridization is denaturation or melting: an increase of the temperature or the presence of particular concentrations of denaturing agents (e.g., urea or formamide) both destroy the nucleic acid hybrid. Hybridization can be made highly specific by modulation of the experimental conditions. Depending on temperature, the presence of salts or divalent cations, or the concentration of stabilizing compounds, selection may be made for DNA molecules that are 100% complementary and thereby remain annealed. This is fundamental to molecular diagnostics: hybridization specificity determines whether or not the DNA of a given microorganism can be detected and efficiently identified. Molecules that are used to identify uncharacterized nucleic acids are called probes. It goes without saying that many different formats that employ probe hybridization-specificity at various levels have been developed for application in the medical microbiology laboratory.

C. Southern analysis

Southern hybridization is one of the founder technologies of modern recombinant DNA procedures and is an essential component to many of the nucleic acid diagnostics which are relevant to medical microbiology. The principle is relatively simple: DNA for analysis by probe technology is immobilized on a solid phase, e.g., nylon filter. A labeled probe is provided in aqueous solution and allowed to bind specifically to target DNA on the filter. After washing, bound probe can be detected on the basis of the label that is remnant on the solid phase. Color development, chemiluminescence, and fluorescence are most widely used for this latter detection step. Southern hybridization has many applications in diagnostic sciences. For bacteriology, PCR products are frequently identified on the basis of Southern hybridization with sequence-specific DNA oligonucleotide probes. This can be performed alternatively with immobilized oligonucleotides that can be probed essentially with the PCR product that is to be identified. By analogy to the Southern procedure, Northern blotting is used to characterize RNA molecules, whereas Western blotting focuses on protein analysis.

D. In situ hybridization

In situ hybridization involves the detection and identification of nucleic acid molecules in their "natural environment". While maintaining the physical integrity of the material in which a certain target molecule is located and where it needs to be detected, hybridization is performed. The ideal protocol combines processes which are focussed on the conservation of structure, while at the same time ensuring that the DNA which is embedded in the same material is adequately accessible to probe hybridization. The balance between the degree of fixation and the accessibility of the target molecules is critical. The conservation of morphological detail allows detection of microbial pathogens in the cellular context of the infected or colonized host. In situ hybridization has shown its value especially in pathology and virology, but is also of value for the detection of intracellular bacteria. Species identification by specific probes, even for closely related bacteria, is feasible with the currently available experimental protocols (2) (Figure 1). Particularly elegant are the studies of bacterial population diversity which make use of

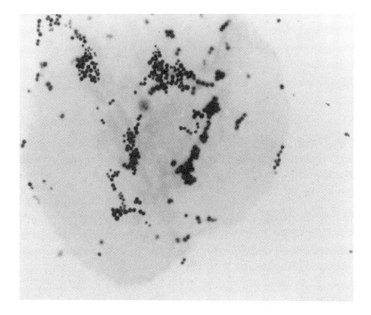

Figure 1   Detection and identification of *Staphylococcus aureus* adherence to a buccal epithelial cell with the use of in situ oligonucleotide hybridization. Cells were fixed in ethanol-containing medium and treated with proteinase K. A DIG-labeled oligonucleotide, precisely complementary to a region in the small subunit ribosomal gene, was used as a probe. Staining was performed with alkaline phosphatase-conjugated anti-DIG monoclonal antibody and a phosphatase sensitive dye.

group-specific 16S rRNA targeted oligonucleotide probes (3). These allow for detailed bacterial species assessment in ecological niches as complex as the human gut and enable assessments of normal biological variation in contrast to those that arise as a consequence of flora-modulating factors such as antibiotics or immuno-suppressive agents.

E. Nucleic acid amplification

Procedures that use small initial quantities of nucleic acid as template in order to synthesize large amounts of the same material, or a part thereof, are referred to as a nucleic acid amplification strategies. The procedures that have been developed over the past years are exquisitely sensitive and with extremely small amounts of template nucleic acid, sometimes in the order of a single or just a few molecules, massive amounts of end-product can be synthesized. Sensitivity is the primary advantage for amplification technologies. Despite this and other intentions, however, problems such as contamination (4), inhibition of the sensitive enzymes which are required (5), and critical dependence on sequence or length of the material to be amplified (6), provide experimental pitfalls that must often be surpassed in order for experimental procedures to translate into robust routine applications. It is requisite that nucleic acid amplification procedures be treated with respect in the clinical laboratory. Careful set-up of laboratory logistics is required to prevent, for instance, contamination problems, and the involvement of dedicated personnel remains a strict necessity, as is training of this personnel. The transition of "in house" protocols into routinely applied assays must also command special attention. The development of fully automated systems has been an industrial priority and several successes have been evident over the past few years. Our discussion herein includes only the most popular of DNA amplification methods. Two classes essentially can be distinguished. The first is broadly one that uses a probe which is specifically attached to a target molecule and which can be amplified post-hybridization (so-called probe amplification). The second class is a category of processes that practically amplify a specific part of the microbial target molecule itself (so-called target amplification).

1. Probe amplification

Two major classes of probe amplification assays have progressed to the point of advancement which is sufficient for introduction to the medical microbiology laboratory. Many alternative procedures have been described in recent literature but these are not yet relevant to daily practice. The two main techniques are highlighted as follows:

Qß replication
The RNA-dependent RNA polymerase that drives replication of the genome of coliform bacteriophage Qß is also capable of exponentially replicating smaller RNA molecules that essentially contain the structural requisites for nucleic acid duplication only (7). These variant RNA molecules have been stripped from any genetic coding potential and are the product of so-called minimizing evolution, a process that can be mimicked in vitro. The fact, that these small molecules can be exponentially replicated, forms the basis for the development of diagnostic tests. A technology which enables the modification of small templates has been developed, and it has been demonstrated that artificial templates, containing non-canonical probe sequences that are useful for the attachment to and identification of other nucleic acid molecules, could be prepared using recombinant RNA technology (8). This recombinant RNA technology was then used to generate RNA probes that could be detected by the replicase after specific hybridization. This technology allows for the synthesis of hundreds of nanograms from starting amounts that were in the order of just a tenth of a femtogram (corresponding to approximately 1000 molecules) (9). These correlate with an amplification factor of approximately 10^9, which can be obtained within 30 minutes of isothermic incubation at 37°C. The probes are termed amplifiable reporter molecules. It is interesting to note as well that this process allows for massive production of large recombinant RNA molecules. Entire mRNA molecules can be included in the constructs, and efficiently reproduced. Massively produced recombinant mRNA can be translated into protein in addition (10).

Several microbiologically relevant diagnostic assays have been developed (as detailed below and in Figure 2).

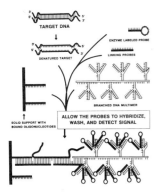

A. Signal amplification scheme including branched DNA molecules. Target nucleic acids are captured onto a solid support which contains sequence-specific capture oligonucleotides. Hybridization proceeds in the presence of labeled probes, linking probes for immobilization, and branched DNA multimers for signal amplification. Hybridization generates arborization: the many individual enzyme-labeled probes generate signals that are easy to detect.

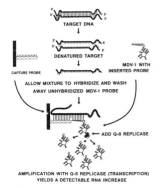

B. Q-beta replicase amplification indirectly amplifies a target molecule by the generation of huge amounts of transcript of a midivariant 1 (MDV-1) derived probe construct. In combination with a capture probing procedure for immobilization of the target and facilitation of post-hybridization washing steps, the RNA amplification yields an easily detectable increase in the probe concentration.

Figure 2 Principles of DNA probe amplification procedures. [Reprinted from Wolcott MJ. Advances in nucleic acid-based detection methods. Clin Microbiol Rev 1992; 5:370-386 and Wolcott MJ. DNA-based methods for the detection of foodborne pathogens. J Food Prot 1990; 54:387-401 with permission of the publishers. Copyright held by the International Association for Food Protection, Inc. (151,152)]

Branched DNA assays

The branched DNA approach capitalizes on the possibilities that organic chemistry has provided. Not only may linear DNA molecules can be synthesized, but also branched molecules can be prepared. These molecules harbor multiple 5'-ends which can all be equipped with detectable haptens or enzymes. Furthermore, branched DNA molecules harbor multiple sites for hybridization of additional labeled probe molecules. As such, a single probe can be coupled to the target molecule. Afterwards, multiple additional probes can be coupled to non-target regions of the primary probe and as such initiate the generation of complex reporter probe networks. Taking advantage of this effective arborization, large amounts of label can be incorporated at a single site of hybridization (see Figure 2). This type of assay can also be categorized as a signal amplification procedure.

2. Target amplification

Procedures that replicate (parts of) nucleic acid molecules in vitro are defined as target amplification techniques. These procedures have been developed over thepast two decades and were strongly stimulated by the development of novel synthetic DNA strategies and the availability of a diversity of pure DNA modifying enzymes, most importantly including the thermotolerant DNA polymerases. The most widely used procedures are described below:

Nucleic acid sequence based amplification (NASBA)

Nucleic acid sequence based amplification (NASBA) is a procedure that was initially intended for RNA amplification and as such found its initial application in the field of virology (11,12). Essentially, three enzymes work in concert and synthetic primers are equipped with extensions that are suited to function as second stage targets for some of these enzymes. Avian myeloblastosis virus (AMV) reverse transcriptase copies RNA target molecules into cDNA in a specific, primer-dependent manner. The 5' extensions on these primers initiate RNA re-synthesis by the RNA polymerase of bacteriophage T7. Finally, RNase H degrades the DNA in the resulting DNA:RNA hybrids. The reaction also allows for straightforward DNA amplification since the RT is a versatile enzyme which is also capable of initiating DNA synthesis from a DNA:DNA template. All reactions occur continuously at a single incubation temperature which facilitates a process where only a simple water bath is required and where no additional specialized laboratory equipment may be needed. Apart from the viral NASBA tests, assays were developed for bacterial species such as mycobacteria and the different *Campylobacter* spp. (13-15). NASBA can also be referred to as self-sustained sequence replication (3SR), and some variants of the basic principle have been described in the past (TAS and TMA are well-known acronyms).

Polymerase chain reaction (PCR)

The polymerase chain reaction (Figure 3) is a highly successful technology (truly deserving of the Nobel Prize) that has had and will continue to have a tremendous impact on all fields of molecular biology. The technique is based on DNA oligonucleotide primer-directed in vitro enzymatic DNA synthesis. Two primers hybridize in opposite polarities on the two strands of a target DNA molecule and they are subsequently extended by a DNA polymerase. This occurs in such a way that the extended primer becomes a hybridization target for both primers in a subsequent round of extension. The process allows for exponential duplication of the target region (16,17). The entire process, described for the first time in 1985, needs to be cycled: repetitions of nucleic acid denaturation, annealing, and enzymatic chain extension are required to drive the replication process into an exponential mode. This approach was enormously facilitated in 1988 upon the discovery, purification, and application of extremely stable DNA polymerases from thermophilic bacterial species, e.g., *Thermus aquaticus* and *Thermus thermophilus* (18). Currently, PCR finds its application in all aspects of molecular diagnostics. PCR is used for the diagnosis of genetic disorders, assessment of oncogene activation, detection of allelic sequence variation, forensic identification, facilitation of cloning, the detection of infectious agents and many other matters of diagnostic importance (see reference (19) and (20) for more detail).

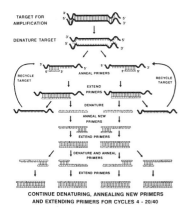

A. PCR. During the polymerase chain reaction (PCR), cycles of denaturation, annealing, and chain extension are alternated. After the denaturation, single-stranded DNA is hybridized to sequence-specific DNA oligonucleotides which direct enzymatic chain extension by a thermo-stable enzyme molecule. After the first cycle, the number of potential molecules is doubled (theoretically, assuming 100% enzyme efficacy); all molecules serve as template in a second round of ampification. After 20-40 cycles, large quantities of template have been copied.

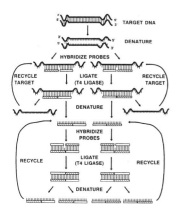

B. LCR. During ligase chain reaction (LCR), oligonucleotide probes are coupled through the action of a DNA ligase enzyme. Due to the precise positioning of the adjacent oligonucleotides, a covalent bond between the two can be generated. Once ligated, the coupled "oligos" serve as template in a second round of amplification. Per successful LCR test, four different oligonucleotides are used in a two-by-two fashion. This system can also be used in combination with a solid phase capturing system (see Figure 2).

Figure 3   Principles of DNA target amplification procedures. [Reprinted from Wolcott MJ. Advances in nucleic acid-based detection methods. Clin Microbiol Rev 1992; 5:370-386 and Wolcott MJ. DNA-based rapid methods for the detection of foodborne pathogens. J Food Prot 1990; 54:387-401 with permission of the publisher. Copyright held by the International Association for Food Protection, Inc. (151,152)]

PCR has been included in many diagnostic microbiology applications and several procedural simplifications have been evaluated over the past years. For example, necessity for pure DNA preparations has been circumvented and crude extracts alone may allow for accurate detection of bacterial pathogens. In combination with a reverse transcriptase enzyme, so-called RT PCR enables the detection of RNA molecules. Multiplex PCR involves the amplification of more thanone (sometimes up to eight!) different targets during a single incubation. When primary PCR products are re-amplified on the basis of additional primer sites that are available within the particular amplicon, the process is referred to as nested PCR. The sensitivity of this application has the potential to exceed that of single step PCR. Finally, PCR can be modified to amplify DNA from a large multitude of microorganisms in one single assay. By choosing primer sequences that are universally present, so-called broad-spectrum PCR is facilitated. Primers such as these are called consensus primers. In the best possible scenario, the consensus PCR products derived from different microorganisms can be identified to the species level on the basis of species specific-sequence elements that are bordered by the two consensus elements.

In situ PCR represents an interesting interplay between PCR and in situ hybridization. Although the pioneering studies of Nuovo et al. (21,22) were met with some skepticism initially, several authors managed to reproduce at least the technical part of the latter findings. Suspensions of single cells, however, appeared to be the best-appreciated target for in situ PCR (23). Whereas most of the developments occurred in the field of virology, some bacterial pathogens, especially the facultative or obligate intracellular ones, remain as interesting diagnostic targets for in situ PCR approaches. Future improvements of this technique will involve the increased suppression of DNA repair activity during the procedure. Since there is a level of background staining that must be eliminated before wide-spread application of this PCR assay can take place.

Ligase chain reaction (LCR)

The ligase chain reaction is a PCR look-alike in the sense that again synthetic oligonucleotides are used (four per test in this case) in combination with thermocycling and a thermostable enzyme. LCR uses DNA ligase to specifically and covalently couple the oligonucleotides that hybridize at immediately adjacent positions in the target (and in the target molecule only) (24). No DNA synthesis is involved generally as a single ligation step is sufficient (Figure 3). LCR is especially suited for the detection of single nucleotide polymorphism because the ligation is very sensitive to mispairing at the site of ligation. The specificity of the LCR can be further enhanced by the introduction of a single nucleotide gap between the primer sites. This gap needs to be completed with the help of the appropriate nucleotide triphosphate and a thermostable DNA polymerase before the ligation can occur. LCR can enable the accurate distinction between wild-types and mutants (25). It must be recognized that LCR is essentially as versatile as PCR and shares many of the advantages but also some of the disadvantages (26).

Rolling circle mechanism as an example of a novel technique

A wide variety of alternative DNA or RNA amplification procedures have been detailed over the past years. Many of these will never reach the diagnostic laboratory but some do seem to have interesting science. A very recently published and patented protocol involves rolling-circle amplification (27) (Figure 4). The primary hybridization involves a linear DNA probe which consists of two target complements, located at the 5' and 3' end of the probe respectively. After correct hybridization, the probe is circularized using free nucleotides and a ligase. Due to this ligation, the probe is secured to the template and after addition of an another primer and phage Φ29 DNA polymerase, the now circular probe can be replicated. Due to the fact that this specific Φ29 DNA polymerase is not inhibited when it encounters aregion of double-stranded DNA on its single stranded template, continuous replication of the circle into a long concatameric stretch of DNA ensures amplification of the probe. Essentially, this procedure combines elements of both probe and target amplification. The technique becomes exponential once additional primers are added. These should be complementary to another region of the circular probe and will allow for the synthesis of hyperbranched DNA complexes. It is perhaps futuristic to determine whether this procedure will finally be incorporated in diagnostic assays, but patent protection and

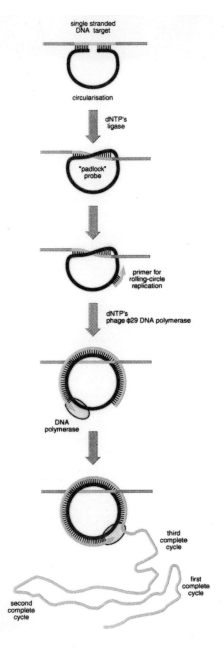

Figure 4   Rolling circle amplification. During rolling circle amplification, a primer is used of which the termini are complementary to a particular sequence in the target DNA. With DNA ligase, the hybrid probe is circularized which then locks the probe to the template. The now circular probe is copied into millions of identical molecules with primer-directed DNA synthesis with the use of a phage DNA polymerase. The sensitivity of the procdure can be enhanced by the addition of additional primers that can be used as recognition signals for the phage DNA polymerase. (Adapted from Bio Neuws, June 12, 1999; courtesy of Jos van den Broek.)

commercialization are likely to drive the applications for the rolling circle procedure in a positive direction.

F. Amplification-associated analysis technology

Quite often, amplification of a DNA molecule in itself is not conclusive with respect to the precise nature of the fragment. Although the size of the amplicon and perhaps even probe reactivity assist in establishing identity, additional studies may yet be required. Some of the most widely used analytical procedures in this regard are mentioned:

1.   Restriction fragment length polymorphism analysis

Amplified DNA molecules of similar size can be identified on the basis of the presence of different recognition and cutting sites for restriction enzymes. The differences in the primary structure can be visualized by incubation with a restriction enzyme and subsequent electrophoretic analysis. The restriction fragment length polymorphisms (RFLP) provide important and easily accessible genetic information (Figure 5). Where there are related amplicons, more than a single restriction enzyme can be used. Especially for broad spectrum PCR, RFLP analysis has been demonstrated to be very useful and as such, the structure analysis of large amplicons is enormously facilitated.

2.   Single strand conformation polymorphism analysis (SSCP)

PCR amplified material consists of double stranded DNA. Since the amplicons are generally quite short, the structure of the DNA is usually rather rigid. If the DNA is denatured and quenched on ice, renaturation into double stranded DNA again, a bimolecular reaction, is less frequent than the monomolecular

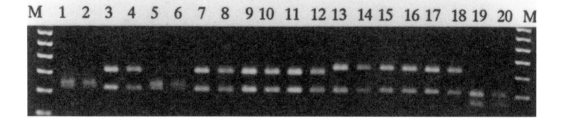

Figure 5   Restriction fragment length polymorphism in the staphylococcal protein A gene. Amplification of the so-called X-region of the protein A gene from *Staphylococcus aureus* yields a DNA fragment that ranges in size between approximately 320 and 600 basepairs in length. This variability is due to the presence of variable numbers of tandem repeats. When the full PCR product is cleaved with the restriction enzyme *RsaI*, the amplicon is cut in three. One of these three fragments contains the repeats, and after gel electrophoresis, length variation in this fragment can be visualized. The Figure shows data from 20 different isolates of *S. aureus*. Isolates were obtained as a series from persistent nasal carriers. Strains 1-2, 3-4, 5-6, 7-12, 13-18, and 19-20 were isolated from 6 different individuals thus showing stability of the repeat region within a single, person-specific strain.

restructuring reaction. Consequently, single stranded DNA molecules start to assume secondary and tertiary structures that heavily depend on their primary structure. Consequently, differences in primary structure may result in a different tertiary structure. These differences can be detected after resolution by native electrophoresis and there may appear sequence variants among the PCR products which are derived from diverse template sources. A particularly successful application involves 16S rDNA amplification, SSCP, and sensitive silver staining of subsequent acrylamide gels (28). This laid the foundation for a bacterial identification system that has been successfully validated for more than 100 strains of 40 different species that belong to 15 different genera. Because of the sensitive PCR step that precedes the SSCP analysis, the procedure requires only 30 bacterial cells for identification purposes.

3.   Denaturing gradient and temperature gradient gel electrophoresis

Nucleic acid melting is severely influenced by the presence of thermodynamically stable GC-rich domains in the sequence. In fact, melting behavior of the DNA double helix strongly depends on the stability of that region which is richest in G and C nucleotides. Thereafter, the addition of artificial regions which consist of GC only may determine the melting temperature to a great extent. If the GC stretch is sufficiently long, however, the overall melting behavior is mainly determined by the remainder of the double helix simply because the so-called GC clamp does not melt at all. Upon complete melting of the remainder molecule a fork-like construct arises that has limited electrophoretic mobility. This results in a characteristic stop of the fragment in a native acrylamide gel. The position of migration is highly characteristic for a given DNA sequence. Besides chemical gradients, temperature gradients can also be used for identification purposes. If the gradient is applied during electrophoresis, perpendicular to the direction of the run, melting curves can be generated. The curves arise because differences in the melting status of the DNA molecules result in differences in electrophoretic mobility.

4.   Allele specific oligonucleotide hybridization

Allele specific oligonucleotides (ASOs) are DNA probes that are used for mapping single nucleotide polymorphism (Figure 6). Sequence heterogeneity among amplified DNA molecules can be determined on the basis of differential reactivity towards the individual ASOs. Again, in case of broad spectrum PCRs, ASOs are very helpful in defining the nature of the amplified DNA. Clinically useful reverse hybridization assays have been developed. Some of these assays are capable of discriminating more that 20 species on the basis of the consensus amplification of a region of DNA as short as 65 basepairs (29).

5.   Molecular beacons and TaqMan technology

Molecular beacons are chemical compounds which structurally resemble simple oligonucleotides (Figure 7). Apart from the nucleotide probe sequences that are required for specific hybridization, however, some additional sequence elementswhich impose a tight secondary hairpin structure are included. During the hybridization procedure and in the native structure of the beacon, a fluorescence moiety is in the immediate vicinity of a quencher group: no fluorescence signal can be detected. Once the oligonucleotide specifically hybridizes, the secondary structure unfolds and the quencher moves away from the fluorescent group. With appropriate illumination, the fluorescent group can now emit light (Figure 1).

Molecular beacons can be used for the detection of hybridization in a very specific and target-concentration dependent manner (30). The first studies which described multiplex molecular beacon approaches that enable high-throughput diagnostics at high speed with correct identification and quantification of multiple virus species have already been published (31).

Another similar major application of this type is in the TaqMan strategy. On-line monitoring of PCR amplification introduces possibilities for the development of semi-quantitative estimation of the amount of template that was initially present. Based on the principle of fluorescence quenching as outlined for the molecular beacons, online generation of fluorescence during the process of PCR amplification has been made possible. Instead of removing the quencher from the fluorescent group by the

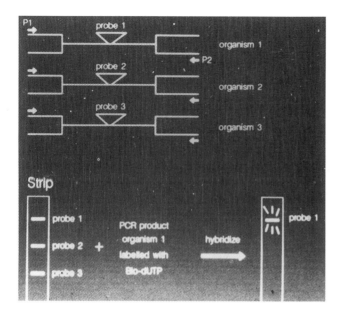

Figure 6 Allele specific oligonucleotides (probe 1 to 3) are capable of recognizing species-specific DNA sequences in PCR products that are generated from a diversity of different micro-organisms, but use consensus sequence motifs (primer P1 and P2). If the probes are immobilized onto a solid support and reverse-hybridized with a labeled PCR product, a simple staining procedure can assess the nature of the PCR product.

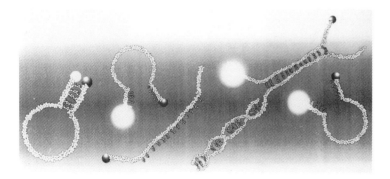

Figure 7 Schematic presentation of the principle of molecular beacon activity. In the native structure, primarily imposed by the base-pairing interaction between the 3' and 5' termini of the oligonucleotide component, the fluorescent and correct template, fluorescence is no longer inhibited by the quenching activity and light is emitted. The light can be detected with spectrophotometry. (Karl Gehrman, Stratagene, LaJolla, California, kindly provided this illustration.)

melting of secondary and tertiary structures of the probe, quencher groups are in close vicinity. If the molecular beacon attaches to the many of the TaqMan assays involve digestion of the probe whereby physical distance between quencher and fluorophore is generated as well.

Although TaqMan technology has its biggest impact in virology, several bacteriological assays have been described recently. In food microbiology, there is an obvious interest in the numbers of bacteria present in food stuffs, and tests for *Salmonella* and *E. coli* O157 in this regard have been published (32,33). In clinical microbiology, there may be an important future role for assays which quantify mycobacteria or tick-borne pathogens such as *Ehrlichia* spp. (34,35).

6. Conventional and automated DNA sequencing

DNA sequencing originates from the initial chemical approaches designed in the 1970s by Maxam and Gilbert. This strategy of base-specific chemical cleavage of end-labeled nucleic acid molecules was replaced by an enzymatic chain termination procedure employing dideoxynucleotidetriphosphates. Inclusion of these compounds during PCR resulted in amplification-based DNA sequencing procedures. Commercial PCR sequencing kits can currently be purchased from various biochemical companies. Over the past five years, the standard slab-gels have been replaced by high-throughput capillary systems thereby enabling longer sequence readings and higher speed determination (36). Continuing improvement, which includes the development of DNA chips for sequencing purposes (see below), has maintained priority especially in the light of the tremendous efforts which have been and continue to be dedicated to the elucidation of whole genome sequences for a variety of organisms, including the human genome project.

Sophisticated sequence analysis programs are essential for adequate data management. Generation of construct maps, sequence comparisons (also known as multiple sequence alignment), and graphic presentations have improved tremendously over the past years, and attractive commercially-available software packages can be purchased or downloaded freely from the Internet, e.g., (37). Finally, large and publicly accessible databases have been generated over the past decades. These form an extremely valuable resource for explorations into the nature of new and uncharacterized DNA sequences including whole genome sequences.

III. DEVELOPMENT, DIVERSITY, AND COMPARATIVE QUALITY ASSESSMENT OF DNA DIAGNOSTICS

Many of the tests that involve DNA diagnostics were initially developed in the molecular research laboratory. These home-brew tests were designed to function in a particular research setting and often generally performed quite well. Adaptation to the high-throughput, high-speed clinical microbiology setting however was clearly indicated. Novel tests are still being developed and these may be based on various molecular principles. Soon after laboratory implementation, the DNA-based assays initially had to compete with the gold standard tests of that time. Currently, studies which focus on the development of alternative tests and then the subsequent comparison of conventional and molecular tests or quality assessment are frequently undertaken.

A. Development of species-specific DNA probes through genetic fingerprinting

Nucleic acid diagnostics depend on the availability of specific DNA sequence motifs. For instance, these can be based on elaborate sequence determinations and comparisons as were performed for ribosomal genes. Alternatively, without prior primary structure knowledge, probes can also be derived from genetic DNA fingerprints. When these fingerprints are generated by random amplification of polymorphic DNA (RAPD), distinct banding patterns can be visualized after electrophoresis. If panels of strains belonging to different species are studied, one can frequently observed so-called consensus fragments. These represent DNA fragments that are amplified for all isolates that belong to a given species [for a literature review see (38)]. For several microbial species, including the medically relevant *Campylobacter* spp. (39), this approach turned out to be very successful. Since streptococci form a heterogeneous group of microbial species, additional means for species identification are often required (40). Genetic polymorphism among strains of the various streptococcal species has been documented on several occasions (41,42). It was demonstrated as well that RAPD could be used to segregate the different groups (43). Figure 8 shows such an analysis and at the same time indicates DNA fragments that could represent species-specific DNA markers. Table 1 shows that many of these putative probes met the specificity criteria: after Southern hybridization with immobilized genomic DNA from the same strains, 8 out of 12 probes displayed correct hybridization properties. Only in case of the apparently closely related species groups, e.g., *S. anginosus* and *S. constellatus*, e.g., *S. salivarius*, *S. thermophilus*, and *S. vestibularis*, cross-hybridization with DNA from streptococcal species other than the original one was observed. This procedure provides the diagnostic microbiologist with novel DNA probe candidates in a high-speed fashion. Recently, it was demonstrated that probes which are suited for the discrimination of strains within a single species can be generated as well (44).

B. Comparison and routine application of techniques

Introduction of a new technique in routine microbiology requires due care and must often occur in a stepwise progression. Several issues deserve investigation and it is critical that the sensitivity and specificity of the new test are at least as good as those of the procedure that is in active use. Furthermore, the complexity of the test should be minimized and its added value should be established. Costs are another important aspect. It has to be emphasized that at present molecular diagnostics are not (yet?) the alternative for all of the historically standard microbiological tests. In the fields of virulence assessment and the determination of antimicrobial resistance for instance, classical techniques are often preferable over the molecular alternatives.

An important area for application of molecular diagnostics in microbiology is that of the non-cultivable or yet unrecognized microbial pathogen. Identificationon the basis of DNA sequences only, without preceding clues that are based on the classical determinants such as Gram character or morphology, has become possible with the advent of molecular technology (45). Although not yet a genuine routine application, it is this kind of approach that paves the way for the development of molecular diagnostics for an even wider array of microorganisms. The basis of this approach lies with molecular phylogeny: targets for the identification of unknown pathogens are to be deduced from those sequence elements that are ubiquitous in other species. The ribosomal genes are a particularly well-known example, but others have been brought forward as well (46,47). The identification of the agents of bacillary angiomatosis (48) and Whipple's disease (49) are two of the main hallmarks of this approach (see Chapter 6). In the near future, additional examples of emerging infections due to previously unknown viruses, bacteria, fungi and parasites will be characterized by molecular approaches.

C. Multicentre studies

The number of intercentre studies of the efficacy of DNA amplification diagnostics in bacteriology is surprisingly small. A sentinel study was performed in the mid-1990s by Noordhoek et al. (50). These authors for the first time essentially demonstrated some of the pitfalls of molecular diagnostics. Seven laboratories each examined 200 different clinical and artificial samples by PCR; the specimens contained variable amounts of *Mycobacterium bovis* BCG. Although all centres employed their own DNA processing and analysis protocol, the PCR step itself was standardized. Percentages of false positives ranged between 3% and 77%, and in addition, the figures for sensitivity ranged widely among laboratories. Cross-contamination or loss of template DNA were frequent phenomena and the results of the publication could be summarized as: "….. implementation of an effective system for monitoring sensitivity and specificity is required before the PCR can be used reliably in the diagnosis of tuberculosis".

Table 1 Survey of Southern hybridization data for potential streptococcal species-specific DNA probes derived from RAPD fingerprints.

Species	Code	1	2	3	4	5	6	7	8	9	10	11	12
S. oralis	LMG14532	1	0	0	0	0	0	0	0	0	0	0	0
S. oralis	LMG14534	1	0	0	0	0	0	0	0	0	0	0	0
S. oralis	LMG14535	1	0	0	0	0	0	0	0	0	0	0	0
S. mitis	LMG14557	0	0	0	0	0	0	0	0	0	0	0	0
S. mitis	LMG14552	0	0	0	0	0	0	0	0	0	0	0	0
S. mitis	LMG14555	0	0	0	0	0	0	0	0	0	0	0	0
S. gordonii	LMG14518	0	0	0	0	0	0	0	0	0	0	0	0
S. gordonii	LMG14515	0	0	0	0	0	0	0	0	0	0	0	0
S. gordonii	LMG14516	0	0	0	0	0	0	0	0	0	0	0	0
S. sanguis	LMG14702	0	0	0	0	0	0	0	0	0	0	0	0
S. sanguis	LMG14656	0	0	0	0	0	0	0	0	0	0	0	0
S. sanguis	LMG14657	0	0	0	0	0	0	0	0	0	0	0	0
S. parasanguis	LMG14537	0	0	1	0	0	0	0	0	0	0	0	0
S. parasanguis	LMG14538	0	0	1	0	0	0	0	0	0	0	0	0
S. parasanguis	LMG14539	0	0	1	0	0	0	0	0	0	0	0	0
S. crista	LMG16320	0	0	0	1	0	0	0	0	0	0	0	0
S. crista	LMG14512	0	0	0	1	0	0	0	0	0	0	0	0
S. anginosus	LMG14502	0	0	0	0	1	0	0	0	0	0	0	0
S. anginosus	LMG14696	0	0	0	0	1	0	0	0	0	0	0	0
S. constellatus	LMG14507	0	0	0	0	2	0	0	0	0	0	0	0
S. constellatus	LMG14504	0	0	0	0	2	0	0	0	0	0	0	0
S. intermedius	LMG14510	0	0	0	0	0	0	0	0	0	0	0	0
S. intermedius	LMG14584	0	0	0	0	0	0	0	0	0	0	0	0
S. salivarius	LMG11489	0	0	0	0	0	1	2	0	0	0	0	0
S. salivarius	LMG13106	0	0	0	0	0	1	2	0	0	0	0	0
S. thermophilus	LMG13102	0	0	0	0	0	0	1	0	0	0	0	0
S. thermophilus	LMG13100	0	0	0	0	0	2	1	2	0	0	0	0
S. vestibularis	LMG13526	0	0	0	0	0	2	2	1	0	0	0	0
S. vestibularis	LMG14647	0	0	0	0	0	2	2	1	0	0	0	0
S. mutans	LMG14558	0	0	0	0	0	0	0	0	0	0	0	0
S. mutans	LMG14560	0	0	0	0	0	0	0	0	0	0	0	0
S. rattus	LMG14650	0	0	0	0	0	0	0	0	1	0	0	0
S. rattus	LMG14559	0	0	0	0	0	0	0	0	1	0	0	0
S. cricetus	LMG14508	0	0	0	0	0	0	0	0	0	0	0	0
S. bovis	LMG8518	0	0	0	0	0	0	0	0	0	1	0	0
S. bovis	LMG15062	0	0	0	0	0	0	0	0	0	1	0	0
S. equinus	LMG14891	0	0	0	0	0	0	0	0	0	0	0	0
S. equinus	LMG15115	0	0	0	0	0	0	0	0	0	0	0	0
S. alactolyticus	LMG14808	0	0	0	0	0	0	0	0	0	0	1	0
S. alactolyticus	LMG14588	0	0	0	0	0	0	0	0	0	0	1	0
S. dysgalactiae	LMG15885	0	0	0	0	0	0	0	0	0	0	0	0
S. equi	LMG15886	0	0	0	0	0	0	0	0	0	0	0	0
S. equi	LMG15887	0	0	0	0	0	0	0	0	0	0	0	0
S. canis	LMG15890	0	0	0	0	0	0	0	0	0	0	0	1
S. canis	LMG15893	0	0	0	0	0	0	0	0	0	0	0	1

Note: 0 = no hybridization signal; 1 = strong hybridization signal; 2 = weak hybridization signal. The numbers 1-12 correspond with the numbers indicated in Figure 2.

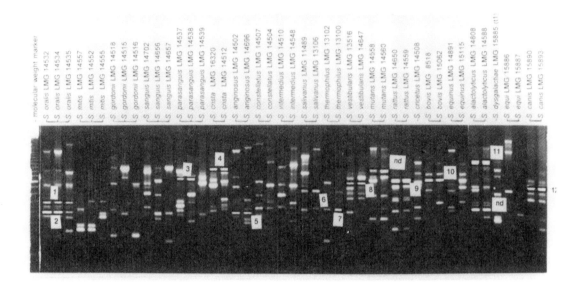

Figure 8   Random amplification of polymorphic DNA (RAPD) analysis for various strains belonging to the genus *Streptococcus*. Above the lanes depicting the DNA fingerprints the species' names are mentioned. The boxed and numbered DNA fragments represent species-specific RAPD consensus moieties. Table 1 describes the hybridization characteristics of these strains, when the fragments interact with whole DNA preparations isolated from the same collection of strains. The lane on the right shows a concatameric array of multiples of 100 base-pair length markers. (Dr. Peter Vandamme, Laboratorium voor Microbiologie, Gent, Belgium, is acknowledged for providing the streptococcal strains that were used to generate Figure 2 and Table 1.)

Much has improved over the years and commercial systems with their inherent standardization have become available. Recent work has provided clear improvements. A multicentre study of the molecular detection of *Chlamydia trachomatis* has documented inter-institutional reproducibility (51). Nevertheless, extreme care still has to be taken with respect to contamination problems. Multicentre studies of molecular diagnosis for *Aspergillus fumigatus* infection have revealed that relatively high frequencies of false-positive testing may occasionally occur (52).

D.   Quality control measures

Like traditional methodology, molecular diagnostics needs to be validated, both qualitatively and quantitatively. Not only do the quality of laboratory procedures need to be monitored but the efficacy of the laboratory worker and the reagents must be guaranteed as well. It is generally accepted by now that the different activities which are involved in DNA amplification technology must be physically separated. The use of an anti-contamination procedure such as the dUTP-UNG system is strongly recommended. Validation of positive results by an alternative assay may be important just as assay inhibition should be monitored with the help of internal control templates. Controls should be scattered along the various steps in the entire procedure. Quality control trials have identified several issues that are of prime importance in achieving a high standard of performance. Technical personnel need to be well-trained and dedicated. Positive control samples should be near the detection limit of the procedure. Tests should be performed on a regular basis and in face of problems, specialized laboratories or companies from which kits were purchased need to be readily available. In the end, interlaboratory standardization and kits were purchased need to be readily available. In the end, interlaboratory standardization and data communication networks may be extremely helpful in establishing high quality molecular diagnostics.

IV. CURRENT STATE OF AFFAIRS OF MOLECULAR DIAGNOSTICS FOR DISTINCT MICROBIAL SPECIES

Commercially available DNA probe tests were among the first to reach the diagnostic market. The GenProbe products represent a successful line of first generation hybridization-based diagnostics. Nearly 20 different assays are available for species confirmation after cultivation of pathogens as diverse as *Neisseria gonorrhoeae* or *Histoplasma capsulatum*. The second generation GenProbe tests could be directly applied to extracts of clinical material, thus enabling the in situ detection of microbial pathogens. Finally, the direct tests were translated in semi-amplified assays: with the help of reverse transcriptase, additional copies of the target nucleic acid were generated. The current set of GenProbe Amplified assays represent the outcome of many years of developmental investigations. Many other assays, including the genuine DNA amplification procedures, have followed the same route from the initial stages of laboratory development into a, sometimes even commercially available, diagnostic kit. The establishment of clinical assays through the developmental routes as described above are reviewed for a limited number of clinically relevant microorganisms:

A. *Chlamydia trachomatis*

C. trachomatis is an obligate intracellular bacterial species and a common sexually transmitted pathogen (see Chapter 27). It can cause a wide variety of clinical illnesses and it is thought to be one of the causal agents of pelvic inflammatory disease (PID), a phenomenon that may lead to female infertility. The gold standard diagnostic for *C. trachomatis* infection has historically been bacterial culture. Clinical samples were inoculated onto mammalian cell-lines and the presence of the pathogen was revealed by its intracellular growth in the cultured target cells. The use of conventional or immunological staining in order to enhance the sensitivity of testing was common practice as well. Any form of bulk diagnostics, however, especially for a high through-put Sexually Transmitted Diseases clinic for instance, can be cumbersome and expensive to perform. This is precisely the reason why the diagnostics for *C. trachomatis* were among the first ones to be translated into molecular assays.

The first DNA amplification assays for *C. trachomatis* were described in the late 1980s and did not only focus on the detection of genital infections. Also, clinically overt ocular infections were an immediate target (53). The latter early study did not actually employ the PCR as it currently stands, but rather described the use of a densely labeled DNA probe as generated with the help of PCR. Secondly, it was demonstrated that PCR could be used to increase the sensitivity of culture by post-cultivation DNA amplification of cell-lysates (54). A sensitivity of detection for a single chlamydial chromosome in a background of DNA from 10^5 eukaryotic cells was documented. Soon after, the first genuine diagnostic PCR studies were published [e.g., (55)]. These initial studies demonstrated that PCR was sensitive and specific, and indeed proved to be superior when compared to the conventional techniques. PCR was further adapted to suit clinical demands. The possibility of performing the assay on voided urine samples was considered to be a major step ahead in the sense that it allows the patient to provide a clinical sample easily. Not all early studies were equally successful, but these preliminary attempts paved the way for future success (56), even for the clinical diagnostics relating to other species of *Chlamydia* (57). Another interesting advance was the combination of diagnostics (detecting a pathogen) and bacterial genotyping (identification of a strain below the species level). When the major outer membrane protein (MOMP) gene was selected as a target for example, the use of post-amplification DNA digestion with a restriction enzyme allowed for the discrimination of MOMP subtypes on the basis of the observed RFLPs (58). Assays that define genetic heterogeneity can potentially be used for the in depth analysis of microbial spread; evolutionary change may be associated with antigenic diversity and hence changes in immunogenicity. Finally, the amplification component of these assays is not the only important area for improvement. It has been demonstrated that the assay's sensitivity could be improved by the addition of steps for both the sample processing and DNA purification protocol. The capture of bacterial cells with immobilized C1q, a complement factor with affinity for bacterial surface components, clearly enhanced versatility (59), whereas variation in the amount of clinical material that is assessed had an obvious effect as well (60).

After the first wave of useful PCR tests, the ligase chain reaction was also implemented in direct diagnostic tests for *C. trachomatis* (61,62). LCR development has followed the progressive success of PCR in the sense that LCR was also considered a clear improvement when compared to the old gold standards of culture and staining. The Qß replicase amplified hybridization assay, a probe amplification system, has also found its way to the clinical laboratory (63). Currently, many high quality molecular tests are available to the clinical microbiology laboratory, and some may find it difficult to come to a consensus on either the right choice of procedure or instrument. This is especially true given the complete and automated diagnostic systems that have become commercially available. For this reason, many comparative studies have been undertaken. Quite often it is difficult to evaluate assays in that no absolute "non-sense" tests exist. When the Qß test is compared to PCR, the tests are comparable and they detect equal numbers of culture-positive or culture-negative samples. A major difference however is that it appears that PCR is more affected by the activity of inhibitors, whereas the Qß system seems to be relatively unscathed by this problem (64). A recent study from our laboratory revealed that for three commercially available test systems, the specificity exceeded 99%. When the GenProbe transcription-mediated amplification assay (AMP CT) was compared to the Roche COBAS AMPLICOR (PCR) and the Abbott LCx assay (LCR) for *C. trachomatis,* somewhat clearer differences in the sensitivities were calculated (65). The sensitivities were 84%, 93% and 85%, respectively, and for all three assays, the sensitivity dropped comparably when tests were performed on urine samples. Applicability of one test versus another may differ from laboratory to laboratory on the basis of differences in sample trafficking, numbers of tests per annum, qualifications of personnel or otherwise. In many laboratories, however, the current gold standard technique for the detection of *C. trachomatis* involves DNA amplification techniques.

B. *Mycobacterium tuberculosis*

Tuberculosis is still one of the major infectious diseases of our day; millions of people are infected every year and a significant proportion of these individuals finally succumb to their infection (see Chapter 14). Recently, another threat has arisen: some *M. tuberculosis* strains have become multi-drug resistant thus rendering the infections difficult to treat. Obviously, once DNA diagnostics became generally available, there was an immediate impetus for an improvement of the lengthy and complicated gold standard culture techniques. Despite investments in increased speed and automation of culture procedures, even the briefest of protocols are still considered prolonged in comparison to theoretical gains from molecular techniques. Again, similar molecular developments were initiated as described previously for *C. trachomatis*. Various test systems have been marketed, including amplified direct tests [GenProbe amplified, see (66)], a Q-beta replicase-amplified assay (67) and an AMPLICOR system for detection of *M. tuberculosis* in clinical samples (68). All systems held promise for exquisite sensitivity and specificity, but although the specificities are generally acceptable, sensitivity was somewhat disappointing in many trials. In some of the earlier studies, frequent inhibition was documented for the AMPLICOR test, for instance. In a preliminary trial, 15 out of 23 samples, known to contain *M. tuberculosis* cells, were inhibited in the PCR thus giving rise to falsely negative results (68). For the DNA diagnostics of a pathogen such as *M. tuberculosis*, the preferred commercial test should perform optimally with two categories of specimens: 1) culture positive but microscopy negative, and 2) samples from patients that are suffering from clinically evident tuberculosis but that remain culture negative should preferably yield a positive result (69). What has been presented for *M. tuberculosis* in a very convincing manner is that DNA technology can be efficiently used for the identification of the diverse nontuberculous species. Recent sequencing studies on heatshock protein genes have identified additional targets which are suited for the expansion of this technology (70). It should be acknowledged that the typing of strains of *M. tuberculosis* below the species level has been internationally standardized to a large extent (71,72). Efforts on attaining a similar level of inter-laboratory agreement on the (molecular) diagnosis of this important pathogen should receive high priority.

C. *Candida albicans*

Candida albicans is one of the major fungal pathogens for humans. Especially in the context of the immunocompromised host, infection with this yeast may have devastating consequences. For this reason, a wide array of different diagnostic techniques has become available over the past few decades (73). Among these procedures, the molecular analyses are continuously gaining in importance and impact. For the clinical microbiology laboratory, those studies that aim towards identification of fungal species that are cultivated on synthetic media are currently most important. What initially started with Southern hybridization-based identification tests with for instance actin probes (74), gradually developed into PCR RFLP (75) or PCR-probe hybridization assays (76,77). Other assays focussed on the amplification of species specific size-variable regions of homologous genetic loci such as the chitin synthetase or cytochrome P-450 lanosterol-α-demethylase genes for discrimination of medically important yeasts (78,79). Recently, fluorescent *in situ* hybridization with the use of rRNA specific oligonucleotides has been described as a diagnostic approach for invasive *Candida* infection (80). These probes have displayed excellent performance, and yeast cells could be identified in many different tissues of systemically infected mice. Moreover, the assay could be performed directly on a filter, enabling FISH-mediated detection of three *C. albicans* cells in 0.5 ml of blood.

Clinically more relevant are the studies which describe the use of molecular diagnostics for detecting candidemia in animal models or humans. Again, various PCR tests were designed and validated (81-83). In our laboratory, we designed a PCR which focussed on the specific amplification of the *C. albicans* 18S rRNA gene which is subsequently confirmed with a DNA oligonucleotide probe (84) (Figure 9). Using the immunocompromised mouse as a model for infection, we were able to demonstrate that between 10 and 15 yeast cells could be detected in 100 μl of blood. PCR appeared to be more sensitive than blood culture and the detection signal increased with progression of the infection. Mere gastrointestinal colonization did not lead to a positive PCR for peripheral blood samples (85). Furthermore, it was demonstrated that PCR results correlated well with the therapeutic efficacy of antifungal regimens (86). Detailed clinical studies in humans are now eagerly being awaited, and in that respect, it may prove to be that serum will be the specimen of choice for the PCR-mediated diagnosis of candidemia (87). Preliminary studies reveal that for patients with hematological malignancies, PCR may have a high negative predictive value (>97%) and the use of restriction analysis may facilitate concerted *Candida* spp. identification without a culture step (88). The molecular diagnosis of fungi in general poses some problems to the laboratory; in many cases the fungal cells are ubiquitous, either as colonizers on healthy people or as spores in the air. This implies that contamination of clinical material is a realistic concern (89), but also that the introduction of competitive DNA should be avoided. In this respect, it was stunning to notice that the source of this type of contaminating DNA frequently is the enzyme preparation to be used for the lysis of fungal cells to begin with (90).

D. Some selected species

For several other microbial species, molecular tests have been developed. In many cases the developments followed the same route as described for *C. trachomatis*. In the case of *Neisseria gonorrhoeae*, for instance, probes were initially developed to identify the species and some of its characteristics (91,92). These were rapidly followed by non-amplification in vitro diagnostics for clinical materials (93), and soon after different classes of amplification tests were designed (94,95). Other developments were initiated specifically on the basis of an overt clinical necessity. In the case of meningococcal

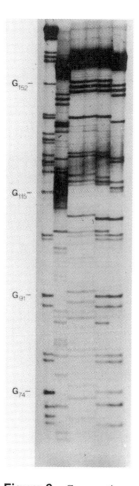

Figure 9   Comparative sequence analysis of the V9 region of the small subunit ribosomal RNA gene for several *Candida* species. From left to right the experimental data for determination of the position of the guanosine residues is shown for *C. glabrata*, *C. krusei*, *C. parapsilosis*, *C. pseudotropicalis*, *C. tropicalis*, and *C. stellatoidea*. Based on the heterogeneity observed, it was shown that species-specific DNA probes which differentiate the medically relevant *Candida* species could be developed.

meningitis, for example, rapid turnaround and high sensitivity are of utmost importance when a patient is likely to be infected. Pioneering studies have shown that PCR can be a useful asset even though the rapidity of results could not yet be delivered as desired in the early nineties when cerebrospinal fluid was used as the clinical material (96,97). Even more recently, however, with the advent of DNA testing- for meningococci in peripheral blood, the immediate usefulness of "bed-side" PCR has not yet been made completely clear and accessible for meningococcal meningitis (98).

It goes without saying that for the so-called emerging infectious agents, PCR diagnostics are developed instantaneously after the first nucleic acid sequences have become available. For *Helicobacter pylori*, the major cause for ulceration and cancerous transformation of the human stomach, many assays were recently designed. The use of molecular assay has been applied to studies of fecal shedding (99,100). PCR also enables the detection of virulence factors in *H. pylori*; the *vac* and *cag* genes may be important examples of factors that are associated with the propensity to cause disease (101). In other microbial species, e.g., *E. coli*, many other examples of PCRs that enable the detection of virulence factors such as toxins have been described in great detail (102). How the current molecular procedures can be applied in order to assess antimicrobial resistance has recently been reviewed and requires no additional in depth discussion in this chapter (103). Assays which aim at the detection of individual resistance traits however are designed, clinically validated, and published at an exponential rate (104).

V. CURRENT TECHNOLOGICAL DEVELOPMENTS

In microbiological research, enormous advances in our knowledge of species diversity and molecular aspects in the infectious disease process have surfaced in the past years. As technology has improved, several spectacular achievements have been instrumental in continuously adapting our way of thinking about microbial life. Instruments for automated DNA extraction, pipetting, and processing have been developed and are in a constant trend towards optimization. Efforts which aim at the improvement of molecular diagnostics rely on increasing the speed, miniaturization of equipment, and increasing the number of specimens that can be handled at once. Some of the major recent and current developments will be reviewed below.

A. Whole genome sequencing

In 1995, the first full-genome sequence for a living organism was presented (105). With shotgun cloning of genomic DNA fragments and massive random sequencing and computer-assisted assembly of these data into a single chromosome, a complete catalogue of genes for *Haemophilus influenzae* could be presented. A little later, the entire chromosome for one of the smallest bacteria, *Mycoplasma genitalium*, was elucidated as well (106) (Figure 10). What followed were examples of an archaeon (107), *Escherichia coli* K-12 (108), and many other bacterial species of which several additional examples are

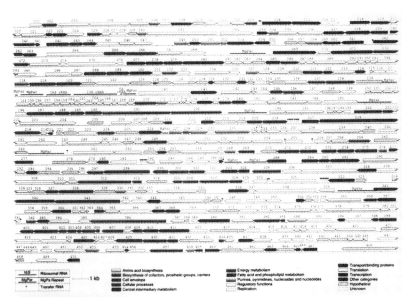

Figure 10 Gene map of the *Mycoplasma genitalium* genome. All predicted coding regions in the 580,070 nucleotide long genome ae shown, and arrowheads indicate the direction of transcription. Each line in the Figure represents 24,000 base-pairs. Gene categories are shade-coded (colour-coded in the original), and several operons and the positions of tRNA genes are labeled. [Reprinted with permission from Fraser et al. (106) The minimal gene complement of *Mycoplasma genitalium*. Science 1995; 270:397-403; copyright 1995, American Association for the Advancement of Science]

still underway (109). For *Helicobacter pylori*, two isolates have been sequenced in full thus allowing for an accurate comparison of genetic diversity within a species (110,111). Much was learned during the early stages of prokaryote sequencing and many of the developments have been extrapolated to eukaryote projects as well. *Saccharomyces cerevisiae* was the first eukaryotic microorganism for which all of its approximately 6000 genes were categorized (89). The first multicellular organism, *Caenorhabditis elegans*, has also gone through the various stages of whole genome sequencing (112). The current database which contains the whole genome sequence is expanding rapidly and within a few years, at least one but probably more whole genome sequences will be available for all of the medically important species of microorganisms including parasites and fungi.

It is obvious that future microbial diagnostics will be heavily influenced by spin-offs from these genome studies. Many additional diagnostic targets are being uncovered at an amazing rate whereas a great diversity of additional virulence genes are being defined on the basis of primary DNA structure. Sequence data will be instrumental in tracing evolutionary networks (113). The novel data will assist in the development of sequence-based diagnostic schemes that enable concerted detection of microorganisms, microbial resistance, and virulence factors from individual clinical specimens even those that contain mixtures of different pathogens. A tremendous amount of work is yet required to enable the translation of voluminous sequencing data into relevant biological models. Many of the genes so identified are still without function, and mutation analysis for instance has to precede definite conclusions on functional and, consequently, potentially pathogenic features. Obviously, genetic information needs to be associated with well-defined phenotypic traits. Furthermore, the availability of whole genome sequences may also shed light on the biology of the host: as a derivative, novel host-specific markers for ongoing or latent infection may be yet recognized (114,115).

Whole genome technology has already had a major impact on economies and this will further increase once the medical microbiology diagnostic market is targeted. In 1996, more than 500,000 patent applications involving DNA sequences entered the patent offices, and many pharmaceutical industries have invested large amounts of money in microbial genomics. The availability of whole genome sequences provides new means for the identification of suitable targets for new generations of antimicrobial agents as well (116). Microbial genes can be analyzed for their ubiquity and lack of analogous genes (and gene products!) in the human genome. The protein products of those genes that are represented in all microbes but absent from the human sequence database, may prove to be promising candidates for the targeting of potential therapeutics in the end. The use of proteomics, the methodology used to identify and characterize complex mixtures of microbial proteins, may also turn out to be very helpful in this respect. The generation of gene knock-outs, in vitro expression of the proteins involved, and assay development for high-throughput screening of libraries with putative antimicrobial compounds can be performed in a limited time-span due to the availability of the massive and detailed DNA sequence information. Bioinformatics is becoming an extremely important discipline, just as robotics, nanotechnology, high-throughput screening, and combinatorial chemistry (117).

B. DNA chip technology

DNA chips are small physical entities, generally made out of glass or silica, and may contain large arrays of immobilized nucleic acids. These can be oligonucleotides, genome fragments, and cDNA molecules. Proteins and peptides can also be successfully immobilized onto solid templates (148,149). Essentially, DNA chips are miniature blots that allow for hybridization studies which employ (extremely) large numbers of individual probes. Many different procedures have been described for the manufacturing of DNA chips. Using a variety of spotting methods, probes can be printed onto various matrices. Several intelligent combinatory chemistry approaches have been developed. One of these very elegant procedures for the manufacturing of DNA chips employs a process called photolithographic oligonucleotide synthesis (118). A solid phase (the chip) is completely covered with a chemical compound that can be photo-activated into a reactive form. The activation can be limited to a small part of the chip thus allowing for chemical coupling of one of the four bases which in itself is photo-protected again. In four chemical steps, the entire chip surface is covered with a first layer of nucleotide derivatives. In a similar fashion, a second layer can be applied. In this way, if the synthesis domains are chosen to be perpendicularly oriented, all sixteen possible dinucleotides are being synthesized. In conclusion, in 4n chemical steps, 4^n different oligonucleotides are synthesized on the DNA chip surface, n equaling the length of the oligonucleotides. The capacity of the current technology is to synthesize several hundred thousands of oligonucleotides on a square centimeter of chip surface (Figure 11). Lengths of up to 20 bases per oligonucleotide can be achieved. These chips can be used to access large quantities of genetic information in such a way that the entire human mitochondrial genome can be sequenced by hybridization (SBH) (119). SBH surveys sequences on the basis of 4 different probes per individual nucleotide position in a given DNA molecule. Whether the probe with the A, C, T or G base in the variable position hybridizes most effectively will determine the base present in the particular site of the molecule under surveillance. The SBH principle is important in microbiology because it allows for the detailed, high speed sequence confirmation of microbial variants that differ in natural antibiotic resistance for example (120). Furthermore, the DNA chips can be used for the monitoring of gene expression in minute detail (121,122).

With the advent of successful production techniques for the DNA chips as mentioned above, broad application of the technology is within scope of the average scientist and massive comparative sequencing projects can, in the future, be rooted in chip technology (123). A multitude of different products is in development, many of which are based on the technology as outlined above. Affymetrix, the founding industry of the photolithographic procedure, has strategic alliances with many pharmaceutical companies for the development of different sorts of molecular diagnostics. In the field of infectious diseases, Affymetrix has teamed with Glaxo-Wellcome for the development of HIV diagnostics and with Hoffman-La Roche in regards to the development of gene-expression screening chips for *H. influenzae* and *S. pneumoniae*. Of prime importance for bacteriology and retrovirology is the interaction with the French biotechnology firm bioMerieux. Within this consortium, diagnostic kits for bacterial identification and antibiotic resistance determination are being developed. Microbial typing is another industry priority. Also, other companies are developing infectious disease diagnostics in a concerted action. Nanogen Inc (San Diego, CA, USA) collaborates with Becton Dickinson Co (Franklin Lakes, NJ, USA) in order to develop infectious disease diagnostics on the basis of Nanogen's proprietary electrochips. Prefabricated 20-mer oligonucleotides are captured via electro-active spots on silicon wafers. With polarization of the spots, hybridization speed and efficacy are greatly enhanced thus resulting in high-speed, high-specificity signaling.

The first examples of the diagnostic use for DNA chip technology have already begun to reach the scientific literature. In diagnostic microbiology, DNA chips which contain immobilized oligonucleotide probes for nitrifying soil bacteria have appeared very useful for assessing the nature of composite bacterial communities (124). The first genuine DNA chip technology application suited forimplementation in the clinical laboratory was presented recently. A micro-array which is suited for the re-sequencing of ribosomal genes and of the *rpo*B gene which encodes a β subunit of the RNA polymerase has been developed. It was demonstrated that antibiotic resistance could be predicted on the basis of the *rpo*B sequence whereas the nature of the mycobacterial species could be pinpointed on the basis of the ribosomal sequences (125) (Figure 11). Similar developments are ongoing in the field of diagnostic virology, of course. Especially for the detection of HIV and its resistant derivatives, major advances have already been presented (126).

VI. FUTURE DEVELOPMENTS

It has to be recognized that not all workers in the field are equally optimistic with respect to the future of DNA diagnostics in microbiology. Some remain circumspect (127,128), whereas others cannot hide their enthusiasm and remain highly optimistic (129,130). As usual, the truth will probably be some-

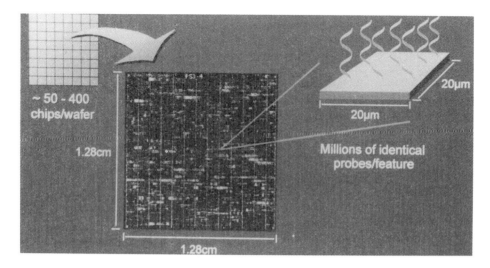

A.   DNA chips can be generated with the help of photolithographic procedures (see text). This enables the manu-
      facturing of between 50 and 400 chips from a single wafer in a co-ordinated manner. The individual chip
      elements are 1.28 X 1.28 cm. and contain 20 X 20 mcm. surfaces with separate oligonucleotide probes. Cur-
      rent technology allows for the synthesis of approximately 400,000 probes per square cm., but numbers of
      over a million are anticipated once technology improves further.

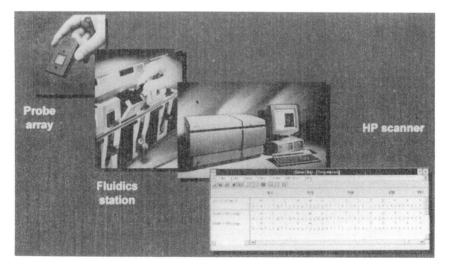

B.   Automated chip processing. The arrays are manufactured in a plastic case. These cases can be inserted di-
      rectly into the fluidics hybridization station, where probe binding and subsequent washing occurs. Signal can
      be read out with the use of Hewlett-Packard confocal microscope scanners. Data need to be processed by
      specific and dedicated software. (Figures were kindly provided by Dr. Patrice Allibert, bioMerieux, Lyon,
      France.)

Figure 11 DNA chip technology.

where in the middle. As a matter of fact, the current technology clearly has its drawback: sometimes false-positive and false-negative results are frequent, whereas costs and versatility are generally considered to be sub-optimal at present. Efforts which focus on the elimination of any such problems are intense, and novel developments may in the end solve many of the current controversies. Some activities that are worth mentioning are highlighted as follows:

A. Multispecific analyses from single specimens

Many PCR assays target consensus sequence elements in order to expand the diagnostic coverage. Targeting the conserved regions of ribosomal genes for instance allows for the amplification of DNA for all of the bacterial species present in a given (clinical) material. By characterization of the amplified material, insight can be obtained in regards to the diversity of bacteria that inhabit certain sites. For several clinical circumstances, this approach has proven to be the method of choice for unraveling complex populations of microorganisms (131-133). A pertinent example is the recent development of a panel of PCR tests for the diagnosis of bacterial infections of the upper respiratory tract (134). In addition, a set of broad range PCR primers which target the 16S rRNA gene have been recently described (135) and may be applied for accurate species classification of more than 60 clinically relevant microorganisms. Environmental model studies have also shown that quantitative approaches are feasible (136). This may in the end enable the precise determination of different species at a given locus, and also the precise ratio in which the species share the same ecological niche.

B. Sample processing facilities

The microbiology laboratory that performs molecular diagnostics should be equipped appropriately. Technical expertise and (robotic) machinery should be available for all steps in the diagnostic protocol. When clinical materials are received, storage should be fast and efficient. In processing the samples for the ultimate goal, the quantitative isolation of high quality DNA preparations could start with an enrichment procedure. Several simple separation techniques have been used in the past which vary from sedimentation and filtration to lyophilization or dialysis. A novel procedure makes use of (immuno)magnetic separation: small paramagnetic particles can be covered with monoclonal antibodies that are specific for a given bacterial species. After capturing these bacteria in a specific manner from a complex matrix, the particles can be physically separated by magnetic force. In the most optimal instances, this process completely purifies the bacteria to be used as templates in future molecular diagnostics (137). Obviously, after this type of pre-purification, accurate DNA purification protocols are yet required. An example of a frequently applied procedure, generally rendering templates well suited for molecular analyses, is the guanidinium-celite affinity protocol, for which a recent up-dated protocol is available (138). The near future will see the introduction of various novel robots for sample processing, hands-on time and problems with contamination will be minimized in this way.

C. Microbiology and the clinical chemistry way of working

The introduction of automated PCR equipment into the diagnostic microbiology laboratory is a continuous activity. Comparisons between "old-fashioned" methods and the COBAS AMPLICOR approach, for instance, have revealed that true automation, which is cost saving and labour reducing, is feasible in clinical bacteriology as well as virology (139). Further automation and miniaturization will take place in the molecular diagnostic laboratory. At this moment, PCR equipment equaling the size of a 3x3 cm. glass plate has been developed (140). By drilling holes in an etched glass plate and applying regions of constant temperature (denaturation, annealing, and extension temperature) across the holes, a sample containing the DNA to be amplified can be pushed in a constant flow over the different temperature regions. The equipment accommodates for very small volumes (up to 10 μl.) and run times can in the optimal circumstances be limited to less than one minute. The sensitivity of these amplifications is still rather limited: testing is essentially confined to nested PCR assays. Another interesting development is the fabrication of portable equipment. Using TaqMan technology high-speed assays, completion in less than 10 minutes and detection limits of five bacteria can be achieved. Ten reaction modules, which can be activated by a laptop computer, are housed in a single protective casing (141-143). In the end, integrated systems for processing of clinical samples, nucleic acid extraction, amplification and analysis of the amplified material will become commercially available. Systems that integrate PCR and microchip technology in a small format have been already described and their successful use in the detection of various nucleic acid target molecules has been demonstrated (144).

D. Integration of microbial diagnostics and host susceptibility testing

The vulnerability of a human individual towards infection is not only determined by the pathogenicity of the disease-causing organism, but also by predisposing factors that are encoded in the host genome. Relevant genetic polymorphism among humans that influences the opportunities for a given pathogen to infect has been recently presented in the scientific literature. A distinct example is provided by promoter polymorphism in the human plasminogen activator inhibitor gene. It was shown that individuals with an increased expression of this gene, associated with a certain promoter sequence, were at a greater risk for the development of serious meningococcal infection (145). By affecting the coagulation cascade, disease may progress into a more severe form. It was also shown that variability of promoters that regulate the expression of immuno-regulatory genes, like the one encoding interleukin-10, is associated with susceptibility to Epstein-Barr virus infection (150). Moreover, susceptibility towards the disease-causing potential of superantigens, as produced by several species of mainly gram-positive bacteria, was shown to be dependent on major histocompatibility complex (MHC) gene variability (146). Even dynamic processes such as persistent or short term colonization of a host by a bacterial strain are determined partly by host factors (147).

The examples discussed concisely herein illustrate that, in the future, the microbiology laboratory may also need to consider the host for assessing those characteristics that may predispose to an infectious disease. One can imagine that a person at risk for the development of serious meningococcal infections, based on his or her genetic make-up, should receive even more attention than a person shown to be of another genotype. In the end, combined analysis of both microbial and host parameters may not only lead us to improved insight in infectious diseases, but may even guide the way to more adequate treatment modalities.

REFERENCES

1. Kricka LJ. Nucleic acid detection technologies – labels, strategies and formats. Clin Chem 1999; 45:453-458.
2. Krimmer V, Merkert H, Von Eiff C, Frosch M, Eulert J, Lohr JF, Hacker J, Ziebuhr W. Detection of *Staphylococcus aureus* and *Staphylococcus epidermidis* in clinical samples by 16S rRNA directed in situ hybridization. J Clin Microbiol 1999; 37:2667-2673.
3. Franks AH, Harmsen HJM, Raangs GC, Jansen GJ, Schut F, Welling GW. Variations of bacterial populations in human feces measured by fluorescent in situ hybridization with group-specific 16S rRNA targeted oligonucleotide probes. Appl Environ Microbiol 1998; 64:3336-3345.
4. Rys PN, Persing DH. Preventing false positives: quantitative evaluation of three protocols for inactivation of polymerase chain reaction amplification products. J Clin Microbiol 1993; 31:2356-2360.
5. Wilson IG. Inhibition and facilitation of nucleic acid amplification. Appl Environ Microbiol 1997; 63:3741-3751.
6. Espy MJ, Smith TF, Persing DH. Dependence of polymerase chain reaction product inactivation on amplicon length and sequence composition. J Clin Microbiol 1993; 31:2361-2365.
7. Kacian DL, Mills DR, Kramer FR, Spiegelman S. A replicating RNA molecule suitable for detailed analysis of extracellular evolution and replication. Proc Natl Acad Sci USA 1972; 69:3038-3042.
8. Miele EA, Mills DR, Kramer FR. Autocatalytic replication of a recombinant RNA. J Mol Biol 1983; 171:281-295.

9. Lizardi PM, Guerra CE, Lomeli H, Tussie-Luna I, Kramer FR. Exponential amplification of recombinant-RNA hybridisation probes. Biotechnol 1988; 6:1197-1202.

10. Wu Y, Zhang DY, Kramer FR. Amplifiable messenger RNA. Proc Natl Acad Sci USA 1992; 89:11769-11773.

11. Compton J. Nucleic acid sequence based amplification. Nature 1991; 350:91-92.

12. Kievits T, Van Gemen B, Van Strijp D, Schukkink R, Dircks M, Adriaanse H, Malek L, Sooknanan R, Lens P. NASBA isothermal enzymatic in vitro nucleic acid amplification optimized for the diagnosis of HIV-1 infection. J Virol Methods 1991; 35:273-286.

13. Van der Vliet GME, Schukkink RAF, Van Gemen B, Schepers P, Klatser PR. Nucleic acid sequence based amplification (NASBA) for the identification of mycobacteria. J Gen Microbiol 1993; 139:2423-2429.

14. Uyttendaele M, Schukkink R, Van Gemen B, Debevere J. Identification of *Campylobacter jejuni*, *Campylobacter coli* and *Campylobacter lari* by the nucleic acid amplification system NASBA. J Appl Bacteriol 1994; 77:694-701.

15. Uyttendaele M, Schukkink R, Van Gemen B, Debevere J. Detection of *Campylobacter jejuni* added to foods by using a combined selective enrichment and nucleic acid sequence-based amplification (NASBA). Appl Environ Microbiol 1995; 61:1341-1347.

16. Mullis KB, Faloona FA. Specific synthesis of DNA in vitro via a polymerase catalysed chain reaction. Meth Enzymol 1987; 155:335-350.

17. Saiki RK, Scharf S, Faloona FA, Mullis KB, Horn GT, Erlich HA, Arnheim N. Enzymatic amplification of ß-globin genomic sequences and restriction site analysis for diagnosis of sickle cell anemia. Science 1985; 230:1350-1354.

18. Saiki RK, Gelfand DH, Stoffel S, Scharf SJ, Higuchi R, Horn GT, Mullis KB, Erlich HA. Primer-directed enzymatic amplification of DNA with a thermostable DNA polymerase. Science 1988; 239:487-491.

19. Erlich HA, Gelfand DH, Saiki RK. Specific DNA amplification. Nature 1988, 331:461-462.

20. Tan YW, Procop GW, Persing DH. Molecular diagnosis of infectious diseases. Clin Chem 1997; 43:2021-2038.

21. Nuovo GJ, Gallery F, MacConnell P, Becker J, Bloch W. An improved technique for the in situ detection of DNA after polymerase chain reaction amplification. Am J Path 1991; 139:1239-1244.

22. Nuovo GJ, Forde A, MacConnell P, Fahrenwald R. In situ detection of PCR amplified HIV-1 nucleic acids and tumor necrosis factor cDNA in cervical tissues. Am J Path 1993; 143:40-48.

23. Patterson BK, Till M, Otto P, Goolsby C, Furtado MR, McBride LJ, Wolinsky SM. Detection of HIV-1 DNA and messenger RNA in individual cells by PCR-driven in situ hybridization and flow cytometry. Science 1993; 260:976-979.

24. Barany F. Genetic disease detection and DNA amplification using cloned thermostable ligase. Proc Natl Acad Sci USA 1991; 88:189-193.

25. Barany F. Single nucleotide genetic disease detection using cloned thermostable ligase. In: Ahmad F - ed. Advances in Gene Technology: The Molecular Biology of Human Genetic Disease. Oxford, UK: Oxford University Press, 1991.

26. Barany F. The ligase chain reaction in a PCR world. PCR Meth Appl 1991; 5:5-16.

27. Lizardi P, Huang X, Zhu Z, Bray-Ward P, Thomas DC, Ward DC. Mutation detection and single molecule counting using isothermal rolling circle amplification. Nature Genet 1998; 19:225-232.

28. Widjojoatmodjo MN, Fluit AC, Verhoef J. Rapid identification of bacteria by PCR-single-strand-conformation polymorphism. J Clin Microbiol 1994; 32:3002-3007.

29. Kleter B, Van Doorn LJ, Schrauwen L, Molijn A, Sastrowijoto S, Ter Schegget J, Lindeman J, Ter Harmsel B, Burger M, Quint W. Development and clinical evaluation of a highly sensitive PCR reverse hybridization line probe assay for detection and identification of anogenital human papillomavirus. J Clin Microbiol 1999; 37:2508-2517.

30. Konstrikis LG, Tyagi S, Mhlanga MM, Ho DD, Kramer FR. Spectral genotyping of human alleles. Science 1998; 279:1228-1229.

31. Vet JAM, Majithia AR, Marras SAE, Tyagi S, Dube S, Poiesz BJ, Kramer FR. Multiplex detection of four pathogenic retroviruses using molecular beacons. Proc Natl Acad Sci USA 1999; 96:6394-6399.

32. Kimura B, Kawasaki S, Fujii T, Itoh T, Flood SJ. Evaluation of TaqMan PCR assay for detecting *Salmonella* in raw meat and shrimp. J Food Prot 1999; 62:329-335.

33. Oberst RD, Hays MP, Bohra LK, Phebus RK, Yamashiro CT, Paszko-Kolva C, Flood SJ, Sargeant JM, Gillespie JR. PCR-based DNA amplification and presumptive detection of *Escherichia coli* O157:H7 with an internal fluorogenic probe and the 5' nuclease (TaqMan) assay. Appl Environ Microbiol 1998; 64:3389-3396.

34. Desjardin LE, Chen Y, Perkins MD, Teixeira L, Cave MD, Eisenach KD. Comparison of the ABI 7700 system (TaqMan) and competitive PCR for quantification of IS6110 DNA in sputum during treatment of tuberculosis. J Clin Microbiol 1998; 36:1964-1968.

35. Pusterla N, Huder JB, Leutenegger CM, Braun U, Madigan JE, Lutz H. Quantitative real-time PCR for detection of members of the *Ehrlichia phagocytophila* genogroup in host animals and *Ixodes ricinus* ticks. J Clin Microbiol 1999; 37:1329-1331.

36. Mathies RA, Huang XC. Capillary array electrophoresis: an approach to high-speed, high throughput DNA sequencing. Nature 1992; 359:167-169.

37. Rajagopal I. All-in-one sequence analysis. Science 1999; 283:652-653.

38. Giesendorf BAJ, Quint WGV, Vandamme P, Van Belkum A. Generation of DNA probes for detection of microorganisms by polymerase chain reaction fingerprinting. Zbl Bakt 1996; 28:417-430.

39. Giesendorf BAJ, Van Belkum A, Koeken A, Stegeman H, Henkens MHC, Van der Plas J, Goossens H, Niesters HGM, Quint WGV. Development of species specific DNA probes for *Campylobacter jejuni, Campylobacter lari* and *Campylobacter coli* by polymerase chain reaction fingerprinting. J Clin Microbiol 1996;31:1541-1546.

40. Coykendall AL. Classification and identification of viridans streptococci. Clin Microbiol Rev 1989;2:315-328.

41. Hookey JV, Saunders NA, Clewly JP, Efstratiou A, George RC. Virulence regulon polymorphism in group A streptococci revealed by long PCR and implications for epidemiological and evolutionary studies. J Med Microbiol 1996; 45:285-293.

42. Chatellier S, Huet H, Kenzi S, Rosenau A, Geslin P, Quentin R. Genetic diversity of rRNA operons of unrelated *Streptococcus agalactiae* strains isolated from cerebrospinal fluid of neonates suffering from meningitis. J Clin Microbiol 1996; 34:2741-2747.

43. Bert F, Picard B, Branger C, Lambert-Zechovsky N. Analysis of genetic relationships among strains of groups A, C and G streptococci by random amplified polymorphic DNA analysis. J Med Microbiol 1996; 45:278-284

44. Van Leeuwen W, Sijmons M, Sluijs J, Verbrugh H, Van Belkum A. On the nature and use of randomly amplified DNA from *Staphylococcus aureus*. J Clin Microbiol 1996; 34:2770-2777.

45. Fredricks DN, Relman DA. Sequence-based identification of microbial pathogens: a reconsideration of Koch's postulates. Clin Microbiol Rev 1996; 9:18-33.

46. Wilson KH. Detection of culture-resistant bacterial pathogens by amplification and sequencing of ribosomal DNA. Clin Infect Dis 1994; 18:958-962.

47. Relman DA, Falkow S. Identification of uncultured microorganisms: expanding the spectrum of characterized microbial pathogens. Infect Agents Dis 1992; 1:245-253.

48. Relman DA, Loutit JS, Schmidt TM, Falkow S, Tompkins LS. The agent of bacillary angiomatosis: an approach to the identification of uncultured pathogens. New Engl JMed 1990; 323:1573-1580.

49. Relman DA, Schmidt TM, McDermott RP, Falkow S. Identification of the uncultured bacillus of Whipple's disease. New Engl J. Med 1992; 327:293-301.

50. Noordhoek GT, Kolk AHJ, Bjune G, Catty D, Dale JW, Fine PEM, Godfrey-Faussett P, Cho SN, Shinnick T, Svenson SB, Wilson S, Van Embden JDA. Sensitivity and specificity of PCR for detection of *Mycobacterium tuberculosis*: a blind comparison among seven laboratories. J Clin Microbiol 1994; 32:277-284.

51. Chernesky MA, Lee H, Schachter J, Burczak JD, Stamm WE, McCormack WM, Quinn TC. Diagnosis of *Chlamydia trachomatis* urethral infection in symptomatic and asymptomatic men by testing first-void urine in a ligase chain reaction assay. J Infect Dis 1994; 170:1308-1311.

52. Loeffler J, Hebart H, Bialek R, Hagmeyer L, Schmidt D, Serey FP, Hartmann M Eucker J, Einsele H. Contaminations occurring in fungal PCR assays. J Clin Microbiol 1999; 37:1200-1202.

53. Dean D, Pant CR, O'Hanley P. Improved sensitivity of a modified polymerase chain reaction amplified DNA probe in comparison with serial tissue culture passage for detection of *Chlamydia trachomatis* in conjunctival specimens from Nepal. Diagn Microbiol Infect Dis 1989; 12:133-17.

54. Pollard DR, Tyler SD, Ng CW, Rozee KR. A polymerase chain reaction (PCR) protocol for the specific detection of *Chlamydia* spp. Mol Cell Probes 1989; 3:383-389.

55. Griffais R, Thibon M. Detection of *Chlamydia trachomatis* by the polymerase chain reaction. Res Microbiol 1989; 140:139-141.

56. Sellors JW, Mahony JB, Jang D, Lickard L, Goldsmith CH, Gafni A, Chernesky MA. Comparison of cervical, urethral and urine specimens for the detection of *Chlamydia trachomatis* in women. J Infect Dis 1991; 164:205-208.

57. Gaydos CA, Roblin PM, Hammerschlag MR, Hyman CL, Eiden JJ, Schachter J, Quinn TC. Diagnostic utility of PCR-enzyme immunoassay, culture and serology for detection of *Chlamydia pneumoniae* in symptomatic and asymptomatic patients. J Clin Microbiol 1994; 32:903-905.

58. Lar J, Walboomers JMM, Roosendaal R, Van Doornum GJJ, MacLaren DM, Meijer CJLM, Van den Brule AJC. Direct detection and genotyping of *Chlamydia trachomatis* in cervical scrapes by using polymerase chain reaction and restriction fragment length polymorphism analysis. J Clin Microbiol 1993; 31:1060-1065.

59. Herbrink P, Van den Munckhof HAM, Niesters HGM, Goessens WHF, Stolz E, Quint WGV. Solid-phase C1q-directed bacterial capture followed by PCR for detection of *Chlamydia trachomatis* in clinical specimens. J Clin Microbiol 1995; 33:283-286.

60. Goessens WHF, Kluytmans JAJW, Den Toom N, Van Rijsoort-Vos TH, Niesters HGM, Stolz E, Verbrugh HA, Quint WGV. Influence of volume of sample processed on detection of *Chlamydia trachomatis* in urogenital samples by PCR. J Clin Microbiol 1995; 33:251-253.

61. Dille BJ, Butzen CC, Birkenmeyer LG. Amplification of *Chlamydia trachomatis* DNA by ligase chain reaction. J Clin Microbiol 1993;31:729-731.

62. Chernesky MA, Lee H, Schachter J, Burczak JD, Stamm WE, McCormack WM, Quinn TC. Diagnosis of *Chlamydia trachomatis* urethral infection in symptomatic and asymptomatic men by testing first-void urine in a ligase chain reaction assay. J Infect Dis 1994; 170:1308-1311.

63. Shah JS, Liu J, Smith J, Popoff S, Radcliffe G, O'Brien WJ, Serpe G, Olive DM, King W. Novel, ultrasensitive Q-beta replicase-amplified hybridization assay for detection of *Chlamydia trachomatis*. J Clin Microbiol 1994; 32:2718-2724.

64. Liu QA, O'Brien W, Radcliffe G, Buxton D, Popoff S, King W, Vera-Garcia M, Lu L, Shah J, Klinger J, Olive DM. Comparison of characteristics of Qß replicase-amplified assay with competitive PCR assay for *Chlamydia trachomatis*. J Clin Microbiol 1995; 33:58-63.

65. Goessens WHF, Mouton JW, Van der Meijden WI, Deelen S, Van Rijsoort-Vos TH, Lemmens-den Toom N, Verbrugh HA, Verkooyen RP. Comparison of three commercially available amplification assays, AMP CT, LCx and COBAS AMPLICOR for detection of *Chlamydia trachomatis* in first-void urine. J Clin Microbiol 1997; 35:2628-2633.

66. Miller N, Hernandez SG, Cleary TJ. Evaluation of Gen-Probe amplified mycobacterium tuberculosis direct test and PCR for direct detection of *Mycobacterium tuberculosis* in clinical specimens. J Clin Microbiol 1994; 32:393-397.

67. Shah JS, Liu J, Buxton D, Stone B, Nietupski R, Olive DM, King W, Klinger JD. Detection of *Mycobacterium tuberculosis* directly from spiked human sputum by Q-beta replicase-amplified assay. J Clin Microbiol 1995; 33:322-328.

68. Schirm J, Oostendorp, Mulder JG. Comparison of Amplicor, in-house PCR and conventional culture for detection of *Mycobacterium tuberculosis* in clinical samples. J Clin Microbiol 1995; 33:3221-3224.

69. Dawson DJ. Comparison of nucleic acid amplification tests for tuberculosis. J Clin Microbiol 1999; 37:1236.

70. Ringuet H, Akoua-Koffi C, Honore S, Varnerot A, Vincent V, Berche B, Gaillard JL, Pierr-Audiger C. *hsp65* Sequencing for identification of rapidly growing mycobacteria. J Clin Microbiol 1999; 37:852-857.

71. De Beenhouwer H, Liang Z, De Rijk P, Van Eekeren, Portaels F. Detection and identification of mycobacteria by DNA amplification and oligonucleotide-specific capture plate hybridisation. J Clin Microbiol 1995; 33:2994-2998.

72. Kamerbeek J, Schouls L, Kolk A, Van Agterveld M, Van Soolingen D, Kuijper S, Bunschoten A, Molhuizen H, Shaw R, Goyal M, Van Embden J. Simultaneous detection and strain differentiation of *Mycobacterium tuberculosis* for diagnosis and epidemiology. J Clin Microbiol 1997; 35:907-914.

73. Reiss E, Morrison CJ. Nonculture methods for diagnosis of disseminated candidiasis. Clin Microbiol Rev 1993; 6:311-323.

74. Mason MM, Lasker BA, Riggsby WS. Molecular probe for identification of medically important *Candida* species and *Torulopsis glabrata*. J Clin Microbiol 1987; 25:563-566.

75. Maiwald M, Kappe R, Sonntag HG. Rapid presumptive identification of medically relevant yeasts to the species level by polymerase chain reaction and restriction enzyme analysis. J Med Vet Mycol 1994; 32:115-122.

76. Miyakawa Y, Mabuchi T, Kagaya K, Fukazawa Y. Isolation and characterisation of a species-specific DNA fragment for detection of *Candida albicans* by polymerase chain reaction. J Clin Microbiol 1992; 30:894-900.

77. Elie CM, Lott TJ, Reiss E, Morrison CJ. Rapid identification of *Candida* species with species specific DNA probes. J Clin Microbiol 1998; 36:3260-3265.

78. Jordan JA. PCR identification of four medically important *Candida* species by using a single primer pair. J Clin Microbiol 1994; 32:2962-2967.

79. Burgener-Kairuz P, Zuber JP, Jaunin P, Buchman TG, Bille J, Rossier M. Rapid detection and identification of *Candida albicans* and *Torulopsis (Candida) glabrata* in clinical specimens by species-specific nested PCR amplification of a cytochrome P-450 lanosterol-α-demethylase (L1A1) gene fragment. J Clin Microbiol 1994; 32:1902-1907.

80. Lischewski A, Kretschmar M, Hof H, Amann R, Hacker J, Morschhäuser. Detection and identification of *Candida* species in experimentally infected tissue and human blood by rRNA-specific fluorescent in situ hybridisation. J Clin Microbiol 1997; 35:2943-2948.

81. Kan VL. Polymerase chain reaction for the diagnosis of candidemia. J Infect Dis 1993; 168:779-783.

82. Rand KH, Houck H, Wolff M. Detection of candidemia by polymerase chain reaction. Mol Cell Probes 1994; 8:215-222.

83. Fujita SI, Lasker BA, Lott TJ, Reiss E, Morrison CJ. Microtitration plate enzyme immunoassay to detect PCR amplified DNA from *Candida* species in blood. J Clin Microbiol 1995; 33:962-967.

84. Van Belkum A, Niesters HGM, Goessens WHF, Meis JFGM, Quint WGV. Rapid polymerase chain reaction based identification assays for *Candida* species. J Clin Microbiol 1993; 31:904-910.

85. Van Deventer AJM, Goessens WHF, Van Belkum A, Van Vliet HJA, Van Etten EWM, Verbrugh HA. Improved detection of *Candida albicans* by PCR in blood of neutropenic mice with systemic candidiasis. J Clin Microbiol 1995; 33:625-628.

86. Van Deventer AJM, Goessens WHF, Van Belkum A, Van Etten EWM, Van Vliet HJA, Verbrugh HA. PCR monitoring of response to liposomal amphotericin B treatment of systemic candidiasis in neutropenic mice. J Clin Microbiol 1996; 34:25-28.

87. Bougnoux ME, Dupont C, Mateo J, Saulnier P, Faivre V, Payen D, Nicolas-Chanoine MH. Serum is more suitable than whole blood for diagnosis of systemic candidiasis by nested PCR. J Clin Microbiol 1999; 37:925-930.

88. Morace G, Pagano L, Snaguinetti M, Posteraro B, Mele L, Equitani F, D'Amore F, Leone G, Fadda G. PCR restriction enzyme analysis for detection of *Candida* DNA in blood from febrile patients with hematological malignancies. J Clin Microbiol 1999; 37:1871-1875.

89. Goffeau A, Barrell BG, Bussey H, Davis RW, Dujon B, Feldman H, Galibert F, Hoheisel JD, Jacq C, Johnston M, Louis EJ, Mewes HW, Murakami Y, Philippsen P, Tettelin H, Oliver SG. Life with 6000 genes. Science 1996; 274:546-567.

90. Rimek D, Garg AP, Haas WH, Kappe R. Identification of contaminating fungal DNA sequences in zymolyase. J Clin Microbiol 1999; 37:830-831.

91. Lewis JS, Kranig-Brown D, Trainor DA. DNA probe confirmatory test for *Neisseria gonorrhoeae*. J Clin Microbiol 1990; 28:2349-2350.

92. Sanchez-Pescador R, Stempien MS, Urdea MS. Rapid chemiluminescent nucleic acid assays for detection of TEM-1 β-lactamase-mediated penicillin resistance in *Neisseria gonorhoeae* and other bacteria. J Clin Microbiol 1988; 26:1934-1938.

93. Panke ES, Yang LI, Leist PA, Magevney P, Fry RJ, Lee RF. Comparison of Gen-Probe test and culture for the detection of *Neisseria gonorrhoeae* in endocervical specimens. J Clin Microbiol 1991; 29:883-888.

94. Limberger RJ, Biega R, Evancoe A, McCarthy L, Slivienski L, Kirkwood M. Evaluation of culture and the Gen-Probe PACE 2 assay for detection of *Neisseria gonorrhoeae* and *Chlamydia trachomatis* in endocervical specimens transported to a state health laboratory. J Clin Microbiol 1992; 30:1162-1166.

95. Stary A, Ching SF, Teodorowicz L, Lee H. Comparison of ligase chain reaction and culture for detection of *Neisseria gonorrhoeae* in genital and extragenital specimens. J Clin Microbiol 1997; 35:239-242.

96. Kristiansen BE, Ask E, Jenkins A, Fermer C, Radstrøm P, Skold O. Rapid diagnosis of meningococcal meningitis by polymerase chain reaction. Lancet 1991; 337:1568-1569.

97. Ni H, Knight AI, Cartwright K, Palmer WH, McFadden J. Polymerase chain reaction for diagnosis of meningococcal meningitis. Lancet 1992; 340:1432-1434.

98. Newcombe J, Cartwright K, Palmer WH, McFadden J. PCR of peripheral blood for diagnosis of meningococcal disease. J Clin Microbiol 1996; 34:1637-1640.

99. Van Zwet AA, Thijs JC, Kooistra-Smid AMD, Schirm J, Snijder JAM. Use of PCR with feces for detection of *Helicobacter pylori* infections in patients. J Clin Microbiol 1994; 32:1346-1348.

100. Enroth H, Engstrand L. Immunomagnetic separation and PCR for detection of *Helicobacter pylori* in water and stool specimens. J Clin Microbiol 1995; 33:2162-2165.

101. Van Doorn LJ, Figueiredo C, Sanna R, Plaisier A, Schneeberger P, De Boer W, Quint W. Clinical relevance of the *cagA*, *vacA* and *iceA* status of *Helicobacter pylori*. Gastroenterol 1998; 115:58-66.

102. Blanco M, Blanco JE, Gonzalez EA, Mora A, Jansen W, Gomes TAT, Zerbini LF, Yano T, De Castro AFP, Blanco J. Genes coding for enterotoxins and verotoxins in porcine *Escherichia coli* strains belonging to different O:K:H serotypes: relationship with toxic phenotypes. J Clin Microbiol 1997; 35:2958-2963.

103. Cockerill III FR. Genetic methods for assessing antimicrobial resistance. Antimicrob Agents Chemother 1999; 43:199-212.

104. Anthony RM, Connor AM, Power EGM, French GL. Use of the polymerase chain reaction for rapid detection of high-level mupirocin resistance in staphylococci. Eur J Clin Microbiol Infect Dis 1999; 18:30-34.

105. Fleischmann RD, Adams MD, White O, Clayton RA, Kirkness EF, Kerlavage ER, Bult CJ, Tomb JF, Dougherty BA, Merrick JM, McKenney K, Sutton G, FitzHugh W, Fields C, Gocayne JD, Scott J, Shirley R, Liu L, Glodek A, Kelley JM, Weidman JF, Phillips CA, Spriggs T, Hedblom E, Cotton MD, Utterback TR, Hanna MC, Nguyen DT, Saudek DM, Brandon DC, Fine DL, Fritchman JL, Fuhrmann JL, Geoghagen NSM, Gnehm CL, McDonald LA, Small KV, Fraser CM, Smith HO, Venter JC. Whole-genome random sequencing and assembly of *Haemophilus influenzae* Rd. Science 1995; 269:496-512.

106. Fraser CM, Gocayne JD, White O, Adams MD, Clayton RD, Fleischmann RD, Bult CJ, Kerlavage AR, Sutton G, Kelley JM, Fritchman JL, Weidman JF, Small KV, Sandusky M, Fuhrmann J, Nguyen D, Utterback TR, Saudeck DM, Phillips CA, Merrick JM, Tomb J, Dougherty BA, Bott KF, Hu P, Lucier TS, Peterson SN, Smith HO, Hutchinson III CA, Venter JC. The minimal gene complement of *Mycoplasma genitalium*. Science 1995; 270:397-403.

107. Bult CJ, White O, Olsen GJ, Zhou L, Fleischmann RD, Sutton GG, Blake JA, FitzGerald LM, Clayton RA, Gocayne JD, Kerlavage AR, Dougherty BA, Tomb JF, Adams MD, Reich CI, Overbeek R, Kirkness EF, Weinstock KG, Merrick JM, Glodek A, Scott JL, Geoghagen NSM, Weidman JF, Fuhrmann JL, Nguyen D, Utterback TR, Kelley JM, Peterson JD, Sadow PW, Hanna MC, Cotton MD, Roberts KM, Hurst MA, Kaine BP, Borodovsky M, Klenk HP, Fraser CM, Smith HO, Woese C, Venter JC. Complete genome sequence of the methanogenic archaeon, *Methanococcus jannaschii*. Science 1996; 273:1058-1068.

108. Blattner FR, Plunkett III G, Bloch CA, Perna NT, Burland V, Riley M, Collado-Vides J, Glasner JD, RodeCK, Mayhew GF, Gregor J, Davis NW, Kirkpatrick HA, Goeden MA, Rose DJ, Mau B, Shao Y. The complete genome sequence of *Escherichia coli* K-12. Science 1997; 277:1453-1462.

109. Strauss EJ, Falkow S. Microbial pathogenesis: genomics and beyond. Science 1997; 276:707-712.

110. Tomb JF, White O, Kerlavage AR, Clayton AR, Sutton GG, Fleischmann RD, Ketchum KA, Klenk HP, Gill SR, Dougherty BA, Nelson K, Quackenbush J, Zhou L, Kirkness KA, Peterson S, Loftus B, Richardson D, Dodson R, Khalak HG, Glodek A, McKenney K, Fitzgerald LM, Lee N, Adams MD, Hickey EK, Berg DE, Gocayne JD, Utterback DR, Peterson JD, Kelly JM, Cotton MD, Weidman JM, Fujii C, Bowman C, Watthey L, Wallin E, Borodovsky M, Hayes WS, Karp P, Smith HO, Fraser CM, Venter JC. The complete genome sequence of the gastric pathogen *Helicobacter pylori*. Nature 1997; 338:539-547.

111. Alm RA, Ling LSL, Moir DT, King BL, Brown ED, Doig PC, Smith DR, Noonan B, Guild BC, DeJonge BL, Carmel G, Tummino TJ, Carusa A, Uria Nickelsen M, Mills DM, Ives C, Gibson R, Merberg D, Mills SD, Jiang Q, Taylor DE, Vovis GF, Trust TJ. Genomic sequence comparison of two unrelated isolates of the human gastric pathogen *Helicobacter pylori*. Nature 1999; 397:176-180.

112. The *C. elegans* Sequencing Consortium. Genome sequence of the nematode *C. elegans*: a platform for investigating biology. Science 1998; 282:2012-2018.

113. Doolittle RF. Microbial genomes opened up. Nature 1997; 392:339-342.

114. Oliver SG. From DNA sequence to biological function. Nature 1996; 379:597-600.

115. Jenks PJ. Sequencing microbial genomes – what will it do for microbiology? J Med Microbiol 1998; 47:375-382.

116. Moir DT, Shaw KJ, Hare RS, Vovis GF. Genomics and antimicrobial drug discovery. Antimicrob Agents Chemother 1999; 43:439-446.

117. Enriquez J. Genomics and the world's economy. Science 1998; 281:925-926.

118. Fodor SPA, Read JL, Pirrung MC, Stryer L, Lu AT, Solas D. Light-directed, spatially addressable parallel chemical synthesis. Science 1991; 251:767-773.

119. Chee M, Yang R, Hubbell E, Berno A, Huang XC, Stern D, Winkler J, Lockhart DJ, Morris MS, Fodor SPA. Accessing genetic information with high-density DNA arrays. Science 1996; 274:610-614.

120. Kozal MJ, Shah N, Shen N, Yang R, Fucini R, Merigan TC, Richman DD, Morris D, Hubbell E, Chee M, Gingeras TR. Extensive polymorphisms observed in HIV-1 clade B protease gene using high density oligonucleotide arrays. Nature Med 1996; 2:753-759.

121. Lockhart DJ, Dong H, Byrne MC, Follettie MT, Gallo MV, Chee MS, Mittmann M, Wang C, Kobayashi M, Horton H, Brown EL. Expression monitoring by hybridisation to high-density oligonucleotide arrays. Nature Biotech 1996; 14:1675-1680.

122. DeRisi JL, Iyer VR, Brown PO. Exploring the metabolic and genetic control of gene expression on a genomic scale. Science 1997; 278:680-686.

123. Fodor SPA Massively parallel sequencing. Science 1997; 277:393-395.

124. Guschin DY, Mobarry BK, Proudnikov D, Stahl DA, Rittmann BE, Mirzabekov AD. Oligonucleotide microchips as genosensors for determinative and environmental studies in microbiology. Appl Environ Microbiol 1997; 63:2397-2402.

125. Troesch A, Nguyen H, Miyada CG, Desvarenne S, Gingeras TR, Kaplan PM, Cros P, Mabilat C. *Mycobacterium* species identification and rifampin resistance testing with high-density DNA probe arrays. J Clin Microbiol 1999; 37:49-55.

126. Vahey M, Nau ME, Barrick S, Cooley JD, Sawyer R, Sleeker AA, Vickerman P, Bloor S, Larder B, Michael NL, Wegner SA. Performance of the Affymetrix genechip HIV PRT 440 platform for antiretroviral drug resistance genotyping of human immunodeficiency virus type 1 clades and viral isolates with length polymorphisms. J Clin Microbiol 1999; 37:2533-2537.

127. Vaneechoutte M. A plea for caution with regard to applicability of PCR for direct detection. J Clin Microbiol 1999; 37:3081.

128. Vaneechoutte M, Van Eldere J. The possibilities and limitations of nucleic acid amplification technology in diagnostic microbiology. J Med Microbiol 1997; 46:188-194.

129. Bergeron MG, Ouelette M. Preventing antibiotic resistance through rapid genotypic identification of bacteria and their antibiotic resistance genes in the clinical microbiology laboratory. J Clin Microbiol 1998; 36:2169-2172.

130. Martineau F, Picard FJ, Roy PH, Ouelette M, Bergeron MG. Species-specific and ubiquitous DNA-based assay for rapid identification of *Staphylococcus epidermidis*. J Clin Microbiol 1996; 34:2888-2893.

131. Post JC, Preston RA, Aul JJ, Larkins-Pettigrew M, Rydquist-White J, Anderson KW, Wadowsky RM, Reagan DR, Walker ES, Kingsley LA, Magit AE, Ehrlich GD. Molecular analysis of bacterial pathogens in otitis media with effusion. JAMA 1995; 273:1598-1604.

132. Dymock D, Weightman AJ, Scully C, Wade WG. Molecular analyses of microflora associated with dentoalveolar abscesses. J Clin Microbiol 1996; 34:537-542.

133. Millar MR, Linton CJ, Cade A, Glancy D, Hall M, Jalal H. Application of 16S rRNA gene PCR to study bowel flora of preterm infants with and without necrotizing enterocolitis. J Clin Microbiol 1996; 34:2505-2510.

134. Post JC, White GJ, Aul JJ, Zavoral T, Wadowsky RM, Zhang Y, Preston RA, Ehrlich GD. Development and validation of a multiplex PCR-based assay for the upper respiratory tract bacterial pathogens *Haemophilus influenzae*, *Streptococcus pneumoniae* and *Moraxella catarrhalis*. Mol Diagn 1996; 1:29-39.

135. Klausegger A, Hell M, Berger A, Zinober K, Baier S, Jones N, Sperl W, Kofler B. Gram type specific broad range PCR amplification for rapid detection of 62 pathogenic bacteria. J Clin Microbiol 1999; 37:464-466.

136. Voordouw G, Shen Y, Harrington CS, Telang AJ, Jack TR, Westlake DWS. Quantitative reverse sample genome probing of microbial communities and its application to oil field production waters. Appl Environ Microbiol 1993; 59:4101-4114.

137. Olsvik Ø, Popovic T, Skjerve E, Cudjoe KS, Hornes E, Ugelstad J, Uhlén M. Magnetic separation techniques in diagnostic microbiology. Clin Microbiol Rev 1994; 7:43-54.

138. Boom R, Sol C, Beld M, Weel J, Goudsmit J, Wertheim-van Dillen P. Improved silica-guanidinium thiocyanate DNA isolation procedure based on selective binding of bovine alpha-casein to silica particles. J Clin Microbiol 1999; 37:615-619.

139. Jungkind D, Direnzo S, Beavis KG, Silverman NS. Evaluation of automated COBAS AMPLICOR PCR system for detection of several infectious agents and its impact on laboratory management. J Clin Microbiol 1996; 34:2778-2783.

140. Kopp MU, De Mello AJ, Manz A. Chemical amplification: continuous-flow PCR on a chip. Science 1998; 280:1046-1048.

141. Belgrader P, Bennett W, Hadley D, Richards J, Stratton P, Mariella R, Milanovich F. PCR detection of bacteria in seven minutes. Science 1999; 284:449-450.

142. Northrup MA. A miniature analytical instrument for nucleic acids based in micromachined silicon reaction chambers. Anal Chem 1998; 70:918-922.

143. Ibrahim MS, Lofts RS, Jahrling PB, Henchal EA, Weedn VW, Northrup MA, Belgrader P. Real-time micro-chip PCR for detecting single-base differences in viral and human DNA. Anal Chem 1998; 70:2013-2017.

144. Belgrader P, Bennett W, Hadley D, Long G, Mariella R, Milanovich F, Nasarabadi S, Nelson W, Richards J, Stratton P. Rapid pathogen detection using a microchip PCR array instrument. Clin Chem 1998; 44:2191-2194.

145. Hermans PW, Hibberd ML, Booy R, Daramola O, Hazelzet JA, De Groot R, Levin M. 4G/5G promoter poly-morphism in the plasminogen-activator-inhibitor-1 gene and outcome of meningococcal disease. Lancet 1999; 354:556-560.

146. Kotb M. Superantigens of gram positive bacteria: structure – function analyses and their implications for bio-logical activity. Curr Opin Microbiol 1998; 1:56-65.

147. Blaser MJ, Kirschner D. Dynamics of *Helicobacter pylori* colonization in relation to the host response. Proc Natl Acad Sci USA 1999; 96:8359-8364.

148. Wallace RW. DNA on a chip: serving up the genome for diagnostics and research. Mol Med Today 1997; 3:384-389.

149. Marshall A, Hodgson J. DNA chips: an array of possibilities. Nature Biotech 1998; 16:27-31.

150. Helminen M, Lahdenphja N, Hurme M. Polymorphism of the interleukin-10 gene is associated with suscepti-bility to Epstein-Barr Virus infection. J Infect Dis 1999; 180:496-499.

151. Wolcott MJ. Advances in nucleic acid detection methods. Clin Microbiol Rev 1992; 5:370-386.

152. Wolcott MJ. DNA-based rapid methods for the detection of foodborne pathogens. J Food Prot 1990; 54:387-401.

6

Searching for the Unknown

David N. Fredricks
Division of Infectious Diseases, Department of Medicine, Stanford University Medical Center, Stanford, California

I. INTRODUCTION

The task of detecting a known bacterial pathogen in a known infectious disease can sometimes be challenging even when our knowledge of the pathogen is extensive. For instance, the entire genome of the uncultivated bacterium *Treponema pallidum* has been sequenced and yet the diagnosis of active syphilis remains dependent on non-specific serological tests (VDRL or RPR) that employ a generic phospholipid (cardiolipin) as antigen. The task of detecting unknown or previously undescribed bacterial pathogens in suspected infectious diseases presents an even greater technical and philosophical challenge. What does it mean to search for the unknown? In the context of bacterial infection, it means searching for a bacterial pathogen that is associated with a disease without *a priori* knowledge of the characteristics of the microbe. The implication is that the microbe is occult and defies detection by conventional methods. Such a search should have the broadest scope and should be based on the detection of highly conserved bacterial features.

For established infectious diseases, the etiological microbes are known, and diagnostic tests are available for detection and diagnosis. For instance, a rash which is consistent with erythema migrans leads the clinician to order a Lyme serology thus confirming the diagnosis of Lyme disease. In this scenario, knowledge of a pathogen leads to the development of a specific diagnostic test such as serology or cultivation.

Other diseases may have characteristics which suggest a microbial etiology in the absence of having detected an infectious agent with the use of conventional methods; their causes remain unknown. Does the failure to cultivate a microbe from diseased tissue mean that a disease is not infectious? This chapter discusses the limitations of conventional diagnostic methods in bacteriology, the possible role of microbes in idiopathic diseases, and methods for novel pathogen discovery.

II. WHIPPLE'S DISEASE: A PARADIGM FOR PATHOGEN DISCOVERY

Whipple's disease was meticulously described by George Hoyt Whipple in 1907 when he noted the clinical and pathological features of what was then an idiopathic disease (1). Whipple's disease can affect multiple organs including the intestines, lymph nodes, brain, heart, and musculoskeletal system (2). It is characterized histologically by the infiltration of tissues with foamy histiocytes that stain with periodic acid-Schiff reagent. Although Whipple suggested that the disease was a disorder of fat metabolism ("intestinal lipodystrophy"), he also noted the presence of structures that resembled small bacteria in a lymph node from his patient. The utility of antibiotics in curing this previously fatal disease gave further credence to the hypothesis that Whipple's disease is caused by a bacterium (3). Decades later, a bacterial etiology for Whipple's disease was again suggested by electron microscopic studies of Whipple's disease tissue which revealed rod-shaped organisms with a plasma membrane, a cell wall, and a membrane external to the cell wall (4,5). Proving that Whipple's disease is caused by a specific bacterium, however, was not a trivial undertaking. Multiple attempts have been made to grow the Whipple bacillus in the laboratory on artificial media, in cell culture, and in animal hosts. These attempts at propagation had failed except for some recent reported successes using cell cultivation techniques (6). It is difficult to characterize a microbe without cultivation. Propagation on artificial media allows one to study the metabolic requirements, cell composition, and antigenic properties of a microbe. How can one characterize a microbe and prove that it is the cause of a disease when the microbe resists attempts at cultivation?

The approach that was used to identify the Whipple bacillus was based on phylogenetic analysis of the 16S rRNA gene that was directly amplified from infected tissue through the use of the polymerase chain reaction (PCR) (see below) (7,8). This approach does not depend on either cultivation or serology. Phylogenetic relationships that were inferred from this amplified gene sequence suggested that the Whipple bacillus is a novel actinomycete (see Chapter 14), and the name *Tropheryma whippelii* was proposed. Furthermore, primers were designed that are complementary to unique portions of this 16S rDNA sequence thus leading to the development of a specific PCR assay for the Whipple bacillus. Using this technique, investigators have shown that the Whipple bacillus is present in the tissues of patients with Whipple's disease but not in uninfected tissues (9). Although conventional methods failed to identify the Whipple bacillus, identification and detection of this novel pathogen were successful using a broad sequence-based approach.

III. LIMITATIONS OF CONVENTIONAL DIAGNOSTIC APPROACHES

In medical microbiology, cultivation on artificial media has been a very successful broad range approach for detecting pathogens in clinical samples. Routine laboratory media are able to grow a large variety of bacterial pathogens from different phylogenetic groups. Yet, we know that routine cultures can be negative even when these samples contain bacteria that are normally amenable to cultivation. Antibiotics that are administered to patients may hinder bacterial growth in the laboratory. Sample volumes may be too small to yield viable organisms, or suboptimal transport conditions may kill bacteria (e.g., anaerobes). Some bacteria may be too fastidious to grow on routine media, and unless these organisms are suspected, special isolation methods will not be employed and these microbes will not be detected. Finally, some bacterial pathogens do not grow at all on artificial media. These cultivation-resistant bacteria must be isolated in cell culture (*Chlamydia*), or they must be detected using such methods as serology (*Treponema pallidum*), microscopy (*Mycobacterium leprae*), or sequence-based techniques (*Tropheryma whippelii*).

Other evidence suggests a more basic problem with cultivation for the detection of bacteria. Surveys of bacteria in environmental niches reveal a discrepancy between the large numbers of microbes that are detected using cultivation independent methods (e.g., microscopy) and the smaller numbers of microbes that are detected using cultivation technology (10). This discrepancy has been termed the "great plate count anomaly" (11). What accounts for this discrepancy? Some of these bacteria may be known organisms that are in a temporary unculturable state, and some of these bacteria may be unknown organisms that defy all cultivation attempts. It is estimated that only about 1% of bacteria present on earth can be cultivated using the existing technology. Investigators have analyzed bacterial 16S rDNA sequences to study bacterial diversity in environmental niches, and have discovered novel bacteria that were not otherwise detected by cultivation (12-14). About one-third of the known bacterial divisions consist entirely of uncultivated members that have been identified through sequence-based methods (15). The failure of cultivation to reveal the full extent of microbial diversity has also been noted in human microbiology. A study of bacterial diversity in the human subgingival crevice compared the representation of bacteria as determined by cultivation with that determined by PCR amplification and phylogenetic analysis of bacterial 16S rRNA genes (16). The bacteria that were identified with the sequence-based approach were more divergent than those which were revealed by cultivation. Numerous previously unidentified bacteria were detected using the molecular approach. In a study of human fecal flora, investigators found that 76% of the 16S rDNA sequences generated from a fecal sample did not match known bacteria in public databases (34). It is clear that molecular methods are providing new insights about the diversity of microbes that colonize man. Do some of these microbes also cause disease?

IV. IDIOPATHIC VERSUS INFECTIOUS DISEASES

Many diseases have no clear etiology. Some of these unexplained diseases are classified as autoimmune since tissues show evidence of inflammation, but microbes or other sources of inciting antigens have not been detected. Nevertheless, several of these idiopathic diseases have features which suggest a role for microbes in their pathogenesis. For instance, there is some evidence that patients with the necrotizing granulomatous vasculitis (Wegener's granulomatosis) improve when treated with the antibiotic trimethoprim-sulphamethoxazole (17,18). Is this salutary effect due to the antibacterial action of this antibiotic or due to some anti-inflammatory property? As another example, patients with tropical sprue develop chronic diarrhea and intestinal inflammation after travel or residence in endemic areas. The disease is cured with antibiotic treatment (tetracycline) yet no credible pathogen has been clearly linked to this syndrome. It has been suggested that other idiopathic inflammatory diseases may be infectious including Crohn's disease, ulcerative colitis, Kawasaki's disease, sarcoidosis, rheumatoid arthritis, scleroderma, and psoriasis.

Is it possible that some or all of these idiopathic diseases are caused by microbes? The skeptic would argue that the failure to detect bacterial pathogens in these idiopathic diseases with the use of conventional technologies argues against microbial involvement. Conventional diagnostic modalities, however, may not detect unconventional or fastidious bacterial pathogens as noted above. Recent history shows that bacterial pathogens may lurk in the shadows of "idiopathic diseases." Lyme disease and peptic ulcer disease are examples of diseases that were recently linked to novel bacteria.

A. *Borrelia burgdorferi* and Lyme disease

In the 1970s, a cluster of children from Lyme, Connecticut were noted to have oligoarticular arthritis and were initially diagnosed as having juvenile rheumatoid arthritis (19). The association of this disease with tick bites and the subsequent improvement seen after antibiotic therapy suggested that this illness is caused by a bacterium that is transmitted by ticks. It took seven years to isolate the etiological bacterium, *Borrelia burgdorferi*, from *Ixodes* ticks and to prove that this illness is an infectious disease. Chronic Lyme disease has characteristics of other systemic inflammatory illnesses, and may affect the joints, heart, skin, and nervous system (see Chapter 25).

B. *Helicobacter pylori* and peptic ulcer disease

In the recent past, peptic ulcer disease was considered a metabolic disease. The factors that were considered as contributing to peptic ulcer disease included everything from psychological stress and spicy food to excessive acid production and defective mucosal protection. In the last decade, it has become clear that the primary factor that is responsible for causing peptic ulcer disease is infection with the bacterium *Helicobacter pylori* (see Chapter 20). Eradication of infection by treatment with antibiotics cures patients of the disease whereas treatments aimed solely at acid secretion or mucosal protection usually provide only short term benefits (20). *Helicobacter pylori* is an example of a bacterial pathogen that is capable of producing chronic infection and chronic disease. We are reminded that our understanding of disease pathogenesis is sometimes flawed, and clarification awaits discovery of a novel etiological factor such as a microbe.

V. SEQUENCE-BASED DETECTION AND IDENTIFICATION OF BACTERIA

Bacteria contain conserved nucleic acid sequences that can be used as targets in assays that are based on nucleic acid amplification. Detection of these conserved sequences in a clinical sample suggests that bacteria are present. Detailed knowledge of the bacteria, their antigens, and cultivation requirements is not necessary for detection. In addition, these genes contain regions of sequence variability which can be used to identify bacteria or infer phylogenetic affinities.

The small subunit (16S) and large subunit (23S) ribosomal RNA genes have proven to be the most valuable and widely used targets for bacterial detection and identification. These rRNA genes contain numerous regions of highly conserved sequence which can be targeted with PCR primers. These highly conserved regions of the gene probably encode segments of rRNA which are functionally important for protein synthesis, and hence are evolutionarily conserved. Amplification generates sequence between the two priming sites in the gene, and this more variable sequence can be used for bacterial identification (Figure 1). The rRNA genes accumulate mutations over time, and therefore can be used as a molecular chronometer to measure evolutionary distances between bacteria. Two bacteria that are distant evolutionary relatives are likely to have larger sequence differences in the rRNA genes than two bacteria that are close evolutionary neighbors. Other targets for broad range PCR include genes that encode heat shock proteins, elongation factors, and ATPases. Each of these targets contains less phylogenetic information than the 16S rRNA gene. Although the 23S rRNA gene contains more phylogenetic information than the 16S rRNA gene, it is less useful currently due to the relative paucity of these sequences in databases.

The development of 16S rDNA consensus sequence PCR arose due to a confluence of theoretical and technological advancements. Carl Woese and colleagues established a useful phylogeny of prokaryotes by using the 16S rRNA gene as a molecular chronometer to gauge evolutionary distances between organisms (21). Although the information contained in the 16S rRNA gene sequence is sufficient to identify most bacteria, access to this information was limited by the difficulty in obtaining this sequence from large numbers of different bacteria. In 1985, Norm Pace and colleagues used conserved oligonucleotide primers and reverse transcriptase to generate copies of the bacterial 16S rRNA for subsequent sequencing (22). The ability to rapidly sequence 16S rDNA, however, expanded with the later application of the polymerase chain reaction for the enzymatic copying of this gene. Several groups proposed using consensus sequence 16S rDNA PCR for the detection of uncultivated or fastidious bacteria (23-26). Consensus sequence PCR of the 16S rRNA gene has been successfully used to detect and identify novel bacterial pathogens in such diseases as bacillary angiomatosis (*Bartonella henselae*) (25), Whipple's disease (*Tropheryma whippelii*) (7,8), and human ehrlichiosis (*Ehrlichia chaffeensis*) (27).

How might one apply this technology in the search for an unknown bacterial pathogen that is associated with an idiopathic disease such as sarcoidosis? Tissue samples such as sarcoid lymph nodes

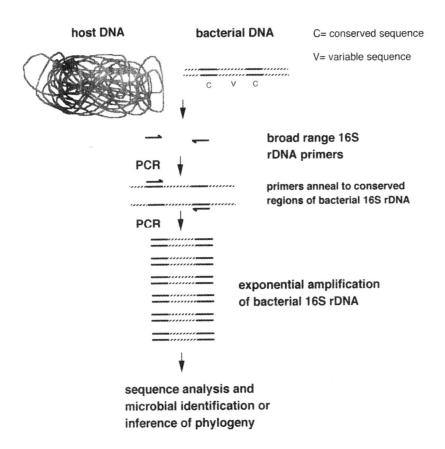

Figure 1 Diagram of broad range PCR for the detection of microbial DNA in tissue samples. Oligonucleotide primers anneal to highly conserved segments of microbial DNA, but fail to anneal to host DNA. PCR amplifies the microbial DNA which spans the priming sites and produces large amounts of DNA which can be sequenced or probed to confirm the identity of the microbe.

could be digested to liberate DNA from host tissue and any bacteria that might be present. Control tissues should be processed in parallel with the query tissue. The DNA is then added to a broad-range 16S rDNA PCR assay. If an amplification product is detected, as with gel electrophoresis, the product can either be directly sequenced, or cloned and then sequenced. If multiple 16S rRNA gene sequence types are present in the sample, these must then be distinguished with cloning or other methods. Once a sequence is obtained, it is compared to other 16S rDNA sequences in a database such as Genebank with the use of a search algorithm such as BLAST. If the sequence matches a known bacterium (and is sufficiently long to provide discrimination between bacterial types), then the bacterium is identified. If there is no match in the database, an understanding of the phylogeny of the bacterium can then be obtained by determining relationships to other bacteria based on 16S rDNA sequence similarity.

VI. OTHER APPROACHES FOR NOVEL PATHOGEN DISCOVERY

Although consensus sequence PCR has been the most widely applied approach in the search for novel bacteria pathogens, other approaches are feasible. Representational difference analysis (RDA) had been successfully used to identify novel viral pathogens such as human herpesvirus 8 (HHV-8 or KSHV)

(28) and novel transfusion-associated viruses (GVB and TTV). This technique uses subtractive hybridization and PCR-based kinetic enrichment to isolate segments of microbial DNA that are present in infected tissue but that are absent from uninfected tissue (29). This technique is limited by the need for a relatively high concentration of microbes in the infected tissue. In addition, the segment of microbial DNA that is isolated with this procedure may not be phylogenetically informative especially if it comes from a large microbial genome such as a bacterium.

Other possible methods for pathogen discovery include differential display, serial analysis of gene expression, screening of expression libraries with immune serum, mass spectroscopy for conserved microbial molecules, hybridization of tissue DNA to microarrays that contain microbial genes or gene fragments, and in situ hybridization of conserved oligonucleotide probes which target microbial sequences in infected tissue samples (30). For example, one could screen tissue for bacterial pathogens by using a fluorescent-labeled oligonucleotide probe that targets highly conserved regions of bacterial 16S rRNA. Bacteria which are present in the tissue could be visualized using fluorescence microscopy. Application of this fluorescence in situ hybridization assay to tissues from patients with idiopathic diseases could help to prove that bacteria are involved in pathogenesis.

VII. MOLECULAR KOCH'S POSTULATES

Identification of a novel microbial sequence in diseased tissue is merely the first stage of pathogen discovery using sequence-based methods. Once a microbe is identified as a possible pathogen, it is critical to collect evidence of causal association to support or reject the hypothesis that the microbe is a cause of disease. When the microbe is fastidious or uncultivated, Koch's postulates for establishing disease causation do not apply. Koch's postulates demand that the candidate pathogen should be isolated from diseased tissue, cultivated in vitro, and then inoculated into a susceptible host where it should produce the characteristic disease (31). If the pathogen cannot be cultivated in vitro, the microbe cannot meet the criteria for causality delineated by Koch's postulates. How can one prove that an uncultivated microbe is the cause of a disease?

Hill's epidemiological criteria for causal association serve as a useful template for collecting evidence that an uncultivated microbe is the cause of a disease (32). Hill's criteria have been adapted to create some sequence-based guidelines for microbial disease causation (33). Meeting the criteria set forth in these molecular guidelines helps to prove that a microbe is causally linked to a disease. There is no single experiment, however, that absolutely proves that a microbe is a pathogen. Evidence for causality comes from the concordance of scientific evidence that is collected over many experiments and observations, in different locations, and at different times.

VIII. CONCLUSIONS

Modern molecular methods have created an opportunity to search for novel bacteria which may colonize humans and/or cause disease. These methods do not rely on cultivation in the laboratory. Several novel bacterial pathogens have been identified using a sequence-based approach to pathogen discovery. Future application of this technology will undoubtedly identify new bacteria as causes of human disease thus creating known pathogens from the unknown.

REFERENCES

1. Whipple GH. A hitherto undescribed disease characterized anatomically by deposits of fat and fatty acids in the intestinal and mesenteric lymphatic tissues. Johns Hopkins Hosp Bull 1907; 18:382-391.
2. Dobbins WO. Whipple's Disease. Springfield, Ill:Charles C. Thomas, 1987.

3. Paulley JW. A case of Whipple's disease (intestinal lipodystrophy). Gastroenterology 1952; 22:128-133.

4. Silva MT, Macedo PM, Nunes JFM. Ultrastructure of bacilli and the bacillary origin of the macrophagic inclusions in Whipple's disease. J Gen Microbiol 1985; 131:1001-1013.

5. Dobbins WO, Kawanishi H. Bacillary characteristics in Whipple's disease: an electron microscopic study. Gastroenterology 1981; 80:1468-1475.

6. Schoedon G, Goldenberger D, Forrer R, Gunz A, Dutly F, Hochli M, Altwegg M, Schaffner A. Deactivation of macrophages with interleukin-4 is the key to the isolation of *Tropheryma whippelii*. J Infect Dis 1997; 176:672-677.

7. Wilson KH, Blitchington R, Frothingham R, Wilson JA. Phylogeny of the Whipple's disease-associated bacterium. Lancet 1991; 338:474-475.

8. Relman DA, Schmidt TM, MacDermott RP, Falkow S. Identification of the uncultured bacillus of Whipple's disease. N Engl J Med 1992; 327:293-301.

9. Ramzan NN, Loftus EJ, Burgart LJ, Rooney M, Batts KP, Wiesner RH, Fredricks DN, Relman DA, Persing DH. Diagnosis and monitoring of Whipple's disease by polymerase chain reaction. Ann Intern Med 1997; 126:520-527.

10. Amann RI, Ludwig W, Schleifer K-H. Phylogenetic identification and in situ detection of individual microbial cells without cultivation. Microbiol Rev 1995; 59:143-169.

11. Staley JT, Konopka A. Measurement of in situ activities of nonphotosynthetic microorganisms in aquatic and terrestrial habitats. Ann Rev Microbiol 1985; 39:321-346.

12. Ward DM, Weller R, Bateson MM. 16S rRNA sequences reveal numerous uncultured microorganisms in a natural community. Nature 1990; 345:63-65.

13. Giovannoni SJ, Britschgi TB, Moyer CL, Field KG. Genetic diversity in Sargasso Sea bacterioplankton. Nature 1990; 345:60-63.

14. Schmidt TM, DeLong EF, Pace NR. Analysis of a marine picoplankton community by 16S rRNA gene cloning and sequencing. J Bacteriol 1991; 173:4371-4378.

15. Pace NR. A molecular view of microbial diversity in the biosphere. Science 1997; 276:734-740.

16. Kroes I, Lepp PW, Relman DA. Bacterial diversity within the human subgingival crevice. Proc Natl Acad Sci USA 1999; 96:14547-14552.

17. DeRemee RA, McDonald TJ, Weiland LH. Wegener's granulomatosis: observations on treatment with antimicrobial agents. Mayo Clin Proc 1985; 60:27-32.

18. Stegeman CA, Cohen TJ, de JP, Kallengerg CG. Trimethoprim-sulfamethoxazole (co-trimoxazole) for the prevention of relapses of Wegener's granulomatosis. Dutch Co-trimoxazole Wegener Study Group. N Engl J Med 1996; 335:16-20.

19. Steere AC, Malawista SE, Snydman DR, Shope RE, Andiman WA, Ross MR, Steele FM. Lyme arthritis: an epidemic of oligoarticular arthritis in children and adults in three Connecticut communities. Arthritis Rheum 1977; 20:7-17.

20. Hentschel E, Brandstatter G, Dragosics B, Hirschl AM, Nemee H, Scutze K, Taufer M, Wurzer H. Effect of ranitidine and amoxicillin plus metronidazole on the eradication of *Helicobacter pylori* and the recurrence of duodenal ulcer. N Engl J Med 1993; 328:308-312.

21. Fox GE, Stackebrandt E, Hespell RB, Gibson J, Maniloff J, Dyer TA, Wolfe RS, Balch WE, Tanner RS, Magrum LJ, Zablen LB, Blakemore R, Gupta R, Bonen L, Lewis BJ, Stahl DA, Luersen KR, Chen KN, Woese CR. The phylogeny of prokaryotes. Science 1980; 209:457-463.

22. Lane DJ, Pace B, Olsen GJ, Stahl DA, Sogin ML, Pace NR. Rapid determination of 16S ribosomal RNA sequences for phylogenetic analyses. Proc Natl Acad Sci USA 1985; 82:6955-6959.

23. Bottger EC. Rapid determination of bacterial ribosomal RNA sequences by direct sequencing of enzymatically amplified DNA. FEMS Microbiol Lett 1989; 53:171-176.

24. Wilson KH, Blitchington RB, Greene RC. Amplification of bacterial 16S ribosomal DNA with polymerase chain reaction. J Clin Microbiol 1990; 28:1942-1946.

25. Relman DA, Loutit JS, Schmidt TM, Falkow S, Tompkins LS. The agent of bacillary angiomatosis. An approach to the identification of uncultured pathogens. N Engl J Med 1990; 323:1573-1580.

26. Weisburg WG, Barns SM, Pelletier DA, Lane DJ. 16S ribosomal DNA amplification for phylogenetic study. J Bacteriol 1991; 173:697-703.

27. Anderson BE, Dawson JE, Jones DC, Wilson KH. *Ehrlichia chaffeensis*, a new species associated with human ehrlichiosis. J Clin Microbiol 1991; 29:2838-2842.

28. Chang Y, Cesarman E, Pessin MS, Lee F, Culpepper J, Knowles DM, Moore PS. Identification of herpesvirus-like DNA sequences in AIDS-associated Kaposi's sarcoma. Science 1994; 266:1865-1869.

29. Lisitsyn N, Lisitsyn N, Wigler M. Cloning the differences between two complex genomes. Science 1993; 259:946-951.
30. Carulli JP, Artinger M, Swain PM, Root CD, Chee L, Tulig C, Guerin J, Osborne M, Stein G, Lian J, Lomedico PT. High throughput analysis of differential gene expression. J Cell Biochem 1998; 31:S286-S296.
31. Koch R. Die Aetiologie der Tuberculose. In: Clark DH - ed. Source Book of Medical History. New York NY:Dover Publications, Inc., 1882:392-406.
32. Hill AB. The environment and disease: association or causation? Proc R Soc Med 1965; 58:295-300.
33. Fredricks DN, Relman DA. Sequence-based identification of microbial pathogens: a reconsideration of Koch's postulates. Clin Microbiol Rev 1996; 9:18-33.
34. Suau A, Bonnet R, Sutren M, Godon JJ, Gibson GR, Collins MD, Dore J. Direct analysis of genes encoding 16S rRNA from complex communities reveals many novel molecular species within the human gut. Appl Environ Microbiol 1999; 65:4799-4807.

7

Molecular Epidemiology

Marc Struelens
Department of Microbiology, Center for Molecular Diagnostics, Hôpital Erasme, and Infectious Diseases Epidemiology Unit, School of Public Health, Université Libre de Bruxelles, Bruxelles, Belgium

I. DEFINITIONS

Molecular epidemiology may be defined as the study of microbial pathogens with the use of high resolution genotyping methods which generate and test hypotheses regarding the mode of acquisition and the transmission of these infectious agents among human populations. Microbial isolates that are part of the same chain of transmission (and replication) from host to host or from the environment to host are clonally related, i.e., they are the recent progeny of the same ancestor (1-2). Although isolates of a given bacterial species share a common phylogeny and ecological niche(s) (see Chapter 2), epidemiologically unrelated isolates exhibit a considerable amount of genomic and phenotypic diversity, whereas epidemiologically (and clonally) related isolates are significantly more homogeneous. Polymorphic characters, called *epidemiological markers*, are scored by typing systems that are designed to optimize discrimination of epidemiologically related and unrelated pathogenic isolates. Thus, *epidemiological typing systems* are composed of a *typing method* and the cognate *classification system* which allocates isolates to a type that is based on their markers. When a complex set of characters is generated (e.g., a DNA restriction fragment pattern), the term *fingerprint* is used, and the comparison of patterns is called *fingerprinting*.

In this chapter, definitions will follow consensus recommendations (1-2). The term *isolate* is used for a single-cell derived culture that is obtained from picking one colony on primary isolation medium. A *strain* comprises one or more isolates which share phenotypic and/or genotypic characteristics that are distinctive of other isolates of the same species. A *reference strain* is a well-characterized strain that is preserved in culture collection and that is included in further studies for comparison. A *clone* (or clonal group of isolates or strains) is a set of isolates that show a significantly higher level of marker similarity than is expected for randomly occurring isolates of that species, and it is inferred therefore that they are derived recently from the same cell. Identification of clones in this epidemiological sense requires the characterization of isolates with the aid of multiple discriminatory markers. The threshold of similarity that is used for the delineation of a clone needs to be empirically adjusted to the typing system(s) that is used (and their underlying "molecular clock"), the species studied, the environmental selective pressure, and the time scale of the study. In general, one cannot absolutely demonstrate the clonality of isolates but rather only estimate its likelihood which is proportional to the degree of homogeneity, the amount of genetic information that is compared, and the extent of subspecies diversity at the genetic target(s).

II.   BACTERIAL GENOME DIVERSITY AND EVOLUTION

A.   Composition of the bacterial genome

The bacterial genome is a complex assembly of several self-replicating DNA macromolecules, or replicons, that include a chromosome and plasmids and that are themselves mosaics of vertically inherited and horizontally inserted genetic elements. The bacterial chromosome is typically composed of a single (less commonly multiple) circular (less commonly linear) double-stranded DNA molecule of 0.5 to 10 kb in length. Plasmids are typically circular, double-stranded DNA molecules which range in size from 1 to 200 kb. Other mobile genetic elements of bacterial genomes include insertion sequences, transposons, and lysogenic bacteriophages; all of these can integrate into the chromosomal or plasmid DNA. Plasmids and transposons can carry genetic determinants of virulence and/or antimicrobial resistance.

B.   Evolution and diversity of bacterial genomes

The definition of a bacterial species is the subject of continuing debate among taxonomists (3). The classical criterion of reproductive isolation that is used for sexual organisms does not apply to bacteria. Although it has been accepted that bacteria belong to the same species if they share a DNA/DNA homology in the order of 70% or greater (see Chapter 2), this definition has been criticized as one that imposes an arbitrary division on a continuum (3). An alternative view of the bacterial species is "a condensed node in a cloudy and confluent taxonomic space" that operationally can be described as "an assemblage of isolates which originated from a common ancestor population in which a steady generation of genetic diversity resulted in clones with different degrees of recombination ... characterized by a certain degree of phenotypic consistency and a significant degree of DNA/DNA hybridization and over 97% of 16S rDNA sequence homology" (3).

The generation of genomic diversity in bacteria follows two major routes, and each of these operates by way of multiple mechanisms: the first is vertical evolution through mutagenesis, and the second is horizontal gene transfer (4). Both routes are modulated by the selection of genetic changes that depend on the modification of fitness which is produced by new phenotypic traits. Mutation occurs during DNA replication due to errors that result in nucleotide substitution, or sequence duplications or deletions, as well as by enzyme-mediated processes such as IS transposition and other DNA rearrangements (4). Although the basal rate of mutation is low due to efficient enzymatic DNA repair systems, hypermutator strains may emerge in stressful environments that enhance the mutation rate more than ten-fold (5). It has also been found that pathogenic bacteria possess "hyper-adaptable" loci in regions of short DNA repetitive elements called *variable number tandem repeats* (VNTR) (6). These repeat motifs are hyper-mutatable by slipped strand mispairing that leads to repeat unit deletion or duplication. These VNTR elements are often located upstream from surface-associated virulence determinants, and they modulate the expression of these determinants by frameshift mutations (6).

The importance of horizontal gene transfer in bacterial evolution is increasingly recognized (7). These acquisitions of foreign DNA from related or, less frequently, distant organisms occur by conjugation, transposition, transduction, and transformation. After conjugal transfer, whole plasmid DNA, plasmid-borne genes, or transposons can integrate into the chromosome of the recipient cell to the extent that the chromosome has been viewed as the "genetic necropolis of previously mobile genes" (7). Bacteria possess a number of systems to minimize DNA recombination between distant species: restriction-modification systems which degrade unmodified DNA, mismatch repair systems which abort homologous recombination of divergent DNA, specific receptors that limit susceptibility to transducing phages, and the development of a conjugation tube. Therefore, most DNA exchanges take place between cells of the same or closely related species. Among the key evolutionary steps that are related to the acquisition of large genetic elements are the plasmid-encoded virulence determinants (like the invasion plasmids of *E. coli* and *Shigella*), temperate phage-mediated exotoxin production (like cholera and Shiga toxins), and pathogenicity islands (like PAIs of enteropathogenic *E. coli* and *Salmonella*) that resemble defective phages, plasmid, or compound transposon remnants (8)

The general organization of chromosomal genes and operons (genetic map) is typically conserved within a species, but major variations can be observed in chromosome size and genetic composition. For example, *Escherichia coli* genomes have been extensively characterized by genetic linkage mapping (9), gene sequence polymorphism analysis (10), and the determination of the entire chromosomal nucleotide sequence (11). Genetic diversity is extensive and heterogeneously distributed; large regions of identical sequence are punctuated by clustered polymorphic sites. Diversity derives from multiple mechanisms including point mutations, homologous recombination, site specific recombination, chromosomal rearrangements, short repetitive DNA element variation in copy number and sequence motifs, transposition, intragenic recombination, and gene conversion. Approximately 17% of the *E. coli* genome represents integrated foreign DNA which includes prophage DNA, insertion sequences, tranposons, and pathogenicity islands (10). The comparison of whole genome sequences is now providing new answers regarding the structure and evolution of bacterial genomes. For example, a comparison of the chromosomal nucleotide sequence of two unrelated strains of *Helicobacter pylori*, a genetically diverse human pathogen, has confirmed the general conservation of topology and sequences of housekeeping genes in which the majority of nucleotide substitutions are synonymous (12). Strain-specific genes account for 7% of all structural genes, and approximately one-half of those are concentrated into a single "plasticity zone". The current accumulation of whole bacterial genome sequences will allow for more extensive comparative genomics.

C. Bacterial population genetics

Population geneticists have examined the genetic structure of bacterial species by means of multi-locus enzyme electrophoresis (MLEE), and more recently, multi-primer randomly amplified polymorphic DNA (RAPD) analysis and multi-locus sequence typing (MLST) (13-16). Depending on the species, there appears to be a wide spectrum of structure that ranges between two extremes: (i) a *clonal structure* that is characterized by strong multilocus linkage disequilibrium, i.e., a stable association of alleles of distinct genes that indicates the predominance of vertical gene flow; and, (ii) a *panmictic structure* that is characterized by allele equilibrium, or lack of association of alleles of distinct genes due to frequent lateral gene transfer and recombination (15). The majority of bacterial species that are pathogenic to humans exhibit some degree of clonal structure (e.g., *Haemophilus influenzae*, *E. coli*, and *Salmonella*) whereas other species appear basically panmictic (e.g., *H. pylori* and *Neisseria gonorrhoeae*) (13-15). Clonality can result from the dominant reproduction mode (efficient barriers against inter-genomic recombination), from ecological isolation, or develop as an "epidemic burst of clonality" that is related to the rapid spread of a hyper-successful variant which transiently resists erosion from endemic recombination (14-15). The latter behaviour is well-documented for *Neisseria meningitidis*. This basically panmictic and transformable pathogen has expanded in epidemic waves; these are caused by virulent clones that could be traced by phenotypic and genotypic markers as they spread from China to Africa over several decades (17).

D. Micro-evolution and genetic drift

Micro-evolution (biological evolution at the human time scale that is monitored by epidemiological investigations) and emergence of subclonal variants occur during chronic bacterial infection, replication in an environmental reservoir, or prolonged transmission in human or animal populations. These genetic events appear at a rate that can be recognized by several typing systems, and they complicate the interpretation of results (17-23). Quantitative analysis of polymorphism among epidemiologically-related strains helps define the clonal relationships and helps correct for minor genotype variations due to genetic drift. For example, methicillin-resistant *S. aureus* strains from a two-year long hospital outbreak exhibited up to three *Sst*II fragment pattern variation or 80% pattern relatedness (18). Clonally-related strains of *Pseudomonas aeruginosa* that were recovered over a period of many years from individual cystic fibrosis patients show more than 80% chromosomal macrorestriction pattern similarity, whereas strains from unrelated patients display only 20 to 60% pattern similarity (Figure 1) (19-20). Predominant environmental clones of this organism with conserved phenotypic traits were associated with several epidemics while undergoing similar minor chromosomal rearrangements (20). Likewise, closely related strains of epidemic *Salmonella* serotype Typhi produced different ribotypes as a result of homologous recombination between *rrn* operons (21). In chronic gastric colonization by *H. pylori*, recent observations from extensive genotyping of sequential isolates suggest that a pool of genetic variants (or quasispecies) develops over several years as a result of genetic drift and intergenomic recombination within the host (22).

III. APPLICATIONS OF GENOMIC TYPING

Genomic typing systems are used as tools in biomedical research as well as diagnostic techniques in the clinical and public health microbiology laboratory (1). Rapid technological progress over the past decades in genomic analytical methods has provided a large array of highly discriminating typing methods that have revolutionized our understanding of bacterial infections and that have vastly increased the power of resolving the transmission dynamics of the causative pathogens.

In research, typing has contributed to the determination of the genetic population structure of many bacterial species and has unravelled the natural history of endogenous and exogenous infections by identifying the reservoir and the mode of translocation or transmission of bacteria (1,13,16,17,22).

In the clinical laboratory, genotyping can solve diagnostic ambiguities by distinguishing infection from sample contamination with skin commensals, e.g., in the context of foreign body infection or endocarditis with *Staphylococcus epidermidis* (23). It can also determine the occurrence of polyclonal infections and ensure that representative antimicrobial susceptibility testing is performed in those circumstances (23-25). When isolates from the same bacterial species are recovered repeatedly from the same patient over periods ranging from days to months, genotyping can provide a distinction between relapse (repeat isolation of the same clone pointing to insufficient treatment in order to eradicate the focus of infection) and reinfection (isolation of a new clone indicating new acquisition and possibly decreased host defence capacity against the particular organism) (26).

For public health applications, genotyping has become the gold standard to detect and confirm outbreaks, to delineate the transmission patterns of the epidemic clone(s), to test hypotheses about the sources and vehicles of transmission of these clones, and to monitor the reservoirs of epidemic organisms (1-2,27-31; Table 1). When multiple epidemic and/or sporadic clones are identified, stratification of patients that are infected with distinct pathogens is necessary to analyze specific risk factors for acquisition which would otherwise become obscured by their complexity (28-30). Therefore, molecular typing should guide analytical epidemiology and vice-versa. Molecular typing also contributes to the evaluation of outbreak control measures by documenting eradication, or decreased circulation, of the epidemic clone(s) in the exposed population (1,28-30). Molecular typing can also document that immunization has effectively eliminated a prevalent pathogen rather than having induced its antigenic shift (32). For these outbreak studies, the testing of a limited number of isolates can be achieved by using a number of in-house *comparative genotyping* or *fingerprinting* methods (27; Tables 1 and 2).

In addition, genomic typing is increasingly used for the long term monitoring of the prevalence of particular clones in a population and its geographic distribution as part of long term *surveillance programs* at a local (27,33-34), regional, and international (35-37) or global level (16,38-40). For these

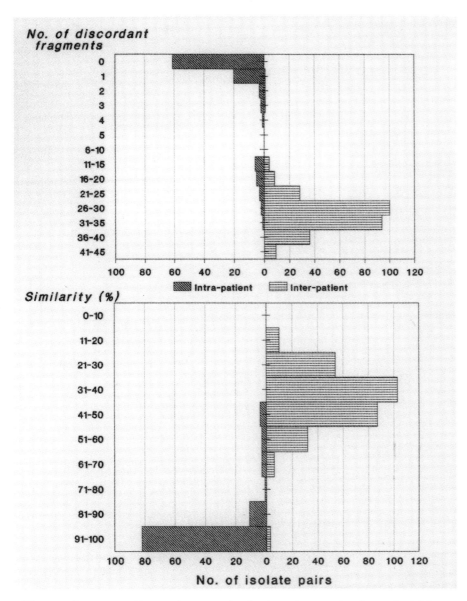

Figure 1 Intra- and inter-patient genomic relatedness (expressed as the number of fragment mismatches in the upper panel and as the Dice co-efficient of pattern similarity in the lower panel) of *Pseudomonas aeruginosa* isolates from cystic fibrosis patients as analyzed by PFGE with *Xba*I. Intra-patient: pairwise pattern comparison of consecutive versus initial isolates from 18 chronically-colonized patients (n=104 pairs). Inter-patient: pairwise pattern comparison (n= 292 pairs) of major PFGE types from these 18 patients (19).

macro-epidemiological applications, *library typing systems* that possess high throughput, standardized methods, and a uniform type nomenclature should be used (27; Table 1). To date, only a few such molecular typing systems are available, although a number of harmonized schemes are in active development for library genotyping of bacterial pathogens of global public health importance (Table 2). One of

Table 1   Purpose of epidemiological typing and requirements for systems that are used in outbreak investigations and surveillance programs (27).

Outbreak investigation

   Rationale: short term control of transmission

   Purpose: compare isolates from suspect outbreak to delineate clonally-related strains (epidemic cases/vehicles) from unrelated strains (sporadic cases)

   Scale: days to months; dozens to hundreds of infected individuals

   Requirements: comparative typing (reproducible in single assay), full typeability, high discrimination (D > 0.95)

Epidemiological surveillance

   Rationale: long-term evaluation of preventative strategies; detection
   and monitoring of emerging and re-emerging infections

   Purpose: monitor the geographic spread and prevalence shifts of epidemic and endemic clones

   Scale: years to decades; thousands of infected individuals

   Requirements: library typing (reproducible over time and between
   laboratories, standard type nomenclature), discrimination balanced against evolutionary stability
   to recognize clonal dispersion through high number of infectious cycles

---

the first international standard genotyping methods to be developed was the IS*6110* RFLP typing scheme for *Mycobacterium tuberculosis* (41); it remains the reference method (36).

IV. EVALUATION OF MOLECULAR GENOTYPING METHODS

Several criteria are applied for evaluating the performance of typing systems (1-2, 42). *Typeability* refers to the proportion of isolates that can be scored in the typing system and assigned a type (ideally all isolates). *Discriminatory power*, or the ability to distinguish unrelated clones, is a key characteristic of a typing system because it conditions the probability that isolates sharing identical or closely-related types are truly clonal and part of the same chain of transmission. Discriminating power can be calculated based on Simpson's Index of diversity (1,42). Ideally, the D index, based on testing a large number of epidemiologically unrelated isolates, should equal 1. In practice, a typing system, or combination of systems, displaying a discrimination index greater than 0.95 is acceptable (1) as this level of discrimination corresponds to a lower than 5% probability of erroneously assigning independent isolates to the same clone (type I error). *Reproducibility* refers to the ability of the typing system to assign the same type on repeat testing of the same strain. This property can differ significantly for testing that is performed by the same investigator, different investigators in the same laboratory, or different laboratories. *Stability* is the property of clonally-derived isolates to express constant markers over the course of time and infectious cycles that are subject to the investigation (27). The stability of markers may be acceptable even in the presence of minor variation provided that the typing system classification

Table 2   Applicability and performance characteristics of genomic typing systems.

Typing system	Application		Versatility	Typeability	Discrimination	Reproducibility
	Outbreak	Surveillance				
Plasmid RFLP	✓		moderate	low	variable	moderate
Genome REA	✓		good	excellent	good	moderate
Ribotyping	✓	✓	good	excellent	moderate	excellent
Southern blot RFLP	✓	✓	poor	excellent	variable	excellent
Macrorestriction (PFGE)	✓	✓	excellent	excellent	excellent	good
PCR gene RFLP	✓	✓	poor	excellent	variable	excellent
Arbitrarily-primed PCR/RAPD	✓		excellent	excellent	good	moderate
Repetitive element PCR	✓		good	variable	good	good
AFLP analysis	✓		excellent	excellent	excellent	excellent
Nucleotide sequence analysis	✓	✓	excellent	excellent	excellent	excellent

enables the recognition of clonal relatedness and does not misclassify subclonal variants as epidemiologically unrelated.

New typing systems must be carefully calibrated by testing well-documented collections of epidemiologically–linked isolates (1). *Epidemiological concordance* is the capacity of a typing system to correctly classify all epidemiologically related isolates from a well-described outbreak into the same clone (1, 43,44-50). Finally, *typing system concordance* is the congruence of clonal grouping by new versus established genotyping systems (1,44-50). This criterion modulates the previous one when interpreting results that are obtained by a combination of several typing methods: isolates initially believed to be part of an outbreak, but that are concordantly shown to be unrelated to an epidemic clone by a number of independent markers, should be re-examined for possible misclassification (1-2,44,47).

Table 2 presents a personal overview of the performance and suitability of genomic typing systems for micro and macro-epidemiological studies. As only a limited number of studies have rigorously compared the performance of typing systems according to the above criteria, additional comparative studies are needed to establish the relative value of many systems already in use or in development. Moreover, Table 2 is a broad generalization of average performance, whereas in reality, there are important variations in the performance of a given method depending on the bacterial species and on the modifications of the procedure as applied by different investigators.

Optimal typing systems should have practical advantages in addition to their intrinsic performance when applied to a particular microbial pathogen. Versatility, or the ability to type any pathogen, given minor modifications of the method, is an important advantage for use in the study of nosocomial infections. Conventional phenotypic typing systems often necessitate specific reagents (antisera, phage panels, etc.) for each particular species. In contrast, many molecular methods are of broader applicability because they analyze the structure of DNA by using similar reagents (e.g., enzymes) and equipment

Table 3   Infrequently cleaving endonucleases that are suitable for macrorestriction analysis of selected bacteria.

Bacterium	Enzymes
Acinetobacter baumannii	*Sma*I, *Apa*I
Bacteroides spp.	*Not*I
Bordetella pertussis	*Xba*I, *Asn*I, *Dra*I
Campylobacter spp.	*Sma*I
Clostridium difficile	*Sma*I, *Sst*II
Enterobacter spp.	*Xba*I, *Spe*I
Enterococcus spp.	*Sma*I, *Apa*I
Escherichia coli	*Xba*I, *Not*I, *Sfi*I
Haemophilus influenzae	*Sma*I, *Rsr*II
Klebsiella pneumoniae	*Xba*I, *Asn*I
Legionella pneumophila	*Sfi*I, *Not*I
Mycobacterium spp.	*Ase*I, *Xba*I, *Dra*I, *Asn*I
Neisseria meningitidis	*Not*I, *Bgl*II
Pseudomonas aeruginosa	*Spe*I, *Dra*I, *Ssp*I, *Xba*I
Staphylococcus aureus	*Sma*I, *Sst*II, *Csp*I
Staphylococcus epidermidis	*Sma*I, *Sst*II, *Kpn*I
Stenotrophomonas maltophilia	*Xba*I
Streptococcus pneumoniae	*Sma*I, *Apa*I

(e.g., electrophoresis) (Tables 2 and 3). Other important aspects of typing systems include ease of performance and of result interpretation, as well as cost of reagents and equipment. Moreover, results should be obtained rapidly enough to be useful for outbreak control interventions. Problems that require rapid typing include confirmation of a suspect outbreak and identification of carriers or an environmental source of the epidemic in order to implement carrier isolation and decolonization or environmental disinfection. Rapid screening systems can be used for preliminary assessment of clonality. If the clonal link hypothesis appears to hold, confirmation can be obtained, if required, by using more reliable but less efficient typing systems (1).

Historically, epidemiological typing has long relied on phenotypic traits, like serotyping, antimicrobial susceptibility testing, biotyping, phage or colicin typing, and later on, molecular phenotypic analysis of cell components including protein electrophoretypes and Western blot profiles (1). Some of these methods are still widely used for epidemiological studies. Serotyping monitors antigenic properties that are associated with variation in virulence and specific herd immunity. Antibiograms allow the detection and routine surveillance of emergence and dissemination of multi-resistant bacteria (1-2). Conventional typing, however, has many intrinsic limitations. Many isolates may be untypeable with standard reagents due to the development of new variants. Reagents are often costly and available only to a few reference laboratories with variable responsiveness to requests of rapid outbreak investigations. Expression of phenotypic traits depends on environmental conditions, and therefore clonally related isolates can exhibit diverse phenotypic characters, like surface antigens. In addition, phenotypic characters that influence fitness in stressful environments such as a human host may be rapidly selected. For example, unrelated clones of nosocomial pathogens that are exposed to antimicrobial selective pressure show evolutionary convergence to the same adaptative resistance phenotype through mutations and multiple genetic exchanges. Horizontal transfer of virulence, antigenic, or resistance determinants explains how bacteria of distantly related lineages can share identical phenotypes (14,51).

The explosion of nucleic acid technology, combined with high resolution molecular separation and detection instruments that are interfaced with computer data acquisition and analysis systems, have offered the widespread availability of sophisticated genotyping methods to clinical and public health laboratories. Most conventional typing is now performed by genotyping methods that are clearly more reliable than phenotypic methods, but they are nevertheless in a constant state of technological flux. In this overview of currently available molecular typing techniques, we will highlight their basic principles, major advantages and limitations, and current range of applications.

V. MOLECULAR GENOTYPING METHODS

A. Plasmid analysis

In the 1970s, rapid and simple methods of plasmid DNA extraction and of size profile determination by agarose electrophoresis led to the application of plasmid profiling as the first DNA-based typing method that was available for epidemiological studies of bacterial infection (52). It proved useful for the investigation of infections that are caused by bacterial species which harbour multiple plasmids (e.g., *Staphylococcus epidermidis* and *Klebsiella pneumoniae*), but many species with low diversity of plasmids were less typeable or poorly discriminated. In addition, technical and biological limitations of plasmid typing have made it obsolete as a clonal marker. Technical variability results from a number of factors including: variable yield and inaccurate size determination of large plasmids, and unreliable determination of number and size of plasmids which are migrating with different mobility as polymeric, supercoiled, open-circular, and linear forms. Restriction endonuclease analysis of plasmid DNA (REAP) improves reproducibility and discrimination, and it is currently the preferred method of plasmid typing. Secondly, many plasmids are unstable. They can be lost in nature or in vitro during storage and

replication. They can be acquired by conjugation with other bacteria, and they can recombine internally or into the chromosome by transposition. Thus, identical plasmid profiles may indicate horizontal plasmid spread rather than clonal relatedness, and distinct plasmid profiles do not rule out clonal spread. For example, the rate of in vivo plasmid instability is high in organisms such as *S. aureus*. Changes in the restriction endonuclease pattern of plasmid DNA can occur in 15% of sequential isolates from patients who have chronic colonization with methicillin-resistant *S. aureus* (53). Plasmid analysis is of particular interest for the epidemiological study of institutional infections with multiple-antibiotic resistant organisms. Used in conjunction with clonal delineation by chromosomal DNA typing, plasmid content analysis is essential for tracing dissemination of mobile antibiotic resistance genes like those that encode extended-spectrum beta-lactamases (54).

B. Restriction endonuclease analysis and RFLP analysis by Southern hybridization of genomic DNA

In the 1980s, simple techniques were developed for genomic DNA extraction from lyzed bacterial cells and for cleavage into many small (1 to 50 kb) fragments by restriction endonucleases that have frequent recognition sites. These fragments are partly resolved into complex patterns by agarose or polyacrylamide gel electrophoresis, and then the gel is stained with ethidium bromide or silver (55). The number and length of restriction fragments is affected by sequence variations that create or delete recognition sites and by insertion, duplication, inversion, and other recombinational events that occur at or between restriction sites. This simple and rapid DNA typing method showed good typeability and discrimination with optimal selection of enzymes and electrophoresis conditions for a given species (18,55). Interpretation is hindered, however, by the complexity of patterns with numerous overlapping DNA fragments. Between-gel reproducibility is difficult to achieve, which seriously limits the analysis of large samples.

To improve the resolution and "readability" of genomic restriction fragment length polymorphisms (RFLPs), two practical solutions have been developed: (i) transfer of restriction fragments onto membranes, followed by Southern-blot hybridization with DNA probes, and (ii) restriction with endonucleases that recognize infrequent (< 30) sites in the chromosome, followed by separation of these macrorestriction fragments by pulsed-field gel electrophoresis (PFGE).

Four types of nucleic acid probes were developed for RFLP analysis (55): (i) randomly cloned chromosomal fragments, (ii) genes encoding metabolic, virulence, or resistance functions, (iii) multicopy elements, including insertion sequences and transposons, and, (iv) ribosomal RNA or DNA (ribotyping). *Randomly cloned DNA fingerprinting* has been evaluated for a few pathogens, including *Legionella pneumophila*, but it is less discriminatory than PFGE, AP-PCR, and AFLP (47). *Southern blot analysis of gene polymorphism* is moderately discriminating but highly reproducible. Examples include *mecA* probe polymorphisms for the typing of methicillin-resistant *S. aureus* and the exotoxin A probe used for the typing *P. aeruginosa* strains from cystic fibrosis patients. Both of these systems, however, are less discriminating than PFGE and AP-PCR (44,46). *IS-fingerprinting*, or Southern blot analysis of genomic DNA with insertion sequences as probes, provides a very reproducible and highly discriminating typing tool. Discrimination is related to the presence of these elements in multiple copies at diverse locations in the chromosome. IS-fingerprinting has been validated and standardized for the epidemiological typing of *M. tuberculosis* (36,41) and *Salmonella* serotype Typhimurium (56). These techniques are slow, however, and each pathogen requires careful selection of the appropriate IS element, probe sequence, restriction endonucleases, electrophoresis, and hybridization conditions.

Ribotyping is the most versatile and the most widely used strategy of Southern blot RFLP analysis of bacterial genomes. The evolutionary conservation of ribosomal RNA makes *E. coli* rRNA applicable as a universal bacterial probe. Many important pathogens, including *Enterobacteriaceae, Pseudomonas* spp., *Listeria monocytogenes*, and staphylococci have more than five ribosomal operons per chromosome and thus yield ribotype patterns of 5 to 15 bands (57). Ribotypes exhibit two levels of polymorphism: some hybridized fragments are species-specific while others are strain-specific, thus making ribotyping useful for both taxonomic and epidemiological applications (57). Ribotyping is a robust method that exhibits excellent reproducibility and stability. It is only moderately discriminating, however, at a level that is equal or inferior to that of MLEE (57). The latter is due to the fact that ribosomal operons cover less than 0.1% of the chromosome and tend to cluster in a particular region of the genome. Discrimination of ribotyping depends on species and on choice and number of restriction endonucleases used. No general consensus has been achieved on the rules for interpretation of pattern variations and ribotype designation. The first fully automated and commercially-available genotyping system was developed for standardized ribotyping (Riboprinter, Qualicon). This system can be used conveniently as a first major clonal lineage discriminating step with high efficiency for large scale analysis in macro-epidemiological studies (58).

C.   Genome macrorestriction analysis by pulsed-field gel electrophoresis (PFGE)

This method has emerged in the 1990s as a gold standard fingerprinting technique for microbial pathogens (1-2). Low-frequency cleaving restriction endonucleases that are selected on the basis of genomic G+C content of the species of interest cut the bacterial chromosome into less than 30 fragments that range from 10 to 700 kb in size. To avoid mechanical shearing, genomic DNA preparation and macrorestriction are conducted on bacteria that are embedded in agarose plugs. Using special programmable electrophoresis units, periodic orientation changes of the electric field, or pulsed field gel electrophoresis, allows the separation and size determination of macrorestriction fragments (59). The whole procedure takes 2 to 4 days. DNA fragments can be transferred from PFGE gels or directly analyzed in dried gels with DNA probes by Southern hybridization for analysis of polymorphism of gene locations (20).

PFGE can be applied to a wide range of bacteria by selecting one or two of a dozen enzymes and by minor modifications of "pulsing protocols" (Table 3). A few species present difficulties with untypeable strains. For example, *H. pylori* strains may not be typed due to modification of the DNA, and some strains of *Clostridium difficile* produce DNA degradation due to endogenous nuclease activation (2,48,59). Although direct probing by rare cutting recognition sequences detects variation in less than 0.01% of the chromosome, PFGE analysis scans >90% of the chromosome for large size rearrangements such as sequence duplications, deletions, or insertions that are detected as a shift in fragment size and/or number. In comparison with other typing methods, PFGE has shown equal or greater discriminatory power than conventional REA (18,47), ribotyping and RFLP analysis by Southern blotting (44,46-47), MLEE (44), and AP-PCR (47). Due to its broad versatility, excellent discrimination and good intra-laboratory reproducibility, genome macrorestriction analysis by PFGE is currently a method of choice for clinical and reference laboratories that study the molecular epidemiology of nosocomial pathogens (1-2,59).

D.   PCR analysis of whole genome polymorphism

In the 1990's, a number of PCR-based strategies were developed for strain discrimination of microbial pathogens (60-61). *Arbitrarily-primed PCR (AP-PCR),* and similar methods like *random amplified polymorphic DNA (RAPD),* are based on low-stringency PCR amplification by using a single, 10 to 20-mer primer of arbitrary sequence. In the early cycles of the PCR reaction, the primer anneals to multiple sequences with partial homology, and fragments of DNA lying within less than 2 kb between annealing sites on opposite DNA strands are amplified. After additional cycles, a strain-specific array of amplified DNA segments of various sizes is obtained (60-62).

This efficient and rapid technique has been successfully applied to the genotyping a broad range of microbial pathogens, including bacteria, fungi, and protozoans (14,60-64). All isolates are typeable, and no prior knowledge of target genome sequences is necessary. Discrimination depends on the number and sequence of arbitrary primers and amplification conditions, and correlates well with other genotyping techniques (60-61,63-64). In spite of its attractive power and simplicity, AP-PCR typing currently suffers from problems in reproducibility and from the lack of consensus rules for the interpretation of pattern differences (60,62). A number of technical factors need to be strictly standardized for optimal reproducibility (62). In general, differences in protocols, equipment, or even the batch of reagent that is used result in different AP-PCR patterns, but the overall clustering of isolates into identical, similar, or divergent patterns is reproducible (65).

that are due to minor variations of reagent concentration or due to thermal cycles that influence the first rounds of low-stringency annealing of primers to partly homologous genomic sequence motifs (1,47,62). An inter-centre comparison of AP-PCR protocols for *S. aureus* typing revealed divergent patterns, which, however, concordantly grouped strains into epidemiologically relevant clusters (65). Better inter-centre reproducibility was achieved for AP-PCR typing of *Acinetobacter baumannii* and rep-PCR typing of *S.aureus* through the use of single batch reagents and a standardized protocol (50,66). Further improvement was obtained by the analysis of fluorescent DNA products with laser densitometry (50,60).

Repetitive elements PCR, or rep-PCR typing, targets repetitive and dispersed genetic elements with the use of outwardly-directed primers that amplify arrays of inter-repeat spacers. It operates at higher stringency than RAPD/AP-PCR, and it is therefore a more reproducible method, albeit more specialized. Short and repetitive elements that are targeted for rep-PCR typing include the repetitive extragenic palindromes (REPs), the enterobacterial repetitive intergenic consensus (ERIC) sequences, insertion sequences, and other species-specific repeat elements. Rep-PCR strategies produce fewer amplified DNA fragments than AP-PCR, and they have moderate discriminatory power. For example, rep-PCR typing of *S. aureus* strains that are based on the RepMP3 motif, 16S-23S rDNA spacer, and the insertion element IS*256* produce patterns that are less dicriminating than PFGE (50,67). Laser scanning of fluorescence-labeled DNA products which are separated on denaturing polyacrylamide gels (Figure 2) enhances the resolution and reproducibility of inter-IS PCR fingerprinting (50,60).

E. Amplified fragment length polymorphism (AFLP) analysis

The *amplified fragment length polymorphism* (AFLP) analysis is an increasingly used method that combines the efficiency of PCR and the accuracy of restriction polymorphism analysis (68). It is based on the double restriction of genomic DNA which is followed by ligation with special oligonucleotide adapters and then by selective PCR amplification of various subsets of these fragments as determined by primers that are complementary to these adapters and a variable number of adjacent nucleotides. The *infrequent-restriction-site amplification*, or IRS-PCR, is another variation of this approach that is based on selective amplification of DNA sequences which flank infrequent restriction sites (69). Both methods

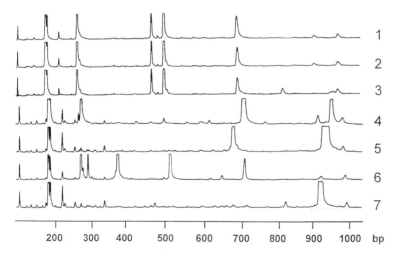

Figure 2   Laser densitogram patterns of inter-IS 256 spacer elements from methicillin-resistant *Staphylococcus aureus* genomes (ALF Express automated DNA sequencer, Amersham Pharmacia Biotech, Uppsala, Sweden). Products in lanes 1-3 are derived from clonally-related strains and those in lanes 4-7 are from unrelated strains of distinct origin (27).

perform very well; there is a high and easily adjusted discriminating power and a very good level of pattern reproducibility for a wide range of bacterial pathogens including Gram positive and Gram negative bacteria as well as *M. tuberculosis* (47,68–76). In general, AFLP typing proved faster, more reproducible, easier to perform, and equally or more discriminating when compared to macrorestriction analysis. More studies are needed to determine the stability of these markers over time, to establish criteria for the interpretation of pattern differences, and to evaluate inter-laboratory reproducibility.

F. Single locus PCR fingerprinting

In *PCR-gene RFLP typing*, a 1 to 2 kb target sequence that is known to show polymorphism among strains of the species of interest, is amplified at high stringency. The amplified product is then cut with restriction endonucleases, and isolates are compared by RFLP pattern. This approach requires the careful identification of polymorphic gene sequences and the selection of discriminant enzymes for each species that are to be studied. PCR-RFLP typing is a rapid, simple, and reproducible technique that has shown moderate discrimination, e.g., coagulase gene polymorphism among *S. aureus* (44), e.g., urease gene polymorphism for *H. pylori* (48).

One of the applications of this method is *PCR-serotyping*. It takes advantage of the conserved sequences at each end of protein antigen genes, e.g., flagellin and outer membrane proteins of Gram negative pathogens, for PCR-amplification of allelic variant sequences that encode the central and antigenically variable portion of these proteins (77-79). The polymorphic alleles can be determined by amplicon characterization with suitable restriction endonucleases [PCR-RFLP serotyping; (77-78)], conformational analysis [e.g., single strand conformation analysis, or PCR-SSCP serotyping; (79)], or nucleotide sequencing. The advantages of these methods over classical serotyping include the unlimited availability of reagents, universality of techniques, typeability of variants with cryptic antigens [e.g., non-motile *E. coli*; (77)], and direct typing from clinical specimens of non-viable organisms from those patients who were treated with antimicrobials (22). Nevertheless, genetic serotyping has important limitations that must be acknowledged. Like conventional serotyping, it is susceptible to the evolutionary instability of antigens. For example, rapid rearrangement of antigen determinants can occur during the infectious process, and horizontal gene exchanges introduce mosaic gene structures that are not valid clonal markers (80).

Apart from antigen structural genes, the genetic mechanisms and the evolutionary pace of variation at any single locus that is used as a target for PCR-RFLP need to be determined before one infers clonal relationships from allelic variation. Among *S. aureus*, for example, a variable number of direct repeats in the *spa* gene, as determined by PCR-RFLP analysis, appear to evolve quickly as *spa* variants are randomly scattered across clones delineated by PFGE analysis (81). In contrast, *Alu*I polymorphisms of the coagulase gene appear to closely match clonal groups as defined by macrorestriction analysis (81). Whereas PCR-RFLP of single polymorphic loci has relatively low discriminatory power, resolution can be increased by sequencing (see below) and/or by combined analysis of multiple loci (82).

G. Binary probes and oligotyping schemes

Multi-locus, sequence-based genotyping fulfills the requirements of library typing methods that are suitable for surveillance systems. By use of a panel of clone-specific DNA probes for high stringency hybridization, patterns of binary results which have positive and negative matches are produced with each probe. Reverse dot blot or line blot hybridization with immobilized DNA probes has been developed for binary typing of *S. aureus* (83-84), *M. tuberculosis* (49,85), *H. pylori* (86), and *N. gonorrhoeae* (87). Although these probe typing schemes tend to provide less resolution than RFLP-based techniques, they nevertheless provide the type of unambiguous and numeric clonal signatures that are required for the surveillance of major pathogens. The power and efficiency of these genotypic hybridization schemes should greatly benefit from the use of high density DNA probe assays, also known as "DNA chips".

H. Single and multi-locus sequence typing

As the logical next step, sequencing of PCR-amplified gene(s) is the most sensitive and accurate means of indexing localized yet genomically representative DNA polymorphisms for strain typing. Sequence analysis of ~700 bp PCR products, including variable repeat units of the coagulase gene (88) and of the protein A gene (89-90), provides strain discrimination of *S. aureus* that is more limited than PFGE but that has the advantages of shorter turnaround time, ease of interpretation, and complete inter-laboratory portability. Other types of gene targets that are successfully used for PCR sequence typing include the gene of an outer membrane protein of *Chlamydia trachomatis* (91) and the toxin regulatory gene of *Vibrio parahaemolyticus* (92).

The ultimate approach in sophistication for molecular epidemiology thus far is arguably the *multi-locus sequence typing* (MLST) scheme that was recently developed at the University of Oxford (16,93-96). The basic concept of multi-allele scoring with MLEE as a population genetics tool was transposed to the direct analysis of the nucleotide sequences from internal fragments of seven housekeeping genes. This method was validated for *N. meningitidis*, *Streptococcus pneumoniae*, and *S. aureus* (93-95). It is a biologically meaningful, accurate, and precise method that can index genomic polymorphism at representative and evolutionary neutral loci. The data are relevant for population genetics, evolutionary genetics, and global epidemiology (16, 93-96). Perfect exchangeability allows for database sharing between laboratories over the internet (http://mlst.zoo.ox.ac.uk). The usefulness of MLST for local and regional epidemiological studies remains to be ascertained. Despite improved automation and high throughput of nucleotide sequencers, the cost of the procedure is still limiting the use of this method.

VI. ANALYSIS AND INTERPRETATION OF MOLECULAR TYPING DATA

Like any scientific discipline, molecular epidemiology necessitates the formulation of clear and testable questions and hypotheses in order to provide useful data to the microbiologist, epidemiologist, and/or clinician. Although the question typically is narrowed down to the deceivingly simple: "are these microbial isolates clonally-related and does this means that they are part of the same chain of transmission?", the answer more often than not is much more complex and perhaps elusive. Therefore, one should avoid applying rigid interpretation rules. Instead, all of the biological, clinical, and epidemiological information that is available must always be considered simultaneously in order to arrive at an answer to these questions.

Among the practical issues that are to be considered include the possibility that composite populations made of several clones co-colonize an environmental reservoir or a human host. Therefore, three to five colonies of each morphological type should, as a rule, be picked from primary isolation plates and subcultured in parallel for identification, archival, and typing (1). This precaution minimizes the risk of erroneously rejecting the clonal link hypothesis, as a result of sample bias which leads to the typing of non-representative isolates from epidemic cases and/or suspected sources of infection.

Another important issue is that of the interpretation of minor differences in RFLP/amplification polymorphism (1-2). When a set of isolates show identical DNA banding patterns, this clue to clonality is proportional to the number of typing systems that are used and their discriminatory power. A problem arises when patterns are similar but not identical. What level of pattern similarity can be used to define clonally or epidemiologically related organisms? Again, there are no fixed rules; this threshold needs to be adjusted to the resolving power of the system, the genomic plasticity of the organism under study, and the time scale of the investigation (1-2). In practice, PFGE or AP-PCR pattern variation of three bands or less is likely to result from at least one genetic event, and the variation can be safely assumed to reflect subclonal evolution that occurs during an outbreak or as a consequence of persistent infection.

Table 4   Tenover's criteria for the interpretation of PFGE patterns for small isolate sets that are related to a putative outbreak (2).

Number of fragment differences versus the epidemic strain	Number of genetic differences	Category of genetic relatedness	Epidemiological interpretation
none	0	indistinguishable	part of the outbreak
2-3	1	closely related	probably part of the outbreak
4-6	2	possibly related	possibly part of the outbreak
>6	3 or more	different	not part of the

This level of variation is equivalent to coefficients of pattern similarity $\geq 80\%$ in many cases (1). Tenover and colleagues have published widely-accepted rules for interpretation of differences in PFGE patterns (Table 4) as applied to outbreak investigations whereby the gradual increase in the number of restriction fragment mismatches is equated with an increasing number of genetic differences and with a decreasing probability of epidemiological relatedness (2). For PFGE analysis, most polymorphisms appear related to large rearrangements rather than mutations which affect restriction sites (97).

Calculation of restriction pattern similarity coefficients and graphical display of pattern relatedness as dendrograms are also useful for interpretation, particularly for large scale studies (1,18,35,38,70). Such quantitative analysis, however, is invalid for phylogenetic inferences, because DNA fragment pattern variation does not reflect independent genetic events. Practically, this requires computer-assisted gel image acquisition, quality control check, pattern normalization, and calculation of a pair-wise matrix of pattern matching coefficients (Figure 3). These are calculated either from the comparison of densitometric curves or from fragment number and size, for which the Dice co-efficient is the formula most widely used, as previously described (1). From the similarity matrix, tree construction algorithms can be applied to display inter-type relatedness. The most neutral algorithm which is commonly used is the unweighted pair group method which uses arithmetic averages (UPGMA) (Figure 3).

VII. SELECTING AND IMPLEMENTING MOLECULAR TYPING SYSTEMS

Novel typing methods are being published at an amazing pace, and most "established" techniques and instruments undergo rapid evolution. Few methods have been rigorously evaluated and compared for their performance and efficiency. Any consensus as to the ideal typing method (1-2), or combination thereof, for a given pathogen is bound to become rapidly obsolete. In selecting methods for a clinical laboratory so that it can assist with surveillance and outbreak investigations, several criteria should be borne in mind. Firstly, the combined use of at least two methods is currently required for the confident assessment of clonality of bacterial isolates. Secondly, broad range typing systems that are great advantages to clinical or public health laboratories should be capable of typing a variety of bacterial or fungal pathogens. Thirdly, the method that is used should be highly discriminatory and should have excellent reproducibility at least within a single assay for outbreak studies and between assays for surveillance.

Molecular methods which have demonstrated epidemiological usefulness and rules for interpretation of results are to be preferred for routine use. Besides antimicrobial susceptibility testing and, where appropriate, serotyping, the methods that are currently best suited for hospital epidemiology are: PFGE, AP-PCR, rep-PCR, and AFLP genotyping methods. With increasing automation of PCR based techniques and with improving computer-assisted pattern recognition, automated DNA sequence-based microbial identification and typing systems are gaining a strong foothold in the clinical microbiology laboratory and are opening a new era of "microbial genodiagnostics".

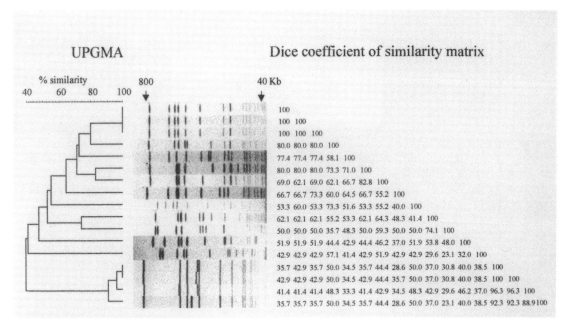

Figure 3   PFGE analysis of 17 strains of methicillin-resistant *Staphylococcus aureus* with various degrees of relatedness as assessed by *Sma*I restriction patterns (middle panel). The matrix of pairwise Dice similarity coefficient (right panel) was determined based on the basis of normalized patterns with the Bionumerics software and using 0.8% band matching tolerance. The left panel shows the dendrogram of similarity that was constructed from the matrix by the UPGMA method.

VIII. CONCLUSIONS AND PERSPECTIVES

Molecular typing systems are rapidly expanding our understanding of the epidemiology of endemic and epidemic infections. Phenotypically difficult-to-type bacterial pathogens are now demonstrated by molecular typing to cause common-source or cross-infection in the community and in hospitals (20,30,31,48). They are revealing a more complex epidemiology that is characterized by polyclonal infections and outbreaks that are due to multiple clones of the same species (22-29). The precision of techniques that index genomic polymorphism allows us to study in vivo micro-evolution of microorganisms (19,22,96).

From a public health perspective, molecular typing is now a standard laboratory service for hospital and community epidemiologists, and is applicable to outbreak studies and increasingly for local surveillance (1-2,27). Molecular genotyping is also becoming a key component of the large scale surveillance of infectious diseases and contributes to a description of their global epidemiology (35-39,54,92-

96). Future refinements of genotyping methods and their wider application will further unveil the epidemiology of bacterial infections and improve our preparedness to cope with emerging infections.

REFERENCES

1. Struelens MJ, and the Members of the European Study Group on Epidemiological Markers (ESGEM), of the European Society for Clinical Microbiology and Infectious Diseases (ESCMID). Consensus guidelines for appropriate use and evaluation of microbial epidemiologic typing systems. Clin Microbiol Infect 1996; 2:2-11.
2. Tenover FC, Arbeit RD, Goering RV, the Molecular Typing Working Group of the Society for Healthcare Epidemiology of America. How to select and interpret molecular typing methods for epidemiological studies of bacterial infections: a review for healthcare epidemiologists. Infect Control Hosp Epidemiol 1997; 18:426-439.
3. Vandamme P, Pot B, Gillis M, De Vos P, Kersters K and Swings J. Polyphasic taxonomy, a consensus approach to bacterial systematics. Microbiol Rev 1996;60:407-438.
4. Arber W. The generation of variation in bacterial genomes. J Mol Evol 1995; 40:7-12.
5. LeClerc J.E, Li B, Payne WL, Cebula TA. High mutation frequencies among *Escherichia coli* and *Salmonella* pathogens. Science 1996; 274:1208-1211.
6. Deitsch KW, Moxon ER, Wellems TE. Shared themes of antigenic variation and virulence in bacterial, protozoal, and fungal infections. Microbiol Mol Biol Rev 1997; 61:281-293.
7. De la Cruz F, Davies J. Horizontal gene transfer and the origin of species: lessons from bacteria. Trends Microbiol 2000; 8:128-133.
8. Hacker J, Blum-Oehler G, Müldorfer I, Tschäpe H. Pathogenenicity islands of virulent bacteria: structure, function and impact on microbial evolution. Mol Microbiol 1997; 23:1089-1097.
9. Berlyn MK. Linkage map of *Escherichia coli* K-12, edition 10: the traditional map. Microbiol Mol Biol Rev 1998; 62:814-984.
10. Lawrence JG, Ochman H. Molecular archaeology of the *Escherichia coli* genome. Proc Natl Acad Sci USA. 1998; 95:9413-9417.
11. Blattner FR, Plunkett III G, Bloch CA, Perna NT, Burland V, Riley M, Collado-Vides J, Rode GCK, Mayhew GF, Gregor J, Davis NW, Kirkpatrick HA, Goeden MA, Rose DJ, Mau B, Shao Y. The complete genome sequence of *Escherichia coli* K12. Science 1998; 277:1453-1474.
12. Alm, RA, Ling LSL, Moir DT, King BL, Brown ED, Doig PC, Smith DR, Noonan B, Guild BC, de Jong B, Carmel G, Tummino PJ, Caruso A, Uria-Nickelsen M, Merberg D, Mills SD, Jiang Q, Taylor DE, Vovis GF, Trust T. Genomic-sequence comparison of two unrelated isolates of the human gastric pathogen *Helicobacter pylori*. Nature 1999; 397:176-180.
13. Whittam TS, Ochman H, Selander RK. Multilocus genetic structure in natural populations of *Escherichia coli*. Proc Natl Acad Sci USA 1983; 80:1751-1755.
14. Tibayrenc M. Towards a unified evolutionary genetics of microorganisms. Ann Rev Microbiol 1996; 50:401-429.
15. Maynard-Smith J, Smith NH, O'Rourke M, Spratt BG. How clonal are bacteria? Proc Natl Acad. Sci USA 1993; 90:4384-4388.
16. Enright M, Spratt G. Multilocus sequence typing. Trends Microbiol 1999; 7:482-487.
17. Caugant DA, Froholm LO, Bovre K, Holten E, Frasch CE, Mocca LF, Zollinger WD, Selander RK. Intercontinental spread of a genetically distinctive complex of clones of *Neisseria meningitidis* causing epidemic disease. Proc Natl Acad Sci USA 1991; 83:4927-4931.
18. Struelens MJ, Deplano A, Godard C, Maes N, Serruys E. Epidemiologic typing and delineation of genetic relatedness of methicillin-resistant *Staphylococcus aureus* by macrorestriction analysis of genomic DNA by using pulsed-field gel electrophoresis. J Clin Microbiol 1992; 30:2599-2605.
19. Struelens MJ, Schwam V, Deplano A, Baran D. Genome macrorestriction analysis of diversity and variability of *Pseudomonas aeruginosa* strains infecting cystic fibrosis patients. J Clin Microbiol 1993; 31:2320-2326.
20. Römling U, Wingender J, Müller H, Tümmler B. A major *Pseudomonas aeruginosa* clone common to patients and aquatic habitats. Appl Environ Microbiol 1994; 60:1734-1738.
21. Echeita MA and Usera MA. Chromosomal rearrangements in *Salmonella enterica* serotype Typhi affecting molecular typing in outbreak investigations. J Clin Microbiol 1998; 36:2123-2126.

22. Kuipers EJ, Israel DA, Gerrits M, Weel J, van der Ende A, van der Hulst RWM, Wirth HP, Höök-Nikanne J, Thomson SA, Blaser M. Quasispecies development of *Helicobacter pylori* observed in paired isolates obtained years apart from the same host. J Infect Dis 2000; 118:273-282.

23. Van Wyngaerden E, Peetermans WE, Van Lierde S, Van Eldere J. Polyclonal staphylococcus endocarditis. Clin Infect Dis 1997; 25:69-71.

24. Hakim A, Deplano A, Maes N, Kentos A, Rossi C, Struelens MJ. Polyclonal coagulase-negative staphylococcal catheter-related bacteremia documented by molecular identification and typing. Clin Microbiol Infect 1999; 5:224-227.

25. de Viedma DG, Rabadan PM, Diaz M, Cercenado E, Bouza E. Heterogeneous antimicrobial resistance patterns in polyclonal populations of coagulase-negative staphylococci isolated from catheters. J Clin Microbiol 2000; 38:1359-1363.

26. Wendt C, Shawn A, Messer A, RJ Hollis, Pfaller MA, Wenzel RP, Herwaldt LA. Molecular epidemiology of Gram-negative bacteremia. Clin Infect Dis 1999; 28:605-610.

27. Struelens MJ, De Gheldre Y, Deplano A. Comparative and library epidemiological typing systems : outbreak investigations versus surveillance systems. Infect Control Hosp Epidemiol 1998; 19:565-569.

28. Struelens MJ, Rost F, Deplano A, Maas A, Schwam V, Serruys E, Cremer M. *Pseudomonas aeruginosa* and *Enterobacteriaceae* bacteremia after biliary endoscopy : an outbreak investigation using DNA macrorestriction analysis. Am J Med 1993; 95:489-498.

29. Villers D, Espaze E, Caste-Burel M, Giauffret F, Ninin E, Nicolas F, Richet H. Nosocomial *Acinetobacter baumannii* infections: microbiological and clinical epidemiology. Ann Intern Med 1998; 129:182-189.

30. Johnson S, Samore MH, Farrow KA, Killgore GE, Tenover FC, Lyras D, Rood JI, DeGirolami P, Baltch AL, Rafferty ME, Pear S, Gerding DN. Epidemics of diarrhea caused by a clindamycin-resistant strain of *Clostridium difficile* in four hospitals. N Engl J Med 1999; 341:1645-1651.

31. Aureli P, Fiorucci C, Caroli D, Marchiaro G, Novara O, Leone L, Salmosa S. An outbreak of febrile gastroenteritis associated with corn contaminated *by Listeria monocytogenes*. N Engl J Med 2000; 342:1236-1241.

32. Van Loo I, van der Heide GJ, Nagelkerke NJD, Verhoef J, Mooi FR. Temporal trends in the population structure of *Bordetella pertussis* during 1949-1996 in a highly vaccinated population. J Infect Dis 1999; 179: 915-924.

33. Hartstein AI, LeMonte AM, Iwamoto PKL. DNA typing and control of methicillin-resistant *Staphylococcus aureus* at two affiliated hospitals. Infect Cont Hosp Epidemiol 1997;18: 42-48.

34. Webster CA, Towner KJ. Use of RAPD-ALF analysis for investigating the frequency of bacterial cross-transmission in an adult intensive care unit. J Hosp Infect 2000; 44:254-260.

35. Deplano A, Witte W., Van Leewen WJ, Brun Y, Struelens MJ. Clonal dissemination of epidemic methicillin-resistant *Staphylococcus aureus* in Belgium and neighbouring countries. Clin Microbiol Infect 2000; 6:1-7.

36. Bauer J, Yang Z, Poulsen S, Andersen AB. Results from 5 years of nationwide DNA fingerprinting of *Mycobacterium tuberculosis* complex isolates in a country with a low incidence of *M. tuberculosis* infection. J Clin Microbiol 1998; 36:305-358.

37. Van Looveren M, Vandamme P, Hauchecorne M, Wijdooghe M, Carion F, Caugant DA, Goossens H. Molecular epidemiology of recent Belgian isolates of *Neisseria meningitidis* serogroup B. J Clin Microbiol 1998; 36:2828-2834.

38. Tassios PT, Gazouli M, Tzelepi E, Milch H, Kozlova N, Sidorenko S, Legakis NJ, Tzouvelekis LS. Spread of a *Salmonella* Typhimurium clone resistant to expanded-spectrum cephalosporins in three European countries. J Clin Microbiol 1999; 37:3774-3777.

39. De Sousa MA, Sanches IS, Ferro ML, Vaz MJ, Saraiva Z, Tendeiro T, Serra J, De Lencastre H. Intercontinental spread of a multidrug-resistant methicillin-resistant *Staphylococcus aureus* clone. J Clin Microbiol 1998; 36:2590-2596.

40. Davies T, Goering RV, Lovgren M, Talbot JA, Jacobs MR, Appelbaum PC. Molecular epidemiological survey of penicillin-resistant *Streptococcus pneumoniae* from Asia, Europe and North America. Diagn Microbiol Infect Dis 1999; 34:7-12.

41. Van Embden JDA, Cave MD, Crawford JT, Dale JW, Eisenach KD, Gicquel B, Hermans PWM, Martin C, Mcadam R, Shinnick TM, Small PM. Strain identification of *Mycobacterium tuberculosis* by DNA fingerprinting : recommendations for a standardized methodology. J Clin Microbiol 1993; 31:406-409.

42. Hunter PR. Reproducibility and indices of discriminatory power of microbial typing methods. J Clin Microbiol 1990; 28:1903-1905.

43. Rabkin CS, Jarvis WR, Anderson RL, Govan J, Klinger J, LiPuma J, Martone WJ, Monteil H, Richard C, Shigeta S, Sosa A, Stull T, Swenson J, Woods D. *Pseudomonas cepacia* typing systems: collaborative study to assess their potential in epidemiologic investigations. Rev Infect Dis 1989; 11:600-607.

44. Tenover FC, Arbeit R, Archer G, Biddle J, Byrne S, Goering R, Hancock G, Hébert A, Hill B, Hollis R, Jarvis WR, Kreiswirth B, Eisner W, Maslow J, McDougal LK, Miller MJ, Mulligan M, Pfaller MA. Comparison of traditional and molecular methods of typing isolates of *Staphylococcus aureus*. J Clin Microbiol 1994; 32:407-415.

45. Marcos MA, De Anta JMT, Vila J. Correlation of six methods for typing nosocomial isolates of *Acinetobacter baumannii*. J Med Microbiol 1995; 42:328-335.

46. Grundman H, Schneider C, Hartung D, Daschner FD, Pitt TL. Discriminatory power of three DNA-based typing techniques for *Pseudomonas aeruginosa*. J Clin Microbiol 1995; 33:528-534.

47. Fry NK, Alexiou-Daniel S, Bangsborg JM, Sverker B, Pastoris MC, Etienne J, Forsblom B, Gaia V, Helbig JH, Lindsay D, Lück C, Pelaz C, Uldum SA, Harrison TG. A multicenter evaluation of genotypic methods for epidemiologic typing of *Legionella pneumophila* serogroup 1: results of a pan-European study. Clin Microbiol Infect 1999; 5:462-477.

48. Burucoa C, Lhomme V and Fauchere JL. Performance criteria of DNA fingerprinting methods for typing of *Helicobacter pylori* isolates: experimental results and meta-analysis. J Clin Microbiol 1999; 37:4071-4080.

49. Kremer K, van Sollingen D, Frothingham R, Haas WH, Hermans PWM, Martin C, Palittapongarnpim P, Plikaytis BB, Riley LW, Yakrus MA, Musser JM, van Embden DA. Comparison of methods based on different molecular epidemiological markers for typing of *Mycobacterium tuberculosis* complex strains: interlaboratory study of discriminatory power and reproducibility. J Clin Microbiol 1999; 37:2607-2618.

50. Deplano A, Schuermans A, Van Eldere J, Witte W, Meugnier H, Etienne J, Grundmann H, Jonas D, Noordhoek GT, Dijkstra J, van Belkum A, van Leeuwen W, Tassios PT, Legakis NJ, van der Zee A, Bergmans A, Blanc DS, Tenover FC, Cookson BC, O'Neil G, Struelens MJ and the European Study Group on Epidemiological Markers of ESCMID. Multi-center evaluation of epidemiological typing of methicillin-resistant *Staphylococcus aureus* strains by repetitive element-PCR analysis. J Clin Microbiol 2000; 38:3527-3533..

51. Musser JM, Kapur V. Clonal analysis of methicillin-resistant *Staphylococcus aureus* strains from intercontinental sources: association of the *mec* gene with divergent phylogenetic lineages implies dissemination by horizontal transfer and recombination. J Clin Microbiol 1992; 30:2058-2063.

52. Mayer LW. Use of plasmid profiles in epidemiologic surveillance of disease outbreaks and in tracing the transmission of antibiotic resistance. Clin Microbiol Rev 1998; 1:228-243.

53. Hartstein AI, Phelps CL, Kwok RYY, Mulligan ME. In vivo stability and discriminatory power of methicillin-resistant *Staphylococcus aureus* typing by restriction endonuclease analysis of plasmid DNA compared with those of other molecular methods. J Clin Microbiol 1995; 33:2022-2026.

54. Wiener J, Quinn P, Bradford PA, Goering RV, Nathan C, Bush K, Weinstein RA. Multiple antibiotic-resistant *Klebsiella* and *Escherichia coli* in nursing homes. JAMA 1999; 281:517-523.

55. Owen RJ. Chromosomal DNA fingerprinting – a new method of species and strain identification applicable to microbial pathogens. J Med Microbiol 1989; 30:89-99.

56. Stanley J, Chowdry-Baquar N, Threlfall EJ. Genotypes and phylogenetic relationships of *Salmonella typhimurium* are defined by molecular fingerprinting of IS*200* and 16S *rrn* loci. J Gen Microbiol 1993; 139:1133-1140.

57. Bingen EH, Denamur E, Elion J. Use of ribotyping in epidemiological surveillance of nosocomial outbreaks. Clin Microbiol Rev 1994; 7:311-327.

58. Hollis RJ, Bruce JL, Fritschel SJ, Pfaller MA. Comparative evaluation of an automated ribotyping instrument versus pulsed-field gel electrophoresis for epidemiological investigation of clinical isolates of bacteria. Diagn Microbiol Infect Dis 1999; 34:263-268.

59. Struelens MJ, De Ryck R, Deplano A. Analysis of microbial genomic restriction patterns by pulsed-field gel electrophoresis (PFGE typing). In: Dijkshoorn L, Towner KJ, Struelens MJ - eds. New Approaches for the Generation and Analysis of Microbial Fingerprints. Amsterdam:Elsevier Science, (In press).

60. Towner K, Grundmann H. Generation and analysis of RAPD fingerprinting profiles. In: Dijkshoorn L, Towner KJ, Struelens MJ - eds. New Approaches for the Generation and Analysis of Microbial Fingerprints. Amsterdam:Elsevier Science, (In press).

61. Power EGM. RAPD typing in microbiology – a technical review. J Hosp Infect 1996; 34:247-265.

62. Tyler KD, Wang G, Johnson WM. Factors affecting reliability and reproducibility of amplification-based DNA fingerprinting of representative bacterial pathogens. J Clin Microbiol 1997; 35:339-346.

63. Louie M, Jayaratne P, Luchsinger I, Devenish J, Yao J, Schlech W, Simor A. Comparison of ribotyping, arbitrarily primed PCR, and pulsed-field gel electrophoresis for molecular typing of *Listeria monocytogenes*. J Clin Microbiol 1996; 34:15-19.

64. De Gheldre Y, Maes N, Rost F, De Ryck R, Clevenbergh P, Vincent JL, Struelens MJ. Molecular epidemiology of an outbreak of multidrug-resistant *Enterobacter aerogenes* infections and in vivo emergence of imipenem resistance. J Clin Microbiol 1997; 35:152-160.

65. van Belkum A, Kluytmans J, van Leeuwen W, Bax R, Quint W, Peters E, Fluid A, Vandenbroucke-Grauls C, van den Brule A, Koeleman H, Melchers W, Meis J, Elaichouni A, Vaneechoutte M, Moonens F, Maes N, Struelens M, Tenover F, Verbrugh H. Multicenter evaluation of arbitrarily primed PCR for typing of *Staphylococcus aureus* strains. J Clin Microbiol 1995; 33:1537-1547.

66. Grundmann HJ, Towner KJ, Dijkshoorn, Gerner-Smidt P, Maher M, Seifert H, Vaneechoutte M. Multicenter study using standardized protocols and reagents for evaluation of reproducibility of PCR-based fingerprinting of *Acinetobacter* spp. J Clin Microbiol 1997; 35:3071-3077.

67. Deplano A, Vaneechoutte M, Verschraegen G, Struelens MJ. Typing of *Staphylococcus aureus* and *Staphylococcus epidermidis* strains by PCR analysis of inter-IS256 spacer length polymorphisms. J Clin Microbiol 1997; 35:2580-2587.

68. Vos P, Hogers R, Bleeker M, Reijans M, Vandele T, Hornes M, Frijters A, Pot J, Peleman J, Kuiper M, Zabeau M. AFLP: a new technique for DNA fingerprinting. Nucleic Acids Res 1995; 23:4407-4414.

69. Mazurek GH, Reddy V, Marston BJ, Haas WH, Crawford JT. DNA fingerprinting by infrequent-restriction-site amplification. J Clin Microbiol 1996; 34:2386-2390.

70. Savelkoul PHM, Aarts HJM, de Haas J, Dijkshoorn L, Duim B, Otsen M, Rademaker JLW, Schouls L, Lenstra JA. Amplified-fragment length polymorphism analysis : the state of an art. J Clin Microbiol 1999; 37:3083-3091.

71. Desai M, Tanna A, Wall R, Efstratiou A, George R, Stanley J. Fluorescent amplified-fragment length polymorphism analysis of an outbreak of group A streptococcal invasive disease. J Clin Microbiol 1998; 36:3133-3137.

72. Gibson JR, Slater E, Xerry J, Tompkins DS, Owen RJ. Use of an amplified-fragment length polymorphism technique to fingerprint and differentiate isolates of *Helicobacter pylori*. J Clin Microbiol 1998; 36:2580-2585.

73. Goulding JN, Stanley J, Saunders N, Arnold C. Genome-sequence-based fluorescent amplified-fragment length polymorphism analysis of *Mycobacterium tuberculosis*. J Clin Microbiol 2000; 38:1121-1126.

74. Van Eldere J, Janssen P, Hoefnagels-Schuermans A, Van Lierde S, Peetermans WE. Amplified-fragment length polymorphism analysis versus macro-restriction fragment analysis for molecular typing of *Streptococcus pneumoniae* isolates. J Clin Microbiol 1999; 37:2053-2057.

75. Riffard S, Lo Presti F, Vandenesch F, Forey F, Reyrolle M, Etienne J. Comparative analysis of infrequent-restriction-site PCR and pulsed-field gel electrophoresis for epidemiological typing of *Legionella pneumophila* serogroup 1 strains. J Clin Microbiol 1998; 36:161-167.

76. Speijer H, Savelkoul PHM, Bonten MJ, Stobberingh EE, Tjhie JHT. Application of different genotyping methods for *Pseudomonas aeruginosa* in a setting of endemicity in an intensive care unit. J Clin Microbiol 1999; 37:3654-3661.

77. Fields PI, Blom K, Hughes HJ, Helsel LO, Feng P, Swaminathan B. Molecular characterization of the gene encoding H antigen in *Escherichi coli* and development of a PCR-restriction fragment length polymorphism test for identification of *E. coli* O157:H7 and O157:NM. J Clin Microbiol 1997; 35:1066-1070.

78. Nachamkin I, Ung H, Patton CM. Analysis of HL and O serotypes of *Campylobacter* strains by the flagellin gene typing system. J Clin Microbiol 1996; 34:277-281.

79. Newcombe J, Dyer S, Blackwell L, Cartwright K, Palmer WH, McFadden J. PCR-single stranded conformational polymorphism analysis for non-culture-based subtyping of meningococcal strains in clinical specimens. J Clin Microbiol 1997; 35:1809-1812.

80. Harrington CS, Thomson-Carter FM, Carter PE. Evidence for recombination in the flagellin locus of *Campylobacter jejuni*: implications for the flagellin gene typing scheme. J Clin Microbiol 1997; 35:2386-2392.

81. Hoefnagels-Schuermans A, Peetermans WE, Struelens MJ, Van Lierde S, Van Eldere J. Clonal analysis and identification of epidemic strains of methicillin-resistant *Staphylococcus aureus* by antibiotyping and determination of protein A gene and coagulase gene polymorphisms. J Clin Microbiol 1997; 35:2514-2520.

82. Calderwood SB, Baker MA, Carroll PA, Michel JL, Arbeit RD, Ausubel FM. Use of cleaved amplified polymorphic sequences to distinguish strains of *Staphylococcus epidermidis*. J Clin Microbiol 1996; 34:2860-2865.

83. van Leeuwen W, Sijmons M, Sluijs J, Verbrugh H, van Belkum A. On the nature and use of randomly amplified DNA from *Staphylococcus aureus*. J Clin Microbiol 1996; 34:2770-2777.

84. van Leeuwen W, Verbrugh H, van der Velden J, van Leeuwen N, Heck M, van Belkum A. Validation of binary typing for *Staphylococcus aureus* strains. J Clin Microbiol 1999; 37:664-674.

85. Kamerbeek J, Schould L, Kolk A, van Achterveld M, van Soolingen D, Kuijper S, Bunschoten A, Molhuyzen H, Shaw R, Goyal M, van Embden J. Simultaneous detection and strain differentiation of *Mycobacterium tuberculosis* for diagnosis and epidemiology. J Clin Microbiol 1997; 35:907-914.

86. van Doorn LJ, Figueiredo C, Rossau R, Jannes G, van Asbroeck M, Sousa JC, Carneiro F, Quint WGV. Typing of *Helicobacter pylori vacA* gene and detection of *cagA* gene by PCR and reverse hybridization. J Clin Microbiol 1998; 36:1271-1276.

87. Thomson DK, Deal CD, Ison CA, Zenilman J, Bash M. A typing system for *Neisseria gonorrhoeae* based on biotinylated oligonucleotide probes to PIB gene variable regions. J Infect Dis 2000; 181:1652-1660.

88. Schwarzkopf A, Karch H. Genetic variation in *Staphylococcus aureus* coagulase genes: potential and limits for use as epidemiological marker. J Clin Microbiol 1994; 32:2407-2412.

89. Shopsin B, Gomez M, Montgomery SO, Smith DH, Waddington M, Dodge DE, Bost DA, Riehman M, Naidich S, Kreiswirth BN. Evaluation of protein A gene polymorphic region DNA sequencing for typing of *Staphylococcus aureus* strains. J Clin Microbiol 1999; 37:3556-3563.

90. Tang YW, Waddington MG, Smith DH, Manahan JM, Kohner PC, Highsmith LM, Li H, Cockerill III FR, Thomson RL, Montgomery SO, Persing DH. Comparison of protein A gene sequencing with pulsed-field gel electrophoresis and epidemiologic data for molecular typing of methicillin-*resistant Staphylococcus aureus*. J Clin Microbiol 2000; 38:1347-1351.

91. Dean D, Schachter J, Dawson CR, Stephens RS. Comparison of the major outer membrane protein variant sequence regions of B/Ba isolates : a molecular epidemiologic approach to *Chlamydia trachomatis* infections. J Infect Dis 1992; 166:383-392.

92. Matsumoto C, Okuda J, Ishibashi M, Iwanaga M, Garg P, Rammamurthy T, Wong HC, Depaola A, Kim YB, Albert MJ, Nishibuchi M. Pandemic spread of an 03:K6 of *Vibrio parahaemolyticus* and emergence of related strains evidenced by arbitrarily primed PCR and *toxRS* sequence analyses. J Clin Microbiol 2000; 38:578-585.

93. Maiden MCJ, Bygraves JA, Feil E, Morelli G, Russel JE, Urwin R, Zhang Q, Zhou J, Zurth K, Caugant DA, Feavers IM, Achtman M, Spratt BG. Multilocus sequence typing: a portable approach to the identification of clones within populations of pathogenic microorganisms. Proc Natl Acad Sci USA 1998; 95:3140-3145.

94. Shi ZY, Enright MC, Wilkinson P, Griffiths D, Spratt BG. Identification of three major clones of multiply antibiotic-resistant *Streptococcus pneumoniae* in Taiwanese hospitals by multilocus sequence typing. J Clin Microbiol 1998; 36:3514-3519.

95. Enright MC, Day NP, Davies CE, Peacock SJ, Spratt BG. Multilocus sequence typing for characterization of methicillin-resistant and methicillin susceptible clones of *Staphylococcus aureus*. J Clin Microbiol 2000; 38:1008-1015.

96. Feil EJ, Maiden MC, Achtman M, Spratt BG. The relative contributions of recombination and mutation to the divergence of clones of *Neisseria meningitidis*. Mol Biol Evol 1999; 16:1496-1502.

97. Hall LMC, Duke B. Conservation of restriction sites in isolates of *Streptococcus pneumoniae* with diverse restriction fragment patterns. J Clin Microbiol 1998; 36:1805-1807.

8

Determination of Resistance to Antibacterials

John D. Turnidge and Jan M. Bell
Department of Microbiology and Infectious Diseases, Women's and Children's Hospital, North Adelaide, South Australia, Australia

I. INTRODUCTION

Susceptibility testing of bacteria is a routine practice in diagnostic microbiology among both medical and veterinary disciplines. Most modern routine methods evolved from those that were developed soon after antibiotics became part of clinical practice, and they involve either antibiotic dilution in liquid or solid media, an extension of the measurement of minimum inhibitory concentrations, or diffusion through agar. In recent times, these have been supplemented with tests to detect enzymes or resistance genes for specific organisms and resistance problems.

The performance of susceptibility testing requires discipline and strict adherence to written guidelines. Unlike culture and identification, the steps of susceptibility testing involve a large number of steps where error can be introduced. In addition, some methods are highly prone to interpretive error. These errors can be greatly compounded by misidentification of the organism.

The choice of methods for an individual laboratory is driven by a number of factors including staff resources, cost of consumables, volume of throughput, and level of access to expertise. Disc diffusion tests are the simplest and cheapest, while the semi-automated dilution breakpoint commercial systems are of the highest quality and can be the most rapid, but are considerably more expensive due to the cost of consumables. Many laboratories use two methods to cover the full range of common bacteria that require testing. It is important that each laboratory maintain expertise in more than one method, as well as ensure ready access to a reference laboratory to resolve problems or unusual results.

The title of this chapter has been deliberately chosen. Instead of 'susceptibility testing', laboratories need to come to terms with the idea that they are really testing for the presence of resistance. To emphasize this concept, Sanders has coined the phrase 'antimicrobial resistance testing (ART)' (1). It is a play on words which conveys that there are elements of art/craft as well as science in the practice of susceptibility testing.

II. BASIC CONSIDERATIONS

The importance of susceptibility is not confined to the generation of results which fall into susceptibility categories. Indeed, the four principal objectives for susceptibility testing are to:

1.   Provide guidance to the treating practitioner on appropriate therapy for the condition under treatment.
2.   Accumulate data on susceptibility patterns and local trends. Data generated should be able to feed into regional or national surveillance programs without major reinterpretation.
3.   Detect new or emerging resistances.
4.   Assist in the confirmation of isolate identification through the recognition of antibiograms.

The first objective is the most important to understand, and it revolves around the term 'guidance'. Susceptibility test results are not absolute; the result 'susceptible (S)' or 'sensitive' predicts success using that antibiotic for treatment, but does not guarantee it. Likewise, the result 'resistant (R)' does not imply that use of that antibiotic will always result in failure. It should be obvious that there are many other clinical factors that influence outcome of treatment, especially the natural resolution rate of the infection (there are very few diseases that are always fatal), the immunological status of the patient, whether there is a role for bacterial toxins in the disease process, and the presence of foreign bodies. The result 'S' really means "there is a high likelihood of treatment success with this antibiotic if there are no detrimental patient factors", and the result 'R' means "there is a variable likelihood of failure depending on how frequently this disease resolves without treatment".

Most antibacterial susceptibility test methods also employ the category 'intermediate (I)', which has a more complex meaning. For drugs with a large safety margin, the result 'intermediate' means that the agent is likely to be efficacious if higher doses are used or if it is concentrated at the site of infection (e.g., in urine). In the development of antifungal susceptibility tests, this meaning has been incorporated into the term 'susceptible dose-dependent' rather than' intermediate' (2). As a corollary, 'intermediate' means that the efficacy will be reduced compared to susceptible strains if standard doses are used. 'Intermediate' also serves a purpose in the conduct of the test. It provides a buffer zone to control for inherent errors in testing by ensuring that truly resistant strains are not falsely categorized as susceptible, and vice versa.

III. THEORETICAL BACKGROUND

Susceptibility testing is ultimately based on the minimum inhibitory concentration (MIC). The MIC as a concept was spawned early-on in the development of antimicrobials. It is defined simply as the lowest concentration of antimicrobial that inhibits the growth of a strain of organism in culture over a defined period of incubation (most often 24 hrs). In its simplest (and original) form, the MIC is measured by: a) performing a number of serial two-fold dilutions of an antibiotic (often 8-12) in series in a culture medium from a known starting concentration, b) adding a high inoculum of bacteria that is insufficient to impart turbidity, and c) incubating at 35°C for 16-24 hrs. At the end of incubation, the MIC is the lowest concentration that inhibits growth as demonstrated by the prevention of turbidity. The MIC as a concept has been often maligned but never improved upon.

As it is performed in an artificial system, the measurement of the MIC cannot mimic the environment in which a bacterium finds itself during an infection. Significant differences between the test system and the environment in vivo include the substantially lower in vitro inoculum, the non-fluctuating nature of the antimicrobial concentration in vitro, and the time over which the MIC test is conducted as compared to antibiotic treatment intervals. These discrepancies are generally irrelevant. The MIC is simply a measure of activity of an antimicrobial against a strain of a bacterium in the same way that a measure such as the metre or the foot is used as a reference for measurement of length. This measurement has proven to be a meaningful variable in the maturing science of antimicrobial pharmacodynamics (3).

The MIC is a value ascribed to an individual strain of a bacterium, and is not identical for all susceptible strains of a species with the same resistance mechanism. Instead, each species will demonstrate a range of MICs for susceptible strains and different ranges for each resistance mechanism. These ranges are 'lognormally' distributed, as one might expect for any drug-receptor interaction. Thus, the two-fold dilution method of measuring MICs – a base 2 logarithmic series and devised for reasons of convenience and simplicity – turns out to be the 'correct' method.

The importance of this 'log-normal' distribution should not be underestimated. It is widely accepted that the 'error' of the test is one two-fold dilution. At very low MICs, such 'errors' have trivial effects. At higher MICs, however, especially those close to levels that are achievable during treatment, the 'error' can lead to serious misclassification of susceptibility. For instance, an antibiotic with normal intravenous doses gives a peak concentration of 30 mg./L. and a trough concentration of 10 mg./L. A strain of a bacterium with a MIC of 1 mg./L. implies that the MIC is in the range of 0.5 to 2 mg./L.; both values being well below those achieved clinically. If another strain has a MIC of 16 mg./L., the true value lies in the range of 8-32 mg./L. Given the upper end of this range, one would be very uncertain about whether this organism is covered by normal antibiotic doses. To compensate for this problem, many methods attempt to keep breakpoint values a reasonable number of dilutions lower than clinically achievable drug levels (see later for a discussion of breakpoints).

IV. MIC TESTING

Unfortunately, there is no internationally-agreed reference method for performing MICs despite efforts 30 years ago to achieve this (4). The most widely accepted methods at present are those that are recommended by the NCCLS of the U.S. in a dedicated guideline (5). The NCCLS guidelines describe broth macrodilution, broth microdilution, and agar dilution methods using Mueller-Hinton media which may have specialized supplements in some cases. Other media, such as Sensitest (6), Isosensitest (7), and PDM-ASM (8) are recommended for methods in other countries. Whether these media give comparable results for all organism-antimicrobial combinations is not known. Many countries have adopted methods very similar to the NCCLS guidelines as reference methods.

The broth macrodilution method is the original method, performed in standard laboratory tubes in broth volumes of 1 mL. The simplest dilution technique for this method, starting with 2 mL. at the highest concentration, and serially transferring 1mL volumes to subsequent tubes containing 1 mL. of broth, is not recommended because there can be a compound error at the end of the dilution series. Instead, it is preferred to use four or five starting concentrations from stock solutions (5). Ideally two controls are used: one with broth but neither drug nor inoculum (broth control), and one with broth and inoculum but no drug (growth control). The preferred inoculum is 5×10^5 colony-forming units (CFU) per mL.

The broth microdilution test is performed in 100 µL. volumes in microtitre trays, but in most other ways, it resembles the broth macrodilution test. The agar dilution method involves the incorporation of the antibiotic dilutions into molten agar, and the pouring of plates which contain the individual drug concentrations. The inoculum is placed directly onto the plates, from the lowest to the highest concentration in the agar dilution method, usually with the use of a device with multiple 'pins' called a replicator.

The two methods differ from the broth macrodilution method in having lower inocula. The total inoculum in the broth microdilution is one-tenth that of broth macrodilution, while for agar the inoculum it is around 10^4 per spot.

In most cases, the inoculum for MIC tests can be prepared from either a short-term subculture to initiate log-phase growth, or directly from plate culture. The most common method of inoculum standardization is by comparison to a turbidity standard, usually 0.5 McFarland, or the photometric/nephelometric equivalent. For most organisms, incubation at 35°C for 18-24 hrs. is adequate to reach a readable endpoint.

V. DEFINITIONS OF RESISTANCE

The term *resistance* has several meanings in relationship to susceptibility testing and antibiotic use. Ambiguities can result particularly at the interface of the laboratory and the clinician.

Intrinsic resistance (natural or inherent resistance) to an antibiotic in a bacterial species means that the antibiotic will never be able to cover the species with treatment doses because the normal MIC range is near or above the levels of drug that are reached in vivo. Intrinsic resistance is the corollary of the spectrum of an antibiotic. Those species that are normally outside the spectrum are intrinsically resistant. Most intrinsic resistance comes about because the species possesses a target with reduced affinity for the antibiotic, or because the antibiotic is prevented from reaching the target. In some cases, it results from the possession of a naturally-degrading enzyme. By way of example, *Enterobacteriaceae* and non-fermentative Gram negative bacteria are resistant to many antibiotics as the result of their specialized outer membranes that are capable of excluding the penetration of many antibiotic classes. In some instances, intrinsic resistance is due to mechanisms that are analogous or identical to those that are seen in acquired resistance. For example, several genera in the family *Enterobacteriaceae* such as *Klebsiella* and *Enterobacter* naturally possess ß-lactamases. A more complete list of intrinsic resistances is provided in Table 9 of Section XIV.

Acquired resistance means that the bacterium has acquired a resistance mechanism (coded by one or more new or mutated genes) that has raised the MIC to a greater or lesser extent above the normal range. Occasionally, the acquisition of the resistance mechanism may have no discernible effect at all on the MIC. The clinical significance of this phenomenon is mostly unknown, and as one would expect, the presence of the resistance [gene(s)] will go undetected in routine susceptibility testing. In relationship to bacteria that have acquired resistance mechanisms that are similar or identical to those seen as intrinsic in other species, a species with intrinsic resistance would be the original source of the resistance gene in most instances.

Ambiguity also arises between the research laboratory and the routine laboratory when describing resistance. For research purposes, the term resistance is normally used to imply the presence of a resistance mechanism whether shown phenotypically (raised MIC) or genotypically. In the routine testing, resistance means that the resistance breakpoint, as defined by the method, has been exceeded, and it indicates the clinical meaning described under II. Basic Considerations, above, which relates to the result with the likely outcome of treatment using that antibiotic. These two different meanings can be summarized as *microbiological resistance* and *clinical resistance*. In Section VII below, the focus is microbiological resistance, while in the discussion of breakpoints in Section VIII and the interpretation of test results in Section X, clinical resistance is implied.

VI. ANTIBIOTIC CLASSIFICATION

Table 1 details antibacterial agents that are generally available in various countries around the world. It is important for the laboratory to be familiar with the agents in this list that are available in any individual country so that appropriate interpretations and extrapolation of results are made.

VII. MECHANISMS OF ACTION AND RESISTANCE

In order to understand the basis of susceptibility testing, a brief overview of mechanisms of action and resistance to the various groups of antimicrobials is required. Resistance can be generated in one of seven ways:

(i)   production of an inactivating enzyme (by degrading or modifying),
(ii)   alteration of target site by mutation in the coding gene,
(iii)   alteration of target site by enzymatic modification,
(iv)   production of an additional functional target with poor drug affinity,
(v)   overproduction of the target,
(vi)   active afflux of the drug from the cell, and
(vii)   reduced uptake of drug into cell or onto binding site.

A. ß-lactams

The ß-lactams in clinical use include the penicillins (penams), the cephalosporins (cephems and carbacephems), the monobactams and the carbapenems. All are based on the 4-membered cyclic entity called the ß-lactam ring. ß-lactams act on the cell wall synthetic and modelling enzymes, often called penicillin-binding proteins (PBPs) (9). Each species has a different complement of PBPs, 3-6 in number usually. The most important PBPs are the transpeptidases which are responsible for the cross-linking of the pentapeptide side chains of the peptidoglycan backbone. ß-lactams mimic the D-alanine ends of these pentapeptides and therefore attach to the active binding site of the transpeptidases thereby inhibiting their action.

1. *β-lactamases*

ß-lactamases are enzymes that break the ß-lactam ring between the nitrogen and carboxyl group and result in complete loss of activity (10). There is a vast array of ß-lactamases now recognized, and there are formal systems of classification (11). ß-lactamases can be either acquired or intrinsic; that is, the genes can be acquired from other bacteria or are a natural part of the species. Some ß-lactamases are excreted extracellularly in large amounts which thus makes them relatively easy to detect directly by routine methods, while others remain trapped behind outer membranes and are difficult to detect directly in routine testing. For the latter, their presence can be often be inferred by antibiograms and response to inhibitors of ß-lactamase. Like antibiotics themselves, ß-lactamases have a spectrum of activity. Some affect predominantly penicillins, while others prefer cephalosporins as a target. ß-lactamases may also differ in their response to inhibitors of ß-lactamase.

2. *Altered penicillin-binding proteins*

Altered penicillin-binding proteins are usually encoded by acquired resistance genes rather than occurring because of mutations in the normal PBP genes (12). Altered PBPs retain their function but have significantly reduced binding affinity for ß-lactams. This reduced affinity will affect most or all ß-lactams simultaneously, but will not necessarily generate resistance to all ß-lactams as some agents with high potency will still be reasonably active despite raised MICs. ß-lactamase inhibitors have no effect on altered PBPs.

B. Aminoglycosides

Aminoglycosides act by inhibiting protein synthesis at the ribosomal level. In addition, they cause misreading of the genetic code and result in the production of nonsense proteins. Unlike other classes that act at the ribosomal level, these agents are bactericidal (13).

Table 1   Members of antibiotic classes that are used for the therapy of infections due to bacteria.
This list excludes specific antimycobacterial agents.

Class	Subclass	Group	Members
ß-lactams	Penicillins (Penams)	Narrow spectrum penicillins	Benzylpenicillin (penicillin G) Phenoxymethylpenicillin (penicillin V) Phenethicillin Procaine penicillin Benzathine penicillin
		Moderate spectrum penicillins	Ampicillin (and its esters) Amoxycillin Cyclacillin Hetacillin Mecillinam (amdinocillin)
		Antistaphylococcal (including isoxazoyl penicillins[a])	Methicillin[a] Oxacillin[a] Cloxacillin[a] Flucloxacillin[a] Dicloxacillin[a] Nafcillin
		Antipseudomonal (including carboxypenicillins[b] and ureidopenicillins[c])	Carbenicillin[b] Ticarcillin[b] Azlocillin[c] Mezlocillin[c] Piperacillin[c]
		Beta-lactamase inhibitor combinations	Amoxycillin-clavulanate Ampicillin-sulbactam Ticarcillin-clavulanate Piperacillin-tazobactam
	Cephalosporins (Cephems and Carbacephems)	1st generation	Cephalothin Cephalexin Cephaloridine Cefadroxil Cefazolin Cephapirin Cephradine
		2nd generation (including carbacephems[d])	Cefamandole Cefaclor Cefuroxime Ceforanide Cefonicid Cefprozil Cefmetazole Loracarbef[d]
ß-lactams	Cephalosporins	Cefamycins	Cefoxitin Cefotetan
		3rd generation	Cefotaxime Ceftriaxone Cefoperazone Cefpodoxime Cefixime

Table 1 cont'd.

Class	Subclass	Group	Members
			Ceftibuten
			Ceftizoxime
			Ceftazidime
			Cefdinir
		4th generation	Cefpirome
			Cefepime
	Carbapenems		Imipenem
			Meropenem
			Panipenem
	Monobactams		Aztreonam
Aminoglycosides and aminocyclitols (topical only[e])			Streptomycin
			Neomycin (includes framycetin)[f]
			Kanamycin
			Gentamicin
			Tobramycin
			Paromomycin
			Netilmicin
			Amikacin
			Dibekacin
			Arbekacin
Quinolones		1st generation	Nalidixic acid
			Oxolinic acid
			Cinoxacin
		2nd generation (fluoroquinolones)	Norfloxacin
			Ciprofloxacin
			Enoxacin
			Fleroxacin
			Lomefloxacin
			Ofloxacin
			Levofloxacin
			Pefloxacin
			Rufloxacin
			Balofloxacin
		3rd generation (fluoroquinolones)	Sparfloxacin
			Grepafloxacin
			Tosufloxacin
			Trovafloxacin
			Moxifloxacin
			Gatifloxacin
MLSK	Macrolides	14-membered	Erythromycin
			Troleandomycin
			Roxithromycin
			Clarithromycin
			Dirithomycin
		15-membered	Azithromycin
		16-membered	Spiramycin
	Lincosamides		Lincomycin
			Clindamycin
	Streptogramins	Streptogramins B	Pristinamycin I

Table 1 cont'd.

Class	Subclass	Group	Members
			Quinupristin
		Streptogramins A (combined with Streptogramins B)	Pristinamycin II Dalfopristin
	Ketolides		Telithromycin
Tetracyclines			Tetracycline Chlortetracycline Oxytetracycline Methacycline Doxycycline Minocycline Demeclocycline (not used as an antibacterial)
Glycopeptides			Vancomycin Teicoplanin
Sulphonamides (topical only[f], used in combination with a dihydrofolate reductase inhibitor[g])			Sulfamethizole Sulfamethoxazole[g] Sulfadiazine Sulfadoxine[g] Sulfisoxazole Silver sulfadiazine[f] Sulfacetamide[f]
Dihydrofolate reductase inhibitors			Trimethoprim Pyrimethamine
Polymyxins			Polymyxin B Colistin Colistin methanesulfonate
Polypeptides (topical only)			Bacitracin
Nitroimidazoles			Metronidazole Tinidazole Ornidazole
Phenicols			Chloramphenicol Thiamphenicol
Rifamycins			Rifampicin Rifabutin Rifaximin
Nitrofurans			Nitrofurantoin Furazolidone
Fosfomycins			Fosfomycin and esters
Fusidanes			Fusidic acid (sodium fusidate)
t-RNA inhibitors (topical only)			Mupirocin
Oxazolidinones			Linezolid
Coumermycins			Novobiocin

1. Aminoglycoside-modifying enzymes

The most common mechanism of resistance to aminoglycosides is the production to enzymes that modify their structure through the addition of molecules to active attachment sites thus rendering them inactive (12). There are three basic types of aminoglycoside-modifying enzymes: phosphoryltransferases (APH), acetyltransferases (AAT), and nucleoside transferases (ANT). Some enzymes are bifunctional. A strict nomenclature exists for each of these enzyme types, and it defines the sites of action of the enzyme (12). Each enzyme has a spectrum of activity against different aminoglycosides. Both Gram positive and Gram negative bacteria can harbour aminoglycoside-modifying enzymes. Unlike ß-lactamases, there are no routine methods that are available to detect the activity of the aminoglycoside-modifying enzymes. For some bacteria, their existence is inferred from the phenotype of resistance (MIC).

2. Reduced uptake

Reduced uptake of aminoglycosides is found as a mechanism of resistance in some bacteria, especially non-fermentative Gram negative bacilli (12). It is a natural phenomenon within small subpopulations of all susceptible strains of *Pseudomonas aeruginosa* and *Stenotrophomonas maltophilia*.

C. Quinolones

Quinolones, including the fluoroquinolones, affect DNA synthesis by inhibiting topoisomerases which are the enzymes that are involved in the coiling and uncoiling of DNA so that it can be packaged and read. The principal topoisomerase target in most susceptible bacteria is DNA gyrase, which possesses two subunits: GyrA and GyrB. Quinolones attack the GyrA subunit. In some bacteria, such as *S. pneumoniae*, a second target, topoisomerase IV which also has two subunits (ParC and ParE), is the primary target of quinolone action. Resistance can be either due to mutations in topoisomerases or to drug efflux (12).

1. Altered topoisomerases

The most common form of quinolone resistance follows mutations in the genes and encodes the topoisomerase subunits GyrA, ParC, or ParE. Mutations occur in a region of the genes that encode these subunits called the quinolone-resistance determining region (QRDR). Resistance results from reduced quinolone binding to the subunit. In bacteria which are highly susceptible to the fluoroquinolones, multiple mutations in either a single gene or more commonly multiple subunit genes are required for clinical resistance to be achieved. This type of resistance can be found in a wide range of bacteria.

2. Efflux

More recently, resistance due to drug efflux has been described in Gram negatives and staphylococci. Some are related to multiple antibiotic resistance operons as noted for tetracyclines above. Other specific efflux genes have been described.

D. Macrolides, lincosamides, streptogramins B, and ketolides

Macrolides, lincosamides, streptogramins B, and ketolides (MLS$_B$K) all act at the same site, namely the 50S ribosomal level. They inhibit protein synthesis and are generally bacteriostatic, but are bactericidal against the streptococci. 14- and 15-membered macrolides are generally equally affected by the same resistance mechanisms while 16-membered macrolides are often unaffected (14).

1. Ribosomal binding site methylation

The best-described mechanism of resistance to the MLS$_B$K group is through the acquisition of a gene that encodes for an enzyme that methylates the ribosomal binding site of these drugs (14). All these genes have the *erm* epithet. There are many different *erm* genes and each predominate in different species of bacteria. Due to methylation, some or all of the class are unable to bind. In some strains, an additional gene codes for a control peptide that controls the expression of the methylation gene and leads to inducible resistance. Mutations in the control peptide gene results in constitutive, and generally broader, resistance to the group.

2. Efflux

Recently, resistance to the MLS_BK group through active efflux of the drug has been described (12). This type of resistance turns out to be quite common in some bacteria, especially in streptococci, where it is coded for by the *mef* class of genes.

3. Inactivation

Although MLS_BK have no clinically useful activity against enteric Gram negative bacilli, high-level resistance that results from macrolide inactivation has been described (12). Mostly, inactivation is due to the presence of esterases.

E. Tetracyclines

Tetracyclines act by inhibiting protein synthesis at the level of the 30S ribosomal subunit. Resistance can result from antibiotic efflux, ribosomal protection, or reduced uptake (12).

1. Efflux

The only common mechanism of resistance to tetracyclines is active efflux of the drug. A number of different efflux pumps are involved and are coded for by a range of efflux genes that are widely dispersed in pathogenic and commensal bacteria. All of these genes have the *tet* epithet, but the epithet is not confined to this mechanism of resistance.

2. Other resistance mechanisms

Tetracycline resistance may also result from ribosomal protection due to the production of a protein that reverses the tetracycline effect on the ribosome or due to reduced uptake from induction/mutation of the multiple antibiotic resistance op eron (*marRAB*) in Gram negative bacteria.

F. Glycopeptides

Glycopeptides act on cell-wall peptidoglycan synthesis. These agents bind to the D-alanine-D-alanine terminus of the pentapeptide side chains of peptidoglycan thus preventing cross-linking by steric interference. A small number of Gram positive bacteria are naturally resistant to vancomycin, because their pentapeptide ends in D-alanine-D-serine to which glycopeptides bind poorly.

1. Target modification

Acquired glycopeptide resistance in enterococci results from target modification (15). A proportion of pentapeptides that end in D-alanine-D-lactate are produced, to which glycopeptides bind poorly, and pentapeptides ending in D-alanine-D-alanine are degraded by a complex series of genes. Five types of resistance in enterococci have been described (VanA to VanE), of which only VanA and VanB are common, while VanC is important for the intrinsic resistance (from D-alanine-D-serine) in the less common enterococcal species, *Enterococcus casseliflavus* and *Enterococcus gallinarum*.

2. Target overproduction

Resistance to glycopeptides in *Staphylococcus* species has recently been discovered. The putative mechanism is the overproduction of peptidoglycan (16).

G. Folate antagonists (sulfonamides and trimethoprim)

Folate antagonists act by inhibiting the production of tetrahydrofolate (THF), an essential co-factor for enzymes that are involved in a range of cell reactions, especially the synthesis of thymidylate (and hence DNA synthesis). All cells require THF; human cells can take up exogenous folate, but bacteria and some parasites cannot and must synthesize their own. Sulfonamides and trimethoprim inhibit sequential steps in THF synthesis, dihydropteroate synthetase (of which p-aminobenzoic acid is a substrate), and dihydrofolate reductase respectively, and thus their combination can be synergistic. There are three well-described mechanisms of resistance (17).

1.   Overproduction of target enzyme

One common form of sulfonamide resistance follows mutations that result in overproduction of p-aminobenzoic acid which competes with sulfonamides.

2.   Altered target enzyme

Some trimethoprim resistance follows mutations which lead to the production of a dihydrofolate reductase that has reduced trimethoprim affinity.

3.   Additional less-susceptible target

Enterobacteriaceae with high-level trimethoprim resistance usually have acquired a new plasmid-borne gene that codes for a reduced affinity dihydrofolate reductase. Similar types of genes are found in staphylococci. Resistance to sulfonamides can also be due to the acquisition of plasmid-borne genes which encodes a reduced affinity dihydropteroate synthetase.

H. Other agents

1.   Phenicols

Chloramphenicol acts on protein synthesis at the ribosomal level by binding to the 50S subunit and inhibiting peptidyltransferase. Resistance to chloramphenicol is most often due to the acquisition of degrading enzymes called chloramphenicol acetyltransferases (CAT) (12). Both Gram negative bacteria and staphylococci have been shown to harbour varieties of CAT. Multiple antibiotic resistance operons can also result in chloramphenicol resistance among Gram negative bacteria. Decreased permeability also accounts for resistance in some species.

2.   Rifamycins

Rifamycins directly inhibit DNA-dependent RNA polymerase. Resistance to these agents results from mutations, often already present in low numbers among populations of bacteria being targeted, in the gene that encodes the target enzyme, and these consequently result in a major reduction of drug affinity.

3.   Nitroimidazoles

Nitroimidazoles act to disrupt DNA after intracellular conversion to a short-lived, highly toxic metabolic intermediate by nitroreductase. Resistance may result from reduced uptake, failure to convert to the toxic metabolite, or the production of enzymes that are able to scavenge free radicals such as the active metabolic ingredient.

4. Nitrofurans

The mechanism of action of nitrofurans is poorly understood, but appears to involve damage to DNA (18). There are little data on mechanisms whereby bacteria become resistant to these agents.

5. Fusidanes

The action of fusidic acid relates to its ability to inhibit protein synthesis at the level of the ribosome by inhibiting an enzyme called elongation factor G. Resistance occurs through a number of mechanisms, the most common being alteration of elongation factor G. Plasmid-encoded altered permeability may account for some resistance as well (19).

VIII. DETERMINATION OF BREAKPOINTS

Breakpoints are defined values that categorize susceptibility test results into 'susceptible', 'intermediate', and 'resistant'. They may or may not vary for different bacteria with each antibiotic. Reference breakpoints are concentrations of antibiotic within the two-fold dilution series as discussed above. For dilution and gradient diffusion susceptibility testing, these reference breakpoints are the same as those used in testing. For disc diffusion testing, zone diameters are calibrated to the reference dilution concentrations.

A. Reference dilution and gradient diffusion breakpoints

The setting of reference breakpoints is a somewhat arcane process for the average user of susceptibility testing. Usually, a variety of different data are examined and applied for their determination. The different methods that are developed in different countries around the world use all or only some of the data sets that are described here.

1. MIC distributions

Each species of bacterium has its own individual MIC distribution for an antibiotic which is influenced by that species' version of the antibiotic's target, by any mechanisms that promote or inhibit the antibiotic's access to the target, and by the presence of any strains within the species that harbour an acquired resistance mechanism. When an acquired resistance is present in some strains, their MICs are usually high enough to result in a bimodal MIC distribution. A natural 'breakpoint' is thus defined between the upper end of the MIC distribution of normal strains and the lower end of the MIC distribution of strains with the acquired resistance mechanism. If there is a range of concentrations between the upper and lower ends of the two distributions, a natural 'intermediate' category is defined. Alternatively, the MICs of those with acquired resistance may overlap to a greater or lesser extent with normal strains, leading to a skewing of the upper tail of the distribution. In the latter case, the authority which sets the breakpoints may need to weigh up the value of including susceptible strains into an intermediate or resistant category against the problem of classifying intermediate or resistant strains as susceptible. This situation is analogous to that which is seen with biochemical and hematological tests where a value that is used to define abnormality intersects the distribution of both normal and abnormal values, and thus leads to a sensitivity and specificity of the test with that intersecting value.

2. Pharmacokinetics

Pharmacokinetics describes the time-related movement of drug through the body – absorption, distribution, metabolism, and elimination. Outputs of pharmacokinetics are parameters such at plasma peak levels, areas-under-the-curve (AUC), elimination half-lives, and tissue penetration into certain body compartments. Some international methods (e.g., those of Britain and Japan) apply formulas that employ pharmacokinetic values directly in the calculation of breakpoints.

3. Pharmacodynamics

Pharmacodynamics describes the time-related action of antibiotics on bacteria. Parameters of interest include MIC, bacteriostatic versus bactericidal activity, concentration-dependent inhibition or killing, and delayed re-growth after drug removal (the post-antibiotic effect). Recently, these pharmacodynamics and pharmacokinetics have been integrated to develop parameters that predict bacteriological efficacy during treatment. Three parameters are now defined: peak/MIC ratio, AUC/MIC ratio, and time above MIC. Each drug class has one of these parameters as its principal parameter of efficacy, and there are increasingly better-defined optimum values for each antibiotic class/parameter pair. Since these parameters involve the MIC, it is possible to define pharmacodynamic breakpoints from the optimum values for the antibiotic class/parameter pair.

4. Clinical and bacteriological response rates

During antibiotic development, extensive clinical studies are conducted with several dosing schedules. Clinical outcomes (rates of cure, improvement, or failure) and bacteriological outcomes (rates of eradication or persistence) are the primary determinants of such studies. If the MIC of the infecting pathogen is measured as part of the study, it is possible to relate the clinical and bacteriological response rates to the MIC.

5. Other data

For some bacteria, a particular resistance mechanism may increase MICs to levels that are well within achievable levels during treatment. Nevertheless, failure may have been observed in clinical studies or may be feared such that we might consider clinical studies unethical and the consequences of failure too serious to risk. Detection of this resistance mechanism may thus take precedence over other considerations.

Unfortunately, there are no fixed algorithms for the application of these data sets to the setting of breakpoints. For each antibiotic, breakpoints as determined independently from these data sources may be weighed, and final values may be set to conservative values so as to ensure at least a small margin of error in testing.

IX. REPRESENTATIVE TESTING AND EXTRAPOLATIONS

It is not possible for the routine laboratory to test every antibiotic that is available to their clients. Fortunately in several instances, single agents can be used to represent a group or even a class of antibiotics as listed in Table 1. Table 2 provides guidance on these test agents, the results that may be extrapolated, the agents to which they may be extrapolated, and the species for which these extrapolations are valid.

X. ROUTINE SUSCEPTIBILITY TESTING METHODS

A range of options is available to the diagnostic laboratory for routine susceptibility testing. Over the last 30 years, several countries have developed local standardized methods for dilution and diffusion testing (Table 3). The choice of methods has therefore been driven somewhat by local influences. Despite efforts in the early 1970s, there are no agreed international standards. Readers are referred to the 1971 ICS publication for an excellent description of the basis of susceptibility testing as it was understood at the time (4). Since then, the broader range of considerations in setting breakpoints has been included into the improvement of many of the methods.

Of all methods, the NCCLS and the CASFM are the only ones that have a structured regular update process. The NCCLS methods are the reference standards, and NCCLS breakpoints the default,

Table 2   Antibacterial agents for which susceptibility can be extrapolated.

Test agent	Result[a]	Mechanism of resistance[b]	Species for which inference is valid	Agents for which results can be inferred (see Table 1 for groups)
Benzylpenicillin	S,I,R	ß-lactamase	*Staphylococcus* spp. *N. gonorrhoeae*	Narrow spectrum penicillins Moderate spectrum penicillins Antipseudomonal penicillins
Oxacillin	S,I,R	altered PBP	*Staphylococcus* spp.	Narrow spectrum penicillins, Moderate spectrum penicillins Antipseudomonal penicillins Antistaphylococcal penicillins Beta-lactamase inhibitor combinations All cephalosporins Carbapenems
Ampicillin	S,I,R	ß-lactamase	*Haemophilus* spp. *Enterobacteriaceae*	Moderate spectrum penicillins
Cephalothin	S	-	*Enterobacteriaceae*	All cephalosporins (S)
Cephalothin	I,R	ß-lactamase	*Enterobacteriaceae*	1st generation cephalosporins except cefazolin
Cefotaxime	S	-	*Enterobacteriaceae*	3rd and 4th generation cephalosporins (S) (except *Klebsiella oxytoca*)
Erythromycin	S,I,R	*erm* and *mef* encoded resistance	*Staphylococcus* spp. *Streptococcus* spp.	14-membered macrolides 15-membered macrolides
Clindamycin	S,I,R	various mechanisms	*Staphylococcus* spp. *Streptococcus* spp.	Lincosamides
Tetracycline	S,I,R	various mechanisms	*Enterobacteriaceae* *Streptococcus* spp.	Tetracyclines
Sulfisoxazole or other sulfa agent	S,I,R	various mechanisms	all species	Sulphonamides
Nalidixic acid	S	-	*Enterobacteriaceae*	Quinolones (S)
Chloramphenicol	S,I,R	various mechanisms	all species	Phenicols
Vancomycin	S	-	*Staphylococcus* spp. *Streptococcus* spp. *Enterococcus* spp.	Glycopeptides (S)

[a] S – susceptible; I – intermediate susceptibility; R – resistant; [b] PBP – penicillin-binding protein.

Table 3   International standards for routine susceptibility testing methods.

Method name and reference	Country	Organization	Type	Main medium	Comments
BSAC (7,20)	Great Britain and Ireland	British Soc. for Antimicrobial Chemotherapy	Breakpoint dilution	Iso-Sensitest	for high throughput laboratories
			Comparative and Stoke's	Iso-Sensitest	no longer recommended
			Disc diffusion	Iso-Sensitest	new standard
CASFM (21,22)	France	Société Francaise de Microbiologie	Dilution and disc diffusion	Mueller-Hinton	regular updates
DIN (23)	Germany	Deutches Institut fur Normung	Dilution and disc diffusion	Mueller- Hinton (other media if calibrated)	irregular updates
WRG (24)	Netherlands	Werkgroep Richtlijnen Gevoeligheids-bepalingen	Dilution and disc diffusion	Iso-Sensitest	
SIR (8,25-27)	Sweden	Swedish Reference Group for Antibiotics	Disc diffusion	PDM-ASM	zone diameter (microbiological) breakpoints
Neo-sensitabs (28)	Denmark (+Belgium)	commercial product	Diffusion using compressed tablets	Mueller-Hinton	irregular updates
JSC (29)	Japan	Japan Soc. for Chemotherapy	Dilution	Mueller-Hinton	clinical breakpoints(30-32)
CDS (6,33)	Australia	none	Disc diffusion	Sensitest	regular updates, no Intermediate category, annular radii measured
NCCLS (5,34)	USA	National Committee for Clinical Laboratory Standards	Dilution and disc diffusion	Mueller-Hinton	yearly updates

for most of the commercial semi-automated methods to be described below. NCCLS methods involve a significant amount of input from pharmaceutical firms and reagent manufacturers, giving them the greatest access to the data sets that are required for setting breakpoints. For this reason, the NCCLS methods might be considered the de facto international standard for susceptibility testing.

A. Range of organisms that can be tested

It is not widely appreciated that there are limitations to the range of rapidly-growing bacteria that can be confidently tested using the standard methods as described above. The accompanying table (Table 4) shows which bacteria can be assessed by adequately standardized routine laboratory tests, and those that cannot. Whichever method or methods a laboratory chooses, these limitations must be recognized. Documentation on an individual method must be checked carefully to ensure that susceptibility tests are not applied inappropriately to non-standardized species. There is a range of bacteria for which breakpoints (and therefore zone diameters) have not yet been set. Some advice will be provided about testing these.

B. Maintenance of quality control strains

Regardless of method, QC testing (QC) with organisms of known and stable pedigree is essential practice. All QC organisms should be sourced from a reputable supplier. It is important that the strains are handled in such a way that viability is maintained and that the opportunity for resistant mutants to develop is minimized. Stock cultures should be stored at –80°C, or lyophilized. Ideally, there should be both primary and secondary stock cultures. Only secondary stock cultures should be accessed routinely. At least monthly, fresh working cultures are prepared from the secondary stocks. These working cultures can be stored at 2-8°C on tryptic soy agar (non-fastidious) or chocolate agar (fastidious) slants, and then they may be subcultured weekly to provide strains for the routine QC.

C. Dilution methods

There are three variations on routine dilution testing. All of them are adaptations of the standard dilution methods for measuring MICs. Instead of the full 8-12 two-fold dilution series of a MIC test, these routine tests use either a restricted range of 1 to 5 dilutions that cover the breakpoint concentrations, or just the one to two breakpoint concentrations.

1. Common elements of dilution testing

All bacterial susceptibility tests have features in common. Attention to detail is a vital part of susceptibility, and the attention must be given to all steps in the procedure.

Table 4   Bacteria to consider for routine susceptibility testing.

Standardized	Not standardized
Staphylococcus aureus	Corynebacterium spp.
Coagulase-negative staphylococci	Bacillus spp.
Streptococcus pneumoniae	Listeria monocytogenes
Streptococcus spp.	Other Gram positive cocci
Enterococcus spp.	Vibrio spp.
Enterobactericeae	Aeromonas spp.
Pseudomonas aeruginosa	Pasteurella spp. and other fastidious Gram negative bacteria
Acinetobacter spp.	
Stenotrophomonas maltophilia	
Haemophilus influenzae	
Moraxella catarrhalis*	
Neisseria gonorrhoeae	
Neisseria meningitidis*	
Helicobacter pylori	
Vibrio cholerae	
Anaerobes	
Other non-glucose-fermenting Gram negative bacilli	

* No NCCLS breakpoints.

Stock antibiotic solutions

Recommendations for the preparation of stock solutions, including the use of appropriate solvents, ideal storage conditions, and shelf life, are available in a number of reputable references (5,35). The potency of the powder that is being used must be known. Unless there is no other choice, it is unwise to use pharmacy stocks of injectable products because their content can legitimately vary from that which is stated on the label by as much as 15%. A suitable method for QC of stock solutions is mandatory. If preparing your own laboratory material, incorrect stock concentration is one of the most common errors. All stock solutions should be stored at -80°C.

Medium preparation

Culture media should be prepared according to the manufacturer's instructions. Each method provides instructions for when additives are required and at what stage during preparation they should be added. Some additives are heat-labile, and must be added after partial or complete cooling of the medium.

Inoculum preparation

The single greatest source of error in susceptibility testing is incorrect preparation of the inoculum. Some antibiotics are particularly vulnerable to the 'inoculum effect' and yield higher MICs at higher inocula. It is vital that the method's instructions for inoculum preparation are followed exactly. There are two methods of inoculum preparation: subculture and direct. In both methods, about 4 to 5 colonies of the test organism on the primary plate should be sampled. The colonies may either be subcultured into a suitable broth and incubated for a small number of hours to ensure logarithmic growth, or put directly into saline or broth that is warmed to room temperature. Direct preparation is preferred for staphylococci when testing methicillin or oxacillin. The broth or saline, prepared either way, is then diluted to a turbidity/optical density standard that is most commonly a 0.5 McFarland barium sulfate standard.

Inoculation procedures

To avoid a significant increase in bacterial numbers, inoculation of the test system should occur within 15 minutes of inoculum preparation if suspended in broth or within 30 minutes if suspended in saline. After inoculation, a fixed volume, such as that obtained with a calibrated loop, should be subcultured to check the inoculum size and purity.

Growth and sterility controls

A tube, well, or agar plate containing no antibiotic should be included in every run to act as a growth control. A second tube or well that does not contain an antibiotic and which is not inoculated, should be included to act as a sterility control for broth methods.

Incubation

Most aerobic bacteria grow sufficiently and rapidly such that the test can be read the next day. The following durations of incubation are recommended: most facultative bacteria, 16-20 hrs.; enterococci and vancomycin, 24 hrs.; staphylococci and methicillin, oxacillin, and vancomycin, 24 hrs.; and anaerobes, 48 hrs. Air is the appropriate atmosphere for aerobic bacteria. Use of increased CO_2 for incubation is not recommended unless essential for growth of the organisms. The optimum temperature for all tests is 35°C.

Control organisms

Each test run should include one or more control organisms. Reference control strains are nominated for each method. For NCCLS methods, these organisms are essential for dilution testing: *Escherichia coli* ATCC 25922, *Staphylococcus aureus* ATCC 29213, *Enterococcus faecalis* ATCC 29212, *Pseudomonas aeruginosa* ATCC 27853, *Haemophilus influenzae* ATCC 49247 and ATCC 49766, *Streptococcus pneumoniae* ATCC 49619, *Neisseria gonorrhoeae* ATCC 49226, and *Helicobacter pylori* ATCC 43504. *E. coli* ATCC 35218 is recommended if the laboratory is routinely testing ß-lactamase inhibitor combinations.

Interpretation

The growth control, the sterility control, and the subculture which confirms the correct inoculum density should be checked first. For most antibiotics, all tubes, wells, or plates are read as growth or no growth. If there is more than one concentration of antibiotic that is being tested, the result is read as the lowest concentration showing no growth. For sulphonamides, trimethoprim, chloramphenicol, and tetracyclines, the endpoint is an abrupt change or 80% reduction in turbidity rather than no growth. Occasionally, 'skip' dilutions are encountered. These are concentrations that show no growth, but that are associated with growth at concentrations both immediately below and above. They should be ignored unless there are only two dilutions in the series, in which case the test must be repeated. If there is more than one 'skip' dilution in an MIC series, the test may be invalid and should be repeated. All results are compared to reference tables of breakpoints that are published as part of the method.

Quality control procedures

For commercially-manufactured media such as microtitre trays, QC procedures are usually performed on batches prior to shipping. Each batch should be tested on arrival with appropriate QC strains to ensure that they have been adequately handled during shipping.

All home-made antibiotic stocks must undergo QC for potency following preparation. For home-made tests, all freshly-prepared trays or plates should be QC tested to ensure correct content and sterility. Stored trays or plates should have a QC check at each test run, or at least weekly. Out-of-range values generally mean that the results should be disregarded and that the batch should be discarded. Reference strains with known reproducible MIC ranges are recommended for each method. All QC results must be stored for later review.

2.   *Broth macrodilution*

This method is least used for routine purposes since it requires a considerable amount of glass/plastic ware in order to include the necessary range of antibiotics. It is, however, the original method for performing MIC tests, and thus it merits detailed description.

Stock solutions

To simplify the process, stock concentrations should be 200-fold that of the starting concentration.

Medium preparation

The manufacturer's instructions for preparation of liquid media should be followed. Prepared sterile liquid media may be stored at 4°C in air-tight bottles for several weeks prior to use. If supplements are recommended, they should be added at this point. When setting up for testing, tubes with dimensions of about 13 by 100 mm. are filled initially with sterile broth. The most common choice of initial volume is 1 mL.

Dilutions

Antibiotics are added to each tube in order to achieve a concentration that is twice that of the desired final concentration. A tube without antibiotic, to act as a growth control, should also be made. Preferably, tubes should be freshly-prepared prior to use. If the desire is to perform a full range MIC test, dilutions can be prepared from a single stock solution. The NCCLS provides methods for achieving this (5). The scheme is designed to minimize the error of repeated two-fold dilution. The choice of range for a dilution series for MIC testing should take into account the expected MIC(s) of the test organism(s). The aim is to have the expected MIC of the test organism near the middle of the series.

Inoculum preparation

Most methods aim to achieve a final bacterial concentration in the test system of 5×10^5 CFU/mL. To achieve this, a broth culture or direct suspension is matched to a 0.5 McFarland turbidity standard. This should result in an inoculum concentration of about 1×10^8/mL.

Inoculation procedures

The turbidity-adjusted broth or saline is then diluted 100-fold in fresh sterile test medium (without additives). One mL. of this diluted medium is then added to each tube. To minimize further growth, this should be done within 30 min. of preparing the inoculum. Recently, it has been recognized that a 0.5 McFarland standard overestimates the size of the inoculum for some bacteria. Consequently, some methods recommend different dilutions for different bacteria. If the NCCLS method is being followed, the single 100-fold dilution is recommended. A 10 µL. aliquot from the growth control tube should be diluted 1:100, and 10 µL. of this should be subcultured to an agar plate to confirm inoculum density and purity.

Incubation

Tubes should be loosely capped and incubated in air, except for anaerobes, where anaerobic chambers or jars must be used. Added CO_2 is not required for this method of testing. Durations of incubation are as recommended under Common Elements above (B1).

Interpretation

Tubes are read as growth or no growth, and the concentrations compared to the method's published breakpoints. A single large 'button' or multiple small colonies at the base of the tube should be interpreted as growth.

3.   Broth microdilution

Broth microdilution is almost identical to broth macrodilution except that the test is performed 96-well microtitre trays; thus, the volumes of test liquid are smaller, usually 100 µL. The significant advantage of this method over broth macrodilution is that several MIC or many breakpoint tests may be performed in a single tray. Since the volume in which the test is conducted is one-twentieth that of the macrodilution test, however, the total number of bacteria that are exposed during the test is also one-twentieth. If there is interest in detecting resistant mutants to a particular antibiotic within the test population, then the broth macrodilution test is more sensitive.

Stock solutions

Stock antibiotic solutions are prepared according to the recommended methods.

Medium preparation

The appropriate broth culture medium is prepared according to the manufacturer's instructions.

Dilutions

Stock antibiotic solutions are diluted appropriately into the culture medium. The choice of dilution depends on how the test volumes are set up. The two common options are: (i) to dispense antibiotics in 100 µL. volumes into the wells at the desired final concentration and then add 1-5 µL. of inoculum, or (ii) to dispense antibiotics in 50 µL. volumes at twice the desired final concentration and then add 50 µL. of inoculum. Automated dispensers are available to deliver these fixed volumes. One well should be left free of antibiotic to act as a growth control, and a further one for sterility control.

Plate storage

Microtitre trays may be stored after preparation of the antibiotic dilutions. They should be stacked, and then an empty tray should be placed on top of the uppermost tray prior to sealing in plastic bags before freezing at –20 to –70°C. Plates are stable for 6 weeks at –20°C and many months at –70°C, except for those that contain cefaclor, clavulanic acid (in combination with amoxycillin or ticarcillin), or imipenem which readily degrade during storage. Plates that contain these antibiotics should be stored for no longer than 2 weeks. Alternatively, plates may be freeze-dried for storage at room temperature. Freeze-dried plates generally have a shelf-life of at least 6 months.

Inoculum preparation and procedures

The inoculum is prepared to ensure that the final bacterial concentration is 5×10^5 CFU/mL. (5×10^4 CFU in 100 µL.), and it thus depends on the choice of dilution procedure as described above. A broth culture or direct suspension is matched to a 0.5 McFarland turbidity standard. If the inoculum is intended to be 1-5 µL., a 1:10 dilution in broth or saline is made, and this is used to deliver the necessary volume to the wells. For 50 µL. inoculum volumes, a 1:100 dilution is made into broth and used directly.

Incubation

Each tray should be covered with a plastic adhesive (preferably transparent) or a tightly-fitted lid to avoid evaporation during incubation. Trays should be stacked no more than four high. They are incubated in air (not CO_2) for durations as described above under Common Elements (B1).

Interpretation

It is best to employ a specific viewing device for microtitre trays. The most widely available is one with a parabolic mirror that improves light conditions over which the tray is suspended. Growth is compared to the growth control, but generally appears as turbidity or a single 'button' to multiple 'colonies' at the bottom of the well.

4. Agar dilution (and breakpoint) testing

Stock solutions

Stock antibiotic solutions are prepared according to the recommended methods. Only a limited number of stock solutions are required if performing breakpoint agar dilution testing. The most common method for this type of testing is to prepare working stock solutions that are 10 times concentrated from the master stock.

Medium preparation

The appropriate agar culture medium is prepared according to the manufacturer's instructions. Usually, it is dispensed into screw cap bottles of suitable volume to which stock solutions are added (e.g., 90 mL. to take 10 mL. of antibiotic stock solution if prepared at 10 times concentration). Bottles are then sterilized and placed in a water bath to cool and to be held at 48-50°C in readiness for the addition of stock antibiotic solutions. Any required supplements, including defibrinated sheep or horse blood that should be used for testing streptococci, may then be added.

Dilutions

Antibiotic working stock solutions are added to the molten agar. To avoid localized setting of agar while adding the stock solution, the stocks must be at room temperature prior to the addition. Each bottle is mixed to ensure even distribution of antibiotic (but avoid a froth), and then poured into suitably-sized Petri dishes to a depth of 3 to 4 mm. The depth of the agar does not have to be precise. The pH of the agar should be checked after pouring and setting to ensure it is between 7.2 and 7.4. This can be done either with a surface electrode or with an electrode that has been immersed into a small aliquot that has been poured separately and allowed to set around it.

Plate storage

Plates may be stored after preparation. They should be held at 4-8°C, in sealed plastic bags or containers, and used within one week of preparation, or longer if it has been established that the MICs of control strains do not change.

Inoculum preparation

The inoculum is prepared in either subcultured broth or directly, and it is adjusted to the 0.5 McFarland standard (i.e., around $1x10^8$ CFU/mL.). A 1:10 dilution is then made. The objective is to apply about $1x10^4$ CFU per spot onto the plate surface.

Inoculation procedures

This inoculum may be applied directly to the surface of the plate with a loop or pipette. More commonly, it is applied using a replicator [a multi-pinned device that allows more precise multiple surface application (1-4 μL. depending on device)] after placing the inoculum into a well of the replicator holding block. For MIC dilution series, the inoculum should be applied from the lowest to the highest concentration to avoid any possible carry-over of drug by the replicator. Plate surfaces should be dry before inoculation. Plates should be allowed to absorb the inoculum prior to commencing incubation.

Incubation

Plates are inverted into their lids and incubated for recommended times (above under Common elements). Additional CO_2 should be avoided unless fastidious organisms are being tested.

Interpretation

Spots should be examined for growth after checking for adequate growth on the growth control plate. In general, a single colony or a faint haze caused by the inoculum is ignored and interpreted as growth inhibition. More difficulty will be experienced with sulfonamides, trimethoprim, chloramphenicol, and to a lesser extent tetracyclines, where growth tends to 'trail off' rather than cease abruptly above the MIC. The MIC (or inhibition on a breakpoint plate) should be interpreted as a sudden decrease in growth or 80% inhibition.

Quality control

All freshly-prepared plates should be QC tested to ensure correct content and sterility. Reference strains with known reproducible MIC ranges are recommended for each method. These strains should be included in each test run, and the results should be stored for later review.

D. Semi-automated systems

A number of commercial systems are now available that are adapted from dilution or dilution breakpoint methods. All of these systems have adopted the basic principles that are involved in broth microdilution and have automated some of the steps involved. Many different commercial systems have been developed over the last 20 years, but only a few have stood the test of time. The two most popular of these are the Vitek® from bioMérieux and the autoSCAN®/WalkAway® from Dade Behring. A recent entrant in the field is the Phoenix™ system from Becton Dickinson, while Trek Diagnostic Systems also have the SENSITITRE® system.

Essentially, these methods use dilution series or breakpoint concentrations of antibiotics that are incorporated into plastic wells in a system-specific format. Around that are built methods for inoculum preparation and standardization, manual or automated inoculation of the wells, and fixed interval or semi-continuous monitoring of growth in the wells until specified end-points are reached. The main advantage of these systems are:

(i)   improved discipline in inoculum preparation and standardization;
(ii)   when used, automatic comparison of species identification and susceptibility test results;
(iii) in some formats, results within hours rather than the next day; and
(iv)   so-called expert systems which examine the identification and susceptibility patterns and provide feedback about unusual patterns, possible errors, and hidden resistances.

All of these systems generate a considerable amount of plastic waste, and most importantly have significantly more expensive consumables than the manual methods described in this section.

The Vitek® system was the first of the semi-automated systems, and it continues to be enhanced (as the Vitek® 2). It employs a playing card-sized plastic card inside of which are found small wells that contain antibiotics at breakpoint and some additional concentrations. After inoculum preparation with the use of a colorimeter that is supplied with the system for optimizing the inoculum density, cards are filled with a dedicated device (inside the machine in the case of the Vitek® 2). The system accepts the card, commences incubation inside its chamber, and regularly reads the optical density of the wells. When the machine has detected adequate growth in the control, it examines the growth curves in the different antibiotic-containing wells and interprets the susceptibility categories with its specialized software. An expert system then examines the output and provides additional interpretations. The number of wells in the card, 30 or 45 for the Vitek® and 64 for Vitek® 2, determines the number of antibiotics that can be tested, but 12 to 20 per isolate is normal. Cards can be custom-made to suit the client's antibiotic testing needs if the size of the order is sufficient. Common panels for several laboratories is the best way to deal with this.

The autoSCAN® and WalkAway® systems use a format which is similar to that of the microtitre tray. Trays come in a variety of types: combined identification and susceptibility testing, identification only, or susceptibility testing only. For straight susceptibility testing plates, the number of antibiotics that can be tested is obviously higher. The Phoenix® and Sensititre® systems are similar to the Walk-Away®.

E. Diffusion methods

Diffusion methods of susceptibility testing are the most widely used internationally. The predominant reasons for this are that they are simple to use, comparatively inexpensive, and very flexible. The tests rely on the natural effect of antibiotic diffusion from a small carrier through agar over time. The standard method involves the use of a paper disc which contains antibiotic, and which is placed onto a lawn of test bacterium that is applied to the surface of the agar – so-called disc diffusion. Recently, a variant has been developed (Etest®) that applies antibiotic via a gradient on a carrier strip and that can generate a MIC value for the test strain.

The most common form of disc is made from a 6mm. special grade paper that is available commercially from several manufacturers. One method employs a larger compressed tablet of inert carrier into which the antibiotic has been incorporated.

1. Principles of diffusion testing

The two most important aspects of diffusion methods are the rate at which the test bacterium grows and the rate at which the antibiotic diffuses through agar. For most routine testing, organisms commence growing rapidly soon after the lawn is applied, and antibiotics diffuse rapidly immediately after the disc is applied to the surface. Some bulky or highly-charged antibiotics such as vancomycin or colistin diffuse more slowly. A combination of the rates of growth and diffusion defines the 'critical time' at which the final zone of inhibition is established, usually within an hour of application. The rest of the incubation time in the test is the time that is required for sufficient growth in order to visualize the zone of inhibition. Other influences on the size of the zone include the temperature of incubation, the depth of the agar, the nutritive content of the medium, the presence of growth enhancers (e.g., blood) which may bind highly-protein bound antibiotics, and the incubation atmosphere (e.g., additional CO_2).

For disc diffusion tests, it is theoretically possible to calculate the MIC from the zone diameter. Indeed, there is at least one commercial zone diameter reader that undertakes this function (37). This calculation is rarely made, however, because of its proven inaccuracy. Instead, the disc diffusion method is used for categorization of results into susceptible, intermediate, and resistant. This is achieved by correlating zone diameters with MIC using a variety of mathematical techniques. The most widely applied is that of Metzler and DeHaan (38), or modifications of this method (39). Regression lines are often calculated as well, but are of no direct value in the correlation, and are in many cases statistically invalid. The categorization is made as shown in the Figure 1. The objective is to select zone diameters for the three categories that will minimize the number of errors of categorization using the MIC breakpoints as previously set. In choosing zones, very major errors should be avoided. Major errors might be tolerated to a small degree, and minor errors will be tolerated more. It is often possible, however, to choose zone diameters with few or no errors at all.

2. Disc diffusion

Plate preparation

Plates of the appropriate agar medium for the chosen method must be prepared carefully. Notice should be taken of any required additives for certain test species, but only those additives recommended in the method. Most importantly, the depth of the agar must be consistent, and close to 4 mm. is ideal. This can be achieved by calibrated molten agar pouring equipment or by dispensing known volumes into each plate with a volumetric pipette or burette. The appropriate volume depends on the size of the plate: 20-22 mL. for 90 mm. plates, 25-30 mL. for 100 mm. plates, and 60-70 mL. for 150 mm. plates. Plates should not be free-poured. After the agar has set, the pH of the medium should be checked with a pH meter, and should be between 7.2 and 7.4 at room temperature.

Plate storage

Plates can be stored by refrigeration for up to 8 weeks in sealed plastic bags. After removal from storage prior to use, plates should have their lids removed, and the plates should be dried by inversion in an incubator for 10-30 min.

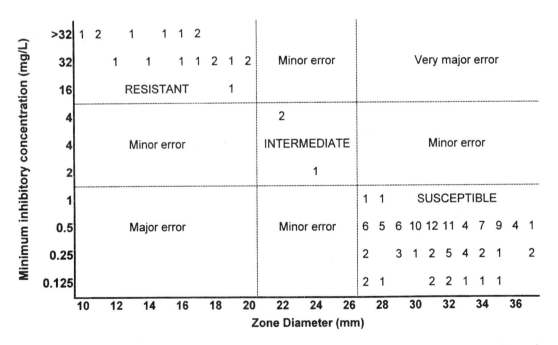

Figure 1 Comparison of zone diameters (ZD) with MICs for a hypothetical antimicrobial agent. Very major error = ZD susceptible, MIC resistant; major errors = ZD resistant, MIC susceptible; minor errors = ZD intermediate, MIC susceptible or resistant, or MIC intermediate, ZD susceptible or intermediate.

Disc storage

Discs must be stored according to the manufacturer's instructions and always sealed with a desiccant. In general, stock discs should be stored frozen (-20°C) while regular working discs can be stored with desiccants at standard refrigerator temperature. Mechanical dispensers that contain disc cartridges must be sealed tightly with desiccant and kept at 2-8°C between uses. Care must be taken to avoid using discs that have an expired date.

Prior to opening the containers/dispensers for plate application, all required discs should be brought to room temperature for at least 30 min. to avoid condensation which can result in rapid antibiotic degradation.

Inoculum preparation

Standardized preparation of the inoculum is described for each method. In general, the inoculum may be prepared directly from the primary culture plate or from a pre-incubated broth, although direct preparation is the most common. Usually, inocula are prepared to a turbidity standard, and then diluted with sterile water, normal saline, or broth at different rates according to species so to produce the final inoculum. Methods of inoculum preparation cannot be used interchangeably between methods as differences in bacterial concentration have a significant effect on zone diameters. Several disc diffusion methods have different instructions for inoculum preparation depending on the species being tested. These instructions must be followed to avoid interpretive errors.

Inoculation procedures

After plates have been dried, the inoculum is applied to the surface. The inoculum should be applied within 15 min. of inoculum preparation. Methods differ on the technique of application. The NCCLS method employs a sterile cotton swab which is immersed in the final inoculum, squeezed against the side of the tube to remove excess moisture, and then swabbed over the whole plate three times by rotating the plate approximately 60° on each occasion. For other methods, an aliquot of the final inoculum is poured over the surface, and thereafter, the excess is removed with a pipette thus allowing a few minutes for drying of the surface before disc application.

Disc placement

After the inoculum has had time to absorb, discs are placed on the agar surface at evenly spaced intervals of at least 24 mm. (centre to centre). Different sized plates have different capacities: 90-100 mm. round plates should have a maximum of 6 discs (5 only in some methods); 150 mm. round plates can take up to 12 discs; and 120 mm. square plates can take up to 16 discs. Discs may be placed by hand using sterile forceps, and then pressed gently onto the surface to ensure even contact. The best application technique uses a mechanical disc dispenser which automatically places the discs at appropriate intervals and tamps them onto the agar surface. Most manufacturers supply suitable mechanical dispensers for their discs. When discs touch the surface, even edge-on, antibiotic will commence diffusion immediately. Thus, once a disc has touched the surface, it should not be moved. If this results in discs being too close to each other, re-inoculate a fresh plate and re-dispense the discs.

Incubation

Inverted plates are placed into the incubator within 15 min. of disc placement and incubated in air at 35°C for 18-24 hrs. Fastidious organisms should be incubated in 5% CO_2. A full 24 hrs. incubation is required before reading if antistaphylococcal penicillins or glycopeptides are being tested.

Reading and interpretation

Depending on the method, growth should be confluent or semi-confluent at the completion of incubation. If there are discrete colonies, the inoculum has been too light; the test cannot be interpreted, and it must be repeated. The principles of reading the zones of inhibition are outlined above. Zones should be examined in bright reflected light, either from the back of the plate if the test medium is clear, or from the plate surface for opaque test media. Ideally, all zones should be measured to the nearest millimetre, preferably with sliding callipers, and recorded. Interpretation is made by comparison of values with the interpretative table for the appropriate method. Alternatively, a template may be constructed to match the distribution of the discs, and it may be marked with the critical zone diameters for easy interpretation. Zones must never be measured by 'eye'.

Several semi-automated zone readers are available. Plates are placed onto the scanning plate one at a time; the zones are determined by a variety of sophisticated scanning techniques and are recorded automatically. All zone diameter values can be adjusted and over-ridden manually. All semi-automated readers have interpretative software to translate the zone diameters into susceptibility categories according to the chosen method.

Quality control

Each method has QC recommendations and strains. In addition, QC zone diameter ranges for the appropriate QC organism(s) are published for each method. At a minimum, each batch of plates must be tested with all nominated QC organisms after they have been newly prepared and weekly thereafter. Ideally, QC organisms should be run with every test batch as well. All QC zone diameters need to be recorded. If results are out of range, they should be repeated. If repeatedly out-of-range, investigations should be initiated into the possible cause. Of course, out-of-range results may occur from problems with disc content, especially those arising from improper storage. If so, it is possible/likely that this will be obvious for more than one QC organism (if tested).

For NCCLS methods, these organisms are essential for diffusion testing: *Escherichia coli* ATCC 25922, *Pseudomonas aeruginosa* ATCC 27853, *Haemophilus influenzae* ATCC 49247 and ATCC 49766, *Streptococcus pneumoniae* ATCC 49619, and *Neisseria gonorrhoeae* ATCC 49226. *E. coli* ATCC 35218 is recommended if routinely testing ß-lactamase inhibitor combinations. An alternative strain of *Staphylococcus aureus* to that used for dilution testing, ATCC 25923, is recommended for QC of disc diffusion testing. Other methods have similar QC organisms.

3. *Common interpretive issues in diffusion testing*

For disc diffusion tests, lower disc strengths are more discriminatory than higher disc strengths. Disc strengths need to be sufficient, however, to yield an obvious gap, at least 4 mm. and preferably more, between the disc edge and the zone edge for susceptible organisms. Different disc diffusion methods often make use of different disc strengths. Discs cannot be interchanged between methods if the disc strengths are different since the interpretive zone diameters will necessarily be different.

Zone diameters are measured at the point where there is complete inhibition of growth. This method of interpretation is adequate for most tests, but problems can be encountered. It is common for there to be a narrow 'shoulder' of incomplete inhibition; between a zone of complete growth and no growth over a millimetre or so. The inner zone of complete inhibition (no growth) is the correct zone for interpretation. With the exception of those examples listed below, fine growth inside the zone up to or near the disc should be interpreted as resistance.

Occasionally, this 'shoulder' of incomplete inhibition can be wide. The most common examples of this are *Proteus mirabilis* which frequently swarms as a very thin film over the zone of inhibition up to the disc edge. In this instance, it is the edge of heavy growth that is used for measurement. Wide 'shoulders' are also common with the folate antagonists: trimethoprim and the sulfonamides. With these drugs, there is usually a readily discernible margin of heavy growth; with growth inside this margin being reduced by at least 80% compared to that outside of the margin. This margin is the one chosen for measurement.

Another frequently encountered problem is the presence of colonies inside the zone of inhibition. This phenomenon implies that there are resistant variants in the test population and should result in a 'resistant' interpretation. It can also mean that the test culture is mixed so that careful observation of colony morphology is required. A strong clue to a mixed test culture is the finding of colonies inside the zone for several antibiotics.

Particular care must be exercised with alpha- and beta-hemolytic organisms when testing on blood-containing media. Hemolysis often occurs inside the zone of inhibition and can be easily misread as the inhibition zone itself.

4. Gradient diffusion

A recent application of diffusion technology is the so-called gradient diffusion technique. This has been developed commercially by AB BIODISK as the Etest® which has found a broad range of uses for common, uncommon, and otherwise difficult-to-test organisms (40). It consists of an inert plastic strip, onto the underside of which has been applied an array of small 'dots' containing antibiotic that are aligned in such a way as to generate a continuous gradient of antibiotic concentrations when applied to the test plate. The test result that is generated is a MIC which is read from the upper side scale.

Test plates are prepared as per standard disc diffusion, and the test organism inoculum is prepared and applied in the routine manner. Test strips are then applied to the surface, tamped down, and incubated to the recommended time for the organism/antibiotic combination. Following incubation, an ellipse of inhibition is generated. The point where the ellipse intersects the strip is the MIC of the organism. The caveats on interpretation about zone edges, colonies inside the zone, and hemolysis apply equally to this test as they do for conventional disc diffusion. The Etest® has been evaluated extensively against a very broad range of organisms and appears to produce comparable results to routine MIC tests. Before use, however, the user should check with the manufacturer about the extent of experience with the particular organism/antibiotic combination.

Gradient diffusion has supplanted most MIC tests when these need to be performed. We recommend its use for the common bacteria when an MIC value is required for optimum treatment, such as in endocarditis or pneumococcal meningitis.

F. Direct testing

Direct testing refers to susceptibility testing straight from the original specimen. It is not a practice that is endorsed by any of the standardized methods. Nevertheless, it can be extremely useful as a preliminary screen as it shortens the time to produce at least qualitative susceptibility information one day earlier (7,41).

It is prone to a number of problems. The greatest of these is the lack of control on the size of the inoculum. Mixed cultures are a problem with some specimens such as urines, and interference by antibiotics in the specimen if the patient is already undergoing treatment can also be troublesome. Blood and protein in the specimen can also result in error.

Typical specimens on which direct testing may be considered include urines that have evidence of pyuria and a single bacterial morphology on microscopy, cerebrospinal fluid in which bacteria have been demonstrated microscopically, and positive blood cultures. Tests on CSF may be limited by the availability of sufficient volume. Choice of test panel is based on the Gram stain and presumptive identification of the organism.

The simplest test method to apply to direct testing are disc and gradient diffusion. The specimen may be applied directly to the agar surface, or if possible, a spun deposit (supernatant discarded) can be re-suspended and then used as the inoculum. This latter method of preparation can also be used to generate sufficient volume for dilution testing, including semi-automated methods.

Any results so generated must be repeated on isolated colonies the next day, unless the laboratory has undertaken extensive validation procedures to confirm the accuracy of the direct tests (for certain antibiotic-organism combinations) as compared to the standard methods.

Table 5   Recommended routine chromogenic cephalosporin tests.

Species tested	Isolates worth testing	ß-lactamase(s) detected	Antibiotic resistances predicted from a positive result
Haemophilus influenzae	All	TEM-1 and ROB-1	Moderate spectrum and anti-pseudomonal penicillins
Neisseria gonorrhoeae	All	TEM-1	Narrow spectrum, moderate spectrum and anti-pseudomonal penicillins
Moraxella catarrhalis	All	BRO-1 and BRO-2	Narrow spectrum, moderate spectrum and anti-pseudomonal penicillins
*Enterococcus faecalis**	Blood and CSF	PEN	Narrow spectrum, moderate spectrum and anti-pseudomonal penicillins

* - ß-lactamase production is rare

G. Supplementary tests

A number of antibiotic degrading or modifying enzymes can be detected in the laboratory by direct phenotypic testing. Some of these tests are sufficiently simple and meaningful to be of value in routine testing.

1.   Enzyme detection

Direct tests for conventional ß-lactamases

Many different methods have been developed for detecting ß-lactamases over the years. In general, the tests that are most valuable on a routine basis are those that detect ß-lactamases that are produced in large amounts and which are excreted extracellularly. Two of the methods depend on the fact that cleavage of the ß-lactam ring results in the production of penicilloic acid which is an acidic molecule that results in a significant drop of pH. These methods are called acidometric tests. If the detection relies on a pH indicator such as phenol red, the method is called colorimetric. If the indicator is the starch-iodine complex, the method is called iodometric.

While both of these methods have been popular in the past, they have been essentially replaced by the chromogenic cephalosporins, nitrocefin, and cefesone (42). These molecules change colour from a pale clear yellow colour to a pink colour when the ß-lactam ring is broken by a ß-lactamase. We recommend the use of chromogenic cephalosporins for all direct ß-lactamase tests as they cover a wider range of ß-lactamases than the acidometric tests. Application of colonies picked directly from the primary or subculture plates will result in detection of clinically-significant ß-lactamases within minutes. Table 5 is a guide to chromogenic cephalosporin tests that should be applied to routine testing.

These tests can also be applied to *Staphylococcus aureus*, *Prevotella* and *Porphyromonas* species. For *S. aureus* in particular, penicillin resistance may be so frequent that the test may not be considered worthwhile.

ß-lactamase inhibitor potentiation testing for extended-spectrum ß-lactamases

Extended-spectrum ß-lactamases (ESBLs) are enzymes that capable of degrading 3rd generation, and to a lesser extent, 4th generation cephalosporins (10). They are found predominantly in species of *Enterobacteriaceae* that do not naturally possess chromosomal cephalosporinases; *Klebsiella pneumoniae* and *E. coli* being the most common. Their presence is likely if these bacteria test resistant to a 3rd generation cephalosporin, and additional tests mentioned here are unnecessary unless the laboratory is keen to confirm the inference. There are a proportion of strains, however, that possess ESBLs which test as susceptible or intermediate by routine methods.

The presence of ESBLs should be suspected if the strain tests resistant to a 1st generation cephalosporin, gentamicin, or ciprofloxacin. The reason for suspecting strains to be resistant to gentamicin or ciprofloxacin relates to the frequent association of ESBLs with these additional resistances. Strains with MICs to cefotaxime, ceftriaxone, ceftazidime, or aztreonam greater than 1 mg./L. should also be suspected of harbouring ESBLs. This concentration may be included in screening tests as part of routine testing.

β-lactamase inhibitor potentiation testing relies on the fact that almost all ESBLs are inhibited by clavulanate. Detection of ESBLs is achieved by a comparison of a test for a 3rd generation cephalosporin with a test where a 3rd generation cephalosporin is combined with clavulanate. There are two variants of the test: the disc approximation test as originally described by Jarlier et al. (43) and sequential disc placement as described by Casals (28). In the current version of the former method, a disc of a 3rd generation cephalosporin, usually ceftazidime or cefotaxime, and a disc containing clavulanate are placed 20 mm. apart (edge-to-edge) on a plate inoculated with the test organism. If the strain possesses an ESBL, there will be an increase in the inhibition zone of the 3rd generation cephalosporin on the side facing the disc that contains clavulanate, or a 'keyhole' between the two discs, after overnight incubation. In the NCCLS version of the second test, 10 μg. of clavulanate is added to the standard 3rd generation cephalosporin discs and allowed to dry (34). Both the clavulanate-impregnated discs and the straight 3rd generation cephalosporin discs are placed on a lawn of the test culture. After overnight incubation, the presence of an ESBL will be confirmed if the zone diameter around the clavulanate-impregnated disc is >4 mm. larger than the non-impregnated disc.

ESBLs may also be detected using MIC-based methods. In these methods, the potentiation by clavulanate is demonstrated with a >2 two-fold dilution reduction in MIC compared to the drug alone (5). This technique has also been applied to some of the semi-automated systems.

It is important to understand that no one method detects all ESBLs, and knowledge of the local enzyme types will assist in choosing which methods and substrates are most suitable.

Disc approximation test for inducible β-lactamases

Chromosomally-encoded and inducible β-lactamases are found naturally in almost all strains of *Enterobacter* species, *Serratia marcescens*, *Citrobacter freundii*, *Acinetobacter* species, *Proteus vulgaris* and *penneri*, *Providencia* species, *Pseudomonas aeruginosa*, and *Morganella morganii* (the so-called ESCAPPPM group) (10). They are clinically significant because they confer natural resistance to 1st and 2nd generation cephalosporins and cefamycins in these species. In addition, many of these enzymes can be produced at very high levels after exposure to 3rd generation cephalosporins which then also result in resistance to them. Their presence can be confirmed by their inducible property with the use of a disc approximation technique between a 3rd generation cephalosporin and an inducing β-lactam such as imipenem. As the vast majority of strains of the above-mentioned species possess the inducible enzyme, however, routine testing for its presence offers little additional information, and therefore, we do not recommend its use for routine testing.

2.   *Screening tests*

A number of tests to screen for resistance have been developed for routine laboratory testing (Table 6). Their value lies principally in their greater sensitivity by providing additional information about the presence of a resistance mechanism that in diffusion or dilution testing may generate a borderline or susceptible result. They are most useful when certain resistances are emerging for the first time locally because they reduce the chance of missing an important resistance in standard tests.

High-level aminoglycoside resistance in enterococci

Optimum treatment of enterococcal endocarditis usually includes a combination of a penicillin (usually benzylpenicillin, ampicillin, or amoxycillin) or a glycopeptide (vancomycin or teicoplanin) with an aminoglycoside (gentamicin or streptomycin) (44). Strains of enterococci with high-level aminoglycoside resistance, rather than the natural borderline to low-level resistance, are now common.

Table 6 Useful screening tests for resistance.

Genus	Resistance	Isolates worth testing	Mechanism	Test	Interpretation
Enterococcus species	High-level aminoglycoside	Endocarditis	Aminoglycoside-modifying enzymes	High-conc. plate or high-strength disc	Resistant to the synergistic action of aminoglycoside with a cell-wall active agent
	Vancomycin	All	VanA-E	Screening plate	Resistant to vancomycin but not teicoplanin necessarily
Streptococcus pneumoniae	Penicillin	All	Altered PBPs	Oxacillin disc or low strength penicillin disc	Intermediate or resistant to narrow spectrum penicillin
Staphylococcus species	Anti-staphylococcal penicillins	All	Additional insensitive PBP (*mecA* gene)	Screening plate	Resistant to anti-staphylococcal penicillins

High-level resistance is mostly due to the possession of aminoglycoside-modifying enzymes. The chances of cure are substantially reduced if the strain has high-level resistance to the chosen aminoglycoside. Resistance to gentamicin and streptomycin is due to two entirely different aminoglycoside-modifying enzymes. Thus, a strain can be resistant to high levels of gentamicin but not streptomycin, and vice versa, as well as being resistant to both through the possession of both enzymes. Due to the nature of the aminoglycoside-modifying enzyme that confers high-level gentamicin resistance, almost all other aminoglycosides except streptomycin will also be inactive in combination therapy. Thus, it is necessary only to screen for resistance to these two agents.

High-level resistance may be detected by the use of agar screening plates, broth microdilution, or high strength discs (5,34). The recommended agar plates contain 500 mg./L. of gentamicin and 2000 mg./L. of streptomycin in brain-heart infusion agar (5). Plates are inoculated by spotting with 10 µL. of a 0.5 McFarland suspension of the test strain, and results are read after a full 24 hrs. of incubation. Strains showing more than a single colony or a fine growth are considered as high-level resistant. This test can also be conducted in broth, but the concentration of streptomycin of 1000 mg./L. is used instead. The disc method employs the standard test method for disc diffusion, but uses high-strength discs of gentamicin (120 µg.) and streptomycin (300 µg.) (34). Zone diameters around these discs of <7 mm. confirm high-level resistance. Zone diameters of 7-9 mm. are inconclusive, and an agar or broth method should be performed. *E. faecalis* ATCC 29212 (susceptible to both agents) and *E. faecalis* ATCC 51299 (resistant to both agents) should be used as controls for each test. It is recommended that all confirmed endocarditis isolates of enterococci have high-level aminoglycoside testing. There is also value in screening all blood culture isolates, because it is common at the time of the positive blood culture that endocarditis may not yet be clinically apparent.

Vancomycin resistance in enterococci

Vancomycin resistance among enterococci is now seen at a low frequency in many countries, and it is common in the United States (45). These bacteria are presently considered important nosocomial pathogens. Most major routine diffusion and dilution tests have been modified to ensure detection of these strains. Thus, there is usually no need for additional screening tests to ensure detection. If there is concern that the routine methods that are used by a laboratory may have weaknesses in detection, a screening method such as the one described here should be instituted for all enterococci. One recommended screening method is a plate of brain heart infusion agar that contains 6 mg./L. of vancomycin, is inoculated with 10 µL. of a 0.5 McFarland suspension of the test strains, and is incubated for a full 24 hrs. (5). More than one colony, or a fine growth, should be interpreted as presumptively resistant. This method will detect many strains of the enterococcal species that have natural low-level vancomycin resistance (VanC). Thus, the full identification of resistant strains is essential. Vancomycin and teico-planin MIC testing of screen-positive strains will enable tentative phenotype categorization (VanA, VanB, or VanC). We recommend that all presumptive vancomycin-resistant enterococci have their identity and vancomycin resistance confirmed genetically (see below).

Penicillin resistance in *Streptococcus pneumoniae*

In many disc diffusion methods, the standard disc strength of penicillin is such that zone diame-ters for *Streptococcus pneumoniae* are poorly correlated with MICs. Instead, these methods employ an oxacillin disc in place of a penicillin disc which functions as a screen for reduced susceptibility to peni-cillin (20,34). This approach is effective because oxacillin is intrinsically less active than penicillin against pneumococci. Strains that are resistant to oxacillin may be intermediate or resistant to benzyl-penicillin and other narrow spectrum penicillins. If there is a clinical need to know whether they are intermediate or resistant, MIC testing will be required. Occasional penicillin-susceptible strains test as resistant in the oxacillin screen.

Staphylococcal resistance to antistaphylococcal penicillins

Resistance to antistaphylococcal penicillins is almost always the result of the acquisition of an ad-ditional penicillin protein, called PBP2a or PBP2', that is encoded by the *mecA* gene. Although other types of resistance have been described, they are rare. Routine methods have been fine-tuned over many years to ensure detection of resistance, and they now work well for *Staphylococcus aureus*. Problems are often encountered, however, with some coagulase-negative staphylococci, mostly due to their poor and slower growth. Consequently, some authorities recommend the use of a screening test in addition to routine testing. The best developed of these is the oxacillin screen for *S. aureus* (5). In this method, Mueller-Hinton agar, which incorporates 4% sodium chloride (to enhance detection) and 6 mg./L. of oxacillin, is spotted with the test strains. The spots are applied with a swab which has been dipped into a 0.5 McFarland suspension and which is then squeezed against the side of the tube to remove excess fluid prior to application.

A recent innovation is a commercial latex agglutination test that detects the *mecA* gene product, PBP2a (46). This test has high sensitivity and specificity when applied to *S. aureus*, and it is currently being evaluated for coagulase-negative staphylococci.

Reduced susceptibility to glycopeptides in staphylococci

The recent emergence of reduced vancomycin susceptibility in *Staphylococcus aureus* has fo-cussed attention on this worrying problem (47). There is good circumstantial evidence that this resis-tance is clinically meaningful, and that it is very troublesome as strains are almost always resistant to multiple other antibiotics including ß-lactams. At present, there are insufficient strains to permit recali-bration of routine dilution or diffusion tests to ensure detection, and this is further complicated by fact that the resistance is often initially hetero-resistance; MIC increases are small (4-8 mg./L. compared to susceptible strains at ≤ 2 mg./L.). Disc diffusion methods are currently unable to detect this low-level resistance. We recommend that any strains of staphylococci with MICs to vancomycin of ≥ 4 mg./L. should be sent to a reference laboratory for further testing.

If there is local concern about the presence of this type of resistance, in *S. aureus* or coagulase-negative staphylococci, a screening test should be introduced. Currently, the most widely-examined method is an agar screen (48). Brain heart infusion agar that incorporates 6 mg./L. of vancomycin (as for enterococci) is spotted with 10 µL. of a 0.5 McFarland suspension of the test strain. Plates are incu-bated for a full 24 hrs. before reading. It is likely that better screening methods will be developed. An-tagonism between certain ß-lactams and vancomycin has been shown to be able to predict heteroresistance, while synergy between certain cephalosporins and vancomycin has been used to detect homo-resistance (49). All screen-positive isolates should have formal MIC testing against vancomycin and teicoplanin. A teicoplanin MIC of ≥16 mg./L. is strongly suggestive of reduced glycopeptide susceptibility.

XI. RESISTANCE GENE DETECTION

Some genetic molecular methods are now well within the capability of diagnostic laboratories. In particular, polymerase chain reaction (PCR)-based methods are attractive because of the rapid (same-day) turn-around and the ability to provide a definitive answer for antibiotic/organism combinations where routine tests are poorly discriminatory. At present, resistance gene detection may be of value to the routine laboratory in only two circumstances: the detection of resistance to antistaphylococcal penicillin in staphylococci, and the detection and characterization of vancomycin resistance in enterococci. We do not recommend that these tests be performed routinely unless there is a specific clinical need, e.g., for infection control purposes to prevent or control outbreaks.

The detection of *mecA* in staphylococci by gene probe or PCR methods is well described (50). The most popular method is PCR. It is usually combined with the simultaneous detection of the gene that encodes the thermostable nuclease (*nuc* gene). Results are often available within 4 hrs. of setup.

Vancomycin resistance in enterococci is more complex and may be assessed by multiplex PCR which covers the common resistance genotypes (*vanA*, *vanB*, and *vanC*) (51). It is often useful to combine these assessments with PCR tests for the identification of *Enterococcus faecalis* and *Enterococcus faecium* since standard biochemical tests can give ambiguous results with vancomycin-resistant strains. Unless vancomycin-resistant enterococci are common in the institution, it is valuable to have all presumptive strains confirmed by a reference laboratory with the use of PCR methods.

XII. SPECIALIZED TESTS

There are a number of specialized tests that are available and occasionally requested or considered for use in the diagnostic microbiology laboratory.

A. Minimum bactericidal concentration

Antibiotics can be classified as either bactericidal or bacteriostatic. That is, they demonstrate killing or inhibition in vitro only. Standardized methods are available for examining the property that describes this difference termed the minimum bactericidal concentration (MBC) (52). The MBC is defined as the minimum concentration of antibiotic that is required to achieve a 1000-fold reduction in the inoculum during the test interval, usually 24 hrs. It is measured via an additional step in the performance of the MIC in broth dilution systems; by subculture of at least one tube that demonstrates growth and by subculture of all those that show no growth at the end of incubation. Standardized ways of counting a 1000-fold reduction are described in at least one standard method (53). In most instances, the MBC is the same or only one dilution higher than the MIC for bactericidal agents, whereas the MBC is many dilutions higher than the MIC for bacteriostatic agents. Tolerance is present in strains of a species when bactericidal agents fail to kill, and therefore the MBC is substantially higher than the MIC.

In almost all circumstances, there is no clinical value in measuring the MBC. Theoretically, we may wish to recognize tolerant strains in circumstances where there is great dependence on the killing power of the antibiotic, e.g., septicemia, endocarditis, or meningitis. Studies of tolerance, however, even when strains have been described with some frequency, have generally shown no distinct relationship to failure of treatment when that drug is used. Thus, there are no conditions or antibiotic/organism combinations for which the MBC should be measured as a matter of course. Laboratories might consider using this test when there is a question of antibiotic failure in a serious infection and when there are few other antibiotic choices in order to determine whether tolerance might be contributing to failure.

B. Tests for synergy

Antibiotic combinations are common in clinical medicine, but they are almost always used to ensure coverage of pathogens. In a very small number of infections, they are used to ensure optimum outcome: streptococcal and enterococcal endocarditis, serious *Pseudomonas aeruginosa* infections, and tuberculosis. Tests for synergy in endocarditis and *P. aeruginosa* infections have occasionally been recommended, but they are of dubious value.

Combinations of a ß-lactam or glycopeptide and gentamicin or streptomycin are standard in the management of streptococcal and enterococcal endocarditis. With the former species, the combination shortens the duration of treatment. For the latter, it is essential to confidently achieve bacteriological eradication. In enterococcal endocarditis, synergy or lack of it can be inferred from the results of high-level aminoglycoside resistance tests as described above.

Combinations of agents with different mechanisms of action are essential for serious *P. aeruginosa* infections. The principal reason for combinations is to prevent the emergence of resistance during treatment rather than for true synergy. The relationship between synergy and outcome has never been clearly demonstrated for this organism.

Tests for synergy or antagonism of antibiotic combinations, such as the 'checkerboard' technique, and methods for interpretation are well described, but they are essentially research tools (44). Requests for such tests from clinicians should be dealt with by communicating their lack of value over and above that which is already known from research.

C. Serum inhibitory and bactericidal titres

Serum inhibitory and bactericidal titres (SITs and SBTs) are assays of bacteriostatic and bactericidal activity that are performed for a patient who is undergoing treatment. They have been used for many years in selected, difficult to treat, conditions such as osteomyelitis and endocarditis. Over the years, methods for performing this test have evolved and have become more standardized. The best standardized method is that described by the NCCLS (53).

The principle of the SBT is the examination of bactericidal activity of serum which is collected at specified times from the patient (usually a peak and trough level). Serum is incorporated into the growth medium and then diluted in a two-fold series after which a standardized inoculum of the patient's own organism is added. Thus, the test is independent of the antibiotic or combination that may being used for treatment, and it has the advantage of including the actual pathogen in the test. Performance and reading of the test has much in common with broth macro- and micro-dilution testing for the determination of MIC values.

Tests results have been shown to correlate with outcome (54). The role of this test, however, is still not clearly established, and with the advent of pharmacodynamic studies which draw a relationship of treatment schedules to outcomes, the need for this test is diminishing. Instead, antibiotic levels themselves, if timed correctly, can be used to ensure adequacy of treatment, and they are generally easier to perform.

If used, we recommend the NCCLS method (53). If possible, serum from the same patient prior to the commencement of antibiotics should be included as part of the test broth as it corrects for possible variation or defects in protein binding. Alternatively, a method for performing this test on serum ultrafiltrate is recommended as it also overcomes protein binding variation (55).

D. Anaerobes

Currently, no authority recommends routine testing of anaerobes. The principal reasons for this are the lack of simple methods, the rarity of resistance to common anti-anaerobic agents such as metronidazole, and the fact that many anaerobic or mixed infections respond to surgical treatment as much as to treatment with antibiotics. Resistances are starting to emerge now to some of the more important anti-anaerobic agents, and as such, laboratories should consider anaerobe testing, even in occasional batches, in order to predict problems with certain agents. In the future, a simple standardized method of anaerobe testing may be developed that will allow it to become part of routine laboratory practices.

There is a range of standardized methods that are available for testing. Of these, the best-evaluated methods are those published by the NCCLS (56). The NCCLS document provides detailed guidance on the set-up and reading of tests as well as recommendations on when to test. Gradient diffusion is a well-established alternative, particularly for one-off tests (57).

XIII. RANGE OF ORGANISMS AND LIMITATIONS

Table 7 is a summary of bacteria and testing methods that should be included in the routine diagnostic laboratory. Most of these recommendations are adopted from widely-used methods such as those of the NCCLS. As well, we have added our recommendations for regular use of supplementary tests and when isolates should be referred to reference laboratories.

We also provide some guidance about what to do for species where there are currently no standardized breakpoints. This is a common and problematic area. Technically, if the standardized methods that are being used in the laboratory do not specifically cover the organisms in question, then one should not test by a dilution breakpoint or disc diffusion method. For the occasional circumstance where treatment is definitely indicated, however, it is better to have some information about possible resistances than none at all. Consultation with the clinician may in the first instance clarify whether testing will be of any value. Furthermore, results from published studies may provide sufficient information to guide therapy without the need for testing.

When tests are considered important, extrapolation of methods and breakpoints from other species can at least provide qualitative information for the prescriber. If there is serious uncertainty, then the performance of a MIC, most simply by gradient diffusion, will increase the confidence of the laboratory and the prescriber. As a rule, for bacteria that do not have standardized methods or breakpoints, it is essential if extrapolating from the recommended species that growth is relatively rapid. It must be stressed that the following recommendations (Table 8) are entirely those of the authors, and are not recognized officially in any standardized methods.

XIV. RECOMMENDATIONS ON WHICH AGENTS TO TEST AND REPORT

Many methods provide recommendations for which antibiotics to test routinely and which to report routinely. For large laboratories, testing of a wide range of agents creates little additional work and cost. Most of the semi-automated methods generate results on 12 or more antibiotics per isolate.

Ultimately, the choice of what to test and what to report depends on the needs of the institution or other clientele, the availability locally or nationally of antimicrobials, and the wish of the laboratory to control prescribing by a restriction of the number of the agents that are reported.

Nevertheless, some general recommendations can be made:

1. test at least 6 agents (except perhaps enterococci where 4 may be adequate as a routine).

2. report at least 2 to 4 agents.

3. report all important resistances (including those that are predicable and not necessarily tested, e.g., cephalosporins and enterococci).

Table 7   Recommendations for testing where standardized tests and breakpoints exist. Abbreviations are those referred to in Table 3.

Group, genus, or species	Routine methods exist		Supplemental methods
	Dilution	*Disc*	
Staphylococcus species	Yes	Yes	Oxacillin screen plate or *mecA* PCR when considered valuable
Streptococcus pneumoniae	Yes	Yes	–
Other *Streptococcus* species	Yes	Yes	–
Enterococcus species	Yes	Yes	High level aminoglycoside resistance and nitrocefin/cefesone ß-lactamase test for all blood isolates, confirm presumptive vancomycin resistance by full identification and PCR genotyping
Enterobacteriaceae	Yes	Yes	ESBL screening *K. pneumoniae*, *E. coli*
Pseudomonas aeruginosa	Yes	Yes	–
Acinetobacter species	Yes	Yes	–
Stenotrophomonas maltophilia	Yes	Yes	–
Burkholderia cepacia	Yes	Yes	–
Haemophilus influenzae	Yes	Yes	Nitrocefin/cefesone ß-lactamase
Neisseria gonorrhoeae	Yes	Yes	Nitrocefin/cefesone ß-lactamase
Neisseria meningitidis	Yes (CASFM, BSAC, CDS)	Yes (CASFM, BSAC, CDS)	–
Moraxella catarrhalis	Yes (BSAC, CDS)	Yes (BSAC, CDS)	–
Helicobacter pylori	Yes	No	–
Anaerobes	Yes (NCCLS, CASFM)	No	Test only if isolated from invasive disease where antibiotics essential to achieve cure

Table 8   Recommendations for testing where standardized tests and breakpoints are not available.

Group, genus, or species	Recommendation of which group, genus, or species method and breakpoints to use
Facultative Gram positive cocci other than staphylococci, streptococci and enterococci	Other *Streptococcus* species
Corynebacterium species	*Staphylococcus* species
Listeria monocytogenes[a]	*Enterococcus* species
Lactobacillus species, *Erysipelothrix rhusiopathiae*	Other *Streptococcus* species
Bacillus species	*Staphylococcus* species
Aeromonas species	*Enterobacteriaceae*
Vibrio species	*Enterobacteriaceae*
Pasteurella multocida[b] and other species	*Haemophilus influenzae*[b]
Other fastidious Gram negative bacilli	*Haemophilus influenzae*[b]
Campylobacter species	Disc methods have been described (33,58)

[a] CDS method available
[b] use Mueller-Hinton with defibrinated (±) lysed sheep or horse blood.

4. report at least 2 agents showing susceptibility.

5. report at least one oral agent to which the organism is susceptible.

6. report what the patient is on (if such information is readily available and within reason).

XV. ANTIBIOGRAMS, INTERPRETATIONS, AND EXPERT SYSTEMS

The greatest challenge faced by the routine laboratory is the recognition of unusual or unexpected results. Some are due to errors in testing, some to the local rarity of a genuine resistance type, and some to the incompatibility of certain result combinations. Some of the more common examples are discussed below.

A. Natural resistances (normal antibiograms)

As a starting point, the laboratory must have an intimate knowledge of the intrinsic resistances of the common species that they are testing; Table 9 lists these. When factored into testing, they provide us with the expected antibiograms of a fully susceptible member of the species.

Some of the resistances noted here do not show up in susceptibility testing of every strain. For instance, a small proportion of *Klebsiella* spp. test as susceptible to ampicillin as do a small proportion of *Proteus mirabilis* to tetracycline. There is no definitive answer as to whether these strains are truly susceptible clinically, and most authorities suggest that these strains be reported as resistant. In general, for resistances listed in Table 9, all strains should probably be reported as resistant (if tested) no matter what the result of the test.

B. Predictable acquired resistances

Some acquired resistances are so common that knowledge of the organism's identification gives a high likelihood that the resistance will be present. Unlike the situation with natural resistances, strains testing as susceptible to the antibiotic should be reported as such, and the result should not be over-ridden. Important examples in this category are penicillin resistance in *Staphylococcus aureus* (~10% of strains are susceptible), penicillin/ampicillin resistance in *Moraxella catarrhalis* (~10% of strains are susceptible), and tetracycline resistance in *Streptococcus agalactiae* (~20% of strains are susceptible).

C. 'Impossible' resistances

There are also certain combinations of results that might be considered 'impossible'. If such results are obtained, serious scrutiny of the susceptibility test and the identification of the organism are required, and the susceptibility test should be repeated. Examples are:

- Resistance to an anti-pseudomonal penicillin and susceptibility to ampicillin (except enterococci)
- *Staphylococcus aureus* susceptible to penicillin and resistant to antistaphylococcal penicillins
- Resistance to amoxycillin-clavulanate and susceptibility to ampicillin (has been documented rarely as a genuine pattern in *Citrobacter freundii*)
- Resistance to 3rd generation cephalosporin and susceptibility to a 1st generation cephalosporin
- Resistance to one macrolide and susceptibility to another
- Resistance to one tetracycline and susceptibility to another (with the possible exception of staphylococci)
- Resistance to penicillin and susceptibility to ampicillin in enterococci. This will confuse many readers as it has been the dogma for years, and is a continuation from the days when enterococci were in the *Streptococcus* genus. It is merely, however, that penicillin MICs in entero-

cocci are higher than those of streptococci. When correct breakpoints are used for enterococci, the results should be concordant, and patients with susceptible strains can be equally well-treated with penicillin in high doses.

D. Difficult or controversial interpretations

Some areas of result interpretation are difficult, and the application of certain rules remains confusing or controversial. Some important examples are listed below:

- Many authorities recommend that staphylococci which test as resistant to erythromycin should be reported as resistant to lincosamides, regardless of the test result. The difficulty here revolves around the phenomenon of inducible resistance, which is common in staphylococci, whereby resistance to lincosamides can be induced in the presence of erythromycin (14). This phenomenon is quite easy to demonstrate in the laboratory by a disc approximation test. Whether it has clinical importance, given that the drugs are never given together clinically, remains unclear.

- There is no universal agreement on how to report the susceptibility test results for 3rd generation cephalosporins for *Enterobacteriaceae* that naturally possess chromosomal cephalosporinases. This group of organisms includes *Enterobacter* spp., *Serratia* spp., *Citrobacter freundii*, *Proteus vulgaris* and *penneri*, *Providencia* spp. and *Morganella morganii*. Many recommend reporting them as resistant regardless of the test result, because of the known ability of 3rd generation cephalosporins to select for resistance strains during treatment (33). The propensity to select for resistant mutants, however, varies widely between these different species. We recommend reporting the true result, but making note in a comment on the report about the propensity for resistance selection if the test result is 'susceptible'.

- Most methods do not explicitly suggest extrapolating results for cefotaxime to ceftriaxone, or vice versa. Normally, the laboratory would choose to test the agent that is used by clientele, but both agents may be in use, or there may be a formulary switch, or there may even be difficulty in acquiring a panel with the correct agent if purchasing through a consortium. In almost all circumstances, results for these two agents are interchangeable. The one important exception is the hyperproduction of the K1 enzyme in *Klebsiella oxytoca*, which makes the strain resistant to ceftriaxone but still susceptible to cefotaxime (on testing at least) and ceftazidime (10). Therefore, if cefotaxime is used for testing, it may fail to detect hyper-producing strains of *K. oxytoca* which may resist treatment with ceftriaxone.

- At least one method recommends that ampicillin-resistant *Enterobacteriaceae* be reported as resistant to cephalothin (6). This relates to a demonstrable inoculum effect that can be shown in ß-lactamase-producing *Enterobacteriaceae* (mainly *E. coli* with cephalothin). By contrast, there is a paucity of data to show whether these strains fail to respond to cephalothin in vivo.

- With current breakpoints, many strains of *Staphylococcus saprophyticus* test resistant to penicillin and anti-staphylococcal penicillins. The reason for this is that the breakpoints which are used straddle the normal MIC distribution for this species, rather than the presence of a true resistance mechanism. Many strains have a ß-lactamase that is detectable using nitrocefin, but its presence does not correlate with changes in MIC, and thus, it is of dubious significance. As this is a urinary pathogen, and levels of penicillins achieved in urine are many fold higher than the MICs of this species, we recommend that *S. saprophyticus* be reported as susceptible to penicillins whatever the result of the test. Unfortunately, there are no prospective clinical data to confirm or to deny the validity of this approach.

Table 9   Intrinsic resistances that are anticipated.

Species	Natural resistances (borderline resistance in square brackets)
Gram positive bacteria	
All	Mecillinam, aztreonam, 1st generation quinolones, polymyxins
Bacillus cereus	Penicillins, cephalosporins
Corynebacterium jeikeium and *C. urealyticum*	ß-lactams, aminoglycosides, macrolides, lincosamides, sulfonamides
Erysipelothrix rhusiopathiae	Glycopeptides
Enterococcus species	Anti-staphylococcal penicillins, 1st, 2nd, and 3rd generation cephalosporins [4th generation cephalosporins], pefloxacin, fosfomycin
Enterococcus faecalis	Lincosamides
Lactobacillus species	Sulfonamides
Heterofermentative *Lactobacillus* species	Glycopeptides
Listeria monocytogenes	Anti-staphylococcal penicillins, cephalosporins, lincosamides, 2nd generation quinolones
Nocardia species	Trimethoprim, glycopeptides, rifampicin, 2nd and 3rd generation quinolones
Pediococcus and *Leuconostoc* species	Glycopeptides
Rhodococcus equi	Streptogramins
Staphylococcus saprophyticus	Novobiocin, fosfomycin
Staphylococcus cohnii and *S. xylosis*	Novobiocin, lincomycin
Streptococcus species	Pefloxacin [aminoglycosides]
Gram negative bacteria	
All	Glycopeptides
Acinetobacter baumannii and *A. calcoaceticus*	Moderate spectrum penicillins, 1st and 2nd generation cephalosporins, fosfomycin, trimethoprim, nitrofurans
Aeromonas species	Moderate spectrum penicillins (except *A. rota*), 1st and 2nd generation cephalosporins (except *A. veronii*)
Burkholderia cepacia	Carboxypenicillins, ticarcillin-clavulanate, cefotaxime and ceftriaxone, carbapenems, quinolones, amphenicols, trimethoprim, fosfomycin, polymyxins
Campylobacter spp.	Aztreonam, novobiocin, streptogramins, trimethoprim
C. jejuni ss *jejuni, C. coli,* and *C. lari*	Cephalosporins
C. lari and *C. fetus*	Quinolones
Enterobacteriaceae	Narrow spectrum penicillins, anti-staphylococcal penicillins, MLSK group, fusidic acid
Enterobacter spp. and *Citrobacter freundii*	Moderate spectrum penicillins, amoxycillin-clavulanate, 1st and 2nd generation cephalosporins, cefamycins
Haemophilus species	16-membered macrolides [14- and 15-membered macrolides]
Klebsiella spp., *Citrobacter diversus* (*koseri*), and *Yersinia enterocolitica*	Moderate spectrum and anti-pseudomonal penicillins
Moraxella species	Trimethoprim
Moraxella catarrhalis	Lincosamides
Neisseria species	Trimethoprim
Neisseria meningitidis and *N. gonorrhoeae*	Lincosamides, polymyxins
Non-fermentative Gram negative bacilli	Narrow spectrum penicillins, anti-staphylococcal penicillins, fusidic acid, MLSK group
Proteus mirabilis	Tetracyclines, polymyxins, nitrofurans
Providencia stuartii	Moderate spectrum penicillins, 1st generation cephalosporins, polymyxins
Pseudomonas aeruginosa	Moderate spectrum penicillins, 1st and 2nd generation cephalosporins, cefotaxime, ceftriaxone, ceftizoxime, tetracyclines, amphenicols, folate antagonists, 1st generation quinolones, nitrofurans
Serratia marcescens, Proteus vulgaris, Proteus penneri and *Morganella morganii*	Moderate spectrum penicillins, amoxycillin-clavulanate, 1st and 2nd generation cephalosporins, cefamycins, polymyxins, nitrofurans
Stenotrophomonas maltophilia	Anti-pseudomonal penicillins, cefotaxime, ceftriaxone, carbapenems, trimethoprim, fosfomycin

Table 9 cont'd.

Species	Natural resistances (borderline resistance in square brackets)
Anaerobic bacteria	
All	Aminoglycosides, aztreonam (except *Fusobacterium* species), folate antagonists, 1st and 2nd generation fluoroquinolones
Bacteroides fragilis group	Narrow and moderate spectrum penicillins, 1st and 2nd generation cephalosporins, polymyxins, glycopeptides, fosfomycin
Clostridium spp., *Eubacterium* spp. and *Peptostreptococcus* spp.	Polymyxins, fosfomycin
Clostridium difficile	Cephalosporins
Clostridium innocuum	Glycopeptides
Fusobacterium spp.	Macrolides
Fusobacterium mortiferum and *F. necrophorum*	Rifamycins
Porphyromonas spp.	Fosfomycin, polymyxins
Prevotella spp.	Glycopeptides, fosfomycin

E. Expert systems

A combination of antibiograms, natural resistances, and 'impossible' results is used by the expert systems and is incorporated into the operating systems of some modern semi-automated systems (36). They remove the tedium of having to remember all the rules for all of the organisms. They also remove the skill of the tester, however, to understand resistances and their mechanisms, and to spot errors in the procedures.

XVI. HANDY HINTS

A. Enteric pathogens

It is common practice not to test bacterial enteric pathogen isolates based on the fact that the great majority of gastroenteritides that are caused by these pathogens are self-limiting and do not require antibacterial treatment. Furthermore, susceptibility testing is generally focussed on treatment of systemic infection, and no correlates for outcome of treatment with enteric infections has ever been made.

   Of course, none would argue about testing blood culture isolates of these organisms. Up to 10% of bacterial diarrheas, however, will eventually be treated with antibacterials, and it may not be obvious to the laboratory at the time of isolation that antibacterials will be required. We would argue that many of the common pathogens should be tested routinely, such that treatment can be administered in a more informed way for complicated local, bacteremic, or metastatic infection. Current guidelines for *Enterobacteriaceae* can be readily applied to *Salmonella* spp., *Shigella* spp., and *Yersinia enterocolitica*. There are no guidelines at present in most methods for *Campylobacter* spp. In addition, those laboratories that contribute regularly to surveillance programs will be generating valuable epidemiological data for the region or the nation.

B. Mucoid *Pseudomonas aeruginosa*

Patients with cystic fibrosis and other chronic bronchiectactic lung conditions often become colonized with *Pseudomonas aeruginosa*. Mostly in these circumstances, the *P. aeruginosa* produces an alginate capsule that confers a mucoid colony phenotype. Acute exacerbations of infection in these patients require sputum culture and susceptibility testing. It is more difficult to standardize an inoculum for susceptibility testing with mucoid *P. aeruginosa* than their non-mucoid counterparts. Nevertheless, if the standard methods are used, it has been shown, at least for NCCLS methods, that reproducible results can be obtained (59). Whether this applies to other methods is not known.

C. Topical antibiotics

The relevance of testing antibiotics that are used topically against localized infections is not known. Nevertheless, requests for testing still arise for such infections as bacterial conjunctivitis and otitis externa which are almost always managed by topical rather than systemic antibiotics. Antibiotic choices for these infections fall into two groups. There are a number of antibiotics that are used topically, and not systemically, such as neomycin, framycetin, bacitracin, and gramicidin. There are also systemic antibiotics that also enjoy extensive topical use including chloramphenicol, the sulfonamides, gentamicin, tobramycin, ciprofloxacin, colistin, and polymyxin B. Two problems arise when contemplating the assessment of isolates from topical infections. Firstly, no breakpoints have been established with the topical (only) agents in particular because there have been no correlations to clinical outcome. Secondly, topical concentrations of antibiotics are many fold higher (100- to 1000-fold is not uncommon) than can be achieved systemically; thus, using systemic breakpoints seems inappropriate as again there has been no correlation with outcome. We would recommend either not testing at all, or testing for those agents that are used systemically with systemic breakpoints and with a comment on reports that resistance cannot easily predict failure due to the very high topical concentrations.

XVII. UNSOLVED PROBLEMS

There are a number of less common but important pathogens for which there are no routine standardized methods or which present particular problems for testing. Bacteria in this category include *Nocardia* spp., *Campylobacter* spp., *Brucella* spp., other fastidious Gram negative pathogens such as *Eikenella corrodens*, rapid-growing *Mycobacteria*, *Mycoplasma* spp., and *Ureaplasma urealyticum*. Methods exist for all of these organisms, but they are mostly applied to research. For some of them, it is possible to generate MICs or to include them in routine tests. For others, special growth requirements or prolonged incubation are needed, and thus specialized methods must be used. Difficulties arise, however, in the interpretation of any values that are generated by including them in routine tests since legitimized breakpoints have not been developed. It is hoped that relatively simple methods and/or breakpoints will be developed for these organisms in the future. In the meantime, if susceptibility results are important for patient management, the best option is to refer isolates to a reference laboratory that has established methods for these organisms where this is possible.

REFERENCES

1. Sanders CC. ARTs versus ASTs: where are we going? J Antimicrob Chemother 1991; 28:621-623.
2. Rex JH, Pfaller MA, Galgiani JN, Bartlett MS, Espinel-Ingroff A, Ghannoum MA, Lancaster M, Odds FC, Rinaldi MG, Walsh TJ, Barry AL for the Subcommittee on Antifungal Susceptibility Testing of the National Committee for Clinical Laboratory Standards. Development of interpretive breakpoints for antifungal susceptibility testing: conceptual framework and analysis of in vitro-in vivo correlation data for fluconazole, itraconazole, and *Candida albicans* infections. Clin Infect Dis 1997; 24:235-247.
3. Craig WA. Pharmacokinetic/pharmacodynamic parameters: rationale for antibacterial dosing of mice and men. Clin Infect Dis 1998; 26:1-12
4. Ericcson JM, Sherris JC. Antibiotic sensitivity testing. Report of an international collaborative study. Acta Pathol Microbiol Scand [B] 1971; 217:S1-S90.
5. NCCLS. Methods for dilution antimicrobial susceptibility tests for bacteria that grow aerobically. Approved Standard – Fifth Edition M7-A5. Wayne, Pa.:NCCLS, 2000.

6. Bell SM. The CDS method of antibiotic sensitivity testing (calibrated dichotomous sensitivity test). Pathology 1975; 7:S1-S48.

7. British Society for Antimicrobial Chemotherapy. Report of the working party on antibiotic sensitivity testing of the British Society for Antimicrobial Chemotherapy: a guide to sensitivity testing. J Antimicrob Chemother 1991; 27 (Suppl D):1-50.

8. The Swedish Reference Group for Antibiotics. A revised system for antibiotic sensitivity testing. Scand J Infect Dis 1981; 13:148-152.

9. Waxman DJ, Strominger JL. Penicillin-binding proteins and the mechanism of action of beta-lactam antibiotics. Ann Rev Biochem 1983; 52:825-869.

10. Livermore DM. Beta-lactamases in laboratory and clinical resistance. Clin Microbiol Rev 1995; 8:557-584.

11. Bush K, Jacoby GA, Medeiros AA. A functional classification scheme for beta-lactamases and its correlation with molecular structure. Antimicrob Agents Chemother 1995; 39:1211-1233.

12. Quintiliani R Jr, Sahm DF, Courvalin P. Mechanisms of resistance to antimicrobial agents. In: Murray PR, Baron EJ, Pfaller MA, Tenover FC, Yolken RH, eds. Manual of Clinical Microbiology. 7th Edition. Washington, DC:ASM Press, 1999:1505-1525.

13. Davies JE. Resistance to aminoglycosides: mechanism and frequency. Rev Infect Dis 1983; 5 (Suppl 2):261-267.

14. Leclerq R, Courvalin P. Bacterial resistance to macrolide, lincosamide and streptogramin antibiotics by target modification. Antimicrob Agents Chemother 1991; 35:1267-1272.

15. Arthur M, Courvalin P. Genetics and mechanisms of glycopeptide resistance in enterococci. Antimicrob Agents Chemother 1993; 37:1563-1571.

16. Kuroda M, Kuwahara-Arai K, Hiramatsu K. Identification of the up- and down- regulated genes in vancomycin-resistant *Staphylococcus aureus* strains Mu3 and Mu50 by cDNA differential hybridization method. Biochem Biophys Res Commun 2000; 269:485-490.

17. Huovinen P, Sundstrom L, Swedberg G, Skold O. Trimethoprim and sulfonamide resistance. Antimicrob Agents Chemother 1995; 39:279-289.

18. McCalla DR. Biological effects of nitrofurans. J Antimicrob Chemother 1977; 3:517-520.

19. Turnidge J, Collignon P. Resistance to fusidic acid. Int J Antimicrob Agents 1999; 12:S35-S44.

20. Working Party on Sensitivity Testing. BSAC standardized disc sensitivity testing method. Newsletter of the British Society for Antimicrobial Chemotherapy, Summer, 1998.

21. Courvalin P, Soussy C-J. 1996 Report of the Comite de l'Antibiogramme de la Societe Francaise de Microbiologie. Clin Microbiol Infect 1996; 2 (Suppl 1):1-49.

22. Comite de l'Antibiotique de la Societe Francaise de Microbiologie. Communique 1999. http://www.sfm.asso.fr/Sect4/atbuk/.html

23. Deutches Institut fur Normung. Methoden zur Empfindlichkeitssprufung von Bakteriallen Krankheitserregern (auber Mycobacterien) gegen Chemotherapeutika. DIN 58940. Berlin, Germany:Beuth Verlag GmbH, 1983.

24. Werkgroep Richtlijnen Gevoeligheidsbepalingen. Satndaardisatie van Gevoeligheidsbepalingen. Bilthoven, The Netherlands:Werkgroep Richtlijnen Gevoeligheidsbepalingen, 1981.

25. Ringertz S, Olsson-Liljequist B, Kahlmeter G, Kronvall G. Antimicrobial susceptibility testing in Sweden. II. Species-related zone diameter breakpoints to avoid interpretive errors and guard against unrecognized evolution of resistance. Scand J Infect Dis 1997; 105:S8-S12.

26. Olsson-Liljequist B, Larsson P, Walder M, Miorner H. Antimicrobial susceptibility testing in Sweden. III. Methodology for susceptibility testing. Scand J Infect Dis 1997; 105:S13-S23.

27. Kahlmeter G, Olsson-Liljequist B, Ringertz S. Antimicrobial susceptibility testing in Sweden. IV. Quality assurance. Scand J Infect Dis 1997; 105:S24-S31.

28. Casals JB, Pringler N. Antibacterial/antifungal senstivity testing using Neo-sensitabs. Rosco Diagnostica, Taastrup, Denmark, 1991.

29. Report of the committee for Japanese Standard for Antimicrobial Susceptibility Testing for Bacteria. Japan Society for Chemotherapy 1993; 41:183-189. (in Japanese)

30. Saito A. clinical breakpoints for antimicrobial agents in pulmonary infections and sepsis: report of the Committee for Japanese Standards for Antimicrobial Susceptibility Testing for Bacteria. J Infect Chemther 1995; 1:83-88.

31. Arakawa S, Matsui T, Kamidono S, Kawada Y, Kumon H, Hirai K, Hirose T, Matsumoto T, Yamaguchi K, Yoshida T, Watanabe K, Uueno K, Saito A, Teranishi T. Derivation of a calculation formula for breakpoints of antimicrobial agents in urinary tract infections. J Infect Chemother 1999; 5:223-226.

32. Saito A, Inamatsu T, Okada J, OguriT, Kanno H, Kusano N, Kumon H, Yamagichi K, Watanabe A, Watanabe K. Clinical breakpoints in pulmonary infections and sepsis: new antimicrobial agents and supplemental information for some agents already released. J Infect Chemother 1999; 5:223-226.
33. Bell SM, Gatus BJ, Pham JN. Antibiotic sensitivity testing by the CDS method. Sydney, Australia:South Eastern Area Laboratory Services, 1999.
34. NCCLS. Performance standards for antimicrobial disk susceptibility tests. Approved Standard – 7th Edition M2-A7. Wayne, PA:NCCLS, 2000.
35. Shungu DL. Chemical and physical properties of antibiotics: preparation and control of antibiotic susceptibility disks and other devices containing antibiotics. In: Lorian V, ed. Antibiotics in Laboratory Medicine, 4th Edition. Baltimore, MD:Williams and Wilkins, 1996:765-792.
36. Ferraro MJ, Jorgensem JH. Susceptibility testing instrumentation and computerized expert systems for data analysis and interpretation. In: Murray PR, Baron EJ, Pfaller MA, Tenover FC, Yolken RH, eds. Manual of Clinical Microbiology. 7th Edition. Washington DC, ASM Press, 1999:1593-1600.
37. D'Amato RF, Hochstein L, Vernaleo JR, Thornsberry C. Evaluation of BIOMIC antimicrobial test system. J Clin Microbiol 1985; 22:793-798.
38. Metzler DM, DeHaan RM. Susceptibility tests for anaerobic bacteria: statistical and clinical considerations. J Infect Dis 1974; 130:588-594.
39. Brunden MN, Zurenko GE, Kapik B. Modification of the error-bounded classification scheme for use with two MIC breakpoints. Diagn Microbiol Infect Dis 1992; 15:135-140.
40. Brown DF, Brown L. Evaluation of the Etest, a novel method for quantifying antimicrobial activity. J Antimicrob Chemother1991; 27:185-190.
41. Doern GV, Vautour R, Gaudet M, Levy B. Clinical impact of rapid in vitro susceptibility and bacterial identification. J Clin Microbiol 1994; 32:1757-1762.
42. Leitch C, Boonlayangoor. ß-lactamase tests. In: HD Isenberg, ed. Clinical Microbiology Procedures Handbook. Washington, DC: ASM Press. 1992: 5.3.1-5.3.8.
43. Jarlier V, Nicolas MH, Fournier G, Philippon A. Extended broad-spectrum beta-lactamases conferring a transferable resistance to newer beta-lactam agents in *Enterobacteriaceae*: hospital prevalence and susceptibility patterns. Rev Infect Dis 1988; 10:867-878.
44. Eliopoulos GM, Moellering RC. Antimicrobial combinations. In: Lorian V, ed. Antibiotics in Laboratory Medicine. Baltimore, MD:Williams and Wilkins, 1996:330-396.
45. Woodford N. Glycopeptide-resistant enterococci: a decade of experience. J Med Microbiol 1998; 47:849-862.
46. Cavassini M, Wenger K, Jaton K, Blanc DS, Bille J. Evaluation of MRSA-Screen, a simple anti-PBP 2a slide latex agglutination kit, for rapid detection of methicillin-resistance in *Staphylococcus aureus*. J Clin Microbiol 1999; 37:1591-1594.
47. Hiramatsu K, Hanaki H, Ino T, Yabuta K, Oguri T, Tenover FC. Methicillin-resistant *Staphylococcus aureus* clinical strain with reduced vancomycin susceptibility. J Antimicrob Chemother 1997; 40:135-136.
48. Tenover FC, Lancaster MV, Hill BC, Steward CD, Stocker SA, Hancock GA, O'Hara CM, Clark NC, Hiramatsu L. Characterization of staphylococci with reduced susceptibility to vancomycin and other glycopeptides. J Clin Microbiol 1998; 36:1020-1027.
49. Hiramatsu K. Vancomycin resistance in staphylococcus. Drug Resistance Updates 1998; 1:135-150.
50. Muramaki K, Minamide W, Wada K, Nakamura E, Teraoka H, Watanabe S. Identification of methicillin-resistant strains of staphylococci by polymerase chain reaction. J Clin Microbiol 1991; 29:2240-2244.
51. Dutka-Malen S, Evers S, Courvalin P. Detection of glycopeptide resistance genotypes and identification to the species level of clinically relevant enterococci. J Clin Microbiol 1995; 33:24-27.
52. NCCLS. Methods for determining bactericidal activity of antimicrobial agents. Approved Guideline M26-A. Wayne, PA:NCCLS, 1999.
53. NCCLS. Methodology for the serum bactericidal test. Approved Guideline M21-A. Wayne, PA:NCCLS, 1999.
54. Reller LB. The serum bactericidal test. Rev Infect Dis 1986; 8:803-808.
55. Leggett JE, Wolz SA, Craig WA. Use of serum ultrafiltrate in the serum dilution test. J Infect Dis 1989; 160:616-623.
56. NCCLS. Methods for antimicrobial susceptibility testing of anaerobic bacteria. Approved Standard M11-A4. Wayne, PA:NCCLS, 1997.
57. Citron DM, Oostovari MI, Karlsson Å, Goldstein EJC. Evaluation of Etest susceptibility testing of anaerobic bacteria. J Clin Microbiol 1991; 29:2197-2203.
58. Huysmans MB, Turnidge JD. Disc susceptibility testing for thermophilic campylobacters. Pathology 1997; 29:209-216.

59. Burns JL, Saiman L, Whittier S, Larone D, Krzewinski J, Liu Z, Marshall SA, Jones SN. Comparison of agar diffusion methodologies for antimicrobial susceptibility testing of *Pseudomonas aeruginosa* isolates from cystic fibrosis patients. Antimicrob Agents Chemother 2000; 38:1818-1822.

9

Blood Culture Systems

W. Michael Dunne, Jr.
Barnes-Jewish Hospital and Washington University School of Medicine, St. Louis, Missouri

Mark LaRocco
Department of Pathology, St. Luke's Episcopal Health System, Houston, Texas

I. INTRODUCTION

The ability to rapidly detect the presence of microorganisms in the bloodstream of a patient with an invasive, life-threatening infection is truly one of the most important functions of the clinical microbiology laboratory. This responsibility was recognized early in the 20th century but from an historical perspective, the report of Scott in 1951 (1), which described a modification of the Casteneda blood culture technique (2), is considered to represent the birth of the modern day blood culture method. Numerous adaptations of this protocol have been reported since Scott's publication but the basic design, that consists of two complementary bottles of broth media and head-space atmospheres so fashioned to optimize the recovery of aerobic and anaerobic microorganisms from blood, remains the mainstay of blood culture technology today. The evolution of blood culture systems has advanced considerably over the past fifteen years but the basic principles have not changed. During this most recent period of development, greater emphasis was placed on instrumentation and automation of the blood culture process. With the advent of immunosuppressive therapy, opportunistic infections, and biomedical implants, however, a new responsibility has been placed on the microbiology laboratory, i.e., to determine whether microorganisms recovered from blood are actually involved in the disease process or were accidentally introduced into the culture media during specimen procurement or inoculation.

During the course of this chapter, the newest concepts in blood culture collection, incubation, and interpretation will be reviewed. In order to keep the topic contemporary, the discussion that follows will be limited to applications that have been developed within the past two decades. The reader is referred to two previous publications for a review of blood culture systems that were developed prior to 1980 (3,4).

II. COLLECTION OF BLOOD CULTURES

The frequent association of indigenous skin and mucosal microflora with infected transcutaneous catheters, biomedical implants, and heart valves, necessitates strict attention to the process of skin antisepsis and venipuncture during the collection of blood for culture. The venipuncture site is prepared by scrubbing with 70% alcohol for 30 sec. or longer and is followed by the concentric application of an iodine solution over the site. Both tincture of iodine (1-2%) or 10% povidone-iodine have been used with success although the latter requires a longer contact time (60 sec. or more) to achieve antisepsis. A variety of commercially prepared skin antisepsis kits are available for this purpose. The phlebotomist must avoid reintroduction of skin flora at the puncture site as a consequence of palpating the vein with a contaminated finger or glove after the area has been disinfected. The appropriate volume of blood is then collected with the use of either a syringe and needle or a transfer set, and the iodine is removed from the skin site with a terminal alcohol scrub (5).

In addition to the skin site, the rubber septum of the blood culture bottle(s) must also be disinfected prior to inoculation. This is accomplished by applying 70% alcohol or iodine solution to the septum for at least 1 min. of contact time or until the solution dries. If an iodine solution is used, it is best to remove the excess with an alcohol wipe or sterile gauze prior to inoculation in order to prevent the introduction of iodine into the culture medium (5).

The volume of blood that is collected for each blood culture set must take into consideration the appropriate blood-to-broth ratio (see below) and the age of the patient. For pediatric patients, volumes ranging from 1-5 ml. per draw (depending on age) are sufficient to detect significant bacteremia whereas larger volumes (10-30 ml. per draw or 5-15 ml. per bottle) are required to achieve the same sensitivity in adults (5). In the case of a child, if 1 ml. of blood or less is obtained, the entire sample should be inoculated into an aerobic blood culture bottle or collected in a pediatric Isolator™ tube (see lysis-centrifugation) as the likelihood of anaerobic bacteremia in children is considerably less (6).

The number of blood cultures that are required to detect clinically significant episodes of bacteremia and the timing of the collection schedule still remain somewhat controversial. In the past, the timing of blood culture collection was initiated at the point in which the patient developed characteristic symptoms of sepsis, i.e., chills, fever, hypotension, etc. The greatest magnitude of bacteremia, and therefore the most productive time to obtain blood cultures, usually precedes the expression of symptoms by an hour or more (5). In the absence of psychic powers, it is reasonable to obtain two or three independent blood specimens for culture as soon as the patient is symptomatic and before the administration of antimicrobial agents. Generally, three independent blood culture sets within a 24 hr. period are sufficient for the diagnosis of bacteremia and/or endocarditis. After the initial sets of blood cultures are obtained, the timing of subsequent blood cultures is totally arbitrary and does not increase the overall yield. From a practical sense, orders for 30, 45, or 60 min. timing intervals between draws often creates a logistical nightmare for the phlebotomy service and could delay the diagnosis of significant bacteremia and/or the institution of appropriate therapy. In fact, it is the total volume of blood collected per culture rather than the timing that contributes most to the detection of a septic event (7).

III. THE ANATOMY OF A BLOOD CULTURE

At the foundation of all blood culture systems (with the exception of lysis-centrifugation) is the visually monitored or 'conventional' broth culture. The basic blood culture generally consists of a pair of bottles that contain various media combinations which cover the nutritional and respiratory needs of the wide spectrum of microorganisms that invade the bloodstream of humans. Brain heart infusion (BHI), Columbia, tryptic and Trypticase soy, thiol and thioglycollate broth formulations with or without supplements have all been successfully employed. A variety of broth volumes are also commercially available ranging from 18 to 100 ml. The volume of broth in the bottle coincides with the anticipated draw volume of blood so that an ideal blood-to-broth ratio of 1:5 to 1:10 is maintained (4). The anticoagulant, anticomplement, and anti-lysosomal activities of sodium polyanethol sulphonate (SPS) and its utility as a blood culture additive were recognized in the early 1930s (8,9). SPS, however, was also found to inhibit the growth of fastidious organisms such as *Neisseria gonorrhoeae* when concentrations exceeded 0.05% (8). Currently, many blood culture broth formulations contain SPS in concentrations ranging from 0.006 to 0.05%. Supplements such as vitamin K_1, hemin, L-cysteine, gelatin, and hypertonic sucrose have been preferentially added to broth media to enhance the recovery of selected pathogens. Polymeric adsorbent or ionic exchange resins have been incorporated into blood culture media in an attempt to inactivate antimicrobial agents that might be present in the blood specimen. The atmosphere within commercially prepared blood culture bottles is evacuated to remove O_2 and is enriched with CO_2. After injection of the blood specimen, one bottle may be vented to generate an aerobic atmosphere.

In the absence of an automated bacterial growth detection system, both bottles are examined visually for signs of bacterial growth, i.e., macroscopic colonies, turbidity, hemolysis, gas production, or a change in the color of blood. This ritual is performed initially after 6-18 hrs. of incubation and daily thereafter for a total of seven days (10). In addition, routine subcultures and/or Gram or acridine orange stain of the cultures at the time of the initial examination have proven useful for early detection of growth in conventional cultures (11,12). Blind or terminal subcultures and microscopic examination of blood cultures performed thereafter are of little value (13,14). With rare exceptions, such as for patients with suspect brucellosis or with infections caused by slowly growing microorganisms, extension of the incubation of basic blood cultures beyond seven days is fruitless. Over a two-year period, 76 conventional blood cultures at Henry Ford Hospital were held for a total of four weeks by special request. Bacteria were recovered from five cultures, four of which grew *Propionibacterium* species and one which yielded coagulase-negative staphylococci. None of these were considered clinically significant.

With the advent of automated, continuously-monitored blood culture systems and the lysis-centrifugation technique, the manual blood culture procedure has been replaced in many high volume laboratories but still finds limited application when the capacity of an automated system is exceeded or when the daily volume of blood cultures received does not justify the purchase of an automated system.

IV. BIPHASIC BLOOD CULTURE MEDIA

The use of a solid-liquid medium interface or biphasic culture system was first described by Casteneda in 1947 (2) for the recovery of *Brucella* species from blood but the versatility of this format for rapid detection of bacteremia in general and fungemia was quickly recognized. Unfortunately, the advantages of using biphasic media for blood cultures were offset by the difficulty in producing the bottles. Commercially prepared biphasic blood culture bottles, however, have appeared on the market including the Opticult® and Septi-Chek™ systems from Becton-Dickinson Microbiology Systems (Sparks, Maryland). The former product has been discontinued but the latter is still available and consists of a standard broth culture bottle and a cylindrical housing which contains a paddle that is coated with chocolate, MacConkey, and malt agars (Figure 1). Bottles are available with either 20 or 70 ml. of broth in four different formulations to accommodate the correct blood-broth ratio; they can be purchased with antimicrobial removal resins in order to facilitate the recovery of organisms from patients who receive concomitant antibiotic therapy. A more recent version of the Septi-Chek™ product has been formulated specifically for culture of mycobacteria. After inoculation of the broth bottle with blood, the agar device is attached to the top of the bottle. Routine subculture is accomplished by simply inverting the assembly which will allow the blood-broth mixture to flood over the surface of the agar. Due to the ambient atmospheric interface between the bottle and the agar, neither of the biphasic systems described here has an anaerobic component.

In side-by-side comparisons with conventional blood culture bottles, biphasic media have generally provided enhanced recovery of clinically significant aerobic and facultatively anaerobic organisms, including fungi, with a decreased time to detection of positive cultures and isolated colonies (15-24). Conversely, two-bottle blood culture sets retain an advantage over biphasic media with attachable agar devices in that there are lower contamination rates and that the isolation of anaerobic bacteria from blood is improved (19,20,22,24).

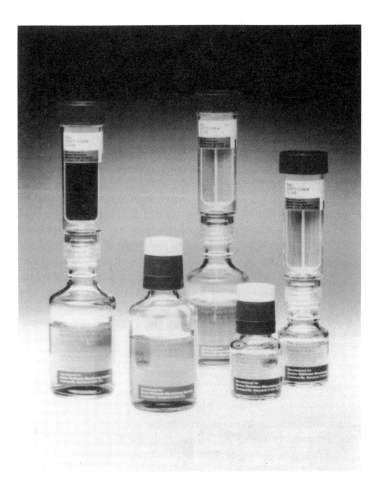

Figure 1   The Septichek™ system from Becton-Dickinson Microbiology Systems (Sparks, Maryland) consists of a standard broth culture bottle and a cylindrical adapter that contains an agar-coated paddle with chocolate, Mac-Conkey, and malt agars. After inoculation of the broth with blood, the adapter is attached to the top of the bottle. Subculture is accomplished by inverting the bottle and allowing the blood-broth mixture to wash over the agar surface.

V.   LYSIS-CENTRIFUGATION

In 1917, Mildred Clough (25) first demonstrated the value of a lysis-centrifugation method for the isolation of *Mycobacterium tuberculosis* from blood. Using a forbearer of the current technique, she was able to obtain isolated colonies of mycobacteria within two weeks of plating the processed blood on solid agar media. Despite these encouraging results, the evolution of lysis-based blood culture techniques proceeded at a glacial pace over the next 60 years.

In 1976, Dorn et al. (26) reported on a modification of the lysis-centrifugation procedure in which microorganisms were extracted from lysed blood into a sucrose-gelatin or Ficoll density layer. The device was eventually modified to reduce contamination and to enhance recovery by the use of a fluoro-chemical density layer and a fixed-angle centrifuge rotor (27). The improved apparatus was found to exceed the performance of conventional blood cultures in both total recovery of microorganisms and in time to detection of a positive blood culture (28). This work led to the development of the Isolator™ 10 by the E.I. du Pont de Nemours & Co., Inc. but that is now owned and marketed by Wampole Laboratories (Cranbury, New Jersey; Figure 2). The commercial product consists of a 10 ml. glass vacutainer-type tube containing saponin as a lysing agent, polypropylene glycol as an antifoaming agent, SPS, EDTA as an anticoagulant, and an inert fluorochemical density layer. After the addition of blood, the tube is thoroughly mixed and is thereafter centrifuged at 3,000 x g for 30 min. in a fixed-angle rotor. Following centrifugation, the rubber septum is pierced by a plastic adapter and the high density/microorganism phase is removed from the bottom of the tube with a pipette. The latter is then directly plated onto solid media. The media repertoire and incubation conditions are selected to optimize the recovery of fastidious and anaerobic bacteria, yeasts, and/or mycobacteria. This system also provides for direct quantitation of isolated organisms which may prove useful for risk assessment and for the evaluation of intravascular device-associated infections (29-31). The Isolator™ is also available in a 1.5 ml. tube for use with pediatric patients.

The strengths of this system are somewhat similar to biphasic blood culture methods in that isolated colonies for identification and susceptibility testing are available sooner than broth-based methods while the rate of recovery of yeasts and filamentous fungi from blood appears equal to or superior to biphasic media (32-36). Most clinical evaluations have demonstrated that the Isolator™ has proven to be comparable or superior to other methods for the recovery of bacteria and fungi from blood, especially *Enterobacteriaceae, Staphylococcus aureus,* and yeasts (32-37). The advantages of lysis-centrifugation seem to be negated, however, when media containing antimicrobial resins or saponin are used (38,39). For the recovery of mycobacteria from blood, the Isolator™ has proven comparable or superior to conventional or radiometric methods (40,41). The weakness of the lysis-centrifugation method is a propensity for higher contamination rates (33-35,37).

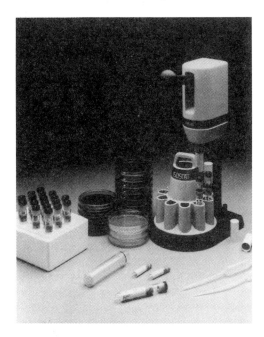

Figure 2   The Isolator™ lysis-centrifugation blood culture system as distributed by Wampole Laboratories. The product consists of a 10 ml. or 1.5 ml. vacutainer-type tube which contains a lysing agent, polypropylene glycol, SPS, EDTA, and an inert fluorochemical density layer. After the addition of blood, the tube is mixed and centrifuged in a fixed-angle rotor. Following centrifugation, the rubber septum is pierced by a plastic adapter and the fluorochemical/micro-organism phase is removed and cultured directly on solid media.

The enhanced performance of automated, continuous monitoring blood culture (CMBC) systems (see below) has, by most published accounts, diminished the advantages of lysis-centrifugation for the recovery of bacteria from bloodstream infections. The automated features of these systems as compared to the manual processing times that are required by lysis-centrifugation is attractive to most busy clinical microbiology laboratories. Moreover, performance comparisons of the Isolator lysis-centrifugation system to BacTAlert (42-44), BACTEC 9240 (45,46), and ESP (47) showed equivalent or superior recovery of Gram positive and Gram negative bacterial pathogens by the automated systems, and also often showed lower median times to detection as well as lower contamination rates. The Isolator^{TM} remains an effective device for the recovery of some fungi from blood, and in some studies, it performed better than CMBC systems for the detection of fungemia. A comparison of Isolator^{TM} to BacTAlert with standard aerobic media showed superior performance of Isolator for the detection of fungemia as caused by *Candida* spp., *Histoplasma capsulatum*, and *Malassezia furfur* (48). Another study compared Isolator^{TM} to the ESP 80A blood culture bottle and found better recovery of *C. albicans* and *C. glabrata* by Isolator^{TM} (49). A third study compared the performance of Isolator^{TM} to the BACTEC 9240 with Myco/F lytic medium (50). Although the number of fungal bloodstream infections was too small for statistical evaluation, the overall performance trends of the two systems were comparable.

VI. CONTINUOUS MONITORING BLOOD CULTURE (CMBC) SYSTEMS

Prior to 1990, all blood culture systems, whether manual or semi-automated, suffered from similar deficiencies. The frequency for daily inspection of blood culture bottles in regards to providing evidence of microbial growth was limited by staffing constraints. At best, each culture in a high volume laboratory could be examined thrice daily either by visual inspection or by loading an instrument for batch processing. This type of quantum inspection was not only labor intensive, but it also significantly delayed the detection of positive cultures and, therefore, the institution of appropriate therapy. With this impediment in mind, several companies initiated the development of fully automated CMBC systems. The fruit of these competitive endeavors is a new generation of instrumentation that has evolved with diverse growth detection technology. For the sake of correctness, the term 'continuous monitoring' is a misnomer that should be more aptly named high frequency monitoring. Systems that support CMBC technology have emerged as the new standard in blood culture instrumentation and differ from other automated blood culture devices in several ways (51). Firstly, the systems are fully automated and incorporate the detection system incubator and agitation mechanism into a single unit. Once the bottles are loaded, there is no need for further manual manipulation unless growth is detected or unless the culture is terminated. Secondly, each individual bottle is monitored electronically on an almost continuous basis (typically once every ten minutes) and in a noninvasive manner. This eliminates the chance of cross-contamination of bottles. Thirdly, culture bottle data is stored in a microcomputer that determines when growth has occurred through a series of sophisticated algorithms. The algorithms allow for an earlier detection of growth and minimize the number of false positive signals. Finally, these systems incorporate software that provides data management capability to the user.

A. BacT/Alert blood culture systems

The BactT/Alert blood culture system (Organon Teknika Corporation, Durham, North Carolina) was the first instrument approved by the FDA to offer continuous monitoring blood culture capability. The BacT/Alert utilizes a microbial detection system that is based on the colorimetric detection of CO_2 (52). A sensor that is bonded on the inside bottom of each bottle is separated from the liquid contents by a membrane that is permeable only to CO_2. As actively growing microorganisms liberate CO_2 into the blood-broth mixture, the gas interacts with water that has been incorporated in the sensor thus causing a release of hydrogen ions. The hydrogen ions acidify the sensor and lead to colorimetric change from a green to yellow. A light-emitting diode projects light on the sensor every ten minutes and the light which is reflected is measured by a photodetector. The amount of light so reflected is proportionate to the amount of yellow colour change in the sensor and which in turn is proportionate to the amount of CO_2 in the bottle. Data is transferred to a microcomputer where it is analyzed as reflectance units per time. Software algorithms employ three criteria to determine bottle status: an initial reading in comparison to an arbitrary threshold, a sustained linear increase in CO_2 production, and an increased rate of CO_2 production. Organon Teknika has used this detection technology to also develop a system for mycobacterial detection called the MB/BacT.

Several media formulations for the BacT/Alert blood culture systems are available. The standard aerobic and anaerobic media consist of tryptic soy broth with a supplementation of complex amino acids and carbohydrates that are designed to support growth and to ensure optimal CO_2 production. Bottles contain 30 ml. of media with 0.035% sodium polyanetholesulfonate as an anticoagulant and can accommodate the introduction of up to 10 ml. of blood. The aerobic and anaerobic FAN media include brain-heart infusion broth base which contains Ecosorb (a proprietary substance that is composed of adsorbent charcoal, Fuller's earth, and other components). The FAN media are designed to enhance the recovery of micro-organisms from patients who receive antimicrobial therapy. Finally, there are the Pedi-BacT media which have been developed to accommodate smaller volume samples from pediatric patients.

The configuration of the "classic" BacT/Alert blood culture system consists of incubator cabinets which are linked to a microcomputer. Two cabinet sizes are available, including a 240-bottle or 120-bottle capacity (Figure 3). The bottles are contained in blocks, each holding 24 bottles that rock back-and-forth at a rate of 34 cycles per minute. As many as six incubator cabinets can be monitored by the microcomputer. The Microsoft Windows-based data management system (BacT/View) is menu driven with touch screen operation. The software supports all routine operating functions of the system and has bi-directional interface capability. User-defined data reporting functions include incidence by source or location, percent positive blood cultures, and contamination rates.

A more recent configuration of the system, the BacT/Alert 3D, offers a more compact and modular design, and allows the user to integrate blood culture and mycobacterial testing into a single platform. The BacT/Alert 3D consists of one to six stackable incubation drawers, each holding 60 bottles that are directed by a controller module (Figure 4). The controller module has a touch-activated operator panel for text-free user interface to direct random loading and unloading of samples. The controller also supervises the reading of the sensors and contains the decision-making algorithms in order to determine which specimens are positive. The basis for microbial detection and overall system performance, however, are identical to the "classic" BacT/Alert.

The first published evaluation of the BacT/Alert by Thorpe et al. (52) involved in vitro seeding experiments and a limited clinical evaluation which compared the performance of the prototype instrument to detection by the radiometric BACTEC method (see below). Results were sufficiently encouraging to warrant full-scale controlled clinical trials. The results of the first trial were published in 1992 by Wilson et al. (53). The BacT/Alert was comparable to the nonradiometric BACTEC method (see below) for microbial recovery but had earlier detection of bacterial growth and fewer false positive instrument signals.

B. BACTEC blood culture systems

The origins of BACTEC blood culture systems (Becton-Dickinson Microbiology Systems) can be traced back to work that was performed by Johnston Laboratories Inc. in the late 1960s. The company, having developed a tritium monitor for the detection of radiolabeled CO_2 on a flow-through basis, designed the first semi-automated systems for measuring bacterial growth that is based on the metabolic utilization of ^{14}C-labeled substrates. Designed primarily for research applications, the BACTEC Model 225 incubated, mixed, and tested 25 culture bottles as held in a circular lift-out tray. The bottles were moved to a detection platform at predetermined intervals where two needles penetrated the rubber

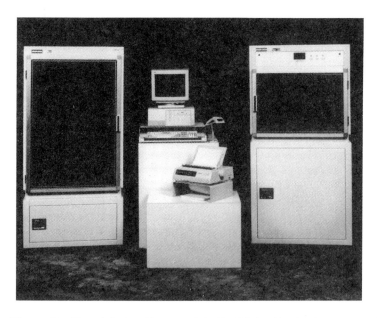

Figure 3   The original architecture of the BacT/Alert blood culture system that was developed by the Organon Teknika Corporation. The 240-bottle (left) and 120-bottle (right) capacity incubator cabinets are shown. Bottles are placed in blocks that rock back and forth at a rate of 34 cycles per minute. As many as six incubator cabinets can be monitored by the microprocessor (center).

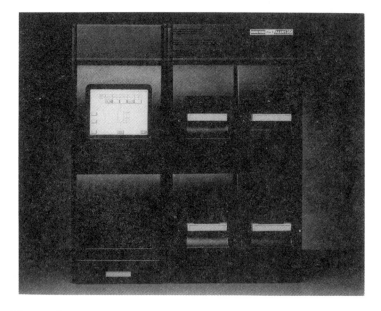

Figure 4   The BacT/Alert 3D is the most recent blood culture system that has been produced by the Organon Teknika Corporation. It provides a more compact and modular design which consists of one to six stackable incubation drawers each holding 60 blood culture bottles which are monitored by a single microprocessor.

septum at the top of each bottle, withdrew the gas that had collected in the head space, and replaced it with a fresh mixture. Radiolabeled CO_2 detected by the instrument was presumed to be the end-product of bacterial utilization of the ^{14}C-labeled substrates that were incorporated in the growth medium. The measured gas was expressed as an arbitrary "growth index" which, upon exceeding a predetermined threshold, was considered evidence of microbial growth. The application of the BACTEC 225 for the more rapid detection of microorganisms in blood specimens soon became apparent (54-56). The less expensive BACTEC Model 301 was marketed in 1972 and, for the first time, offered instrumented blood culture technology to small- and medium-sized hospital laboratories. Three media types were available: the aerobic medium [6A], the anaerobic medium [7A] and a hypertonic medium [8A]. As a manual system, the Model 301 was quite labour intensive. To accommodate the workflow needs of laboratories with larger blood culture volumes, the automated BACTEC Model 460 was introduced in 1976. The Model 460 allowed users to load the instrument with up to 60 bottles and essentially walk away. Individual bottles were moved by conveyor belt to a position under a needle assembly that automatically sampled the bottle gas. The needles were sterilized in an electrical furnace between each bottle. A printout recorded the growth indices for each bottle and an LED display alerted the user when a positive bottle was detected. The instrument processed 60 bottles in one hour. With the design of a special biosafety hood, the BACTEC Model 460 also became a popular system for processing mycobacterial cultures, and it continues to function in that capacity in many laboratories today.

In the early 1980s, Becton Dickinson Diagnostic Instrument Systems introduced the BACTEC 16B Aerobic and 17D Anaerobic Resin Media. These media incorporated cationic and anionic resin beads which are designed to adsorb antibiotics that are present in blood samples. The intent of these new formulations was to improve the detection of bacteremia in patients who receive antimicrobial therapy. The cost-benefit of these media has often been the subject of lively debate among clinical microbiologists.

Also in the 1980s, with many clinical laboratories becoming increasingly sensitive to the disposal of all radioisotopes, Becton Dickinson directed research efforts toward the development of a non-radiometric detection system. A promising and economically favorable method proved to be infrared analysis of "cold" CO_2 in the head-space gas. The method was sensitive and robust when tested with a wide range of clinically significant micro-organisms. The BACTEC Model NR660, introduced in 1983, replaced radiometric detection with infrared detection. Like the Model 460, the NR660 tested 60 bottles so held in a custom molded tray per test sequence. The NR660, however, was designed to test bottles more rapidly (35 versus 60 sec. per bottle). Rudimentary data processing and bottle-tracking were provided. The system initially included reformulated aerobic (NR6A) and anaerobic (NR7A) media but the resin counterparts, NR16A and NR17A, soon became available. The NR Plus Aerobic and Anaerobic media were launched in 1988; NR Peds Plus medium for pediatric specimens was offered in 1989, followed by NR Lytic medium in 1990 and NR Fungal medium in 1991. A smaller version of the NR660, the NR730, was made available in 1986. The NR730 processed 30 bottles. The introduction of the BACTEC NR860 in 1990 offered users the first fully automated, non-radiometric system with incubator, shaker, and detector all in one instrument.

As data management capabilities became important considerations to clinical microbiologists in the 1980s, manufacturers of microorganism identification and antimicrobial susceptibility test systems began to use desktop computers to handle test interpretation and reporting. The first BACTEC Data Management Center was provided on an Apple computer in June of 1983. It provided data management and epidemiology functions for the Model 460 instrument base. The hardware platform was changed to Digital Equipment computers in 1984. The NR 660 High Performance System, linking multiple 660 instruments for combined data management, was introduced in 1986. Once the IBM personal computer became well-established, data management applications were migrated to a PC platform.

In 1992, Becton Dickinson launched the first of three instrument configurations comprising the BACTEC 9000 series. The BACTEC 9000 series differs substantially from its predecessors in that it utilizes CMBC technology. Detection of microbial growth by the BACTEC 9000 series blood culture systems is facilitated by the presence of a gas-permeable fluorescent sensor on the bottom of each blood culture bottle. As CO_2 diffuses into the sensor and dissolves in water that is present in the sensor matrix, hydrogen ions are generated. This causes a decrease in pH, which, in turn, increases the fluorescence output of the sensor. Cultures are recognized as positive by computer algorithms that measure an increasing rate of change as well as a sustained increase in CO_2 production. The BACTEC 9000 series consists of the BACTEC 9240 (240-bottle capacity; Figure 5a), the BACTEC 9120 (120-bottle capacity), and the BACTEC 9050 (50-bottle capacity; Figure 5b). Media formulations include standard aerobic and anaerobic media (Aerobic/F, Anaerobic/F), their resin counterparts (Plus Aerobic/F, Plus Anaerobic/F), and a medium designed for pediatric patients (PEDS Plus) (Figure 5c). In addition, two lytic media are available. The first (Lytic/10 Anaerobic F) is formulated to enhance the recovery of intracellular bacteria while the second (MYCO/F Lytic) is intended for the recovery of fungi and mycobacteria from blood.

The BACTEC VISION Information Management Program facilitates data management for the BACTEC 9000 series. The software operates in a Microsoft Windows environment and has bi-directional interface capability. The software allows the user to generate a variety of epidemiological reports and permits expanded log-in fields, multiple user-definable fields, and comment fields.

The first published evaluation of the BACTEC 9240 by Nolte et al. (57) compared the performance of standard Aerobic/F and Anaerobic/F media to BACTEC NR6A and NR7A bottles that were processed on the NR 660 instrument. The 9240 recovered significantly more *S. aureus*, coagulase-negative staphylococci, and *Enterobacteriaceae*. The 9240 also detected significantly more septic episodes and had a significantly shorter time to detection of microbialgrowth. Contamination rates and proportions of false positive instrument signals were similar.

C. bioMérieux VITAL and miniVITAL

The VITAL blood culture system developed by bioMérieux, Inc. has been marketed extensively in Europe and Asia but not in the United States and has not received American FDA [1999] clearance. Similar to the design of other CMBC instruments, the VITAL is a component system which consists of incubator/monitor modules and a microprocessor. The basic incubator unit houses 100 blood culture bottles. Starter systems are available in 200-, 300-, or 400-bottle capacities and up to three 400-bottle modules can be monitored by a single microprocessor thus giving a maximum capacity of 1200 bottles without the need for an additional microprocessor (Figure 6a). The miniVITAL, as the name implies, is a compact, bench-top version of the VIDAS which was designed for use in smaller volume laboratories. It carries all the same features and functions of the full-sized instrument but with a maximum capacity of 100 blood culture bottles per unit (Figure 6b).

As with the BACTEC 9000 series instrument, the VITAL uses a fluorescent sensor to monitor microbial growth. There are however two distinct differences. Firstly, the sensor molecule is incorporated directly into the broth medium. Secondly, changes in the redox potential, pH, or CO_2 content of the broth which result from microbial growth combine to reduce the fluorescent intensity of the sensor. Blood culture bottles are agitated in a sinusoidal motion at 150 cycles per minute, and the fluorescence of each bottle is monitored once every 15 min. by a noninvasive light-emitting diode/photon detector system. The degree of fluorescence reduction is analyzed with time by a programmed computer algorithm. The VITAL also utilizes a minimum fluorescence threshold value to immediately detect microbial growth in bottles by extended off-line incubation.

A single volume (40 ml.) bottle size for aerobic and anaerobic cultures has been developed for use in conjunction with this system. The broth is an enriched soybean-casein digest formulation with 0.025% SPS as an anticoagulant. Bottles can be inoculated with up to 10 ml. of blood for a minimum dilution of 1:5. Neither bottle requires post-inoculation processing such as venting prior to incubation.

Very few clinical studies involving the VITAL have been published since its introduction, but a review of the available literature provides a reasonable degree of insight into the performance of this CMBC system. In a report of the performance kinetics of the VITAL over an 11 month period,

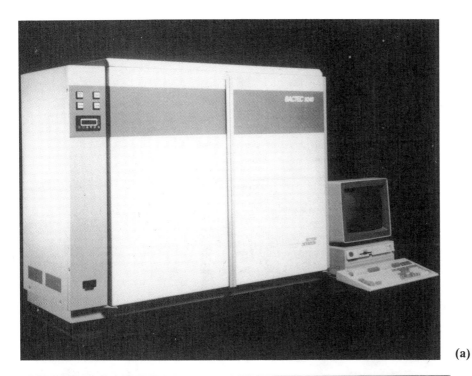

(a)

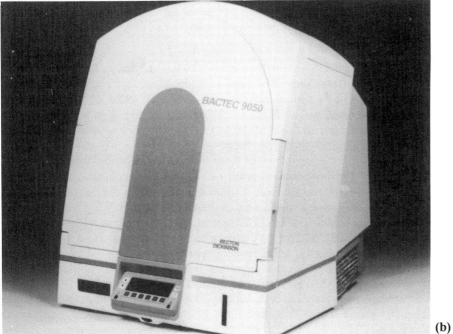

(b)

Figure 5 a,b   The BACTEC 9000 series blood culture system marketed by Becton-Dickinson includes a variety of incubator modules: the 9240 (a), 9120 and 9050 (b) versions have capacities of 240, 120, and 50 per unit respectively.

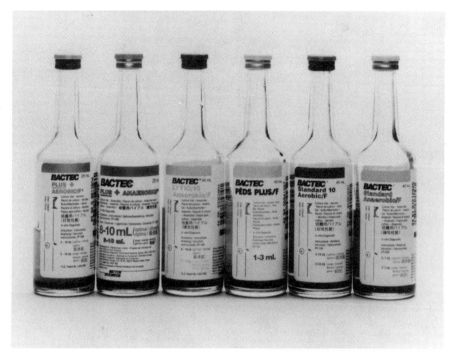

Figure 5c A variety of media formulations have been developed for use with this system including aerobic and anaerobic versions of standard, resin-containing, pediatric, and lytic bottles.

Marchandin et al. (58) identified a 1% false-positivity and a 0.05% false-negativity rate for the 19,706 blood cultures that were examined. Two-thirds of all positive blood cultures were signaled within the first 24 hrs. of incubation and 83% of all positive cultures were recognized within 48 hrs. The authors determined that a 5-day incubation cycle was sufficient for the detection of all clinically significant isolates. Perez et al. (59) compared the performance of the VITAL system using a 7-day protocol to a Septi-Chek biphasic aerobic and anaerobic bottle set (Becton-Dickinson) with a 14-day protocol, and essentially found no difference in the performance of these methods. The same cannot be said for evaluations which compare the VITAL with two different BACTEC systems. Zaidi and colleagues (60) performed a parallel trial of the VITAL and the BACTEC NR-660 systems for the detection of bacteremia in children. For this study, only aerobic media were evaluated (the standard VITAL and the resin-containing PEDS PLUS BACTEC bottle). The BACTEC system out-performed the VITAL for the recovery of all microorganisms ($p < 0.001$) and for the detection of clinically significant episodes of sepsis ($p < 0.01$). The BACTEC system also had fewer falsely negative cultures than did the VITAL, but when both systems identified a positive culture, the mean time to detection of the VITAL system was 1.6 hours earlier than the BACTEC. When the same two systems were compared in a study that involved an adult patient population and that used both aerobic and anaerobic culture sets, similar results were observed (61). Finally, Leliévre et al. (62) contrasted the performance of the VITAL system which used standard media to the BACTEC 9240 CMBC system that used resin-containing aerobic and anaerobic bottles. The BACTEC system out-performed the VITAL in both mean time to detection (10.65 hrs. vs. 18.41 hrs. respectively) and the detection of clinically significant isolates ($p < 0.001$). It is unclear from these comparisons whether the difference in performance between the BACTEC and VITAL

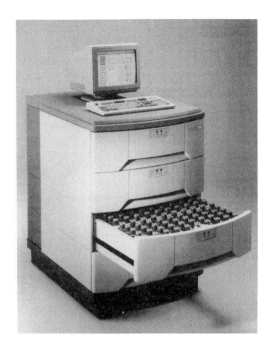

Figure 6a The VITAL blood culture system developed by bioMerieux, Inc. which has a 400-bottle capacity incubator/monitor capacity incubator/monitor module and a microprocessor. Each drawer of this system houses 100 blood culture bottles. Starter systems are also available in 100, 200, and 300 bottle modules.

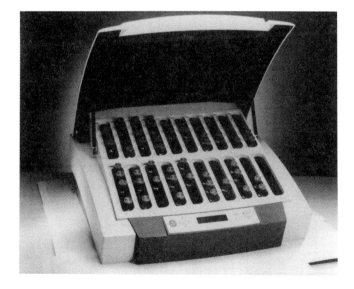

Figure 6b The miniVITAL, as the name implies, is a compact bench-top version of the VITAL that carries all of the same features and functions of the full-sized instrument but with a maximum capacity of 100 blood culture bottles/unit.

systems is a function of hardware, software, detection, or media formulation, but it is clear that the VI-TAL system will require continued evolution to remain competitive in the CMBC system market.

D. TREK Diagnostic Systems ESP

The ESP blood culture system was originally developed by Difco Laboratories (Detroit, MI, USA), purchased by AccuMed International, Inc. (Westlake, OH, USA), and ultimately acquired by TREK Diagnostic Systems, Inc. (Westlake, OH, USA). This was the last of the major CMBC systems to receive FDA clearance for commercial use and the first to receive FDA clearance to support continuously-monitored mycobacterial cultures. The hardware configuration of the ESP is also divided into incubator/monitor modules and a microprocessor, but the similarities between the ESP, BacT/Alert, BACTEC 9000, and VITAL systems ends there. Unlike the CMBC systems that preceded it, the ESP senses changes in the head space pressure of the blood culture bottle that are attributable to microbial O_2 consumption and/or H_2, N_2, or CO_2 production as a sign of growth.

The incubator/monitor units of the ESP are currently available in 128 (Figure 7a), 256 (Figure 7b), or 384 bottle capacities. Up to five units can be commanded by a single microprocessor for a maximum capacity of 1920 bottles per system. Regardless of capacity, each unit is subdivided into pull-out drawers with each drawer housing up to sixteen bottles (Figure 7c). Each bottle station consists of a spring-loaded cup on the bottom and a T-bar with a pressure transducer on the top. Blood culture bottles are placed into the cup and connected to the pressure transducer via a sterile plastic adapter. The adapter is a cylinder with a recessed needle in the bottom which penetrates the rubber septum of the bottle, a 2 μm. filter in the middle to prevent aerosols, and a rubber "O" ring at the top to seal the connection to the pressure transducer (Figure 7d). The lower drawers of each ESP module (50% of the total) are reserved for aerobic cultures and are continuously agitated at 160 cycles/minute. The upper drawers are stationary for anaerobic bottles. Aerobic and anaerobic bottles are monitored once every twelve and twenty-four minutes respectively. Pressure readings are translated into growth curves over time by a computer algorithm which also corrects for changes in atmospheric pressure. Quality control of the detection system is currently accomplished by the generation of an acceptable warm-up pressure curve when bottles are initially loaded into the system. A positive culture is signaled by a light atop the module, a light in front of the drawer, and a light above and below the station, an audio alarm on the microprocessor, and a screen on the microprocessor.

Currently, two media formulations in two bottle sizes are approved for use with the ESP. The aerobic A medium is a supplemented soy-casein peptone broth with 0.006% SPS and is available in 40 or 80 ml. bottles which accommodate up to 5 and 10 ml. of blood respectively. The anaerobic N medium is a supplemented proteose peptone broth with 0.07% trisodium citrate instead of SPS as an anticoagulant, and is also available in 40 or 80 ml. bottles. With the adapter attached, an anaerobic gradient is formed within the N medium which allows for the recovery of both aerobic and anaerobic organisms.

A number of clinical evaluations of the ESP system and comparison trials with other blood culture methodologies have appeared in the literature since this product was launched in the early 1990s with mixed results. A multi-centre comparison of the ESP with the BACTEC NR660 was coordinated by Morello et al. (63) and demonstrated that the former was statistically superior to the latter for the recovery of *S. pneumoniae*, *Candida* species, "single system isolates", and aerobic Gram positive bacteria. The former detected also more episodes of bacteremia and had a reduced mean time to detection. Zwadyk et al. (64) showed that the ESP detected significantly more positive cultures than the first generation BacT/Alert system although there was no difference between the systems in the overall detection of clinically significant bacteremia. More recent studies comparing the BacT/Alert FAN and ESP 80A aerobic media in both pediatric (65) and adult (66) patient populations highlighted the strengths of either medium: the former being superior for the recovery of *S. aureus* and detecting clinically significant isolates from patients who received antimicrobial therapy, and the latter for detecting bacteremia caused by streptococci and enterococci.

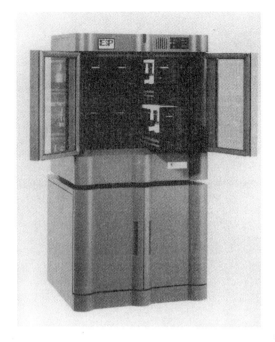

(a)

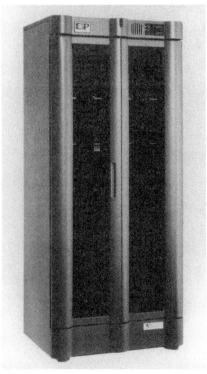

(b)

Figure 7 a,b   The ESP blood culture system by Trek Diagnostic Systems, Inc.: (a) 128 bottle capacity module and (b) 256 bottle capacity module. A 384-bottle unit is also available.

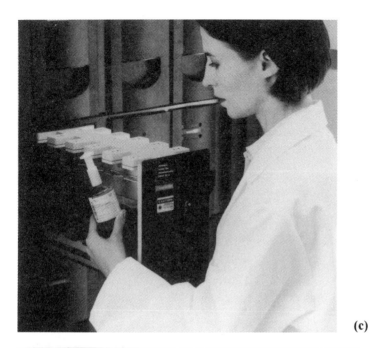

(c)

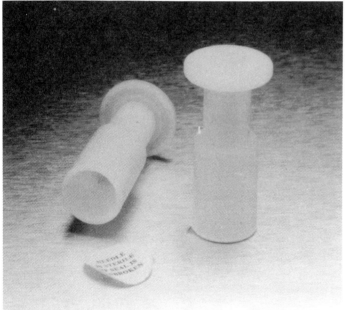

(d)

Figure 7 c,d   The ESP blood culture system: (c) Each unit is subdivided into pull-out drawers with each drawer housing up to 16 bottles. Each bottle station consists of a spring-loaded cup on the bottom and a T-bar with a pressure transducer on the top. Blood culture bottles are placed into the cup and are connected to the pressure transducer via a sterile plastic adapter. (d) The adapter is a cylinder which contains a recessed needle in the bottom to penetrate the rubber septum of the bottle, a filter in the middle to prevent aerosols, and a rubber "O" ring at the top to seal the connection to the pressure transducer.

In a clinical study which compared the performance of the ESP 80A with the Septi-Chek™ biphasic system, there was no difference with regard to the total recovery of aerobic organisms between the two, but the ESP system demonstrateda statistically significant shorter mean time to detect a positive culture (47). Two independent studies (47,49), however, suggested that the Wampole Isolator™ lysis-centrifugation method identified significantly more positive cultures and more episodes of bacteremia than did the ESP using the 80A medium. Many of the infections identified only by the Isolator™ system were attributable to episodes of bacteremia and fungemia caused by *S. aureus* and *Candida* species respectively.

While the ESP received FDA clearance based on performance that included a five-day incubation cycle, two recent publications have suggested that a four and possibly three-day protocol could be instituted without adversely affecting the recovery of clinically significant microorganisms from blood (67,68).

VII. PROCESSING POSITIVE BLOOD CULTURES

The first and most important manipulation to be performed on any signal-positive blood culture is the Gram stain. The information provided by the Gram stain, combined with patient information, will likely determine the choice of empiric antimicrobial therapy and, therefore, should be as accurate and descriptive as possible. A report of "Gram positive cocci in pairs" as opposed to "Gram positive cocci" for example narrows the selection of empiric therapy chosen by the clinician until a definitive identification is made. Descriptive terms, however, such as "diphtheroid" rather than "pleomorphic Gram positive rod" should be avoided because organisms such as *Rhodococcus equi* or *Mycobacterium* species, which share morphological characteristics of coryneform bacteria, are becoming increasingly prevalent as agents of bacteremia in immunosuppressed individuals. Additionally, organisms previously considered as reliable indicators of blood culture contamination such as coagulase-negative staphylococci are now recognized as agents of catheter-related bacteremia (69,70).

If the Gram stain of a signal-positive blood culture is negative, it is often useful to repeat the microscopic examination using an acridine orange stain before resuming incubation. This technique has been helpful in cases of *Campylobacter* bacteremia or brucellosis where the poor counter-staining quality of the organism might prevent detection by Gram stain (71,72).

Regardless of the microscopic results, all signal-positive blood cultures should be subcultured to appropriate microbiological media. The selection of media should minimally include 5% sheep blood and chocolate agars (which are incubated in CO_2 at 35° C for 48 hours) and a CDC anaerobic blood agar plate, or equivalent (which is incubated in an anaerobic atmosphere for 48-72 hours). MacConkey's, colistin-nalidixic acid (CNA), or mycologic agar can be preferentially added if the Gram stain dictates. Vancomycin or methicillin screening agar can be included if resistance among nosocomial enterococci or *S. aureus* is a concern.

In the case of a Gram stain-positive bottle, several opportunities exist to provide rapid preliminary information. Protocols have been developed for identification and direct susceptibility testing using either commercial kits or in-house reagents. For this, the organism is concentrated from 10 ml. of the blood culture broth by centrifugation and adjusted to a standardized turbidity prior to the inoculation of a identification or susceptibility panel (73). Additional direct identification procedures can also be performed from the pelleted material or the resulting supernatant (74,75).

In contrast to broth-based systems, those that utilize a solid medium component such as lysis-centrifugation or biphasic medium provide isolated colonies as a "signal". Consequently, the Gram stain result can (and should) be supplemented with additional biochemical reactions to influence the selection of appropriate therapy.

Blood cultures that are positive for coagulase-negative staphylococci (CONS) pose a particular challenge for clinical microbiologists. Over the past three decades, CONS have become a major cause of bacteremia and sepsis that is associated with infected biomedical implants and transcutaneous catheters (70). Unfortunately, because of their cutaneous habitat, they are also a leading cause of blood culture contamination. In the absence of pertinent patient data, it is difficult to distinguish clinically significant isolates of CONS from contaminants. The following protocol was instituted in one author's laboratory (WMD) in order to avoid excessive evaluation of insignificant CONS while retaining the ability to provide clinically relevant data if necessary. Firstly, a single patient isolate of CONS is reported and saved in the freezer for future reference. Speciation and susceptibility testing is not performed on this initial isolate. Upon recovery of a second or subsequent strain(s) of CONS from the same patient within a five-day period, the primary isolate is subcultured, and identification and susceptibility studies are performed on all strains. Although it is difficult to ensure clonality of CONS based on common laboratory assays, most clinically significant isolates are *S. epidermidis*, are multiply resistant in vitro to antimicrobial agents, demonstrate in vitro adhesion to glass or plastic surfaces, and are recovered from more than one culture. The molecular typing techniques that are required to definitively classify strains of CONS as clonal is generally beyond the workload constraints of most clinical laboratories.

While it has become possible recently to identify microorganisms and their resistance determinants directly from blood cultures using genomic amplification, the practical and cost-effective use of this technology for routine application is far from standard practice.

VIII. REPORTING BLOOD CULTURES

A positive blood culture is almost universally recognized to be a critical value by microbiology laboratories and, therefore, warrants an immediate verbal report to the patient's physician or designee. The time and date of notification as well as the name of the recipient should be noted in the specimen log. At that time, the clinician should be provided with all salient information including the Gram stain morphology, the number of bottles or sets that are positive, the atmosphere of the positive bottle(s), and any rapid biochemical results if the organism was isolated on solid media. All verbal reports should be followed by a written report (electronic and/or hard copy) which are to be included in the patient's chart. Subsequent verbal updates are unnecessary unless preliminary information is found to be in error or when additional findings might alter patient management, e.g., uncovering a second organism from a subcultured bottle. Additional written reports should be issued as new information becomes available and when a culture is finalized.

For negative blood cultures, written preliminary reports should be issued after twenty-four and forty-eight hours of incubation and when the culture is finalized. The forty-eight hour report is used by some facilities as a milestone for patient discharge when the admitting diagnosis included possible sepsis. All negative blood culture reports should include the length of incubation at the time of issue, e.g., "No growth after 5 days."

REFERENCES

1. Scott EG. A practical blood culture procedure. Am J Clin Pathol 1951; 21:290-294.
2. Casteneda MR. A practical method for routine blood cultures in brucellosis. Proc Soc Exp Biol Med 1947; 64:114-115.
3. Bartlett RC, Ellner PD, Washington II JA. Blood Cultures. Cumitech 1. Washington, DC: American Society for Microbiology, 1974.
4. Reller LB, Murray PR, MacLowry JD. Blood Cultures II. Cumitech 1A. Washington, DC: American Society for Microbiology, 1982.
5. Dunne, Jr. WM, Nolte FS, Wilson ML. Blood Cultures III. Cumitech 1B. Washington, DC: American Society for Microbiology, 1997.

6. Dunne, Jr. WM, Tillman J, Havens PL. Assessing the need for anaerobic medium for the recovery of clinically significant blood culture isolates in children. Pediatr Infect Dis J 1994; 13:203-206.

7. Li J, Plorde J, Carlson L. Effects of volume and periodicity on blood cultures. J Clin Microbiol 1994; 32:2829-2831.

8. von Haebler T, Miles AA. The action of sodium polyanethol sulphonate ("liquoid") on blood cultures. J Pathol Bacteriol 1938; 46:245-252.

9. Hoare ED. The suitability of "liquoid" for use in blood culture media with particular reference to anaerobic streptococci. J Pathol Bacteriol 1939; 48:573-577.

10. Blazevic DJ, Stemper JE, Matsen JM. Comparison of macroscopic examination, routine Gram stains, and routine subcultures in the initial detection of positive blood cultures. Appl Microbiol 1974; 27:537-539.

11. McCarthy LR, Senne JE. Evaluation of acridine orange stain for detection of microorganisms in blood cultures. J Clin Microbiol 1980; 2:107-111.

12. Tierney BM, Henry NK, Washington II JA. Early detection of positive blood cultures by the acridine orange staining technique. J Clin Microbiol 1983: 18:830-833.

13. Campbell J, Washington II JA. Evaluation of the necessity for routine terminal subcultures of previously negative blood cultures. J Clin Microbiol 1980; 12:576-587.

14. Gill VJ. Lack of clinical relevance in routine terminal subculturing of blood cultures. J Clin Microbiol 1981; 14:116-118.

15. Roberts GD, Washington II JA. Detection of fungi in blood cultures. J Clin Microbiol 1975; 1:309-310.

16. Caplan LM, Merz WG. Evaluation of two commercially prepared biphasic media for recovery of fungi from blood. J Clin Microbiol 1978; 8:469-470.

17. Hall MM, Mueske CA, Ilstrup DM, Washington II JA. Evaluation of biphasic medium for blood cultures. J Clin Microbiol 1979; 10:673-676.

18. Bille J, Roberts GD, Washington II JA. Retrospective comparison of three blood culture media for the recovery of yeasts from clinical specimens. Eur J Clin Microbiol 1983; 2:22-25.

19. Bryan LE. Comparison of a slide blood culture system with a supplemented peptone broth culture method. J Clin Microbiol 1981; 14:389-392.

20. Pfaller MA, Sibley TK, Westfall LM, Hoppe-Bauer JE, Keating MA, Murray PR. Clinical laboratory comparison of a slide blood culture system with a conventional broth system. J Clin Microbiol 1982; 16:525-530.

21. Kiehn TE, Capitolo C, Mayo JB, Armstrong D. Comparative recovery of fungi from biphasic and conventional blood culture media. J Clin Microbiol 1981; 14:681-683.

22. Henry NK, Grewell CM, McLimans CA, Washington II JA. Comparison of the Roche Septi-Chek blood culture bottle with a brain heart infusion biphasic medium bottle and with a tryptic soy broth bottle. J Clin Microbiol 1984; 19:315-317.

23. Weckbach LS, Staneck JL. Performance characteristics of a commercially prepared biphasic blood culture bottle. J Clin Microbiol 1986; 23:700-703.

24. Weinstein MP, Reller LB, Mirrett S, Wang WL, Alcid DV. Controlled evaluation of trypticase soy broth in agar slide and conventional blood culture systems. J Clin Microbiol 1985; 21:626-629.

25. Clough MC. The cultivation of tubercle bacilli from the circulating blood in miliary tuberculosis. Am Rev Tubercul 1917; 1:598-621.

26. Dorn GL, Haynes JR, Burson GG. Blood culture technique based on centrifugation: developmental phase. J Clin Microbiol 1976; 3:251-257.

27. Dorn GL, Smith K. New centrifugation blood culture device. J Clin Microbiol 1978;7:52-54.

28. Dorn GL, Land GA, Wilson GW. Improved blood culture technique based on centrifugation: clinical evaluation. J Clin Microbiol 1979;9:391-396.

29. Campos JM. Detection of bloodstream infections in children. Eur J Clin Microbiol Inf Dis 1989; 8:815-824.

30. Sullivan TD, LaScolea LJ, Neter E. Relationship between the magnitude of bacteremia in children and the clinical disease. Pediatrics 1982; 69:699-702.

31. Raucher HS, Hyatt AC, Barzilai A, Harris MB, Weiner MA, LeLeiko NS, Hodes DS. Quantitative blood cultures in the evaluation of septicemia in children with broviac catheters. J Pediatr 1984; 104:29-33.

32. Bille J, Stockman L, Roberts GD, Horstmeier CD, Ilstrup DM. Evaluation of a lysis- centrifugation system for recovery of yeasts and filamentous fungi from blood. J Clin Microbiol 18:469-471.

33. Kiehn TE, Wong B, Edwards FF, Armstrong D. Comparative recovery of bacteria and yeasts from lysis-centrifugation and a conventional blood culture system. J Clin Microbiol 1983; 18:300-304.

34. Kellogg JA, Manzella JP, McConville JH. Clinical laboratory comparison of the 10-ml Isolator blood culture system with BACTEC radiometric blood culture media. J Clin Microbiol 1984; 20:618-623.

35. Brannon P, Kiehn TE. Large-scale comparison of the lysis-centrifugation and radiometric systems for blood culture. J Clin Microbiol 1985; 22:951-954.

36. Walker RC, Henry NK, Washington II JA, Thompson RL. Lysis-centrifugation blood culture technique: clinical impact in *Staphylococcus aureus* bacteremia. Arch Intern Med 1986; 146:2341-2343.

37. Henry NK, McLimans CA, Wright AJ, Thompson RL, Wilson WR, Washington II JA. Microbiological and clinical evaluation of the Isolator lysis-centrifugation blood culture tube. J Clin Microbiol 1983; 17: 864-869.

38. Brannon P, Kiehn TE. Clinical comparison of lysis-centrifugation and radiometric resin systems for blood culture. J Clin Microbiol 1986; 24:886-887.

39. Murray PR, Spizzo AW, Niles AC. Clinical comparison of the recoveries of bloodstream pathogens in Septi-Chek brain heart infusion broth with saponin, Septi-Chek tryptic soy broth, and the Isolator lysis-centrifugation system. J Clin Microbiol 1991; 29:901-905.

40. Gill VJ, Park CH, Stock F, Gosey LL, Witebsky FG, Masur H. Use of lysis-centrifugation (Isolator) and radiometric (BACTEC) blood culture systems for the detection of mycobacteremia. J Clin Microbiol 1985; 22:543-546.

41. Salfinger M, Stool EW, Piot D, Heifets L. Comparison of three methods for recovery of *Mycobacterium avium* complex from blood specimens. J Clin Microbiol 1988; 26:1225-1226.

42. Frank U, Malkotsis D, Mlangeni D, Daschner FD. Controlled clinical comparison of three commercial blood culture systems. Eur J Clin Microbiol Infect Dis 1999; 18:248-255.

43. Hellinger WC, Cawley JJ, Alverez S, Hogan SF, Harmsen WS, Ilstrup DM, Cockerill III FR. Clinical comparison of the Isolator and BacT/Alert aerobic blood culture systems. J Clin Microbiol 1995; 33:1787-1790.

44. Pickett DA, Welch DF. Evaluation of the automated BacT/Alert system for pediatric blood culturing. Am J Clin Pathol 1995;103:320-323.

45. Cockerill III FR, Reed GS, Hughs JG, Torgerson CA, Vetter EA, Harmsen WS, Dale JC, Roberts GD, Ilstrup DM, Henry NK. Clinical comparison of BACTEC 9240 Plus aerobic resin bottles and the Isolator aerobic culture system for detection of blood stream infections. J Clin Microbiol 1997; 35:1469-1472.

46. Pohlman JK, Kirkley BA, Easley KA, Washington II JA. Controlled clinical comparison of Isolator and BACTEC 9240 Aerobic/F resin bottle for detection of blood stream infections. J Clin Microbiol 1995; 33:2525-2529.

47. Cockerill III FR, Torgerson CA, Reed GS, Vetter EA, Weaver AL, Dale JC, Roberts GD, Henry HK, Ilstrup DM, Rosenblatt JE. Clinical comparison of Difco ESP, Wampole Isolator, and Becton Dickinson Septi-Chek aerobic blood culturing systems. J Clin Microbiol 1996; 34:20-24.

48. Lyon R, Woods G. Comparison of BacT/Alert and Isolator blood culture systems for recovery of fungi. Am J Clin Pathol 1995; 103:660-662.

49. Kirkley BA, Easley KA, Washington II JA. Controlled clinical evaluation of Isolator and ESP aerobic blood culture systems for detection of blood stream infections. J Clin Microbiol 1994; 32:1547-1549.

50. Waite RT, Woods GL. Evaluation of the BACTEC Myco/F lytic medium for the recovery of mycobacteria and fungi from blood. J Clin Microbiol 1998; 36:1176-1179.

51. Reimer LG, Wilson ML, Weinstein MP. Update on the detection of bacteremia and fungemia. Clin Microbiol Rev 1997; 10:444-465.

52. Thorpe TC, Wilson ML, Turner JE, DiGuiseppi JL, Willert M, Mirrett S, Reller LB. BacT/Alert: an automated colorimetric detection system. J Clin Microbiol 1990; 28:1608-1612.

53. Wilson ML, Weinstein MP, Reimer LG, Mirrett S, Reller LB. Controlled comparison of the BacT/Alert and BACTEC 660/730 nonradiometric blood culture systems. J Clin Microbiol 1992; 30:323-329.

54. DeBlanc Jr. HJ, Deland F, Wagner HN. Automated radiometric detection of bacteria in 2,967 blood cultures. Appl Microbiol 1971; 22:846-849.

55. Renner ED, Gatheridge LA, Washington II JA. Evaluation of radiometric system for detecting bacteremia. Appl Microbiol 1973; 26:368-372.

56. Thiemke WA, Wicher K. Laboratory experience with a radiometric method for detecting bacteremia. J Clin Microbiol 1975; 1:302-308.

57. Nolte FS, Williams JM, Jerris RC, Morello JA. Multicenter clinical evaluation of a continuous monitoring blood culture system using fluorescent-sensor technology (BACTEC 9240). J Clin Microbiol 1993; 31:552-557.

58. Marchandin H, Compan B, Simeon De Buochberg M, Despaux E, Perez C. Detection kinetics for positive blood culture bottles using the VITAL automated system. J Clin Microbiol 1995; 33:2098-2101.

59. Perez C, Marchandin H, Compan B, Bonifacj C, Despaux E, Mion P. Comparative evaluation of blood culture using the VITAL automated system and the Becton-Dickinson Septi-Chek BHI-S biphasic and Sch bottles. Ann Biol Clin (Paris) 1996; 54:159-163.

60. Zaidi AK, Mirrett S, McDonald J, Rubin EE, McDonald LC, Weinstein MP, Gupta M, Reller LB. Controlled comparison of bioMérieux VITAL and BACTEC NR-660 systems for detection of bacteremia and fungemia in pediatric patients. J Clin Microbiol 1997; 35:2007-2012.
61. Wilson ML, Mirrett S, McDonald LC, Weinstein MP, Fune J, Reller LB. Controlled clinical comparison of bioMérieux VITAL and BACTEC NR-660 blood culture systems for detection of bacteremia and fungemia in adults. J Clin Microbiol 1999; 37:1709-1713.
62. Leliévre H, Gimenez M, Vandenesch F, Reinhardt A, Lenhardt D, Just HM, Pau M, Ausina V, Etienne J. Multicenter clinical comparison of resin-containing bottles with standard aerobic and anaerobic bottles for culture of microorganisms from blood. Eur J Clin Microbiol Infect Dis 1997; 16;669-674.
63. Morello JA, Leitch C, Nitz S, Dyke JW, Andruszewski M, Maier G, Landau W, Beard MA. Detection of bacteremia by Difco ESP blood culture system. J Clin Microbiol 1994; 32:811-818.
64. Zwadyk Jr. P, Pierson CL, Young C. Comparison of Difco ESP and Organon Teknika BacT/Alert continuous-monitoring blood culture systems. J Clin Microbiol 1994; 32:1273-1279.
65. Welby-Sellenriek PL, Keller DS, Ferrett RJ, Storch GA. Comparison of the BacT/Alert FAN aerobic and the Difco ESP 80A aerobic bottles for pediatric blood cultures. J Clin Microbiol 1997; 35:1166-1171.
66. Doern GV, Barton A, Rao S. Controlled comparative evaluation of BacT/Alert FAN and ESP 80A aerobic media as means for detecting bacteremia and fungemia. J Clin Microbiol 1998; 36:2686-2689.
67. Doern GV, Brueggemann AB, Dunne WM, Jenkins SG, Halstead DC, McLaughlin JC. Four-day incubation period for blood culture bottles processed with the Difco ESP blood culture system. J Clin Microbiol 1997; 35:1290-1292.
68. Han XY, Truant AL. The detection of positive blood cultures by the AccuMed ESP-384 system: the clinical significance of three-day testing. Diagn Microbiol Infect Dis 1999; 33:1-6.
69. Brook I, Frazier EH. Infections caused by *Propionibacterium*. Rev Infect Dis 1991; 13:819-822.
70. Rupp ME, Archer GL. Coagulase-negative staphylococci: pathogens associated with medical progress. Clin Infect Dis 194; 19:231-245.
71. Chusid MJ, Warmann DW, Dunne WM. *Campylobacter upsaliensis* sepsis in a boy with acquired hypogamma-globulinemia. Diagn Microbiol Infect Dis 1990; 13:367-369.
72. Chusid MJ, Perzigian RW, Dunne WM, Gecht EA. Brucellosis: an unusual cause of a child's fever of unknown origin. Wis Med J 1989; 88:11-13.
73. Almon R, Pezzlo M. Processing and interpretation of blood cultures. In: Isenberg HD - ed. Clinical Microbiology Procedure Handbook. Washington, DC:American Society for Microbiology, 1992:1.7.1-1.7.11.
74. Knight RG, Shales DM. Rapid identification of *Staphylococcus aureus* and *Streptococcus pneumoniae* from blood cultures. J Clin Microbiol 1983; 17:97-99.
75. Gordon LP, Damm MAS, Anderson JD. Rapid presumptive identification of streptococci directly from blood cultures by serologic tests and the L-pyrrolidonyl-β naphthylamide reaction. J Clin Microbiol 1987; 25:238-241.

10

The Quality Laboratory

Nevio Cimolai
Children's and Women's Health Centre of British Columbia, Vancouver, British Columbia, Canada

I. INTRODUCTION

What makes a quality laboratory? A simple answer would negate the necessary consideration for the varied contexts of diagnostic bacteriology. From bedside to clinic to laboratory to reference centre, a spectrum of complexity emerges (Figure 1). Yet, each requires a basic set of ingredients which are fundamental to all operations. Perhaps it is better to acknowledge that the discussion of a particular laboratory in isolation detracts from the reality that all of these diagnostic functions, from simple to complex, are part of a system, and that this system needs to be an effective participant in the provision of patient care. Laboratory function is as integral a part of medicine as any other area. It is the loss of this vision which will isolate the laboratory and lead to its devaluation, and indeed demise.

What is 'quality'? In essence, quality will always be fundamentally defined in the eye of the beholder. Nevertheless, quality infers the provision of the best possible service with the best possible balance of resource utilization and patient care. Quality diagnostic service will ensure the utmost in standards, yet in a cost effective manner. Both patient and provider are beneficiaries in an altruistic sense.

Technology has changed much of medicine, and the diagnostic bacteriology laboratory has been no less influenced. In the 1980s, it was prognosticated by some that the revolution in molecular biology would reduce the diagnostic bacteriology laboratory to automated robotics in short order. Yet, much of the routine diagnostics in this area are still of the traditional format. Nonetheless, molecular tools, new pathogens, and changing diseases have fostered new approaches and new challenges. We have more tools but we also have more work and an ever increasing frontier. How many new pathogens are yet to found? How many known pathogens will re-emerge ?

Every area of laboratory medicine has worked its way down (or up) to the molecule. Seemingly this would imply convergence of these disciplines, perhaps to the point of amalgamation. If the laboratory were only to serve in balancing an equation, of input and output, such melding would have long taken place. What has continued to provide strength and emphasis, however, is the truth that the knowledge base, of microbes and infection, is a driving force which pushes diagnostic bacteriology ahead and in relevant form. This knowledge base and its application from a quality laboratory are no less a form of medical practice than an ambulatory patient visit or a surgical procedure.

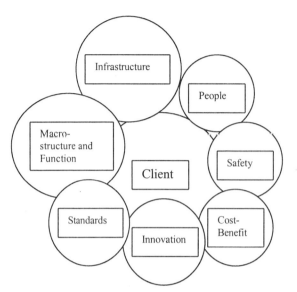

Figure 1   Essential ingredients that define the quality laboratory.

The physical resources for a quality laboratory will no doubt vary from region to region, and we cannot pretend that all will have the same opportunity to provide. Emphases must shift to meet priority, and so too we must acknowledge that the balance of quality in work will need to adjust. It is far better, however, to provide less with quality than much with none since the effect on patient care of good work may be overshadowed by the contrary.

Whereas the comments herein are being made in the midst of a diagnostic bacteriology laboratory textbook, it is evident that they are transferable to diagnostic microbiology in general and laboratory medicine otherwise.

II. PEOPLE

Conceptually, it is most direct to agree that the bacteriology laboratory should have the best possible people performing the best possible work. This sentiment in large part denies the necessary infrastructure that is requisite - people are the most essential of the infrastructural components.

It is tempting to quantitate a required personnel pool based on the numbers of tests or work-load unitage. Work-load unitage (1-4) can be standardized to reflect the quantitation of given work per technologist unit time. Such assessments of work-load may allow for laboratory-to-laboratory comparisons or for estimations of efficiency. Perhaps these tools are most relevant for routine specimen handling, especially where there is little diversity, when classical methods are used, and when volume (relating to specimen number) is relatively high. The use of work-load measurements is less likely to be of relevance when the technical diversity is greater and when infrastructural support is more complex. This consideration is especially pertinent when a larger component of research and development is required. Nevertheless, the work-load instruments are likely to be requested by bureaucrats and perhaps by laboratorians when the politic dictates. It is critical that such measurements be viewed as quantitative measures, not performance ratings.

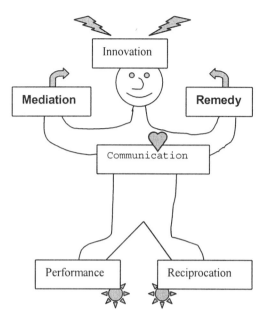

Figure 2   Multi-skilling of people in the quality laboratory.

Perhaps it is better to view quantitative personnel resources from the perspective of relevancy to patient care-oriented needs and development and from the perspective of capacity fulfillment. The filling of capacity requires individuals who are multi-skilled (Figure 2).

From a purely industrial perspective, multi-skilling requires that the individual be capable of performing many tasks. These tasks may be of varying needs for classical bacteriology or for variation from very simple to complex. Beyond the completion of standard laboratory requests, multi-skilling by necessity must include performance, communication, reciprocation, mediation, remedy, and innovation. Performance requires a knowledge base, a systematic approach or methods, precision, and efficiency. Communication skills are important within the laboratory at different levels but are perhaps most important in relationship to the laboratory consumer, i.e., patient and direct care-giver. Reciprocation places the laboratory in a win-win relationship analogous to a reciprocal industry-consumer relationship. Mediation and remedy are problem-solving skills. Innovation facilitates adaptation to a never-ending change. Education standards need to be heightened from early training. It may be difficult to have the same standard for all that participate in laboratory endeavors, but this approach is nevertheless suitable for most. A minimum degree or certification should be a goal but not necessarily an absolute limitation. The education standards need to reflect recruitment and training of the multi-skilled individual who is able to cope with change and who is able to adapt to special environments. By necessity, these standards will be a hybrid of clinical bacteriology and newer molecular advancement. Personnel should strive for continuing education; the goals should reflect general and specific needs for personal development. Learning tools will include access to literature and didactic sessions. A periodic review of standards, achievement, and future aims should be routine although the focus on work intensity and reporting often overshadow such a desirable approach. The review may act as a formal process to activate positive change.

Morale is reflected in acceptance of compensation, positive feedback, cordial consumer-provider relationships, realization of participation in the overall pro-patient processes, and opportunity to innovate. Only too often do these facets become mired in change, politics, and over-work.

III. THE CLIENT

In a politically-correct present, the 'client' represents the individual(s) at the receiving end of a laboratory service. In a practical sense, the term refers to health provider, provider institution or organization, and above all the patient. The latter are all beneficiaries whose needs and directed impact must be understood in order to provide quality.

From the patient's perspective, the best possible service should provide the most prompt and accurate answer in the least costly fashion and with the potential to diminish morbidity. Providers of the laboratory service as a structure must therefore have some understanding of the patient care process. This process will include patient assessment, short term care, and long term impact. Necessarily then, the best possible avenue will be for the laboratory service to directly and pro-actively participate in patient care functions (5,6). This may consist of discussion relating to active care such as differential diagnosis among other things. An audit of past impact or a prospective study exemplify two active look-see approaches. Research and development are certain to open doors towards insight in these regards.

The caregiver's role is the necessary link with greater or lesser participation depending on the nature of the issue. The dominant, subordinate, or equal role in the applications process will vary from one context to another. In many circumstances, the care-giver may have the best view on how the laboratory functions can best be applicable (7,8). On the hand, the mere complexity of procedures in current day bacteriology may necessitate a dominant role for the laboratory to provide direction, perhaps even as it relates to the bed- or clinic- side (9). A direct participation of both the laboratory service and caregiver in active patient care, audit and review, and developmental aspects is likely to ensure effective translation into quality.

Infection control services and public health authorities are also client beneficiaries of a quality laboratory (10,11). Both must obtain timely and accurate information in order to translate documentation into prevention (12).

The clinical bacteriology laboratory has the potential to affect the care of large populations. The laboratory's choice of offerings and their accuracy, as well as their delivery, can impact with broad-ranging effects. In this sense, the laboratory is a community and public provider. On the hand, it is care of individuals that make up the demand for the majority of specific laboratory requests. How will the laboratory then define its client? The key here is flexibility. The laboratory must define an acceptable standard that is broadly applicable on a population basis. Some of these services will be more or less independent of specific patient details. In order to provide quality hereafter, the laboratory must then cater to individual variation, at times using knowledge of specific contexts to make the best fit. The latter will only transpire when incremental knowledge is made available. In a negativistic sense, some may choose the adage "garbage-in, garbage-out ". Perhaps in the new millennium, we will accept this adage to be reconfigured into "knowledge in, quality out".

Adaptation to patient needs can occur at several levels. Initial information may support a standard approach which may be modified by incremental information, initial results, and perhaps later contributions. The creation of clinical utilization and then laboratory paradigms is an example of such adaptation. Paradigms must not be used as a mechanism to exclude or to create rigidity, but rather as a mechanism to introduce fluidity.

Communication strategies are at the heart of providing good client service. At one level, these communications relate to an open atmosphere of dialogue. At a more fundamental level, communication implies timely and useful reporting of results and value-added information which enhances utilization and patient care. From a strictly business sense, the clinical bacteriology laboratory must also develop strategies to effectively translate communication into a positive force. Whether private or public, the laboratory should be earnestly building a private business sensibility of how the customer is treated.

Again, the context will determine what relevance and emphasis these approaches should have.

IV. INNOVATION

Innovation to many may imply novelty, with a creation of new services and new applications. The most important innovation will necessarily relate to a reformation of existing service. Seeking efficiency, refining applications, filling of capacity, and enhancing existing staff among other things necessitate a change from within. A better product in its delivery should emerge. Some may translate internal change into a tumultuous restructuring. The quality laboratory already recognizes that an effective structure is in place but that it can be improved. The existing functions will be near peak productivity, capacity, and value because effort has been adequately directed to these issues on a ongoing basis. The more important facet of innovation to most therefore will be renovation.

In the present and future of microbiology, new products and new science are inevitable (13). New science is emerging at a pace unparalleled in history. The science must be available, reviewed, and placed in the appropriate context (14). Although the intensity of review in this area will be dictated by the complexity of the laboratory services, it cannot be denied that the review of new science in the current era requires sufficient time. Again, depending on the complexity of the laboratory, it may directly participate in creating new science. Ultimately decisions are required as to whether it should be done and then how it should be done. The positive end-product is not always measured by a variable contribution in the form of new science. The processes of creating new science and their spin-off benefits may be as beneficial or more beneficial than the prospect of new science in itself. In this regard, the interaction with career scientists, who are perhaps remotely affiliated with a clinical bacteriology, will generate new thoughts and approaches.

Development will translate science into patient care equivalents and will include process as well as output. Development will depend on priority and may in some circumstances represent a major portion of the diagnostic laboratory. Development is by definition a function for every laboratory service whether more or less. Development requires space, an appropriate fluid resource allocation (budget), infrastructure for accomplishment and translation, and integration with knowledge-based personnel who can effect a synthesis with clinical medicine.

Research and development may be truly clinical, purely basic science, or varied mixes of the two. It is obviously an impractical extension to believe that any laboratory, great or small, should be able to capture research and development to its fullest in regard to all topics that it may directly relate to. The quality laboratory may be limited by its resource to be focal. Yet, the more broad-ranging the voyage into research and development, the more applicable and insightful the service.

What innovation is therefore applicable to the diagnostic bacteriology laboratory? Improvements should be sought with respect to obtaining resource in all of its dimensions, the enhancement of infrastructure, client relationships, specimen acquisition, applications, patient care, and utilization. These are not formidable tasks when patient benefit is the main outcome.

V. INFRASTRUCTURE

Infrastructure is essentially the glue that binds all elements that are individually required to deliver the quality service. No matter how small or large the operations, infrastructure to some extent will be a basic minimum. Infrastructure will be required to provide a simple answer; it will also be required to provide the most complex. Infrastructure is less flexible than other elements of laboratory operations. The fluidity of service provision and an adjustment of related resources must be viewed in a context where minimum infrastructure supports are maintained. Above and beyond this minimum, service capacity will then bear the brunt of dynamic change. Although variation in capacity relates more to service, the appropriate infrastructure allows for a realization of capacity that exists, how it should be filled, and how it should alter depending on the variation of internal and external forces. Whereas it is desirable to maximize capacity utilization, an effective infrastructure recognizes that full capacity may not be possible at all times and that buffers must be readily available to accommodate ad hoc variation in either a positive or negative direction.

When the health of a patient population is placed first, the mission of the clinical diagnostic laboratory becomes readily apparent (15). The glossy mission statement is meaningless if it is only provided to imply that a clinical service has direction. Most often, diagnostic services will follow the general mission of patient or public health care as detailed by clinics, institutions, and public health authorities. These will generally have similiar primary intentions with some variations. The clinical bacteriology laboratory will be led astray if it believes that individual patients only are the beneficiaries of its work in contrast to the general public. Conversely, the laboratory will also be missing the mark if it believes, even as a reference or large public health laboratory, that public health is the sole beneficiary rather than the individual patient. Rather than dwell overly in regards to mission, the definition of some practical goals and objectives with realistic potential represents a more tangible form of enterprise. The prioritization of these aims may be the subject of change in the short term, however, given the rapidity of novelty in the science.

Infrastructure defines appropriate feedback loops. These loops complete what some may term total quality management. Appropriate infrastructure attends to the assurance of adequate or superior standard. Standards describe a basic minimum, perhaps below which a service should not be provided. Standards detail the basic minimum, above which service strives the utmost in excellence. Effective infrastructure rationalizes emphases. Not all services require the same depth in intensity of standard and assurance; infrastructure acts as a fulcrum in the balance. Infrastructure will also help manage risk (16).

Resources can be rigidly defined as people, space, capital, equipment, and materials. As some purists will assert, however, these essentially arise from money. It is impossible to affix a standard label of money per amount of work since clinical bacteriology operations are so varied in their complexity. Nevertheless, quality is difficult to achieve without adequate operating budgets. The mix of people ingredients is dependent on the complexity of work, multi-skilling, degree of development, supervisory requirements, among other things. The trick in achieving quality is to find the appropriate balance and to allow for sufficient flexibility rather than to define a fixed ratio of work per personnel. Confinement or aspiration to fixed productivity ratios will be applicable only when there is a straight forward input-output view of service. The provision of capital equipment is evermore so a problem in the age of computerization. It is a fallacy to believe that automation in itself leads to efficiencies in a grand sense. New dilemmae have been encountered, and the trend has been to facilitate more utilization. Depreciation of capital equipment is proceeding at a rate unprecedented in the history of clinical bacteriology; a view of change in the computer industry itself serves as a quick reminder. The provision of materials or supplies must take into account numerous variables. Rather than determining a supply budget per test, work unit, or personnel quota, the goal should be to provide sufficient resource which will be well-managed and which will be subject to accountability.

The provision of space for laboratory functions is no less a complex issue. There undoubtedly will evolve new automation with lesser space requirements. Such has already been realized by larger microbiology laboratories in the areas of blood culture technology, microbial identification and susceptibility testing, serodiagnostics, and genetic amplification among others. Clinical bacteriology, however, continues to have a strong manual component and to some extent, it is inevitable that this approach to work will continue in the foreseeable future. In the mid 1980s, there were many who predicted the demise of traditional bacteriology within the decade. Where are we now? Whereas automation has contributed immensely, much of the so called routine bacteriology is performed by the same traditional methods, more or less, and with the same demands for space and people. Perhaps some individuals will predict that automation should further facilitate a shrinkage of space requirements - what would we all predict for ten to twenty years into the new millennium? Molecular diagnostics and computer use have both created new uses for space. Niche services may necessitate the availability of slightly modified versions of automation despite that fundamental techniques may remain relatively the same. Newer expectations and higher expectations have led to greater space needs despite innovation and automation. Worker demands for enhanced standards of the work-place have added to the overall complexity, and this is coupled with the employer's realization that the work environment affects productivity and quality. The quality laboratory will challenge convention in regards to space requirements and utilization.

Organizational structure and management will facilitate the service of the quality laboratory when patient care is viewed as a primary focus. By necessity, there must be individuals who will make decisions of fundamental impact, who will take responsibility for infrastructure, and who will be accountable to provide quality (17). Such individuals need to have specific laboratory management skills (18). There will also be a basic need for individuals that will provide laboratory and medical service. How these are admixed and the outcomes are a function of the structure, management, and context. The strata of personnel and their managerial roles will be affected by the complexity of operations, the degree of innovation expected, and labor agreements. A rigid view of hierarchical structures that deliver management determines two major views — vertical and horizontal. The vertical approach maintains a more traditional totem pole, hand-me-down pattern of decision-making responses. This system is capable of making quick decisions but vests authority (and hence responsibility) in few. The horizontal approach is not built on echelons of authority but is seemingly more interactive and interdependent, and more likely to widely distribute directive responsibility. This system may seem more democratic but it is not necessarily more likely to provide quality if it becomes inefficient or slow to respond. Realistically, it is both approaches which must co-exist more or less in order to reach a maximization of quality. Like the needle in a compass, the service must have direction. In striving to reach direction, the needle (service) will vary to and fro on its axis until North is found. Whereas in the end, a pattern of needle pointing and compass orientation will emerge, the needle system will have rotated back and forth both vertically and horizontally. Each time the compass is needed, a similiar reconfiguring but ultimate direction will emerge. Again, quality and accountability must reign supreme. Hardwick and Morrison have provided a succinct view of directing the clinical laboratory (19).

Somewhere in the system of providing service, it must be acknowledged that a scientific service must translate into effective patient care. As well, the laboratory must provide value-added, patient-oriented service either before any actual direct laboratory service is provided or well after the service is seemingly completed. This translation of bacteriology into medical bacteriology requires individuals who can effectively acquire, maintain, and develop the related knowledge base and its applications. How this translation may be achieved will obviously vary in a given context, but it nevertheless implies a higher level of education and synthesis.

Informatics is the direct language that translates work into practice. Informatics may be verbal or written. Verbal forms cater to client relationships. They may transfer critical results or provide value-added information. Written informatics consumes the majority of effort in these regards and in contemporary times are mainly represented by computerized laboratory information systems (20,21). The latter should be capable of receiving information, recording, storing, reporting, and reviewing. The patient/client side of the information system must be user friendly — it needs to be simple, informative, and timely. From the laboratory perspective, it must facilitate quality by assisting the infrastructure otherwise to deliver its goods in a palatable fashion, efficiently, accurately, and with reasonable cost. Interface engineering will allow for a more intricate interaction of technology service automation and information systems (22,23). It would seem that the use of computers should especially facilitate this aspect of the quality laboratory, but who would have imagined the new era of associated concerns as a result? These concerns include information burn-out, systems failure and down-time, need for greater systems capacity, need for a bureau of computer technocrats, physical personal problems of repetitive over-use, deforestation and paper trail, among others (24). The laboratory information system should facilitate accountability, and it is perhaps the benefits in this dimension that will outweigh current and future headaches that such a system and its development may impose.

VI. MACRO-STRUCTURE AND FUNCTION

The configuration of the bacteriology laboratory has emerged from traditional emphases which were predominantly based on the nature of clinical specimens and their associated work-up. In sufficiently large services, compartmentalization to blood cultures, enterics, urine bacteriology, respiratory specimens, wound and special fluids, antimicrobial susceptibility, etc. is all too familiar. This compartmentalization is likely to continue as efficiencies are sought to rapidly deal with common specimens. Nevertheless, common foci among these areas and the continued transition to molecular and more complex is likely to provide reason to change. Integration of molecular techniques, quality measures, and filling of capacity are examples of this trend.

The relationships with other laboratory services should be viewed both with interest and concern. An overall structure which seeks efficiency by reciprocation of ideas and sharing of managerial duties has the potential to benefit all. Topics relating to labor, safety, quality assurance, among others benefit from a greater voice. Of concern, however, is the fragmentation of the body of knowledge when benchtop integration occurs mainly as a result of common technology. For example, enzyme immunoassay technology may be performed on a common instrument for microbiology and chemistry services. As an input-output level of service, this will lead to a result being generated, reported, and used by the client. As a complete service, however, value-added components have the potential to be short-cut. The quality laboratory, given sufficient complexity, offers a greater package of benefit beyond the mere result. It recognizes the need for advancement in the specific science or body of knowledge and clinical impact of applications.

As new relationships are forged with client or other laboratory services, so too are new relationships emerging with larger patient services, administration, regional links, and reference services. These changing interactions have in their short history been both of benefit and of detriment to the quality laboratory. Economic and political movements of themselves may be short-sighted. Change for the sake of change has a habit of being embraced if not only for novelty. The quality laboratory thrives because the patient and the system of delivery are balanced in priority. It is the quality laboratory that the understands the application of its body of knowledge and that acts as the provider of direction.

Laboratory restructuring on a greater scale has impacted most services if not all. Laboratory evolution, renewal, and progression are all to be striven for in a time of dynamic change (25). Regionalization (26) in itself however may not be progressive if quality is it be the major trade-off for economic concern. So too, the use of decentralized or point-of-care testing, while appealing initially, may not be as truly workable as desired (27-29). A direct measure of cost for labor and supplies, and infrastructure and its reassortment, are tangible tools for the bureaucratic manager/administrator. The net equation of input and patient/societal benefit is the effective tool for the quality laboratory. The quality laboratory should provide leadership; leadership should not be primarily provided by accountants, consultants, or bureaucrats.

VII. STANDARDS

The quality laboratory will be performing at a level that in a practical manner meets or exceeds the established national or local standards. Indeed, its functions participate in creating those standards. The internal creation of standard provides assurance that a minimal competency is continued as the laboratory's emphases shift. It also acts as a buffer for complacency and change. The entrenchment of standards must however be viewed with caution since an unbalanced investment in this area may usurp other functions (30). The quality laboratory recognizes the necessary balance within such investment, and it reprioritizes as required. On an international basis, we may avoid promulgation of standards which are capably supported in a society with considerable resource, but where the standards may be obviously fiscally unbearable, and hence inappropriate, in an underdeveloped or under-resourced society. Priorities may require a shift in the balance given these specific contexts.

The vocabulary of standards is based on convention, much of which does not have roots in classic bacteriology. The principles however do have a fundamental history in medical microbiology. Different terms, connotations, and appreciations have in fact provided much in the way of what industry in general and contemporary clinical bacteriology in particular has referred to as quality control, quality assurance, proficiency, accreditation, quality improvement, continuous quality improvement, and total quality management (31-36). It is a misunderstanding of contemporary proponents that these standard applications have never been in place. It will be evident to those who explore history that, whether such specific terms have been used or not, their effective practice has been a complacent reality in various forms in many quality laboratories.

Quality control (Table 1) provides methods for direct control of day-to-day activities, more so in regard to technical services. The stringency of these activities may be variable. There must be a reasonable minimum; quality will be enhanced with quality control improvements, but excessive burden may have a negative influence if taken to the extreme. Quality control is predominantly an internal task. External quality control will have some impact, and essentially it is comprised of proficiency testing programs which are provided by centralized authorities. Quality control will monitor work within predefined limits of tolerance. Such limits and the procedures to which they apply will necessarily be written as policy within an acceptable manual form. Records of quality control must be an accepted component of routine work, and the records must be retained for review. A critical reporting of laboratory results to the care-giver must be conducted as necessary. Specimen receipt and the details thereof require close attention. Specimens may be unlabeled or mislabeled, of inappropriate quality, registered in permanent documentation, and received and processed on a timely basis. Errors in interpretation and analysis require a system for review in order that they be ascertained. Biohazard concerns may present another item for review. Incidents and complaints should be accepted for review. At a more fundamental level, quality control places tolerance limits for acceptability of bacteriological media (37), quality control bacterial isolates, stains, reagents, purchased resources (e.g., kits), susceptibility testing, amplification technology wares, and equipment and large automated instruments. Specific laboratory technical staff issues such as work plans, accidents, incidents, meetings, and continuing medical education are lesser recognized but nevertheless important components of quality control.

External proficiency testing has historically had merit as a third party arbiter of competence at a given level (38-40). A few large laboratory systems may have sufficient participants in order to create in-house proficiency testing programs. In the past, some external proficiency programs have had considerable value in defining major problem areas. Often, these programs have functioned by routinely sending examples of bacteria which may have had problems associated with their identification and susceptibility testing. Such programs seem initially rudimentary, but their value is nonetheless considerable especially in the early phases of enhancing quality. Some such programs have recognized the need to evolve towards including incremental components that in part address interpretation rather than straightforward identification and susceptibility testing. The latter concept more directly addresses quality and furthermore follows a natural progression especially when identification and susceptibility testing methods become considerably harmonized and externally provided. There continue to be trends whereby quality can be improved by this approach. In some areas, this mode may be the only external form of partial review. We must appreciate, however, limitations of this approach. It makes little sense to have a laboratory service mired in an extensive search for identification when on a practical basis, the laboratory would normally refer out a complicated specimen or isolate. An external program will have limited ability to truly appreciate the quality of a service given what it uses as instruments and given that it never truly places a context or comes necessarily on-site. External proficiency testing will mainly identify major dilemmae on an all-or-none basis. Perhaps, though, it will continue at least to provide a route for information updates. Proficiency testing is a quality control tool – it must not be depended on extraordinarily or with the risk of jeopardizing the requisite time for other quality activities or, for that

Table 1   A sample structure for quality control activities.

A.   Policy and procedure
>   establish goals and limits for methods
>   written procedures, i.e., manuals

B.   Records
>   maintenance of quality control records
>   retention of quality control records
>   critical reporting of service results
>   results log and databasing
>   timeliness of reporting
>   reporting errors

C.   Specimen handling
>   unlabelled
>   mislabeled
>   quality of specimen
>   biohazardous incidents
>   log-in errors

D.   Interpretive error

E.   Reagents
>   media – storage, preparation, expiry, sterility, performance
>   indicator bacteria
>   stains
>   reagents
>   antisera
>   genetic amplification

F.   Tools
>   purchased kits
>   instruments, e.g., blood culture, incubators, freezers, autoclaves, centrifuges
>   equipment – maintenance standards, record checks, pipettes, calibrated loops, autoclave, sterility

G.   Service staff
>   work plans
>   accidents
>   incidents
>   in-service, continuing medical education
>   staff meetings

H.   External proficiency testing

matter, routine service work. To be of value, specimens for proficiency testing should be approached as if they are the next clinical specimens for the routine day's work. They should provide a test to the system and not draw extraordinary attention from a set of highly knowledgeable few. It remains to be seen whether organizations such as the International Standards Organization will have the ability to ensure that basic standards are achieved globally.

Quality assurance to some will imply an enhancement of activities which are focused on patient care. Whereas this belief is fundamentally true, quality assurance on a grander scale is a completed loop of accountability, efficiency, and improvement. The laboratory service has responsibility for simple or complex functions. These functions are monitored through quality control; an acknowledged standard or expectation is pre-set. The service has delegated responsibility for this program; obviously it is pertinent to all, but individuals may be selectively chosen to direct. Service improvement areas are identified as are specific problems. Solutions are made available, and there is a mechanism to assure the effective implementation or correction. These activities follow in a carefully structured and acknowledged systematic plan. Records of such activities are maintained and reviewed. It must be re-emphasized that quality assurance which seems narrowly pertinent to a particular laboratory endeavor always has a direct or indirect potential impact on patient care. Quality assurance can be pertinent to individuals or populations.

As proficiency testing is an external quality control tool, laboratory accreditation provides an external quality assurance measure. Accreditation is variably practiced (41-44). Many countries fail to endorse this quality assurance item; others claim not to afford them. The regulation, structure, depth of review, and impact of accreditation programs are all too variable. Essentially, accreditation is a third-party review of quality as a whole. It must, to be of value, examine a context from both the patient/delivery and laboratory/service perspectives. The accreditation must be accountable but in order to be so, it must have some degree of autonomy and authority. The quality laboratory should be performing at a level whereby accreditation is able to provide suggestion for some useful adjuncts, not revolution. Again, it remains to be seen whether global standards can be achieved in this area through influential bodies such as the International Standards Organization (45,46).

Much may be written about continuous quality improvement and total quality management, and indeed a complex area of philosophy and managerial programs may be the subject of theses and dissertations (47-49), but the sum effect may be a simple net gain in a positive direction. Continuous quality improvement is a systematic approach towards making a client better or more happy with the system or overall approach. Continuous quality improvement may be thought of as pro-active development; development of culture and process rather than strictly a research application taken to fruition. Total quality management is seemingly an inter-related system of planned and multi-faceted management which will facilitate quality. Perhaps these are newer terms as arisen in the last decade for the bacteriology laboratory, but the practical side of their impact or intent is not new. We need to know who the patient is and what his/her needs are. We need to recognize the care-giver, his/her clinical service, and what the needs are. We need to appreciate the overall context for how patient and care-givers achieve maximal benefit, given an understanding of resource utilization and the practicalities of reality. These needs, as inter-related as they are, were no less a part of the quality laboratory existence in the past, during the present, or for the future.

VIII. SAFETY

The quality laboratory assures a relevant work which will provide for patient safety. At a routine level, however, safe practices refer more directly to specimen acquisition and processing, and their immediate work environments.

A safety program requires structure (Figure 3), often provided best with the delegation to a safety officer and/or committee. In a multi-disciplinary laboratory, there is some benefit to the pooling of resources in this regard and to the recognition of essential commonalities so that efficiencies will be sought. The structure of a safety program will facilitate minimum standards, provide orientation and continuing education, monitor prevention and incidents, participate with higher safety committees, and be accountable. A safety manual which addresses common concerns and educational items should be established; the manual will be practical and useful. Records of safety incidents and concerns should

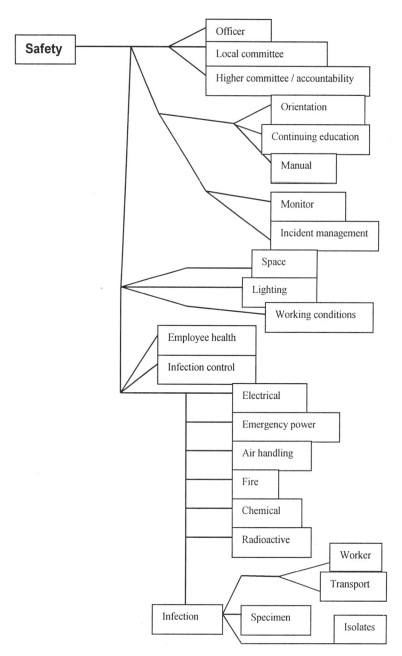

Figure 3   The safety dendrogram.

facilitate documentation in the program. Participation in safety exercises must be mandatory although allowing for some realism with respect to emphasis and spectrum.

Safety will be supported by the provision of adequate space and reasonable working conditions. Routine microbiology services will require sufficient lighting given the variables which may relate to visualized color changes and colonial growth and morphology. Given the potential for infectious hazards, appropriate apparel must be worn. Apart from more typical versions of electrical safety, it should also be considered that an emergency power supply be required depending on the complexity of operations and their needs for incubation and storage. Adequate air handling must be considered for specimen set-up and subsequent follow-through as is appropriate. The provision of handling cabinets with acceptable air flow will meet the latter needs. Attention to fire safety in all of its aspects, provision of first aid and eye wash stations, and safety in the handling of compressed gases are all relevant to the operations of the diagnostic bacteriology laboratory.

Chemical hazards and their control can be a complex task, but consistent uses have been the norm for bacteriology laboratories. There should be a knowledge of the presence of chemicals in the workplace and their potential to harm. Records of chemicals and potential hazards should be readily available especially when a diverse array of individuals may be confronted with a medical emergency. Records and reviews of incidents should be maintained. Radioactive hazards are becoming much less, if any, of a problem for the diagnostic bacteriology laboratory, but a shift towards molecular technologies may reverse this trend for a select few laboratories that delve heavily into research and development.

Safety and infection no doubt receive much attention (50,51). These concerns begin with the collection of the specimen and its transport to the laboratory. Most clinical specimens can be processed on the open bench, but notable exceptions (e.g., *Brucella*, *Coccidioides*) do exist (52,53). A classification for infectious hazards and conditions of their handling should be recognized; indeed these are often defined by higher regulatory authorities, e.g., federal. Safe waste handling facilities for both bacteria and specimens are needed. A protocol for transportation of dangerous goods to reference or other laboratories is essential; this may be applicable to local, inter-territorial, and international concerns. The quality laboratory necessarily has a strong liaison with the infection control services of the patient/care facility, and the laboratory subscribes to the institutional standards in this regard. Furthermore, there is reasonable accessibility to employee health services given that an infection occurs and that an employee's personal health is at risk. The employee health service may facilitate prevention via administration of pertinent vaccines for example. Contemporary concerns about employee health in the context of clinical samples is best exemplified by current knowledge and practice regarding potential HIV exposure. Health care worker acquisition of HIV from patients is a sobering reminder of the need to be vigilant (54) with respect to prevention. Possible exposure to HIV in a high risk situation, e.g., needle-stick injury or mucosal contamination, necessitates a cascade of events which include First Aid, reporting of the incident, assessment of risk, counseling, antiviral prophylaxis, and follow-up (Figure 4).

IX. COST AND BENEFIT

Cost-benefit analyses are among the most complex of endeavors that may be considered in the area of medical economics. In relevance to a laboratory procedure, the complete picture is not simply one of test output and focal patient impact (55). Consider only the reality of diagnostic test accuracy. A given assay may seemingly perform very well if applied to a patient population for whom the result and its correlation with a true indication of infection is very highly probable. The same assay, though, performed with the same technical input and accuracy, may have much lesser impact for another patient population for whom the frequency of disease is much different. That is, predictive values of a diagnostic test will vary for different populations, and this accuracy or inaccuracy itself may have major impact outcomes.

The numerous variables that may affect cost-benefit analyses deserve careful deliberation. Assays which are performed in high volume are amenable to efficiencies of multiple testing. The filling of capacity is economically sensible. Yet the relevance of a single assay for a given patient may outweigh the relevance of multiple similar tests which have been provided in an efficient and automated approach. The cost may include reagents, automation and equipment, personnel, infrastructure (with the many facets as detailed in this chapter), requisites for repeat testing, requisites for associated and subsequent

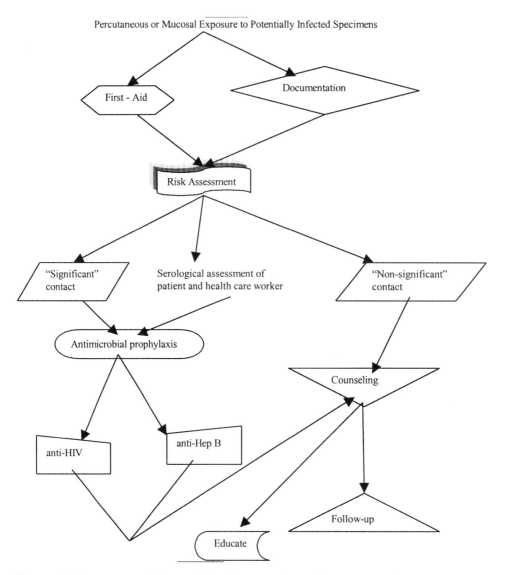

Figure 4   Post-exposure follow-up for health care workers who suffer from an accidental exposure to patient specimens.

other tests, impact of false negative misdiagnosis (e.g., morbidity, institutional care, investigation, additional visits, etc.), and impact of false positive misdiagnosis (e.g., morbidity, institutional care, treatments, complacency over other diagnoses, etc.). Benefits will hopefully include decreased morbidity (mainly) and thereafter decreased mortality. Benefits will also include more appropriate treatment (e.g., improved antibiotic use and its benefits for both the individual and society), a reduction in care visits or institutional admissions, a reduction in other investigations, more accurate understanding of a disease process, and perhaps an enhancement in prevention for both the individual and the general population.

Accurate and useful diagnostic information from the quality laboratory will enhance the education of care-givers. The results and the relevant discussion which will follow should facilitate the development of good practices. Education in itself may necessarily lead to a change in the requirement for diagnostic support. For example, an effective diagnostic assay may initially be required to elucidate difficult clinical circumstances but may lead to decreased utilization of the same when knowledge is sufficiently heightened.

With the advancement of both traditional and new molecular techniques, it is conceivable that several diagnostic technologies could be co-applicable for a single infection. The combination of microbe-specific and non-specific (e.g., blood chemistry and hematology) tests may be relevant. Alternatively, a given diagnostic assay may be desirable in a context when other individual or multiple pathogens may be sought simultaneously. The medical context may dictate.

There is no doubt a trend to establish paradigms for laboratory or clinical services (56,57). The initial focus in these endeavors has been predominantly utilization. Whether inside or outside the laboratory, there may be rational needs for such approaches. In the end, however, there must be sufficient knowledge to address medical relevance. The quality laboratory will have sufficient depth and insight to understand when such paradigms will be applicable and which patients will especially require advanced deliberation.

REFERENCES

1. Ackerman VP, Berriman PS. Assessment of workload in the microbiology laboratory. Pathology 1977; 9:207-212.
2. Elin RJ, Robertson EA, Sever GA. Workload, space, and personnel of microbiology laboratories in teaching hospitals. Amer J Clin Pathol 1984; 82:78-84.
3. Forward KR, Digout GL. Non-unit producing activities in a large microbiology laboratory. Amer J Clin Pathol 1992; 98:287-290.
4. Cartwright RY, Davies JR, Dulake C, Hart RJ, Morris CA, Wilkinson PJ. A study of workload units in five microbiology laboratories. J Clin Pathol 1985; 38:208-214.
5. Thomson RB, Peterson LR. Role of the clinical microbiology laboratory in the diagnosis of infections. Cancer Treat Res 1998; 96:143-165.
6. LaRocco MT, Burgert SJ. Infection in the bone marrow transplant recipient and role of the microbiology laboratory in clinical transplantation. Clin Microbiol Rev 1997; 10:277-297.
7. Philips G, Senior BW, McEwan H. Use of telephone inquiries to a microbiology laboratory as a proxy measure of reporting efficiency. J Clin Pathol 1992;45:250-253.
8. Dupont PF. Automation in microbiology: a physician's viewpoint. Amer J Med Tech 1983; 49:323-325.
9. Neu HC. What should the clinician expect from the microbiology laboratory? Ann Intern Med 1978; 89 (Suppl):781-784.
10. Gaunt PN. Information in infection control. J Hosp Infect 1991; 18 (Suppl A):397-401.
11. Gordts B, Van Landuyt H. Epidemiology as a tool for hospital infection control. Acta Clin Belg 1998; 53:75-82.
12. Emori TG, Gaynes RP. An overview of nosocomial infections, including the role of the microbiology laboratory. Clin Microbiol Rev 1993; 6:428-442.
13. O'Sullivan MB. Changing technologies in the reference laboratory. Arch Pathol Lab Med 1987; 111:657-661.
14. Jenkins SG. Evaluation of new technology in the clinical microbiology laboratory. Diagn Microbiol Inf Dis 1995; 23:53-60.
15. Kelly DL. Reframing beliefs about work and change processes in redesigning laboratory services. Joint Commission J Qual Improvement 1998; 24:154-167.
16. Lord JT. Risk management in pathology and laboratory medicine. Arch Pathol Lab Med 1990; 114:1164-1167.
17. Thomson RB. The changing role of the clinical microbiology laboratory director: results of a survey. Diagn Microbiol Inf Dis 1995; 23:45-51.
18. De Cediel N, Fraser CG, Deom A, Josefsson L, Worth HG, Zinder O. Guidelines (1988) for training in clinical laboratory management. Clin Chim Acta 1989; 185:S4-15.
19. Hardwick DF, Morrison JI. Directing the Clinical Laboratory. New York:Field & Wood Medical Publishers, Inc., 1988.
20. Kunz KJ. Computerization in microbiology. Hum Pathol 1976; 7:169-175.
21. Cowan DF, Gray RZ, Campbell B. Validation of the laboratory information system. Arch Pathol Lab Med 1998; 122:239-244.

22. Willard KE, Shanholtzer CJ. User interface re-engineering: innovative applications of bar coding in a clinical microbiology laboratory. Arch Pathol Lab Med 1995; 119:706-712.

23. Evangelista AT. The clincal impact of automated susceptibility reporting using a computer interface. Adv Exp Med Biol 1990; 263:131-142.

24. Smith MJ, Conway FT, Karsh BT. Occupational stress in human computer interaction. Ind Health 1999; 37:157-173.

25. Chapin K, Baron EJ. Impact of CLIA 88 on the clinical microbiology laboratory. Diagn Microbiol Inf Dis 1995; 23:35-43.

26. Matsen JM. The regionalization of laboratory services at the University of Utah Medical Center. Arch Pathol Lab Med 1988; 112:957-959.

27. Kost GJ, Ehrmeyer SS, Chernow B, Winkelman JW, Zaloga GP, Dellinger RP, Shirey T. The laboratory-clinical interface: point-of-care testing. Chest 1999; 115:1140-1154.

28. Ehrmeyer SS, Laessig RH. Regulatory requirements for decentralized testing. Amer J Clin Pathol 1995; 104 (Suppl 1):40-49.

29. Howanitz PJ. College of American Pathologists Conference XXVIII on alternate site testing: What must we do now? Arch Pathol Lab Med 1995; 119:979-983.

30. Sonnenwirth AC. Constraints under which the microbiology laboratory functions. Ann Intern Med 1978; 89:S785-S788.

31. Baron EJ. Quality management and the clinical microbiology laboratory. Diagn Microbiol Inf Dis 1995; 23:23-34.

32. Schifman RB. Strategies for quality management in clinical microbiology. Clin Lab Med 1995; 15:437-446.

33. Bartlett RC. Trends in quality management. Arch Pathol Lab Med 1990; 114:1126-1130.

34. Libeer JC. Total quality management for clinical laboratories: a need or a new fashion? Acta Clin Belg 1997; 52:226-232.

35. Dorsey DB. Evolving concepts of quality in laboratory practice: a historical overview of quality assurance in clinical laboratories. Arch Pathol Lab Med 1989; 113:1329-1334.

36. Wakefield DS, Cyphert ST, Murray JF, Uden-Holman T, Hendryx MS, Wakefield BJ, Helms CM. Understanding patient-centered care in the context of total quality management and continuous quality improvement. Joint Commission J Qual Improvement 1994; 20:152-161.

37. Shanholtzer CJ, Peterson LR. Laboratory quality assurance testing of microbiologic media from commercial sources. Amer J Clin Pathol 1987; 88:210-215.

38. Shahangian S. Proficiency testing in laboratory medicine: uses and limitations. Arch Pathol Lab Med 1998; 122:15-30.

39. Richardson H, Wood D, Whitby J, Lannigan R, Fleming C. Quality improvement of diagnostic microbiology through a peer-group proficiency assessment program: a 20-year experience in Ontario. Arch Pathol Lab Med 1996; 120:445-455.

40. Von Graevenitz A. External quality assessment programs in microbiology. Med Microbiol Lett 1994; 3:129-154.

41. Anonymous. Royal College of Pathologists' United Kingdom pilot study of laboratory accreditation. J Clin Pathol 1990; 43:89-91.

42. Menditto A, Morisi G. National and regional regulations on minimal requirements, quality control and accreditation for clinical laboratories in Italy. Ann Ist Super Sanita 1995; 31:149-155.

43. Lawson NS. Quality assurance programs in the United States. Ann Ist Super Sanita 1995; 31:21-35.

44. Kailner A. Quality management in the medical laboratory: a comparison of draft standards. Clin Chim Acta 1998; 278:111-119.

45. Dunavant DW, Jones KR. ISO 9000 laboratory accreditation. Qual Assur 1995; 4:41-59.

46. Royal PD. Harmonization of good laboratory practice requirements and laboratory accreditation programs. Qual Assur 1994; 3:312-315.

47. Bartlett RC, Mazens-Sullivan M, Tetreault JZ, Lobel S, Nivard J. Evolving approaches to management of quality in clinical microbiology. Clin Microbiol Rev 1994; 7:55-88.

48. Nardella A, Farrell M, Pechet L, Snyder LM. Continuous improvement, quality control, and cost containment in clinical laboratory testing: enhancement of physicians' laboratory-ordering practices. Arch Pathol Lab Med 1994; 118:965-968.

49. Haeckel R, Bohm M, Capel PJ, Hoiby N, Jansen RT, Kallner A, Kelly A, Kruse-Jarres JD, Kuffer H, Libeer JC. Concepts for a model of good medical laboratory services. Clin Chem Lab Med 1998; 36:399-403.

50. Anonymous. Safety from infection in the microbiology laboratory. J Infect 1980; 2:101-104.

51. Anonymous. Safety measures in microbiology: minimum standards of laboratory safety. WHO Chron 1980; 34:144-146.

52. Harrington JM, Shannon HS. Incidence of tuberculosis, hepatitis, brucellosis, and shigellosis in British medical laboratory workers. Br Med J 1976; i:759-762.

53. Staszkiewicz J, Lewis CM, Colville J, Zervos M, Band J. Outbreak of *Brucella melitensis* among microbiology laboratory workers in a community hospital. J Clin Microbiol 1991; 29:287-290.

54. Chiarello LA, Cardo DM, Panlilio AL, Bell DM, Kaplan JE, Martin LS. Public health service guidelines for the management of health-care worker exposure to HIV and recommendations for post-exposure prophylaxis. MMWR Morb Mortal Wkly Rep 1998(Suppl); 47:RR-7.

55. Washington JA. The clinical microbiology laboratory: utilization and cost-effectiveness. Am J Med 1985; 78:8-16.

56. Nardella A, Pechet L, Snyder LM. Continuous improvement, quality control, and cost containment in clinical laboratory testing: effects of establishing and implementing guidelines for preoperative tests. Arch Pathol Lab Med 1995; 119:518-522.

57. Wu AH. Improving the utilization of clinical laboratory tests. J Eval Clin Pract 1998; 4:171-181.

11

Staphylococcal Infections

Nevio Cimolai
Children's and Women's Health Centre of British Columbia, Vancouver, British Columbia, Canada

Frank Espersen
Division of Microbiology, Statens Serum Institut, Copenhagen, Denmark

I. HISTORICAL BACKGROUND

Staphylococcus aureus has been an important human pathogen whose contribution to infections outside of hospitals has been relatively constant while its role in hospital-acquired infections has increased over the last several decades (1-5). Although perhaps more prominent prior to the era of antibiotics and among normal populations, e.g., nurseries, the bacterium has been able to persist as a major cause of human infection and has adapted quickly to antibiotic pressure. The advent of a large number of medical devices as well as structural and immune compromise has ensured that *S. aureus* will continue to be a major cause of human infection. Infections range from the most simple, e.g., superficial skin infection, to complex, e.g., endocarditis, brain abscess, and osteomyelitis. Given that the bacterium is often a component of the normal flora, given its continuing possession of several virulence factors, and given the many opportunities that arise for it to gain an advantage, it is not surprising that the actual numbers of infections among humans are many and that the infections affect both ambulatory patients and those who are admitted to hospitals. During the late 1970s and early 1980s, the exponential increase in the occurrence of staphylococcal toxic-shock syndrome proved to be a function of human engineering; whereas this systemic illness had indeed been described in other words for as long as *S. aureus* was so recognized, the use of tampons, which enhanced toxin production, was largely implicated in an epidemic that has now essentially passed.

Methicillin resistance among staphylococci developed soon after the introduction of antistaphylococcal semi-synthetic penicillins, but the severe impact on human health was not felt until that last two decades (6). Entering the new millenium, however, methicillin-resistant *S. aureus* (MRSA) is commonly mentioned in medical and lay circles and is a global problem (6,147). Apart from methicillin resistance, the bacterium is developing resistance as well to most other anti-staphylococcal agents (8), thus justly deserving the lay term 'superbug'. In areas where MRSA is highly endemic, vancomycin and a few other antibiotics remain effective for treatment, but borderline vancomycin resistance has become evident (VISA = vancomycin intermediate [susceptible] *S. aureus*) and poses a real threat that is of major concern (9,10).

Outside of the recognition that *S. saprophyticus* is a cause of urinary tract infections (11), albeit in a small proportion, coagulase-negative staphylococci (CoNS) mainly cause infection as opportunists. Immunocompromise in itself is not a sufficient risk, but the presence of foreign medical devices poses the greatest threat. Accordingly, CoNS have become important comtemporary pathogens due to the many advances in medical procedures which carry with them the risk of new infections (12). Thus, serious CoNS infections have increased in frequency during the modern medical era (13). In addition, there continues to be a problem with distinguishing infection and contamination.

Although not staphylococci proper, there are several other catalase-positive Gram positive cocci that deserve some discussion in this context, e.g., micrococci, *Stomatococcus* sp., and *Alloiococcus otitidis*. In general, these behave much like CoNS and are associated largely with the same sorts of infections although to a lesser frequency. It is also relevant to consider them here since they often pose some difficulty with appropriate categorization in the laboratory where the confusion occurs in the context of considering CoNS.

II. CLINICAL ASPECTS

A. *S. aureus*

S. aureus infections among humans range from silent carrier states to severe life-threatening infections such as bacteremia or endocarditis. The primary infections may either be self-limiting or may progress to bacteremia with a risk of secondary (i.e., hematogenous spread) infections (Figure 1). In addition to these, *S. aureus* is also associated with toxin-related diseases.

S. aureus is commonly carried in the nasopharynx, and carriage rates have ranged from 5-50% depending on the population (14). In addition to nasal carriage, the bacterium may be found in the bowel and female genital tract. Some individuals carry *S. aureus* commonly on the skin analogous to

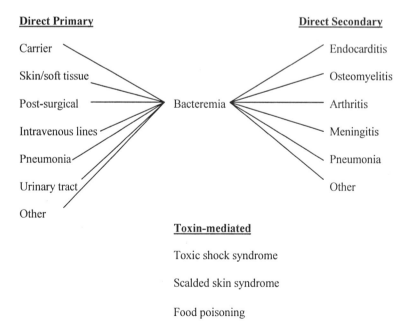

Figure 1   The spectrum of *S. aureus* infections.

the frequent carriage of CoNS (15). All of these areas, but particularly the nasopharynx, serve as reservoirs for human infection. Asymptomatic carriage may be intermittent or prolonged, and different strains may be acquired over many years.

Essentially every possible body site has been infected by *S. aureus*, and there is a voluminous literature which details patient series for many of the systems that are so affected (1-3). Among this myriad of potential infections, the most common primary infections include those of skin, soft tissue, postsurgical sites, intravenous lines, and lung, while the most common secondary infections are endocarditis, osteomyelitis, and septic arthritis.

Infections of the skin present with a diverse array of clinical manifestations. Direct infection may lead to superficial illnesses such as impetigo and folliculitis or may be involved in deeper structures thus giving rise to carbuncles, furuncles, or cellulitis. In scalded skin syndrome, the presence of the bacterium is not sufficient in itself; a toxin is liberated which cleaves the skin in the epidermal layer thus giving the appearance of a desquamating rash (16). Surgical skin sites are familiar targets for *S. aureus*, and it is the most common pathogen in infections of these areas. Burns, ulcers, and decubiti are also among the favourite targets for this bacterium.

Deep tissues may be involved as a direct consequence of superficial invasion, and mastitis and breast abscesses among females exemplify the latter. Bacteremia may be spontaneous or as a consequence of the interruption of normal barriers, e.g., especially skin. In-dwelling vascular access devices are major risk factors for infection regardless of whether they are placed in superficial veins or deep vessels, e.g., arteries or central veins. Given the frequency of *S. aureus* colonization and given that spontaneous bacteremias from oral and gut sources are probably not uncommon, there is plenty of opportunity for the bacterium to enter circulation apart from the breaches of host defences that may otherwise occur.

Primary pneumonia may occur in patients with varied risk factors (e.g., intubated patients in intensive care units, patients with cystic fibrosis), and a secondary pneumonia not uncommonly complicates viral lower respiratory diseases (e.g., during influenza especially among the elderly). Pediatric bacterial tracheitis is most often due to this bacterium. Complications of respiratory infection include lung abscess and empyema. Secondary pneumonia may also be seen among intravenous drug addicts who have right-sided endocarditis.

S. aureus is among the most common causes of osteomyelitis and septic arthritis (among both pediatric and adult populations), endocarditis (especially among damaged valves or among intravenous drug users), pericarditis, graft infections, infectious bursitis, tropical pyomyositis, brain abscesses, and ambulatory peritoneal dialysis-associated peritonitis. Patients who suffer from neutrophil dysfunction are at increased risk for infection.

Pre-formed toxin from some strains is responsible for staphylococcal food poisoning which can occur in early and late forms (17,18). Within several hours, the toxin can be a potent emetic, whereas 6-12 hrs. later, the toxin produces a diarrheal illness. When tetracyclines were commonly used, it was postulated that staphylococcal overgrowth due to resistant bacteria could lead to an antibiotic-associated diarrhea. When *Clostridium difficile* became recognized as an important etiological agent of antibiotic-associated diarrhea, the latter entity was thereafter not often considered.

Toxic shock syndrome is also a toxin-associated systemic illness (19,20). Patients develop a relatively sudden onset of fever, macular rash, and hypotension. Other organs may become involved: diarrhea, myositis, mucous membrane hyperemia, renal failure, hepatitis, thrombocytopenia, and neurological illness have all been reported. The rash often desquamates during resolution. The bacterium is present at a particular site and liberates a toxin which is absorbed. In 'menstrual' toxic-shock syndrome, the disease occurred as a result of the use of hyperabsorbent tampons which promoted toxin production. The latter illness has essentially disappeared as innovations in the industry have promoted the production of adsorbents that are not susceptible to this problem. 'Nonmenstrual' toxic shock occurs as a consequence of toxin production at other sites. Quite often, the latter include surgical sites, but toxic shock can also occur during the course of bacteremias or deep-seated infections otherwise (21).

MRSA are capable of causing all of the aforementioned illnesses. It has been proposed that MRSA in general are no more virulent than methicillin-susceptible *S. aureus*. Nevertheless, whether methicillin-resistant or methicillin-susceptible, it has been long recognized that particular strains of *S. aureus* are more likely to be associated with infection and specific forms of infection than other strains. This should be anticipated if not only on the basis for strains to vary in their potential to produce toxins.

B. Coagulase-negative staphylococci

With few exceptions, CoNS are opportunists and as such are major causes of nosocomial infection (12,22). Most bonafide infections occur as a consequence of the presence of vascular access devices. Bacteremias are often seen as a result of the latter among patients in neonatal intensive care, other inten-sive care settings, oncology wards, and those who require prolonged intravenous access, e.g., total par-enteral nutrition therapy. Prosthetic devices such as grafts, artificial joints, and heart valves (23) are prime targets as are central nervous system shunts and peritoneal catheters that are used for ambulatory dialysis. Native heart valves are less often targets for CoNS infection. Infections can occur in surgical wounds such as sternal osteomyelitis after open heart surgery or ophthalmological procedures. When sampled from superficial wounds, most CoNS isolates are obtained as a consequence of site contamina-tion rather than from true infection. The mere presence of these bacteria in a context where superficial infection is present and where no other cause of an apparent infection is isolated should not imply that there is a cause-and-effect relationship.

The occurrence of the above infections is particularly a function of the normal presence of CoNS in abundance on normal skin and the subsequent entry through breached skin or mucosal barriers or via direct entry from a surgical procedure itself. The common presence on skin also translates into having these bacteria become common contaminants in blood cultures. Although disinfection reduces the num-ber of CoNS on the skin surface prior to venipuncture, the reduction does not usually occur on an all-or-none basis. In a neonatal intensive care setting where blood acquisition through skin is often difficult at best, the potential for contamination is high; despite a major role for CoNS in nosocomial bacteremia, the majority of positive blood cultures for these bacteria represent specimen contamination.

As there are a large number of species within the CoNS group (12), some have attempted to ex-amine whether particular species are more likely to infect than others. In general, however, the distribu-tion of species causing infection, e.g., predominantly *S. epidermidis*, is consistent with the frequency of these respective species as normal flora. One exception to this rule is the role of *S. saprophyticus* in urinary tract infections. These infections typically occur among adolescent or young women and mainly present in the form of a simple cystitis (11). Initially, this species was considered to be a biotype of *S. epidermidis* that was highly tropic to the urinary tract. Its designation as a species is somewhat helpful in identifying a more likely urinary pathogen. Nevertheless, under the appropriate circumstances, other CoNS are also capable of causing urinary tract infections, but the patients so affected often have com-plicating factors such as catheterization or an anomalous urinary tract.

C. Other gram positive cocci

1.   Micrococcus spp.

These bacteria are opportunists like CoNS but quite rarely cause infection. There are several species that have been isolated from human infection. Like CoNS, many are merely contaminants when found in blood cultures, and they are not uncommonly isolated in combination with either salivary contaminants or CoNS. Nevertheless, infections have been cited including line-associated bacteremias, peritoneal dialysis-associated peritonitis, central nervous system shunts, endocarditis, among others (24).

Kocuria spp. are new designations for some former *Micrococcus* spp. (25); their role in infection is essentially as above therefore, and historic citations of infection will more often be captured by searching under the *Micrococcus* genus name.

2. *Stomatococcus*

As well an opportunist, *S. mucilaginosus* is a rare cause of bacteremia and other infections. The most common presentations of infection include: intravenous device-related sepsis, presence of other foreign devices, bacteremia with unknown focus but often among neutropenic cancer patients, endocarditis, and meningitis (again mainly in oncology patients) (24,26-29). A number of other extremely rare infections are cited in the medical literature.

3. *Alloiococcus otitidis*

This bacterium has been found in middle ear effusions, but its role in otitis media is not certain. It has not been isolated outside of specimens from the external ear (30).

III. EPIDEMIOLOGY OF INFECTION

A. *S. aureus*

Chronic carriage of *S. aureus* by humans is a well-recognized phenomenon and has been intensively studied. The bacterium is most commonly harboured in the anterior nares although the entire upper respiratory tract may serve as a reservoir (31). Essentially, there is a tropism between the bacterium and mucous membranes but with a preference for the nares. Skin and sweat glands may also carry the bacteria but to a lesser degree. Vaginal cultures for this bacterium are positive in up to 1/10 of the female population. Shortly after birth, newborns are often colonized with bacterium that has been acquired from mother, care-giver, or environment. The bacterium is able to survive in the inanimate environment (e.g., manual objects, clothing, and linens). Food may become contaminated and then allow for growth. All of these areas act as mechanisms for the bacterium to persist and then have the potential to cause infection when the opportunity arises. Shedding from the nares and skin is frequent, and the burden of bacterium in the neighboring environment is a direct reflection of the quantity and distribution of carriage. The majority of carriers are intermittent rather than chronic, and the duration of carriage is quite variable (many weeks to years). As well, both intermittent and chronic carriers may be colonized by new strains. The risk for carriage of *S. aureus* is increased as a consequence of chronic dermatological problems, renal failure and dialysis, participation in health care, in-hospital status, among other factors.

S. aureus carriage poses a greater (2-10X) risk for subsequent *S. aureus* infection (32). In the surgical setting, infections are most often due to bacterium of endogenous origin. The recognition of this endogenous risk has led many to investigate the impact of *S. aureus* eradication from the nares and skin with antibiotics as a mechanism to reduce subsequent infection. Consistently, the risk of infection has been reduced with a concomitant reduction in carriage (31,33,34). A range of risk factors for the development of *S. aureus* bacteremia has been described including recent surgery or trauma, dialysis, intravenous drug use, and previous hospital admission in addition to nasal carriage (35). For hospital-acquired bacteremia, logistic regression analysis has found associations with the presence of a central venous cathether, anemia, and hyponatremia (36). Effective infection control practices in hospitals are of major importance in preventing spread of the bacterium. Overall, person-to-person transmission is of greatest importance in facilitating spread, and the value of handwashing cannot be overstated.

MRSA is now a major dilemma in many regions and has extended from major health care centres to long-term care facilities (37,38) and the general community, although some regions have been effective in controlling these bacteria and indeed have reported a decline in their frequency (39). Even though hospitals and the setting of acute medical care offer the greatest risk for spread, these expanding reservoirs in the community serve to allow for an ongoing cycle of transmission. In endemic areas, there are often several strains that circulate in the population. Person-to-person spread is again of major importance, but the potential role of chronic health care worker carriage and a persistence in the environment of the infected patient are often not emphasized. Risk factors for colonization and infection with MRSA are published (40), and there is reason to believe that antibiotic abuse is but one such factor (41). Apart from appropriate treatment of active MRSA infections, there is a potential role for eradication of the carrier state, but good infection control practices are again of utmost value (38,42). The degree of MRSA spread (i.e., carriage rates in an institution) is often an indicator of the standard of infection control in general. The impact of changing health care structures on MRSA control and the actual costs of MRSA infection and control must be taken seriously (43). Of interest, Kluytmans and colleagues (44) detail the transmission of MRSA in outbreak form via food.

Toxic shock syndrome continues to be seen, but there has obviously been a decline since the early 1980s (20).

Other coagulase-positive staphylococci can infect humans but appear to do so rarely, e g , *Staphylococcus intermedius* is acquired from animals.

B. Coagulase-negative staphylococci

There is a preferential colonization of different body areas by some CoNS (12). For example, heavier quantities are not uncommonly associated with areas of increased sweat or sebum. Dependent areas of the body are most heavily colonized. Quantitations of the bacterium may reach 10^3-10^6/cm.^{2}. Skin shedding of the bacterium is therefore extremely common. In addition, there may be some degree of species specificity for particular sites, e.g., *S. capitis* in the scalp area and *S. auricularis* in the external ear.

Given the heavy burden of bacterium at the site where diagnostic and therapeutic procedures are initiated, infection is most often of endogenous origin. It is only natural though that cross-infection should take place given the strong opportunity for bacterium to be mobilized via hands (45). There are increasing reports of such cross-transmission among neonatal and cardiac surgical units now that molecular fingerprinting techniques have facilitated investigations (46).

A role for CoNS in nosocomial infections have been increasing over the last three decades. Perhaps this has been best exemplified by the increasing importance of CoNS in nosocomial bacteremia (47).

IV. NATURE OF THE BACTERIUM, PATHOGENESIS, AND CLINICAL MANIFESTATIONS

Staphylococci are facultative Gram positive cocci that characteristically cluster when stained from cultures and often clinical specimens. The Gram stain appearances of other catalase-positive Gram positive cocci may be variable and may differ by forming packets of tetrads or other not typically staphylococcal arrangements. Nevertheless, the latter appearances are not always clearly apparent, and therefore, confusion with staphylococci in the laboratory not uncommonly occurs at least on a preliminary basis. Catalase-positive, medically important Gram positive cocci include staphylococci, *Micrococcus* spp., *Kocuria* spp., *Alloiococcus*, and some *Stomatococcus* isolates. On a genetic basis, there is considerable distance between members of the staphylococci and *Micrococcus* spp. (and new taxonomic variants) (25). Such distance is exemplified by the C+G% contents: staphylococci ~ 35%, micrococci ~ 70%.

Staphylococci are hardy and grow on a variety of simple media that are otherwise used in diagnostic bacteriology. Some auxotrophs of *S. aureus* are recognized such as thymidine-dependent strains which grow less well (48) and which may arise as a consequence of specific antibiotic exposure, e.g., cotrimoxazole use. Although staphylococci are facultative, micrococci as a group grow much better aerobically.

Staphylococci often bear multiple plasmids, and these are often important in the context of antimicrobial resistance (49).

There are now in total well over thirty *Staphylococcus* spp. known, but only about a dozen or so are associated with human infection (12). Among the CoNS, *S. epidermidis* proper is associated with most infections and indeed isolations. The group of CoNS have often been collectively referred to as 'S. epidermidis', but 'CoNS' is preferable given the implications of some species, e.g., *S. saprophyticus* as a urinary pathogen. The former collection of micrococci has been investigated for genetic homology, and these studies have led to the definition of several new species (Figure 2). From a phylogenetic perspective, these latter species have more in common with members of the actinomycetes than staphylococci.

A. *S. aureus*

This species is characterized by the frequent production of a gold-yellow pigment by growing colonies on blood agar, although this criterion has become less reliable for identification. The bacterium produces a coagulase (of sera), a DNAase, and produces acid from mannitol.

Rather than rely on one or a few virulence factors, it appears that there are several products or structures of the bacterium which have a major or minor role in pathogenesis. A large component of bacterial cell wall weight is composed of teichoic acid and peptidoglycan; there may be some role for the latter in facilitating responses that are clinically manifest as sepsis. Over ten immunotypes of capsule have been described, although there appears to be a random distribution of these among patients (50). The bacterium possesses surface proteins which may function as adhesins and which may bind the organism to various components of tissue matrix (51). As well, the bacterium produces a number of tissue lytic enzymes which may therefore serve to allow for spread of infection.

Specific toxin-mediated illnesses occur in several forms. Up to 50% of isolates produce one or more of a variety of enterotoxins. These are relatively resistant to heat and may serve as the basis for food poisoning when they are preformed in foods. The toxins are capable of affecting gastrointestinal motility and also have central nervous systems effects, e.g., emetic. One of these toxins, termed TSST-1 and which is the same as the formerly designated enterotoxin F, is the major virulence factor for *S. aureus* isolates that are linked with toxic shock syndrome (52,53). Investigation of this syndrome and

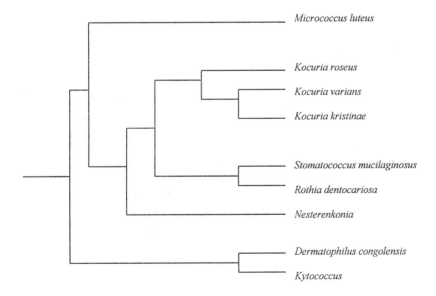

Figure 2   Phylogenetic positioning of micrococci and related species [compiled from (25)].

the associated toxin have been highly influential in stimulating research in the area of 'superantigens' (54). In contrast to the standard handling of antigens by macrophages which involves processing and presentation, superantigens like TSST-1 are capable of binding directly to MHC Class II antigens and thereafter trigger a massive release of cytokines and also induce T cell proliferation. The clinical manifestations of the latter events are those that constitute toxic shock syndrome. TSST-1 can be absorbed from a distal site and then activate these events on a systemic basis; up to 5% of all clinical *S. aureus* may be capable of producing TSST-1, but the ability to produce toxic shock is also a function of the host since pre-existing anti-TSST-1 antibody may mitigate the illness or prevent it entirely. Exfoliative toxins A and B are capable of cleaving the epidermis (55); again the bacterium may be at a focal site rather than over the entire area that is involved in the disease process. A variety of other toxins including a leucocidin are produced variably by isolates (56).

The polymorphonuclear response is critical to the containment of active infection, although it may be of little value in dealing with *S. aureus* toxins. It appears that cell wall peptidoglycan plays a key role in the recognition of the bacterium by these phagocytic cells (57). Sites of active infection draw a strong polymorphonuclear response. After these bacteria are opsonized, they are ingested by neutrophils. The bacterium has some ability to resist intracellular degradation. The presence of foreign materials in the body may serve to interfere with phagocytosis, and defects in phagocytic function, e.g., chronic granulomatous disease, may increase susceptibility to *S. aureus* infection. Almost uniformly, isolates possess protein A which is capable of binding the Fc portion of immunoglobulins such as IgG; a definitive role for protein A in pathogenesis is yet to be established.

Despite the above knowledge, there is much yet to be learned about the entire sequence of host-bacterial interactions during *S. aureus* infections (58,59).

B. CoNS

Regardless of species diversity in this group, there a number of attributes which are common (12). Most work in the area of pathogenesis has been accomplished with *S. epidermidis* since it is responsible for the majority of CoNS infections.

These bacteria often have differential expression of extracellular polysaccharides which may interfere with host defences such as opsonization or the triggering of antibody production. Although strains that are associated with infection are more likely to produce these substances, their presence does not absolutely correlate with disease-causing potential (60). Capsule-like material serves to resist phagocytosis (61). For *S. epidermidis*, there are currently several different immunotypes of capsule. Adhesion for CoNS is not as well characterized as it is for *S. aureus*, but in elementary form, it is apparent that surface proteins do foster attachment to biofilms (62). The presence of impaired host defences, breached anatomic barriers, and foreign devices (63,64) are important for initiating infection. Thus, both immunosuppression and aggressive medical and surgical therapy, which include central venous infusion and monitoring, are major host risk factors. Neonatal intensive care is also a major risk factor (65).

V. IMMUNOLOGY OF INFECTION

A. *S. aureus*

Given the frequency of permanent or temporary *S. aureus* colonization, it is not surprising that pre-existing antibody to this bacterium should be recognized in the sera of most patients. The presence of such antibody then complicates the appreciation of antibody increments during the course of infection. Most *S. aureus* infections are acute, and there will not be sufficient time in order for an antibody response to be measured during the course of active infection. Serodiagnosis will then be either of retrospective value if it were available or suited more for the diagnosis of chronic infection. For example, the measurement of teichoic acid antibodies were touted at one time to provide for such diagnosis (66,67), but this approach has largely been abandoned. Either way, the predictive values of any such serology are likely to be compromised due to the common presence of the bacterium as normal flora and due to the high likelihood that an individual will have experienced a *S. aureus* infection at some point in time.

Given the presence of protein A which binds Fc fragments, the differentiation of true versus Fc-mediated binding can be difficult when whole bacterial cells are used as the substrate. Antigenic variation among isolates also poses potential problems in regard to finding a stable and representative antigen for serological studies. Despite active infection, the immune response to varied toxins, e.g., TSST-1 and enterotoxins A, B, and C, is also variable (68).

Immunoblotting for diagnostic purposes is also complicated due to the presence of pre-existing antibody. The evolution of greater antibody quantities during the course of infection seems of limited value. Nevertheless, immunoblotting of different bacterial isolates with common sera has been of some value for the purposes of typing *S. aureus* (69). The latter has been found to be of nearly equivalent value to some PFGE methods for typing purposes.

Immunization against *S. aureus* continues to be a subject for research. Immunization does not necessarily augment the bactericidal activity of sera against this bacterium however (70). Recent studies have focused on the use of capsular polysaccharides for vaccination, and the immunogenicity has been enhanced by the development of capsule conjugates (71). The presence of several capsular types, however, will complicate even this strategy.

Alterations in the immune response to the bacterium have been proposed as possible mechanisms which allow for increased colonization of patients with atopic dermatitis who are particularly at risk for *S. aureus* infection (72).

B. CoNS

Innate immune responses to surface-exposed proteins have been studied (73). Although rises in such responses can be appreciated after acute infection, the increments are not dramatic (e.g., by immunoblotting, there is not much in the way of increased numbers of polypeptides that are recognized).

Local cellular immune responses are relatively suppressed at the site of some infections, e.g., Dacron graft (74). The presence of bacterial "slime" significantly reduces the lymphoproliferative response of mononuclear cells, and this effect is dose-related (75).

Rises in antibody status to CoNS have been used for the purpose of documenting chronic infection, e.g., shunt infection and endocarditis (76,77), but this approach is not widely used, and there continues to be concern regarding the predictive value of such an approach given the high frequency of human exposure to these bacteria on skin and mucosal sites.

VI. LABORATORY DIAGNOSIS

A. Staining

In clinical specimens, the classic staphylococcal clustering may not always be apparent or may be apparent for only a minority of the cocci. The cocci of staphylococci, when present in singles, tend to be smaller than those of streptococci in general. Morphology may be altered after antibiotic exposure; usually this effect leads to considerable variation in the size of the cocci, and some may not retain the Gram stain consistently.

The predictive value for determining the presence of staphylococci, or for that matter more strictly *S. aureus* as the likely pathogen, is dependent on the site of acquisition and the nature of the specimen. Morphology in itself does not allow for distinction of *S. aureus* from CoNS in Gram-stained smears of clinical material. When Gram positive cocci in clusters are identified in a Gram stain, the probability that *S. aureus* is present is diminished when the specimen has been acquired from skin, mouth, and mucous membranes (especially genital). The presence of the same Gram positive cocci in privileged sites such as cerebral abscess, bone, or joint is very likely to be indicative of the presence of *S. aureus*. For CoNS, the high density normally on skin also complicates the potential to implicate these bacteria in an infection when superficial samples are collected. When sterile fluids are examined and there are evidently Gram positive cocci in clusters, previous knowledge in the field should be used to alter the probability that either *S. aureus* or CoNS are being dealt with, e.g., Gram stain as such from a central nervous system shunt fluid is more likely to imply presence of CoNS, whereas a Gram stain with the same from cerebrospinal fluid of a patient with post-traumatic meningitis is more likely to be indicative of *S. aureus*.

True invasive infections with other catalase-positive Gram positive cocci are rare, and it is unlikely that they will be considered on the basis of a Gram stain of clinical material since *S. aureus* and CoNS are much more common pathogens.

B. Culture

Staphylococci, micrococci, and other catalase-positive Gram positive cocci are relatively hardy and do not require special transport mechanisms or storage conditions. Bacterial survival is adequate in commonly-used transport kits regardless of whether charcoal is added to the basal medium.

Bacterial growth generally takes place within 24 hrs. but may be delayed or prevented altogether when antibiotics have been used. Uncommon isolates of *S. aureus* may be delayed in growth when there are nutritional deficits, e.g., thymidine dependency. The growth of some CoNS may also be delayed. The presence of CoNS in delayed growth from enrichment in the absence of antibiotic use should raise the possibility of contamination. For example, a positive blood culture after 24 hrs. which yields CoNS is most likely a function of contamination at the time of collection. The latter probability is in large part owing to the fact that the bacterium is being enriched. Samples from skin, blood, and urine are especially prone to contamination with CoNS.

S. aureus can be selected with a variety of commonly-used media for this purpose, and these include mannitol-salt agar, colistin-nalidixic acid agar, and media with phenylethyl alcohol. The isolation of *S. aureus* from food is often achieved with the use of other media (78). Selective media for *S. aureus* are not often used when routine clinical samples are analyzed, since the bacterium is not difficult to find in most circumstances of pure or mixed infection. When culture for *S. aureus* only is desirable, e.g., nasal screening for carriage or screening for MRSA, mannitol-salt agar is most often used, and the addition of oxacillin (4 mg./L.) provides a good medium for MRSA selection (79). Growth on mannitol-salt agar may be delayed, and media should be held for several days. CoNS occasionally also appear on mannitol-salt agar, and mannitol-positive (colour indicator-changed) colonies other than *S. aureus* may be present. Staphylococci also grow on MacConkey's medium when the crystal violet is deleted. The use of selective enrichment is not necessary in most circumstances, but in theory has some advantage when MRSA are being sought thoroughly or when antibiotics have been given.

As previously indicated, the finding of CoNS is not uncommonly associated with specimen contamination. For blood cultures, timing may be suggestive of a greater likelihood for contamination but so too may the frequency of positive cultures. For example, the positivity in one of two blood culture bottles from a set or from bottles sporadically from several sets is suggestive of contamination. Growth only from enrichment of other specimens is also likely to be indicative of contamination from almost every site. Sterile fluids can often be contaminated when the acquisition is percutaneous regardless of whether the procedure has occurred during a sterile surgery. The finding of few colonies on primary media is also more likely to be associated with contamination. In the latter context, it is critical to ensure that the few colonies which are observed are obtained from the region of the medium that is directly inoculated. The presence of two or more colonial variants, and hence isolates, of CoNS from an otherwise sterile site, e.g., blood, is also highly suggestive of contamination, albeit not absolute.

C. Identification

1. S. aureus

Colonial size, morphology, and pigmentation are all soon recognized for this bacterium given its frequency among clinical specimens. Some isolates may appear non-pigmented and more like CoNS. On sheep blood agar, a narrow band of beta-hemolysis is often apparent especially when the colonies are well developed or after the growth has been held for several days. Non-hemolytic variants do, however, occur and again, confusion may be had with CoNS on a preliminary basis. Traditionally, identification has been based on the presence of coagulase, DNAase, and mannitol fermentation; variations in each of these is possible, and therefore, it is prudent to use a combination of them if not all three for definitive identification.

Coagulase activity is best demonstrated with EDTA-treated rabbit plasma in a test tube. This assessment determines the presence of 'cell-free' coagulase. Inoculation of a tube with rabbit plasma usually results in full or partial clot formation within 4-6 hrs. Some isolates manifest coagulase activity by delayed clotting up to 18-24 hrs. later, but care must be taken to observe the tube on the same day of inoculation since some clots may lyse overnight due to proteases, and hence be perceived as a false-negative reaction on the next day. The presence of cell-free coagulase remains the standard for determining coagulase status. The presence of 'cell-bound' coagulase correlates very well with the former but not in an absolute sense. Cell-bound coagulase, also termed clumping factor, is determined usually by slide agglutination whereby plasma and bacterium are admixed on a glass slide, and microbial agglutination is determined visually. A control for autoagglutination should be had. Determination of clumping factor is used by many laboratories for convenience especially when high volumes of specimens are handled, and since the results of slide agglutination may be available in minutes in contrast to the tube coagulase which may require many hours. Presence of clumping factor should be viewed as a screening test, however, since false-negative assessments have long been recognized. In addition, a few CoNS [e.g., *S. lugdunensis* and *S. schleiferi* (80)] may agglutinate under these conditions. A number of commercial assays for slide agglutination have become available, and these perform equal or slightly better than the traditional slide agglutination (81-83). Variations of the latter have also included antibodies for protein A such that bacterial agglutination is a function of both cell-bound coagulase and protein A presence. It is clear that the rapid slide agglutination assays do not work well for isolates directly in blood cultures (83). Coagulase-negative *S. aureus* do occur, but they are exceedingly rare (84). Other coagulase-positive staphylococci include *S. intermedius*, *S. hyicus*, and rare isolates of *S. schleiferi*; all of these are very uncommon human isolates, and the first two especially are mainly animal pathogens.

With so few tests required to identify *S. aureus* in the vast majority of circumstances, complex commercial identification schemes are often not needed on a practical basis. Nevertheless, these other identification methods do perform well in defining *S. aureus*. Heat-stable DNAase has been touted as a method to presumptively identify *S. aureus* from blood cultures when Gram positive cocci which resemble staphylococci are identified (85,86), although DNAase-negative *S. aureus* have been found albeit uncommonly. Direct genetic probes to confirm *S. aureus* speciation have also been commercialized [Accuprobe™ (87) and Evigene™ (88)] and the application of this technology to centrifugates of positive blood cultures has met with some success. The use of the latter must be tempered by the pre-test probability of finding CoNS versus *S. aureus*. For example, if most positive blood cultures with Gram positive cocci in clusters prove to be CoNS, it may be more appropriate to apply the technology selectively. Cost considerations are usually also a factor in determining whether the latter assay should be incorporated. On a referral or tertiary basis, there are a number of molecular methods which could ultimately be used to confirm the species, but it is very uncommon for these to be required.

The diagnosis of *S. aureus* food poisoning should initially depend on identifying an epidemiologically-compatible circumstance (17). The nature of the illness and a consistent incubation period are often all that are needed to highly suspect such food poisoning. The finding of the bacterium in high quantities through quantitative culture of the implicated food is also supportive (18). Vomitus may also be cultured, but stool cultures are not often of value. Several methods are also available to assess whether a given isolate is capable of producing an enterotoxin, but it must be recognized that many isolates of S. aureus are capable of producing one or more enterotoxins regardless of source of isolation. Enterotoxin determinations on the food isolates are therefore not commonly of value. Circulating enterotoxins are not identified systemically. Assays for enterotoxins in implicated foods are hampered by the complexity of available methods but seem appealing as adjuncts (89)

TSST-1 determination [reference laboratory (90) or now via commercial kit, e.g., Oxoid (91)] may be of some value, but again, the opportunities for using this assay are limited. Toxic shock syndrome is defined by a set of predominantly clinical criteria, and the presence of a scenario for S. aureus infection or local overgrowth may suffice to impart a high probability for the diagnosis. For example, in the absence of tampon-associated toxic shock, it would not be uncommon to find toxic shock syndrome in the presence of a post-surgical S. aureus wound infection. The determination of TSST-1 producing capability in the latter circumstance would not be of much value. Like for enterotoxins otherwise, but to a lesser degree, TSST-1 may be found in a small percentage of isolates, and thus TSST-1 genotype does not absolutely prove that a multi-system illness with some similarity to toxic shock syndrome has been necessarily diagnosed. TSST-1 is not identified systemically, and presumably little actual toxin is necessary to effect superantigen activity.

On a generic basis, it does not appear that the determination of enterotoxin status has prognostic significance in most clinical diseases (92).

2. CoNS

For fresh cultures of CoNS, there is often little in the way of appreciable difference between colony morphology among isolates, although subtle differences may become apparent after prolonged culture (12). Mixed cultures are not uncommon and are more likely to be found when skin contamination has occurred. It is nevertheless worth pursuing whether mixed cultures are present from sterile sites since their presence will support in large part the likelihood that contamination was had and that the microbial growth is not likely relevant. Growth rates among clinically-relevant CoNS are often not sufficiently variable. Hemolysis is uncommon but possible among some isolates.

Despite the large number of staphylococci that have been defined, there are fourteen human pathogens of note and they include:

S. auricularis	S. capitis	S. caprae
S. cohnii	S. epidermidis	S. haemolyticus
S. hominis	S. lugdunensis	S. saccharolyticus
S. saprophyticus	S. schleiferi	S. simulans
S. warneri	S. xylosus	

S. cohnii, S. capitis, and S. schleiferi have been divided into two subspecies each (12). Only a handful of these are regularly isolated from clinical specimens, and S. epidermidis is by far the most common clinical isolate in most settings. The use of the term 'S. epidermidis' to denote all members of this group should be abandoned in favour of using the more correct 'CoNS' when presumptive identification is based on few assessments including the coagulase test. The need to speciate CoNS when they are obtained from clinical samples is somewhat debatable, but it is clear that such speciation has little to offer in most clinical settings. First, many isolations reflect contamination so that extra work is not warranted given that the clinician is unlikely to act on the positive information. Even when a CoNS is isolated from a sterile site and is believed to be responsible for infection, the designation of CoNS already carries with it enough implications with respect to source, clinical course, complicating features, and therapy such that definitive speciation carries little or no consequence. If CoNS are obtained from special sites, e.g., blood, prosthetic joint, or CSF shunt, the isolates may be preserved for future use and speciation if it is warranted. For example, there may be some merit in speciating two isolates obtained many weeks or months apart if issues relating to recurrent infection arise. For blood cultures, most positive isolations of CoNS are dealt without knowledge of speciation; speciation may play a limited role in identifying whether isolates in a serious situation, e.g., suspect endocarditis, are similar. Despite the latter potential for speciation, it must be re-emphasized that the vast majority of such isolates prove to be speciated as *S. epidermidis*, and thus, even when repeat isolation occurs, it is likely that the *S. epidermidis* species will again be identified. There is also the potential for speciation to be of some value when the epidemiology of an outbreak requires investigation; again, maintenance of key isolates is likely to be of value.

Commercial systems for the species identification of CoNS are available, and numerous of these perform reasonably well; up to 60-90% of isolates may be reliably speciated especially including *S. epidermidis*, *S. saprophyticus*, and *S. haemolyticus*. Representative systems include API Staph, Vitek GPI Card, MicroScan Pos ID set, StaphZym, and RapiDEC Staph (93-97). In addition to speciation, these systems also provide biotype numbers which in themselves may assist epidemiological investigations even though not all may be speciated per se (98). Data regarding performance should be reviewed when less common CoNS are of concern, and supplemental tests may be of assistance (99). Tests that may be of value for CoNS speciation include: coagulase (cell-free and clumping factor), DNAase, alkaline phosphatase, arylamidase activity for pyrrolidonyl and arginine bases, urease, acetoin production, nitrate reduction, esculin hydrolysis, novobiocin resistance, ornithine decarboxylation, and acid production from varied sugars (12). The presumptive identification of *S. saprophyticus* is the best known exception to the need for speciation. This bacterium is a recognized cause of urinary tract infection in particular contexts. Presumptive identification is usually achieved on a practical basis solely with the recognition that the isolate is a CoNS and that it is resistant to the antibiotic novobiocin. The latter can be achieved easily in broth, agar dilution, or by the modified Kirby-Bauer method. A high quantity and relatively pure growth of novobiocin-resistant CoNS in the context of a symptomatic urinary tract infection gives a reasonable probability that *S. saprophyticus* has been isolated. It must be recognized that this approach is presumptive and that several pitfalls must be considered. Firstly, other CoNS may be novobiocin resistant (e.g., some *S. hominis*, *S. cohnii*, and *S. xylosus*). Secondly, significant quantities of *S. saprophyticus* from a symptomatic urinary tract infection may be less than 100×10^6/L., and a meagre amount of information is provided on most laboratory requisitions to know whether the patient is symptomatic and to what extent. Thirdly, *S. saprophyticus* is not the only CoNS that can be a urinary tract pathogen; the presumptive identification is but added information that significantly increases the probability that it is pathogenic in a given circumstance. Such presumptive identification should only be applied to urine isolates since it is likely that other novobiocin-resistant species are more often found in samples of blood or other sites; for the uncommon situations where speciation is needed, a more definitive approach should be considered.

It is likely that genotypic methods for CoNS speciation will emerge (100).

3. *Micrococci and other catalase-positive Gram positive cocci*

On a preliminary basis, the differentiation of micrococci from staphylococci may poses some difficulty, but reference methods are detailed (101). Micrococci are often positive for oxidase when the tetramethyl- reagent is used (102). When inoculated into a broth medium, they grow best at the top of the tube in contrast to staphylococci which grow throughout the liquid medium. On a generic basis, staphylococci are susceptible to the lytic effects of lysostaphin, whereas micrococci are resistant (103,104). Some micrococci may be deeply pigmented, e.g., pink or yellow. Staphylococci and micrococci are tolerant to salt (6.5%), but *Stomatococcus* isolates are not. Stomatococci form a 'gummy' colony that is adherent to the solid medium surface.

Alloiococcus otitidis is aerobic, oxidase-negative, salt-tolerant, and may be alpha-hemolytic on blood agar (30).

D. Epidemiological typing

1. S. aureus

Interest in the epidemiology of *S. aureus* infections has long been maintained due to epidemic spread of this bacterium in surgical and dermatology wards as well as epidemic spread among newborns in nurseries. The need to control antibiotic-resistant *S. aureus*, especially MRSA, has also given impetus to the development of new typing methods. On a preliminary basis, colony morphology and culture characteristics are not commonly of value here. A distinctive antibiogram may be of assistance, but most *S. aureus* that are isolated from putative epidemics have historically been relatively antibiotic susceptible. Phage typing became available decades ago and for those isolates that were typeable, this approach was of considerable utility for many years. Unfortunately, the method is time-consuming and does not lend itself to application beyond a few reference centres. It was not surprising that investigators would choose to trial other techniques, especially molecular, when they became available. Plasmid profiling was of some help given the likelihood that isolates would possess multiple plasmids, but the value of this approach was furthered when enzyme digests of plasmids were then assessed. Despite the presence of multiple plasmids, there may be a limited number of restriction digest bands for identity so that the potential for differentiation is low; some isolates may have plasmids that are unstable in vitro.

Within the last 10-15 years, the availability of new technology in general provided ample opportunity for new molecular methods to be developed. These latter have included: analysis of whole cell protein profiles (after standard electrophoresis by SDS-PAGE), multilocus enzyme electrophoresis (MLEE), immunoblotting of protein profiles, ribotyping (conventional and PCR based), pulsed field gel electrophoresis (PFGE; or variations thereof), PCR typing (e.g., randomly amplified for polymorphic DNA, e.g., coagulase gene typing) (105-110), and more recently multilocus sequence typing (111) (see Chapter 7). Numerous variations have since been published for several of these methods. Some of them are sufficiently discriminative of strains, but there is considerable variation in the perceived suitability to apply them on a practical basis. For example, immunoblotting of protein profiles compares very well with PFGE which, when optimized, may serve as a standard for comparison for all other techniques. Yet, the former is complicated by the need for standard sera and is laborious. PFGE may also be considered laborious, but it can be standardized. PCR techniques offer a simple and rapid alternative, but may not be as discriminatory as PFGE. PFGE has been studied in large multi-national settings; interlaboratory variations are evident despite standardized protocols, although the general concordance is good (112). Some have chosen to combine several methods, and this is best seen with the combination of PCR techniques which utilize different primer sets. In all of these assessments, one must bear the specific need in mind. At a local level, a rapid and less discriminatory method may suffice, and reference strains per se may not be required if the comparisons are simply internal. On the other hand, the designations of fixed 'types' in larger collections or reference centres may require comparison to reference strains. Fingerprinting patterns can now be analyzed by automated and computerized methods which will further reduce variability (111). The application of typing methods for *S. aureus* will continue to have use for the foreseeable future, and molecular technologies have ensured that these methods will be widely available.

2. CoNS

The evolution of typing methods for CoNS has essentially followed those for *S. aureus* (12). Conceivably, the available techniques will allow for 'typeability' of any staphylococcal species. Most methods have been applied to *S. epidermidis* since it is the most common clinical isolate. In general, RAPD and PCR ribotyping are not as discriminatory as PFGE (113). MLEE, plasmid analysis, and protein profiles (with or without immunoblotting) are not favoured for various reasons. Figure 3 illustrates an example of *S. epidermidis* typing by ERIC-PCR.

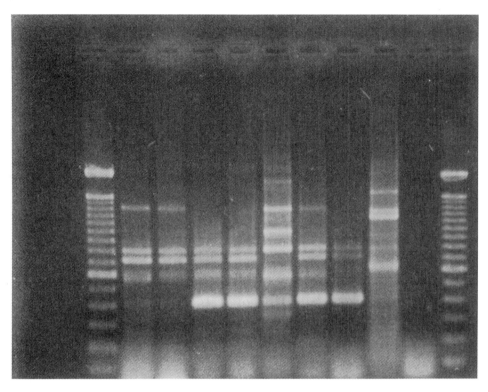

Figure 3 Application of ERIC PCR to provide discrimination among isolates of *S. epidermidis* that were isolated from the blood cultures of newborns in neonatal intensive care. Concerns were expressed that a common strain may have been circulating. The Figure shows at least three different types among 7 isolates. The left-most lane is the molecular marker.

Whereas antibiograms are relatively predictable for most *S. aureus* isolates, there is considerably more variation among antibiograms for CoNS. Given the latter and given also that *S. epidermidis* may have various biotypes (e.g., as assessed by conventional biochemical tests for CoNS speciation or as assessed by differences in numerical codes for commercial systems), a time-honoured method for typing has included the combination of biotyping and antibiogram (114).

Although there may be some obvious differences among some isolates, this approach has been limited by the frequent shift in susceptibility when critical concentrations for testing are used. The latter may result in run-to-run variation. Overall, this simple method for strain discrimination may be of value when the differences are obvious and multiple, but it is better to resort to a molecular method for the few circumstances when such information is needed.

VII. SUSCEPTIBILITY TESTING

A. S. aureus

Given the hardy growth of this bacterium in vitro, susceptibility testing can be performed by a wide array of standardized methods including modified Kirby-Bauer, critical agar dilution, broth dilution, and

E test (115,116). The method chosen will be influenced by existing automation for identification, cost, volume of isolates to be assessed, among other things.

1.   Beta-lactamase

The presence of beta-lactamase among staphylococci and *S. aureus* in particular was evident among isolates even before penicillin became widely used, but the frequency of apparent beta-lactamase positivity was low. By the late 1950s, the frequency of beta-lactamase positive strains markedly increased after penicillin became widely used (117). As a consequence, beta-lactamase resistant synthetic analogues such as methicillin, oxacillin, cloxacillin, and nafcillin were created and rapidly became the primary anti-staphylococcal agents. By the early 1960s, however, MRSA had already emerged. Beta-lactamase positive *S. aureus* comprise up to 80-95% of isolates depending on whether these are from inpatient or out-patient sources, and depending on region. *S. aureus* beta-lactamase is a serine protease which is inducible by exposure to beta-lactam antibiotics and which is produced by expression of plasmid-borne genes. There are some structural variations in these enzymes, and a few have been determined by chromosomal genes rather than those on plasmids. This enzymatic activity is largely extracellular and can be detected by acidometric, iodometric, and chromogenic cephalosporin assays; the activity is best detected after prior stimulation for enzyme induction by passage on media with low subinhibitory concentrations of penicillin. Some chromogenic cephalosporin paper methods may not be as sensitive as other approaches, and the applicability of the former for the purposes of detecting *S. aureus* beta-lactamase should be confirmed (118). Beta-lactamase negative and penicillin-sensitive *S. aureus* infections respond well when penicillin is used for treatment.

2.   MRSA

S. aureus with intrinsic resistance to beta-lactamase resistant semi-synthetic penicillins are termed MRSA. These will also have nearly the same likelihood of producing beta-lactamase as non-MRSA. The major mechanism of resistance for MRSA is the production of an altered penicillin-binding protein (PBP2a) which has reduced affinity for the beta-lactam and hence resistance to antibiotic inhibition at the active site (119). The *mecA* gene is responsible for PBP2a production, but other genes may be involved in modulating expression. Indeed, whereas the vast majority of obvious MRSA possess *mecA* and express its product, there are nevertheless some *S. aureus* which appear phenotypically as MRSA but do not have the *mecA* gene.

Resistance in these regards is defined as a minimum inhibitory concentration (MIC) to oxacillin >4 mg./L. (115). Resistance is heterogeneously expressed, and a variable proportion of cells among the population of a particular isolate appear resistant. The degree of such expression varies considerably among different MRSA; some show high level resistance among nearly all colonies from subculture, whereas others may have only a small fraction that are apparently resistant. Although many MRSA are very easy to identify by conventional susceptibility testing methods, some isolates with marked heterogeneous populations and low level resistance may be difficult to identify. Factors which enhance the expression of the resistance phenotype include the addition of sodium chloride (2-4%) to the solid susceptibility testing medium, reduced temperature for incubation (30°C rather than 35-37°C), prolonged incubation (minimum 24 hrs.), and increased inoculum. The difficulties with ensuring that the MRSA phenotype is detected have led to the need for a tandem approach for laboratory investigation whereby a screening method for such resistance is initially used, and confirmatory testing then follows. Some MRSA may grow slower than other *S. aureus*, and occasionally, the colony phenotype may not be typical for *S. aureus*, i.e., indistinguishable from CoNS. It is critical, before considering the following discussion, that an isolate be deemed pure and not mixed.

When using disc diffusion, an oxacillin (1 um.) disc is employed and a standard zone of inhibition is applied (116). In order to maximize resistance determination, the disc diffusion assay should be observed after a full 24 hrs. of incubation. Apparent resistance by this method should be followed by an MIC determination especially if this is the first occasion that MRSA has been identified for a given patient; a resistant isolate from a known positive patient, especially when there are other clear markers of multiple antibiotic resistance that identifies a strain with high likelihood, may receive less attention. Some have shown that more prolonged incubation, up to 48-72 hrs., may help in identifying even more MRSA, but the gain from this extended approach appears to be marginal.

Critical agar dilution screening includes 6 mg./L. oxacillin in Mueller-Hinton medium and spot inocula of approximately 5×10^5 bacteria (115). The medium has 4%-added NaCl, and it should be incubated for a full 24 hrs. Isolates which clearly grow or manifest a haze of growth should be further screened for oxacillin MIC. Some have historically used a slightly greater inoculum or a critical concentration of 4 mg./L., but both of these approaches add to the numbers which then require confirmation, and the incremental gain is again meagre. The lower critical concentration will allow 'hyper-beta-lactamase' producing isolates to appear resistant.

A broth microdilution assay for these same purposes also uses added salt (148) and incubation for up to 24 hrs. (115). Such an assay in the microtitre fashion has enjoyed use for over two decades, and automated methods generally take the same approach but in a miniaturized format. Initial productions of these microformats and automated methods were reknowned for missing low level MRSA, but years of experience and modification have improved these assays. Furthermore, the choice of a breakpoint for MRSA, whether based on oxacillin or methicillin as the testing antibiotic, underwent some change in the 1970s and 1980s, and this flux in itself provided some confusion as to how MRSA should be best appreciated.

Confirmation of resistance generally is accomplished by either broth microdilution or E-test (120). The use of the latter method for routine screening of MRSA is complicated by the cost of the test strips and the fact that a single antibiotic is being tested at one time. Nevertheless, the E-test is an excellent method for confirming MRSA. Those isolates with MICs >8 mg./L. are undisputed as MRSA on most occasions. Those with MICs in the 4-8 mg./L. range, however, may provide some challenge. Isolates with the latter somewhat indeterminate MICs have been variously labeled, but the term 'BORSA' (borderline oxacillin-resistant *S. aureus*) has been popularized in the last decade. Although this term may well designate a group of bacteria with intermediate-resistance phenotype, it is apparent that the group is heterogeneous and that perhaps this term is being applied too broadly to a cluster of bacteria that have different mechanisms of resistance despite having the initial resistance phenotype in common (121).

Isolates with intermediate resistance should initially be assessed as candidates for hyper-beta-lactamase production (122). These bacteria have a full induction of beta-lactamase activity, perhaps as a consequence of in vivo antibiotic exposure. The MIC may decrease after in vitro passage, and indeed initially resistant bacteria may not be confirmed as such when the screen, e.g., critical agar dilution plate, is repeated; the MIC may be in the 2-6 mg./L. range. The differentiation of hyper-beta-lactamase or intrinsic resistant bases for intermediate MICs has often depended on the ability to demonstrate that beta-lactam resistance in this context can be nullified by the presence of a beta-lactam inhibitor, e.g., clavulanic acid or sulbactam (122,123). For example, intermediate-resistant isolates can be assessed for susceptibility to amoxycillin/clavulanic acid. Those which are susceptible (disc diffusion zone >20 mm. for 20ug./10 ug. discs) would be deemed hyper-beta-lactamase producers while amoxycillin/clavulanate resistant isolates would be assumed to have an intrinsic mechanism for intermediate resistance which is identical to or somewhat analogous to that of typical MRSA. This latter approach seems convenient for practical purposes, but there are limitations. For example, some isolates do indeed produce beta-lactamase, but the zone of inhibition to amoxycillin/clavulanic acid is intermediate. Other isolates, although not common, may actually be beta-lactamase negative and appear to be amoxycillin/clavulanic acid susceptible (124); there may truly be an intrinsic resistance mechanism for the latter, but due to the lack of beta-lactamase and due to the high concentration of amoxycillin in the diffusion disc, they appear phenotypically (sensitive) as putative hyper-beta-lactamase producers when the assessment includes only oxacillin MIC determination and amoxycillin/clavulanic acid testing. The beta-lactamase test should thus be performed in this context.

Given that the *mecA* gene is largely associated with typical MRSA (i.e., high level resistance), it has been proposed that determination of the gene may serve as a reliable confirmatory assay for MRSA (119). *MecA* presence can be determined by direct probing but is often now determined by a genetic amplification method. Commercial products for these purposes have already been produced [e.g., Evigene™ (88)]. In addition to genetic detection of *mecA*, immunological detection of PBP2a by agglutination methods on live bacterium from culture has also been developed and indeed also commercialized (125,126). Care should be exercised in applying the latter agglutination methods since some will also react with *mecA*-positive CoNS; thus, speciation should be ensured in order to not falsely identify a resistant CoNS as a MRSA (126). Some have assumed that the presence or absence of *mecA*, all-or-none, correlates with the absolute definition of MRSA; this belief is probably correct, but it must be tempered with the following considerations. High level MRSA (>16 mg./L.) invariably have *mecA*, but the determination of *mecA* presence in this context is of little added value once the resistance phenotype (i.e., MIC) is determined. For *S. aureus* with intermediate MICs, the demonstration of *mecA* presence may be helpful to confirm the intrinsic resistance that is perceived after the isolate's oxacillin MIC and amoxycillin/clavulanic acid testing are consistent with the latter. Unfortunately, there is a sizeable proportion of these that will be *mecA* negative and yet have seemingly an intrinsic mechanism of resistance; failure to demonstrate *mecA* does not rule out the possibility of intrinsic resistance. Obviously one must also ensure that methodological issues do not falsely lead to a conclusion about *mecA* status.

Other antibiotic resistances should also be considered as markers for MRSA. During the early evolution of MRSA, isolates not uncommonly expressed beta-lactam resistance only. These isolates often maintained susceptibility to other good antistaphylococcal agents such as erythromycin, clindamycin, cotrimoxazole, chloramphenicol, and aminoglycosides. As these alternate antibiotics were used, however, MRSA strains began to acquire mechanisms of resistance to match the selective pressure. Currently, many MRSA, especially those that have been circulating in epidemic form, have many associated resistances, and their presence should raise concern that a MRSA is at hand. The number of accompanying resistances among MRSA is often highly influenced geographically and will range from none to almost all non-vancomycin antistaphylococcal agents. Thus, while multi-resistance may be a marker for MRSA, its absence does not rule MRSA out. In addition, it is generally accepted that MRSA are cross-resistant to other beta-lactam agents regardless of in vitro susceptibility; isolates of MRSA should thus be reported as having resistance to other beta-lactam agents.

Treatment options for MRSA are dependent on the spectrum of other resistances, but vancomycin is most often touted for serious infections. Vancomycin is effective for treatment, but it must be remembered that treatment failures can occur due to various clinical factors which do not relate to the actual in vivo susceptibility. Vancomycin-intermediate susceptible *S. aureus* (VISA) have become recent concerns (10,38). The MICs have ranged from 4 to 16 mg./L. These strains have typically emerged in areas where MRSA are highly endemic and where vancomycin use is therefore considerable. As with almost any other drug-'bug' combination, resistance will tend to emerge if there is sufficient selective pressure from frequent antibiotic use. In addition to vancomycin alone, some have assessed the addition of rifampin and other antibiotics for complicated circumstances, but the net synergistic effects are clinically dubious. Teichoplanin is a glycopeptide antibiotic like vancomycin and is effective in MRSA infections. Topical antibiotics such as bacitracin and mupirocin often prove of value even when the MRSA is multi-resistant. Fusidic acid and chloramphenicol also may serve as alternate therapies and should be tested.

3. Tolerance

'Tolerance' to anti-staphylococcal beta-lactam agents is defined by a wide variation between antibacterial killing (minimum bactericidal titre; MBC) and inhibitory (MIC) effects (127). One such definition uses a minimum difference in titre of 32X. Thus, bacteria which are deemed to show tolerance to cloxacillin are inhibited by conventional concentrations of antibiotic that would classify the isolate as being susceptible, but there is an apparent great difference between the concentration that is required to lyse the bacterium and that which simply prevents its growth. The latter phenomenon would be analogous to the differences between MIC and MBC that are seen for antibiotics that are referred to as 'static', e.g., macrolides, e.g., co-trimoxazole.

The relevance of tolerance is still a subject for debate. While some differences can be shown in vitro and in animal models between tolerant and non-tolerant bacteria (128,129), these effects are not always reproducible, and proof for clinical impact of tolerance has been difficult to find. On a practical basis, the search for tolerance cannot be recommended routinely even in serious infections. It is questionable whether the phenomenon is simply an in vitro artifact (130).

4. Non-beta-lactam antibiotics

There are few circumstances where combination antibiotics are used for treating *S. aureus* infections. For cloxacillin- (i.e., methicillin, nafcillin, and oxacillin) susceptible strains, some choose to add an aminoglycoside for the early part of treating serious infections, e.g., endocarditis. In vitro data support a synergistic effect of aminoglycoside and beta-lactam, and there may be some clinical benefit in reducing bacterial load quickly in early disease. Nonetheless, the vast majority of infections will respond satisfactorily to single agents whether orally or intravenously administered.

For most *S. aureus* that are acquired in the general community, susceptibility to a large number of alternate agents persists – these may include aminoglycosides, chloramphenicol, fluoroquinolones, co-trimoxazole, fusidic acid, erythomycin, clindamycin, rifampin, bacitracin, mupirocin, and tetracyclines. The resistance rate to these agents may range from < 2% for fusidic acid to 5% for cotrimoxazole. Fluoroquinolone resistance has increased among *S. aureus* (MRSA or not) due to the increased use of this drug class for *S. aureus* infections and due to the considerable general use in the community. Tetracycline resistance became very common when this agent and its analogues were commonly used in the 1960s and 1970s for various purposes; such resistance was temporarily associated with a putative staphylococcal enterocolitis (i.e., antibiotic-associated overgrowth of *S. aureus* and suppression of enteric flora). Mechanisms for resistance to these non-beta-lactam agents have been studied (Table 1). Erythromycin and clindamycin resistances are often linked.

The use of topical agents like mupirocin and bacitracin for the eradication of nasal MRSA carriage has been associated with the emergence of resistance to these (131); their use for such purposes must be closely restrained and monitored.

The development of multi-resistant MRSA and the threat of pending vancomycin resistance has driven industry and the medical community to seek new antistaphylococcal antibiotics. One such novelty, quinupristin/dalfopristin, has become available and has been already used in the context of MRSA and vancomycin-resistant enterococcal infections (132). Linezolid has also recently been approved for such use (149).

Overall, the genetic ability to acquire and transfer resistance genes within and between species is evident (133).

B. CoNS

Despite the many differences between *S. aureus* and CoNS, what have emerged as major commonalities between these two groups are the similarities among their resistance mechanisms. For example, both have intrinsic resistance potential which is mainly *mecA* dependent. Sequencing of *mecA* genes from these two groups shows considerable homology (134). *MecA* has been found among several CoNS species (135).

Penicillin resistance is also common for CoNS, and they may produce beta-lactamase. In contrast to *S. aureus*, oxacillin resistance among CoNS is very common, and up to 60-80% of nosocomial isolates may have this phenotype. The methods which are recommended for susceptibility testing of CoNS are similar to those that are recommended for *S. aureus* including conditions which drive the expression of heterogeneous resistance (115,116).

Table 1 Major mechanisms of resistance among *S. aureus* isolates for non-beta-lactam antibiotics. 'Frequency' reflects a general estimate for community-acquired isolates.

Antibiotic	Mechanism	Frequency	Characteristics
aminoglycosides	modifying enzymes	1-5%	especially acetyltransferases and phosphotransferases; especially plasmid-borne
erythromycin	*ermC, ermA* (erythromycin resistance methylase)	2-10%	inducible or constitutive; often plasmid-borne
clindamycin	*ermC* (as above)	1-5%	cross-resistance with erythromycin due to MLS$_B$ phenotype
trimethoprim	altered dihydrofolate reductase	1-5%	transposon-mediated; plasmid or chromosomal
chloramphenicol	acetyl transferases (CATs)	1-5%	>5 variants of inactivating enzymes; plasmid-borne
fusidic acid	elongation factor G alteration	< 2%	also altered permeability
quinolones	alteration of DNA gyrase (*gyrA*)	< 2%	also possible enhanced efflux
mupirocin	isoleucyl-tRNA synthetase modification	< 2%	can confer very high level resistance; plasmid-borne

It has been recognized that CoNS infections may not respond as well as might be anticipated to beta-lactam antibiotics, including the synthetic antistaphylococcal agents such as cloxacillin and analogues, on the basis of susceptibility testing when conventional methods (i.e., those used for *S. aureus*) are used. In these circumstances, the particular problem appeared to be persistent infection despite cloxacillin susceptibility and the use of this antibiotic. Such failure could in many circumstances be associated with various factors that typically complicate CoNS infections (e.g., persistence of central venous lines or prosthetic devices which would protect CoNS in their milieu), but nevertheless many clinicians had reservations about treating CoNS infections with beta-lactams; vancomycin was used as the agent of choice for most. It is now apparent that such concern was indeed valid and that conventional testing for oxacillin resistance among CoNS significantly underestimated the frequency of true resistance even when salt is added to solid testing media and despite incubation for up to 24 hrs. (136). More extensive assessment may facilitate the finding of up to 25% more resistant strains than determined by routine testing, e.g., critical agar dilution. The E-test facilitates the recognition of heteroresistance (136). Whereas the majority of organism on the agar medium appears to yield an MIC, small colonies within the apparent susceptible zone emerge. These should be subcultured and then retested; a resistant MIC will then be found which truly reflects the underlying resistance potential. This method can make a major contribution to the understanding of CoNS, since the opportunity to encounter a difference between conventional testing and true resistance is more common. This approach nevertheless is also applicable to *S. aureus*, and overall, it simply represents a method to enhance the finding of heteroresistant populations which have resistance expressed among a small fraction of the organism. In addition to using the E-test for these purposes, it is also possible to examine for *mecA* by PCR or by direct hybridization (88,137). Oxacillin-resistant, *mecA*-negative isolates have, however, been determined (135). Like *S. aureus*, the finding of other antibiotic resistance increases the probability that oxacillin resistance is present (138). Oxacillin-resistant CoNS should be considered resistant to other beta-lactam agents. Automated methods are as susceptible to errors in detecting oxacillin resistance as are standard methods (139).

Another approach has been recommended recently to overcome the problem with underestimating CoNS oxacillin resistance: the critical oxacillin concentration breakpoint has been reduced to 0.5 mg./L. (140,141) This change certainly enhances the sensitivity for finding oxacillin-resistant strains, but it is not clear that universal application of this criterion to all CoNS is correct (142). Furthermore, the break-point may prove applicable to ensuring safety of cloxacillin use for CoNS infections at invasive sites, but it may not be as applicable to urinary tract isolates, i.e., the criterion may excessively lead to the designation of resistance. It may very well prove that the application of this new breakpoint will undergo some further alterations which may be site- or species- specific.

Other antibiotic resistance is also more common among CoNS than *S. aureus*. Resistance to mac-rolides and lincosamides is among the more common of these, and the linkage of the latter resistances bears similarity to that of *S. aureus* (144). Vancomycin intermediate-resistant *S. haemolyticus* have been previously found, and perhaps these are the critical antecedents of VISA (143). Teichoplanin resistance among CoNS has also been reported.

C. Other

Micrococcus spp. and *Kocuria* spp. are usually very penicillin susceptible (140,145). For practical pur-poses, these can be assessed for susceptibility with the same general methods and criteria that are used for Gram positive cocci otherwise. Due to the rarity of serious infections, relevant and scientifically valid in vivo/in vitro correlations may require many years to accumulate. In the interim, it is apparent that such serious infections have responded to beta-lactam therapy.

Stomatococcus infections are also susceptible to beta-lactam agents (140,145), but relatively peni-cillin-resistant stomatococci have been described (146).

REFERENCES

1. Sheagren JN. *Staphylococcus aureus*: the persistent pathogen (part I). N Engl J Med 1984; 310:1368-1373.
2. Sheagren JN. *Staphylococcus aureus*: the persistent pathogen (part II). N Engl J Med 1984; 310:1437-1442.
3. Lowy FD. *Staphylococcus aureus* infections. N Engl J Med 1998; 339:520-532.
4. Espersen F, Frimodt-Moller N, Thamdrup Rosdahl V, Jessen O. *Staphylococcus aureus* bacteraemia in children below the age of one year. Acta Paediatr Scand 1989; 78:56-61.
5. Frimodt-Moller N, Espersen F, Skinhoj P, Thamdrup Rosdahl V. Epidemiology of *Staphylococcus aureus* bacte-remia in Denmark from 1957 to 1990. Clin Microbiol Infect 1997; 3:297-305.
6. Mulligan ME, Murray-Leisure KA, Ribner BS, Standiford HC, John JF, Korvick JA, Kauffman CA, Yu VL. Methicillin-resistant *Staphylococcus aureus*: a consensus review of the microbiology, pathogenesis, and epi-demiology with implications for prevention and management. Am J Med 1993; 94:313-328.
7. Cookson B. Aspects of the epidemiology of MRSA in Europe. J Chemother 1995; 7:93-98.
8. Corso A, Santos Sanches I, Aires de Sousa M, Rossi A, de Lencastre H. Spread of a methicillin-resistant and multiresistant epidemic clone of *Staphylococcus aureus* in Argentina. Microb Drug Resist 1998; 4:277-288.
9. Anonymous. Update: *Staphylococcus aureus* with reduced susceptibility to vancomycin – United States, 1997. MMWR 1997; 46:813-815.
10. Perl TM. The threat of vancomycin resistance. Am J Med 1999; 106:S26-S37.
11. Wallmark GI, Anemark I, Telander B. *Staphylococcus saprophyticus*: a frequent cause of urinary tract infec-tions among female outpatients. J Infect Dis 1978; 138:791-797.
12. Kloos WE, Bannerman TL. Update on clinical significance of coagulase-negative staphylococci. Clin Microbiol Rev 1994; 7:117-140.
13. Nafziger DA, Wenzel RP. Coagulase-negative staphylococci: epidemiology, evaluation, and therapy. Infect Dis Clin North Am 1989; 3:915-929.

14. Kluytmans J, van Belkum A, Verbrugh H. Nasal carriage of *Staphylococcus aureus*: epidemiology, underlying mechanisms, and associated risks. Clin Microbiol Rev 1997; 10:505-520.

15. Noble WC. Skin bacteriology and the role of *Staphylococcus aureus* in infection. Br J Dermatol 1998; 139:S9-S12.

16. Ladhani S, Joannou CL, Lochrie DP, Evans RW, Poston SM. Clinical, microbial, and biochemical aspects of the exfoliative toxins causing staphylococcal scalded-skin syndrome. Clin Microbiol Rev 1999; 12:224-242.

17. Crane JK. Preformed bacterial toxins. Clin Lab Med 1999; 19:583-599.

18. Wieneke AA, Roberts D, Gilbert RJ. Staphylococcal food poisoning in the United Kingdom, 1969-1990. Epidemiol Infect 1993; 110:519-531.

19. Chesney PJ, Bergdoll MS, Davis JP, Vergeront JM. The disease spectrum, epidemiology, and etiology of toxic-shock syndrome. Ann Rev Microbiol 1984; 38:315-338.

20. Stevens DL. The toxic shock syndromes. Infect Dis Clin North Am 1996; 10:727-746.

21. Broome CV. Epidemiology of toxic shock syndrome in the United States. Rev Infect Dis 1989; 11:S14-S21.

22. Pfaller MA, Herwaldt LA. Laboratory, clinical, and epidemiological aspects of coagulase-negative staphylococci. Clin Microbiol Rev 1988; 1:281-299.

23. Edmiston CE, Schmitt DD, Seabrook GR. Coagulase-negative staphylococcal infection in vascular surgery: epidemiology and pathogenesis. Infect Control Hosp Epidemiol 1989; 10:111-117.

24. Magee JT, Burnett IA, Hindmarch JM, Spencer RC. *Micrococcus* and *Stomatococcus* spp. from human infections. J Hosp Infect 1990; 16:67-73.

25. Stackebrandt E, Koch C, Gvozdiak O, Schumann P. Taxonomic dissection of the genus *Micrococcus*: *Kocuria* gen. nov., *Nesterenkonia* gen. nov., *Kytococcus* gen. nov., *Dermacoccus* gen. nov., and *Micrococcus* Cohn 1872 gen. emend. Int J Syst Bacteriol 1995; 45:682-692.

26. Ascher DP, Zbick C, White C, Fischer GW. Infections due to *Stomatococcus mucilaginosus*: ten cases and review. Rev Infect Dis 1991; 13:1048-1052.

27. Kaufhold A, Reinert RR, Kern W. Bacteremia caused by *Stomatococcus mucilaginosus*: report of seven cases and review of the literature. Infection 1992; 20:213-220.

28. Gruson D, Hilbert G, Pigneux A, Vargas F, Guisset O, Texier J, Boiron JM, Reiffers J, Gbikpi-Benissan G, Cardinaud JP. Severe infection caused by *Stomatococcus mucilaginosus* in a neutropenic patient: case report and review of the literature. Hematol Cell Ther 1998; 40:167-169.

29. Goldman M, Chaudhary UB, Greist A, Fausel CA. Central nervous system infections due to *Stomatococcus mucilaginosus* in immunocompromised hosts. Clin Infect Dis 1998; 27:1241-1246.

30. Bosley GS, Whitney AM, Pruckler JM, Moss CW, Daneshvar M, Sih T, Talkington DF. Characterization of ear fluid isolates of *Alloiococcus otitidis* from patients with recurrent otitis media. J Clin Microbiol 1995; 33:2876-2880.

31. Perl TM, Golub JE. New approaches to reduce *Staphylococcus aureus* nosocomial infection rates: treating *S. aureus* nasal carriage. Ann Pharmacother 1998; 32:S7-S16.

32. Perl TM, Roy MC. Postoperative wound infections: risk factors and role of *Staphyloccus aureus* nasal carriage. J Chemother 1995; 7:S29-S35.

33. Casewell MW. The nose: an underestimated source of *Staphylococcus aureus* causing wound infection. J Hosp Infect 1998; 40:S3-S11.

34. Kluytmans J. Reduction of surgical site infections in major surgery by elimination of nasal carriage of *Staphylococcus aureus*. J Hosp Infect 1998; 40:S25-S29.

35. Espersen F. Identifying the patient risk for *Staphylococcus aureus* bloodstream infections. J Chemother 1995; 7:S11-S17.

36. Jensen AG, Wachmann CH, Poulsen KB, Espersen F, Scheibel J, Skinhoj P, Frimodt-Moller N. Risk factors for hospital-acquired *Staphylococcus aureus* bacteremia. Arch Intern Med 1999; 159:1437-1444.

37. Bradley SF. Methicillin-resistant *Staphylococcus aureus* in nursing homes: epidemiology, prevention and management. Drugs Aging 1997; 10:185-198.

38. Bradley SF. Methicillin-resistant *Staphylococcus aureus*: long-term care concerns. Am J Med 1999; 106:S2-S10.

39. Espersen F, Rosdahl VT, Frimodt-Miller N, Skinhoj P. Epidemiology of *Staphylococcus aureus* bacteremia in Denmark. J Chemother 1994; 6:219-225.

40. Doebbling BN. The epidemiology of methicillin-resistant *Staphylococcus aureus* colonisation and infection. J Chemother 1995; 7:99-103.

41. Monnet DL. Methicillin-resistant *Staphylococcus aureus* and its relationship to antimicrobial use: possible implications for control. Infect Control Hosp Epidemiol 1998; 19:552-559.

42. Herwaldt LA. Control of methicillin-resistant *Staphylococcus aureus* in the hospital setting. Am J Med 1999; 106:S11-S18.

43. Casewell MW. New threats to the control of methicillin-resistant *Staphylococcus aureus*. J Hosp Infect 1995; 30:S465-S471.

44. Kluytmans J, van Leeuwen W, Goessens W, Hollis R, Messer S, Herwadlt L, Bruining H, Heck M, Rost J, van Leeuwen N, van Belkum A, Verbrugh H. Food-initiated outbreak of methicillin-resistant *Staphylococcus aureus* analyzed by pheno- and genotyping. J Clin Microbiol 1995; 33:1121-1128.

45. Hubner J, Kropec A. Cross infections due to coagulase-negative staphylococci in high-risk patients. Zentralbl Bakteriol 1995; 283:169-174.

46. Bialkowska-Hobrzanska H, Jaskot D, Hammerberg O. Evaluation of restriction endonuclease fingerprinting of chromosomal DNA and plasmid profile analysis for characterization of multiresistant coagulase-negative staphylococci in bacteremic neonates. J Clin Microbiol 1990; 28:269-275.

47. Thylefors JD, Harbarth S, Pittet D. Increasing bacteremia due to coagulase-negative staphylococci: fiction or reality? Infect Cont Hosp Epidemiol 1998; 19:581-589.

48. Gilligan PH, Gage PA, Welch DF, Muszynski MJ, Wait KR. Prevalence of thymidine-dependent *Staphylococcus aureus* in patients with cystic fibrosis. J Clin Microbiol 1987; 25:1258-1261.

49. Skurray RA, Rouch DA, Lyon BR, Gillespie MT, Tennent JM, Byrne ME, Messerotti LJ, May JW. Multiresistant *Staphylococcus aureus*: genetics and evolution of epidemic Australian strains. J Antimicro Chemother 1988; 21:S19-S39.

50. Albus A, Fournier JM, Wolz C, Boutonnier A, Ranke M, Hoiby N, Hochkeppel H, Doring G. *Staphylococcus aureus* capsular types and antibody response to lung infection in patients with cystic fibrosis. J Clin Microbiol 1988; 26:2505-2509.

51. Foster TJ, McDevitt D. Surface-associated proteins of *Staphylococcus aureus*: their possible roles in virulence. FEMS Microbiol Lett 1994; 118:199-205.

52. Parsonnet J. Mediators in the pathogenesis of toxic shock syndrome: overview. Rev Infect Dis 1989; 11:S263-S269.

53. Kass EH, Parsonnet J. On the pathogenesis of toxic shock syndrome. Rev Infect Dis 1987; 9:S482-S489.

54. Johnson HM, Torres BA, Soos JM. Superantigens: structure and relevance to human disease. Proc Soc Exp Biol Med 1996; 212:99-109.

55. Gemmell CG. Staphylococcal scalded skin syndrome. J Med Microbiol 1995; 43:318-327.

56. Krakauer T. Immune response to staphylococcal superantigens. Immunol Res 1999; 20:163-173.

57. Peterson PK, Wilkinson BJ, Kim Y, Schmeling D, Douglas SD, Quie P. The key role of peptidoglycan in the opsonization of *Staphylococcus aureus*. J Clin Invest 1978; 61:597-609.

58. Cunningham R, Cockayne A, Humphreys H. Clinical and molecular aspects of the pathogenesis of *Staphylococcus aureus* bone and joint infections. J Med Microbiol 1996; 44:157-164.

59. Villavicencio RT, Wall MJ Jr. The pathogenesis of *Staphylococcus aureus* in the trauma patient and potential future therapies. Am J Surg 1996; 172:291-296.

60. Wadstrom T. Molecular aspects on pathogenesis of wound and foreign body infections due to staphylococci. Zentralbl Bakteriol Mikrobiol Hyg [A] 1987; 266:191-211.

61. Hancock IC. Encapsulation of coagulase-negative staphylococci. Zentralbl Bakteriol 1989; 272:11-18.

62. Fleer A, Timmerman CP, Besnier JM, Pascuual A, Verhoef J. Surface proteins of coagulase-negative staphylococci: their role in adherence to biomaterials and in opsonization. J Biomater Appl 1990; 5:154-165.

63. Von Eiff C, Heilmann C, Herrmann M, Peters G. Basic aspects of the pathogenesis of staphylococcal polymer-associated infections. Infection 1999; 27:S7-S10.

64. Goldmann DA, Pier GB. Pathogenesis of infections related to intravascular catheterization. Clin Microbiol Rev 1993; 6:176-192.

65. St Geme JW, Harris MC. Coagulase-negative staphylococcal infection in the neonate. Clin Perinatol 1991; 18:281-302.

66. Wheat J, Kohler RB, Garten M, White A. Commercially available (ENDO-STAPH) assay for teichoic acid antibodies: evaluation in patients with serious *Staphylococcus aureus* infections and in controls. Arch Intern Med 1984; 144:261-264.

67. Wise KA, Tosolini FA. Detection of teichoic acid antibodies in *Staphylococcus aureus* infections. Pathology 1992; 24:102-108.

68. Kunstmann G, Schroder E, Hasbach H, Pulverer G. Immune response to toxic-shock syndrome toxin-1 (TSST-1) and to staphylococcal enterotoxins A, B, and C in *Staphylococcus aureus* infections. Zentralbl Bakteriol 1989; 271:486-492.

69. Tenover FC, Arbeit R, Archer G, Biddle J, Byrne S, Goering R, Hancock G, Hebert GA, Hill B, Hollis R, Jarvis WR, Kreiswirth B, Eisner W, Maslow J, McDougal LK, Miller JM, Mulligan M, Pfaller MA. Comparison of traditional and molecular methods of typing isolates of *Staphylococcus aureus*. J Clin Microbiol 1994; 32:407-415.

70. Traub WH, Bauer D, Leonhard B. Immunobology of methicillin-resistant *Staphylococcus aureus*: immune response of rabbits and patients to systemic infection. Chemotherapy 1996; 42:118-132.

71. Fattom A, Li X, Cho YH, Burns A, Hawwari A, Shepheerd SE, Coughlin R, Winston S, Naso R. Effect of conjugation methodology, carrier protein, and adjuvants on the immune response to *Staphylococcus aureus* capsular polysaccharides. Vaccine 1995; 13:1288-1293.

72. Hauser C, Wuethrich B, Matter L, Wilhelm JA, Schopfer K. Immune response to *Staphylococcus aureus* in atopic dermatitis. Dermatologica 1985; 170:114-120.

73. Plaunt MR, Patrick CC. Identification of the innate human immune response to surface-exposed proteins of coagulase-negative staphylococci. J Clin Microbiol 1991; 29:857-861.

74. Henke PK, Bergamijni TM, Garrison JR, Brittian KR, Peyton JC, Lam TM. *Staphylococcus epidermidis* graft infection is associated with locally suppressed major histocompatibility complex class II and elevated MAC-1 expression. Arch Surg 1997; 132:894-902.

75. Gray ED, Peters G, Verstegen M, Regelmann WE. Effect of extracellular slime substance from *Staphylococcus epidermidis* to the human cellular immune response. Lancet 1984; i:365-367.

76. Bayston R, Rodgers J. Role of serological tests in the diagnosis of immune complex disease in infection of ventriculoatrial shunts for hydrocephalus. Eur J Clin Microbiol Infect Dis 1994; 13:417-420.

77. Espersen F, Wilkinson BJ, Wheat LJ, White A, Bayer AS, Hopper DC. Antibody response to *Staphylococcus epidermidis*: comparison of ultrasonic extract and cell wall antigens for serological diagnosis of coagulase-negative staphylococcal endocarditis. Serodiagn Immunother 1987; 1:367-378.

78. Baird RM, Lee WH. Media used in the detection and enumeration of *Staphylococcus aureus*. Int J Food Microbiol 1995; 26:15-24.

79. Lally RT, Ederer MN, Woolfrey BF. Evaluation of mannitol salt agar with oxacillin as a a screening medium for methicillin-resistant *Staphylococcus aureus*. J Clin Microbiol 1985; 22:501-504.

80. Fleurette J, Bes M, Brun Y, Freney J, Forey F, Coulet M, Reverdy ME, Etienne J. Clinical isolates of *Staphylococcus lugdenensis* and *S. schleiferi*: bacteriological characteristics and susceptibility to antimicrobial agents. Res Microbiol 1989; 140:107-118.

81. Wilkerson M, McAllister S, Miller JM, Heiter BJ, Bourbeau PP. Comparison of five agglutination tests for identification of *Staphylococcus aureus*. J Clin Microbiol 1997; 35:148-151.

82. Personne P, Bes M, Lina G, Vandenesch F, Brun Y, Etienne J. Comparative performance of six agglutination kits assessed by using typical and atypical strains of *Staphylococcus aureus*. J Clin Microbiol 1997; 35:1138-1140.

83. Cooke RP, Jenkins CT. Comparison of commercial slide agglutination kits with a tube coagulase for the rapid identification of *Staphylococcus aureus* from blood culture. J Clin Pathol 1997; 50:164-166.

84. Vandenesch F, Bes M, Lebeau C, Greenland T, Brun Y, Etienne J. Coagulase-negative *Staphylococcus aureus*. Lancet 1993; 342:995-996.

85. Madison BM, Baselski VS. Rapid identification of *Staphylococcus aureus* in blood cultures by thermonuclease testing. J Clin Microbiol 1983; 18:722-724.

86. Megson GM, Law D, Ganguli LA. Problems of thermonuclease detection for identifying *Staphylococcus aureus* in blood culture broths. J Clin Pathol 1991; 44:772-774.

87. Skulnick M, Simor AE, Patel MP, Simpson HE, O'Quinn KJ, Low DE, Phillips AM, Small GW. Evaluation of three methods for the rapid identification of *Staphylococcus aureus* in blood cultures. Diagn Microbiol Infect Dis 1994; 19:5-8.

88. Skov RL, Palleson LV, Poulsen RL, Espersen F. Evaluation of a new 3-h hybridization method for detecting the *mecA* gene in *Staphylococcus aureus* and comparison with existing genotypic and phenotypic susceptibility testing methods. J Antimicrob Chemother 1999; 43:467-475.

89. Rasooly L, Rose NR, Shah DB, Rasoolly A. In vitro assay of Staphylococcus aureus enterotoxin A activity in food. Appl Environ Microbiol 1997; 63:2361-2365.

90. Mehrotra M, Wang G, Johnson WM. Multiplex PCR for detection of genes for Staphylococcus aureus enterotoxins, exfoliative toxins, toxic shock syndrome toxin 1, and methicillin resistance. J Clin Microbiol 2000; 38:1032-1035.

91. Schumacher-Perdreau F, Akatova A, Pulverer G. Detection of staphylococcal enterotoxin B and toxic shock syndrome toxin: PCR versus conventional methods. Zentralbl Bakteriol 1995; 282:367-371.

92. Roder BL, Eriksen NH, Nielsen LP, Slotsbjerg T, Rosdahl VT, Espersen F. No difference in enterotoxin production among *Staphylococcus aureus* isolated from blood compared with strains isolated from healthy carriers. J Med Microbiol 1995; 42:43-47.

93. Kellogg JA, Hanna MD, Nelsen SJ, Sprenkle LS, Thomas ML, Young KS. Predictive values of species identifications from the Vitek Gram-Positive Identification Card using clinical isolates of coagulase-negative staphylococci. Am J Clin Pathol 1996; 106:374-377.

94. Ieven M, Verhoeven J, Pattyn SR, Goossens H. Rapid and economical method for species identification of clinically significant coagulase-negative staphylococci. J Clin Microbiol 1995; 33:1060-1063.

95. Janda WM, Ristow K, Novak D. Evaluation of RapiDEC Staph for identification of *Staphylococcus aureus*, *Staphylococcus epidermidis*, and *Staphylococcus saprophyticus*. J Clin Microbiol 1994; 32:2056-2059.

96. Perl TM, Rhomberg PR, Bale MJ, Fuchs PC, Jones RN, Koontz FP, Pfaller MA. Comparison of identification systems for *Staphylococcus epidermidis* and other coagulase-negative *Staphylococcus* species. Diagn Microbiol infect Dis 1994; 18:151-155.

97. Grant CE, Sewell DL, Pfaller M, Bumgardner RV, Williams JA. Evaluation of two commercial systems for identification of coagulase-negative staphylococci to species level. Diagn Microbiol Infect Dis 1994; 18:1-5.

98. Bannerman TL, Kleeman KT, Kloos WE. Evaluation of the Vitek Systems Gram-Positive identification card for species identification of coagulase-negative staphylococci. J Clin Microbiol 1993; 31:1322-1325.

99. Rhoden DL, Miller JM. Four-year prospective study of STAPH-IDENT system and conventional method for reference identification of *Staphylococcus*, *Stomatococcus*, and *Micrococcus* spp. J Clin Microbiol 1995; 33:96-98.

100. Gribaldo S, Cookson B, Saunders N, Marples R, Stanley J. Rapid identification by specific PCR of coagulase-negative staphylococcal species important in hospital infection. J Med Microbiol 1997; 46:45-53.

101. Rhoden DL, Hancock GA, Miller JM. Numerical approach to reference identification of *Staphylococcus*, *Stomatococcus*, and *Micrococcus* spp. J Clin Microbiol 1993; 31:490-493.

102. Faller A, Schleifer KH. Modified oxidase and benzidine tests for separation of staphylococci from micrococci. J Clin Microbiol 1981; 13:1031-1035.

103. Geary C, Stevens M. Rapid lysostaphin test to differentiate *Staphylococcus* and *Micrococcus* species. J Clin Microbiol 1986; 23:1044-1045.

104. Poutrel B, Caffin JP. Lysostaphin disk test for routine presumptive identification of staphylococci. J Clin Microbiol 1981; 13:1023-1025.

105. van der Zee A, Verbakel H, van Zon JC, Frenay I, van Belkum A, Peeters M, Buiting A, Bergmans A. Molecular genotyping of *Staphylococcus aureus* strains: comparison of repetitive element sequence-based PCR with various typing methods and isolation of a novel epidemicity marker. J Clin Microbiol 1999; 37:342-349.

106. Tambic A, Power EGM, Talsania H, Anthony RM, French GL. Analysis of an outbreak of non-phagetypeable methicillin-resistant *Staphylococcus aureus* by using a randomly amplified polymorphic DNA assay. J Clin Microbiol 1997; 35:3092-3097.

107. Hookey JV, Richardson JF, Cookson BD. Molecular typing of *Staphylococcus aureus* based on PCR restriction fragment length polymorphism and DNA sequence analysis of the coagulase gene. J Clin Microbiol 1998; 36:1083-1089.

108. Cuny C, Witte W. Typing of *Staphylococcus aureus* by PCR for DNA sequences flanked by transposon Tn*916* target region and ribosomal binding site. J Clin Microbiol 1996; 34:1502-1505.

109. Olmos A, Camarena JJ, Nogueira JM, Navarro JC, Risen J, Sanchez R. Application of an optimized and highly discriminatory method based on arbitrarily primed PCR for epidemiologic analysis of methicillin-resistant *Staphylococcus aureus* nosocomial infections. J Clin Microbiol 1998; 36:1128-1134.

110. del Vecchio VG, Petroziello JM, Gress MJ, McCleskey FK, Melcher GP, Crouch HK, Lupski JR. Molecular genotyping of methicillin-resistant *Staphylococcus aureus* via fluorophore-enhanced repetitive-sequence PCR. J Clin Microbiol 1995; 33:2141-2144.

111. Enright MC, Day NPJ, Davies CE, Peacock SJ, Spratt BG. Multilocus sequence typing for characterization of methicillin-resistant and methicillin-susceptible clones of *Staphylococcus aureus*. J Clin Microbiol 2000; 38:1008-1015.

112. van Belkum A, van Leeuwen W, Kaufmann ME, Cookson B, Forey F, Etienne J, Goering R, Tenover F, Steward C, O'Brien F, Grubb W, Tassios P, Legakis N, Morvan A, El Solh N, de Ryck R, Struelens M, Salmenlinna S, Vuopio-Varkila J, Kooistra M, Talens A, Witte W, Verbrugh H. Assessment of resolution and intercenter reproducibility of results of genotyping *Staphylococcus aureus* by pulsed-field gel electrophoresis of *Sma*I macrorestriction fragments: a multicenter study. J Clin Microbiol 1998; 36:1653-1659.

113. Kluytmans J, Berg H, Steegh P, Vandenesch F, Etienne J, van Belkum A. Outbreak of *Staphylococcus schleiferi* wound infections: strain characterization by randomly amplified polymorphic DNA analysis, PCR ribotyping, conventional ribotyping, and pulsed-field gel electrophoresis. J Clin Microbiol 1998; 36:2214-2219.
114. Carlos CC, Ringertz S, Rylander M, Huovinen P, Faxelius G. Nosocomial *Staphylococcus epidermidis* septicaemia among very low birth weight neonates in the an intensive care unit. J Hosp Infect 1991; 19:201-207.
115. National Committee for Clinical Laboratory Standards. Methods for dilution antimicrobial susceptibility tests for bacteria that grow aerobically. Wayne, PA:NCCLS, 1997.
116. National Committee for Clinical Laboratory Standards. Performance standards for antimicrobial disk susceptibility tests. Wayne, PA:NCCLS, 1997.
117. Thornsberry C. The development of antimicrobial resistance in staphylococci. J Antimicrob Chemother 1988; 21:S9-S17.
118. Petersson AC, Eliasson I, Kamme C, Miorner H. Evaluation of four qualitative methods for detection of beta-lactamase production in *Staphylococcus* and *Micrococcus* species. Eur J Clin Microbiol Infect Dis 1989; 8:962-967.
119. Chambers HF. Methicillin resistance in staphylococci: molecular and biochemical basis and clinical implications. Clin Microbiol Rev 1997; 10:781-791.
120. Petersson AC, Miorner H, Kamme C. Identification of *mecA*-related oxacillin resistance in staphylococci by the E test and the broth microdilution method. J Antimicrob Chemother 1996; 37:445-456.
121. Michel M, Gutmann L. Methicillin-resistant *Staphylococcus aureus* and vancomycin-resistant enterococci: therapeutic realities and possibilities. Lancet 1997; 349:1901-1906.
122. McDougal LK, Thornsberry C. The role of beta-lactamase in staphylococcal resistance to penicillinase-resistant penicillins and cephalosporins. J Clin Microbiol 1986; 23:832-839.
123. Montanari MP, Massidda O, Mingoia M, Varaldo PE. Borderline susceptibility to methicillin in *Staphylococcus aureus*: a new mechanism of resistance? Microb Drug Resist 1996; 2:257-260.
124. Zaher A, Al-Thawadi S, Cimolai N. Beta-lactamase negative, methicillin-resistant *Staphylococcus aureus* lacking the *mecA* gene determinant. J Antimicrob Chemother 1997; 39:108-109.
125. van Griethuysen A, Pouw M, van Leeuwen N, Heck M, Willemse P, Buiting A, Kluytmans J. Rapid slide latex aggutination test for detection of methicillin resistance in *Staphylococcus aureus*. J Clin Microbiol 1999; 37:2789-2792.
126. van Leeuwen WB, van Pelt C, Luijendijk A, Verbrugh HA, Goessens WH. Rapid detection of methicillin resistance in *Staphylococcus aureus* isolates by the MRSA-screen latex agglutination test. J Clin Microbiol 1999; 37:3029-3030.
127. Ishida K, Guze PA, Kalmanson GM, Albrandt K, Guze LB. Variables in demonstrating methicillin tolerance in *Staphylococcus aureus* strains. Antimicrob Agents Chemother 1982; 21:688-690.
128. Goessens WH. Basic mechanisms of bacterial tolerance of antimicrobial agents. Eur J Clin Microbiol Infect Dis 1993; 12:S9-S12.
129. Voorn GP, Thompson J, Goessens WH, Schmal-Bauer WC, Broeders PH, Michel MF. In vitro developemnt and stability of tolerance to cloxacilin and vancomycin in *Staphylococcus aureus*. Eur J Clin Microbiol Infect Dis 1994; 13:741-746.
130. Sherris JC. Problems in in vitro determination of antibiotic tolerance in clinical isolates. Antimicrob Agents Chemother 1986; 30:633-637.
131. Ramos RL, Teixeira LA, Ormonde LR, Siqueira PL, Santos MS, Marangoni D, Figueiredo AM. Emergence of mupirocin resistance in multiresistant *Staphylococcus aureus* clinical isolates belonging to Brazilian epidemic clone III::B:A. J Med Microbiol 1999; 48:303-307.
132. Carbon C. Costs of treating infections caused by methicillin-resistant staphylococci and voncomycin-resistant enterococci. J Antimicrob Chemo 1999; 44:S31-S36.
133. Lacey RW, Kruczenyk SC. Epidemiology of antibiotic resistance in Staphylococcus aureus. J Antimicrob Chemother 1986; 18:S207-S214.
134. Ryffel C, Tesch W, Birch-Machin I, Reynolds PE, Barberis-Maino L, Kayser FH, Berger-Bachi B. Sequence comparison of *mecA* genes isolated from methicillin-resistant *Staphylococcus aureus* and *Staphylococcus epidermidis*. Gene 1990; 94:137-138.
135. Suzuki E, Hiramatsu K, Yokota T. Survey of methicilin-resistant clinical strains of coagulase-negative staphylococci for *mecA* gene distribution. Antimicrob Agents Chemother 1992; 36:429-434.
136. Cimolai N, Trombley C, Zaher A. Oxacillin susceptibility of coagulase-negative staphylococci: role for *mecA* genotyping and E-test susceptibility testing. Int J Antimicrob Agents 1997; 8:121-125.

137. Predari SC, Ligozzi M, Fontana R. Genotypic identification of methicillin-resistant coagulase-negative staphylococci by polymerase chain reaction. Antimicrob Agents Chemother 1991; 35:2568-2573.

138. Cimolai N. Ciprofloxacin and multiresistant staphylococci. Lancet 1997; 349:1030.

139. Ramotar K, Bobrowska M, Jessamine P, Toye B. Detection of methicillin resistance in coagulase-negative staphylococci initially reported as methicillin susceptible using automated methods. Diagn Microbiol Infect Dis 1998; 30:267-273.

140. Rochette A, Chomarat M, de Montclos M. Sensitivity to antibiotics of 64 strains of *Stomatococcus mucilaginosus* isolated in human clinical cases. Pathol Biol 1988; 36:394-397.

141. Marshall SA, Wilke WW, Pfaller MA, Jones RN. *Staphylococcus aureus* and coagulase-negative staphylococci from blood stream infections: frequency of occurrence, antimicrobial susceptibility, and molecular (*mecA*) characterization of oxacillin resistance in the SCOPE program. Diagn Microbiol Infect Dis 1998; 30:205-214.

142. Hussain Z, Stoakes L, Massey V, Diagre D, Fitzgerald V, El Sayed S, Lannigan R. Correlation of oxacillin MIC with *mecA* gene carriage in coagulase-negative staphylococci. J Clin Microbiol 2000; 38:752-754.

143. Schwalbe RS, Stapleton JT, Gilligan PH. Emergence of vancomycin resistance in coagulase-negative staphylococci. N Engl J Med 1987; 316:927-931.

144. Jenssen WD, Thakker-Varia S, Dubin DT, Weinstein MP. Prevalence of macrolides-lincosamides-streptogramin B resistance and *erm* gene classes among clinical strains of staphylococci and streptococci. Antimicrob Agents Chemother 1987; 31:883-888.

145. von Eiff C, Herrmann M, Peters G. Antimicrobial susceptibilities of *Stomatococcus mucilaginosus* and of *Micrococcus* spp. Antimicrob Agents Chemother 1995; 39:268-270.

146. Pinsky RL, Piscitelli V, Patterson JE. Endocarditis caused by relatively penicillin-resistant *Stomatococcus mucilaginosus*. J Clin Microbiol 1989; 27:215-216.

147. Ayliffe GA. The progressive intercontinental spread of methicillin-resistant *Staphylococcus aureus*. Clin Infect Dis 1997; 24:S74-S79.

148. National Committee for Clinical Laboratory Standards. Performance standards for antimicrobial susceptibility testing: ninth information supplement, vol. 19, no. 1. NCCLS document M100-S9. Wayne, PA, USA:NCCLS.

149. Noskin GA, Siddiqui F, Stosor V, Hacek D, Peterson LR. In vitro activities of linezolid against important gram-positive bacterial pathogens including vancomycin-resistant enterococci. Antimicrob Agents Chemother 1999; 43:2059-2062.

12

Streptococcal and Enterococcal Infections

Graziella Orefici, Roberto Nisini, and Christina von Hunolstein
Laboratory of Bacteriology and Medical Mycology, Instituto Superiore di Sanitá, Rome, Italy

I. HISTORICAL BACKGROUND

The term "streptococcos" was used by Billroth (1874) to describe chain forming, coccoid bacteria that were found in wounds or discharge from animals. Later, Rosenbach (1884) used the name of "streptococcus" to describe organisms, growing in chains, that were isolated from suppurative lesions in man. In the following years, the association of streptococci with different diseases in man and animals was firmly established, and numerous attempts to classify and identify the different forms were undertaken. Early classifications of these bacteria were made on the basis of pathogenicity, cultural characteristics, cell morphology, reactions on blood agar, and growth temperature.

An early important classification of streptococci based on morphological observations together with fermentation of sugars, reduction of neutral red, and growth characteristics in milk was detailed by Andrews and Horder (1906), but the first systematic classification of streptococci was achieved by Sherman (1937). He observed that fermentation tests were valuable for differentiating closely related types, but when applied to streptococci as a whole and without previous subdivisions via other methods, they were unable to give a useful classification. Therefore, he divided streptococci into four preliminary groups: pyogenic, viridans, lactics, and enterococci. It is interesting to note that Sherman excluded pneumococci (on the basis of the extreme sensitivity to bile) and strictly anaerobic streptococci in his classification although he included enterococci.

When Lancefield described the presence of the group polysaccharides in 1933, it appeared that a very good correlation existed between the streptococcus species that were characterized on the basis of physiological and biochemical properties of Sherman and serological groups. Since the serological grouping was relatively easy and fast to perform, it became 'the' identification system and in some circumstances the group was used as a synonym for the species name (e.g., group A for *S. pyogenes*, group B for *S. agalactiae*). This fact had two consequences: a) the acceptance of serological groups as taxonomic entities for streptococci which had not been extensively studied by other criteria, and b) the inclusion in the same group (e.g., group D) of well-known and characterized species (e.g., *S. bovis* and *S. equinus*) together with species that were physiologically dissimilar (e.g., enterococci).

The introduction of molecular methods in taxonomic studies resulted in broad changes in the classification of streptococci. Presently, the *Streptococcus* genus includes more than thirty species. There is agreement that no single classification scheme is entirely satisfactory, but that the classification should be made on a combination of features: growth characteristics, biochemical properties, hemolytic pattern on blood agar, antigenic composition, and genetic analysis. While no relevant changes have been introduced in the classification of better known beta-hemolytic species or pneumococci, many changes have been achieved for the classification of viridans streptococci. The different species have been divided in six groups on the basis of 16s rRNA sequence determination, and new species have been described.

Moreover, enterococci, formerly belonging to group D streptococci, are now classified in the separate genus *Enterococcus* and include at least 16 different species. A new genus *Abiotrophia*, which includes three species, has been recently proposed to accommodate nutritionally variant or satellitic bacteria previously belonging to the viridans streptococci (1). Lactococci and vagococci, previously considered group N streptococci, have been excluded from the *Streptococcus* genus and presently belong to two separate genera, *Lactococcus* and *Vagococcus* (2). *S. morbillorum* was previously included among the 'anaerobic'streptococci, but has been transferred to the new genus *Gemella* (3).

A. *Streptococcus pyogenes*

S. pyogenes (Group A streptococcus; GAS) is one of the most important and intriguing human pathogens. It is an ubiquitous Gram positive bacterium that is responsible for a wide array of human diseases ranging from minor skin or throat infections to severe invasive disease (including necrotizing fasciitis and toxic shock). Moreover, it may cause non-suppurative sequelae such as acute rheumatic fever (ARF) and acute glomerulonephritis (AGN).

The description of some of the major clinical manifestations of post-streptococcal disease preceded the demonstration of the micro-organism in clinical isolates: chorea was described by Sydenham in 17th century, and Charles Wells in 1812 pointed out the association of rheumatism and carditis, and also gave the first description of subcutaneous nodules in rheumatic fever. The relationship between sore throat with rheumatic fever was reported by Fowler in 1880. In the last part of the 19th century, several different observations indicated an association of streptococci with severe human disease. Chain-forming organisms were isolated from wound infections and erysipelas by Billroth in 1874, and from blood in a case of puerperal sepsis by Pasteur. In 1884, Rosenbach designated these organisms as *S. pyogenes*.

The study of GAS has long fascinated investigators in different parts of the world: Shötmuller in 1903, by the use of blood agar, provide the way to differentiate hemolytic from non-hemolytic streptococci, and Brown, in 1919, introduced the terms α, β, and γ hemolysis. The Lancefield classification on the basis of the Group polysaccharide (1933) (4) showed that most strains from human disease belonged to the Group A and that this serogroup was practically synonymous with *S. pyogenes*. Moreover, Lancefield developed the key typing system for GAS on the basis of M protein and demonstrated the critical role of this antigen in virulence as well as the type specificity of the immune response.

The relationship between scarlet fever and streptococcal infection was reported by Dicks in 1920 and Todd, some years later, described the still widely-used method for titration of anti-streptolysin O antibodies.

B. *Streptococcus agalactiae* (Group B streptococci)

S. agalactiae is also known as the Group B Streptococcus (GBS) on the basis of the Lancefield classification of hemolytic streptococci of 1933 (4).

GBS was first reported as a veterinary pathogen causing bovine mastitis long before its human clinical importance was recognized. In 1935, Lancefield and Hare identified this organism in vaginal cultures from asymptomatic post-partum women, but the first description of human GBS disease was made in 1938 by Fry who reported three cases of fatal puerperal sepsis. GBS infections were infrequently reported until the early 1960s when, both in Europe and in the United States, GBS was recognized to be more frequently associated with maternal and neonatal infections than appreciated in the past. During the 1970s, it became clear that both the incidence of GBS septicemia and meningitis in neonates and that of infections in pregnant or non-pregnant adults were increasing (5). The reason for this increase remains unclear. After a first period in which its emergence did not replace the predominant neonatal pathogen *Escherichia coli*, in the United States GBS became the most common cause of sepsis and meningitis in newborns (early-onset syndrome) with an incidence ranging from 1.8-3.7 per 1,000 birth and a case fatality ratio of 50% or more. In the 1990s, the incidence of early-onset neonatal infection decreased by 65% (6). This decrease reflects the enormous efforts undertaken by prevention strategies promoted by the US Centres for Disease Control, the American College of Obstetricians and Gynecologists, and the American Academy of Pediatrics which, through routine GBS screening of pregnant women, lead to the adoption of a selective intrapartum chemoprophylaxis to prevent early-onset neonatal disease (7,8). As not all GBS diseases can be prevented by this strategy, however, (in utero infections and late-onset disease seemingly cannot be prevented), and the costs of acute care or that of infections with meningitis remain high, alternative strategies such as vaccination of pregnant women have been evaluated in recent years. Moreover, vaccination can also be helpful in preventing severe disease in non-pregnant adults which have shown an increasing trend during the past decade (9). While the current understanding of neonatal GBS infection pathogenesis received a remarkable contribution by in vitro, animal model, and molecular genetic studies, the knowledge of GBS pathogenesis in older infants and adults remains to be achieved (10).

C. Beta-hemolytic Groups C and G streptococci

Beta-hemolytic streptococci that bear the C and G Lancefield antigens constitute a heterogeneous group of unrelated organisms in which some of the species produce small β-hemolytic colonies on blood agar and are strictly related with species belonging to the viridans group, while other species, forming large β-hemolytic colonies, are more similar to *S. pyogenes*. Therefore, it is very important to differentiate these large colony forming, Lancefield group C and G streptococci from β-hemolytic members of the 'S. anginosus group'.

Beta-hemolytic streptococci bearing G antigen, isolated from parturient women, were described by Lancefield and Hare in 1935 (11). Originally this group of organisms were not considered pathogenic, since they were part of the skin and mucosal flora of healthy population. Nevertheless, in more recent years, they have been shown to cause severe infections in humans and in animals. In the past, members of this group that were isolated from humans have been divided into species on the basis of carbohydrate fermentation. More recently, genetic studies have shown that marked similarities exist between human Groups C and G strains and have suggested that they should be classified into the same species. Presently, this group of organisms includes the following species: *S. dysgalactiae*, divided in 2 variants (*S. equisimilis* and *S. dysgalactiae*); *S. equi* also divided in 2 variants (*S. equi* and *S. zooepidemicus*), and *S. canis* (12,13).

D. Viridans streptococci

Viridans streptococci are among the most numerous residents of the oral cavity where they may be isolated from saliva, gingiva, cheeks, and tongue; they may also be found in the nasopharynx, genital tract, and on the skin.

This group of bacteria have traditionally been difficult to identify. The name (viridans, "green" from Latin) comes from the color, due to incomplete hemolysis, of the blood agar that surrounds the colonies, but many of the species or some isolates of particular species in this group may be non-hemolytic; others are definitely beta-hemolytic. Moreover, the second traditional method of identification (i.e., the possession of a Lancefield group antigen) has also limited usefulness, since several species or strains do not have such antigens or may show more than one of them.

Several classifications of these organisms have been proposed in the last century. Since 1906, Andrewes and Horder recognized, among the others, three species whose names are still valid: *S. mitis*, *S. salivarius*, and *S. anginosus* (14). *S. mitis* is a resident organism of the mouth and intestine, is rarely pathogenic, and ferments or hydrolyses few of the substrates commonly used to identify streptococci. With the name of *S. salivarius*, it was indicated as a well-defined species that is common in saliva; it fermented sucrose, lactose and raffinose. They also described a third (hemolytic) species, *S. anginosus*, which ferments sucrose, lactose, and often raffinose. Although beta-hemolytic, *S. anginosus* is now regarded as a member of the viridans group, since many non-hemolytic variants (*S. milleri*, *S. constellatus*, and *S. intermedius*) presently included in this species have been described later. *S. bovis* was described by Orla-Jensen in 1919 (15). The organism, common in the bovine gut, fermented several sugars but not mannitol. In 1922, J.K. Clarke described *S. mutans*, a species often associated with dental caries which fermented several sugars and produced a pH of 4.2 in glucose broth (16).

In the 1930s and 1940s, Sherman et al. reviewed the characteristics of several streptococci and noted that the "mitis" group contained different entities given that a group of strains, at difference with other members, hydrolyzed arginine and esculin, and fermented salicin. This new species, frequently found in endocarditis, which produced a strong green discoloration of blood agar and an extracellular polysaccharide (glucan) in media containing sucrose, was later named *S. sanguis* (17).

In the 1970s, two important new classifications, the Colman and Williams (18) and the Facklam classifications (19) were published. These two classification systems were only partially equivalent since Colman and Williams preferred to call *S. mitior* a species formerly defined as *S. mitis*. *S. mitior* in the Facklam classification, however, corresponded to two different species: *S. mitis* and *S. sanguis* II. Moreover, Colman and Williams included in *S. milleri* several hemolytic streptococci with minute colonies and some non-hemolytic streptococci bearing Lancefield A, C, or G antigens, while Facklam separated these organisms in two species. *S. MG-intermedius* and *S. anginosus-constellatus* (Table 1). At the present time, no unequivocal classification has been established. This makes it difficult for clinical laboratories to assign a strain to a particular species. Following the scheme suggested by Kawamura (20), five groups (*mitis*, *anginosus*, *mutans*, *salivarius*, and *bovis*) include the species commonly isolated from humans. Nevertheless, this scheme cannot be intended as definitive, since new species or inclusion of well-known species may alter it in the future.

Chemotaxonomic and the recent genetic techniques have led to a considerable increase in the number of species that are recognized, and an improved identification scheme has been developed to accommodate these new species (Table 2).

E. *Streptococcus pneumoniae*

S. pneumoniae is an important human pathogen. It frequently causes community-acquired pneumonia, meningitis, sinusitis, and otitis media, and less often septic arthritis and endocarditis. Since its first isolation in 1881, *S. pneumoniae* has been one of the most extensively studied organism and its name is linked to many important scientific developments in microbiology and immunology.

Described independently in the same year by Louis Pasteur in France who called it "Microbe septicemique du salive" (21) and by George Sternberg in the United States who named it *Micrococcus Pasteuri* (22,23); the bacterium was eventually referred to as "Pneumococcus" by Fraenkel (1886) for its capacity to cause lobar pneumonia and subsequently "Diplococcus pneumoniae" (Winslow, 1920) because of the appearance in pathologic samples. Only in 1974 did the bacterium receive the present name, *Streptococcus pneumoniae* (24), which is based on its growth in chains in liquid media. The role of pneumococci in the etiology of pneumonia was established before 1885 by several investigators, and before the end of the 19th century, their role as causes of meningitis and otitis media had also been demonstrated (25). Studies on pneumococci resulted in other important discoveries: Hans Christian Gram, while studying techniques for the visualization of bacteria in lungsections, observed that these microorganisms were capable of retaining Crystal violet stain while other species did not; this was one of the basic principles for the Gram stain (26). In addition, the therapeutic efficacy of penicillin (27), the role of capsules in resistance to phagocytosis (28), the role of DNA in inducing transformation of pneumococcal types (29), the ability of capsular polysaccharides to induce antibodies (30), and therefore the

Table 1   Past and present classifications for viridans streptococci.

Colman and Williams*	Facklam**	Present classification***
S. mitior	S. mitis S. sanguis II	'S. mitis group'
S. sanguis	S. sanguis I	
S. salivarius	S. salivarius	'S. salivarius group'
S. mutans	S. mutans	'S. mutans group'
S. milleri	S. MG-intermedius S. anginosus- constellatus	'S. anginosus group'

(From: * - ref. 17; ** - ref. 18; *** - ref. 19)

Table 2 Groups and species of viridans streptococci.

'S. anginosus group'	'S. mitis group'	'S. salivarius group'
S. anginosus	S. oralis	S. salivarius
S. constellatus	S. pneumoniae	S. vestibularis
S. intermedius	S. mitis	
	S. gordonii	
	S. sanguis (sanguinis)	
'S. bovis group'	S. parasanguis (parasanguinis)	
	S. crista (cristatus)	
S. bovis	S. infantis	'S. mutans group'
S. equinus	S. peroris	
S. alactolyticus		S. mutans
		S. rattus
		S. cricetus
		S. sobrinus
		S. macacae
		S. downei

(Modified from ref. 19)

possible use of polysaccharides as vaccines and many other important observations came from the study of pneumococci.

F.   Enterococci

In 1899, Thiercelin proposed the name of "enterococque" to designate a new Gram positive diplococcus with an intestinal habitat (31). In the same year, a case of endocarditis caused by an organism called "Micrococcus zymogenes", later presumptively identified as an enterococcus, was described by McCallum and Hastings. The designation *Streptococcus faecalis* was coined by Andrews and Horder to indicate that the characteristic habitat of the organism was the intestine (14), while the name *S. faecium* was used in 1919 by Orla-Jensen (15).

In 1937, Sherman proposed the use of the term of "enterococcus" on physiological bases to indicate a separate division of streptococci having, beside other characteristics, well-defined resistance to adverse pH, temperature, and salt content of media; many of these characteristics are still in use to distinguish enterococci from streptococci such as *S. bovis* (32). The Sherman classification correlated with the Lancefield serological scheme since enterococci reacted with group D antisera (despite the presence of group D polysaccharide in the cell wall, *S. bovis* was classified by Sherman as a viridans streptococcus). A number of other enterococci were isolated from humans, food, and environment in the following years. In 1957, *Streptococcus faecium* was accepted as a separate species since numerous reports had shown that its technical characteristics were different from those of *S. faecalis* (33).

In 1970, Kalina suggested that, on the basis of phenotypic characteristics and cell arrangement, a different genus from *Streptococcus*, that of *Enterococcus*, should be created to accommodate enterococcal streptococci (*S. faecium* and other different species or subspecies) (34). By1984, Schleifer and Kilper-Balz provided genetic evidence that *S. faecium* and *S. faecalis* merit a separate genus (35). Since that time, several other species have been proposed for inclusion in the genus *Enterococcus* on the basis of DNA:DNA and DNA:rRNA hybridization and of 16S rDNA sequencing. By the latter technique, some species have moved to other genera, e.g., *Tetragenococcus* and *Lactococcus*.

Enterococci are increasingly appreciated as causative agents of urinary tract infections, bacteremia, intra-abdominal infections, endocarditis, and endophthalmitis.

II. CLINICAL ASPECTS

A. *S. pyogenes*

1. *Pharyngitis*

GAS pharyngitis is one of the most common bacterial infections of childhood, but may develop in patients of all ages. Fever (38°C or more), malaise, sore throat and headache are the most common symptoms of this disease which is characterized by an exudative pharyngitis and lymphadenopathy. Both symptoms and signs are quite variable, and range from a mild sore throat, to severe manifestations that are associated with purulent exudate over the posterior pharyngeal wall and tonsillar pillars along with erythema and swelling. Throat culture represents the gold standard for the diagnosis of GAS pharyngitis. Total white blood cell count is usually higher than 12×10^9/L. with an increase in the polymorphonuclear leukocytes. The natural course of the disease is a resolution of symptoms in 3-5 days, but it may be shortened by antibiotic treatment that is aimed to prevent suppurative consequences and non-suppurative sequelae, such as ARF and AGN. The treatment of choice with penicillin is aimed not only towards the reduction of symptoms but also to the eradication of the organism from the pharynx as a primary prevention measure for ARF.

2. *Scarlet fever*

Scarlet fever is usually a complication of pharyngitis and is defined by the characteristic rash which occurs when the infecting GAS isolate produces a pyrogenic exotoxin, but may also follow streptococcal infections at other sites (e.g., wound infections). Within 1-2 days after onset of pharyngitis, a diffuse erythematous rash develops which extends from the upper trunk to the extremities, but spares palms and soles. The rash is characterized by minute papules that give a typical 'sandpaper' feel to the skin. Associated findings include the same symptoms of pharyngitis, circumoral pallor, 'strawberry tongue' (enlarged papillae on a coated tongue which may later become denuded) and Pastia's lines (an accentuation of the rash in the skin folds as is best seen over the abdomen). The rash subsides after 5-9 days and is followed by desquamation. The diagnosis is confirmed by a throat culture for *S. pyogenes*, and the treatment is the same as the pharyngitis. Suppurative (e.g., otitis media, sinusitis) or non-suppurative complications of pharyngitis and scarlet fever became very rare with the use of effective chemotherapy. Recurrent attacks of scarlet fever have also been described (36).

3. Skin infections

Impetigo is a superficial infection of the skin, which occurs most often in young children who live in poor hygienic conditions. GAS colonizes the unbroken skin and minor trauma may serve to inoculate the organism. Individual lesions begin as red papulae which evolve to vesicular and then pustular lesions; these have a tendency to coalesce and to form 'honey-like' crusts. Infections involving subcutaneous tissues are defined as cellulitis. A traumatic or surgical wound as well as an insect bite may represent the portal of GAS entry, but often no entry site is apparent. Another form of GAS infection is known as erysipelas; it is an acute inflammation with involvement of cutaneous lymphatic vessels and is characterized by an area of erythematous skin which is raised and distinctly differentiated from uninvolved tissues. Patients experience local (pain and warmth) and systemic (chills, fever, and malaise) symptoms, and regional lymphadenopathy and leukocytosis are commonly associated. Lesions develop within few hours; antibiotics (penicillin G) represent the treatment of choice.

4. Necrotizing fasciitis

Necrotizing fasciitis is a deep-seated infection of the subcutaneous tissue that progressively destroys fascia and fat but may spare the skin and muscle (37). Infections begin at the site of seemingly irrelevant or inapparent trauma. Within a few hours from the initial lesion, signs of inflammation rapidly develop. During the next 24 to 48 hrs., blisters and bullae, containing clear yellow fluid, appear; some areas become gangrenous with sharply defined lines of demarcation, and the dead skin begins to separate thus revealing an extensive necrosis of the subcutaneous tissue. In more severe cases, the process advances rapidly until large areas of skin become gangrenous and the intoxication renders the patient mentally confused or even delirious. Necrotizing fasciitis caused by GAS is invariably associated with severe manifestations of systemic illness and a high mortality rate despite the absence of underlying chronic diseases and the use of antibiotics and life care support techniques.

5. Streptococcal toxic shock syndrome (STSS)

The portal of entry of streptococci cannot be proven in at least 50% (38) and may only be presumed in many others. Patients with symptomatic pharyngitis rarely develop streptococcal TSS although such cases have been reported in recent years. Most commonly, infection begins at a site of a minor local trauma which frequently does not result in a visible break in the skin. Numerous cases have developed within 24 to 72 hrs. of minor non-penetrating trauma. In other cases, virus infections, such as varicella and influenza, may facilitate entry. The use of non-steroidal anti-inflammatory agents may either mask the early symptoms or predispose the patient to more severe streptococcal infection and shock. For the most part, these infections occurred sporadically and have not been associated with clusters of cases or minor epidemics, though outbreaks of severe GAS infections in closed environments such as nursing homes have been reported (39). Initial symptoms depend on the site of infection and may vary from an influenza-like syndrome to an abrupt onset of pain in patients who develop deep soft tissue infections. Within the following 24-72 hrs., the patient develops high fever, local pain, prostration, and erythema. Fever (>38°C) is the most common sign. Shock syndrome is characterized by hypotension, increased heart rate, and multi-organ failure (e.g., renal failure, toxic cardiopathy, hepatic dysfunction). Blood cultures are positive in about 60% of cases.

6. Bacteremia

Streptococcal bacteremia occurs most commonly in very young children and in the elderly. Among children, predisposing factors include scarlet fever, burns, varicella, malignant neoplasm, immunosuppression, and age less than 2 years. In patients with scarlet fever, the pharynx is the most common source of GAS. Frequently, these patients have complications, such as extension of infection to sinuses, peritonsillar tissue, or mastoids. In elderly patients, the source of bacteremia is invariably the skin and is associated with cellulitis or erysipelas; in these patients sepsis may be associated with diabetes, peripheral vascular disease, malignancy, and corticosteroid use, and there may be mortality rates of 35%-80%. In the past, puerperal sepsis accounted for the majority of bacteremias among those 14-40 yrs. of age. Recently, intravenous drug abuse has emerged as a leading cause of GAS bacteremia in this age group.

7. Non-suppurative post-streptococcal sequelae

Rheumatic fever and glomerulonephritis are the two major non-suppurative post-streptococcal sequelae. Studies from outbreaks of pharyngitis and rheumatic fever reveal that some M serotypes are commonly associated with ARF and that they are different from serotypes that cause glomerulonephritis in the same population (40,41). Strains causing pyoderma are not associated with ARF even though they may colonize the throat (42).

Acute rheumatic fever (ARF)

ARF is an inflammatory disease which occurs as a delayed sequel of pharyngeal *S. pyogenes* infection. Most patients with ARF have a history of streptococcal pharyngitis or scarlet fever. Moreover, tests for antistreptococcal antibodies usually show high titres. ARF involves the heart, joints, central nervous system, skin, and subcutaneous tissues. Usual manifestations are migratory polyarthritis, fever, and carditis, but chorea, subcutaneous nodules, and erythema marginatum may also occur. No single sign, symptom, or laboratory finding, however, is sufficient to make the diagnosis of ARF, but several combinations of them (Jones criteria) are diagnostic. Major manifestations that are reported in the Jones criteria include: polyarthritis, carditis, chorea, erythema marginatum, and subcutaneous nodules, while arthralgia and fever are considered minor manifestations. Common laboratory findings include increases in acute phase reactants, erythrocyte sedimentation rate, and C-reactive protein. Throat culture may be positive. Elevated antistreptococcal antibody titres support the hypothesis of a previous streptococcal infection. The disease is caused by specific serotypes of GAS that are associated with pharyngitis but not cutaneous infections. The mechanism by which GAS initiates the disease is fundamentally unknown (43). A genetic predisposition to the disease is suggested by the relatively small percentage of subjects who develop ARF following a GAS sore throat (44). A direct involvement of the organism in the development of lesions has never been confirmed; *S. pyogenes* is not demonstrable in tissue, and no GAS products has been shown to produce the lesions. Several GAS antigens, however, have been shown to induce the production of antibodies that cross-react with host tissues (45,46). Antibodies to M proteins of strains that are associated with ARF cross-react with myosin, keratin, laminin, and other proteins that are found in cardiac tissue (47,48). In addition, autoantibodies that are reactive with host hyaluronic acid and GAS capsule have been demonstrated. Such findings suggest an autoimmune pathogenesis as a consequence of 'molecular mimicry'.

The classical presentation of ARF includes an acute arthritis which follows a streptococcal pharyngitis after 1-4 weeks. Arthritis occurs with pain and swelling, and usually of a large joint of the extremities. Joint effusions occur but are not persistent. As clinical manifestations subside in one joint, others tend to be involved. This subsequent joint involvement defines the "migratory arthritis" that is characteristic of ARF.

Although arthritis is the most common manifestation, carditis is the most serious. All of the heart tissues (i.e., pericardium, myocardium, and endocardium) may be involved. The endocardial involvement is characterized by a verrucous valvulitis that may heal with fibrous thickening and adhesion of valve commissures and chordae tendinae; the net result may be valvular impairment such as regurgitation or stenosis. Cardiac impairment may become evident by the appearance of heart murmurs of aortic or, most frequently, mitral regurgitation. Signs and symptoms of pericarditis and of heart failure may become evident in more severe cases. Permanent valvular damage may develop and result in serious disability.

Chorea (Sydenham's chorea; chorea minor; Saint Vitus' dance) is a disorder of the central nervous system defined by sudden aimless and irregular movements which are often accompanied by muscle weakness and emotional instability. Chorea is a delayed manifestation of ARF and develops several months after an antecedent GAS infection usually when other manifestations of ARF have abated.

The diagnosis of ARF is established according to the diagnostic Jones criteria and is highly supported by the presence of serological evidence of a recent GAS infection. The anti-streptolysin O test (ASOT) is the best-standardized and most widely-used test in this regard.

Acute glomerulonephritis (AGN)

Post-streptococcal acute glomerulonephritis is a disease that is due to alterations of the structural and functional integrity of the glomerular capillary circulation, and it consists of hematuria and proteinuria; there may be azotemia and renal salt and water retention causing hypertension and edema. A recent streptococcal infection is the main cause of AGN, although non-streptococcal forms have been described. In contrast to ARF, both cutaneous and pharyngeal GAS infections may preceed AGN. Moreover, AGN is reportedly associated with poor personal hygiene and concomitant cutaneous diseases such as scabies infestation (49). Nephritogenic strains of GAS are different from those of ARF and are believed to induce an antibody response that favors the deposition of IgG and complement in the glomerulus with a consequent inflammation that impairs its function. The diagnosis relies on symptoms, abnormal laboratory assay, possibly kidney biopsy, and the evidence of a recent GAS infection.

No precise mechanism by which *S. pyogenes* may cause AGN has been reported, but there is some evidence that renal damage is immunologically mediated. In favor of this are the latent period between the infection and the clinical manifestations, the frequent hypocomplementemia, and the presence in the glomerulus of immunoglobulins and antigens that react with streptococcal antigens.

On the other hand, the frequent presence of IgG and complement components in the glomeruli suggest that the renal injury may be due to the deposition of preformed immunecomplexes between streptococcal antigens and host antibody.

8.   *Other manifestations*

Infection with GAS has also been hypothesized as a possible cause of some forms of psoriasis and PANDAS. The acronym of PANDAS (Pediatric Autoimmune Neuropsychiatric Disorders Associated with Streptococcal infection) has been used in recent years to define a group of neuropsychiatric disorders, particularly obsessive-compulsive disorders and Tourette Syndrome (TS), with onset prior to puberty for which a possible relationship to recent GAS infections has been postulated on the basis of several similarities to Sydenham's chorea (SC). For PANDAS, as for SC, an autoimmune pathogenesis has been suggested (50). Antibodies against GAS components putatively cross-react with neuronal cells, particularly with tissues of the basal ganglia to produce the disease. In favor of this mechanism are the positive results obtained with plasma exchange or intravenous immunoglobulins (51). In difference with SC, patients do not show typical manifestations of rheumatic fever (i.e., carditis, polyarthritis). Moreover, investigators have been unable to find any correlation between the presence or degree of autoantibodies and the severity of symptoms.

The greatest challenge for future investigators is to establish a direct and etiological relationship between the neuropsychiatric syndrome and the streptococcal infections. Although GAS infections are among the inclusion criteria, no accurate microbiological or serological confirmation method for previous infection is recognized. There is not a clear consensus on which laboratory assays are evidence of infection versus colonization or mere exposure. It is, however, interesting that a significant difference in ASOT between patients and controls is evident and that a positive correlation between the severity of tics and ASOT has been reported (52).

B. *S. agalactiae*

1. Neonatal diseases

Two distinctive clinical syndromes related to newborns are described: 'early-onset' or acute infection and 'late-onset' (or delayed infection). The early-onset disease occurs in the first week of life but mostly within a few hours after birth (53), while 'late-onset' infection is seen between 1 week and 3 months of age. Newborns with early–onset disease may become infected in utero as a consequence of GBS-contaminated amniotic fluid aspiration or intrapartum by transmission from mothers who are colonized at the genital tract. Obstetric maternal complications are known to be associated with increased risk of neonatal sepsis. Amniotic infection may lead to spontaneous abortion or stillbirth; premature infants are significantly more often affected than infants at term. The most common manifestations of early-onset infection are pneumonia (35-55% of cases), septicemia (25-40%), and meningitis (5-15%) (53). Sometimes, signs and symptoms of pulmonary insufficiency overshadow clinical manifestations of meningitis. Late-onset syndrome characteristically develops in previous healthy, full-term infants several days or weeks after discharge from the nursery, or, less frequently, in premature infants growing normally. In some cases, nosocomial or community sources, or transmission from mother to infant are probably involved. Nevertheless, the precise mechanism has not been identified. Bacteremia with meningitis is the most common clinical expression of late-onset disease and serotype III GBS is most frequently isolated (95%) in this setting. Initial symptoms of late-onset disease are non-specific (i.e., lethargy, poor feeding and irritability, generally occurring in association with fever). In these cases hospitalization and the acquisition of blood and cerebrospinal fluid cultures are mandatory. Pending laboratory results, empirical antimicrobial therapy should be started.

Both in the early and late syndromes, the incidence of permanent neurological sequelae after meningitis is high and of varying severity (e.g., global or profound mental retardation, spastic quadriplegia, cortical blindness, deafness, uncontrolled seizures, hydrocephalus).

Other common clinical forms of late-onset disease are bacteremia without a detectable focus of infection and bone or joint foci or both. Although septic arthritis and osteomyelitis are considered manifestations of late-onset disease, several features suggest that osteomyelitis represents "early-onset acquisition" and "late-onset expression" of infection. Other clinical manifestations of GBS infections are cellulitis/adenitis, urinary tract infection, omphalitis, shock, fasciitis, otitis, conjunctivitis, endophthalmitis, cardiovascular infection, brain abscesses, etc. (53). Relapse or recurrence of both forms of diseases have been reported. Since infants treated for invasive infections frequently remain colonized by GBS at mucous membrane sites, nasopharyngeal or gastrointestinal tract may be the source of re-infection. A possible explanation for relapse or recurrence of infection may be related to inappropriate dosage or prematurely terminated penicillin therapy. Penicillin-tolerant strains have also been reported (about 4%).

2. Infections in adults

Maternal infections

GBS rectal-vaginal colonization of pregnant women ranges from 25% to 30% (54). In this population, GBS causes clinical illness ranging from mild (asymptomatic) urinary tract infection to life-threatening sepsis and meningitis. Non-invasive syndromes in pregnancy and the postpartum period include amnionitis, endometritis, wound infections (post-Caesarean and post-episiotomy), cellulitis, and fasciitis.

Non-pregnant adults

GBS is an important cause of severe invasive disease also in non-pregnant adults in which, moreover, it is associated with a very high mortality rate. It commonly affects the elderly and persons with chronic underlying diseases such as diabetes mellitus, cancer, hepatic failure, HIV infections, decubitus ulcer, and neurogenic bladder. In a population-based study of 219 cases (55), the most common clinical presentation was bacteremia (42%) followed by skin and soft tissue infections (21%) including cellulitis, infected peripheral ulcer, osteomyelitis, arthritis, and infected decubitus ulcers. Others infections were seen less frequently: pneumonia (12%), urinary tract infection (9%), endocarditis (6%), peritonitis (4%), meningitis (4%) and empyema (1%). Recently, necrotizing fasciitis, which is a severe and uncommon infection usually caused by group A streptococci involving subcutaneous tissues, has been described also for GBS (10).

The association between decubitus ulcer and invasive disease suggest that endogenous skin colonization, supported by integument impairment, is the source of infection. In women, who had mastectomy for breast cancer, the destruction of lymphatic drainage may determine cellulitis, which can lead to bacteremia. GBS pneumonia among survivors of neurologic disorders may be due to the aspiration following the lack of a gag reflex.

C. Beta-hemolytic Groups C and G streptococci

Some Group C and G streptococci have been associated with outbreaks of pharyngitis, even though their role in causing the disease has not been firmly demonstrated. *S. equisimilis* is part of the common commensal flora in humans and the transmission is likely to occur from person-to-person thus yielding sporadic infections rather than being associated with a common source of infection. In general, outbreaks are associated with close contacts. In a study of college students who report to health services with pharyngitis, large colony Group C streptococci were isolated at higher rate in patients with pharyngitis than controls; patients with positive cultures showed evidence of exudative tonsillitis and cervical lymphadenopathy. Their strains were resistant to phagocytosis and contained genomic DNA that encoded for M protein that is similar to that of Group A streptococci (56,57).

Pharyngitis due to Group G streptococci are often related to a common source, usually a food product. These epidemics are characteristic because they occur in general in a short period of time, and it is possible in many cases to recognize a common food vehicle. Episodes with a high attack rates have been reported (58).

There are no significant differences between pharyngitis that is caused by *S. pyogenes* and Group C or G streptococci for symptoms, severity, or duration of the disease. Moreover, in many cases caused by Group G streptococci, a significant increase in antistreptolysin O titres may be found (59).

S. dysgalactiae var. *equisimilis* has been reported to cause both maternal and neonatal hospital infections following the transmission via common objects of use and/or associated with obstetrical complications. Skin and soft tissue infections among individuals with underlying diseases (e.g., diabetes mellitus, venous or lymphatic compromise) are reported. Clinical manifestations include pyoderma, cellulitis, erysipelas, and surgical wound infections (60).

Serious invasive disease and bacteremia due to *S. zooepidemicus* may occur among patients following the exposure to animals or animal products (61). In other instances, the portal of entry was likely the skin, since bacteremia followed postoperative wound infections or transcutaneous procedures.

D. Viridans streptococci

Species belonging to the "viridans" group are major causes of endocarditis. Several different species have been reported to cause endocarditis including *S. mitis*, *S. bovis*, *S. mutans*, *S. sanguis*, and others, but there does not appear that a single streptococcal species is significantly associated with particular clinical manifestations or outcomes of disease.

Due to its participation in the plaque-forming process, *S. mutans* is thought to be involved in dental caries. *S. bovis* has been frequently found in patients with bowel malignancies. All members of the group can be isolated from blood cultures, but only a minority of the episodes are thought to be clinically significant due to the transient nature of the bacteremia and the low virulence of the organism.

Moreover, viridans streptococci are an emerging cause of bacteremia in patients undergoing intensive chemotherapy for acute leukemia or allogenic bone marrow transplantation.

Endocarditis and bacteremia are the most relevant clinical illnesses caused by viridans streptococci. Virtually all the species belonging to the viridans group may cause endocarditis, but due to the continuous changes in taxonomy, it is difficult to attribute greater causation to any particular species. There does not appear to be a significant correlation between the different streptococcal species and the extent of clinical manifestations. In the past, rheumatic fever or congenital heart disease were the main predisposing factors for endocarditis (37-76% and 6-24% respectively). Presently, in countries where rheumatic fever has declined, the main predisposing factors are degenerative valvular lesions (21%) and initial valve prolapse (29%) (62). While infective endocarditis from viridans streptococci is not common in drug users (6%), it occurs frequently in patients known to have heart disease (55%), and with a rate significantly higher than that found in patients not known to have heart disease (29%) (63). The onset of subacute endocarditis is generally insidious. Symptoms may develop within two weeks from the presumed onset, but often the diagnosis will be established after 5-6 weeks or more (64). The most common finding is fever (present in all patients except in those who receive a concomitant antibiotic treatment) (65) which may be accompanied by general symptoms such as fatigue, anorexia, weightloss, and malaise. Splenomegaly is observed in about 50% of patients (66). Osler's nodes, petechiae, splinter hemorrhages, and other manifestations of immune complex circulation may be present. Cardiac murmurs are almost uniformaly present. The diagnosis is achieved on the basis of a continuous low grade bacteremia (1-30 CFU/ml. of blood), in the absence of a recent antibiotic therapy, among 96% of patients at their first blood culture (67). Echocardiography is also commonly used to confirm the diagnosis of endocarditis.

E. S. pneumoniae

S. pneumoniae causes infection of the middle ear, sinus, trachea, bronchi, and lungs by direct spread of organisms from upper respiratory tract colonization. Hematogenous spread is thought to be responsible for the infection of the central nervous system, and occasionally of heart valves, bones, joints, and peritoneal cavity. Several conditions predispose to pneumococcal infection: in addition to primary or secondary immunodeficiencies and to an excess likelihood of exposure, patients suffering from pneumococcal infections often have a history of respiratory infections (influenza or other) or inflammatory conditions such as asthma, chronic obstructive pulmonary disease, or cigarette smoking.

1. Pneumonia

Pneumococcal pneumonia usually begins in the right lower, right middle or left lower lobe which are areas where gravity is most likely to carry upper respiratory secretions that are aspirated during sleep. The usual lesion is segmental or lobar in extension, but in children or in elderly, there may be patchy involvement. Pneumococcal pneumonia evolves in defined stages of lung involvement. These stages represent the evolution of the inflammatory response as determined by the effects of pneumococcal components on the immune system.

The outcome of the infection depends, at least in part, on the ability of the host to withstand the inflammation that is associated with bacterial death. With the arrest of infection, the exudate undergoes liquefaction, and inflammatory debris is removed by expectoration and via lymphatic channels. Due to the relatively low toxin-mediate damage, resolution of the disease is associated with restoration to a normal state of lung architecture.

A common respiratory disease (e.g., viral) often precedes the pneumonia. A rapid onset of fever and chills occurs in more than 80%, and may be accompanied by tachycardia, tachypnea, severe pleuritic pain, and cough. The intense chest pain may inhibit deep inspiration and thus respiration can become rapid and superficial. As a result of hypoxia, caused by abnormal ventilation-perfusion match, patients may become mildly cyanotic. They appear acutely ill and have a cough that is productive of a pinkish "rusty" mucoid sputum. After 7-10 days, diaphoresis, abrupt defervescence (crisis), and a dramatic improvement in well-being characterize the resolution. Less commonly, patients can recover through a more gradual return of temperature to normal (lysis). Death in some patients is associated with one or more complications. The most frequent complication is pleural effusion that is detectable in nearly one-half of all patients, while empyema occurs in less than 1% of patients. The quantity of exudate may become large enough to displace mediastinal structure and contribute to the worsening of oxygenation. Lung abscess is a rare sequel to pneumococcal infection, but pneumococcal infection. Metastatic infections may result in arthritis, endocarditis and meningitis.

2. Otitis media

S. pneumoniae is the most common isolate from the middle ear of patients with otitis media (approximately 35%). It frequently follows a viral infection of upper respiratory tract. Pneumococci reach the middle ear trough the Eustachian tube. Clinical manifestations include a sense of fullness, hearing loss, vertigo, and/or tinnitus, but the hallmarks of middle ear infection are fever, pain and purulent otorrhea if the tympanic membrane undergoes perforation. Almost invariably there is an involvement of the mastoid, because of the direct communication with the middle ear.

3. Meningitis

Pneumococcal meningitis can develop as a primary disease without signs of infection elsewhere, as a complication of pneumococcal pneumonia, or by extension from otitis, mastoiditis, or sinusitis. The mechanisms underlying the pneumococcal migration from circulation across the blood-brain barrier and into the subarachnoid space, in the absence of a skull fracture, are poorly understood. The role of choline on pneumococcal cell wall and its ability to bind PAF receptors have been recently highlighted. Once pneumococci enter and replicate in the cerebrospinal fluid (CSF), subarachnoid space inflammation results as a consequence of the bacterial release of cell wall components and DNA. Inflammation is largely responsible for the pathophysiologic consequences that contribute to the clinical manifestations of pneumococcal meningitis.

Clinical manifestation include headache, chills, fever, and meningismus, with nuchal rigidity. Cranial nerve palsies and cerebral dysfunction that is manifested by confusion, delirium, or a declining level of consciousness may also occur. CSF is under increased pressure, appears cloudy, and shows a high protein and low glucose content. Stained smears reveal Gram positive diplococci and increased polymorphonuclear cells.

With appropriate therapy, full recovery can be obtained in more than 70-90% of patients.

F. Enterococci

Most enterococcal infections occur among hospitalized patients. Major risks for acquiring nosocomial enterococcal infections include a serious underlying disease, the presence of urinary or vascular catheters, and prior antibiotic therapy. Use of advanced therapeutic or diagnostic invasive procedures in an environment where antibiotics are commonly used may allow enterococci to invade debilitated patients after by-passing natural mucosal barriers.

1. Bacteremia

Patients with bacteremia usually develop abrupt fever, chills, tachycardia, tachypnea, and hypotension. The occurrence of enterococcal bacteremia in previously ill patients may develop in the absence of fever or even with hypothermia. In these cases, manifestation of encephalopathy such as disorientation or confusion may be early signs of bacteremia. Following enterococcal bacteremia, metastatic infections rarely occur. Mortality rates after bacteremia are high, but this may be a function of the tendency to infect debilitated patients.

2. Urinary tract infections

Enterococcal urinary tract infections are closely associated with the use of catheters which lead to increased colonization of the urinary tract. The frequency of isolation of enterococci from urinary tract in hospitalized patients shows an increasing trend and has risen from 6% to 16% through 1973-1984 in one study (68) and from 11.1% to 20.8% over 1980-85 in another study (69). The nature of enterococcal interaction with uroepithelial cells is complex and not well understood. In vitro studies, however, have emphasized the potential role played by the sex pheromone system. In particular, the aggregation substance was shown to mediate adhesion not only between different *E. faecalis* strains but also between *E. faecalis* and eukaryotic cells. Enterococci may cause cystitis, pyelonephritis, perinephric abscesses, and prostatitis in hospitalized patients. Symptoms may be minimal unless pyelonephritis develops. Typical symptoms of cystitis such as dysuria, frequency, and urgency may be diminished by the presence of a catheter.

3. Endocarditis

Enterococci cause about 6-15% of native valve endocarditides, and are usually associated with a left-sided endocarditis. Diagnosis is confirmed by echocardiography and positive blood cultures. Patients complain of arthralgias while splenomegaly and petechiae are frequently observed in diseases of long duration. There may be a normocytic, normochromic anemia. In general, the clinical course of enterococcal endocarditis is subacute, and the clinical picture is indistinguishable from that of viridans streptococcal endocarditis.

4. Other infections

Enterococci have also been isolated, alone or in combination with other microrganisms, in intra-abdominal infections, neonatal sepsis, and endophthalmitis, but their role as primary pathogens is controversial.

III. EPIDEMIOLOGY OF INFECTION

A. *S. pyogenes*

Pharyngeal carriage rates have been reported as high as 15-20% among children, but this may be dependent on the season and the geographical area. Carriage is less frequent among adults.

Pharyngitis is one of the most common infections among children, and a majority of such infections caused by bacteria are due to group A streptococci, although groups C and G are occasionally reported as causative agents. The peak incidence is in school children but all age groups are susceptible. As spreading occurs by direct contact or via large salivary droplets, crowding may favor epidemic spread. Large outbreaks of pharyngitis from contaminated food are also reported while personal objects (clothing, blankets) do not seem to play a role.

In untreated patients, the organism may persist for several weeks after the end of the symptomatic disease. During the first days of illness, GAS may be isolated in large numbers from the nose and pharynx, while organisms decrease in number during the convalescence and virulence. Antibodies to the infecting strain or its products are detectable in patients 3-8 weeks after the infection.

In contrast to pharyngitis, purulent streptococcal infections of the skin (pyoderma) occur more frequently in pre-school aged children. The level of hygiene and ambient temperature influence the prevalence of the disease. Transmission, likely by direct contact, is preceded by colonization of the intact skin in many cases. Strains that cause skin infections are different from those that cause throat infections; they belong to a multiplicity of M protein serotypes and may easily lose their M protein thus making it difficult to type them by the commonly used laboratory methods. These strains are able to colonize the throat but, in general, do not cause symptoms.

The epidemiology of severe *S. pyogenes* infections and their sequelae has widely changed in the last 50 years in several parts of the world, while it has not changed at all in many developing countries. Particular serotypes are more commonly associated with particular non-suppurative sequelae (Table 3).

The rate of rheumatic fever in Minnesota was 100/100,000 in the mid-1950s (70). This rate had remarkably decreased in the following two decades in many U.S. states. A survey in Memphis, Tennessee indicated a frequency of 0.5/100,000/year in the early 1980s (71), but in Baltimore, Maryland the incidence of rheumatic fever in the same period was reported to be lower than 1/100,000 (72).

In contrast to industrialized countries, where the primary manifestations of group A streptococcal infection were mainly pharyngitis and superficial skin infections, no significant changes had been seen in many developing countries where the magnitude of the problem of rheumatic fever on rheumatic heart disease remained unchanged. On the basis of a WHO survey conducted during 1986-1990, the prevalence of severe rheumatic fever in children was 12.6/1000 in Zambia, 10.2/1000 in Sudan, and 7.9/1000 in Bolivia (73). It has been estimated that 25-40% of all cardiovascular diseases in developing countries have a rheumatic origin. It should be noted, however, that the incidence of GAS upper respiratory tract infections and the circulation of the microorganism had probably not decreased in industrialized countries where an easier access to medical treatment prevented severe streptococcal disease and post-streptococcal sequelae, In the mid-1980s, new events occurred and for the first time in U.S., individual cases and outbreaks of acute rheumatic fever were reported (74). Even though the number of the cases was limited in comparison with developing countries, it represented a remarkable change for several U.S. states. It is interesting to note that this resurgence of rheumatic fever was not reported by other countries, and it seemed to be limited to North America. During the late 1980s, after the reemergence of episodes of rheumatic disease, severe and suppurative systemic infections were reported (e.g., necrotizing fasciitis, malignant scarlet fever, streptococcal toxic shock) (75). In contrast to rheumatic fever, these diseases were not limited to North America and reports from Europe were also published (76,77).

The reasons for the re-emergence of these GAS severe infections have not been fully realized. It seems, however, enticing to attribute them to an enhanced but undefined virulence of circulating strains.

Originally, only a limited number of M serotypes (e.g., M1, M3) seemed to be associated with severe infections, but further observation showed that several different M serotypes were isolated from serious systemic diseases in different geographical areas. Therefore, some specific properties of these virulent strains rather than a specific serotype seemed to be responsible for the enhanced virulence.

Table 3 Predominant *S. pyogenes* M serotypes that are associated with non-suppurative sequelae.

Acute rheumatic fever	Acute glomerulonephritis
1	1
3	2
5	4
6	12
14	25
18	49
19	55
24	57
	59
	60
	61

Moreover, the low attack rate of severe infections (estimated by the Centres for Disease Control to be 1/100,000) suggests that, in addition to the spread of highly virulent clones, predisposing host factors such as the lack of specific anti-M and anti-pyrogenic toxin antibodies were necessary for the development of such disease.

B. *S. agalactiae*

According to recent data from an active surveillance system for invasive GBS infections in Maryland, the annual incidence of early and late-onset disease is 1.3/1000 and 0.5/1000 live births respectively, and the total case-fatality ratio corresponds to 8% (78). Data from the same study, relative to the annual incidence of GBS diseases for non-pregnant adults reported 6.5/100,000 cases with a case fatality ratio of 12%.

The gastrointestinal tract is the most likely human reservoir of GBS, with the genitourinary tract being the most common site of secondary spread. GBS can also be carried in the throat. Asymptomatic GBS infections of the genital tract occur both in men and in women. Among sexual partners of genitally-colonized women, urethral isolation of GBS can be found in nearly one-half. During pregnancy, GBS may colonize the urinary tract causing asymptomatic bacteriuria. Vaginal colonization rates can differ among ethnic groups, geographical areas and age, but are similar for pregnant and non-pregnant women. In a recent study performed in the United States (54) among 546 mothers, a colonization rate of 28% was found; the prevalence being higher in blacks and Hispanics than in whites (40.6% and 26.9%, respectively vs. 20.3%) and was not influenced by socioeconomic factors. One to 2% of neonates born to colonized mothers develop a symptomatic early-onset septicemia, but the relative risk of invasive infection is considerably increased when one or more of the risk factors reported in Table 4 are present. GBS vertical transmission to neonates can be significantly reduced when mothers receive intrapartum antibiotics (0% vs 52%) (54) according to the protocol for prevention of perinatal GBS diseases (7). Horizontal transmission from hospital staff may account for some late-onset diseases.

In the United States since the early 1990s, the analysis of capsular serotypes (see below) in GBS isolates from invasive pediatric and non-pregnant adult diseases has shown the emergence of a new serotype, namely type V. In early-onset disease, there is no predominance of a particular serotype, while in the late-onset disease, serotype III predominates (60% of the isolates). The frequency with whichdifferent serotypes were isolated in the last decade from early-onset diseases varies depending on the studies (Ia, 36-40%; Ib, 1-9%; II, 6-11%; III, 27-38%, V, 13-15%). In the late 1990s, type V was also

Table 4   Risk factors for invasive newborn GBS diseases.

GBS urinary tract infection	GBS carriage in late pregnancy
Heavy colonization with GBS	Premature delivery
Fever during labor	Labor or rupture of membranes before 37 wks.
Rupture of membranes 18 hrs. or more before delivery	Prolonged obstetrical manipulation
Low level of antibody to type-specific capsular polysaccharide	Previous baby with GBS disease
Caesarean section	

the most frequent type isolated from cases of invasive disease in non-pregnant adults, and accounted for 29% of the isolates. Other serotypes commonly found among non-pregnant adults included Ia (27% of isolates), III (14%), Ib, and II (13% each) (78).

In Japan, serotypes VI and VIII (rarely isolated in other parts of the world) were the predominant serotypes among pregnant women (VIII, 35.6%; VI, 24.7%) (79).

C. Beta-hemolytic Groups C and G streptococci

Human isolates of *S. dysgalactiae* were originally recognized as part of the normal human flora of the nasopharynx, skin, and genital tract and have also been cultured from umbilical specimens of healthy neonates, but in recent years, several reports have indicated that these organisms are important pathogens (80). In many of these patients, underlying conditions have been noted (e.g., age, alcoholism, immunosuppressive therapy, underlying malignancy); in those patients infections are in general of endogenous origin. Group C and G streptococcal suppurative infections are often severe, and resemble those caused by Groups A and B beta-hemolytic streptococci (59,61). Group C organisms are common pathogens in domestic animals. Some human infections may be traced to an animal source and have also been associated with the consumption of homemade cheese or unpasteurized milk.

D. Viridans streptococci

Viridans streptococci are common inhabitants of the respiratory and intestinal tract of various animals and humans. Some species are amongst the earliest colonizers of the oral cavity after birth; some such as *S. sanguis* and *S. mutans* are found only after the first deciduous teeth have erupted. These bacteria are common inhabitants of the upper respiratory tract, the female genital tract, and the gastrointestinal tract, and they are the prevalent flora in the oral cavity. Viridans streptococci account for 45% of the total viable bacterial count of the tongue surface, 46% in saliva, 28% in dental plaque, and 29% in gingival crevices (81). Depending on their selective adherence to various oral tissues, *S. salivarius* predominates on the tongue, *S. mitis* on the buccal mucosa, and *S. mutans* and *S. sanguis* are often associated with teeth. In healthy individuals, the colonization by viridans streptococci prevents the establishment of more pathogenic bacteria such as enterococci or Gram negatives. Fibronectin, a protein found on the surface of mucosal cells, promotes the attachment of *S. salivarius*, *S. mutans*, and *S. mitis*; when fibronectin is lost or decreased as in chronically ill patients, the adherence of Gram negative organisms to oral mucosa increases (82). Therefore, the selective adherence of viridans streptococci can be regarded as a protective mechanism for the host to prevent of Gram negative respiratory infections.

Although viridans streptococci are considered organisms of low virulence, they can be the causes of serious life-threatening diseases. Infections with viridans streptococci are in general caused by the spread of endogenous organisms outside of their natural habitat in predisposed or immunocompromised hosts. Electrophoretic fingerprinting techniques have demonstrated a connection between oral isolates and isolates from blood or heart valve lesions. Dental extractions allow for entrance of micro-organisms into the circulation. In the pre-antibiotic era, viridans sreptococci were responsible for 75% of cases of infective endocarditis (83). In the current era, their frequency has decreased to 30-40 %. The most commonly identified organisms in endocarditis belong to *S. sanguis*, *S. oralis*, or *S. gordonii*. This is due to the increased numbers of patients who acquire staphylococcal endocarditis due to risk factors which included presence of prosthetic valves or injection drug use (84). Viridans streptococci account for 2-5% of positive blood cultures (although only 21% of these are considered as clinically significant). Conversely, despite the frequency with which they cause bacteremia or endocarditis, they are not frequent causes of meningitis (0.3-2.4%) (85,86).

While *S. sanguis*, *S. mitis*, *S. oralis*, and *S. gordonii* are frequently isolated from cases of subacute endocarditis (87,88). *S. intermedius* may be found as a member of polymicrobial infections including abscesses in liver and brain, and other members of the '*S. anginosus* group' may be isolated from oral abscesses and female genital infections.

Among neutropenic patients, viridans streptococci are increasing as causes of bacteremia and endocarditis which can be complicated by acute respiratory distress syndrome and shock. Species such as *S. oralis*, *S. mitis*, and *S. salivarius* are frequently isolated. *S. bovis*, (particularly biotype I), besides being a cause of endocarditis, is frequently isolated from patients with malignancies of the gastrointestinal tract (89). A strong association between *S. bovis* bacteremia and underlying malignancy of the colon has been noted. In a survey of patients with colon cancer, 56% of the patients in comparison with 10% of the healthy controls and 28% of patients with inflammatory bowel diseases were found to have *S. bovis* in their feces (90), and other studies have later confirmed this observation (91). Patients with *S. bovis* bacteremia are now currently examined for colon disease.

E. *S. pneumoniae*

The pneumococcus is a common inhabitant of naso- and oro-pharynges of healthy people; by appropriate methods, it can be detected in 20-40% of healthy children and 5-10% of the adults. Children become transiently colonized as early as six months of age. There is a decrease in the duration of the carriage for each successive acquired serotype. This high rate of carriage contributes to the difficulty for interpreting positive sputum cultures.

In developed countries where conjugate vaccines have strongly reduced *H. influenzae* invasive disease, pneumococci are the major causes of meningitis (43,000 cases/yr. in the U.S.) (92). About 7,000,000 illnesses of otitis media, 500,000 pneumonias, and 50,000 bacteremias per year are attributed to *S. pneumoniae*. The rate of infection is estimated to be 20/100,000 in young adults and 280/100,000 in elderly populations that have low levels of specific protective antibodies (93).

Although strains can be transferred by airborne droplets, epidemics are rare. Risk for infection is increased among those with low socioeconomic status and in overcrowded living conditions e.g. prisons, homeless shelters, mines, and military corps. The incidence of infection appears to be seasonally related with clear increase in cold months. Pneumococcal disease usually occurs when organisms spread from the initial natural site of colonization (throat, nasopharynx) to distal loci such the lung, ear, meninges, and paranasal sinus. Bacteremia can occur following all of these infections.

At risk are individuals with impairment of bacterial clearance from the respiratory tract (e.g., viral respiratory diseases), or from blood (e.g., asplenic) patients, and those with hematological disorders (e.g., malignancy, sickle cell disease).

Increased resistance of pneumococci to penicillin had been reported since the 1960s, but only at the end of the 1970s did strains with high level resistance to penicillin (MICs >1 mg./L.) emerge from South Africa and in the early 1980s from Spain (94). After that, a rapid increase in the incidence of penicillin resistance was reported in several countries (e.g., South Africa, Spain, Hungary, Japan, Thailand, and others) where more than 50% of the isolates were resistant (95). In the U.S., the resistance in recent years reached 25% (96), while in Europe, except for Spain, the resistance seemed to be generally lower (e.g., U.K. - 3.6% in 1995) (95). Subsequently, strains with resistance to penicillin and to the extended-spectrum cephalosporins emerged in the U.S. (96). The resistance is predominantly found in some serotypes and in particular those more commonly found in children (6B, 14, 19A, 19F, 23 F). Due to recombination, resistance can easily spread to other serotypes as has happened recently: a new clone has probably emerged by the spread of PBP altered genes from a resistant clone to a susceptible serotype 9V organism (97). In some countries, a rapid increase of resistance has occurred in a short time period (e.g. Hong Kong - 6.6% in 1993 to 55.8% for sputum isolates (98).

Resistance to macrolides, not frequently found in the past, became widely apparent recently in some countries: France - 26% (99), U.S. - 10-23% (100). Other resistances [e.g., to chloramphenicol (due to production of an acetyl transferase), tetracycline, or co-trimoxazole] can be found.

F.   Enterococci

Enterococci are able to survive and grow in a very wide range of conditions of temperature, pH, and salt concentrations, and they can be found in different environments: soil, food, water, plant, animal, birds, and insects (101,102). In humans and in other animals, their normal habitat is the gastrointestinal tract and the female genital tract. Small numbers of enterococci are occasionally found in oropharyngeal secretions and on the skin, especially in the perineal area. The prevalence of different species may be influenced by age, diet, and other changes in physiological conditions (103). While for some species such as *E. faecalis* and *E. faecium* a large body of epidemiological information has been collected over time, but only limited information is available for the others perhaps due to the changes in taxonomy.

Enterococci are normal human commensals and are adapted to the rich, oxygen depleted, complex gastrointestinal environment. They are the predominant Gram positive cocci in feces with concentrations up to 10^8CFU/gm. of feces, but nevertheless they yet account for less than 0.01% of normal bowel flora which is represented for the main part by various obligate anaerobes (104). The ubiquitous nature of enterococci may complicate the clinical significance of a particular isolate. It was thought that enterococci, as a part of normal gut population, were in the majority of cases only causes of endogenous infection, but most enterococcal infections occur in hospitalized patients, and organisms causing infections often appear to be exogenously acquired (105). Evidence of spread between patients and from one institution to another has been reported (106). Even though medical devices have been demonstrated to play some role in the spread of resistant organisms (107), the importance of hospital environment as a source of infection is difficult to assess because the environment may be only passively contaminated by fecal material, and direct cross infection (with the exception of drug addicts) is generally rare (108,109).

In the U.S., enterococci cause 110,000 urinary tract infections, 25,000 epidsodes of bacteremia, 40,000 wound infections, and more than 100 cases of endocarditis per year (15-20% of total cases) (110). About 90% of enterococcal infections are caused by *E. faecalis* and the remaining 10% by *E. faecium* and other enterococcal species (111). Enterococci are responsible for a remarkable number (10-12%) of all hospital-acquired infections :10-20% of urinary tract infections and 5-10% of bacteremias (112). Even if, in the majority of cases, the increasing isolation rate is caused by multiple endogenous strains, epidemic infections do occur most probably due to spread from patient to patient on the hands of hospital staff. Important reasons that allow survival in the hospital environment include resistance to many disinfectants (e.g., such as aqueous chlorhexidine and povidone-iodine used for handwashing) and the intrinsic or acquired resistance to antimicrobials.

Although the spectrum of infections caused by enterococci did not substantially change since 1990 (113,114), the prevalence of these organisms as nosocomial pathogens is clearly increasing. Enterococci are the third common cause of nosocomial bacteremia (behind *Staphylococcus aureus* and coagulase-negative staphylococci) and the second most common cause (after *Escherichia coli)* of urinary tract infections (111). They are intrinsically resistant to different classes of antimicrobials that may be active against other streptococci, and they can acquire high levels of resistance to glycopeptides and aminoglycosides.

Vancomycin-resistant enterococci (VRE) had been isolated in the U.K. and France in 1986 (115,116), and in the U.S. in 1989 (117). VRE has since become a significant problem throughout the world usually affecting immunocompromised hosts. In the U.S., VRE is presently the second most common cause of hospital-acquired infections; the incidence of VRE over1989-1993 increased from 0.3% to 8% (in ICUs, from 0.4 to 13.6%) (116). Data collected by The Surveillance Network (TSN) database - U.S. for years 1995-1997 showed that while ampicillin and vancomycin resistance was still uncommon among *E. faecalis*, an alarming increase was seen for *E. faecium* where 52% of isolates exhibited vancomycin resistance and 83% were resistant to ampicillin (118). In Europe, the incidence of VRE appears to be lower for the time being. In a recent report by an European VRE study group (119) that was performed for 49 hospitals in 27 countries, vancomycin resistance in *E. faecium* was reported to be 2.9% and in *E. faecalis* - 0.03%. Other enterococcal species appear to be more resistant (e.g., *E.*

casseliflavus 4.8%, *E. gallinarum* 48%). Prior treatment with antibiotics is common among patients who become colonized or infected (120). The use of clindamycin, cephalosporins, ciprofloxacin, aminoglycosides, metronidazole, and other broad spectrum antibiotics often has limited or no activity against enterococci, but by reducing the normal anaerobic population, may lead to enterococcal overgrowth at sites with risk of infection and may help select for resistant organisms. In the U.S., oral vancomycin has been used for many years as the first choice therapy for *Clostridium difficile* infections or as a part of gut decontamination regimens. Since 1975, avoparcin, a glycopeptide which may have cross-resistance to both vancomycin and teichoplanin, has been extensively used as growth promoter among animal feeds in Europe. Even if the hypothesis of transmission to man via the food chain has not received firm evidence, it nevertheless appears reasonable that the presence of VRE in the community and environment may facilitate the replacement of or the supplementation to the resident enterococcal population.

IV. NATURE OF THE BACTERIUM, PATHOGENESIS, AND CLINICAL MANIFESTATIONS

A. *S. pyogenes*

S. pyogenes is a Gram positive, non-motile, catalase-negative, non-spore forming organism, showing spherical or ovoid cells (0.6-1μm) in pairs or in short chains from solid media or in pathological samples and long chains in liquid media. Like other streptococci this organism is facultatively anaerobic; colonies are surrounded by a zone of complete hemolysis (β-hemolysis) when grown on blood agar.

Group A streptococci possess a large number of somatic constituents and extracellular products. On the basis of their known functions, some of these products have been categorized as virulence factors. Their function in vivo has not yet been demonstrated for many of them while multiple domains with different functions in the same molecule have been demonstrated for others. The knowledge of the exact role in pathogenesis of the different components is made more complicated by the fact that nature likes to be redundant and that similar functions may be accomplished by different molecules in different serotypes or in different strains.

The most external layer of *S. pyogenes* is formed by a capsule of hyaluronic acid. This capsule has been shown to protect the organism from ingestion by phagocytes and epithelial cells, therefore enhancing its virulence in animal models but also impairing the attachment to human epithelial cells. In a recent study, Wessels and colleagues demonstrated that, in addition to modulating the binding of other bacterial molecules, the capsule may itself act as an adhesin to the hyaluronic acid-binding protein CD44 on human keratinocytes (121).

The Lancefield group polysaccharide is linked to the surface of the peptidoglycan and may be extracted from the cell wall by different methods.

Several proteins protrude from the cell surface. The great majority of them contains domains that can interact with molecules that are found in body fluids such as immunoglobulin, fibrinogen, fibronectin and albumin. Many of these proteins (e.g., M proteins, IgA binding proteins, IgG/fibrinogen binding protein, serum opacity factor, fibronectin binding proteins) are fixed to the cell membrane through a C terminal complex which contains identical or very similar motifs (122). Among these proteins, M protein is probably the most extensively studied. It is thought to be the major virulence factor since strains rich in this protein are capable of initiating disease and multiply actively in fresh human blood by escaping from the phagocytosis of polymorphonuclear leukocytes; M negative strains are avirulent. M proteins have also been demonstrated to mediate the binding of streptococci to keratinocytes through a receptor, the membrane co-factor protein (MCP or CD46), a membrane-bound complement regulatory protein (123). Other two closely related proteins, SfbI and F1, bind fibronectin with high affinity and are considered both adhesins and invasins. Lipoteichoic acid is also thought to play a role in the adherence of the microorganism.

Group A streptococci are currently typed on the basis of their M protein antigens; more than 80 different serotypes are known. The acquired immunity against streptococcal infections appears to be linked to the development of antibodies against the part of the M protein that is responsible for anti-phagocytic activity; it is type specific and long-lasting. The reason for which particular M serotypes are more likely to cause pharyngitis, ARF, skin infections, and/or AGN are not understood.

Another important protein that has been demonstrated to be very useful for typing is the serum opacity factor (OF) which is an α-lipoproteinase that can opacify horse serum. This protein is antigenic and type-specific; its reaction with serum can be inhibited only by homologous serum. Twenty-nine of the known M types produce specific OF that, in addition, can be detected among isolates that lose their M protein. Therefore, OF typing represent a valuable complement to M typing. A third surface protein, not associated with virulence but widely used for typing, is T protein. This protein may be found in more than 90% of isolates and it appears to be very useful for typing when the M protein cannot be detected, but the number of T serotypes is fewer than the number of M types and several M types may correspond to one T type.

In addition, to its cellular components which can be released in the medium during the growth or after the death of the bacterium, GAS release several products which show a variety of toxic properties.

Among these factors, the most widely studied, also due to the recent resurgence in the frequency and severity of streptococcal invasive diseases, are the large family of pyrogenic toxin superantigens (PTSAAgs) including four well-characterized and serologically-distinct pyrogenic exotoxins (SpeA, SpeB, SpeC and SpeF) and other related antigens. These toxins have low molecular weights (below 30 kD), are heat-stable and are relatively resistant to proteolytic degradation. While SpeA and SpeC are encoded by lysogenic phages (124,125) and SpeA in particular is produced by many M1 and M3 (126) strains that have been isolated from cases of TSS, SpeB appears to be different in several regards. In fact, this toxin, which has been shown to be a protease, is released as a precursor of 43 kD and results, after cleavage, in a 28 kD protein (127). SpeB is not encoded by a phage, and its gene (like SPEF but at difference with SpeA and SSA whose genes are variably present in the strains) may be found in all the *S. pyogenes* strains, even though the proteins may be detected in less than 60% of strains. SpeB has been demonstrated to cleave the portion of M protein that is responsible for the strain's serological M type. This makes the strain more easily cleared by the reticuloendothelial system and less resistant to phagocytosis (128). These toxins were formerly called erythrogenic toxins because their expression causes the characteristic rash that is seen in scarlet fever; the rash results from a hypersensitivity reaction likely linked to superantigen properties of these molecules (see below).

Other important GAS products are the cytolytic toxins, better known as streptolysin O (SLO; oxygen-labile) and streptolysin S (SLS; oxygen-stable). Both are produced by all strains of GAS.

Streptolysin O is reversibly inhibited by oxygen and irreversibly by cholesterol; it binds to cholesterol that is present in eukaryotic membranes, and forms transmembrane pores. It is toxic to a variety of cells including erythrocytes, platelets, and mammalian heart. Streptolysin O is antigenic, and anti-SLO antibodies are used as a marker for a recent streptococcal infections (ASOT).

Streptolysin S is responsible for the beta-hemolysis of the strains grown on the surface of blood agar media. It is a non-antigenic cell-bound peptide which is inactivated by phospholipids and may be easily extracted by whole serum, serum albumin, or α-lipoproteins, and may be, by this means, transferred to its final target which is membrane phospholipid. The mechanism by which it results in cell lysis is not completely understood but, at difference with other molecules that are released during cell proliferation, SLS may be produced by resting cells (129).

Other surface or released products include NADase, DNAase, hyaluronidase, streptokinase, amylase, esterase, enolase, among others. Some of these are glycolytic enzymes and are involved in the production of ATP; many of these may be used by the organism to facilitate spreading through tissues and for the liquefaction of pus. Moreover, several of them are antigenic and, like the ASOT, can be used in the serodiagnosis of streptococcal infections. Among the virulence factors of GAS, it is therefore possible to distinguish those which are involved in bacterial adherence to epithelial cells or those which inhibit or retard phagocytosis and thus favor bacterial growth and spread from those which cause host tissue injury or systemic involvement (Table 5). In addition to mechanisms of acute virulence, several components of GAS have been associated with the development of non-suppurative sequelae of GAS infection.

The mechanisms involved in the ability of GAS to cross mucosal or epidermal barriers and cause systemic infeciton are not completely understood. A critical step in systemic invasion seems to be related to the possibility for GAS to be internalized by epithelial cells (130). Thus, molecules involved in its adhesion to and internalization into epithelial cells are thought to be virulence factors that favor col-

Table 5   Virulence factors of GAS.

	Biological effect	Mechanism of action
Interference with phagocytosis		
capsule	interference with opsonization	non-immunogenic component that does not induce specific antibodies
M protein	interference with opsonization	binds Factor H that, in turn, degrades the complement factor C3b bound on the cell surface
C5a peptidase	reduces PMN chemotaxis	enzymatically degrades the chemotactic C5a fragment of complement
Increase of epithelial cell binding		
F protein	binds fibronectin	
lipoteichoic acid	binds fibronectin	
Induction of toxic effects		
streptolysin S	tissue injury	lyses erythrocytes, leucocytes, platelets, and stimulate the release of lysosomal enzymes
streptolysin O	tissue injury	lyses erythrocytes, leukocytes, platelets, and stimulates the release of lysosomal enzymes
streptokinase	spread of bacteria in tissues	lyses blood clots
DNAase	spread of bacteria in tissues	degrades free DNA in pus reducing viscosity of abscess material
pyrogenic exotoxins	systemic effects due to activation of both innate and adaptive immune system; scarlatiniform rash	release of cytokines from macrophages and T lymphocytes

onization. Although adhesion is not sufficient to promote internalization, it is believed to be critical to the initiation of the preocess which is dependent on at least two classes of molecules: fibronectin (Fn) binding proteins (131) and M proteins (132). A large body of evidence indicates Fn as the primary GAS cellular receptor, and several Fn-binding proteins have been identified. Proteins SfbI and F1 represent the prototypes of Fn-binding GAS molecules, but several studies have proposed LTA as another adhesin (133). There is also a potential role for M protein in invasiveness (134).

The GAS capsule is composed of a hyaluronic acid that is identical to that which is found in the connective tissue of hosts. The molecular mimicry of GAS capsule with a common host constituent is believed to obviate an anti-capsular immune response by means of self-tolerance. This results in the absence of anti-capsular antibody and in an anti-phagocytic function exerted by the capsule. M protein and the GAS C5a peptidase are however also involved in inhibiting the phagocyte-mediated clearance of GAS. M protein precipitates fibrinogen directly onto bacterial surface and binds the complement control protein Factor H. C5a peptidase cleaves C5a which is the main PMN chemotactic factor that is released during complement activation (135). These phenomena result in the inhibition of activation of the alternate complement pathway and, consequently, in the lack of opsonization and in complement-mediated PMN chemotaxis. Streptokinase and DNAse are enzymes that are believed to help bacterial spread among tissues by means of digestion of inflammation-induced physical barriers. Streptokinase is a powerful fibrin-digesting enzyme and is currently used in the therapy of myocardial reperfusion (136,137). Pyrogenic exotoxins cause fever in humans and animals and also help in inducing shock by lowering the threshold to exogenous endotoxin (138). Streptococcal pyrogenic exotoxins A and B induce human mononuclear cells to synthesize tumor necrosis factor-α (TNF-α) (139), interleukin-1β (IL-1β), interleukin-2 (IL-2) (140), and interleukin-6 (IL-6). Peptidoglycan, lipoteichoic acid, DNA, and killed organisms (141,142) are also capable of inducing TNF-α production by mononuclear cells in vitro. Exotoxins such as streptolysin O (SLO) are also potent inducers of TNF-α and IL-1b. Pyrogenic exotoxin B, a proteinase precursor, has the ability to cleave pre-IL-1β to release preformed IL-1β (143). All of these mechanisms are likely to contribute to more cytokine release and subsequent tissue damage as well as to the genesis of shock and organ failure. The interaction between these microbial virulence factors and an immune or nonimmune host determines the epidemiology, clinical syndrome, and outcome. Since horizontal transmission of GAS in general is well-documented, a possible explanation for the absence of a high attack rate of invasive infection is a significant herd immunity against one or more of the virulence factors that are responsible for streptococcal diseases (144).

B. *S. agalactiae*

1. *Capsular polysaccharides, lipoteichoic acid, and surface proteins*

GBS are encapsulated Gram positive cocci occurring in chains. Two surface carbohydrate antigens were described by Lancefield (145): the group B polysaccharide which is common to all strains of this serogroup (C carbohydrate) and the type polysaccharide used for the classification into several serotypes: type Ia, Ib, II-VIII. The group B polysaccharide, associated with the cell wall, is composed of rhamnose, N-acetylglucosamine, and galactose (146). The various type capsular polysaccharides, except type VI and VIII, are polymers of repeating units containing glucose, galactose, N-acetylglucosamine, and N-acetylneuraminic acid (sialic acid) which are immunologically distinct since the ratio and the linkages between sugars are peculiar for each serotype (147-152). For instance, type VI polysaccharide lacks N-acetylglucosamine, and type VIII contains rhamnose. Type-specific polysaccharides are localized on the surface of the cell where they form a capsule that can vary in size.

GBS are known to regulate the degree of capsular polysaccharide expression with cell growth rate in relation to nutritional conditions, and with passages in mice increase the virulence and the capsule size (153).

Capsular type-specific polysaccharide is recognized to be the major virulence factor. In fact, hyperimmune rabbit antisera directed against capsule polysaccharide provide passive protection to mice which are challenged with virulent strains from the homologous serotype (154). Sialic acid is a critical element in the epitope of type polysaccharides, since immunization with strains bearing a desialylated capsular polysaccharide fails to elicit protective antibodies against the homologous serotype. In animals models of GBS infections, type III mutants expressing a sialic acid-deficient capsule, or lacking of capsular polysaccharide, were significantly less virulent. The presence of the capsule was also shown to play a major role in the induction of GBS septic arthritis (155).

The sialylated capsule interferes with C3 deposition: type III mutants expressing a sialic acid-deficient capsule, or lacking of capsule, bind C3 in the active form (i.e., C3b), while the inactive form, C3bi, is predominantly bound by the parent strain (156). Therefore, type III capsule mutants are susceptible to opsonophagocytosis in the presence of complement and neutrophils, while the parent strain needs specific antibodies.

Moreover, the capsular polysaccharide plays a role in inducing the release by human monocytes of pro-inflammatory cytokines (TNF-α, IL-1β, IL-6 and IL-8) (157) that are detectable in septic shock and in septic arthritis (158,159). These cytokines are also induced by GBS lipoteichoic acid (LTA) which is an amphiphilic glycolipid polymer that is anchored to the cytoplasmic membrane and which extends through the cell wall and capsule (Figure 1) (160). Clinical isolates of GBS from infants with invasive diseases have higher levels of LTA than strains from asymptomatically colonized infants. Adherence studies performed in vitro demonstrated that GBS attachment to a variety of epithelial cells (fetal, neonatal, and adult) could be mediated by LTA (161). GBS binding to cultured human amnion cells, alveolar epithelial cells, and cultured epithelial cells does not seem to be mediated by LTA, but rather by surface proteins (162). Adherence of GBS to laminin, which is a major component of the basement membrane, is mediated by the surface protein Lmb (laminin-binding) which was recently identified in all serotypes (163).

Many GBS strains possess surface proteins which are believed to contribute to virulence since they elicit protective antibodies in animals and humans (164-166). These include the C and R proteins, and the Rib protein. Strains derived from animals also posses protein X which is uncommon in human strains. The precise role of these proteins in the pathogenesis and protective immunity to GBS infection is not yet clear. Among the best-characterized proteins are those of the C complex (formely Ibc proteins) which consist of four distinct components designated α, β, γ, and δ. C α and β proteins can be detected in the majority of the serotype Ia and II, while all Ib strains possess at least one of the C components. The γ antigen was found to be associated with early-onset sepsis, independent of serotype, and is always expressed together with the α antigen (167). The α and β antigens are very rarely expressed by type III GBS strains, while the δ antigen is only associated with this serotype (167).

2.   GBS hemolysin, enzymes, and other products

A zone of beta-hemolysis surrounds GBS colonies on blood agar. The β-hemolysin was first described by Todd in 1934 as a non-antigenic, oxygen-stable protein. Due to its lability in the absence of stabilizing agents, β-hemolysin has not been isolated and purified. The hemolytic activity is probably related to the amount of an orange carotenoid-like pigment produced by GBS. The hemolysin was shown to have not only a hemolytic activity, but also a cytolytic effect on McCoy cells and on lung epithelial and endothelial cells (168). The expression of β-hemolysin was shown to induce the release of cytoplasmic lactate dehydrogenase both from human alveolar epithelial cells line (A549) and from lung microvascular endothelial cells. Electron microscopy studies indicate that the GBS β-hemolysin acts as a pore-forming toxin and produces membrane disruption, cellular swelling, loss of intracytoplasmic density, and changes in organelles and chromatin which are consistent with water entry into the cell and hypoosmotic damage. The extent of lactate dehydrogenase release induced by HH strains was reduced when the major component of human surfactant was added in a concentration corresponding to the physio-

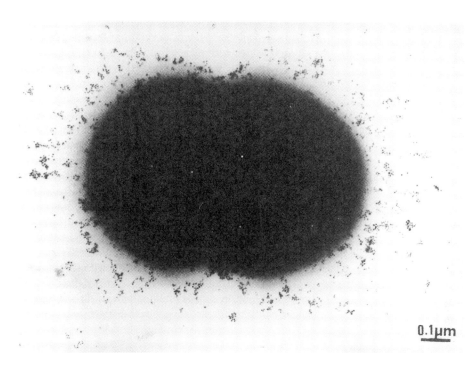

Figure 1   Electron micrograph of unembedded GBS that were incubated with LTA-antibodies and protein A gold complexes thus illustrating LTA about the cell (with permission from Dr. G. Arancia).

logic amount in alveolar fluids during the third trimester of pregnancy.

C5a peptidase, which cleaves the human C5a chemotaxin at histidine residues in the neutrophil binding site, has also been found in GBS strains (169).

Other potential virulence factors for GBS are CAMP factor, hyaluronate lyase (neuraminidase), collagenase, and nucleases for which a clear role in the pathogenesis has not yet been identified.

The CAMP factor (from the name of the original investigators Christie, Atkins and Munch-Peterson) is an extracellular protein that lyses the membranes of erythrocytes which are pre-treated with the beta-hemolysin (sphingomyelinase C) of *Staphylococcus aureus*. CAMP factor binds the Fc portion of human IgG an IgM. The production of this factor is used for a presumptive identification of GBS. The corresponding gene has been recently identified (170) and proposed as a genetic target for PCR assays for the rapid detection of GBS (171).

3.   Pathogenesis of neonatal GBS infection

GBS may asymptomatically colonize the mother while causing very severe invasive diseases in the newborn. Immaturity of newborn host defenses facilitates the onset of GBS diseases. Also, in elderly people and adults with underlying illnesses, the quantitative and qualitative modification of both host-specific and non-specific responses account for GBS disease.

A critical step in the pathogenesis of GBS invasive disease in the newborn is the asymptomatic rectovaginal colonization of pregnant women. The bacterium adheres to vaginal epithelial cells very efficiently as well as to placental membranes, alveolar epithelium and endothelium, and buccal or pharyngeal mucosa; each of these is potentially relevant to vertical transmission and production of invasive diseases in the infant. Binding to cells and to extracellular matrix proteins such as fibronectin, fibrinogen, and laminin is dependent on LTA and surface proteins. Vaginal colonization implies that GBS is able to resist to mucosal immune defenses such as secretory IgA. Heavy maternal colonization has been associated with premature rupture of the membranes as well as with infection of the fetus in utero. Experimentally, GBS has been shown to invade and survive within vacuoles in human cells (172-174); this may account for its ability to overcome host barriers. GBS has been suspected to penetrate into amniotic cavity through intact placental membranes since a fulminant early-onset disease (pneumonia and sepsis) may also develop in infants born by Caesarean section. The aspiration of infected amniotic fluid by the fetus or of infected vaginal secretion by infants while passing through the birth canal allow GBS to reach the lungs. Pneumonia with marked respiratory distress is a hallmark of early-onset. A deficient clearance by the host allows GBS to attain very high concentrations within alveolar spaces. Epithelial and endothelial cell damage, alveolar hemorrhage, interstitial inflammatory exudate, and hyaline formation are present in most pulmonary lesions and may be mediated by the cytotoxic properties of GBS β-hemolysin, which is not inhibited, as in older infants, by the surfactant. GBS can enter alveolar epithelial and pulmonary cells by stimulating their own endocytosis and gain stepwise entry into the bloodstream. All GBS serotypes are capable of invading alveolar epithelial cells. The polysaccharide capsule itself does not appear to be important for invasion. Rather it seems to interfere with it, probably through steric hindrance of receptor-ligand interactions. Direct evidence is accumulating that cellular invasion is a crucial step in the pathogenesis of neonatal disease. Isolates from blood of infected neonates are more invasive than those from vaginal carriers or asymptomatic colonized neonates (173).

Upon entry of GBS into the neonate lung or bloodstream, an immunological response is recruited to clear the bacterium. Newborns, in particular premature infants, have fewer alveolar macrophages than adults and show quantitative deficiencies of the complement system and poor neutrophil chemotaxis. The bacterial capsule plays an important role in limiting the phagocytosis of GBS by lung macrophages, which may, in turn, favor systemic dissemination of the encapsulated microorganism. GBS can survive intracellularly up to 48 hours inside macrophages (174). Moreover, phagocytosis, in the absence of type capsular-specific antibodies and complement, is dramatically reduced. The capsule of type III has been reported to inhibit the deposition of complement C3 and the activation of the alternative pathway. Protein C α and C β retard opsonization by impeding the binding of protective antibodies, and respectively altering their antigenic structure and binding to the Fc portion of immunoglobulins. Neutrophil recruitment to the site of infection is impaired through C5a peptidase which inactivates human complement C5a. Sepsis develops when GBS by bloodstream dissemination reaches multiple body sites where the subsequent tissue penetration results in end-organ disease manifestations such as meningitis, bone and joints infections, etc. The induction of pro-inflammatory cytokines by GBS in the bloodstream and in the cerebrospinal fluid of infants is responsible for the onset of septic shock.

The pathogenesis of the late-onset form is less well understood. Since bacteremia is the presumed first event in the pathogenesis of most late-onset infections, factors promoting the entry of GBS into the bloodstream are of interest. It might be possible that, after colonization of the upper respiratory tract of the infant, GBS bloodstream invasion may be facilitated by mucosal disruption due to intercurrent viral infections which, in fact, are frequently reported to precede late-onset meningitis.

C. Beta-hemolytic Groups C and G streptococci

Adherence is the first step in the process of colonization and infection. As for other Gram positive pathogens, these species produce specific cell wall-associated proteins that are used to bind to host proteins in body fluids or in the extracellular matrix (Table 6). Several bacterial surface proteins are involved in this process such as fibronectin-binding proteins, vitronectin-binding proteins, and collagen-binding proteins (175-177). Another surface protein, C5a peptidase, may function to prevent complement fragment C5a recruitment of phagocytes to the site of infection. Probes that are specific for the peptidase gene from *S. pyogenes* may identify the gene in *S. dysgalactiae* strains of human origin, but fail to identify it in animal isolates (178). M proteins, known to have antiphagocytic effect in *S. pyogenes* and used as reliable antigen for the typing of this microorganism, have been shown on the

Table 6   Virulence factors of human Group C and G beta-hemolytic streptococci.

Function	Bacterial factor
adherence	fibronectin-binding proteins vitronectin-binding proteins collagen-binding proteins
antiphagocytic	M and M-like proteins C5a peptidase
spreading	streptokinase
toxic	streptolysin O

surface of human Group G streptococci; they may play a role in resistance to phagocytosis (179). These antigens have also been shown to cross-react with M typing sera that are raised against group A streptococci (180). Such homology has subsequently been confirmed by genetic studies (181).

Among the proteins that are secreted, streptokinase, an important plasminogen activator (commercially-available), is produced by *S. equisimilis*. Another relevant cytotoxic protein is streptolysin O, whose gene (*slo*), was found in *S. pyogenes*, in *S. dysgalactiae* var. *equisimilis*, and in *S. canis* (182), but not among *S. equi* var. *zooepidemicus*; in both *S. equi* variants, however, there is an oxygen-stable streptolysin which shows a high degree of similarity to group A streptococcal streptolysin S (183). Taken together, these observations show that many of the characteristic factors and mechanisms involved in the colonization and in the pathogenesis of some human Groups C and G streptococci are identical or very similar to those expressed by group A streptococci. Since genomic studies show that Group G streptococci are genetically very different from *S. pyogenes*, however, the most likelyexplanation is that horizontal transfer of the gene coding for M protein has occurred between some Group A and Group G streptococci (184). On the contrary, no pyrogenic exotoxins are produced by Groups C or G streptococci.

D. Viridans streptococci

Viridans streptococci are not known to possess as potent virulence factors as those of beta-hemolytic streptococci nor to produce toxins. Recently, however, a novel cytotoxin, termed intermedilysin and which has some homologies to pneumolysin, has been reported for *S. intermedius* (185). The capacity of these streptococci to cause disease seems to be mainly attributed to the adherence with different substrates and, for some species such as those of the 'S. anginosus group', to the production of degradative enzymes (e.g., glycosidases, nucleases, and hyaluronidases) thus allowing them to multiply in difficult conditions where they must obtain nutrients from host tissue. A peculiarity of the group is their capacity to produce surface polysaccharides in media containing glucose: *S. mutans* and *S. sanguis* produces both water soluble and water insoluble glucan (dextran); *S. salivarius* produce fructan (levan) which may be rapidly metabolized by other components of the oral flora; and many strains of *S. bovis* produce soluble glucan (dextran) and appear to be encapsulated. The two factors which have been most investigated to explain the pathogenicity of this group are the production of polysaccharides and the binding to different substrates, in particular to fibronectin.

By the use of animal models and of a mutant strain of *S. sanguis* which shows reduced binding to fibronectin, it was demonstrated that animals that received the mutant strain showed a significant lower percentage of endocarditis than controls which were inoculated with the parent strain (20% vs. 90%).

Moreover, higher inocula were needed to develop endocardial infections and relevant differences in other virulence markers, including vegetation weight, number of organisms per vegetation and catheter infection rate were seen (186,187).

Endocarditis caused by exopolysaccharide producing strain yields larger vegetations than infection caused by the negative strains. Treatment of experimental endocarditis with penicillin and dextranase results in higher rates of valve sterilization than does the treatment with antibiotic alone. Lipoteichoic acid also seems to play a role in the adherence of viridans streptococci. The exposure of the organism to subinhibitory concentrations of penicillin causes the release of LTA and decreases its ability to produce endocarditis (188). The adherence to the surface of the valves is the first step in the pathogenesis of endocarditis; once adherent, viridans streptococci stimulate the proliferation of infected vegetation by triggering platelet aggregation and the production of tissue factors and cytokines (IL-8, IL-6) from the valvular tissues (189,190).

The production of exopolysaccharides plays also an important role in dental caries because glucans are used to bind to dental enamel and to other bacteria. The cariogenic potential of S. mutans seems to be related both to its capacity to adhere in large masses on teeth and to the production of a local low pH for the fermentation of dietary sugars (191).

Several surface structures like fimbriae, fibrils, and adhesins have been described which can be relevant in the adhesion of viridans streptococci, in particular for S. mitis group, but their role in host tissue colonization or as virulence factors is not always clear (187). Nevertheless, some proteinaceous products such as S. sanguis class I and II adhesins or the IgA1 proteinase, may be relevant in facilitating the infectious process (187).

E. *S. pneumoniae*

S. pneumoniae is a Gram positive, catalase-negative coccus with cells measuring 0.5 to 1.2 μm. in diameter. Colonies of encapsulated organisms are smooth and generally larger on blood agar than on chocolate agar. They appear round, domed, unpigmented, and surrounded by a zone of a greenish hemolysis if incubated aerobically. Non-encapsulated organisms are an uncommon cause of infection; colonies of the latter are smaller and flat.

Like all the other streptococci, the organism does not produce catalase and needs an exogenous source of the enzyme in growth media (e.g., from blood) to overcome the accumulation of hydrogen peroxide. *S. pneumoniae* ferments several carbohydrates but grows poorly in media with high glucose content because lactic acid, the primary metabolic by-product, rapidly reaches toxic levels.

On the surface of pneumococci, three major layers can be distinguished (Figure 2): the plasma membrane, the cell wall, and the capsule. The capsule, which is the thickest layer, completely surrounds the bacterial cell and is constituted by one of the high molecular weight (50-2,000 kD) complex carbohydrates that determine the more than 90 serologically distinguishable types (192). The repeating oligosaccharide units are produced within the cytoplasm and polymerized by transferases that are bound to the cell membrane (193). The polysaccharide is transported to the bacterial surface and remains anchored to the membrane, but is released in the medium following the death of the bacterium. The capsule has long been recognized as the major virulence factor. Encapsulated strains have been demonstrated to be 10^5 times more virulent than those which are unencapsulated (194). The capsular polysaccharides are used for the serological typing of the isolates (see below). Despite the large number of pneumococcal serotypes, only a limited number cause frequent infections in humans. As in other Gram positive cocci, the peptidoglycan consists of alternating subunits of N-acetylglucosamine and N-acetylmuramic acid which are cross-linked by peptide bridges. A main component of the cell wall is teichoic acid (or C substance) which is a species-specific polysaccharide that is unrelated to the group polysaccharides of beta-hemolytic streptococci. This polysaccharide is used for diagnostic purposes because it is able to precipitate a serum globulin that is termed protein C (C reactive protein) and which is present in patients with acute inflammatory diseases. Cell wall integrity is maintained by cross-linking enzymes such as transpeptidases and carboxypeptidases (penicillin binding proteins, PBP). Their active site is the target for beta-lactam antibiotics which, leading to their inactivation, contribute to the disruption of the cell wall with the release of immunologically active fragments. The lipoteichoic acid (Forssman antigen) is a form of teichoic acid which is bound to membrane lipids, and can cross-react with the surface of mammalian cells. Both teichoic and lipoteichoic acid are rich in galactosamine phosphate and choline. The latter plays an important role in cell wall hydrolysis regulation and must be

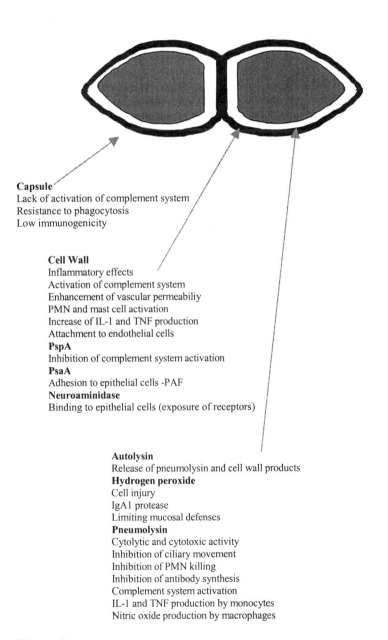

Capsule
Lack of activation of complement system
Resistance to phagocytosis
Low immunogenicity

Cell Wall
Inflammatory effects
Activation of complement system
Enhancement of vascular permeabiliy
PMN and mast cell activation
Increase of IL-1 and TNF production
Attachment to endothelial cells
PspA
Inhibition of complement system activation
PsaA
Adhesion to epithelial cells -PAF
Neuroaminidase
Binding to epithelial cells (exposure of receptors)

Autolysin
Release of pneumolysin and cell wall products
Hydrogen peroxide
Cell injury
IgA1 protease
Limiting mucosal defenses
Pneumolysin
Cytolytic and cytotoxic activity
Inhibition of ciliary movement
Inhibition of PMN killing
Inhibition of antibody synthesis
Complement system activation
IL-1 and TNF production by monocytes
Nitric oxide production by macrophages

Figure 2   Proposed major mechanisms of *S. pneumoniae* virulence.

present for the activity of pneumococcal autolysin which is a crucial component both for the metabolism of the bacterium during the process of cell division and as a virulence factor. An autolysin (n-acetylmuramic-L alanine-amidase) (195) causes the autolysis of the bacterial cell and the subsequent release of pneumolysin, the main pneumococal toxin, and cell wall constituents.

The pneumococcus is a naturally transformable bacterium. Many years ago, it was speculated (196) that autolysis represents a mechanism to facilitate the exchange of genetic material through the release of DNA. The cell wall phosphoryl choline residues are recognition sites for cell wall polysaccharide amidase. The lipoteichoic acid, which is a powerful inhibitor of the autolysin, also contains residues of phosphoryl choline and is released during the stationary phase. It is thought that the loss of this inhibitor is the main cause of the bacterial lysis. Unfortunately, far from being only beneficial, the bacterial lysis involves the release of cell wall fragments and in particular, the cell wall polysaccharide (C substance) that has been found to induce inflammation analogous to that which occurs after infection with the whole organism. Experimental otitis media, meningitis, and pneumonia can be mimicked in animals by the injection of purified cell wall or its degradation products (197). Purified cell wall is a powerful enhancer of the release of inflammatory cytokines (see below) and activate the alternative pathway of complement (198,199).

The main virulence factor is pneumolysin. It is an intracellular protein that is highly conserved among pneumococci, is released after lysis of the bacterium by autolysin, and has a variety of toxic effects on different cell types (200). Pneumolysin shows some sequence homology with C-reactive protein, an acute phase protein with which the enzyme may compete for thebinding of C1q (201). Pneumolysin-negative mutants are less virulent than parent strains, but immunization of mice with pneumolysin is only partially protective against infection with different serotypes (202).

Other pneumococcal proteins whose relevance in infection have not been completely elucidated are IgA1 protease (that might facilitate the infection at mucosal surfaces) (203), neuroaminidase (that may increase the attachment to epithelial cells by cleaving sialic acid from host glycolipids and gangliosides) (204), a peptide permease (that seems to play a role in the adhesion of the organism) (205), hyaluronidase, and a surface trans-membrane protein PspA (that seems to be required for the full virulence of the organism by possibly acting as inhibitor of complement activation) (206).

If compared to Group A streptococci, *S. pneumoniae* produces few toxins, such as autolysin, pneumolysin (207) and a hemolysin with the latter having a proposed minor role in pathogenesis. Disease is rather the outcome of the uncontrolled *S. pneumoniae* replication in host tissues which is associated with an intense inflammatory response that is caused by the release of highly pro-inflammatory *S. pneumoniae* components that are able to activate the innate immune system (Figure 3).

Pharyngeal colonization is mediated by the interaction of bacterial surface adhesins, including pneumococcal surface adhesin A (psaA) (208), with both epithelial cell receptors and extracellular matrix proteins such as fibronectin (209). Receptors for pneumococci have been recognized on human epithelial cells and characterized as carbohydrates that are differentially expressed on cells in the upper respiratory tract (210,211). Infection results if microorganisms reach tissues from which they are not readily cleared, such as lung, where the preferred bacterial target is the type-II pneumocyte (212). Coexisting circumstances may affect normal defense mechanisms which facilitate clearance of microorganisms e.g. allergy, viral infections, or cigarette smoking, and congenital or acquired disturbances of mucociliary physiology (213). Inhaled or aspirated organisms will thus replicate in situ and cause disease. Several factors may contribute to the severity of *S. pneumoniae* disease, but among those more prominent are antibiotic resistance and the increasing number of susceptible hosts, e.g., patients undergoing immunosuppressive therapy, HIV infected, and elderly patients who have various underlying diseases (214).

Pneumolysin causes a variety of cytolytic and cytotoxic effects. It has been shown to bind cholesterol and to form pores on cell membranes thus killing human cells without the restriction of a single receptor. The direct effect of pneumolysin on perfused lung leads to increased alveolar permeability and

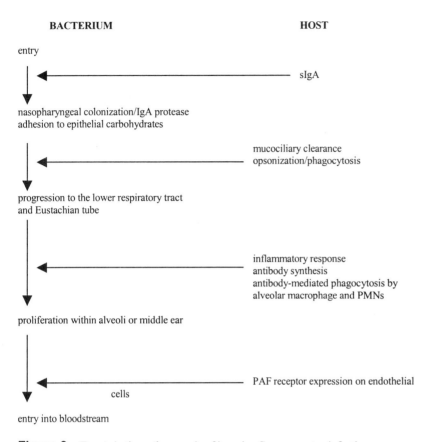

BACTERIUM   HOST

entry

nasopharyngeal colonization/IgA protease
adhesion to epithelial carbohydrates

progression to the lower respiratory tract
and Eustachian tube

proliferation within alveoli or middle ear

entry into bloodstream

sIgA

mucociliary clearance
opsonization/phagocytosis

inflammatory response
antibody synthesis
antibody-mediated phagocytosis by
alveolar macrophage and PMNs

PAF receptor expression on endothelial
cells

Figure 3   Events in the pathogenesis of invasive *S. pneumoniae* infection.

abnormalities of type-1 pneumocytes (215). The lack of toxin liberation until that time that lysis of the bacteria occurs perhaps attenuates pneumolysin activity (216). During the bacterial lysis, released DNA (217) and fragments of the cell wall stimulate the natural immune system and activate complement. Activation occurs at least in part via the stimulation of CD14 and Toll-like receptors (TLR) on monocytes which determine the secretion of huge amounts of locally released cytokines such as IL-1, IL-6 and TNF. With the onset of inflammation, humancells express platelet-activating factor (PAF) receptors. Phosphorylcholine on the pneumococcal teichoic acid has been shown to bind PAF receptors. Attachment of the pneumococcal phosphorylcholine to the PAF receptor enhances adherence and thereafter promotes invasion of epithelial and endothelial cells (218). Virulent pneumococci target the PAF receptor on activated human cells as a necessary step to facilitate subsequent invasion (219).

F.   Enterococci

Enterococci are Gram positive cocci occurring in singles, pairs, or short chains. When gram stains are prepared from thioglycolate broth, cells appear more oval and in chains.

A characteristic of these organisms is their extreme plasticity, i.e., their capacity to adapt and to respond to various environmental conditions. Enterococci tolerate a wide variety of growth conditions including temperatures from 10°C to 45°C, hypotonic or hypertonic media, or acidic or alkaline media. They are facultatively aerobic and may grow under reduced oxygen concentration. In general, they are considered strict fermenters because they lack a respiratory chain and Krebs cycle (220), but *E. faecalis* (as well as *Lactococcus lactis*) is able to express a cytochrome-like respiration when grown in the presence of exogenous hemin (221) thus providing an advantage during aerobic growth. Nearly all strains are homofermentative with lactic acid as the end-product.

As for most bacteria reported to cause human diseases, enterococci also possess properties that can play roles in the pathogenesis. Surprisingly, while great attention has been paid to the complex mechanisms leading to antibiotic resistance in these organisms, little is known about the factors that contribute to the ability of enterococci to cause infection. It is however now generally accepted that, even if enterococci are not as intrinsically as virulent as organisms such as *S. pyogenes* and in many cases only represent a part of the bacterial population found at the site of infection, they possess a number of factors which can be relevant in causing the different types of disease.

Convincing evidence of the presence of polysaccharide capsules on the surface of strains of *E. faecium* and *E. faecalis* has been recently published (222). Suggestive photographs showing *E. faecalis* cells surrounded by a thick capsular material have been obtained also by our group (Figure 4). On the basis of its structure, the polysaccharide described by Hubner proved to be a glycerol teichoic acid containing glucose, galactose, rhamnose, N-acetylgalactosamine, and phosphate (222). It is interesting that the capsular polysaccharide elicits antibodies and that the same polysaccharide has been extracted from both *E. faecium* and *E. faecalis*. About one-third of the *E. faecalis* strains tested were susceptible to killing by antibodies to this polysaccharide. On the other hand, the existence of surface carbohydrates that are linked with survival in vivo had already been observed (223). A gene knock-out for one encoding enzymes of surface carbohydrate synthesis resulted in a strain with normal in vitro growth, but was more rapidly cleared than the wild type parental strain when subcutaneously inoculated (223).

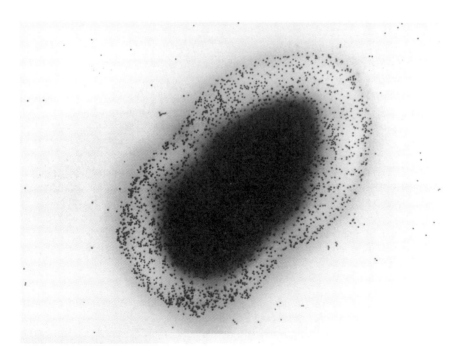

Figure 4   Immunostaining of *E. faecalis* analogous to that demonstrated in Figure 1 for group B streptococci (with permission from Dr. L. Baldassarri).

Aggregation substance is a surface protein which appears to be anchored to the bacterial membrane by its C terminus (224). This protein is encoded by pheromone-responsive plasmids of *E. faecalis* and is expressed in response to pheromone induction (225). *E. faecalis* can exchange plasmids which code for antibiotic resistance or other factors by conjugation. A strain that does not possess a certain plasmid produces and excretes short, hydrophobic peptides (7-8 amino acids) which are sensed by donor organisms carrying the corresponding plasmid. In response to pheromones, the donor strain produces the aggregating substance which leads to clumping of donor with recipient cells and thus facilitates the plasmid transfer. After the transfer, the production of pheromone and that of aggregating substance cease. The new recipient cell is prevented from responding to its own pheromone by a surface exclusion protein which is plasmid encoded (226,227). A strain of *E. faecalis* can harbour two or three sex pheromone plasmids but does not secrete the corresponding pheromone. Sex pheromone plasmids may carry one or more antibiotic resistant genes or may encode for hemolysin/bacteriocin production (227). Even if the original function of this system is the exchange of plasmids among *E. faecalis* strains, it has been observed that the aggregation substance in its amino acid sequence shows motifs that are typically found in the matrix proteins (e.g., fibronectin, fibrinogen) which use this motifs to bind to receptors on eucaryotic cells. Therefore, it was postulated that the aggregation substance may also function as an adhesin to eucaryotic cells that express integrins even if it is not clear whether the adherence is relevant for the virulence of the microorganism.

Lipoteichoic acid is composed of a hydrophilic polyglycerol phosphate backbone that is linked to a hydrophobic glycolipid tail. For enterococci, lipoteichoic acid has been shown to be identical to the Lancefield group D antigen (228). As in *S. pyogenes*, the acyl moiety appears to be essential for binding to red cells (229). Lipoteichoic acid is not only possibly involved in the preliminary reversible stages of adherence, but can inhibit pheromone-induced aggregation of bacterial cells, thus suggesting that lipoteichoic acid acts as a binding substance that is recognized by the aggregation substance on donor cells (230). Moreover, as for other Gram positive organisms, these molecules appear to be active as potent inducers of cytokines.

An extracellular protease (zinc endopeptidase) that is capable of hydrolyzing gelatin, collagen, casein, and hemoglobin is produced by *E. faecalis*. A high percentage (63%) of *E. faecalis* strains that are isolated from surgical intensive care units and 54% of the strains from patients with endocarditis have been shown to produce protease in comparison with 12-14% of enterococcal isolates from uninfected patients or healthy volunteers (231). The enzyme displays amino acid similarities with elastase which is another metalloprotease that is known to be an important virulence factor for *Pseudomonas aeruginosa*.

Enterococci produce this cell-associated enzyme which is known to cleave mucopolysaccharide moieties of connective tissue or cartilage, and has been indicated as a spreading factor for the dissemination of some microorganisms (e.g., *S. milleri*, pneumococci). No studies, however, have adequately addressed this issue for enterococci.

Since 1949 (232), it was known that some "group D streptococci" inhibited the growth of other bacteria. Subsequently, it was found that this activity was due to the fact that cytolytic *E. faecalis* strains produce bacteriocins that have broad activity against Gram positive but not Gram negative bacteria (233). Cytolytic and bacteriolytic activities can be simultaneously lost after UV irradiation (234). Nucleotide sequence determination for the *E. faecalis* cytolysin operon revealed a complex determinant that encodes five gene products (235). Further studies suggested that the cytolysin represents a new branch of lantibiotic family, a group of small secreted proteins with bactericidal activity against Gram positive bacteria. Sequencing of a region that encodes this activity and the components otherwise needed for inactivation resulted in a model for post-translational modification, externalization, and activation (236). Less than 20% of humans are normally colonized with cytolytic enterococci. A study from Japan showed that 60% of the strains from pathological samples in comparison with 17% from carriers were cytolytic (237), and a direct dose dependent correlation between cytolysin expression and *E. faecalis* toxicity in animal models after intraperitoneal injection has been observed. Nevertheless, the exact contribution of the cytolysin to *E. faecalis* pathogenicity has not been established.

The factors that contribute to the capacity of enterococci to cause infections are at the moment poorly understood. Enterococci are commensals of the gastrointestinal tract of many mammals, including man. Due to the dissemination in animal excrement and thereafter the ability to persist in the environment, enterococci are frequently isolated from a variety of sources in hospitals and occasionally found on the hands of medical personnel (238,239). In the establishment of the pathogenetic mechanisms of enterococcal infections, it has to be taken into consideration that enterococci are capable of colonizing without inducing diseases, that they are peculiarly resistant to multiple antimicrobial agents (240), and that infections are mainly limited to hospitalized and debilitated individuals.

To induce a disease, enterococci must first colonize a mucosal surface. From the site of colonization, the organisms must escape the immune defences and finally produce damage. Colonization of the gastrointestinal tract follows oral transmission because enterococci survive the transit through low gastric pH. Moreover, these organisms have been shown to adapt to pH stress since a short incubation at low or high pH renders *E. faecalis* resistant to a subsequent exposure of the same pH stress (241).

Macrophages or intestinal cells may be responsible for translocation of phagocytosed enterococci thus leading to systemic spread. Studies of the pathogenesis of *E. faecalis* have demonstrated that treatment with metronidazole or streptomycin caused intestinal overgrowth in mice which were previously orally inoculated with this organism. By immunofluorescence, *E. faecalis* was localized within columnar epithelial cells, lamina propria, submucosa, and muscularis externa; moreover by transmission electron microscopy, bacteria were shown to be localized within vacuoles in the cytoplasm of intact epithelial cells. These results indicated that *E. faecalis* can translocate across an intact intestinal tract and to cause systemic infection (242). Internalization by cultured epithelial cells has also been shown to increase in the presence of aggregation substance (243). Colonization may be facilitated by diagnostic or therapeutic procedures such as urinary catheterization or intravenous lines (244). Enterococci produce tissue damage through the direct secretion of cytolysin and gelatinase, and through the inflammation that is induced by the release of lipoteichoic acid. Cytolysin posseses both toxin and antimicrobial activities, and is produced at high frequency in clinical isolates. The enterococcal gelatinase may play a role in tissue damage and in bacterial spreading (245); in addition it has been shown that this enzyme can cleave enterococcal pheromones (246) which are potent chemoattractants. Thus, it may be implicated in the ability of enterococci to escape host immune defences (247). As for other Gram positive bacteria, lipoteichoic acid induces inflammation through the activation of the innate immunity and the consequent secretion of cytokines (248), but other bacterial components, such as aggregation and binding substances, may also be involved in this process again via the induction of cytokines (249).

V. IMMUNOLOGY OF INFECTION

A. *S. pyogenes*

Whereas the molecular mimicry of GAS capsule with host hyaluronic acid is believed to prevent an anti-capsular immune response by means of self-tolerance, type-specific antibodies against M protein enhance phagocytosis and are protective. Once internalized in phagocytes, GAS are readily killed and cleared. Opsonic antibodies which are directed against the N terminus of the protein are mostly responsible for type-specific immunity. More than 100 serotypes exist and thus the variability of M proteins accounts for the susceptibility to repeated GAS infections. In addition, it has been demonstrated that some M types contain sequences that elicit cross-reactive antibodies to host tissues that are responsible for autoimmune sequelae in predisposed subjects (250). As a consequence, it seems likely that an effective GAS vaccine would require a M protein antigen that is able to elicit an immune response toward conserved, non-host cross-reactive M protein epitopes. Several laboratories are currently investigating the functionality of such a vaccine in animal models (251-253). Following a GAS infection, antibodies that are specific to several other antigens appear, but their role in protection is controversial if not absent. Among these latter responses is the ASO immune response: if not protective, ASO antibodies are of relevance in monitoring GAS infections. Most of the acute symptoms of local and systemic disorders, as well as the pathogenesis of non-suppurative sequelae of GAS, are believed to be related to the capacity of GAS to secrete pyrogenic exotoxins, the pyrogenic toxin superantigens (SAg) (254). SAg are defined as molecules that can bind MHC Class II molecules on antigen processing cells (APC), thus acquiring the ability to stimulate large families of T lymphocytes whose specificity is not represented by SAg epitopes (255). Conventional protein antigens stimulate specific T lymphocytes only in the form of 10-15 amino acid-long peptides that are bound into the groove of MHC class II molecules and, as a consequence, require internalization, processing and presentation by APC. On the contrary, unprocessed SAg have the ability to bind the outer surface of MHC class II molecules, and they can also bind the β chain of the T cell receptor (TCR) of lymphocytes in its variable region (256). Since a single variable region β (Vβ) of the TCR is shared by T lymphocytes with diverse specificities (257,258), the functional consequence of the aforementioned interaction is that a single SAg can activate a large set of T lymphocytes independently on their specificity (Figure 5). The net effect of SAg is hence to induce T-cell stimulation with production of cytokines that are capable of mediating shock and tissue injury. Alongside their role in acute diseases, SAg are also believed to contribute to the interruption of tolerance that then sustains the pathogenesis of the autoimmune sequelae of GAS infection (259). In fact, it can be postulated that B lymphocytes which produces autoantibodies do not receive help by T lymphocytes, because autoreactive T lymphocytes are negatively selected in the thymus. The SAg-mediated activation of a large set of T lymphocytes could account for a non-specific help that is able to initiate the differentiation of B lymphocytes to plasma cells which secrete antibodies that are specific for GAS molecules mimicking host structures. SAg could therefore bypass the negative selection promoting the secretion

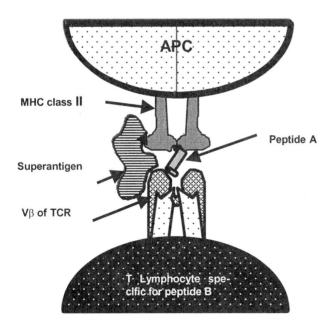

Figure 5 Representation of the interaction of superantigens with APCs and T lymphocytes.

of cross-reacting antibodies that initiate an autoimmune reaction. In predisposed subjects, several other mechanisms, such as the epitope spreading and the emergence of cryptic epitopes (260) may contribute to the maintenance of an autoimmune disease.

B. *S. agalactiae*

Type-specific capsular antibodies play a central role in protecting infants from GBS infection. The first evidence was obtained by Lancefield who demonstrated that mice could be protected from a lethal challenge by the presence of antibodies against the homologous polysaccharide. Baker and Kasper in 1976 demonstrated that infants with very low concentrations of maternally-acquired antibodies to type III capsular polysaccharide in their serum were at risk for invasive diseases (261). Women with GBS colonization at delivery, and whose infants remained healthy had levels of antibody higher than 2 mg./L., significantly more often than women whose infants became ill (261). These data suggest that transplacental transfer of maternal antibody protect infants from invasive infections. Since IgG transfer across the placenta is inefficient until week 34 of gestation, premature infants have proportionally lower levels of passive antibodies. IgG subclasses raised to GBS type polysaccharide are commonly IgG2 (262). Antibodies to group B polysaccharide are not protective.

Although antibodies play a crucial role in determining the onset of GBS disease, other host factors related to the age of the neonate contribute to the incidence of invasive infection. Serotype Ia, differently from type III, can be efficiently opsonized, phagocytosed, and killed by neutrophils via the classic complement pathway also in the absence of antibodies. Preterm infants and neonates show deficits of neutrophil functions (abnormal chemotaxis, adherence, and expression of receptor for C3bi) and quantitative deficit in their complement system (50-60% of the concentration found in adults' sera). In addition, when the infection occurs, neutrophil stores are rapidly depleted and lead to neutropenia. Abnormal neutrophil activity is also encountered in diabetics who are another category of patients prone to such infection.

Due to the relevant role in protection played by type-specific capsular antibodies, polysaccharide vaccines have been prepared several years ago to immunize pregnant women, but since these vaccines did not prove to be highly immunogenic, the preparation of a glycoconjugate vaccine which could be administered at the third trimester of pregnancy was investigated. Purified type polysaccharides of the most frequent serotypes which were conjugated to tetanus toxoid were found to be immunogenic in animals and to confer protection. In humans, they showed to be well-tolerated and to evoke, within 2 weeks, IgG-specific antibodies that persisted at high concentration for one year. These vaccine-induced antibodies were functional in vitro and reached supposedly protective levels (263).

At present, other proteins of bacterial origin (like C α, Rib) are under evaluation in order to prepare vaccines with a wider spectrum of protection.

C. Beta-hemolytic Groups C and G streptococci

Given the similarity among hemolysins with *S. pyogenes*, the cross-reactivity of these must be considered when interpreting ASO titres, and it remains to be seen how reliable the ASO is for facilitating the diagnosis of acute infections due to the large colony Group C and G streptococci.

D. Viridans streptococci

Although antibodies to viridans streptococcal antigens can be detected in humans during the first years of life, there is no definite evidence of their role in affecting the mucosal flora. A role in protecting commensal bacteria from host response may be attributed to IgA1 protease which is produced by *S. sanguis*, *S. mitis*, and *S. oralis* (264).

The study of host responses to bacteria which colonize mucosal surfaces is particularly relevant in the development of novel live recombinant vaccines. Oral lactic streptococci are efficiently transformable, and in particular, *S. gordonii* Challis is used to study the immunogenic effect of the delivery of various heterologous antigens as expressed on the surface of a living member of the commensal flora. Mice colonized orally, intranasally, or vaginally with various antigens were shown to develop significant levels of IgA in saliva, lung, and intestine as well as serum IgG (265,266). Although many questions remain to be answered, such as the duration of protection, the possibility that the vector organism is eliminated by the protective response and the risk of disseminating of recombinant genes in other transformable bacteria (e.g., *S. pneumoniae*), these findings nevertheless open the way to a possible new generation of vaccines.

E. *S. pneumoniae*

When compared to the frequency of nasopharyngeal colonization, the prevalence of *S. pneumoniae* infection appears to be extremely rare. The molecular events that distinguish the simple presence of pneumococci in the nasopharynx from the development of invasive infection have not yet been completely deciphered. Underlying impairments of defence mechanisms are often required for *S. pneumoniae* to cause disease. Host defenses against *S. pneumoniae* rely on the integrity of the mucosal architecture and on humoral factors such as complement, antibodies, and collectins which, opsonizing the bacterial cells, allow their efficient phagocytosis by polymorphonuclear cells (PMNs) and alveolar macrophages. Once internalized in PMN phago-lysosomes, *S. pneumoniae* is easily killed. Since this organism is catalase negative, it is readily killed even in the absence of a normal PMN respiratory burst e.g. in patients affected by chronic granulomatosis disease. Pneumococci are, however, poorly ingested in immunologically naive hosts or in patients with primary or acquired deficiencies of humoral immunity. The ability of *S. pneumoniae* to escape from phagocytosis has been associated with several properties of its capsule such as the absence of specific receptors for *S. pneumoniae* polysaccharides on PMNs and the presence of electro-chemical forces that repel phagocytic cells in addition to the lack of specific anticapsular antibodies. As well, the capsule is supposed to exert a double function in relation to pneumococcal opsonization: at odds with cell wall components, capsular polysaccharides do not activate complement and represent a physical barrier that separates bound and fixed complement components from complement receptors on host phagocytes (267). In this light, the presence of capsular specific antibodies is crucial for an efficient opsonization and ultimately killing of pneumococci. In the presence of anticapsular antibodies, pneumococci are rapidly ingested by phagocytes and cleared. Sera from virtually all normal subjects contain antibodies to cell wall components, these antibodies may limit cell wall induced inflammation, but poorly contribute to opsonization. On the other hand, the rate of reactivity against type-specific polysaccharides was shown to increase from 15% in 19-year-old men to 33% in working adults or elderly populations (268). This observation indicates both that specific anti-capsular antibodies can be elicited following colonization in the absence of disease and that healthy adults of all ages are susceptible to the majority of serotypes of *S. pneumoniae* that commonly cause infection.

Susceptibility to viral infection of upper respiratory tract in infancy and among the elderly are risk factors for pneumococcal infection.

Following pneumonia, antibodies to the infecting serotype appear in about two-thirds of adults, but to a lesser extent in children whether affected by pneumonia, otitis media, meningitis, or primary bacteremia (269).

The purified polysaccharides from the most commonly isolated serotypes are used to prepare polyvalent vaccines: a 14-valent vaccine was licensed in the U.S. in 1977 and this was followed in 1983 by a 23-valent vaccine. After vaccination, IgG and IgM antibodies to an average of 75% of the antigens appear in the serum within 5-7 days (270). IgG rises to a peak in 4-12 weeks after which it subsides gradually and variably over several years. Vaccination studies have identified a group of subjects with low or no response to capsular polysaccharides; this poor response is probably related to yet unrecognized genetic factors. These genetic factors could contribute to the disease susceptibility that is observed in otherwise healthy subjects who suffer from pneumococcal infections In the group of low or non-responders, there are included: children <2 years, elderly subjects, and individuals with immunosuppressive conditions such as multiple myeloma, Hodgkin's disease, lymphoma, splenectomy, nephrotic syndrome, renal failure, cirrhosis, sickle cell disease, bone marrow transplantation, and HIV infection. Recently new conjugate vaccines (which can elicit antibody response in children younger than 2 years of age) have been released in the U.S. and Europe to prevent pneumococcal meningitis (271-273). In these vaccines, a limited number of capsular polysaccharides are covalently linked to a protein carriers. The use of glycoconjugate vaccines, by means of eliciting a T cell response, may contribute to protective immunity in other groups of susceptible individuals as well.

F. Enterococci

The immune system limits enterococcal spread through polymorphonuclear, monocyte, or macrophage phagocytosis of microorganisms after opsonization with complement and/or antibody. Complement seems to be sufficient to mediate effective phagocytosis (274). Sera from normal individuals, however, promote phagocytosis of enterococci at significantly lower titres than sera from hypogammaglobulinemic patients which indicates that enterococcal-specific antibodies are present and act as efficient opsonins. Several studies are in progress to identify molecules that are associated with enterococcal isolates from systemic disease and which show increased resistance to phagocytosis (275,276).

VI. LABORATORY DIAGNOSIS

A. *S. pyogenes*

1.   Collection of the sample and culture methods

Throat culture remains the preferred method to confirm a streptococcal pharyngitis even though a positive throat culture positive alone does not differentiate between asymptomatic carriage and infection.

An accurate laboratory diagnosis begins with an accurate specimen collection. Swabs that are used to collect specimens from throat, nose, skin lesions, and wounds may be made of cotton wool or synthetic fibre. For sampling the throat, the swab should be rubbed over both tonsillar areas and over the posterior wall of the pharynx using gentle pressure and avoiding tongue and buccal mucosa.

For sampling the nose, the swab should be inserted into each of the anterior nares. A nose swab in addition to the throat swab may occasionally help in detecting GAS when they are present in small numbers. To detect carriers in hospital epidemics, other sites (e.g., rectal, perianal, vaginal) may be sampled. Serous material can be collected from skin lesions and wounds. In the case of impetiginous crusts or vesicles, samples should be taken after disinfecting the surface with 70% alcohol. The vesicle may be punctured aseptically or a swab may be taken after removing the crust. If the delay between collection and examination of the sample is longer than a few hours, a transport medium or silica gel transport should be used.

Agar media containing 5% sheep blood are used to grow GAS and to demonstrate the hemolysis. Tryptic soy blood agar or Columbia blood agar base may be used; in any case, blood agar media that are used in the evaluation of the hemolysis should not contain added glucose which inhibits beta-hemolysis. When selective media are needed to avoid overgrowth of other microorganisms, the addition of crystal violet or colistin (10 mg./L.) and nalidixic acid (15 mg./L.) or colistin and oxolinic acid (5 mg./L.) may inhibit staphylococci and coryneforms as well as Gram negative organisms. Sheep blood agar is preferred because clear-cut patterns of hemolysis are obtained (on horse blood agar, other organisms may show beta-hemolysis, and human blood from blood banks may contain antistreptococcal antibodies).

The swab should be rolled on the surface of about 3x2 cm. close to the edge of the plate and spread to obtain separated colonies. Moreover, additional inoculations by a few oblique stabs into the agar by the loop would be useful to obtain a growth or anaerobic conditions in order to enhance the beta-hemolysis from strains that are scarcely hemolytic in aerobic conditions.

Overnight incubation at 35-37°C in 5% carbon dioxide is the method more commonly used, but some laboratories prefer incubation in anaerobic conditions. Plates negative at the first reading should be reincubated for additional 24 hours. A very detailed analysis of the methods used for the culture, identification, and typing is reported (277).

Some laboratories, when an accurate detection of carriers is needed, prefer to briefly suspend the swab in 2-5 ml. of Todd-Hewitt broth and to prepare pour plates by placing a 0.2 ml. suspension into 20 ml. of liquefied Columbia agar which is cooled at 45°C and which also has 0.8 ml. sheep blood. Colistin-nalidixic acid may be added in the usual concentrations to the Todd-Hewitt broth or to the blood agar. This method is less rapid than the usual surface plating method but, in expert hands, often allows the detection of very few (2-5) beta-hemolytic colonies.

After overnight incubation, colonies appear surrounded by a clear hemolysis zone. Group A colonies are round, and 0.5-2 mm. or more in diameters. Colonies from strains that bear large amounts of hyaluronic acid are mucoid. Strains which do not produce capsule show domed colonies that are smaller in size and that are in general thought to be less virulent than mucoid colonies.

2. Identification methods

Group A streptococcal colonies may be indistinguishable from those of other beta-hemolytic streptococci, namely large colonies of group C and G streptococci. Therefore, further characterization is needed to reach the definitive identification. A Gram positive stain showing cocci in short chains and a negative catalase test may be useful to differentiate *S. pyogenes* from other bacteria of the upper respiratory tract such as *Haemophilus* spp., *Corynebacterium* spp., or *Staphylococcus* spp.. A presuntive identification may be performed on isolates in pure culture by bacitracin susceptibility. In fact, Group A streptococci are inhibited by low potency bacitracin disks (0.04 units) on plates that are heavily inoculated with two or three colonies from a pure culture, whereas non-Group A streptococci are generally resistant. It should be noted, however, that some viridans streptococci may be susceptible to bacitracin, and therefore this test should be confirmed by other means.

3. Serological tests

Serological tests are based on the extraction of Lancefield group polysaccharide, and its identification by group-specific sera. Different methods for the extraction may be used: in the Lancefield method, the pellet from 30-40 ml. of a Todd-Hewitt overnight borth culture is extracted by 0.4 ml. of 0.2 mol./L. hydrochloric acid, and boiled in a water bath (100°C) for 10 minutes. The extract is neutralized, centrifuged, and after discarding the pellet, used in identification tests. By this method, not only the group polysaccharide but also the type protein antigens are extracted. Historical methods were based on different types of precipitation tests [e.g., in capillary tubes (278), by double immunodiffusion, and by counter-immuno-electrophoresis]. Rapid methods for grouping pure cultures of groups A, C, G and D streptococci are commercially-available and are based on acid or enzymatic extraction followed by slide agglutination of latex particles that are covered by group-specific immunoglobulins (279) or by coag-glutination (mixing the extract with group specific antibodies (280). The first method is presently the most widely used.

Rapid methods for the detection of group antigen directly from the throat specimens by chemical (nitrous acid) or enzymatic (pronase) extraction, followed by agglutination (281) or enzyme immunoas-say (282) are commercially-available. These methods are very rapid and specific. The false-negative reaction depends on the number of streptococci that are present in the sample. Since in some cases a low number of GAS may be clinically relevant and given the fact that these methods do not allow further studies of the strain (typing), it is recommended that parallel culture be performed.

4.   Physiological tests

Some members of the 'S. anginosus (formerly *S. milleri*) group' may bear group A antigen and be beta hemolytic, but in general colonies are very small. Moreover, other species may occasionally be inhibited in the bacitracin test. In these cases, physiological tests that are commercially-available may help in identification. *S. pyogenes* is the only beta-hemolytic streptococcus that yields a positive PYR (pyrrolidonyl aminopeptidase) test. 'S. anginosus group' are VP-positive (Voges-Proskauer test for the production of acetoin).

5.   Other identification methods

Nucleic acid probe-based tests for the direct detection of GAS directly from the throat specimens are also commercially available (283-285).

6.   Typing methods

Typing of isolates is not commonly performed by clinical laboratories. Nevertheless, typing may be necessary in hospital outbreaks when infections of unusual severity appear in the community population, or in food-borne outbreaks. Moreover, knowledge of the trend of different serotypes in the population over time is essential in order to develop possible type-specific vaccines. Unfortunately, traditional serotyping is time-consuming and needs reagents that are not commercially-available. Therefore, it has always been performed by highly specialized reference centres.

Other non-serologic typing methods have been proposed using new molecular methods: restriction fragments length polymorphism (RFLP), large-fragment DNA pulsed field gel electrophoresis (PFGE), and others. These methods have been successful in particular to detect clonal variations within single M serotypes or to distinguish microbiological persistance or relapses due to treatment failures from recurrences after acquisition of new strains.

The great advantage of M typing in comparison with these molecular methods is that is the only method which correlates with the most important virulent factor of GAS, i.e., the M protein. Due to the large number of M serotypes and the fact that M anti-sera are not commercially-available, typing is performed by steps also using other surface proteins of GAS which can help in a first screening to choose the M sera that are subsequently to be tested. These are T proteins protein and opacity factor (OF). T antigens are produced by most GAS; these proteins are not correlated with virulence, and one single T antigen may correspond to several M proteins. The test consists of a slide agglutination of a suspension (after trypsinization to eliminate M and other proteins) with hyperimmune rabbit antisera (286,287). Pooled sera and single T sera are commercially available. The strain may agglutinate with a single antiserum or give a pattern of agglutination.

Moreover, approximately half of the GAS strains produce OF (apoproteinase), and cause opacification on media with mammalian sera. This antigen also is type-specific and may predict the M type in epidemiological investigations. Different M types will often correspond with particular OF reactions and T types. Therefore, by the combination of these three methods, it is possible to detect the M protein borne by the strain. For instance, a strain identified as T1 will be M1 if OF-negative and M68 if OF-positive. Pattern T4,28 will correspond M types 4, 26, 29, and 46 if the strain is OF-negative and M types 4, 28, 48, 60 and 63 if OF-positive.

Developments in molecular methods are presently changing the approach to typing *S. pyogenes*. M protein is encoded by *emm* gene; the 5' end of *emm* genes that encode for M serotype specificity is highly heterogeneous. On the basis of the sequence of the 5' terminal end of the *emm* gene, two isolates are defined to have identical *emm* sequences if they are ≥ 95% identical over their 5' end 160 nucleotides. The *emm* sequence of many M-type reference strains are presently known and deposited in Gene-Bank. Moreover, more than 30 unknown *emm* sequences have been identified among the 1500 isolates of GAS that have been sequenced. Details on *emm* typing may be found in reference 288.

B. *S. agalactiae*

GBS are catalase-negative Gram positive cocci forming short chains in clinical specimens and longer chains in culture media.

1. *Collection, transport and storage of specimens.*

Specimens suspected of harboring GBS should be collected by classical methods. Special indications in specimen collection have been given for establishing GBS anogenital carriage in pregnant women. The Centres for Disease Control and Prevention recommend that pregnant women should be cultured at 35-37 weeks of gestation. One swab should be obtained from the vaginal introitus and another one from the anorectum.

The swabs should be placed in a non-nutritive moist swab transport system (e.g., Amies medium). In these transport media, GBS maintain their viability for up to 4 days at room temperature or under refrigeration.

2. *Isolation*

Detection of GBS in the genital tracts of pregnant women should be performed by inoculating swabs in Todd-Hewitt broth which is supplemented with colistin (10 mg./L.) and nalidixic acid (15 mg./L.) or with gentamicin (8 mg./L.) and nalidixic acid (15 mg./L.). Selective media are also commercially available (Lim broth or SMB broth). The culture should be incubated for 18-24 hrs. at 35-37°C and then subcultured on to sheep blood (5%) agar. Blood agar plates are incubated in a CO_2 atmosphere.

On blood agar plates, GBS colonies are surrounded by a narrow zone of β-hemolysis which is variable in size from one strain to another. In general, the zone is narrower than that seen with groups A, C, or G streptococci, and a small percentage of GBS strains may be non-hemolytic. Colonies are translucent to opaque, flat, and glossy. If GBS is not detected after 24 hrs., plates should be re-incubated and inspected again at 48 hrs.

GBS grows in 6.5% NaCl broth, on 40% bile agar, on 0.04% tellurite agar, at 10°C (very slowly in comparison to enterococci), and a small percentage of strains (about 12%) also at 45°C.

On special media (Islam's medium) after anaerobic incubation, GBS colonies appear pigmented.

3. *Identification*

Phenotypic identification

For suspected hemolytic or non-hemolytic colonies, the CAMP test may be performed for a presumptive identification. On a blood agar plate, the streptococcus strain is streaked perpendicularly 3-4 mm. apart from the streak of a *Staphylococcus aureus* producer of β-hemolysin. After overnight incubation at 35-37°C, a positive test is characterized by an arrow shaped zone of complete hemolysis in the area into which both staphylococcal β-hemolysin and CAMP factor have diffused.

It is very important to distinguish enterococcal species commonly found in clinical samples (*E. faecalis, E. faecium*) from GBS, because the colonial, and to a certain extent, the cellular morphology of these species, may show great similarity. To this end, the CAMP test is of practical value as enterococci are CAMP negative, while 99% of GBS are positive. Another useful differentiating test is the hydrolysis of esculin since enterococci are positive while GBS are negative. GBS are also able to hydrolyze hippurate.

Identification of GBS can be performed by commercially-available biochemical test systems (API 20 Strep and API ID 32 Strep from Biomérieux, Rapid ID Str System from Remel-Oxoid).

Serological identification

Serological identification of GBS may be performed by detecting the Lancefield's group B antigen using commercial rapid antigen extraction methods and agglutination techniques (Streptococcal grouping kit, Oxoid).

For epidemiological purposes, it may be useful to determine the serotype of the isolate (Ia, Ib, II-VIII). Typing sera are not commercially available, and therefore serotyping is usually performed by streptococcal reference centres.

Molecular identification

Nucleic acid probe for culture-confirmation of GBS are currently available (Accuprobe, Gen-Probe, Inc.). DNA probe-based tests provide practical and rapid alternatives to any confirmatory test which requires subculturing.

4. Rapid detection of GBS

Rapid detection of GBS is based on the detection of the Lancefield antigen (group B polysaccharide) in the sample by different methods (latex agglutination, enzyme immunoassays, etc.).

Methods developed to rapidly identify GBS from the urogenital tract of colonized women at delivery are of limited use since they have been shown to detect only heavily-colonized women (289).

In suspected cases of meningitis, commercial products for detection of the Lancefield group B antigen in CSF may be useful. Some of these methods also include procedures for urine specimens, but these should be used cautiously because of the risk of both false-positive and false-negative results.

C. Beta-hemolytic Groups C and G streptococci

Isolates of large-colony-forming group of β-hemolytic streptococci may be identified on the basis of Lancefield Group C and G antigens and may be separated from the members of 'S. anginosus group' on the basis of colony size (<5 mm. in the anginosus group; ≥5 mm. in the large colony Group C and G species), by their positivity for the production of β-glucuronidase, and the negativity for the production of acetoin (Table 7). Attention should be directed to the bacitracin test that is used to screen for *S. pyogenes* since several strains of C and G group have been shown to be susceptible to bacitracin (290).

D. Viridans streptococci

Viridans streptococci possess the general characteristics that are common to all streptococci. They are catalase-negative Gram positive cocci which form long chains in liquid media. On blood agar, most strains produce a green discoloration of the agar due to the partial hemolysis of erythrocytes but some members may be non-hemolytic or beta-hemolytic.

Until recently, the great majority of the viridans streptococci were identified by a short panel of tests including sugar fermentation, catalase, production of exopolysaccharides from sucrose, hydrolysis of esculin and arginine, and production of acetoin from glucose. With these assessments it was possible to assign isolates to one of the five recognized species: *S. mutans*, *S. salivarius*, *S. mitior*, *S. sanguis*, and *S. milleri*. Due to the large number of species recognized, however, these tests are currently insufficient.

A comprehensive scheme of biochemical tests including the detection of preformed glycosidase activities by chromogenic substrates was described by Kilian (291). The majority of these are presently incorporated in commercial identification tests. Some years later, Beighton et al. in addition to taxonomic changes proposed by Kilian, recognized several additional species in the group of "anginosus" and proposed an identification scheme that was based on the detection of glycosidic enzyme activities and biochemical tests using fluorogenic substrates (292). To accommodate any new described species, the panel of tests to be performed became very wide, and presently for taxonomic studies, the whole set of tests together with accurate genomic studies are necessary to assign an isolate to the correct species.

Table 7 Characteristics of large colony-forming Groups C and G streptococci.

	Lancefield Group	Host	Trehalose	Sorbitol	Acetoin (VP)	β-glucuronidase
S. dysgalactiae (subsp. equisimilis)	C, G	humans	+	+	-	+
S. dysgalactiae (subsp. dysgalactiae)	C, L	animals	+	-	-	+
S. equi (subsp. equi)	C	animals	-	-	-	+
S. equi (subsp. zooepidemicus)	C	animals (humans)	-	+	-	+
S. canis	G	animals	-	-	-	V

For clinical laboratories, it is difficult if not impossible to identify isolates without the use of commercial test kits although the use of these tests is not without problems. The major difficulty is their lack of flexibility which, once the panel has been established, prevents any change of the scheme to include new species following changes in taxonomy. This necessitates, in many cases, the addition of supplementary tests in order to achieve a reliable identification. These systems, however, offer many relevant advantages in the context of serious infections among immunocompromised hosts. In fact, they offer a rapid identification, they are standardized in contrast to 'home-made' laboratory tests, and they are simple to perform. In some instances, they are able to define whether the patient has a relapse or a new infection by their profile index.

If we exclude studies of dental microbiology, the identification of viridans streptococci in clinical samples is only performed from sterile body sites where in general they are present usually as a single infecting species. Some may choose to speciate them from abscesses where they can represent only a part of the infecting population. The main problem with the identification of viridans streptococci is that many different identification schemes have been reported, that several of the tests indicated are not present in the commercial systems, and that, depending on the author and the study, different results for the same test are reported.

The following short schemes are derived in part from references 291 and 292 which are reviewed also on the basis of the expected results reported in commercial tests (API 20 Strep and API 32 Strep. Bio Merieux Vitek, Inc., Hazelwood, Missouri).

1. 'S. anginosus group'

Source and habitat of this group are the human oral cavity, upper respiratory tract, vagina, and purulent infections (293-296). Species included are *S. anginosus*, *S. constellatus*, and *S. intermedius*.

Some isolates of the 'S. anginosus group' may be beta-hemolytic and/or bear Lancefield polysaccharides. They may belong to Lancefield groups A, C, F, or G, or be non-groupable. The appearance of hemolysis before the colony is large is a characteristic trait of the hemolytic members of these species in contrast with the classic beta-hemolytic species such as *S. pyogenes* or *S. equisimilis*. On blood agar, cultures often produce a sweet caramel odor. Non-beta-hemolytic colonies may be separated from non-hemolytic *S. agalactiae* strains by the lack of B polysaccharide, the size of the colony, and negative CAMP and hippurate reactions.

The 'S. anginosus group' may be separated from other viridans streptococci by three important tests: acetoin production or Voges-Proskauer test (VP) (always positive), arginine (always positive), and sorbitol (always negative). If the VP-test is not performed, it could be misidentified as *S. sanguis*. (*S. pyogenes* and *S. equisimilis* are also VP-negative). Among the three species presently included in the group, none produces exopolysaccharide from sucrose-containing media. Some isolates of *S. anginosus* from vaginal samples may ferment mannitol and raffinose. Hyaluronidase is not produced by *S. anginosus*, but it is produced by the majority of *S. constellatus* and *S. intermedius*. Sialidase is produced only by *S. intermedius*, which also produces beta-galactosidase, but usually not beta-glucosidase which is produced by *S. anginosus*. Some of the tests are useful for the identification of the 'S. anginosus group' are shown in Table 8.

2. 'S. mitis group'

This group includes a large number of species (see Table 2) including newly designated ones such as *S. crista* (or *S. cristatus*), *S. infantis*, and *S. peroris* for which a scheme of physiological identification tests has not been yet established. It also includes *S. pneumoniae* since it has been demonstrated to have a close relationship with the commensals *S. mitis* and *S. oralis*. About 60% DNA homology between *S. oralis* and *S. pneumoniae* and 99% 16S rRNA gene sequencing homology among the three species have been reported (297, 298). Other members of the group are *S. gordonii* and *S. sanguis*; a change in nomenclature to *S. sanguinis* and *S. parasanguinis* (to follow Latin form) has been proposed. All members of the group are alpha-hemolytic on blood agar, and they give a strong green discoloration on chocolate agar. Extracellular polysaccharide is produced only by some species (*S. sanguis* and some strains of *S. oralis* and *S. crista*). *S. pneumoniae* (mainly discussed elsewhere) can be easily identified by the typical form of the colonies, bile solubility, and optochin susceptibility.

At difference with the 'S. anginosus group', members of the 'S. mitis group' do not produce acetoin from glucose and in general do not hydrolyze esculin but produce acid from pullulan and lactose. *S. sanguis*, *S. gordonii*, and some isolates of *S. oralis* can produce extracellular polysaccharide on sucrose containing agar and yield hard adherent but smooth colonies. All species produce acid from fructose, galactose, lactose, maltose, melibiose, pullulan, and acetylglucosamine, but not from esculin, glycerol,

Table 8 Relevant identification tests for the 'S. anginosus group'.

	S. anginosus	*S. constellatus*	*S. intermedius*
Acid from:			
arginine	+	+	+
esculin	+	+	+
sorbitol	-	-	-
mannitol	V	-	-
raffinose	V	-	-
Enzyme activity:			
β-D-galactosidase	-	-	+
β-D-glucosidase	+	-	V
β-D-N-acetylglucosaminidase	-	-	+
β-D-N-acetylgalactosaminidase	-	-	+
Production of:			
hyaluronidase	-	V	+
sialidase	-	-	+
acetoin (VP)	+	+	+

Table 9   Relevant identification tests for 'S. mitis group'.

	S. sanguis	S. gordonii	S. mitis	S. oralis	S. parasanguis	S. crista
acid from:						
lactose	+	+	V	+	+	V
raffinose	V	-	V	V	V	-
sorbitol	-	-	-	-	-	-
trehalose	+	+	V	V	V	+
production of:						
α-galactosidase	V	V	V	V	V	V
β-galactosidase	V	V	V	V	+	V
β-glucosidase	-	+	+	+	+	-
hydrolysis:						
arginine	+	+	-	-	+	V
esculin	+	-	-	-	-	-
production of:						
extracellular polysaccharide	+	+	-	V	-	V
alkaline phosphatase	-	+	+	+	+	-
acetoin (VP)	-	-	-	-	-	-
IgA protease	+	ND	V	+	ND	ND

inulin, and mannitol. *S. gordonii* does not usually ferment pullulan. Arginine and esculin are not hydrolyzed by *S. oralis* or *S. mitis*, but are hydrolyzed by *S. sanguis* and *S. gordonii*; *S. parasanguis* and *S. crista* hydrolyze arginine but not usually esculin. Sialidase is produced by *S. oralis* and some isolates of *S. mitis* but not by the other species; alpha-glucosidase is produced by *S. oralis*, *S. parasanguis*, and *S. mitis* but only by a minority of members of *S. sanguis* or *S. gordonii* (Table 9).

3. 'S. salivarius group'

Human species included in this group are presently *S. salivarius* and *S. vestibularis*. Source and habitat is the oral cavity, in particular the tongue and saliva.

   Both species produce large mucoid colonies on sucrose-containing agar and are non-hemolytic on blood agar. Since about 20% of the isolates may grow on 40% bile and nearly all split esculin, *S. salivarius* may be confused with *S. bovis*. At odds with *S. bovis*, *S. salivarius* does not have Group D antigen (about 50% of the strains are Lancefield group K) and does not ferment mannitol. *S. salivarius* produces levan on sucrose agar and has large colonies which do not glide easily across the agar. *S. vestibularis* does not produce exocellular polysaccharide and in contrast to *S. salivarius*, does not produce acid from inulin or raffinose, but it hydrolyzes starch (Table 10).

4. 'S. mutans group'

This group presently includes *S. mutans*, *S. sobrinus*, *S. cricetus*, *S. rattus*, *S. downey*, *S. macacae*, and *S. ferus*. All of these species may be associated to human or animal dental caries.

   S. mutans belongs to the normal flora when specimens are derived from the mouth and throat; even if it is not common in tissue infections, it is frequently one of the causes of endocarditis. Most isolates are non-hemolytic. Large mucoid colonies are produced on sucrose agar. All of the species produce acid from a large range of sugars, and several of them are susceptible to bacitracin (Table 11). Colonies are in general alpha- or non-hemolytic on blood agar. Esculin is hydrolyzed by all members with the exception of *S. sobrinus* and *S. downei*; arginine is hydrolyzed only by *S. rattus*. Acetoin is produced by all the species.

Table 10 Relevant tests for identification of the 'S. salivarius group'.

	S. salivarius	*S. vestibularis*
acid from:		
inulin	+	-
lactose	+	V
raffinose	V	-
production of:		
β-glucosidase	V	-
β-fucosidase	V	-
hydrolysis of:		
arginine	-	-
esculin	+	V
urea	V	-
production of:		
acetoin	+	+
extracellular polysaccharide	+	-

Table 11 Relevant identification tests for the 'S. mutans group'.

	S. mutans	*S. cricetus*	*S. rattus*	*S. downei*	*S. macacae*	*S. ferus*	*S. sobrinus*
production of:							
acetoin (VP)	+	+	+	+	+	+	+
bacitracin resistance	+	-	+	-	-	-	+
hydrolysis of:							
arginine	-	-	+	-	-	-	-
esculin	+	+	+	-	+	+	-
acid from:							
inulin	+	+	+	+	-	+	+
lactose	+	V	V	+	ND	+	V
mannitol	+	+	+	+	+	+	V
raffinose	+	+	+	-	+	-	-
sorbitol	+	+	+	-	+	+	V
trehalose	+	V	+	+	+	+	+
salicin	-	+	+	+	ND	+	-
glycogen	-	-	-	-	ND	+	-

5. 'S. bovis group'

The species which are included in this group are *S. bovis*, *S. equinus*, and *S. alactolyticus*. Only *S. bovis* is commonly found among humans. Recent studies show a clear separation between human and animal strains. Typical human isolates of *S. bovis* (biotype I in API System) ferment mannitol and produce glucan from sucrose, while the variant biotype II is unable to ferment mannitol or to produce glucan. Biotype II may be seen as two variants, II/1 and II/2, because the latter produces β-glucuronidase, β-galactosidase, and β-mannosidase, and ferments trehalose; biotype II/1 gives negative reactions (Table 12). *S. bovis* and *S. mutans* both produce glucan, ferment mannitol, and grow on bile esculin agar, but *S. bovis* does not ferment sorbitol, ferment starch and glycogen, nor possess Lancefield group D antigen. In contrast to *S. salivarius*, *S. bovis* is beta-galactosidase-negative, alpha-galactosidase-positive, urease-positive, and bears Lancefield Group D.

E. S. pneumoniae

1. Microscopic examination

Common specimens that are used for the diagnosis of pneumococcal infections are blood cultures (299,300), sputum, pleural fluid, and cerebrospinal fluid.

Table 12 Relevant identification tests for the 'S. bovis group'.

	S. bovis Biotype I	*S. bovis* Biotype II/1	*S. bovis* Biotype II/2
growth:			
on bile-esculin agar	+	+	+
salt tolerance	-	-	-
at 10°C	-	-	-
acid from:			
mannitol	+	-	-
trehalose	+	- (V)	+
raffinose	+	+	V
sorbitol	-	-	-
hydrolysis of:			
arginine	+	+	-
starch	+	+	-
glycogen	+	-	-
VP test:	+	+	+
Lancefield Group D	+	+	+
Glucan production	+	-	-
production of:			
β-galactosidase	-	-	+
β-glucuronidase	-	-	+
β-mannosidase	V	-	+

A Gram stain of sputum which shows a large number of PMN and lanceolated, Gram positive cocci in pairs or short chains, is strongly suggestive of pneumococcal disease. Bacteria from old cultures tend not to stain well and may appear Gram negative. When appropriately stained, the organism appears surrounded by an unstained capsule. If the patient has already been treated with antibiotics, cell morphology may be distorted.

In general, the diagnosis of pneumococcal pneumonia is often certain unless confirmed by blood cultures. Inadequate sputum specimen collections are often responsible for the lack of reliability of sputum cultures and direct Gram stains. In order to have reliable results, a low power microscopic magnification (100X) of sputum should contain at least 10-20 WBC and no epithelial cells under 1000X magnification. In sputum from infected patients, pneumococci are in general present in large numbers (>25 per field at 1000X magnification). The absence of epithelial cells indicates a low probability for contamination with viridans streptococci that are present in saliva and thus indicate a high level of contamination from the upper respiratory tract.

2. Antigen detection

To detect soluble pneumococcal polysaccharide in infected body fluids, immunological assays such as counterimmunoelectrophoresis (CIE) and latex agglutination can be performed with the use of antibodies that are directed against C polysaccharide (301). Both test are sensitive and specific, but some serotypes (7 and 14) are not detected by these methods. Other tests such as co-agglutination or ELISA have also been used for the same purpose.

3. Culture

S. pneumoniae has fastidious requirements and needs enriched nutrient media. Cultures should preferably be grown on blood or chocolate agar with incubation at 35°-37°C in a 5-10% carbon dioxide atmosphere. Growth in broth that is commonly used for other streptococci such as Todd-Hewitt broth can be used for determination of cellular morphology. Pneumococci can be recovered from sputum cultures in only one-half of the patients who suffer from pneumonia for several reasons: S. pneumoniae can rapidly undergo lysis, it can be overgrown by viridans streptococci which contaminate the specimen, or the culture can become negative when patients are treated with antibiotics. On the contrary, it is relatively easy to isolate the organism from cerebrospinal fluid unless antibiotic treatment has already been started at the time of collecting the specimen: a single dose of antibiotic can make cultures negative for about one-half of all patients.

4. Identification

On solid media, pneumococci produce small, gray colonies, which are transparent and mucoid when the organism bears a large amount of capsular material, and they tend over the time to become umbilicated. Colonies are surrounded by a large area of green (partial) hemolysis.

Even though pneumococci can be identified by the panel of tests that are commercially available for the general identification of streptococci, these methods do not give advantage in respect to the historically-used methods. Suspicious colonies should be assessed for optochin (302) (ethylhydrocupreine hydrochloride) susceptibility by placing a disk that is saturated with optochin in the middle of the inoculum which is obtained by streaking a colony onto a blood agar plate. A large zone of inhibition (usually 20 mm. or more) is seen around the disk after overnight incubation while other streptococci usually show inhibition zones of less than 12 mm. In addition, the organism can be identified by lysis from exposure to bile; isolated colonies of S. pneumoniae are usually solubilized in a few minutes by a drop of bile while viridans streptococci remain unchanged (303). When the test is performed in liquid media, the addition of bile to the culture will clarify the broth.

A definitive identification may be achieved by serological methods using Omniserum, a pooled polyvalent concentrated serum that reacts with all of the known types of pneumococcal capsules (Neufeld test). This reaction was called "Quellung" (swelling) by Neufeld (304), who described it at the turn of the century, and is performed by placing a small drop of bacterial suspension on a slide, mixing with serum, and observation under oil immersion microscopy for capsular reaction and agglutination of bacteria. This reaction is now commonly observed with the contrast microscope. The Neufeld reaction does not lead to a true swelling of the capsule but rather is only a reaction between the type-specific serum and the capsular polysaccharide which results in making the capsule visible. A further serological test that is performed in the same manner with monovalent sera is used for typing. The limits of the latter serological technique are that it can be used only with encapsulated strains, and that it is expensive. Moreover, the availability of sera is limited (Statens Serum Institut, Copenhagen, Denmark). As the typing of strains is not useful for immediate diagnosis or therapy, it is generally performed only by reference centres which use it for specific epidemiological studies of circulating serotypes.

5.   Alternative methods

As many cultures from blood or sputum are falsely negative because of pre-admission antibiotic, there is some need for new and effective rapid diagnostic techniques which give a correct diagnosis also in the absence of a positive culture.

   One of the most useful techniques developed in the last ten years and successfully used in recent epidemics is the polymerase chain reaction (PCR). This technique has been used recently to detect *S. pneumoniae* in sputum, blood, middle ear fluid, and cerebrospinal fluid (305-309). Targets that are used for identification are many; the pneumolysin gene was the first used for the identification of pneumococci. PCR has also been used to identify penicillin resistant strains by using the PBP genes or by comparing the patterns of known sensitive strains to those of unknown strains. By this approach, it has been possible to follow the spread of penicillin-resistant strains (310). Other molecular approaches, such as multilocus enzyme electrophoresis or the field inversion/pulsed field electrophoresis, have already been used to investigate the transmission of clones of resistant organisms within countries. It is expected that these new techniques become routinely available in the next few years and hence radically change the diagnostic techniques for *S. pneumoniae.*

F.   Enterococci

1.   Collection, transport and storage of specimens

Given their remarkable ability to survive and grow under harsh conditions, transport of enterococci can be performed with a large variety of transport media or on dry swabs. On ordinary agar slants, they can survive at 4°C for several months and can be stored at -70°C for several years.

2.   Isolation procedures

Trypticase soy agar, brain heart infusion agar, or other agar base media containing 5% animal blood support the growth of enterococci. Many strains of *E. faecalis* are hemolytic on sheep blood agar. As well, some *E. durans* isolates are hemolytic.

   Media containing chromogenic substrates have been used for samples of urine (311), and cephalexin-aztreonam-arabinose agar has been used for the isolation of *E. faecium* from heavily contaminated sites (312). Vancomycin-containing selective media have been developed in recent years for the isolation of VRE from humans and animals (313,314). Enterococcosel-vancomycin broth and brain-heart infusion-vancomycin agar may be used for the selective isolation of VRE from fecal specimens. When the sample is likely to have Gram negative bacteria, media containing azide, such as bile-esculin azide or Pfizer Selective Enterococcus or other similar commercial products, will facilitate the isolation of enterococci. On these media, enterococci are black colonies due to the hydrolysis of esculin while the Gram negative organisms are inhibited by azide. Other selective media such as Columbia agar with colistin and nalidixic acid and 5% blood (also used for streptococci) or phenylethyl alcohol agar may be used.

Optimum temperature for enterococci is 35-37°C, and they do not usually require a carbon dioxide-enriched atmosphere.

3. Identification

In the past, the typical growth on bile-esculin agar accompanied by a serological test showing that the strain belonged to the Lancefield D group were thought to be sufficient to identify the isolate as an enterococcus. Currently, the knowledge that not all *Enterococcus* species will have the D polysaccharide easily detected and the knowledge that this antigen is present in organisms from other genera and species (e.g., *S. bovis, S. equinus, S. suis, Pediococcus,* and about one-half of the *Leuconostoc* strains from human source) suggest a more cautious interpretation of the serology results.

There are no phenotypic characteristics to unequivocally separate enterococci from other Gram positive, catalase-negative cocci. Enterococci, as other catalase-negative, Gram positive cocci, may be α-, β- or non-hemolytic. The majority of them can grow at 10°C and 45°C, in 6.5% sodium chloride and at pH 9.6, and may survive after heating at 60°C for 30 minutes (315,316). Some strains of *Leuconostoc*, aerococci, pediococci, and lactococci also grow in the presence of 6.5% sodium chloride while *E. cecorum, E. columbae,* and *E. avium* do not. Pediococci and lactococci may grow at 45°C while lactococci and *Leuconostoc* spp. grow at 10°C; moreover, like some enterococci, *Leuconostoc* is vancomycin-resistant.

A presumptive identification of an enterococcus may be made on the basis of the assessments as reported in Table 13 and with the support of serology. Confirmation requires identification to the species level. A complete identification is even more relevant in the case of a vancomycin-resistant organism in hospitals where, given the cost of the measures for preventing VRE spread, laboratories have to perform a complete identification and be sure of the epidemiological importance of the strain before reporting its isolation to the Infection Control team.

Positive reactions with AccuProbe Enterococcus test (GenProbe, Inc., San Diego, California) may be used to identify a strain as an enterococcus. *Vagococcus* sp. strains also give positive reactions in this test.

A preliminary separation of enterococcal species and of some related genera (e.g., *Lactococcus, Vagococcus*) into five groups may be done on the basis of acid formation in mannitol and sorbose broths and the hydrolysis of arginine (Table 14).

Group I include five species: *E. avium, E. malodoratus, E. raffinosus, E. pseudoavium,* and *E. saccharolyticum.* Among them, only *E. raffinosus* and *E. avium* have been reported to cause infections in man (317,318). A short identification scheme of this group is shown in Table 15.

Group II include: *E. faecalis, E. faecium, E. casseliflavus, E. mundtii,* and *E. gallinarum.* In this group, *E. faecalis* and *E. faecium* are the species more frequently isolated from human infections; *E. casseliflavus, E. mundtii,* and *E. gallinarum* have also been isolated from human sources. This group also includes *Lactococcus* because characteristics of *Lactococcus* isolates which are found among humans are similar to those of *Enterococcus* species in this group (Table 16).

E. faecalis tolerate tellurite and utilize pyruvate. Efrotomycin susceptibility (tested by 100 μg. disks), acid formation in methyl-α-D- glucopyranoside, and motility may help to separate *E. faecium* from *E. gallinarum. Lactococcus* gives reactions rather similar to *E. faecium,* but it does not grow at 45°C and does not ferment raffinose.

Among the species included in group III (*E. durans, E. hirae* and *E. dispar*) only the first two have been rarely isolated from human sources. *E. durans* does not utilize pyruvate and has negative reactions for fermentation of arabinose, raffinose, and sucrose; *E. hirae* ferments sucrose and may ferment raffinose. *E. dispar* is resistant to efrotomycin, ferments raffinose and sucrose, and utilizes pyruvate.

Table 13 Characteristics of Gram positive, catalase-negative cocci in chains. Abbreviations and symbols: Van – susceptibility to vancomycin (30 ug. disk); LAP – leucine aminopeptidase; PYR – pyrronidonyl arylamidase; GAS – gas produced from glucose in Mann, Rogosa, Sharpe Lactobacillus broth (MRS); BE – reaction on bile-esculin agar; NaCl – growth in broth containing 6.5% NaCl; MOT – motility; Hem – hemolysis on agar media containing 5% sheep blood; c – cocci; ch – chains; pr – pairs; + - ≥95% positive reactions; - = >95% negative reactions; V – variable; S – susceptible; R – resistant; [a] – some strains are vancomycin resistant under the screening test conditions; [b] – *S. pyogenes* and some isolates of *S. pneumoniae* and of *Abiotrophia* are PYR positive; [c] – 5-10% of viridans streptococci are BE+; [d] – some beta-hemolytic streptococci may grow in 6.5% NaCl broth; NT – not tested. (Modified from ref. 318 and 319)

	Gram	Hem	Van	LAP	PYR	GAS	BE	10°C	45°C	6.5% NaCl	MOT
Abiotrophia	c, ch	alpha	S	V	V	-	-	V	-	-	-
Enterococcus	c, ch	alpha, beta	S[a]	+	+	-	+	+	+	+	V
Streptococcus (all)	c, ch	alpha, beta	S	+	V[b]	-	-[c]	-	V	-[d]	-
S. agalactiae	c, ch	beta, none	S	+	-	-	-	NT	NT	V	-
S. bovis	c, ch	alpha, none	S	NT	-	-	+	-	+	-	-
'viridans strep.'	c, ch	alpha, none	S	+	-	-	V[c]	-	V	-	-
Vagococcus	c, ch	alpha, none	S	+	+	-	+	+	V	NT	+
Lactococcus	c, ch	alpha, none	S	+	+	-	+	+	-	V	-
Globicatella	c, ch	alpha	S	-	+	-	V	-	-	V	-
Leuconostoc	c, pr, ch	alpha	R	-	-	+	V	+	V	V	-

Table 14 Biochemical characterization of enterococcal groups and some related genera. Abbreviations: MAN - mannitol; SOR - sorbose; ARG - arginine; [a] - some atypical strains fail to hydrolyze arginine or to form acid from mannitol.

	MAN	SOR	ARG
Group I	+	+	-
Group II	+[a]	-	+[a]
Group III	-	-	+
Group IV	-	-	-
Group V	+	-	-

Table 15 Identification tests for Group I.

	ARA	RAF	PYU
E. avium	+	-	-
E. malodoratus	-	+	+
E. raffinosus	+	+	-
E. pseudoavium	-	-	-
E. saccharolyticus	-	+	-

Abbreviations: Ara - arabinose; RAF - raffinose; PYR – pyruvate.

Table 16 Relevant identification tests for Group II.

	TEL	PYU	MGP	MOT	EFRO	ARA
E. faecalis	+	+	-	-	R	-
Lactococcus spp.	-	-	-	-	S	-
E. faecium	-	-	-	-	S	+
E. casseliflavus	-	V	+	+	R	+
E. mundtii	-	-	-	-	S	+
E. gallinarum	-	-	-	+	R	+

Abbreviations: TEL - tellurite 0.04%; PYU - pyruvate; MGP – methyl-α-D-glucopyranoside, MOT - motility; ARA - arabinose; EFRO - efrotomycin.

The two species in group IV, *E. sulfureus* and *E. cecorum*, may be differentiated on the basis of pigmentation, MGP (both positive in *E. sulfureus* and negative in *E. cecorum*), and fermentation of SBL (positive among *E. cecorum* but negative for *E. sulfureus*).

Relevant tests which differentiate the two species in group V (*E. columbae* and *V. fluvialis)* are motility, MGP (both positive only in *V. fluvialis),* pyruvate, and fermentation of arabinose and raffinose (positive only in *E. columbae)* (Table 17).

Commercially-available kits, in general, accurately identify only *E. faecalis* and should be used with cautions for other species. Several molecular techniques for the identification and differentiation of typical and atypical *Enterococcus* isolates have been described (320-322), but have yet to be widely used.

The increasing interest in the epidemiology of enterococci due to the spread of enterococcal infections within the hospitals and due to the emergence and dissemination of multiple antimicrobial resistance among these organisms has led to the need for typing of the isolates for epidemiological investigations. Several molecular methods have been described, including multilocus enzyme electophoresis (323), ribotyping (324), and RAPD-PCR (325). *SmaI* restriction digest of genomic DNA and resolution by pulsed-field gel electophoresis (PFGE) has been used to study species exhibiting different resistance patterns (323). PFGE is presently the most widely used typing method for enterococci.

G. Other Gram positive, catalase-negative, and coccoid bacteria

Most of these organisms resemble other more well-known species that are isolated from clinical samples, but they are taxonomically unrelated. Many of them are members of the normal human flora, and they are infrequently isolated either as contaminants in clinical samples or as a component of mixed

Table 17 Relevant identification tests for groups III, IV, and V. Abbreviations: MOT - motility; PIG - pigmentation; RAF - raffinose; SUC - sucrose; ARA - arabinose; PYU - pyruvate; MGP - methyl-α-D glucopyranosyde ; EFRO – efrotomycin.

Group III

	RAF	SUC	PYU	MGP	EFRO
E. durans	-	-	-	-	S
E. hirae	V	+	-	-	S
E. dispar	+	+	+	+	R

Group IV

	PIG	SBL	PYU	MGP
E. sulfureus	+	-	-	+
E. cecorum	-	+	+	-

Group V

	MOT	RAF	ARA	PYU	MGP
E. columbae	-	+	+	+	-
V. fluvialis	+	-	-	-	+

Table 18 Characteristics of catalase-negative, Gram positive coccoid bacteria. Abbreviations and symbols: HEM – hemolysis on 5% sheep blood agar; VAN – susceptibility to vancomycin (30 ug.); LAP – leucine aminopeptidase; NaCl – 6.5% NaCl broth; PYR – pyrrolidonyl arylamidase; BE – bile-esculin; c – coccoid; ch – chains; pr – pairs; cb – coccobacilli; cl – clusters; tet – tetrads. [a] – G. hemolysans is LAP-negative and PYR-positive only using large inocula. V – variable.

	Cellular Arrangement	HEM	VAN	LAP	PYR	BE	NaCl	Growth 10°C	Growth 45°C
Streptococcus-like									
Abiotrophia	c, ch	alpha-	+	V	V	-	-		-	-
Globicatella	c, ch, pr	alpha-	+	-	+	V	V	-	V
Lactococcus	cb, ch	alpha-	+	+	V	+	V	+	V
Leuconostoc	cb, pr, ch	alpha-	-	-	-	V	V	V	V
Staphylococcus-like									
Aerococcus	c, pr, cl	alpha-	+	-	+	V	+	-	-
Alloiococcus	c, pr, tet	none	+	+	+	-	+	-	-
Gemella	c, pr, ch	alpha-	+	V	+[a]	-	-	-	-
Pediococcus	c, pr, tet	alpha-	-	+	-	+	V	-	V
Helcococcus	c, pr, ch, cl	none	+	-	+	+	+	-	-

infections in compromised patients. Table 18 lists some of the organisms which can be encountered in clinical samples and their basic characteristics.

Cell shape and arrangement in Gram-stained samples may help in dividing these organisms into two groups: those with streptococcal-like appearance (coccobacilli in pairs or chains) and those with staphylococcal-like appearance (cocci in pairs, tetrads, clusters).

Some members (*Abiotrophia*) are pleomorphic when grown in non-optimal conditions; others (*Gemella hemolysans*) may appear Gram negative due to the ease of its cells to be decolorized.

All the organisms listed in Table 18 are non-motile, catalase-negative (except *Alloiococcus* which can be weakly catalase-positive) and α- or non-hemolytic.

1. Abiotrophia

Organisms formerly known as 'nutritionally variant streptococci' were thought to belong to viridans streptococci (e.g., *S. mitis*). Two species are described: *A. defectiva* and *A. adjacens*. A third species, *A. elegans*, was described in 1988 (326). All species have been isolated from cases of endocarditis involving native or prosthetic valves and from ophthalmic infections. *Abiotrophia* spp. do not grow on blood agar but can grow on chocolate agar or need media that are supplemented with 0.01% pyridoxal. They may also be cultured in a test of satellitism in the immediate vicinity of a *S. aureus* strain in a CO_2-enriched atmosphere (the reference strain *S. aureus* ATCC 25923 may be used for this test). Disks containing pyridoxal can be used in tests of satellitism and these are commercially available.

2. Globicatella

This species is isolated from patients with bacteremia, urinary tract infections, and meningitis (327). It resembles viridans streptococci in respect to colonial and cellular morphology, but displays PYR positivity, LAP negative reactions, and tolerance to NaCl.

3. Lactococcus

These organisms are difficult to distinguish from streptococci or enterococci. Isolated from blood or urinary tract infections, their growth at 10°C but not at 45°C may help in identification procedures since enterococci grow both at 10°C and at 45°C, and streptococci may grow at 45°C but not at 10°C. Moreover, commercially-available, specific nucleic acid probe tests for *Enterococcus* spp. may be used to rule out enterococci.

4. Leuconstoc and Pediococcus

Members of these genera produce colonies on blood agar which resemble those of alpha-hemolytic streptococci. Thought to have only an environmental habitat, this organism has been recently reported as causing infections in man, but also due to possible misidentifications of the clinical laboratories, there are insufficient data to establish the frequency of these infections (328). Even if many of them occur in severely immunocompromised patients, some cases (including meningitis) have been reported in previously healthy persons. Documented infections include bacteremias, intravenous-line sepsis, neonatal meningitis, and dental abscess.

Leuconostoc, like *Pediococcus*, and some strains of lactococci are vancomycin-resistant and can often be found in the screening tests for VRE. *Leucostonoc* spp. are, in general, cross-resistant to teicoplanin, but susceptible to penicillin, ampicillin, and clindamycin. They may be separated from vancomycin-resistant lactobacilli by the production of gas from glucose and a negative arginine. Clinical significance of pediococci is less well-defined, but they have been isolated from episodes of septicemia and from hepatic abscesses in severely compromised patients (329,330). Pediococci are negative for gas production and usually arginine positive.

5. Aerococcus

Aerococci display weak or no growth when incubated in anaerobic atmosphere. They are rarely isolated from cases of endocarditis and bacteremia (331). *A. urinae* has, in addition, been isolated from urinary tract infections in predisposed patients (332) and from endocarditis cases (333). When grown aerobically they form α-hemolytic colonies similar to those of viridans streptococci or enterococci. Other characteristics are reported in Table 18.

6. Gemella

G. haemolysans has been isolated from patients with endocarditis, meningitis, or septic arthritis. The other member of this genus is *G. morbillorum* (formerly classified among streptococci) which has been isolated from blood, genito-urinary tract, wound, and abscess specimens. All members of the genus are PYR positive. LAP is negative for *G. hemolysans* and positive for *G. morbillorum*. Due to the slow growth of these bacteria, a test for satellitism may be useful to separate *Gemella* from *Abiotrophia*. *G. hemolysans* prefers aerobic atmosphere, while *G. morbillorum* grows well in anaerobic conditions.

7. Helcococcus

Isolated from intact skin and from foot ulcers, the only species of this genus is *H. kunzii*. The clinical significance of these organisms remains to be clearly established. It has been isolated from wound cultures (foot ulcers) containing mixed organisms (334).

By API rapid Strep test, its profile corresponds to a "doubtful" identification of *A. viridans*. It may be differentiated from aerococci by its good growth under anaerobic conditions and because growth is stimulated by the addition of serum or Tween 80 to the medium.

VII. SUSCEPTIBILITY TESTING

A. *S. pyogenes*

Even if penicillin is still considered the drug of choice for *S. pyogenes* infections, other antimicrobials may be chosen on the basis of the site and the severity of the infection. These include cephalosporins, clindamycin, macrolides, some quinolones, and vancomycin.

Penicillin is in general efficacious in the treatment of erysipelas, impetigo, and cellulitis, and for prevention of post-streptococcal sequelae, but it is not uncommon for penicillin to fail in the eradication of the bacteria from the pharynx (335,336). Also an inadequate effect of penicillin in cases of severe invasive disease have been described (337,338).

In fact, even though in laboratory tests the microorganisms appear susceptible, they may change from logarithmic to stationary phase when their number is very high as happens in severe infections. The effect of this change is that some PBPs (PBP1 and PBP4) become undetectable (339) resulting in possible in vivo failures of the antibiotic. This phenomenon, called the Eagle effect (340) has been clearly demonstrated in animal models (339) and is one of the reasons why clindamycin in addition to penicillin is recommended in severe invasive GAS infections (341). Another reason is that clindamycin suppresses the release of immunologically-active components such as lipoteichoic acid from the cell wall.

Some macrolides are used as drugs of choice in the case of pharyngitis. Less than 5% of isolates are generally reported to be resistant to macrolides, lincosamides and streptogramin (MLS). Unfortunately, regional exceptions have been described in several countries such as Japan (342), Finland (343), and the UK (344). In recent large nation wide studies in Italy, 42% resistance to erythromycin as well as to the long acting macrolides, azithromycin and clarithromycin, have been reported (345,346). The resistance to erythromycin may be due to the presence of gene *erm* AM;

resistant strains show two different phenotypes - inducible resistance (in which the strains are erythromycin-resistant but susceptible to miocamycin and clindamycin) and constitutive resistance (in which strains are highly resistant both to macrolides and clindamycin).

A new mechanism of resistance, mediated by an efflux system has been described (347) in strains constitutively showing low levels of resistance to erythromycin, azithromycin, and clarithromycin but susceptible to clindamycin and josamycin. In these strains MICs are in general lower (8-16 mg./L.) in comparison with those of strains expressing the constitutive resistance phenotype (MICs $\geq$128 mg./L.). No clonal diffusion for these strains has been found. (346).

There is no reason for routinely testing the susceptibility of GAS for penicillin. Among beta-hemolytic streptococci (except pneumococci) only sporadic reports of penicillin resistance have been published, but this does not involve Group A streptococci (348). More important, testing for erythromycin and clindamycin resistance may be warranted where high macrolide resistance is reported. When needed the disk diffusion test may be used to test the susceptibility of all beta hemolytic streptococci to penicillin. Other agents may be tested by the MIC or the disk diffusion methods.

According to NCCLS recommendations (349), the zone diameters which define an isolate as resistant to erythromycin are $\leq$15 mm.; for a susceptible isolate, $\geq$21 mm. For clindamycin, a diameter $\geq$19mm. indicates susceptibility. The MIC breakpoints (mg./L.) for erythromycin are $\leq$0.5 for susceptible organisms and $\geq$4 for resistant ones; for clindamycin they are $\leq$0.25 for susceptible isolates and $\geq$1 for resistant ones.

B. *S. agalactiae*

GBS are susceptible to penicillins, and to first, second (with the exclusion of cefoxitin), and third generations of cephalosporins including the oral agents cefixime and cefpodoxime. Ceftriaxone has a very high activity against GBS. Vancomycin and imipenem are also active.

Resistance to macrolides (erythromycin, clindamycin, and clarithromycin) is reported to occur in 1 to 3% of isolates.

Few strains are resistant to chloramphenicol, while they are generally resistant to tetracycline (90% of isolates). All strains are resistant to nalidixic acid, trimethoprim-sulfamethoxazole, metronidazole and aminoglycosides. A synergistic effect is observed in vitro and in vivo between aminoglycosides (gentamicin) and ampicillin.

Penicillin G is considered the therapy of choice, and high doses are recommended for treatment of serious GBS infections. Despite their uniform sensitivity to penicillin, they have a high minimal inhibitory concentration 4 -10 fold higher (range 0.01-0.04 mg./L.) than that of group A streptococci. Furthermore, as high numbers of bacteria are achieved in blood, CSF, and tissue of GBS-infected patients, higher doses of antibiotic are required to provide bactericidal activity. This inoculum effect also has been noted with cefotaxime and imipenem.

Although GBS is always susceptible to penicillin G, in vitro tolerance has been observed among 4-6% of strains. Tolerance has been observed in some strains that were isolated from invasive neonatal infections, but the clinical significance of this in vitro phenomenon is not clear (350).

C. Beta-hemolytic Groups C and G streptococci

These bacteria are generally susceptible to penicillin and macrolides like *S. pyogenes*, and they can be tested in the same manner.

D. Viridans streptococci

Despite the widespread use of penicillin in the community, the susceptibility of viridans streptococci that are isolated from endocarditis infections has not markedly changed over time. Viridans streptococci with MICs $\geq$0.1 mg./L. are considered relatively resistant. The resistance level may vary with the species and the site of isolation. In general, normal oropharyngeal flora display higher MICs than isolates from blood. In some geographic areas like South Africa where the resistance to penicillin has been commonly reported for *S. pneumoniae*, a prevalence of high level-resistant strains with MICs $\geq$4 mg./L. have been found (351). Like pneumococci, these isolates do not produce β-lactamase and are resistant to other beta-lactam drugs (352); resistance is mediated by alterations in PBPs (353). Transfer of resistance determinants between species may be relevant to the dissemination of penicillin resistance.

Although viridans streptococci are usually considered resistant to aminoglycosides, the combination of penicillin with an aminoglycoside has been shown to be synergistic. While the synergistic effect is lost for streptomycin only with very high ($\geq$1000 mg./L.) MICs, the breakpoint is not so clear for gentamicin; isolates with MICs of 16 mg./L. for gentamicin may show synergism and strains with MICs of 64 mg./L. or more may not.

Ceftriaxone has very good in vitro activity against viridans streptococci and may be a good alternative to penicillin for the treatment of endocarditis. Other antibiotics displaying good in vitro activity are: vancomycin, teicoplanin, and imipenem. Macrolides, fluoroquinolones, and clindamycin have variable activity. Although streptococci are considered routinely susceptible to vancomycin, a recent report of resistant *S. bovis* indicated that the strain was found to have acquired the van B enterococcal vancomycin resistance gene. Nevertheless, to date no vancomycin-resistant strains have been isolated from infected sites (354).

E. *S. pneumoniae*

Susceptibility to antimicrobials is a point of major concern that should be taken into account both for epidemiological and treatment purposes.

As for most other streptococci, pneumococci do not produce β-lactamase, but, since the organisms are naturally transformable, can become resistant to penicillin by acquisition of DNA from closely related species such as *Streptococcus oralis* and *Streptococcus mitis* (355). Even though the frequency of this recombination potential is low, a gene that encodes for penicillin-binding proteins that have low affinity to penicillin has evolved. In particular, changes in PBP2X are associated with high levels of cephalosporin resistance (but still low resistance to penicillin). An additional modification in PBP2B results in high level resistance to penicillin (356,357).

Another resistance of increasing importance is that to erythromycin. Two different mechanisms are described: the first causes the efflux of erythromycin from the cell and confers resistance to erythromycin, clarithromycin, and azithromycin. The second, which is the result of ribosomal modification, is the cause of resistance to macrolides, lincosamides and streptogramins (357).

Identification of resistant pneumococci is based on in vitro susceptibility testing. Clinical microbiology laboratories in general screen for susceptibility to penicillin by using disks that contain 1 μg. of oxacillin. This method is cheap and allows for rapid testing of large numbers of strains, but does not differentiate between intermediate- and high- level resistance which may be important for therapeutic decisions. The level of resistance is therefore necessary and this is accomplished by MIC determination. Penicillin-resistant pneumococci are defined as those resistant to $\geq$0.125 mg./L. of penicillin. Strains with MICs $\geq$0.125 mg./L. but $\leq$1mg./L. are termed 'intermediate', while those with MICs $\geq$2 mg./L. are called 'high level resistant strains'.

As for other microrganisms, MICs can be determined in liquid media using the microdilution method or on solid media by E-test. In the first method, serial microdilutions of penicillin are prepared in broth susceptibility media (Mueller-Hinton broth) and a standardized inoculum is added. NCCLS suggests the addition of 5% lysed horse blood. MIC is the penicillin concentration in the first well where, after overnight incubation, no growth is observed.

The E-test (which is commercially-available) consists of a strip that contains a continuous concentration gradient of antibiotic. It is now widely used for many microrganisms. The test is performed in solid media such as Mueller-Hinton agar with additional blood. After inoculation of the organism by streaking or flooding the agar plate, the antibiotic-containing strip is placed on the surface.

streaking or flooding the agar plate, the antibiotic-containing strip is placed on the surface. After overnight incubation, an elliptical zone of inhibition surrounds the strip. The MIC is determined by reading
the level at which the strip is intersected by the area of inhibition.

The NCCLS breakpoints for the interpretation of MICs for several antibiotics are detailed in Table 19. It is suggested that even though many antibiotics including tetracycline, vancomycin, and ceftriaxone can be tested, only the results for penicillin, erythromycin, and trimethoprim/sulfamethoxazole
should routinely be reported while others are selectively reported when needed (358).

Molecular methods can also be used to determine the presence of resistance genes. Fingerprints of
PBP genes can be used to determine the relatedness of specific PBPs. The *Erm* gene can be assessed to
study the epidemiology of strains that are resistant to macrolides, lincosamides, and streptogramins.

F.   Enterococci

The natural ability of enterococci to acquire, accumulate, and share extrachromosomal elements that
encode antibiotic resistance explains in part their increasing importance as nosocomial pathogens. The
recent interest in enterococcal virulence and host-parasite interaction has been influenced by the concern
that increasing antibiotic resistance may render soon chemotherapyinadequate to treat serious enterococcal infections. Although multiresistance has been described for both in *E. faecium* and *E. faecalis*,
the most problematic profile of antibiotic resistance, (i.e., vancomycin and ampicillin resistance) is most
commonly observed among *E. faecium*.

During the past 15 years, the majority of *E. faecium* have become moreresistant to ampicillin
(359). This type of resistance is based on an overproduction of PBP5 in highly resistant strains with a
low capacity for binding penicillin (359,360). In addition to the high MICs, enterococci appear to be
"tolerant" to beta-lactams with MBCs reported for ampicillin and other penicillins that are higher than

Table 19   Interpretation standards for MICs (mg./L.) to be used with S. pneumoniae in microdilution
tests (performed with Mueller-Hinton broth that has been controlled for cation content and which has
2-5% lysed horse blood added).

Antibiotics	Susceptible	Intermediate	Resistant
Amoxicillin	≤ 0.5	1	≥ 2
Amoxicillin/clavulanate	$\leq 0.5/0.25$	1/0.5	$\geq 2/1$
Azithromycin	≤ 0.5	1	≥ 2
Cefepime	≤ 0.5	1	≥ 2
Cefotaxime	≤ 0.5	1	≥ 2
Ceftriaxone	≤ 0.5	1	≥ 2
Cefuroxime	≤ 0.5	1	≥ 2
Chloramphenicol	≤ 4	-	≥ 8
Clarithromycin	≤ 0.25	0.5	≥ 1
Clindamycin	≤ 0.25	0.5	≥ 1
Erythromycin	≤ 0.25	0.5	≥ 1
Imipenem	≤ 0.12	0.25-0.5	≥ 1
Levofloxacin	≤ 2	4	≥ 8
Ofloxacin	≤ 2	4	≥ 8
Penicillin	≤ 0.06	0.12-1	≥ 2
Rifampin	≤ 1	2	≥ 4
Tetracycline	≤ 2	4	≥ 8
Trimethoprim/ Sulphamethoxazole	$\leq 0.5/9.5$	1/19-2/38	$\geq 4/76$
Vancomycin	<1	-	-

100 mg./L. (361). For *E. faecalis*, the production of beta-lactamase by acquisition of a resistance gene from staphylococci has been described. This type of resistance, however, does not seem to be widely spread and thus has not had significant impact on the clinical treatment.

Low level aminoglycoside resistance among *E. faecalis* is intrinsic and appears to be due to a low uptake of these agents. When enterococci are grown in the presence of cell wall synthesis inhibitors (such as penicillin or vancomycin), the uptake of the aminoglycosides is enhanced and results in increased killing of the organism. The high level resistance (HLR) to aminoglycosides is, on the contrary, acquired and may be due both to ribosomal resistance or to the inactivation of the drug by transposon-encoded aminoglycoside-modifying enzymes (362).

Glycopeptide resistance is more often found in *E. faecium* than in *E. faecalis*, and it is genotypically and phenotypically heterogeneous. Acquired resistance is mediated by two classes of genes, *vanA* and *vanB* that encode for closely related ligases. Strains of the *vanB* phenotype are inducibly resistant to vancomycin but remain susceptible to teicoplanin, although vancomycin induces resistance to this antibiotic (363). Enterococci belonging to *vanC* resistance phenotype are intrinsically resistant to low levels of vancomycin (Table 20).

Testing enterococci for susceptibility to antimicrobial agents may depend on the clinical significance of the isolate and on the site of infection. It is superfluous to test enterococci with drugs to which they are intrinsically resistant; these include aminoglycosides at standard concentrations, cephalosporins, aztreonam, clindamycin, and trimethoprim-sulphamethoxazole. Routine testing for enterococci should include penicillin, ampicillin, and vancomycin. For isolates from the urinary tract, ampicillin, quinolones (e.g., ciprofloxacin, levofloxacin, norfloxacin), nitrofurantoin, and tetracycline should be tested (111,364).

Although these infections in general may be treated with ampicillin, isolates from patients with endocarditis, meningitis, or other serious infections should be tested for aminoglycoside susceptibility and for production of beta-lactamase. Resistance to aminoglycoside synergy should be evaluated for those infections for which a combination therapy is indicated. Systemic enterococcal infections such as endocarditis can be treated with a combination of two antimicrobial agents: one acting at the cell walllevel (a beta-lactam drug or a glycopeptide) and an aminoglycoside (gentamicin or streptomycin) which has the potential to act synergistically (365). High levels of resistance to one of the drugs of the

Table 20 Glycopeptide resistance in enterococci [modified from (359)].

	Acquired resistance		Intrinsic resistance
Phenotype	*vanA*	*vanB*	*vanC*
MIC (mg./L.)			
vancomycin	64 - >1000	4 - >1000	2 – 32
teichoplanin	16 – 512	0.5 – 1	0.5 – 1
Expression	inducible	inducible	constitutive
Bacterial species	*E. faecalis*	*E. faecalis*	*E. gallinarum* (*vanC-1*)
	E. faecium	*E. faecium*	*E. casseliflavus* (*vanC-2*)
	E. avium		*E. flavescens* (*vanC-3*)
	E. gallinarum		*E. faecium* (*vanC-4*)
	E. durans		
	E. mundtii		
	E. casseliflavus		

combination prevent the synergistic bactericidal effect (366). Gentamicin and streptomycin are the only aminoglycosides to be tested. Streptomycin resistance is determined by a mechanism that is different from that of other aminoglycosides and consequently resistance to these drugs must be tested independently. *E. faecalis* may be susceptible to gentamicin but resistant to kanamycin and amikacin. *E. faecium,* irrespective of the results of invitro tests for high-level resistance (HLR), do not show synergy between beta-lactams or vancomycin and kanamycin, tobramycin or netilmicin (367).

Methods used to detect vancomycin resistance and HLR to aminoglycosides are reported in Table 21. In the agar dilution method, additional media such as Mueller-Hinton agar with 5% sheep blood may substitute BHI agar (368). The strain is considered resistant if more than 1 colony/spot grow. In the disk diffusion method, strains with no inhibition zone for aminoglycosides are considered resistant while strains giving at least 10 mm zones are considered susceptible. Isolates yielding 7-9 mm. inhibition zones have usually HLR to aminoglycosides, but some strains have only moderately elevated MICs. Therefore, these strains should be retested by agar dilution or broth microdilution methods to determine the effective resistance.

For quality control, *E. faecalis* strain ATCC 29212 is used as a susceptible strain. For disk diffusion tests, the expected inhibition zone for gentamicin (120 µg./disk) is 16-22 mm., for streptomycin (300 µg./disk) is 14-19 mm. The resistant control strain for gentamicin and streptomycin is *E. faecalis* ATCC 51299. The same strains are also used for quality control for vancomycin resistance.

Vancomycin resistance break points, as defined by NCCLS are: susceptible ≤4 mg./L.; intermediate 8-16 mg./L.; resistant ≥32 mg./L. Recommendations published by NCCLS in 1993 include extending the incubation to 24 hrs. and examining the zone under transmitted light to increase the accuracy of the disk diffusion test. The agar screening test adopted by NCCLS displays a very high sensitivity and specificity. Strains of *E. gallinarum* and *E. casseliflavus* may grow on this medium since their MICs for vancomycin are often higher than 4 mg./L., but they may be differentiated from *E. faecalis* and *E. faecium* since they are motile at 30°C.

Enterococci are known to be more resistant to beta-lactams than streptococci. Isolates of *E. faecalis* usually have MICs for penicillin ranging from 2-4 mg./L., while *E. faecium* often range 16-32 mg./L. (with MICs usually one dilution lower for ampicillin for both species). Routine susceptibility tests may detect the resistance due to changes in PBPs but cannot reveal resistance due to the production of beta-lactamase (rather uncommon) for which an inoculum 100-fold greater than that usually

Table 21 Screening methods to detect high-level resistance to aminoglycosides and vancomycin resistance in enterococci. Abbreviations: BHI - Brain Heart Infusion; MHA - unsupplemented Mueller Hinton agar; * - for streptomycin, reincubate for additional 24 hrs. if no growth at 24 hrs. [Modified from (368)].

	Agar dilution	Broth microdilution	Disk diffusion
Medium	BHI agar	BHI broth	MHA
Bacterial	10^6 CFU/spot	5×10^5 CFU/ml.	0.5 McFarland
Incubation	24 hrs.*	24 hrs.*	24 hrs.
Concentrations:			
vancomycin	6 mg./L.	-	-
gentamicin	500 mg./L.	500 mg./L.	120 mg./L.
streptomycin	2,000 mg./L.	1,000 mg./L.	300 µg./disk

recommended (10^7 CFU/ml.) is needed. For resistant strains, a nitrocefin beta-lactamase test is recommended.

In the absence of aminoglycoside resistance, strains of *E. faecium* with MICs for penicillin = 6 mg./L. should be considered still potentially susceptible to the synergy with an aminoglycoside. For beta-lactamase negative strains, MICs may be assessed by agar or broth dilution tests or by E-test (369).

REFERENCES

1. Kawamura Y, Hou X, Sultana F, Yamamoto H, Ezaki T. Transfer of *S. adjacens* and *S. defectives* to *Abiotrophia* gen. nov. as *A. adjacens* comb. nov. and *A. defectiva* comb. nov. respectively. Int J Syst Bacteriol 1995; 45:798-803.
2. Facklam R, Elliott JA. Identification, classification and clinical relevance of catalase-negative, gram-positive cocci, excluding streptococci and enterococci. Clin Microbiol Rev 1995; 8:479-495.
3. Kilpper-Balz R, Schleifer RH. Transfer of *S. morbillorum* to the genus *Gemella* as *G. morbillorum* comb. nov. Int J Syst Bacteriol 1988; 38:442-447.
4. Lancefield RC. A serological differentiation of human and other groups of hemolystic streptococci. J Exp Med 1933; 57:571-595.
5. Baker CJ, Barrett FF. Transmission of group B streptococci among parturient women and their neonates. J Pediatr 1973; 83:919-925.
6. Schrag SJ, Zywicki S, Farley MM, Reingold AL, Harrison LH, Lefkowitz LB, Hadler JL, Danila R, Cieslak PR, Schuchat A. Group B streptococcal disease in the era of intrapartum antibiotic prophylaxis. N Engl J Med 2000; 342:15-20.
7. Schuchat A, Whitney C, Zangwill K. Prevention of perinatal group B streptococcal disease: a public health perspective. MMWR 1996; 45(RR-7):1-24.
8. Gotoff SP. Chemoprophylaxis of early onset group B streptococcal disease in 1999. Curr Opin Pediatr 2000; 12:105-110.
9. Schuchat A. Epidemiology of group B streptococcal disease in the United States: shifting paradigms. Clin Microbiol Rev 1998; 11:479-513.
10. Gardam MA, Low DE, Saginur R, Miller M. Group B streptococcal necrotizing fascitiis and streptococcal toxic shock-like syndrome in adults. Arch Intern Med 1998; 158:1704-1708.
11. Lancefield RC, Hare R. The serological differentiation of pathogenic and non-pathogenic strains of hemolytic streptococci from parturient women. J Exp Med 1935; 61:335-349.
12. Farrow JA, Collins MD. Taxonomic studies on streptococci of serological groups C, G and possibly related taxa. Syst Appl Microbiol 1985; 5:483-493.
13. Vandamme P, Pot B, Falsen E, Kersters K, De Vries LA. Taxonomic studies of Lancefield streptococcal group C, G and L (*S. dysgalactiae*) and proposal of *S. dysgalactiae* subsp. equisimilis subsp. nov. Int J Syst Bacteriol 1996; 46:774-781.
14. Andrewes FW, Horder TJ. A study of the streptococci pathogenic for man. Lancet 1906; ii:708-713.
15. Orla-Jensen S. The lactic acid bacteria. Mem Acad R Sci Dan Sect Sci Ser 1919; 85:81-197.
16. Clarke JR. On the bacterial factor in the aetiology of dental caries. Br J Exp Pathol 1922; 5:141-147.
17. Wittenbury R. Hydrogen peroxide formation and catalase activity in the lactic acid bacteria. J Gen Microbiol 1964; 35:13-26.
18. Colman G, Williams REO. Taxonomy of some human viridans streptococci. In: Wannamaker LW, Matsen JM, eds. Streptococci and Streptococcal Diseases: Recognition, Understanding and Management. New York, NY:Academic Press, 1972:281-299.
19. Facklam RR. Physiological differentiation of viridans streptococci. J Clin Microbiol 1977; 5:184-201.
20. Kawamura Y, Hou XG, Sultana F, Miura H, Ezaki T. Determination of 16S rRNA sequence of *S. mitis* and *S. gordonii* and phylogenetic relationship among members of the genus *Streptococcus*. Int J Syst Bacteriol 1995; 45:406-408.
21. Pasteur L. Note sur la maladie nouvelle provoquee par la salive d'un enfant mort de la rage. Bulletin de l'Academie de Medecine (Paris) (series 2) 1881; 10:94-103.
22. Sternberg GM. A fatal form of septicaemia in the rabbit produced by the subcutaneous injection of human saliva. Annual Reports of the National Board of Health 1881; 3:87-108.

23. Sternberg GM. The pneumonia-coccus of Friedlander (*Micrococcus Pasteuri*, Sternberg). Am J Med Sci 1885; 90:106-123.

24. Deibel RH, Seeley Jr HW. Family II. *Streptococcaceae.* In: Buchanan RE, Gibbons NE - eds. Bergey's Manual of Determinative Bacteriology. Baltimore:Williams & Wilkins, 1974.

25. Netter. De la meningite due au pneumocoque (avec ou sans pneumonia). Arch Generales de Medicine (series 7) 1887; 19:257-277.

26. Austrian R. The Gram stain and the etiology of lobar pneumonia, an historical note. Bacteriol Rev 1960; 24:261-265.

27. Tillet WS, Cambier MJ, McCormack JE. The treatment of lobar pneumonia and pneumococcal empyema with penicillin. Bull NY Acad Sci 1944; 20:142-178.

28. Avery OT, Dubos R. The protective action of a specific enzyme against type III pneumococcus infection in mice. J Exp Med 1931; 54:73-89.

29. Avery OT, MacLeod C, McCarty M. Studies on the chemical nature of the substance inducing transformation of pneumococcal types: induction of transformation by a desoxyribonucleic acid fraction isolated from pneumococcus type III. J Exp Med 1944; 79:137-157.

30. Heidelberger M. Immunologically specific polysaccharides. Chem Rev 1927; 3:403-423.

31. Thiercelin ME. Sur un diplocoque de l'intestin susceptible de devenir pathogene. CR Soc Biol 1899; 5:269-271.

32. Sherman JM. The streptococci. Bacteriol Rev 1937; 1:3-97.

33. Hartmann PA, Renbold GW, Saraswat DS. Indicator organisms- a review. 1. Taxonomy of the fecal streptococci. J Syst Bacteriol 1966; 16:197-221.

34. Kalina AP. The taxonomy and nomenclature of enterococci. Int J Syst Bacteriol 1970; 20:185-189.

35. Schleifer KH, Klipper-Balz R. Transfer of *S. fecalis* and *S. faecium* to the genus *Enterococcus* nom. rev. as *Enterococcus fecalis* comb. nov. and *Enterococcus faecium* comb. nov. Int J Syst Bacteriol 1984; 34:31-34.

36. Chiesa C, Pacifico L, Nanni F, Orefici G. Recurrent attacks of scarlet fever. Arch Pediatr Adolesc Med 1994; 148:656-660.

37. Stevens DL. The flesh-heating bacterium: what's next? J Infect Dis 1999; 179:S366-S374.

38. Stevens DL. Invasive group A streptococcal disease. Infect Agents Dis 1996; 5:157-166.

39. Stevens DL. Streptococcal toxic-shock syndrome: spectrum of disease, pathogenesis, and new concepts in treatment. Emerg Infect Dis 1995; 1:69-78.

40. Bisno AL. The concept of rheumatogenic and non-rheumatogenic group A streptococci. In: Read SE, Zabriskie JB - eds. Streptococcal Diseases and the Immune Response. New York, NY: Academic Press, 1970:789-803.

41. Potter EV, Svartman M, Mohammed I. Tropical acute rheumatic fever and associated streptococcal infections compared with concurrent acute glomerulonephritis. J Pediatr 1978; 92:325-333.

42. Bisno AL, Pearce IA, Wall HP. Contrasting epidemiology of acute rheumatic fever and acute glomerulonephritis: nature of antecedent streptococcal infection. N Engl J Med 1970; 283:561-565.

43. Carapetis JR, Currie BJ, Good MF. Towards understanding the pathogenesis of rheumatic fever. Scand J Rheumatol 1996; 25:127-131.

44. Stollerman GH. Rheumatogenic streptococci and autoimmunity. Clin Immunol Immunopathol 1991; 61:131-142.

45. Senitzer D, Freimer EH. Autoimmune mechanisms in the pathogenesis of rheumatic fever. Rev Infect Dis 1984; 6:832-839.

46. Tsuchiya N, Williams Jr RC. Molecular mimicry-hypothesis or reality? West J Med 1992; 157:133-138.

47. Galvin JE, Hemric ME, Ward K, Cunningham MW. Cytotoxic mAb from rheumatic carditis recognizes heart valves and laminin. J Clin Invest 2000; 106:217-224.

48. Kaplan MH. Cross reaction of group A streptococci with heart tissue antigens: implications for pathogenetic mechanisms in rheumatic fever. In: Bowen WH, Genco RJ, O'Brien TC - eds. Immunologic Aspects of Dental Caries. Washington, DC:Information Retrieval, 1976:171-176.

49. Glurich I, Winters B, Albini B, Stinson M. Identification of *Streptococcus pyogenes* proteins that bind to rabbit kidney in vitro and in vivo. Microb Pathog 1991; 10:209-220.

50. Swedo SE, Leonard HL, Garvey MA. Pediatric autoimmune neuropsychiatric disorders associated with streptococcal infections: clinical description of the first 50 cases. Am J Psychiatry 1998; 155:264-271.

51. Perlmutter SJ, Leitman SF, Garvey MA, Hamburger S, Feldman E, Leonard HL, Swedo S. Therapeutic plasma exchange and intravenous immunoglobulin for obsessive-compulsive disorders and tic disorders in childhood. Lancet 1999; 354:1153-1158.

52. Cardona F, Orefici G. Group A streptococcal infections and tic disorders in an Italian pediatric population. J Pediatr (In press).

53. Baker CJ, Edwards MS. Group B streptococcal infections. In: Remington J, Klein JO - eds. Infectious Diseases of the Fetus and Newborn. Philadelphia, PA:WB Saunders, 1995:980-1054.

54. Hickman ME, Rench MA, Ferrieri P, Baker CJ. Changing epidemiology of group B streptococcal colonization. Pediatrics 1999, 104;203-209.

55. Jackson LA, Hilsdon M, Farley M, Harrison L, Reingold A, Wenger JD, Schuchat A. Risk factors for group B streptococcal disease in adults. Ann Intern Med 1995; 123:415-420.

56. Turner JC, Hayden GF, Kiselica D, Lohr J, Fishburne CF, Murren D. Association of group C streptococci with endemic pharyngitis among college students. JAMA 1990; 264:2644-2647.

57. Bisno AL, Collins CM, Turner JC. M proteins of group C streptococci isolated from patients with acute pharyngitis. J Clin Microbiol 1996; 34:2511-2515.

58. Hill HR, Caldwell GC, Wilson E, Hager D, Zimmerman RA. Epidemic of pharyngitis due to streptococci of Lancefield group G. Lancet 1969; ii:371-374.

59. Stryker WS, Fraser DW, Facklam RR. Foodborne outbreak of group G streptococcal pharyngitis. Am J Epidemiol 1982; 116:533-540.

60. Carmeli Y, Ruoff KL. Report of cases of and taxonomic considerations for large-colony forming Lancefield group C streptococcal bacteremia. J Clin Microbiol 1995; 33:2114-2117.

61. Carmeli Y, Shapiro JM, Neeman D, Yunon AM, Alkan M. Streptococcal group C bacteremia: survey in Israel and analytical review. Arch Intern Med 1995; 155:1170-1176.

62. McRinsey DS, Ratts TE, Bisno AL. Underlying cardial lesions in adults with infective endocarditis. The changing spectrum. Am J Med 1987; 82:681-688.

63. Van der Meer JTM, Thompson J, Valkenburg HA. Epidemiology of bacterial endocarditis in the Netherlands: patient characteristics. Arch Intern Med 1992; 152:1863-1868.

64. Starkenbaum M, Durack D, Beeson P. The "incubation" period of bacterial endocarditis. Yale J Biol Med 1977; 50:49-58.

65. Sussman JI, Baron EJ, Tenenbaum MJ. Viridans streptococcal endocarditis: clinical, microbiological and echo-cardiographic correlations. J Infect Dis 1986; 154:597-603.

66. Von Reyn CF, Levy BS, Arbeit RD. Infective endocarditis: an analysis based on strict case definitions. Ann Intern Med 1981; 94:505-518.

67. Werner AS, Cobbs CG, Kaye D. Studies on the bacteremia of bacterial endocarditis. JAMA 1967; 202:127-131.

68. Morrison AJ, Wenzel RP. Nosocomial urinary tract infections due to enterococcus. Ten years experience at a university hospital. Arch Intern Med 1986; 146:1549-1551.

69. Gross PA, Harkavy L, Barden GE, Flower MF. The epidemiology of nosocomial enterococcal urinary tract infections. Am J Med Sci 1976; 272:75-81.

70. Fleming D, Hirishboeck F, Cosgriff J. Minnesota rheumatic fever survey 1955. Minn Med 1956; 39:208-213.

71. Land MA, Bisno AL. Acute rheumatic fever. A vanishing disease in suburbia. JAMA 1983; 249:895-898.

72. Gordis L. Changing risk of rheumatic fever. In: Shulman S - ed. Management of Streptococcal pharyngitis in an era of declining rheumatic fever. New York, NY: Prager Publishers, 1984; 13-22.

73. World Health Organization. WHO programme for the prevention of rheumatic fever/rheumatic hearth disease in 16 developing countries: Report from Phase 1 (1986-1990). Bull WHO 1992; 70:213-218.

74. Veasy L, Tani L, Hill H. Persistence of acute rheumatic fever in the intermountain area of the United States. J Pediatr 1994; 124:9-16.

75. Stevens DL, Tauner MH, Winship J. Severe group A streptococcal infections associated with a toxic shock-like syndrome and scarlet fever toxin A. N Engl J Med 1989; 321:1-7.

76. Martin P, Hoiby E. Streptococcal serogroup A epidemic in Norway 1987-1988. Scand J Inf Dis 1990; 22(Suppl):421-429.

77. Cherchi GB, Kaplan EL, Schlievert PM, Bitti A, Orefici G. First reported case of *S. pyogenes* infection with toxic shock-like syndrome. Eur J Clin Microbiol Infect Dis 1992; 11:836-838.

78. Harrison LH, Elliot JA, Dwyer D, Libonati JP, Ferrieri P, Billmann L, Schuchat A, and the Maryland Emerging Infections Program. Serotype distribution of invasive group B streptococcal isolates in Maryland: implications for vaccine formulation. J Infect Dis 1998, 177:998-1002.

79. Lachenauer CS, Kasper DL, Shimada J, Ichiman Y, Ohtsuka H, Kaku M, Paoletti LC, Ferrieri P, Madoff LC. Serotype VI and VIII predominate among group B streptococci isolated from pregnant Japanese women. J Infect Dis 1999; 179:1030-1033.

80. Drusin LM, Ribble JC, Topf B. Group C streptococcal colonization in a newborn nursery. Am J Dis Child 1973; 125:820-821.

81. Socransky SS, Manganiello AD. The oral microbiota of man from birth to senility. J Periodontology 1971; 42:485-494.

82. Woods DE, Straus DC, Johanson WG. Role of fibronectin in the prevention of adherence of *P. aeruginosa* to buccal cells. J Inf Dis 1981; 143:784-790.

83. Kaye D, McCormick RC, Hook EW. Bacterial endocarditis: the changing pattern since the introduction of penicillin therapy. Antimicrob Agents and Chemother 1962; 1:37-46.

84. Roberts RB, Kreiger AG, Schiller NI. Viridans streptococcal endocarditis: the role of various species including pyridoxal-dependent streptococci. Rev Infect Dis 1979; 1:955-965.

85. Hoyne AL, Herizon H. *Streptococcus viridans* meningitis. A review of the literature and report of 9 recoveries. Ann Intern Med 1950; 33:879-902.

86. Leiger JF. *Streptococcus salivarius* meningitis and colonic carcinoma. South Med J 1991; 84:1058-1059.

87. Bochud PY, Calandra T, Francioli P. Bacteremia due to viridans streptococci in neutropenic patients: a review. Am J Med 1994; 97:256-264.

88. Beighton DA, Carr AD, Oppenheim BA. Identification of viridans streptococci associated with bacteremia in neutropenic cancer patients. J Med Microbiol 1994; 40:202-204.

89. Ruoff KL, Ferrero MJ, Holden J, Kunz LJ. Identification of *S. bovis* and *S. salivarius* in the clinical laboratory. J Clin Microbiol 1984; 20:223-226.

90. Klein RS, Catalano MT, Edberg SC, Casey JI, Steigbigel NH. Association of *S. bovis* with carcinoma of the colon. N Engl J Med 1977; 91:560-562.

91. Reynolds JG, Silva E, McCormack WM. Association of *S. bovis* bacteremia with bowel disease. J Clin Microbiol 1983; 17:696-697.

92. Anonymous. Defining the public health impact of drug-resistant *Streptococcus pneumoniae*: report of a working group. *MMWR Morb Mortal Wkly Rep* 1996; 45:RR-I.

93. Austrian R. The pneumococcus at the millennium: not down, not out. J Infect Dis 1999 (Suppl 2):338-341.

94. Tomasz A. Antibiotic resistance in *Streptococcus pneumoniae*. Clin Infect Dis 1997; 24:585-588.

95. Crook DWM, Spratt BG. Multiple antibiotic resistance in *Streptococcus pneumoniae*. *Br Med Bull* 1998; 54:595-610.

96. McDougall LK, Rasheed JK, Biddle JW, Tenover FC. Identification of multiple clones of extended-spectrum cephalosporin-resistant *Streptococcus pneumoniae* isolates in the United States. Antimicrob Agents Chemother 1995; 39:2282-2288.

97. Coffey T, Dowson CG, Daniels M. Horizontal transfer of multiple penicillin binding protein genes and capsular biosyntetic genes in natural populations of *Streptococcus pneumoniae*. Mol Microbiol 1991; 5:2255-2260.

98. Lyon DJ, Scheel O, Fung KSC, Cheng AFB, Henrichsen J. Rapid emergence of penicillin-resistant pneumococci in Hong Kong. Scand J Infect Dis 1996; 28:375-376.

99. Geslin P, Buu-Hoi A, Frémaux A, Acar JF. Antimicrobial resistance in *Streptococcus pneumoniae* and epidemiological survey in France, 1970-1990. Clin Infect Dis 1992; 15:95-98.

100. Hofmann J, Cetron MS, Farley MM, Baughman WS, Facklam RR, Elliott JA, Deaver KA, Breiman RF. The prevalence of drug-resistant *Streptococcus pneumoniae* in Atlanta. N Engl J Med 1995; 333:481-486.

101. Dutka BJ, Kwan KK. Comparison of eight media procedures for recovering faecal streptococci from water under winter conditions. J Appl Bacteriol 1978; 45:333-340.

102. Kibbey HJ, Hagedorn JC, McCoy EL. Use of fecal streptococci as indicators of pollution in soil. Appl Environ Microbiol 1978; 35:711-717.

103. Devriese LA, Collins MD, Wirth R. The genus *Enterococcus*. In: Balows A, Truper G, Dworkin M, Harder W, Schleifer KH - eds. The Procaryotes. A Handbook of the Biology of Bacteria: Ecophysiology, Isolation, Identification, Applications. 2nd Edn. New York, NY :Springer-Verlag, 1992; 1465-1481.

104. Vollaard EJ, Clasener HAL. Colonization resistance. Antimicrob Agents Chemother 1994; 38:409-414.

105. Kaye K. Enterococci. Biologic and epidemiologic characteristics and in vitro susceptibility. Arch Intern Med 1982; 142: 2006-2009.

106. Murray BE, Singh RV, Markowitz SM, Lopardo HA, Patterson JE, Zervos MJ, Rubeglio E, Eliopoulos GM, Rice LB. Goldstein FW, and Members of the Study Group. Evidence for clonal spread of a single strain of beta-lactamase producing *E. faecalis* to six hospitals in five states. J Infect Dis 1991; 163: 780-785.

107. Livornese LL, Drus S, Samel C. Hospital acquired infection with vancomycin resistant *E. faecium* transmitted by electronic thermometers. Ann Intern Med 1992; 117:112-116.

108. Hall RW, Bayer AS, Mayer WP. Infective endocarditis following human-to-human enterococcal transmission. Arch Intern Med. 1976; 136:1173-1174.

109. Hall LMC, Duke B, Urwin G. Epidemiology of *E. faecalis* urinary tract infection in a teaching hospital in London, UK. J Clin Microbiol 1992; 30:1953-1957.
110. Megran DW. Enterococcal endocarditis. Clin Infect Dis 1992; 15:63-71.
111. Witte W, Wirth R, Klare I. Enterococci. Chemotherapy 1999; 45:135-145.
112. Schaberg DR, Culver DH, Gaynes RP. Major trends in the microbial etiology of nocosomial infections. Am J Med 1991; 91:725-755.
113. Chenoweth CE, Schaberg DR. *Enterococcus* species. In: Mayhall GG - ed. Hospital Epidemiology and Infection Control. Baltimore, MD:Williams and Wilkins, 1996:334-345.
114. Murray BE. The life and times of the *Enterococcus.* Clin Microbiol Rev 1990; 3:46-65.
115. Uttley AHC, Collins CH, Naidoo J, George RC. Vancomycin-resistant enterococci. Lancet 1988; i:57-58.
116. Leclerc R, Derlot E, Duval J, Courvalin P. Plasmid-mediated resistance to vancomycin and teicoplanin in *E. faecium.* N Engl J Med 1988; 319: 157-161.
117. Sahm DF, Kissinger J, Gilmore MS, Murray PR, Mulder R, Solliday J. In vitro susceptibility studies of vancomycin resistant *E. faecalis.* Antimicrob Agents Chemother 1989; 33:1588-1591.
118. Huycke MM, Sahm DF, Gilmore MS. Multiple-drug resistant enterococci: the nature of the problem and an agenda for the future. Emerg Infect Dis 1998; 4:239-249.
119. Shouten MA, Voss A, Hoogkamp-Korstanje JAA, and European VRE study group. Antimicrob Agents Chemother 1999; 43: 2542-2546.
120. Bates J. Epidemiology of vancomycin-resistant enterococci in the community and the relevance of farm animals to human infections. J Hosp Infect 1997; 37:89-101.
121. Schrager HM, Alberti S, Cywes C, Dougherty GJ, Wessels MR. Hyaluronic acid capsule modulates M protein-mediated adherence and acts as ligand for attachment of group A Streptococcus to CD44 or human keratinocytes. J Clin Invest 1998; 101:1708-1716.
122. Fischetti VA. Surface proteins of gram positive bacteria. In: Fischetti VA, Novick RP, Ferretti JJ, Portnoy DA, Rood JI - eds. Gram Positive Pathogens. Washington, DC:ASM Press, 2000:11-24.
123. Okada N, Liszewski MK, Atkinson JP, Caparon M. Membrane co-factor protein (CD46) is a keratinocyte receptor for the M protein of the group A streptococcus. Proc Natl Acad Sci 1995; 92:2489-2493.
124. Johnson LP, Schlievert PM. Group A streptococcal phage T12 carriers the structural gene for pyrogenic exotoxin type A. Mol Gen Genet 1984; 194:52-56.
125. Goshorn SC, Bohach GA, Schlievert PM. Cloning and characterization of the gene *speC*, for pyrogenic exotoxin Type C from *S. pyogenes.* Mol Gen Genet 1988; 212:66-70.
126. Schlievert PM, Assimacopoulos AP, Cleary PP. Severe invasive group A streptococcal disease: clinical description and mechanisms of pathogenesis. J Lab Clin Med 1996; 127:13-22.
127. Hauser AR, Schlievert PM. Nucleotide sequence of the streptococcal pyrogenic exotoxin B gene and toxin relationship with streptococcal proteinase precursor. J Bacteriol 1990; 172:4536-4542.
128. Reader RH, Woishimik, Podbielski A, Boyle MD. A secreted streptococcal cyteine protease can cleave a surface expressed M1 protein and alters its immunoglobulin-binding properties. Res Microbiol 1998; 149:539-548.
129. Ginsburg I. Streptolysin S. In: Montie TC, Kaddas S, Ajil SJ - eds. Microbial Toxins. New York, NY: Academic Press, 1972:99-171.
130. LaPenta D, Rubens C, Chi E, Cleary PP. Group A streptococci efficiently invade human respiratory epithelial cells. Proc Natl Acad Sci U S A 1994: 91:12115-12119.
131. Jadoun J, Ozeri V, Burstein E, Skutelsky E, Hanski E, Sela S. Protein F1 is required for efficient entry of *Streptococcus pyogenes* into epithelial cells. J Infect Dis 1998; 178:147-158.
132. Berkower C, Ravins M, Moses AE, Hanski E. Expression of different group A streptococcal M proteins in an isogenic background demonstrates diversity in adherence to and invasion of eukaryotic cells. Mol Microbiol 1999; 31:1463-1475.
133. Nealon TJ, Beachey EH, Courtney HS, Simpson WA. Release of fibronectin-lipoteichoic acid complexes from group A streptococci with penicillin. Infect Immun 1986; 51:529-535.
134. Dombek PE, Cue D, Sedgewick J, Lam H, Ruschkowski S, Finlay BB, and Cleary PP. High-frequency intracellular invasion of epithelial cells by serotype M1 group A streptococci: M1 protein-mediated invasion and cytoskeletal rearrangements. Mol Microbiol 1999; 31:859-870.
135. Robinson JH, Kehoe MA. Group A streptococcal M proteins: virulence factors and protective antigens. Immunol Today 1992; 13:362-367.
136. Zeymer U, Neuhaus KL. Clinical trials in acute myocardial infarction. Curr Opin Cardiol 1999; 14:392-402.

137. Gersh BJ. Optimal management of acute myocardial infarction at the dawn of the next millennium. Am Heart J 1999; 138:188-202.

138. Stevens DL. Invasive group A streptococcus infections. Clin Infect Dis 1992; 14:2-11.

139. Fast DJ, Schlievert PM, Nelson RD. Toxic shock syndrome-associated staphylococcal and streptococcal pyrogenic toxins are potent inducers of tumor necrosis factor production. Infect Immun 1989; 57:291-294.

140. Muller-Alouf H, Capron M, Alouf JE, Geoffroy C, Gerlach D, Ozegowski JH, Fitting C, Cavaillon JM. Cytokine profile of human peripheral blood mononucleated cells stimulated with a novel streptococcal superantigen, *SpeA*, *SpeC* and group A streptococcal cells. Adv Exp Med Biol 1997; 418:929-931.

141. Muller-Alouf H, Alouf JE, Gerlach D, Ozegowski JH, Fitting C, and Cavaillon JM. Comparative study of cytokine release by human peripheral blood mononuclear cells stimulated with *Streptococcus pyogenes* superantigenic erythrogenic toxins, heat-killed streptococci, and lipopolysaccharide. Infect Immun 1994; 62:4915-4921.

142. Kotb M, Ohnishi H, Majumdar G, Hackett S, Bryant A, Higgins G, Stevens D. Temporal relationship of cytokine release by peripheral blood mononuclear cells stimulated by the streptococcal superantigen pep M5. Infect Immun 1993; 61:1194-1201.

143. Kapur V, Majesky MW, Li LL, Black RA, Musser JM. Cleavage of interleukin 1 beta (IL-1 beta) precursor to produce active IL-1 beta by a conserved extracellular cysteine protease from *Streptococcus pyogenes*. Proc Natl Acad Sci U S A 1993; 90:7676-7680.

144. Stevens DL. Invasive group A streptococcal infections: the past, present and future. Pediatr Infect Dis J 1994; 13:561-566.

145. Lancefield RC. A serological differentiation of specific types of bovine hemolytic streptococci (group B) J Exp Med 1934; 59:441-458.

146. Michon F, Brisson JR, Dell A, Kasper DK, Jennings HJ. Multiantennary group specific polysaccharide of group B streptococcus. Biochemistry 1988; 27:5341-5351.

147. Jennings HJ, Katzenellenbogen E, Lugoski C, Michon F, Roy R, Kasper DL. Structure, conformation and immunology of sialic acid containing polysaccharides of human pathogenic bacteria. Pure Appl Chem 1984, 56:893-905

148. Wessels MR, Benedì VJ, Jennings HJ, Michon F, DiFabio JL, Kasper DL. Isolation and characterization of type IV group B *Streptococcus* capsular polysaccharide. Infect Immun 1989; 57:1089-1094.

149. Wessels MR, DiFabio JL, Benedì VJ, Kasper DL, Michon F, Brisson JR, Jelínková J, Jennings HJ. Structural determination and immunochemical characterization of type V group B *Streptococcus* capsular polysaccharide. J Biol Chem 1991; 266: 6714-6719.

150. von Hunolstein C, D'Ascenzi S, Wagner B, Jelínková J, Alfarone G, Recchia S, Wagner M, Orefici G. Immunochemistry of capsular type polysaccharide and virulence properties of type VI *Streptococcus agalactiae* (group B streptococci). Infect Immun 1993; 61:1272-1280.

151. Kogan G, Brisson JR, Kasper DL, von Hunolstein C, Orefici G, Jennings HJ. Structural elucidation of the novel type VII group B *Streptococcus* capsular polysaccharide by high resolution NMR. Carbohydr Res 1995; 277:1-9.

152. Kogan G, Uhrin D, Brisson JR, Paoletti LC, Blodget AE, Kasper DL, Jennings HJ. Structural and immunochemical characterization of the type VIII group B streptococcus capsular polysaccharide. J Biol Chem 1996; 271:8786-8790.

153. Orefici G, Recchia S, Galante L. Possible virulence marker for *Streptococcus agalactiae* (Lancefield group B). Eur J Clin Microbiol Infect Dis 1988; 7:302-305.

154. Lancefield RC, McCarty M, Everly WN. Multiple mouse-protective antibodies directed against group B streptococci. Special reference to antibodies effective against protein antigens. J Exp Med 1975; 142:165-179.

155. Tissi L, von Hunolstein C, Bistoni F, Marangi M, Parisi L, Orefici G. Role of group B streptococcal capsular polysaccharides in the induction of septic arthritis. J Med Microbiol 1998; 47:717-723.

156. Marques MB, Kasper DL, Pangburn MK, Wessels MR. Prevention of C3 deposition by capsular polysaccharides is a virulence mechanism of type III group B streptococci. Infect Immun 1992; 60: 3986-3993.

157. von Hunolstein C, Totolian A, Alfarone G, Mancuso G, Cusumano V, Teti G Orefici G. Soluble antigens from group B stretococci induce cytokine production in human blood cultures. Infect Immun 1997; 65:4017-4021.

158. Vallejo JG, Baker CJ, Edwards M. Interleukin-6 production by human neonatal monocytes stimulated by type III group B streptococci. J Infect Dis 1996; 174:332-337.

159. Tissi L, Puliti M, Barluzzi R, Orefici G, von Hunolstein C, Bistoni F. Role of tumor necrosis factor alpha, interleukin-1β and interleukin-6 in a mouse model of group B streptococcal arthritis. Infect Immun 1999; 67:4545-4550.

160. Orefici G, Molinari A, Donelli G, Paradisi, Teti G, Arancia G. Immunolocalization of lipoteichoic acid on group B streptococcal surface. FEMS Microbiol Lett 1986; 34:111-115.

161. Nealon TJ, Mattingly SJ. Association of elevated levels of cellular lipoteichoic acid of group B streptococci with human neonatal disease. Infect Immun 1983; 39:1243-1251.

162. Tamura GS, Kuypers JM, Smith S, Raff H, Rubens CE. Adherence of group B streptococci to cultured epithelial cells: roles of enviromental factors and bacterial surface components. Infect Immun 1994; 62:2450- 2458.

163. Spellerberg B, Rozdzinski E, Martin S, Weber-Heynemann J, Schnitzler N, Lüttiken R, Podbielski A. Lmb, a protein with similarities to the LraI adhesin family, mediates attachment of *Streptococcus agalactiae* to human laminin. Infect Immun 1999; 67:871-878.

164. Madoff LC, Michel JL, Gong EW, Rodewald AK, Kasper DL. Protection of neonatal mice from group B streptococcal infection by maternal immunization with beta C protein. Infect Immun 1992; 60:4989-4994.

165. Fasola EL, Flores AE, Ferrieri P. Immune response to the R4 antigen in streptococcal human sera. In: Pathogenic Streptococci: Present and Future., St. Petersburg, Russia: Lancer Symposium, 1994:172-174.

166. Larsson C, Stålhammer-Carlemalm M, Lindhal G. Experimental vaccination against group B *Streptococcus*, an encapsulated bacterium, with highly purified preparations of cell surface proteins Rib and α. Infect Immun 1996; 64:3518-3523.

167. Chun CSY, Brady LJ, Boyle MDP, Dillon HC, Ayoub EM. Group B streptococcal C protein associated antigens: association with neonatal sepsis. J Infect Dis 1991; 163:786-791.

168. Nizet V, Gibson RL, Chi EY, Framson PE, Hulse M, Rubens CE. Group B streptococcal hemolysin expression is associated with injury of lung epithelial cells. Infect Immun 1996; 64:3818-3826.

169. Hill HR, Bohsack JF, Morris EZ, Augustine NH, Parker CJ, Cleary PP, Wu JT. Group B streptococci inhibit chemotactic activity of the fifth component of complement. J Immunol 1988; 141:3551-3556.

170. Podbielski A, Blankenstein O, Lüttiken R. Molecular characterization of the *cfb* gene encoding group B streptococcal CAMP-factor gene. Med Microbiol Immunol 1994; 183:239-256.

171. Ke D, Menard C, Picard FJ, Boissinot M, Ouellette M, Roy PH, Bergeron MG. Development of conventional and real time PCR assays for the rapid detection of group B streptococci. Clin Chem 2000; 46:324-321.

172. Nizet V, Kim KS, Stins M, Jonas M, Chi EY, Nguyen D, Rubens CE. Invasion of brain microvascular endothelial cells by group B streptococci. Infect Immun 1997; 65:5074-5081.

173. Valentin-Weigand P, Chhatwal GS. Correlation of epithelial cell invasiveness of group B streptococci with clinical source of isolation. Microbial Pathog 1995; 19:83-91.

174. Cornacchione P, Scaringi L, Fettucciari K, Rosati E, Sabatini R, Orefici G, von Hunolstein C, Modesti A, Modica A, Minelli F, Marconi P. Group B streptococci persist inside macrophages. Immunology 1998; 93:86-95.

175. Lindgren PE, Speziale P, Mc Gavin M, Monstein HG, Höök M, Visai L, Kostiainen T, Bozzini S, Lindberg M. Cloning and expression of two different genes from *S. dysgalactiae* encoding fibronecting receptors. J Biol Chem 1993; 267:1924-1931.

176. Chhatwal GS, Preissner RT, Muller-Berghans, Blobel H. Specific binding of the human S protein (vitronectin) to streptococci, *S. aureus* and *E. coli*. Infect Immun 1987; 55:1878-1883.

177. Visai L, Bozzini S, Raucci G, Toniolo A, Speziale P. Isolation and characterization of a novel collagen-binding protein from *S. pyogenes* strain 6414. J Biol Chem 1995; 270:347-353.

178. Cleary P, Peterson J, Chen C, Nelson C. Virulent human strains of group G streptococci express a C5a peptidase enzyme similar to that produced by group A streptococci. Infect Immun 1994; 59:2305-2310.

179. Campo R, Shultz DR, Bisno A. M proteins of group G streptococci: mechanisms of resistance to phagocytosis. J Infect Dis 1995; 171:601-606.

180. Fischetti VA. Streptococcal M protein: molecular design and biological behaviour. Clin Microbiol Rev 1989; 2:285-314.

181. Collins CM, Kimura A, Bisno AL. Group G streptococcal M protein exibit structural features analogous to those of class I M protein of group A streptococci. Infect Immun 1992; 60:3689-3696.

182. Okumura K, Hara A, Tanaka T, Nishiguchi I, Minamide W, Igarashi H, Yutsudo T. Cloning and sequencing the streptolysin O genes of group C and G streptococci. DNA Seq 1994; 4:325-328.

183. Flanagan J, Collin N, Timoney J, Mitchell T, Mumford JA, Chanter N. Characterization of hemolytic activity of *S. equi*. Microb Pathog 1998; 24:211-221.

184. Simpson WJ, Musser JM, Cleary PP. Evidence consistent with horizontal transfer of the gene (*emm* 12) encoding serotype M12 protein between group A and G pathogenic streptococci. Infect Immun 1992; 60:1890-1893.

185. Nagamune H, Ohnisci C, Katsuura A, Fushitani K, Whiley RA, Tsuji A, Matsuda Y. Intermedilysin, a novel cytotoxin specific for human cells secreted by *S. intermedius* UNS46 isolated from a human liver abscess. Infect Immun 1996; 64:3093-3100.

186. Jenkinson HF. Genetics of *Streptococcus sanguis*. In: Fischetti VA, Novick RP, Ferretti JJ, Portnoy DA, Rood JI, eds. Gram Positive Pathogens. Washington, DC:ASM Press, 2000:287-294.

187. Lowrence JH, Baddour LM, Simpson WA. The role of fibronectin binding in the rat model of experimental endocarditis caused by *Streptococcus sanguis*. J Clin Invest 1990; 86:7-13.

188. Lowy FD, Chang DS, Neuhause EG. Effect of penicillin on the adherence of *Streptococcus sanguis* in vitro and in the rabbit model of endocarditis. J Clin Invest 1983; 71:668-675.

189. Drake TA, Rodgers GM, Sande MA. Tissue factor is a major stimulus for vegetation formation in enterococcal endocarditis. J Clin Invest 1984; 73:1750-1753.

190. Vernier A, Diab M, Saell M, Haan-Archipoff G, Beretz A, Wachsmann D, Klein TP. Cytokine production by human epithelial and endothelial cells following exposure to oral viridans streptococci involves interaction between bacteria and cell surface receptors. Infect Immun 1996; 64:3016-3022.

191. Munro CL, Michalek SM, Macrina FL. Cariogenicity of *S. mutans* V 403 glucosyltransferase and fructosyltransferase mutants constructed by allelic exchange. Infect Immun 1991; 59:2316-2323.

192. Watson DA, Musher DM, Verhoef J. Pneumococcal virulence factors and host immune responses to them. Eur J Clin Microbiol Inf Dis 1995; 14:479-90.

193. van Dam JEG, Fleer A, Snippe H. Immunogenicity and immunochemistry of *Streptococcus pneumoniae* capsular polysaccharides. Antonie Van Leeuwenhoek 1990; 58:1-47.

194. Watson DA, Musher DM. Interruption of capsule production in *Streptococcus pneumoniae* serotype 3 by insertion of transposon Tn916. Infect Immun 1990; 58:3135-3138.

195. Paton GC, Andrew PW, Boulnois GJ, Mitchell TJ. Molecular analysis of the pathogenicity of *Streptococcus pneumoniae*: the role of pneumococcal proteins. Ann Rev Microbiol 1993; 47:89-115.

196. Hotchkiss RD. Transfer of penicillin resistance in pneumococci by the desoxyribonucleate derived from resistant cultures. Cold Spring Harbor Symposia in Quantitative Biology 1951; 16:457-461.

197. Riesenfeld-Orn I, Wolpe S, Garcia-Bustos JF, Hoffmann MK, Tuomanen E. Production of interleukin-1 but not tumor necrosis factor by human monocytes stimulated with pneumococcal cell surface components. Infect Immun 1989; 57:1890-1893.

198. Winkelstein JA, Tomasz A. Activation of the alternative pathway by pneumococcal cell walls. J Immunol 1977; 118:451-454.

199. Winkelstein JA, Tomasz A. Activation of the alternative complement pathway by pneumococcal cell wall teichoic acid. J Immunol 1978; 120:174-178.

200. Rubins JB, Duane PG, Clawson D, Charboneau D, Young J, Niewoehner DE. Toxicity of pneumolysin to pulmonary alveolar epithelial cells. Infect Immun 1993; 61:1352-1358.

201. Boulnois GJ. Pneumococcal proteins and the pathogenesis of disease caused by *Streptococcus pneumoniae*. J Gen Microbiol 1992; 138:249-259.

202. Alexander JE, RA Lock, Peeters CCAM, Poolman JT, Andrew PW, Mitchell TM, Hansman D, Paton JC. Immunization of mice with pneumolysin toxoid confers a significant degree of protection against at least nine serotypes of *Streptococcus pneumoniae*. Infect Immun 1994; 62:5683-5688.

203. Kornfeld SJ, Plaut AG. Secretory immunity and bacterial IgA proteases. Rev Infect Dis 1981; 3:521-534.

204. Krivan HC, Roberts DD, Ginsburg V. Many pulmonary pathogenic bacteria bind specifically to the carbohydrate sequence Gae-Nacb1-4 Gal found in some glycolipids. Proc Natl Acad Sci U S A 1988; 85:6157-6161.

205. Cundell DR, Pearce BJ, Sandros J, Naughton AM, Masure HR. Peptide permeases from *Streptococcus pneumoniae* affect adherence to eukaryotic cells. Infect Immun 1995; 63:2493-2498.

206. Briles DE, Yother J, McDaniel LS. Role of pneumococcal surface protein A in the virulence of *Streptococcus pneumoniae*. Rev Infect Dis 1988; 10 (Suppl 2):5372-5374.

207. Rubins JB, Janoff EN. Pneumolysin: a multifunctional pneumococcal virulence factor. J Lab Clin Med 1998; 131:21-27.

208. Berry AM, Paton JC. Sequence heterogeneity of PsaA, a 37-kilodalton putative adhesin essential for virulence of *Streptococcus pneumoniae*. Infect Immun 1996; 64:5255-5262.

209. van der Flier M, Chhun N, Wizemann TM, Min J, McCarthy JB, Tuomanen EI. Adherence of *Streptococcus pneumoniae* to immobilized fibronectin. Infect Immun 1995; 63:4317-4322.

210. Andersson B, Dahmen J, Frejd T, Leffler H, Magnusson G, Noori G, Eden CS. Identification of an active disaccharide unit of a glycoconjugate receptor for pneumococci attaching to human pharyngeal epithelial cells. J Exp Med 1983; 158:559-570.

211. Talbot UM, Paton AW, Paton JC. Uptake of *Streptococcus pneumoniae* by respiratory epithelial cells. Infect Immun 1996; 64:3772-3777.
212. Cundell DR, Tuomanen EI. Receptor specificity of adherence of *Streptococcus pneumoniae* to human type-II pneumocytes and vascular endothelial cells in vitro. Microb Pathog 1994; 17:361-374.
213. Masaki H, Ahmed K, Fujishita M, Takasugi M, Rikitomi M, Iwagaki A, Tao M, Utsunomiya Y, Kobayashi S, Takahashi H. [A case of Kartagener's syndrome with S. pneumoniae lung abscess]. Kansenshogaku Zasshi 1993; 67:355.
214. Reynolds HY. Defense mechanisms against infections. Curr Opin Pulm Med 1999; 5:136-142.
215. Rubins JB, Duane PG, Clawson D, Charboneau D, Young J, Niewoehner DE. Toxicity of pneumolysin to pulmonary alveolar epithelial cells. Infect Immun 1993; 61:1352-1358.
216. Novak R, Tuomanen E. Pathogenesis of pneumococcal pneumonia. Semin Respir Infect 1999; 14:209-217.
217. Schwartz DA, Quinn TJ, Thorne PS, Sayeed S, Yi AK, Krieg AM. CpG motifs in bacterial DNA cause inflammation in the lower respiratory tract. J Clin Invest 1997; 100:68-73.
218. Cundell DR, Gerard NP, Gerard C, Idanpaan-Heikkila I, Tuomanen EI. *Streptococcus pneumoniae* anchor to activated human cells by the receptor for platelet-activating factor. Nature 1995; 377:435-438.
219. Cundell, D. R., C. Gerard, I. Idanpaan-Heikkila, E. I. Tuomanen, and N. P. Gerard. 1996. PAf receptor anchors *Streptococcus pneumoniae* to activated human endothelial cells. Adv Exp Med Biol 416:89.
220. Willett HP. Energy metabolism. In: Joklik WK, Willett HP, Amos DB, Wilfert CM eds. Zinsser Microbiology, 20th ed. East Norwalk, CT:Appleton and Lange, 1992:53-75.
221. Ritchey TW, Seeley HW. Distribution of cytochrome-like respiration in streptococci. J Gen Microbiol 1976, 95:195-203.
222. Hueber J, Wang Y, Krueger A, Madoff LC, Martirosian G, Boisot S, Goldmann DA, Kasper DL, Tzianabos AO, Pier GB. Isolation and chemical characterization of capsular polysaccharide antigen shared by clinical isolates of *E. faecalis* and vancomycin-resistant *E. faecium*. Infect Immun 1999; 67:1213-1219.
223. Hancock LE, Gilmore MS. The contribution of a cell wall associated carbohydrate to the in vivo survival of *E. faecalis* in a murine model of infection. In: Abstracts of the 97th General Meeting of the ASM, Miami Beach, Florida. Washington, DC: ASM, 1997.
224. Muscholl A, Galli D, Wanner G, Wirth R. Sex pheromone plasmid pAD1-incoded aggregation substance of *E. faecalis* is positively regulated in trans by *Tra* E1. Eur J Biochem 1993; 214:333-338.
225. Dunny GM. Genetic functions and cell-cell interactions in the pheromone-inducible plasmid transfer system of *E. faecalis*. Plasmid 1990; 4:689-696.
226. Dunny GM, Leonard BA, Hedberg PJ. Pheromone inducible conjugation in *E. faecalis*: interbacterial and host-parasite chemical communication. J Bacteriol 1995; 177:871-876.
227. Wirth R. The sex pheromone system of *E. faecalis*. More than just a plasmid-collection mechanism? Eur J Biochem 1994; 222:235-246.
228. Toon P, Brown PE, Baddiley J. The lipid-teichoic acid complex in the cytoplasmic membrane of *S. faecalis*. N.C.I.B. 8191. Biochem J 1972; 127:399-409.
229. Beachey EH, Dale JB, Simpson WA, Evans JD, Knox KW, Ofek I, Wicken AJ. Erythrocyte binding properties of streptococcal lipoteichoic acids. Infect Immun 1979; 23:618-625.
230. Bensing BA, Dunny GM. Cloning and molecular analysis of genes affecting expression of binding substance, the recipient-encoded receptor(s) mediating mating aggregate formation in *E. faecalis*. J Bacteriol 1993; 175:7421-7429.
231. Coque FM, Steckelberg JM, Patterson JE, Murray BE. Possible virulence factors of enterococci. 33rd Interscience Conference on Antimicrobial Agents and Chemotherapy. Washington, DC:ASM, 1993:A1166.
232. Sherwood NP, Russell BE, Jay AR, Bowmann K. Studies on streptococci. III. New antibiotic substances produced by beta hemolytic streptococci. J Infect Dis 1949; 84:88-91.
233. Brock TD, Peacher B, Pierson D. Survey of the bacteriocins of enterococci. J Bacteriol 1963; 86:708-712.
234. Brock TD, Davie JM. Probable identity of a group hemolysin with a bacteriocine. J Bacteriol 1963; :708-712.
235. Segarra RA, Booth MC, Morales A, Huycke MM, Gilmore MS. Molecular characterization of the *E. faecalis* cytolysin activator. Infect Immun 1991; 59:1239-1246.
236. Booth MC, Bogie CP, Sahl HG, Siezen RJ, Hatter KL, Gilmore MS. Structural analysis and proteolytic activation of *E. faecalis* cytolysin, a novel antibiotic. Mol Microbiol 1996; 21:1175-1184.
237. Ike Y, Hashimoto H, Clewele DB. High incidence of hemolysin production by *E. faecalis* strains associated with human parenteral infections. J Clin Microbiol 1987; 25: 1524-1528.

238. Zervos MJ, Terpenning MS, Schaberg DR, Therasse PR, Medendorp SV, Kauffman CA. High-level ami-noglycoside-resistant enterococci. Colonization of nursing home and acute care hospital patients. Arch Intern Med 1987; 147:1591-1594.

239. Zervos MJ, Dembinski S, Mikesell T, Schaberg DR. High-level resistance to gentamicin in *Streptococcus faecalis*: risk factors and evidence for exogenous acquisition of infection. J Infect Dis 1996; 153:1075-1083.

240. Pantosti A, Del Grosso M, Tagliabue S, Macri A, Caprioli A. Decrease of vancomycin-resistant enterococci in poultry meat after avoparcin ban. Lancet 1999; 354:741.

241. Flahaut S, Hartke A, Giard JC, Auffray Y. Alkaline stress response in Enterococcus faecalis: adaptation, cross-protection, and changes in protein synthesis. Appl Environ Microbiol 1997; 63:812-814.

242. Wells CL, Jechorek JP, Erlandsen SL. Evidence for the translocation of *Enterococcus faecalis* across the mouse intestinal tract. J Infect Dis 1990; 162:82-90.

243. Olmsted SB, Dunny GM, Erlandsen SL, Wells CL. A plasmid-encoded surface protein on *Enterococcus fae-culis* augments its internalization by cultured intestinal epithelial cells. J Infect Dis 1994; 170:1549-1556.

244. Schaberg DR, Culver DH, Gaynes RP. Major trends in the microbial etiology of nosocomial infection. Am J Med 1991; 91:S72-S75.

245. Coque TM, Patterson JE, Steckelberg JM, Murray BE. Incidence of hemolysin, gelatinase, and aggregation substance among enterococci isolated from patients with endocarditis and other infections and from feces of hospitalized and community-based persons. J Infect Dis 1995; 171:1223-1229.

246. Su YA, Sulavik MC, He P, Makinen KK, Makinen PL, Fiedler S, Wirth R, Clewell DB. Nucleotide sequence of the gelatinase gene (*gelE*) from *Enterococcus faecalis* subsp. *liquefaciens*. Infect Immun 1991: 59:415-420.

247. Sannomiya P, Craig RA, Clewell DB, Suzuki A, Fujino M, Till GO, Marasco WA. Characterization of a class of nonformylated *Enterococcus faecalis*-derived neutrophil chemotactic peptides: the sex pheromones. Proc Natl Acad Sci U S A 1990; 87:66-70.

248. Montravers P, Mohler J, Saint Julien L, Carbon C. Evidence of the proinflammatory role of *Enterococcus faecalis* in polymicrobial peritonitis in rats. Infect Immun 1997; 65:144-149.

249. Schlievert PM, Gahr PJ, Assimacopoulos AP, Dinges MM, Stoehr JA, Harmala JW, Hirt H, Dunny GM. Aggregation and binding substances enhance pathogenicity in rabbit models of *Enterococcus faecalis* endocarditis. Infect Immun 1998; 66:218-223.

250. Kaplan MH. Rheumatic fever, rheumatic heart disease, and the streptococcal connection: the role of streptococcal antigens cross-reactive with heart tissue. Rev Infect Dis 1979; 1:988-986.

251. Brandt ER, Good MF. Vaccine strategies to prevent rheumatic fever. Immunol Res 1999; 19:89-103.

252. Brandt ER, Sriprakash KS, Hobb RI, Hayman WA, Zeng W, Batzloff WR, Jackson DC, Good MF. New multi-determinant strategy for a group A streptococcal vaccine designed for the Australian aboriginal population. Nat Med 2000 6:455-459.

253. Dale JB, Chiang EY, Liu S, Courtney HS, Hasty DL. New protective antigen of group A streptococci. J Clin Invest 1999; 103:1261-1268.

254. Taylor JE, Ross DA, Goodacre JA. Group A streptococcal antigens and superantigens in the pathogenesis of autoimmune arthritis. Eur J Clin Invest 1994; 24:511-521.

255. Herman A, Kappler JW, Marrack P, Pullen AM. Superantigens: mechanism of T-cell stimulation and role in immune responses. Ann Rev Immunol 1991; 9:745-772.

256. Choi YW, Herman A, DiGiusto D, Wade T, Marrack P, Kappler J. Residues of the variable region of the T-cell-receptor beta-chain that interact with *S. aureus* toxin superantigens. Nature 1990; 346:471-473.

257. Nisini R, Fattorossi A, Ferlini C, D'Amelio R. One cause for the apparent inability of human T cell clones to function as professional superantigen-presenting cells is autoactivation. Eur J Immunol 1996; 26:797-803.

258. Nisini R, Matricardi PM, Fattorossi A, Biselli R, D'Amelio R. Presentation of superantigen by human T cell clones: a model of T-T cell interaction. Eur J Immunol 1992; 22:2033-2039.

259. Paliard X, West SG, Lafferty JA, Clements JR, Kappler JW, Marrack P, Kotzin BL. Evidence for the effects of a superantigen in rheumatoid arthritis. Science 1991; 253:325-329.

260. Moudgil KD, Sercarz EE. The T cell repertoire against cryptic self determinants and its involvement in auto-immunity and cancer. Clin Immunol Immunopathol. 1994; 73:283-289.

261. Baker CJ, Kasper DL. Correlation of maternal antibody deficiency with susceptibility to neonatal group B streptococcal infections. N Engl J Med 1976; 294:753-756.

262. Quinti I, Papetti C, von Hunolstein C, Orefici G, Aiuti F. IgG subclasses to group B streptococci in normals, colonized women and IgG2 subclass-deficient patients. Monographs Allergy 1988; 23:148-155.

263. Baker CJ, Paoletti LC, Wessels MR, Guttormsen HK, Rench MA, Hicman ME, Kasper DL. Safety and immunogenicity of capsular polysaccharide-tetanus toxoid conjugate vaccines for group B streptococcal types Ia and Ib. J Infect Dis 1999; 179:142-150.

264. Kilian M, Reinholdt J, Lomholt H, Poulsen K, Frandsen EVG. Biological significance of IgA I protease in bacterial colonization and pathogenesis: critical evaluation of experimental evidence. APMIS 1996; 104:321-338.

265. Medaglini D, Pozzi G, King TP, Fischetti VA. Mucosal and systemic immune response to a recombinant protein expressed on the surface of the oral commensal bacterium S. gordonii after oral colonization. Proc Natl Acad Sci 1995; 92:6868-6872.

266. Medaglini D, Oggioni MR, Pozzi G. Vaginal immunization with recombinant gram-positive bacteria. Am J Reprod Immunol 1998; 39:199-208.

267. Watson DA, Musher DM, Verhoef J. Pneumococcal virulence factors and host immune responses to them. Eur J Clin Microbiol Infect Dis 1995; 14:479-490.

268. Musher DM, Groover JE, Rowland JM, Watson DA, Struewing JB, Baughn RE, Mufson MA. Antibody to capsular polysaccharides of *Streptococcus pneumoniae*: prevalence, persistence, and response to revaccination. Clin Infect Dis 1993; 17:66-73.

269. Prober CG, Frayha H, Klein M, Schiffman G. Immunologic responses of children to serious infections with *Streptococcus pneumoniae*. J Infect Dis 1983; 148:427-435

270. Musher DM, Luchi MJ, Watson DA, Hamilton R, Baughn RE. Pneumococcal polysaccharide vaccine in young adults and older bronchitics: determination of IgG responses by ELISA and the effect of adsorption of serum with non-type-specific cell wall polysaccharide. J Infect Dis 1990; 161:728-735.

271. Eskola J, Takala AK, Kilpi TM, Lankinen KS, Kayhty H. Clinical evaluation of new pneumococcal vaccines: the Finnish approach. Dev Biol Stand 1998; 95:85-92.

272. Lee CJ, Wang TR, Tai SS. Immunologic epitope, gene, and immunity involved in pneumococcal glycoconjugate. Crit Rev Microbiol 1997; 23:121-142.

273. Lindberg AA. Glycoprotein conjugate vaccines. Vaccine 1999; 17:S28-S36.

274. Arduino RC, Murray BE, Rakita RM. Roles of antibodies and complement in phagocytic killing of enterococci. Infect Immun 1994; 62:987-993.

275. Arduino RC, Jacques-Palaz K, Murray BE, Rakita RM. Resistance of *Enterococcus faecium* to neutrophil-mediated phagocytosis. Infect Immun 1994; 62:5587-5594.

276. Bottone EJ. Encapsulated *Enterococcus faecalis*: role of encapsulation in persistence in mouse peritoneum in absence of mouse lethality. Diagn Microbiol Infect Dis 1999; 33:65-68.

277. Johnson DR, Kaplan EL, Sramek J, Bicova R, Havliceck J, Havlickova H, Motlova J, Kriz P. Laboratory Diagnosis of Group A Streptococcal Infections. Geneva: WHO, 1996.

278. Lancefield RC. A microprecipitin-technique for classifying hemolytic streptococci and improved methods for producing antisera. Proc Soc Exp Biol Med 1938; 38:473-478.

279. Gerber MA. Latex agglutination tests for rapid identification of Group A streptococci directly from throat swabs. J Pediatr 1984; 105:702-705.

280. Christensen P. New method for serological grouping of streptococci with specific antibodies adsorbed to protein A-containing staphylococci. Infect Immun 1973; 7:881-885.

281. Hoffman S. Detection of Group A streptococcal antigen from throat swabs with fine diagnostic kits in general practice. Diagn Microbiol Infect Dis 1990; 13:209-215.

282. Drulak M, Bartolomeu W, La Scalea L, Amsterdam D, Gunnersen N, Young J. Evaluation of the modified visuwell Strep A enzyme immunoassay for detection of group-A streptococcus from throat swabs. Diagn Microbiol Infect Dis 1991; 14:281-285.

283. Heelan JS, Wilbur S, Depetris G, Letourneau C. Rapid antigen testing for group A streptococcus by DNA probe. Diagn Microbiol Infect Dis 1996; 24:65-69.

284. Cleary PP. DNA finger prints of *S. pyogenes* are M type specific. J Infect Dis 1988; 158:1317-1323.

285. Single LA, Martin DR. Clonal differences within M serotypes of the group A streptococcus revealed by pulsed field gel electrophoresis. FEMS Microbiol Lett 1992; 70:85-89.

286. Griffith F. The serological classification of *S. pyogenes*. J Hyg 1934; 34:542-584.

287. Efstratiou A. Preparation of *S. pyogenes* suspension for typing by the agglutination method. Med Lab Sci 1980; 37:361-363.

288. Facklam R, Beall B, Efstratiou A, Fischetti V, Johnson D, Kaplan E, Kriz P, Lovgren M, Martin D, Schwartz B, Totollan A, Bessen D, Hollingshead S, Rubin F, Scott J, Tyrrell G. *emm* typing and validation of provisional M types for Group A streptococci. Emerg Infect Dis 1999; 5:247-253.

289. Baker CJ. Inadequacy of rapid immunoassays for intrapartum detection of group B streptococcal carriers. Obstet Gynecol 1996; 88:811-815.
290. Pollock HM, Dahlgren BJ. Distribution of streptococcal groups in clinical specimens with evaluation of bacitracin screening. Appl Microbiol 1974; 27:141-143.
291. Kilian M, Mikkelsen L, Henrichsen J. Taxonomic study of viridans streptococci: description of S. gordonii sp. nov. and emended description of S. sanguis (White and Niven 1946), S. oralis (Bridge and Sneath 1982) and S. mitis (Andrews and Horder 1906). Int J Syst Bacteriol 1989; 39:471-484.
292. Beighton D, Hardie JM, Whiley RA. A scheme for the identification of viridans streptococci. J Med Microbiol 1991; 35:367-372.
293. Ruoff KL, Whiley RA, Beighton AD. Streptococcus. In: Murray PR, Baron EJ, Pfaller MA, Tenover FC, Yolken RH. Manual of Clinical Microbiology. 7th Edn. Washington, DC:ASM Press, 1999:283-286.
294. Whiley RA, Beighton D. Current classification of oral streptococci. Oral Microbiol Immunol 1998; 13:195-216.
295. Coykendale AL. Classification and identification of the viridans streptococci. Clin Microbiol Rev 1989; 2:315-328.
296. Ruoff KL. Streptococcus anginosus (S. milleri) the unrecognized pathogen. Clin Microbiol Rev 1988; 1:102-108.
297. Kilpper-Bälz R, Wenzig P, Schleifer RH. Molecular relationship and classification of some viridans streptococci as S. oralis and emended description of S. oralis (Bridge and Sneath 1982). Int J Syst Bacteriol 1985; 35:482-488.
298. Kawamura Y, Hou X, Sultana F, Miura H, Ezaki T. Determination of 16S rRNA sequences of S. mitis and S. gordonii and phylogenetic relationship among members of the genus Streptococcus. Int J Syst Bacteriol 1995; 45:406-408.
299. Gillespie SH. The diagnosis of Streptococcus pneumoniae infections. Rev Med Microbiol 1994; 5:224-232.
300. Kalin M, Lundberg AA. Diagnosis of pneumococcal pneumonia: a comparison between microscopic examination of expectorate, antigen detection and cultural procedures. Scand J Infect Dis 1983; 15:247-255.
301. Shattner A, Michel-Harder C, Yeginsoy S. Detection of capsular polysaccharide in serum for the diagnosis of pneumococcal pneumonia: clinical and experimental evaluation. J Infect Dis 1991; 163:1094-1102.
302. Forbes BA, Sahm DF, Weissfeld AS, Baron EJ - eds. Bailey and Scott's Diagnostic Microbiology. 10th Edn. St. Louis, MO:Mosby, 1998.
303. Lund E, Henrichsen J. Laboratory diagnosis, serology and epidemiology of Streptococcus pneumoniae. In: Methods in Microbiology, Vol 2. London:Academic Press, 1978.
304. Neufeld F. Ueber die agglutination der pneumokokken und über die theorie der agglutination. Z Hyg Infektionskr 1902; 40:54-72.
305. Gillespie SH, Ullman C, Smith MD, Emery V. Detection of Streptococcus pneumoniae in sputum samples by PCR. J Clin Microbiology 1994; 32:1308-1311.
306. Zhang Y, Isaacman DJ, Wadowsky RM, Rydquist-White J, Post JC, Ehrlich GD. Detection of Streptococcus pneumoniae in whole blood by PCR. J Clin Microbiol 1995; 33:596-601.
307. Virolainen A, Salo P, Jero J, Karma P, Eskola J, Leinonen M. Comparison of PCR assay with bacterial culture for detecting Streptococcus pneumoniae in middle ear fluid of children with acute otitis media. J Clin Microbiol 1994; 32:2667-2670.
308. Hall LMC, Duke B, Urwin G. An approach to the identification of the pathogens of bacterial meningitis by the polymerase chain-reaction. Eur J Clin Microbiol Infect Dis 1995; 14:1090-1094.
309. Rudolph KM, Parkinson AJ, Black CM, Mayer LW. Evaluation of polymerase chain reaction for diagnosis of pneumococcal pneumonia. J Clin Microbiol 1993; 31:2661-2666.
310. Gillespie SH, McHug TD, Hugues JE. An outbreak of penicillin resistant Streptococcus pneumoniae (PRSP) investigated by a PCR-based genotyping method. J Clin Pathol 1997; 50:847-851.
311. Merlino J, Siarakas S, Robertson GJ, Funnel GR, Gottlieb T, Bradbury R. Evaluation of CHROM agar orientation for differentiation and presumptive identification of gram-negative bacilli and Enterococcus species. J Clin Microbiol 1996; 34:1788-1793.
312. Ford M, Perry JD, Gould FK. Use of cephalexin-aztreonam-arabinose agar for selective isolation of E. faecium. J Clin Microbiol 1994; 32: 2999-3001.
313. Edberg SC, Hardalo CJ, Kontnick C, Campbell S. Rapid detection of vancomycin resistant enterococci. J Clin Microbiol 1994; 32:2182-2184.

314. Landman D, Quale JM, Oydna E, Willy B, Ditare V, Zaman M, Patel K, Saurine G, Huang W. Comparison of five selective media for identifying fecal carriage of vancomycin-resistant enterococci . J Clin Microbiol 1996; 34: 751-752.

315. Hardie JM, Whiley RA. Classification and overview of the genera *Streptococcus* and *Enterococcus*. J Appl Microbiol 1997; 83: S1-S11.

316. Morrison D, Woodford N, Cookson B. Enterococci as emerging pathogens of humans. J Appl Microbiol 1997; 83:S895-S995.

317. Chirurgi VA, Oster SE, Goldberg AA, Zervas MJ, Mc Cabe RE. Ampicillin resistant *E. raffinosus* in acute-care hospital: case-control study and antimicrobial susceptibilities. J Clin Microbiol 1991; 29:2263-2265.

318. Facklam RR, Collins MD. Identification of *Enterococcus* species isolated from human infections by a conventional test scheme. J Clin Microbiol 1989; 27:7331-7334.

319. Facklam RR, Sahm DF, Teixeira LM. *Enterococcus*. In: Murray PR, Baron EJ, Pfaller MA, Tenover FC, Yolken RH - eds. Manual of Clinical Microbiology. 7th Edn. Washington, DC:American Society for Microbiology, 1994:297-305.

320. Descheemaeker P, Lammens C, Pot B, Vandamme P, Goossens H. Evaluation of arbitrarily primed PCR analysis and pulsed-field gel electrophoresis of large genomic DNA fragments for identification of enterococci important in human medicine. Int J Syst Bacteriol 1997; 47:555-561.

321. Merquior VLC, Peralta JM, Facklam RR, Texeira LM. Analysis of electophoretic whole cell protein profiles as a tool for characterization of *Enterococcus* species. Curr Microbiol 1994; 28:149-153.

322. Tyrrell GJ, Bethune RV, Willey B, Low DE. Species identification of enterococci via intergenic ribosomal PCR. J Clin Microbiol 1997; 35:1054-1060.

323. Carvalho MGS, Vianni MCE, Elliott JA, Reeves M, Faklam RR, Teixera LM. Molecular analysis of *Lactococcus garviae* and *Enterococcus gallinarum* isolated from water buffaloes with subclinical mastitis. Adv Exp Med Biol 1997; 418:401-404.

324. Kuhn I, Burman LG, Haggeman S, Tullus K, Murray BE. Biochemical fingerprinting compared with ribotyping and pulsed-field gel electrophoresis of DNA for epidemiological typing of enterococci. J Clin Microbiol 1995; 33:2812-2817.

325. Barbier N, Sauinier P, Chachati E, Dumontier S, Andremont A. Random amplified polymorphic DNA typing versus pulsed-field gel electrophoresis for epidemiological typing of vancomycin-resistant enterococci. J Clin Microbiol 1996; 34:1096-1099.

326. Roggenkamp A, Abele-Horn M, Trebesius KH, Tretter U, Autenreith IB, Heesemann J. *Abiotrophia elegans* sp. nov. a possible pathogen in patients with culture-negative endocarditis. J Clin Microbiol 1998; 36:100-104.

327. Collins MD, Aguirre M, Facklam RR, Shallcross J, Williams AM. *Globicatella sanguis* gen. nov. sp. nov. a new gram-positive catalase negative bacterium from human sources. J Appl Bacteriol 1992; 73:433-437.

328. Ruoff KL. *Leuconostoc, Pediococcus, Stomatococcus* and other catalase negative, gram-positive cocci. In: Murray PR, Baron EJ, Pfaller MA, Tenover FC, Yolken RH - eds. Manual of Clinical Microbiology. 7th Edn. Washington, DC:American Society for Microbiology, 1994:306-315.

329. Golledge CL, Stingemore N, Avavena M, Joske K. Septicemia caused by vancomycin-resistant *Pediococcus acidilactici*. J Clin Microbiol 1990; 28:1678-1679.

330. Sure JM, Donnio PY, Mensard R, Ponedras P, Avril JL. Septicemia and hepatic abscess caused by *Pediococcus acidilactici*. Eur J Clin Microbiol Infect Dis 1992; 11:623-625.

331. Kern W, Vanek E. *Aerococcus* bacteremia associated with granulocytopenia. Eur J Clin Microbiol 1987; 6:670-673.

332. Christensen JJ, Vibits H, Ursing J, Karner B. *Aerococcus*-like organism, a newly recognized potential urinary tract pathogen. J Clin Microbiol 1991; 29:1049-1053.

333. Kristensen B, Nielsen G. Endocarditis caused by *Aerococcus urinae*, a newly recognized pathogen. Eur J Clin Microbiol Infect Dis 1995; 14:49-51.

334. Collins MD, Facklam RR, Rodrigues UM, Ruoff KL. Phylogenetic analysis of some *Aerococcus*-like organism from clinical sources: description of *Helcococcus kunzii* gen. nov. sp. nov. Int J Syst Bacteriol 1993; 43:425-429.

335. Kim KS, Kaplan EL. Association of penicillin tolerance with failure to eradicate Group A streptococci from patients with pharyngitis. J Pediatr 1985; 107:681-684.

336. Brook I. Role of beta-lactamase producing bacteria in the failure of penicillin to eradicate Group A streptococci. Pediatr Infect Dis 1985; 4:491-493.

337. Stevens DL, Tanner MH, Winship J, Swarts R, Reis KM, Schlievert PM, Kaplan EL. Reappearance of scarlet fever toxin A among streptococci in Rocky Mountain West: severe Group A streptococcal infections associated with a toxic shock-like syndrome. N Engl J Med 1989; 321:1-7.

338. Holm SE, Norrby A, Bergholm AM, Norgren M. Aspects of pathogenesis of serious group A streptococcal infections in Sweden, 1988-1989. J Infect Dis 1992; 166:31-37.

339. Stevens DL, Yan S, Bryant AE. Penicillin binding protein expression at different growth stages determines penicillin efficacy in vitro and in vivo: an explanation for the inoculum effect. J Infect Dis 1993; 167:1401-1405.

340. Eagle H. Experimental approach to the problem of treatment failure with penicillin. Group A streptococcal infections in mice. Am J Med 1952; 13:389-399.

341. Kaplan EL. The resurgence of group A streptococcal infections and their sequelae. Eur J Clin Microbiol Infect Dis 1991; 101:55-57.

342. Maruyama SH, Yoshioka H, Fujita K, Takimoto M, Sataka Y. Sensitivity of group A streptococci to antibodies: prevalence of resistance to erythromycin in Japan. Am J Dis Child 1979; 133:1143-1145.

343. Seppala H, Nissinen A, Jarvinen H, Huovinen S, Henriksson T, Herve E, Holm SE, Jankola M, Katila ML. Resistance to erythromycin in group A streptococci. N Engl J Med 1992; 326:292-297.

344. Phillips G, Parrait D, Orange GV, Harper I, McEwan H, Yong N. Erythromycin-resistant *S. pyogenes*. J Antimicrob Chemother 1990; 25:723-724.

345. Varaldo PE, Debbia EA, Nicoletti G, Pavesio D, Ripa S, Schito GC, Tempera G, and the Artemis Study Group. Nationwide survey in Italy of treatment of *S. pyogenes* pharyngitis in children: influence of macrolide resistance on clinical microbiological outcomes. Clin Infect Dis 1999; 29:869-873.

346. Cornaglia G, Ligozzi M, Mazzariol A, Valentini M, Orefici G, Fontana R. The Italian Surveillance Group for antimicrobial resistance. Rapid increase of resistance to erythromycin and clindamycin in *S. pyogenes* in Italy, 1993-1995. Emerg Inf Dis 1996; 2:331-334.

347. Sutcliffe J, Talt-Kamrad A, Wondrack L. *S. pneumoniae* and *S. pyogenes* resistant to macrolides but sensitive to clindamycin: a common resistance pattern mediated by an efflux system. Antimicrob Agents Chemother 1996; 40:1817-1824.

348. Traub WH, Leonard B. Comparative susceptibility of clinical group A, B, C, F and G β-hemolytic streptococcal isolates to 24 antimicrobial drugs. Chemotherapy 1997; 43:10-20.

349. National Committee for Clinical laboratory Standards. Performance Standards for Antimicrobial Susceptibility Testing: sixth informational supplement. National Committee for Clinical Laboratory Standards document M100-56. Villanova, PA:National Committee for Clinical Laboratory Standards, 1995.

350. Kim KS, Anthony BF. Penicillin tolerance in group B isolated from infected neonates. J Infect Dis 1981; 144:411-419.

351. Potgeiter E, Carmichael M, Koornhof HJ. In vitro susceptibility of viridans streptococci isolated from blood cultures. Eur J Clin Microbiol Infect Dis 1992; 11:543-546.

352. Farber BF, Eliopoulos GM, Ward JI. Multiple resistant viridans streptococci susceptibility to beta-lactam antibiotics and comparison of penicillin binding protein patterns. Antimicrob Agents Chemother 1983; 24:702-705.

353. Chalkley L, Shuster C, Potgeiter E. Relatedness between *S. pneumoniae* and viridans streptococci: transfer of penicillin resistance determinants and immunological similarities of penicillin binding proteins. FEMS Microbiol Lett 1991; 69:35-42.

354. Poyart C, Pierre C, Quesne G, Pron B, Berche P, Trien-Cuot P. Emergence of vancomycin resistance in the genus of streptococcus: characterization of *vanB* transferable determinant in *S. bovis*. Antimicrob Agents Chemother 1997; 41:24-29.

355. Muñoz R, Coffey TJ, Daniels M, Dowson DG, Laible G, Casal J, Hakenbeck R, Jacobs M, Musser JM, Spratt BG, Tomasz A.. Intercontinental spread of a multi-resistant clone of serotype 23F Streptococcus pneumoniae. J Infect Dis 1991; 164:302-306.

356. Versalovic J, Kapur V, Mason EO, Shah U, Koeuth T, Lupski JR, Musser JM. Penicillin resistant *Streptococcus pneumoniae* strains recovered in Houston: identification and molecular characterization of multiple clones. J Infect Dis 1993; 167:850-856.

357. Grebe T, Hakenbeck R. Penicillin-binding proteins 2b and 2x of *Streptococcus pneumoniae* are primary resistance determinants for different classes of β-lactam antibiotics. Antimicrob Agents Chemother 1996; 40:829-834.

358. National Committee for Clinical Laboratory Standards. NCCLS Methods For Dilution Antimicrobial Suscep-tibility Tests For Bacteria That Grow Aerobically. Approved standard I M7-A4 , vol. 17, n. 2. Villanova, PA:National Committee for Clinical Laboratory Standards.

359. Watakunakorn C. Increasing prevalence of resistance to ampicillin, penicillin and vancomycin of enterococci isolated from blood cultures during 1990-1991. J Antimicrob Chemother 1993; 31:325-326.

360. Fontana R, Ligoziti M, Pittaluga F, Satta G. Intrinsic penicillin resistance in enterococci. Microb Drug Res 1996; 2: 209-213.

361. Krogstad DJ, Parquette AR. Defective killing of enterococci: a common property of antimicrobial agents act-ing on the cell wall. Antimicrob Agents Chemother 1980; 17: 965-968.

362. Eliopoulos GM, Farber BF, Murray BE, Wennerstein C, Moellering RC. Ribosomal resistance of clinical en-terococcal isolates to streptomycin. Antimicrob Agents Chemother 1984; 1528-1532.

363. Krogstad DJ, Korfhagen TR, Moellering RC, Wennerstein C, Swartz MN. Aminoglycoside-inactivating en-zymes in clinical isolates of *S. faecalis*: an explanation for bacterial synergism. J Clin Invest 1978; 62:480-486.

364. Moellering RC, Koraeniowski OM, Sande MA, Wennerstein CB. Species-specific resistance to antimicrobial synergism in *Streptococcus faecium* and *Streptococcus faecalis*. J Infect Dis 1979; 140:203-208.

365. Swenson JM, Ferraro J, Sahm D, Clark NC, Culver D, Tenover FC, and the National Committee for Clinical Laboratory Standards Working Group on Enterococci. Multilaboratory evaluation of screening methods for detection of high-level aminoglycoside resistance in enterococci. J Clin Microbiol 1995; 33: 3008-3018.

366. National Committee for Clinical Laboratory Standards. Performance Standards For Antimicrobial Disk Sus-ceptibility Tests. Approved standards M2-A5. Villanova, PA:National Committee for Clinical Laboratory Standards, 1995.

367. Wiley BM, Kreiswirth BN, Simor AE, Williams G, Scriver SR, Phillips A, Low DE. Detection of vancomycin resistance in *Enterococcus* species. J Clin Microbiol 1992; 30:1621-1624.

368. Swenson JM, Ferraro MJ, Sahm DF, Charache P, Tenover FC, and The National Committee for Clinical Labo-ratory Standards Working Group on Enterococci. New vancomycin disk diffusion breakpoints for enterococci. J Clin Microbiol 1992; 30: 2525-2528.

369. Schulz JE, Sahm DF. Reliability of the E test for detection of ampicillin, vancomycin and high level aminogly-coside resistance in *Enterococcus* spp. J Clin Microbiol 1993; 31:3336-3339.

13

Gram Positive Bacilli: *Corynebacterium, Listeria, Bacillus*, and Others

Nevio Cimolai
Children's and Women's Health Centre of British Columbia, Vancouver, British Columbia, Canada

Kathryn Bernard
Special Bacteriology Laboratory, Canadian Science Centre for Human and Animal Disease, Winnipeg, Manitoba, Canada

I. HISTORICAL BACKGROUND

The discussion in this chapter includes several diverse genera that may or may not have much relationship to each other from a phylogenetic perspective. They are all Gram positive bacilli which grow aerobically and, in general, are not responsible for common infections even on a worldwide basis. Changes in this area of bacteriology are many, but with some exceptions such change has not necessarily taken on great importance in contrast to the many new, emerging, and re-emerging pathogens among other bacterial groups. In this chapter, we review the diagnostic bacteriology for *Corynebacterium* spp., *Listeria* spp., *Bacillus* spp., propionibacteria, *Erysipelothrix rhusiopathiae*, *Arcanobacterium*, and *Gardnerella*, among other Gram positive bacilli that are not strict anaerobes. For a detailed discussion of the actinomycetes and mycobacteria, see Chapter 14. For a detailed discussion of strict anaerobic Gram positive bacilli, see Chapter 25.

The availability of new molecular techniques during the last decade has provided means for refining the applied systematics in this area. There are manyexamples of change in the species and genus nomenclature (Table 1). Many of these changes do not necessarily have much impact on the practice of routine diagnostic bacteriology, but there is certainly a greater appreciation of the biology of these bacteria and their inter-relationships.

Although the total number of *Corynebacterium* spp. has increased, only *C. diphtheriae* has gained attention on a practical basis in contemporary times. In particular, it appeared as if vaccination would prove to markedly diminish diphtheria throughout the globe, and such a trend was evident for several decades especially in industrialized countries where the disease was almost eliminated. In eastern Europe, major social and political changes during the 1990s, however, led to low immunization coverage among the young and to waning immunity in adults such that nearly 100,000 infections were believed to have occurred in the Ukraine and Russia within a relatively short period of time (1). This example served to demonstrate how well a nearly extinct and seemingly 'old' disease could resurge given

Table 1   Examples of nomenclature changes for various bacteria that are discussed in this chapter.

Current designation	Former designation
Actinomyces neuii	CDC group 1
Actinomyces radingae and	CDC group E
Actinomyces turicensis	
Arcanobacterium bernardiae	*Actinomyces bernardiae* (CDC group 2)
Arcanobacterium pyogenes	*Actinomyces* (*Corynebacterium*) *pyogenes*
(some) *Arthrobacter* spp.	(some) CDC groups B-1, B-3
(some) *Brevibacterium* spp.	(some) CDC groups B-1, B-3
Brevibacillus spp.	(some) *Bacillus* spp.
(some) *Cellulomonas* spp.	CDC group A-3
Cellulomonas cellulans	*Oerskovia xanthineolyticum*
Corynebacterium accolens	CDC group 6
Corynebacterium amycolatum	CDC groups F-2, I-2
Corynebacterium auris	some CDC group ANF-1
Corynebacterium macginleyi	CDC group G-1
Corynebacterium propinquum	CDC group ANF-3
Corynebacterium urealyticum	CDC group D-2
(some) *Dermabacter* spp.	CDC groups 3 and 5
Exiguobacterium acetylicum	*Brevibacterium acetylicum*
Leifsonia spp.	'C. aquaticum'
(some) *Microbacterium* spp.	(some) CDC group A-4 and A-5
(some) *Microbacterium* spp.	*Aureobacterium* spp.
Paenibacillus spp.	(some) *Bacillus* spp.
Propionibacterium propionicus	*Arachnia propionica*

the appropriate conditions and stimuli. International supports were needed in order to control the epidemic (2). Some speculated that the role of non-diphtheria *Corynebacterium* species in human illness would increase in the last two decades due to increasing medical intervention and therefore growth in the pool of immunocompromised patients. Such was apparent initially with *Corynebacterium jeikeium* (*Corynebacterium* JK) which proved to be a cause of central venous line-associated bloodborne infections among patients undergoing intensive immunosuppression during the treatment of malignancies (3). Indeed, such infections proved to be markers of the advanced severity of disease in the affected patient. Although these bacteria are still minor but important causes of infection in compromised patients, a continued increase in frequency did not materialize in large part due to significant changes in the improvement of immunosuppressive drugs and the manner in which they are given.

Listeriosis has been a relatively uncommon and usually sporadic illness in the Western World, but a considerable amount of interest was developed in this area during the late 1980s. Several outbreaks fueled renewed endeavours in the study of what was believed to be a preventable illness given that food sources were critical to several of these episodes. Concerns over cook-chill foods and their introduction into hospitals, as well as a further realization of the magnitude of *Listeria* contamination of many foods, continued to give reason for concern (4). Entering the new millenium, it appears that prevention strategies have ensured that listeriosis will continue to be a relatively uncommon human infection at least in developed countries.

Outbreaks of *Bacillus* spp. infections have been increasingly reported in recent times especially in hospital settings, and *B. cereus* continues to be documented as an important cause of toxin-mediated food poisoning (5-8). Concerns have been raised about the safety of *B. thuringiensis* as a pesticidal spray (9) especially when aerosolized over large populated areas. Although adverse safety issues have not been confirmed, there has been an additional need to differentiate this species from other common *Bacillus* spp. in areas where such pesticidal strategies are used. Despite the latter events, the bacterium of this group that has gained most attention, if not notoriety, is *B. anthracis*. Human anthrax continues to be a very uncommon illness in most countries, although disease in the veterinary domain is not uncommonly reported. Historically, anthrax was recognized as an infection that led to heavy losses of cattle and sheep. Such concerns prompted bacteriologists such as Koch and Pasteur to study this illness and furthermore to attempt vaccine production (10). Most of the renewed interest in this area specifically relates to concerns over the potential for *B. anthracis* to be used for biological warfare and its implications for vaccination programs (11). Such concerns, for example, recently prompted a review in the New England Journal of Medicine (12).

Gardnerella vaginalis was temporarily touted as the possible cause of bacterial vaginosis, especially in the 1980s. It became apparent, however, that although the bacterium was closely associated with this gynecological illness, it was not the actual cause (13).

Although many of the other Gram positive bacilli that are discussed in this chapter may be uncommon causes of infection, the slow accumulation of published clinical data has in many circumstances built to the extent where pointed reviews are now available.

II. CLINICAL ASPECTS

A. *Corynebacterium* spp.

1. Corynebacterium diphtheriae

Asymptomatic carriage of *C. diphtheriae* can occur and especially in areas that remain endemic for diphtheria. Carriage most often occurs in the nose, throat, ear, or skin. Most such carriage is fortunately of non-toxigenic strains (14). In developed countries, carriage of *C. diphtheriae* is more likely to be associated with homeless or otherwise underprivileged individuals. Effective immunization prevents the onset of symptomatic disease among those who may carry toxigenic isolates.

After the acquisition of the bacterium from a carrier or an acutely infected individual, the onset of clinical illness requires an incubation period of usually 2-4 days. In general, diphtheria can be seen as a local disease with onset of pathology at either respiratory or skin sites, or as a systemic illness which is essentially toxin-mediated. Bacteremia can occur with either non-toxigenic or toxigenic isolates; this is rare and is more likely to occur with the non-toxigenic form.

Cutaneous infection often presents as non-healing ulceration although such erosion may be minimal for some patients. The ulceration is not uncommonly chronic, and it is often associated with *S. aureus* or beta-hemolytic streptococci. Indeed, when the bacteriology of such ulcers is mixed and the diphtheroid is non-toxigenic, it is doubtful whether it truly has a causative role in the disease process. Apart from the skin pathology, systemic consequences of diphtheria are not seen; many patients are generally well even when the skin isolate is toxigenic. These infections may serve as reservoirs for spread especially given their chronic nature. They are more likely to be seen among populations who reside in the tropics.

Respiratory infection may present as ulceration in the nasal tract without systemic disease; this is very much the same as the chronic skin infection, although perhaps more short-lived. Most respiratory illnesses, however, will occur in the oropharynx. The acute illness is characterized by a relatively sudden onset of pharyngitis that may be associated with fever and odynophagia (15). In the early phase of illness, the pharyngitis cannot be distinguished clinically from viral or other bacterial pharyngitides. The pharyngitis is progressive in diphtheria, however, and the mid-respiratory tract may become involved. Approximately 50% of patients will develop a membrane over the oropharynx, tonsils, and palate; the membrane is seemingly necrotic and maintains a grey-white colouration. When a throat swab is vigorously applied to the membrane, some bleeding is often elicited. The severity of illness correlates with the extent of the membrane. As the membrane extends into the larynx, or even main bronchi, patients will develop stridorous breathing. Respiratory obstruction is an important cause of mortality. As the immediate tissues become involved with the inflammation that occurs during the disease process, the soft tissues of the surrounding neck may become enlarged with edema and hence give the appearance of 'bull neck'. In mild forms or during early disease, diphtheria is not commonly considered in the differential diagnosis of a pharyngitis. Consideration must be heightened in non-endemic areas, therefore, and the diagnosis must be seriously entertained when pharyngitis is present along with a membrane, progressive breathing difficulty (especially in association with apparent laryngeal involvement), paralysis of the palate, and consistent systemic toxicity.

Mortality can occur in 1-10% of those who are infected. Although death from respiratory complications as detailed above is important, patients can also succumb to cardiac disease which is often delayed (15). As a consequence of absorbed toxin from the respiratory tract, patients may develop a myocarditis which occurs usually 1-2 weeks later. The cardiac illness is accompanied by electrical disturbances that are demonstrable by the ECG. Heart block, other arrhythmias, and cardiac failure are among the more common cardiac manifestations. The severity of cardiotoxicity is a function of the severity of the respiratory illness.

The neurological system may also be involved in various ways. As a consequence of toxin absorption in the oropharynx and nearby tissue, patients may develop a paralysis of the soft palate and pharyngeal wall with the subsequent inability to swallow. Cranial nerve dysfunction (e.g., oculomotor nerve palsy) may also occur. In addition, however, involvement of the peripheral nerves may also follow in 2-12 weeks later; this disease is manifest as motor abnormalities of proximal and distal muscle groups. The latter resolves gradually over many weeks.

Infections due to non-toxigenic *C. diphtheriae* are uncommon, although there are several citations of endocarditis (16).

2. Other Corynebacterium spp.

Other *Corynebacterium* spp. are relatively uncommon causes of serious infection with few exceptions. Although some have unique virulence factors, most others cause infection mainly as a consequence of their presence in the milieu of normal flora.

In discussing these bacteria, it must be acknowledged that historical descriptions of disease associations may now be suspect in several circumstances since the taxonomy has changed (17). Several former "CDC groups" have now been given formal species designations, e.g., group F2 now called *C. amycolatum*, e.g., group D2 now called *C. urealyticum*, e.g., group 6 now called *C. accolens*, e.g., groups ANF-1 and ANF-3 now called *C. afermentans* subsp. afermentans and *C. propinquum* respectively. A number of 'CDC groups' remain without formal species designations, e.g., CDC groups 4 and 7. Furthermore, whereas some of these bacteria are relatively distinctive in their phenotypic traits and may be easily distinguished by common biochemical or other tests, some *Corynebacterium* spp. share features to the extent that identification may be confusing. For example, most previously designated *C. xerosis* have subsequently proven to be *C. amycolatum* (18,19). There are several yellow-pigmented species in the *Corynebacterium* genus, and beyond the genus, some other pigmented species are found (e.g., *Leifsonia* spp. (formerly 'C. aquaticum') have been confused with some *Microbacterium* spp. (formerly *Aureobacterium* spp.) (20). *C. afermentans* subsp. lipophilum has been confused with *C. auris* and *Turicella otitidis* (21). There are many diphtheroid Gram positive bacilli which remain to be appropriately categorized.

Many *Corynebacterium* spp. are found as commensals of skin, mucosal membranes, and urinary tract, and therefore the isolation of most of these bacteria commonly evokes an initial suspicion of contamination rather than an etiological agent of infection. Nevertheless, their ubiquity ensures that they will often be present when such sites of colonization are jeopardized by medical procedures or otherwise; the potential for opportunism then arises. Some species, such as *C. argentoratense* (22), *C. durum* (23,24), *C. imitans* (25), *C. kroppenstedtii* (26), and *C. lipophiloflavum* (27), have been found in clinical specimens, but their role in human illness is yet to be confirmed.

The definition of infection must often depend on the isolation of the bacterium from a sterile site or the reproducible isolation of the organism from other sites where other obvious pathogens are not recovered. Table 2 details some disease associations for *Corynebacterium* spp. that are believed to be pathogenic for humans. Although some may be more aggressive pathogens than others, the majority are rare causes of serious infection which includes bloodborne disease, endocarditis (both native and prosthetic valve), line infections, implant infections, and urinary tract infections among others.

Animals are susceptible to several *Corynebacterium* spp., and humans are accidentally infected especially in the context of animal handling. *C. ulcerans*, *C. pseudotuberculosis*, *C. bovis*, and *C. kutscheri* are all commonly found among various mammals, e.g., bovine, equine.

The role of *C. minutissimum* in erythrasma is not absolute (28). It may have a participatory rather than causal role.

B. *Listeria monocytogenes*

Listeria monocytogenes is by far the most important human pathogen in this genus (66). The bacterium may be carried in the intestines of humans ~1-3%. Disease may arise from endogenous flora or through new acquisition from elsewhere. For the newborn or fetus, acquisition is usually from the colonized or infected mother, whereas there has also been documentation of considerable foodborne transmission for other patients.

Although *L. monocytogenes* has often been touted as one of the handful of important newborn pathogens, the occurrence of listeriosis in this age group is a rare event in most countries. Early-onset newborn sepsis may essentially mimic that which is seen with Group B streptococci (see Chapter 12); the illness may begin in utero if membranes are ruptured and the mother experiences a chorioamnionitis or through transplacental spread, or it may begin within 1-5 days after birth as the bacterium is acquired from the contaminated maternal genital tract. Newborns have latent or obvious symptoms and signs which are consistent with newborn sepsis (67). Meningitis can also occur. Late-onset sepsis also mimics that which is seen with late-onset Group B streptococcal infection; it may present with meningitis or bacteremia and occurs either as a late infection after the perinatal acquisition or due to a later encounter with the bacterium.

The fetus may also be infected through an earlier transplacental passage of the bacterium. The mother will become infected during pregnancy usually after a foodborne acquisition (68). She may experience a mild influenza-like illness with fever or minimally no apparent illness at all. In most gravid females, the illness will spontaneously resolve, although some will have a precipitation of labour. Maternal bacteremia without subsequent fetal infection can occur, but in other infections, the mother may be relatively spared despite a bacteremia, and the organism will be capable of crossing the placenta (69). The latter may result in premature delivery and newborn sepsis. In utero, the bacterium will spread quickly throughout the fetus and cause localized infection at many sites, often with abscess formation. In 'granulomatosis infantiseptica', such abscesses may be found in liver, spleen, muscle, central nervous system, and skin; the skin involvement may appear as diffuse papules. Such spread and peripheral involvement is not seen in newborn sepsis whether early or late, and it presumably reflects the pattern of spread in the context of compromised fetal immunity.

Spontaneous infection otherwise occurs mostly in the compromised adult. Usually the illnesses are either spontaneous bacteremia or meningitis. The underlying illness often includes immunosuppression of some type, and high risk illnesses include malignancy (especially), organ transplantation, diabetes, those that are associated with corticosteroid administration, and alcoholic liver disease (70). It is of interest that listeriosis, although more common than in the general population, has not been a frequent opportunistic infection among patients with HIV infection, even in the era prior to the use of intensive anti-viral therapy (71). The bacteremias will often present as fever of unknown focus. Meningitis has a variable onset and is more likely to occur in the immunocompromised adult although immunocompetent adults have also been infected (72). Patients may have mild confusion or may present with advanced illnesses. Occasionally, focal neurological infections may occur. Actual cerebritis may be accompanied early by fever, headache, and emesis, and progression can be followed by cerebellar signs, loss of consciousness, cranial nerve palsies, hemiparesis, or seizures.

Table 2   Disease associations and some characteristics of non-diphtheria *Corynebacterium* spp. infections that are associated with humans.

Ref.	Bacterium	Disease	Other
29	*C. accolens*	rare	normal skin and pharyngeal flora (CDC group 6)
17,30	*C. afermentans* subsp. afermentans	bacteremia	normal skin flora, especially ear (group ANF-1)
21,31	*C. afermentans* subsp. lipophilum	rare	can be mistaken for *Turicella*
19	*C. amycolatum*	bacteremia (esp. catheter associated), wounds, prosthetic devices	normal skin flora (synonym of CDC group F2)
32	*C. auris*	? pathogenic	ear only
17	*C. bovis*	endocarditis, central nervous system, miscellaneous	rare human pathogen, more common veterinary
33	*C. confusum*	rare	
34	*C. coyleae*	bacteremia	rare pathogen
35	*C. falsenii*	rare	
17	*C. glucuronolyticum*	? urethral pathogen	urethral flora
36	*C. jeikeium*	sepsis during neoplasia esp. with skin disruption, endocarditis, foreign body infections, many miscellaneous infections	increased skin colonization in hospitals, often antibiotic resistant, former group JK
17	*C. kutscheri*	miscellaneous	rare human pathogen, animal source
37,38	*C. macginleyi*	? ocular pathogen	found at the eye site during conjunctivitis and corneal abrasions
28,39	*C. minutissimum*	erythrasma (a pruritic skin infection esp. of intertriginous sites; may be of mixed bacterial etiology), rare miscellaneous other	normal skin flora
17	*C. matruchotii*	rare	oropharyngeal flora
40	*C. mucifaciens*	bacteremia	rare
17,41	*C. propinquum*	endocarditis, rare	oropharyngeal, formerly ANF-3
42-47	*C. pseudodiphtheriticum*	respiratory pathogen including pneumonia, tracheitis, bronchitis; endocarditis, lymphadenitis	usually normal pharyngeal flora, respiratory disease especially of compromised tract or immune deficiency
48,49	*C. pseudotuberculosis*	lymphadenitis	established animal pathogen, rare human pathogen, risk for veterinary acquisition
50	*C. riegelii*	? urinary pathogen	urease producer
17	*C. sanguinis*	bacteremia	rare

Table 2 cont'd.

Ref.	Bacterium	Disease	Other
51	C. simulans	rare	role in infection not clearly defined in part due to recent taxonomic change
52	C. singulare	rare	
53,54	C. striatum	miscellaneous, rare	normal skin and nasal flora
55	C. sundvallense	rare	
17	C. thomssenii	rare	
56-59	C. ulcerans	pharyngitis, skin ulcers, may produce diphtheria-like illness with local and systemic disease	animal source esp. bovine and equine, most isolations from asymptomatic state
60-63	C. urealyticum	alkaline-encrusted cystitis, bacteremia, rare others	urease producer which thrives in alkaline pH, common on skin in hospital (formerly group D2)
18,64	C. xerosis	endocarditis, bacteremia, rare others	skin and oropharyngeal flora, usually of compromised patients, most citations are probably of C. amycolatum rather than C. xerosis
17	group F-1	urinary tract pathogen, rare	
65	group G	miscellaneous	

Several other sites of focal infection have been described, although these are generally quite rare. They have included ocular infection (especially conjunctivitis), skin lesions from direct veterinary contact, tissue abscesses, endocarditis, bone and joint infections, vascular infections, and peritonitis (73-77). In some outbreaks of listeriosis from food sources, it has been suggested that *L. monocytogenes* may be a cause of diarrhea although the evidence is minimal. Infections due to other *Listeria* spp. are extremely uncommon if not highly doubtful, and rare isolations of these other listeriae are possibly a function of transient acquisition from the environment.

C. *Bacillus* spp.

1. *B. anthracis*

Interest in anthrax has certainly been rekindled in recent years due to the issues surrounding biological warfare, but the actual frequency of anthrax, including the very mild forms of the illness, have certainly not increased (12,78). Indeed, sporadic illnesses have decreased in areas where improvements have been made in animal husbandry and in the processing of animal products for manufacturing and consumption. Infection is largely of animals, especially those that are herbivores, but humans continue to be infected mainly on a sporadic basis; some areas of the world continue to have endemic illnesses.

Although the potential severity of human anthrax continues to receive much attention, the vast majority of illnesses are cutaneous (well over 90%) and run a relatively benign course (12). Usually the exposed areas of the hands, arms, face, and neck are involved in cutaneous infection since direct contact with contaminated animal furs or carcasses are often the source for the bacterium. Initially, the infection site will merely appear as an itchy papule within 3-5 days of the contact. The site (usually singular) may develop ulceration and may be surrounded by mild edema and vesicles. The lesion is usually entire and painless, and it may progress to a blackened and seemingly necrotic eschar which can measure up to 1-3 cm.; in the latter form, the surrounding edema may be pronounced. A fever, general feeling of unwell, and regional lymphadenopathy may accompany this localized illness. In a very small percentage of these infections, the bacterium may escape the cutaneous boundary and may become systemic with an accompanying bacteremia and the very severe complications as discussed below.

Inhalational anthrax (also called respiratory anthrax) has a very high mortality rate, and it presents as a biphasic illness (12). After the inhalation of spores, patients will often initially develop fever, generalized illness, and cough, although no active pneumonitis per se. The illness is essentially flu-like and tends to improve after a 2-4 day period. This will be followed by a relatively sudden onset of respiratory distress with accompanying evidence of mediastinitis and pleural effusion. As the bacterium becomes bloodborne, patients will develop massive bacillemia with hypotension and then death in an 18-24 hr. period. Other complications of spread such as meningitis may develop.

Gastrointestinal anthrax usually occurs due to the ingestion of contaminated meat from the infected animal (12). After an incubation of 3-7 days, two forms of illness may occur. Firstly, a localized infection of the oropharynx may arise. Patients will have pharyngitis and fever, and may experience difficulty with swallowing. The latter may be due to an actual focal lesion (like for skin) or due to the localized edema and tissue destruction in the nearby area. Spread will occur to blood, and the accompanying toxemia will progress to death. In the other form of illness which follows ingestion, the disease will begin in the intestines. After an initial nausea and fever with or without vomiting, patients will develop abdominal pain, bloody vomitus, and/or bloody diarrhea due to the destructive lesions that arise from direct bacterial invasion. Abdominal involvement may result in peritonitis, bowel wall edema, and possibly bowel perforation. Again, shock and death follow rapidly as the bacterium becomes bloodborne.

Meningitis can accompany any form of anthrax as a consequence of spread from blood. The degree of bacillemia is impressive ($\sim 10^6$-10^8/mL.).

2.   B. cereus food poisoning

As discussed below, there have been numerous infections that have been associated with non-anthrax *Bacillus* spp., but these are nevertheless relatively uncommon. Food poisonings from the pre-formed toxin (79) of *B. cereus*, however, quite likely outnumber all of the latter combined on a yearly basis.

Two forms of food poisoning manifestations are recognized: emetic phase and diarrheal phase (80). For the first of these, the incubation period is short (~1-6 hrs. depending on the individual and the toxin load) after the ingestion of a food that has served as a culture vehicle for germinating spores and the accumulation of toxin from the vegetative bacterium; the illness is mainly one of vomiting and a general feeling of unwell much like the early form of staphylococcal food poisoning (see Chapter 11). The emetic phase may occur alone or in combination with the diarrheal phase. For the latter, the onset is delayed to 10-12 hrs. after ingestion of the contaminated food, and the illness is more like *C. perfringens* food poisoning. Patients may have nausea that is followed by abdominal pain and a watery diarrhea that lasts for up to 12-24 hrs. The diarrheal volume is variable, and some patients may less commonly experience an intestinal illness for several days. The illness is self-resolving without any intervention.

Although it was historically believed that only *B. cereus* possesses the unique toxin that is capable of leading to food poisoning, there have been several reports of food poisoning that have been associated with other *Bacillus* spp. including *B. licheniformis*, *B. pumilus*, and *B. subtilis*; nevertheless, *B. cereus* is by far the most common.

3.   Other Bacillus spp. infections

Most reported *Bacillus* spp. infections have been cited with either *B. cereus* or *B. subtilis* as the offending pathogen (8). While the latter may have been and may continue to be true, it is important to recognize the historic limitations of speciation from past reports. Apart from infection with these two species, other *Bacillus* spp. that are reported in human infections include *B. brevis*, *B. circulans*, *B. coagulans*,

B. licheniformis, *B. pumilus*, *B. sphaericus*, and *B. thuringiensis* (10). Furthermore, some former species have been renamed, e.g., *Brevibacillus* and *Paenibacillus*. These infections are generally rare, and they are usually opportunistic regardless of which of these species are involved.

Bacillus spp. are common in the environment, and hence their presence in clinical specimens, whether of sterile sites or especially of surface samples, must initially be viewed with some suspicion for contamination. Indeed, a sizeable proportion of blood cultures which yield the organism are merely contaminated. Contamination must also be highly suspect when the bacterium is isolated in a mixture with other bacteria. The species that are represented in contamination will generally reflect the distribution that is seen in clinical specimens as the causes of disease. In addition, contamination may be expressed in the form of pseudo-outbreaks which have been related to several vehicles such as alcohol swabs, bronchoscopy equipment, objects susceptible to faulty decontamination procedures, contaminated blood culture bottles, among others. The ability of spores to resist decontamination is critical to the continued presence of these bacteria among these foci.

True infection has been reported for almost every body site even though these citations are uncommon (8,81). Risk factors for infection are similar for all of the *Bacillus* spp. and include intensive hospital care, medical procedures, presence of vascular access devices, intravenous drug use, and immunosuppression (including cancer therapy, corticosteroid use, and AIDS) (82). Trauma and the postsurgical state may allow these bacteria to penetrate sites that are otherwise sterile, e.g., ocular surgery, e.g., burns. The recognition of *B. cereus* as a very serious intraocular pathogen has long been known (83), and the resulting massive destruction may be difficult to stop. There may be a rapid loss of vision. Intravenous spread during drug abuse may lead to a seeding of the intraocular regions with consequent serious endophthalmitis. The intravenous drug user whose injections are contaminated with bacterial spores may also be at risk for endocarditis, bacteremia without focus, and disseminated complications such as osteomyelitis. Respiratory infection may follow the intubation of compromised patients, and spread may be facilitated by the persistence of spores in ventilatory equipment and tubing. Central nervous system infections most often occur as a result of a medical procedure (e.g. spinal anaesthesia, CNS shunts, or neurosurgery) and hematogenous spread can lead to brain abscesses. Other rare infections have included peritonitis, bites, and prosthetic devices (8).

B. thuringiensis has been used in developed countries as an insecticide, and it is delivered to the wild by aerial spraying maneuvers which have led to concerns of infectious hazards for the general public. Such infections have not evidently materialized, although this bacterium has been otherwise cited as a rare cause of human infection (8,84).

D. *Propionibacterium* spp.

Propionibacterium spp. are clearly included among the normal flora of skin and mucous membranes; *P. acnes* is also not uncommonly a component of usual bowel flora. Although there are several propionibacteria that are associated with humans as normal flora or in disease states, *P. acnes* is by far the most common.

The isolation of propionibacteria from clinical specimens is usually a function of contamination via skin. For example, in some series these bacteria are the second most common contaminants in blood cultures next to coagulase-negative staphylococci. By virtue of their frequency on skin, these bacteria are likely to cause infection in the context of medical procedures that breach the integrity of the natural skin barrier (85). They may cause infections of prosthetic devices and CNS shunts. Infections are often post-surgical such as after ocular or neurological procedures (86,87). There is a diversity of uncommon citations for other sites of infection. Risk factors for infection with propionibacteria generally mimic those that are seen with non-diphtheria corynebacteria and non-anthrax *Bacillus* spp. The associations of propionibacteria and human infection should be reconsidered in the light of contemporary identification methods, but it is quite likely that the majority of propionibacteria would be confirmed as such.

E. *Arcanobacterium* spp.

A. haemolyticum has been recognized as a rare cause of bacterial pharyngitis; in large series, the bacterium has been found in the context of symptomatic pharyngitis ~0.3-2% of throat samples, and the frequency among asymptomatic patients is much less. The sore throat resolves without treatment in several days but may be accompanied by a fine macular, almost scarlatinaform, rash in some patients (88); the rash may desquamate during the convalescence of the illness. Therefore, a special search for this bacterium may be considered among patients who experience an association of pharyngitis and macular rash, especially among adolescents and young adults. Other rare citations describe the finding of this microbe in bacteremias without focus, endocarditis, and osteomyelitis.

Other *Arcanobacterium* spp. have been newly assigned to this genus from the genus *Actinomyces* (89). *A. pyogenes* is a rare human pathogen but may been seen among animals. Among humans, it has been found to cause bacteremia, abscesses, wound infections, abdominal infections, and respiratory infections. *A. bernardiae* has been found in blood cultures and abscesses (90).

F. *Erysipelothrix rhusiopathiae*

Infections with this bacterium are quite uncommon among humans but are often seen among farmed animals such as pigs and turkeys. These animals may be normally colonized with this bacterium as may be the surfaces of fish (91).

Most infections in humans are localized and of the skin (erysipeloid; not erysipelas which is due to *S. pyogenes*) (91). The bacterium enters the skin at an inoculation site which is usually due to an inadvertent puncture; often the latter injury will occur in the context of veterinary or food processing work. Within a few days of the injury, a localized cellulitis will evolve which tends to be painful. The site of infection not uncommonly has a violaceous discolouration but will be well-circumscribed. Regional lymphadenopathy occurs in a minority as may a contiguous arthropathy. The lesion often heals untreated over a few weeks. For some patients, there will be nearby spread from the initial lesion, and a more diffuse skin rash may appear as well as constitutional symptoms. Rhomboid or diamond-shaped skin lesions may occasionally be seen which are essentially similar to those that are described among farm animals as 'diamond-back'. Bacteremia is relatively uncommon, and endocarditis (especially native-valve), CNS infection, and bone and joint infections have also been cited (91).

G. *Gardnerella vaginalis*

G. vaginalis is a normal component of body flora and especially of the female genital tract. It has long been recognized as a rare cause of bacteremia and a few other infections, and mostly in the context of obstetrical complications such as post-partum fever (13). Its presence appears to be an independent risk factor for some obstetrical pathology. Nevertheless, its notoriety in large part stems from its association with bacterial vaginosis (13). The bacterium is present in large numbers during symptomatic bacterial vaginosis, but it does not appear to be the causative agent as was once believed. Although the correlation of high numbers of this bacterium in genital samples with active disease is strong, the bacterium may be found in the asymptomatic state, sometimes in equally high numbers.

H. Miscellaneous Gram positive rods

Apart from *Corynebacterium* spp., it had been acknowledged for years that many aerobic non-spore-forming Gram positive bacilli, often diphtheroidal, were obtained from clinical specimens and could not be easily categorized with the techniques at hand. The advent of molecular and other tools as well as the collection of more such isolates led to a flurry of newly-defined genera and species. In general, true infections with these bacteria are rare, and again the concern about their presence as a consequence of contamination must be entertained. Bonafide infections are generally of the same sites and with the same risk factors as non-diphtheria *Corynebacterium* spp. Table 3 provides some description of these

Table 3   Disease associations and some characteristics of miscellaneous non-spore-forming Gram positive bacilli.

Ref.	Bacterium	Disease	Other
92	*Actinobaculum* spp.	rare human isolates	isolated from blood cultures
93	*Actinomyces neuii*	bacteremia, abscesses, skin, urinary	often mixed with other bacteria, not a cause of actinomycosis
94-96	*Actinomyces radingae* and *A. turicensis*	abscesses, abdominal wounds, urinary, genital	often mixed with other bacteria, not a cause of actinomycosis
97,98	*Arthrobacter* spp.	bacteremia, foreign body infection	? normal flora, formerly CDC groups B1 and B3
100	*Bifidobacterium* spp.	respiratory, bacteremia, abscess	very rare pathogens
101, 102	*Brevibacterium* spp.	rare including bacteremia, peritonitis, osteomyelitis, CNS shunt infections	*B. casei* is most common, *B. casei* and *B. epidermidis* are normal skin flora
103	*Cellulomonas* spp.	blood isolate	very rare
104	*Dermabacter* spp.	bacteremia, abscesses, wounds, ocular	normal flora of skin
105	*Exiguobacterium* spp.	rare human isolate	
	Kurthia sp.	endocarditis	very rare human pathogen, found among animals and environment
106-108	*Lactobacillus* spp.	bacteremia, endocarditis	common human flora, often found in foods such as dairy products
20,99, 109	*Leifsonia* spp.	miscellaneous	common contaminant, may be mistaken for some *Microbacterium* spp.; formerly 'C. aquaticum'
99, 110, 111	*Microbacterium* spp.	bacteremia, endocarditis, ocular, rare others	some can be confused with other yellow-pigmented bacteria
112	*Oerskovia* spp. (*Cellulomonas* spp.)	bacteremia, endocarditis, peritonitis, meningitis, soft tissue infection	rare citations; *O. xanthinolyticum* has been referred to as such recently but is a synonym of *Cellulomonas cellulans*
113	*Turicella otitidis*	association with otitis media but not primary etiological agent	isolates from ear source only

bacteria and their association with infection. Several of these bacteria are well-documented to be part of the normal bacterial flora especially of skin, mucosal sites, and oropharynx, but others have yet to be traced to a reservoir whether human or not.

Clostridia, *Bifidobacterium* spp., and lactobacilli are often discussed in the context of anaerobic infections, and indeed some of the latter are strictly anaerobic. Nevertheless, pathogenic species from these genera which are facultatively anaerobic have been documented; most of the current lactobacilli from human sources are facultative.

III. EPIDEMIOLOGY OF INFECTION

A. *Corynebacterium* spp.

1. C. diphtheriae

Humans are the only reservoir for this bacterium, and spread from symptomatic and chronically colonized individuals serves to continue propagation of virulent organisms in endemic areas. Spread will occur from large particle aerosols and from direct contact. Spread and subsequent disease are facilitated by conditions of crowding and poor hygiene; these same conditions are often accompanied by a lack of immunization and other important health care needs. Healthy carriers of *C. diphtheriae* can exist, but this is much more likely to be so in areas where disease is endemic. Vaccination prevents severe symptomatic disease with a high degree of efficiency, but it also appears as if vaccination with toxoid has some, although not fully understood impact, on carriage of toxigenic strains. Nevertheless, it is possible to have disease among the vaccinated, although such individuals are more likely to have been only partially vaccinated or to have lost considerable quantities of protective antibody. Protective antibody levels have been defined, and these are usually of high frequency among fully immunized populations.

Carriage can occur in both oro-/naso- pharynx and on the skin; the latter may be in the form of chronic skin ulcers in endemic areas. In developed countries where there is a high vaccination rate, carriage of toxigenic *C. diphtheriae* is extremely uncommon. Carriage of non-toxigenic strains is more likely in the latter scenario (14), but even so, it is most often seen among derelicts or focal populations; there is some concern that such strains may serve as a mechanism to facilitate expansion of virulent clones if they become lysogenized (114).

Historically, shifts in the biotype (i.e., belfanti, gravis, intermedius, and mitis) have been evident among isolates from diseased populations. It is unclear what has driven these shifts given that the primary virulence factor, i.e., toxin, has been homogeneous. Nevertheless, such shifts have also included significant variation in the frequency of the bacterial biotype population that is toxigenic.

As previously discussed, the massive rise of clinical diphtheria and associated deaths in Russia was a strong signal to the medical community that major reservoirs of the bacterium continue to exist and that they are capable of exploiting the right opportunity in order to cause epidemic disease (115). Although the eastern European epidemic has been contained and has not led to epidemics elsewhere, this episode has confirmed the need to provide full immunization to susceptible populations.

There is little doubt that universal vaccination and the availability of current and effective antibiotic therapy have markedly changed the epidemiology of diphtheria.

2. Other Corynebacterium spp.

Many of these species are among the normal flora of skin, oropharynx, and eye (the latter presumably from saliva). For skin sites, some of these bacteria may be more evident in sites where lipids are more abundant, i.e., some lipophilic and some non-lipophilic. A few may have tropism for the genital tract, e.g., *C. glucuronolyticum* and *C. urealyticum*. Overall, it is apparent that disease is a relative rarity despite the abundance of some of these bacteria on the human body. *C. jeikeium* colonization increases when patients are admitted to hospital which provides some evidence that clinical status, antibiotic use, and person-to-person spread may modify the acquisition and presence of these bacteria. The acquisition and continued presence of this species in hospital is also consistent with the commonality of multiple antibiotic resistance among isolates.

Others such as *C. bovis*, *C. ulcerans*, and *C. pseudotuberculosis* can be acquired from animals. Milk has been a source for the latter two species, whereas *C. pseudotuberculosis* infection has especially been reported from Australia among sheep handlers (49).

The presence of a toxin among some *C. ulcerans* isolates which is similar to that of *C. diphtheriae* toxin raises an interesting question of how toxigenicity has evolved, and whether an animal reservoir for the toxin gene might continue in the absence of clinical diphtheria.

Both *C. auris* and *Turicella otitidis* have been isolated from the middle ear. Although proof for causation of otitis media is lacking and is highly doubtful, these bacteria must presumably enter such a site from the respiratory tract and may therefore be uncommon normal flora.

B. *L. monocytogenes*

Human enteric colonization occurs as previously indicated and is the source for newborn contact in the immediate perinatal period. Nosocomial spread among neonates is rare.

L. monocytogenes is ubiquitous in the environment. It is widespread among animals. It has been documented among the bacteria that contaminate items in the home. Food is also a major source for the bacterium, and many humans illnesses, if not the vast majority, are acquired from foodborne sources (116). The bacterium may be found among vegetables, raw milk (up to ~5%) and hence several dairy products (especially soft cheeses), fresh poultry, other fresh meats, and many processed meat products. Presence in food is likely to be facilitated by the ability of this bacterium to multiply at refrigeration temperatures. Foods that have been implicated in outbreaks include milk products, smoked fish, cole slaw, pate, and shrimp.

Patient groups at risk for listeriosis include the very young (although such infection is very much a rarity in the developed world), the very old, and patients who are immunocompromised, and pregnant females.

C. *Bacillus* spp.

1. *B. anthracis*

Sporulation is the major factor that allows *B. anthracis* to persist in the environment. Spread does not occur from person-to-person, but soil and infected animals are the source for spread by contact, aerosol, or ingestion. Most disease is acquired by direct contact especially in the animal industries including farming where contact may occur with animal fur and fibres during processing.

In endemic areas, anthrax is mainly a serious issue for domestic animals, but the dissemination of vegetative bacteria, which then convert to spores in the environment, may serve to facilitate the ongoing spread to animals that graze in these areas. Thus, it may prove very difficult to eradicate this bacterium from fields where infected animals have acquired the bacterium and hence died.

Currently, outbreaks among animals continue in Africa. Smaller outbreaks have been reported elsewhere in the world.

2. *Other Bacillus spp.*

Again, the ability to create spores is critical to persistence of *Bacillus* spp. in the many environmental niches. *Bacillus* spp. are common in soil and dust, and studies which have examined airborne particles in either buildings or the outdoors have frequently documented the heavy burden of these bacteria. Sporulation provides a mechanism for some of these bacteria to survive decontamination procedures including boiling.

Food-poisoning is often secondary to vegetative bacteria that have formed from spores after the initial cooking process has allowed spores to survive and then to germinate in the food which provides good growth substrates; considerable pre-formed toxin is then accumulated in the food as the bacteria grow. Re-cooked rice and meatloaves are commonly implicated in *B. cereus* food-poisoning. Preventative strategies must target the appropriate handling of cooked foods.

Materials that are used for intravenous drug use as well as the drugs themselves may be contaminated with *Bacillus* spp. Pseudo-outbreaks occur largely as a function of the inability to properly sterilize or decontaminate materials that are used for medical procedures or blood cultures.

D. *Propionibacterium* spp.

These bacteria are common on skin, but they are also commonly present in the oropharynx, in the large bowel, and occasionally on the eyes (117). *P. acnes* not uncommonly resides in skin follicles. Studies of the epidemiology should be viewed with a reconsideration of the possibility that methods for identification may not have been optimal in retrospect.

E. *Arcanobacterium* spp.

A. haemolyticum can be acquired from both humans and domestic farm animals. *A. pyogenes* is found in bovine, ovine, caprine, and porcine reservoirs; humans presumably acquire the bacterium from animals, but it has been recognized that individuals in the rural setting are more often colonized in the oropharynx.

F. *E. rhusiopathiae*

Animals are infected with this bacterium worldwide, and it is clear that humans are not the reservoir. Infection occurs after direct contact with animals, and so it is not surprising that the bacterium causes an occupational illness especially among fish handlers (91).

G. *G. vaginalis*

G. vaginalis is a common component of the healthy vagina, and female populations around the world are so colonized more or less (13). Person-to-person spread via sexual contact must occur given that male sexual partners of a colonized female are also likely to carry the bacterium and that carriage increases accordingly when sexual contacts are multiple.

H. Miscellaneous Gram positive rods

Many of these bacteria reside on the human skin or in the oropharynx. Some are commensals but not yet associated with infection. For others, it is not clear where the reservoirs exist given that so few isolates have been obtained from clinical samples. *Arthrobacter* spp., *Microbacterium* spp., *Oerskovia*, and *Cellumonas* spp. are evidently environmental bacteria; *Leifsonia* spp. are commonly found in water sources. *B. casei* and some *Microbacterium* spp. are found in milk, cheese, and other dairy products.

Lactobacilli are among the predominant flora in the vagina, but they may also be found in the bowel and mouth (including dental crevices). They are also common among various food products either naturally or through direct processing. Whereas it was believed that *L. acidophilus* was the predominant lactobacillus in the vagina, recent findings from molecular studies have indicated that *L. crispatus* and *L. jensenii* are most common; a variety of other lactobacilli including *L. gasseri*, *L. fermentum*, *L. oris*, *L. reuteri*, *L. ruminis*, *L. vaginalis*, and an undesignated lactobacillus L1086V has also been found in this milieu, and it is quite likely that more, although less common, lactobacilli will continue to be identified (118). Vaginal lactobacilli have a beneficial role in acidifying the vagina which serves to lower the pH to an antibacterial level; other organic acids and some bacteriocins may also have some role in modifying the local microbial flora (119). A beneficial effect of lactobacilli in the gastrointestinal tract has long been postulated, and this has led to an interest for developing probiotics with some lactobacilli and *Bifidobacterium* spp. (120).

IV. NATURE OF THE BACTERIUM, PATHOGENESIS, AND CLINICAL FEATURES

Due to the relative rarity of infections with species from many of the genera so discussed in this chapter, it is inevitable that more species will be defined in the future and will be designated with new species names especially with the availability of molecular techniques to discriminate among isolates. As well, it is anticipated that some realignment of species and genera will occur for the existing designates. Perhaps it is fortunate that common infections with these bacteria do not occur since the plethora of species names will undoubtedly confuse the primary physician.

The genera that are discussed in this chapter are aerotolerant, and most are capable of growing under anaerobic conditions as well, i.e., they are variably oxidative or fermentative. They are not acid-fast, and stain variably with the Gram reagents. *Bacillus* spp., *Listeria*, and lactobacilli in particular tend to be regular in their bacillary form. The irregular shape (often tapering to one end and arranged in the classic 'Chinese letter' pattern) of corynebacteria and others has given rise to the terminology of 'diphtheroids' or 'coryneforms'.

As a cluster, *Bacillus* spp. (and *Paenibacillus* and *Brevibacillus*), *Listeria*, lactobacilli, *Gardnerella*, and *Erysipelothrix* have a low GC content, and yet there is considerable distance between these genera in assessments of genomic homology. Higher GC contents are found among *Corynebacterium* spp., *Arcanobacterium*, and *Actinomyces* spp. Nevertheless, it is evident from the GC content variation among *Corynebacterium* spp. (~45-75%) that current taxonomic clustering will be revisited and revised.

The uniqueness of cell wall composition and cellular fatty acid composition among species and genera has been generally exploited for the purposes of classification. Although the actual determination of the latter may require the use of sophisticated techniques that are more likely to be offered on referral, the assessment of such properties has proven to be of considerable value especially as an adjunct to developing genetic molecular techniques as detailed later.

Figures 1, 2, and 3 illustrate the inter-relationships of some genera and species that are discussed within this chapter.

A. *Corynebacterium* spp.

1. *C. diphtheriae*

It is of interest that *C. diphtheriae* appears to be closely related on a genetic basis to *C. argentoratense*, *C. kutscheri*, *C. pseudotuberculosis*, and *C. ulcerans*. *C. diphtheriae* grows modestly well on conventional bacteriological growth media such as blood agar. Resistance to and reduction of tellurite are important features that factor into the derivation of a selective and differential growth medium; a few isolates of *C. diphtheriae* may be inhibited by tellurite, however, and some other bacteria that are obtained from the throat may also reduce tellurite. Metachromatic granules are not uncommonly present among bacteria, and the bacterial morphology on Gram stain especially conforms to the classic diphtheroid shape. Four biotypes can be distinguished on the basis of colony morphology, biochemical assays, and hemolysis: biotypes belfanti, mitis, intermedius, and gravis. These biotypes may vary in the percentage of isolates that are toxigenic. Although such biotyping may have had some value historically, it is of greater importance to accurately identify a suspect isolate and to determine toxigenicity on a timely basis; even a biotype with historically lower potential for toxin production must nevertheless be assessed with a definitive technique.

Toxin production has been very well-characterized and has historically received considerable attention (121). The 58 kD exotoxin gene is mobilized by bacteriophages, and it is capable of integratinginto the bacterial genome (tox+). Tox- isolates lack the lysogenic phage. The toxin is an extremely potent one and is of the classic A/B subunit model. Two peptides are initially linked by sulphydryl groups. There is a binding domain (B) which attaches to the cellular receptor and then interacts with the cell through a transmembrane component. The other fragment (A) enters the cytoplasm and catalyzes

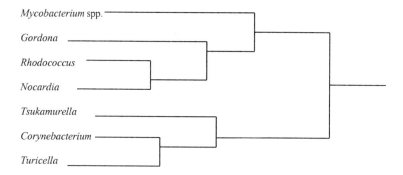

Figure 1   Phylogenetic dendrogram which simplifies the stratification of *Corynebacterium* spp. and other closely related genera based on the comparison of 16S rRNA sequences (123).

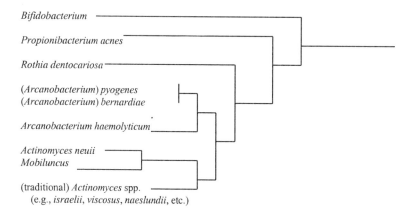

Figure 2   Phylogenetic dendrogram which simplifies the stratification of *Bifidobacterium*, *Propionibacterium*, *Rothia*, and *Actinomyces* based on the comparison of 16S rRNA sequences (89).

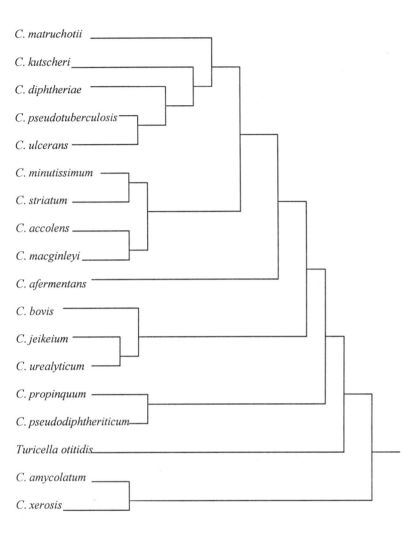

Figure 3 Phylogenetic dendrogram which simplifies the stratification of *Corynebacterium* spp. based on a comparison of 16S rRNA sequences (123).

an interference of protein synthesis at the site of elongation factor 2 activity. Toxin production is iron-regulated through a chromosomal repressor. Biological assays exist for the purposes of detecting toxin production, but PCR assays for the toxin gene have also been devised. Whereas there is a very good correlation between PCR-positive assays and toxigenicity, some PCR-positive non-toxigenic isolates have been found (122). Much work in the area of pathogenesis has rightfully focused on the issue of toxin production, but it unclear what role other virulence factors have in diphtheria.

Toxin can affect a large variety of cells in vitro, but there appears to be a tropism for cells of the heart, nervous system, and kidney even though nephropathy per se is uncommon. The local formation of the classic grey membrane in the respiratory tract is a function of the accumulation of damaged respiratory epithelial cells, red blood cells from local damaged tissue, fibrin exudate, and inflammatory leucocytes. Only rarely do the toxigenic bacteria invade blood, and systemic disease is essentially toxin-mediated alone.

2. Other Corynebacterium spp.

In general, these bacteria grow modestly well on routine media. It is not uncommon to see limited growth within the first 24 hrs., but retention of cultures for 48-72 hrs. usually leads to the formation of 2-3 mm. colonies. As a group, corynebacteria are catalase-positive. Some corynebacteria are lipophilic (e.g., *C. accolens, C. afermentans* subsp. lipophilum, *C. bovis, C. jeikeium,* some *C. diphtheriae, C. macginleyi, C. urealyticum,* CDC group F-1, and CDC group G) and benefit from the addition of serum or Tween 80 to media. For example, in the presence or absence of Tween 80, *C. urealyticum* may yield colonies that are 1-2 mm. and <0.5 mm. respectively at 24 hrs. of incubation. Although blood-supplemented media may have sufficient lipid to allow growth, others (e.g., Mueller-Hinton) may be so limited that growth of the corynebacterium does not occur at all over 2-3 days.

Some corynebacteria (e.g., *C. bovis,* e.g., *C. jeikeium*) are seemingly oxidative in their metabolism, whereas others are fermentative; the variation in sugar fermentation substrates allows for fermentation patterns to be of value in the speciation of these bacteria. Colony morphology can be of incremental value for defining some species when the bacteria are grown on blood agar; particular species attributes are detailed (17). Some species have mild yellow pigmentation, e.g., *C. xerosis.* Others may be moderate or potent urease producers, e.g., *C. pseudodiphtheriticum, C. pseudotuberculosis,* CDC group F-1, *C. ulcerans,* and *C. urealyticum;* a few other species may be variable for this enzyme. Some corynebacteria (e.g., *C. glucuronolyticum*) may show synergistic hemolysis with *S. aureus,* e.g., CAMP test.

On a reference basis, various other features may be exploited to assist in the genus or species identification: variable but particular-sized mycolic acids, presence of *meso*-diaminopimelic acid as the diamino acid of the cell wall, arabinogalactan in the cell wall, and presence of particular major hydrogenated menoquinones [MK-9(H$_2$) + MK-8(H$_2$)]. Within some species, there are clearly multiple genetic groups which may merit further consideration when the taxonomy is again reviewed [e.g., among *C. jeikeium* (124)].

The pathogenesis of non-diphtheria *Corynebacterium* spp. infections is not well-studied, and few animals models of disease exist. *C. pseudotuberculosis* is somewhat unique given the granulomatous reactions that may occur during infection as well as the chronicity of pulmonary infections among animals (hence the 'pseudotuberculosis' designation). The immune response and presumed associated cachexia, which is perhaps due to the local release of soluble mediators (e.g., TNF), have been studied (125). The production of diphtheria-like toxin among a few isolates of *C. ulcerans* and *C. pseudotuberculosis* has been studied; the size and immunological structures are similar, and they exhibit ADP-ribosylating activity (126). There is a strong belief that urease activity of *C. urealyticum* contributes to the pathogenesis of urinary tracts infections by the creation of an alkaline pH which may favour the manifestations of 'alkaline encrusted cystitis'. The issue of adherence has been studied, but there is no clear consensus regarding what role it may have in catheter-associated infections (127).

B. *L. monocytogenes*

The bacilli of this species are generally regular in morphology after initial culture and measure 0.5 X 2 μm. The G+C% content is ~37%. The bacteria are not encapsulated. They grow best at 37°C, but actually are capable of growing in usual refrigeration temperatures; the latter is of benefit for the survival in contaminated food sources even when the food appears to be properly refrigerated. Peritrichous flagella allow for a tumbling motility which is best demonstrated at room temperature; motility may not always be evident at 37°C incubation. Colonies on routine media often resemble those of Group B streptococci and enterococci, and they are associated with a narrow zone of beta-hemolysis on 5% sheep blood agar. Synergistic hemolysis occurs with hemolysins of *S. aureus* and *R. equi* (128). The bacterium is fermentative and catalase-positive.

Antigen diversity has long been studied, and the variation among somatic (lipoteichoic acids) and flagellar antigens has led to the definition of a serotyping scheme. Thirteen serotypes are detailed (1/2a,

1/2b, 1/2c, 3a, 3b, 3c, 4a, 4ab, 4b, 4c, 4d, 4e, and 7), but among human infections, 80-95% of the iso-lates are included within 1/2a, 1/2b, and 4b. The latter fact therefore limits the utility of such a scheme for epidemiological purposes since intraserotype diversity occurs. Some of these serotype antigens are present among other *Listeria* spp. Cross-reactivity of *L. monocytogenes* antigens with other Gram posi-tive bacteria (e.g., enterococci, lactobacilli, beta-hemolytic streptococci, *B. subtilis*, and *A. pyogenes*) has been long appreciated, and it is likely to be in large part a function of the glycerol teichoic acid (Rantz antigen).

The pathogenesis of *Listeria* infection has been and continues to be well-studied. This pathogen is a model for the investigation of intracellular survival, and it can survive ingestion in essentially all cell lines including macrophages. The bacterium facilitates internalization into the cell, but it is able to es-cape the phagosome and enter into the cytoplasm (129). Once inside the cell, it produces proteins that modulate host cell functions (130) and recruits the host actin cytoskeleton to facilitate intracellular movement (131). Cell-to-cell spread occurs thereafter and may be capable of thus avoiding both hu-moral and cellular immunity. These events provide some explanation for the potential to acquire infec-tion from food across the intestinal epithelial barrier, as well as the transfer from mother to fetus across the placenta (132). Listeriolysin O is a hemolysin which has proven to be the most important virulence factor (133), but internalins, actin polymerization proteins, proteases, and phospholipases are also be-lieved to be of necessity.

A factor which stimulates the prolific monocytic response in some infections exists; its effect is variable as witnessed by the inconsistency of monocytic responses in the cerebrospinal fluid of patients with *Listeria* meningitis. The pathology of infection has been studied mainly in animals, but abscess-like formation is evident among some human tissue especially that of the fetus that succumbs to granu-lomatosis infantiseptica.

C. *Bacillus* spp.

The morphology of *Bacillus* spp. is often somewhat distinct among facultative bacteria from clinical specimens in the sense that bacteria are generally larger (0.5-2 μm. in width and 1-10 μm. in length) and regular with 'box-car' shapes. Such consistency is seen after Gram staining, although some will easily decolorize and mimic Gram negative rods even to the experienced. *Bacillus* spp. are most often motile; peritrichous flagellar patterns are evident. Growth on routine media is generally luxuriant even by 18-24 hrs. at 37°C, and the colonies of many species will continue to grow modestly well when culture media are left at room temperature thereafter. Colonies are often rough-edged and crinkled, although there is a tremendous variety of colonial appearances. Hemolysis is variable among and within species. Growth can be facultative, but several species are strictly aerobic. Fermentation patterns of carbohydrates are considerably variable, and this feature can therefore be exploited in part for elucidating the systematics. As a group, these bacteria are catalase-positive.

Sporulation is a key trait of *Bacillus* spp. (Figure 4). The determination of spores among prospec-tively-acquired clinical isolates may occasionally pose some problems, although obvious sporulation can often be seen among blood culture isolates when stained directly after the blood culture bottle has been deemed positive. Sporulation may not always be apparent within the stain of the first subculture on solid media at 18-24 hrs. Furthermore, the inexperienced may have some difficulty in differentiating spores from intracellular granules or other inclusions. In addition to using spore stains, the use of phase-contrast microscopy is often beneficial for determining the presence of spores. Among the different *Bacillus* spp., the spore will have a different impact on the swelling of the vegetative cell. The spore's location within the cell has been used to some extent for the purposes of identification, but to most clinical laboratories, the location will be difficult to use for this purpose, and it is not as useful as it might be when spore location is used in part to facilitate the speciation of clostridia. The germination of spores into vegetative cells can occur in vivo. Spores are heat-resistant (even relatively so to boiling), resistant to ultraviolet light and gamma-irradiation, and variably resistant to most disinfectants, e.g., al-

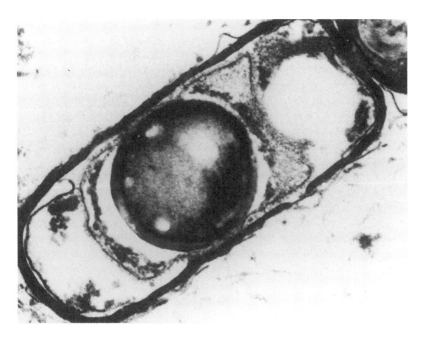

Figure 4   Cross-section of *B. cereus* demonstrating a central spore as seen with electron microscopy.

cohols. Spores are resilient to general environmental conditions, and they may be very resistant to elimination over time as has been clearly witnessed in the case of *B. anthracis* spores.

1.   B. anthracis

The granular colony of *B. anthracis* is somewhat distinctive although not absolutely specific. This bacterium is non-motile, non-hemolytic on blood agars, and produces a capsule. The capsule can be visualized after methylene blue stain and is stimulated by particular culture conditions.

Both toxins and capsule are integral to the pathogenesis of *B. anthracis*. Edema toxin and lethal toxin are encoded by genes on virulence plasmid pXO1. Edema toxin increases cAMP in cells and modifies water transport which may be responsible for the tissue swelling in part. Lethal toxin is a protease which has an effect on eukaryotic protein kinases. The toxins inhibit polymorphonuclear function and thus impair host defences; they may also induce the liberation of cytokines by macrophages which further adds to the cascade of inflammation and other physiological events. Capsule production is dependent on a multigene family which is also plasmid (pXO2)-borne. The capsule is anti-phagocytic and is composed of poly-D-glutamic acid. Transcriptional activators regulate the plasmid genes for toxin and capsule, and loss of any one plasmid results in an avirulent strain (134).

After the uptake of spores from inhalation or ingestion, they may be transported to regional lymph nodes where vegetative forms are released. The local effects of toxin lead to tissue necrosis; systemic pathology may result from the high grade bacteremia and associated toxin. Pathology includes hemorrhagic lymphadenitis, hemorrhagic mediastinitis, pleuritis, and hemorrhagic meningitis. During gastrointestinal anthrax, the bowel wall thickens and there is hemorrhage; there may be associated regional adenitis and peritonitis.

2.   Other Bacillus spp.

Non-anthrax *Bacillus* spp. are many among human isolates, although some species predominate such as *B. cereus* and *B. subtilis*. The species differ in colonial morphology, pigment production, and hemolysis.

Species within this genus may be potent producers of various exoenzymes which may include antibiotic-degrading enzymes that are often liberated when sporulation begins to occur. It is not uncommon to see bacilli with large cytoplasmic inclusions; these are usually made of poly-hydroxybutyrate.

The phylogenetic diversity in the *Bacillus* genus has been studied by 16S rRNA sequencing studies (135,136). There were at least four major clusters, but some of these have subsequently been separated into the *Paenibacillus* and *Brevibacillus* genera. The 'B. cereus group' includes *B. cereus, B. mycoides, B. anthracis,* and *B. thuringiensis* which are considerably homologous when assessed by genetic methods. Some have implied such homology by use of the designation 'B. cereus sensu lato' for this group (137); it may be true that they have evolved from some common ancestry whereby the ecological contexts have promoted the loss or acquisition of current traits (138).

Some *B. cereus* isolates are capable of producing enterotoxins; one of these is an emetic toxin, and the other is a diarrheal toxin which causes fluid accumulation in rabbit ileal loop assays. *B. cereus* is also capable of producing other toxins which may affect the integrity of cell membranes and hence permebilility of vasculature; these may include lecithinases and phospholipases.

B. thuringiensis mimics *B. cereus* in many ways, and it is very difficult to differentiate these by biochemical tests in most laboratories. Some have proposed that these two species may indeed be one. *B. thuringiensis* produces parasporal crystalline bodies, but these bodies may be absent if the bacterium loses the related plasmid (8). *B. thuringiensis* is common in nature and can be divided into more than 50 serovars (139).

Paenibacillus spp. and *Brevibacillus* spp. are differentiated from *Bacillus* spp. mainly by biochemical and some morphological criteria.

D. *Propionibacterium* spp.

Isolates from human specimens commonly include *P. acnes, P. avidum, P. granulosum,* and *P. propionicum. Propioniferax innocua* is a skin resident that has been renamed from its former designation as a propionibacterium. Most *Propionibacterium* isolates have slow growth, and pin-point colonies may appear within 24 hrs. Growth is better in anaerobic or oxygen-reduced environments. In blood culture systems, it may require up to 5-7 days to trigger a positive index. The initial growth pattern of the bacteria on solid media may be suggestive of a strict anaerobe, but often the bacteria will subculture onto media that are placed in an atmosphere that has increased CO_2, i.e., microaerophilic.

In Gram stains, the bacteria are diphtheroidal and not uncommonly manifest short branching. Propionibacteria are catalase-positive except for *P. propionicum* which was formerly an actinomyces. Beta-hemolysis on sheep blood may be weak for isolates of *P. avidum* and *P. granulosum. P. acnes* is indole-positive, and the combination of Gram stain, growth pattern, catalase, and indole are usually sufficient to identify this species accurately.

Propionibacteria have been studied extensively in their putative role as pathogens in acne vulgaris. Extracellular enzymes have been identified. These bacteria are present in high numbers within skin follicles. Overall, the pathogenesis of acne is complex, but a strong role for bacteria is credible.

The potential to stimulate macrophages in vitro and in vivo has led to the use of some strains for the purposes of adjuvant activity.

E. *Arcanobacterium* spp.

Members of this genus are catalase-negative and fermentative. They are share many features with the *Actinomyces* spp., and indeed some were formerly categorized in that genus.

A. haemolyticum maintains a diphtheroid morphology on Gram stain. It is slow-growing. The use of human blood agar, especially in a CO_2-enhanced environment, allows for the demonstration of a beta-hemolysin. This hemolysin contributes to a synergistic hemolysis in a 'reverse' CAMP test. The molecular mechanism for the rash that is occasionally associated with pharyngitis has not be defined.

Phospholipase D, which may be a virulence factor, has homology with enzymes of *C. pseudotuberculosis* and *C. ulcerans* (140).

A. pyogenes also stains as a diphtheroid and yields larger colonies than *A. haemolyticum*. It is often beta-hemolytic on sheep blood agar, and produces a thiol-activated cytolysin (hemolysin) (141). Some isolates will agglutinate with Lancefield serogrouping reagents.

A. bernardiae has somewhat shorter rods and is non-branching.

F. *E. rhusiopathiae*

Thin and sometimes curved rods or filaments are seen from stains (91). The classic diphtheroid morphology is not as apparent. This bacterium is easily overdecolorized in the Gram stain. It is catalase-negative, facultative, and non-motile. It is often alpha-hemolytic on blood agar. The production of H_2S in a TSI slant is a critical reaction for identification. A serotyping scheme has been established.

Studies in the area of virulence factors have mainly been a function of interests from the veterinary area. A neuraminidase and hyaluronidase have been identified. Variability in somatic antigens has allowed for the derivation of a serotyping scheme. The 'diamond-back' pattern of rash in porcine infections and the rash in some humans infections has not been adequately explained, but some histopathological evidence of arteriolar vasculitis has been offered. The sites of focal infections are not uncommonly infiltrated by lymphocytes.

G. *G. vaginalis*

G. vaginalis is catalase-negative. The morphology of bacteria after Gram staining is variable, and the bacteria may easily decolorize. Shapes that are intermediate to rods and coccobacilli are often evident, and the typical diphtheroidal morphology is not always evident. This variability is best reflected by the history of this bacterium when it was formerly designated 'Haemophilus vaginalis' (13). Nevertheless, the cell wall has been studied and is clearly much more like that of Gram positive bacteria; cellular fatty acids more commonly resemble those of corynebacteria. It is non-motile, fermentative, and produces beta-hemolysis on human blood agar rather than with a sheep blood base (13).

H.   Miscellaneous Gram positive rods

Of the many genera and species within this group, there are variable oxidizers and fermenters. Pigment is also variably produced although a yellow pigment is generally consistent among *Exiguobacterium*, some *Microbacterium* spp., and *Leifsonia* spp.. *Exiguobacterium* and *Leifsonia* spp. are motile. Fatty acid profiles can be unique for some species. There is variability in the diamino acid composition of the cell wall.

Brevibacterium spp. yield a scent of cheese. *Turicella otitidis* is positive in the CAMP test. *Oerskovia* has mycelial-like growth that breaks into rod forms. The latter organisms are catalase-positive, fermentative, and have a yellow pigment; *O. xanthineolyticum* is synonymous with *Cellulomonas cellulans*. *Cellulomonas* spp. hydrolyze cellulose. Some *Microbacterium* spp. (formerly *Aureobacterium* spp.) may be confused with *Leifsonia* spp.. *A. neuii* is diphtheroidal and CAMP-positive. Lactobacilli produce lactic acid as the major and dominant peak when organic acid production is assessed by chromatographic methods. More common *Actinomyces* spp. are discussed in Chapter 24.

V. IMMUNOLOGY OF INFECTION

A. *Corynebacterium* spp.

Vaccination against *C. diphtheriae* is a routine component of childhood vaccination programs world-wide, and the formalin-inactivated toxin (toxoid) is usually included within the package of immunogens that contain at least pertussis and tetanus vaccines if not also *H. influenzae* type b conjugate and inactivated polio vaccines. As well, the toxoid, or a smaller component, serves as a very good adjuvant when administered with or conjugated to capsular polysaccharides that are weakly immunogenic otherwise. Vaccination induces a consistent humoral response among the majority (>95%) of recipients. Vaccination appears to effect a decrease in the colonization frequency with *C. diphtheriae* in endemic areas, but there is no such effect on the frequency of non-toxigenic strains. Antitoxin levels are measureable by several methods, and it is accepted that particular levels correlate with protection. Presence of anti-toxin is not an absolute guarantee against diphtheria, however, but the probability that severe diphtheria will result is considerably reduced. Anti-toxin titres decline with increasing age, and subprotective levels may result from this decline; accordingly, it is recommended that the vaccine be given in booster doses every ten years. Infection itself results in much less predictable anti-toxin titres. Cell-mediated immune responses are not apparently critical.

The use of equine anti-toxin, which is administered intravenously, is still believed to be essential in early severe diphtheria. The intent here is to neutralize the circulating toxin before it binds to the target cell receptors.

The immunology of other *Corynebacterium* spp. infections is not studied, although it is apparent that these bacteria are likely to occur among immunocompromised patients.

B. *L. monocytogenes*

As previously detailed, the cross-reactivity of *L. monocytogenes* antigens with other bacteria has hindered serological assays. There is a limited role for serology given that most infections are acute, although serodiagnosis has been studied (142). Antibody responses after infection are not consistent regardless of measure. A seemingly more specific response has been measured with the use of listeriolysin as substrate.

Although listeriae are capable of intracellular multiplication and are relatively resistant to phagocytosis, macrophages may be activated with influence from gamma-interferon and TNF-alpha (143); hence, resistance to primary infection. *L. monocytogenes* antigens are presented by MHC class I-b molecules (144), and antigen processing and T cell responses are well-studied due to the availability of a mouse model (145). These studies have served as valuable precedents in the area of microbial pathogenesis. Affected tissue in humans usually has abscesses or granulomatous responses.

C. *Bacillus* spp.

Serodiagnostic methods have been established, but for anthrax, they will obviously have limited value for prospective diagnoses; they are more likely to be used for retrospective diagnoses and more yet for seroprevalence studies. Seroprevalence to *B. anthracis* antigens is higher in areas that are endemic for clinical anthrax. In EIA methods, both capsule and protective antigen are much better substrates to use than either of lethal or edema factors (146). Serological assays have also been used to assess the response after vaccination.

Vaccination with inactivated anthrax toxin achieves a good response in over 90% of individuals; a series of vaccine doses is followed by annual boosters for those who are deemed to be deserving of protection (147). There are many current controversies regarding the use of the current vaccine formulations (148) in this era where the spectre of anthrax as a weapon of biological warfare is real. In particular, there is some minor controversy over safety, but more importantly, some justified debate over how protective current vaccines are for the most lethal forms of anthrax, i.e., inhalational and gastrointestinal. Challenge studies in the context of vaccination are derived from animal models, and it is very difficult to design a human study with a disease that may be so lethal. It is unclear what impact the vaccine has on cutaneous infection. Vaccine use continues to occur in animal husbandry, albeit limited.

Toxins are known to inhibit polymorphonuclear cell function.

A skin test, which uses an attenuated strain extract and which demonstrates cell-mediated immunity, appears to give evidence of past-infection or active but chronic skin infection; the cellular response is detectable after two weeks.

D.   Other

P. acnes is relatively resistant to phagocytosis.

There is a poor immune response after human erysipeloid, and chronic *E. rhusiopathiae* infection which has relapses can occur. Animal vaccines are available.

The human antibody response has been assessed by immunoblotting for *A. haemolyticum* infection; patients with an illness and isolation of this bacterium have a significantly greater humoral response especially to antigens of 30, 50, 60, and 80 kD (149).

G. vaginalis is effectively killed by human neutrophils in vitro (150). Patients not uncommonly develop a measurable humoral immune response to the bacterium during genital infections. The latter assessment is complicated, however, by the antigenic variability among isolates (13).

VI.   LABORATORY DIAGNOSIS

A.   *Corynebacterium* spp.

1.   C. diphtheriae

This bacterium is maintained reasonably well in usual transport media, and in fact transport media were designed initially by public health laboratories with this and other needs in mind.

Microscopy of direct samples from infection are difficult to evaluate for presumptive *C. diphtheriae* due to the common finding of other corynebacteria in skin and pharyngeal samples.

Both non-selective and selective solid media are preferred for the initial assessment when a directed request for *C. diphtheriae* culture is made. In the past, some bacteriology laboratories, especially referral laboratories or those that provided services in known endemic areas, routinely included a selective agar screen for this pathogen. The remarkable decline in clinical diphtheria led many to abandon such routine screening. Suspect colonies of catalase-positive diphtheroids may be sought on routine blood agar, but a selective medium is desirable due to the overgrowth of normal oral flora. As well, many corynebacteria that are not causes of diphtheria will be sampled from a non-selective plate, and thus it is also useful to provide differential capability. Colistin-nalidixic blood agar provides some selection. Tellurite blood agar or Tinsdale medium are popular selective media that have been time-honoured. The reduction of tellurite on such media produces a black colony, and on Tinsdale medium, cystinase activity results in the appearance of a brown halo around the black colony. Tinsdale medium should be used in 1-2 weeks after preparation depending on the manufacturer's instructions. Given the lack of positive specimens in most regions and given the selective nature of tellurite-containing media, specimens are screened on either one-half or one quarter of an agar plate.

A suspect colony will be catalase-positive, and the Gram stain will show the typical diphtheroid morphology. Essentially all blackened colonies from selective media will be assessed, although it is recognized that a few other bacteria will not be inhibited by tellurite and may reduce it as well. Biochemical characterization of *C. diphtheriae* can be performed by most medium-sized laboratories although serum supplementation of biochemicals may better support some strains. The bacterium ferments glucose and maltose, is nitrate-positive (except biotype belfanti), produces a cystinase, and is negative for the esculin, urease, and pyrazinamidase reactions. The API Coryne biochemical strip provides reliable speciation of *C. diphtheriae*. More recently, 16S rRNA sequencing has been used to speciate corynebacteria, and it is applicable to *C. diphtheriae* (151).

Whereas some of the above methods may require a few days to complete, earlier confirmation of a suspect isolate is desirable given the rarity of this bacterium in non-endemic areas, given the desire to intervene in active diphtheria with antitoxin, and given the cascade that will be required in regards to public health measures. Therefore, a high index of suspicion early on should prompt an assessment of toxigenicity in short order. Historically, animal inoculations were used to assess toxigenicity, and thereafter, some tissue cultures (e.g., Vero cells) could be used for the same purpose. The Elek test, a crude immunoprecipitation assay, became the most commonly-used standard. The latter assay, although simple in principle, was fraught with some difficulty in standardization in particular with respect to base media and antisera. A conventional Elek test may also require up to 48 hrs. to complete. Thus, more timely modifications have been produced and indeed are now recommended (152). Interpretive errors have also been of concern despite controlled reagents. It is not surprising therefore that some have found the method to be fallible in the hands of a concerning number of laboratories when assessed in a proficiency testing context (153). Other methods for toxin testing have thus been assessed including immunoblotting, passive hemagglutination, latex agglutination, immunofluorescence, EIA, and PCR. The EIA has been created in order to obtain a result sooner than that from the Elek test; the published versions are touted to perform as well as the standard method (154-157). PCR testing for toxin also has the potential to generate a rapid answer. The toxin gene (especially the fragment A portion) has been the target for several primer sets (122). There is a very good correlation of PCR-positivity and toxin-positivity by standard methods, but a few reports have confirmed that PCR-positive, biological toxin-negative strains do exist (up to 5-10% of toxin-negative). PCR is thus exquisitely sensitive but not entirely specific for this very serious pathogen; *tox* gene sequences are thus present but not in a sufficient capacity to allow for production of active toxin (158). It is possible nevertheless to use the PCR technique as a rapid screen in acute circumstances; positive assays would be secondarily confirmed with the modified Elek or other assay.

Conventional biotyping has a limited role in epidemiological assessments; phage and serological typing both have their limitations. Given the importance of this infection and the progression in molecular technologies, several more discriminatory approaches have been devised, and these include multilocus enzyme electrophoresis, ribotyping, restriction fragment length polymorphism, pulse-field gel electrophoresis, and PCR typing (159-162). A standardized ribotyping system has been proposed for international comparisons (163).

2. *Other Corynebacterium spp.*

Weakly-growing pin-point colonies of presumptive bacteria that are obtained from specimens that may be contaminated with skin or mucosal flora are not uncommonly and initially suspected as diphtheroids. It is possible therefore that such growth will be confused with coagulase-negative staphylococci and other diphtheroids that are not *Corynebacterium* spp. Among specimens from sites that have mixtures of bacteria, *Corynebacterium* spp. may not appear as dominant flora after the first day of incubation and assessment. The Gram stain appearance of a clinical specimen therefore may serve to guide more extensive consideration for these bacteria. Among sterile sites, the amount of bacterium may be minimal, but these bacteria usually grow well from both solid and enrichment media provided they are maintained for several days. Lipophilic corynebacteria will grow on common blood agars. The actual identification of members from this genus is often confusing given the diversity of species which are currently recognized including those that have been more newly defined. It is accepted that the majority of *Corynebacterium* spp. from all clinical specimens are generally contaminants and are not relevant for an extensive identification exercise. It is appropriate therefore to label many isolates simply as diphtheroid Gram positive bacilli or presumptive *Corynebacterium* spp. A more definitive speciation may then be reserved for isolates from usual sterile sites, suspect *C. diphtheriae*, heavy urinary growths in the context of a urinary tract infection where no other pathogen is found and where the clinical context is suspect, and multiple positive blood cultures.

Although the number of *Corynebacterium* spp. may seem intimidating, the majority of isolates tend to be represented by a handful of species or so. For example, a study from Belgium found that five species (*C. amycolatum*, *C. jeikeium*, *C. striatum*, *C. afermentans*, and *C. minutissimum*) accounted for 87% of all clinical isolates (164). Another study from the U.S. found that three species (*C. jeikeium*, CDC group G2, and *C. minutissimum*) accounted for 67% of isolates (165). These reports should be viewed in the context of methods that were available for speciation and the changes that have subsequently occurred in the applied systematics. Nevertheless, the likelihood of encountering a clinically-relevant *Corynebacterium* spp. that requires full identification and that is especially difficult to speciate is not so common.

Corynebacterium spp. can be speciated usually with the following assessments: catalase, oxidation/fermentation on CTA media, motility, nitrate, urease, esculin, acid from glucose/maltose/sucrose/mannitol/xylose, CAMP test, lipophilia (with and without 1% Tween 80), and pyrazinamidase. The review from Funke and colleagues provides tables for the expected results (17). The latter updates a practical scheme that was previously published by von Graevenitz and Funke (166) and which was originally derived from the CDC schemata of Hollis and Weaver.

Several commercial kits have been produced that are useful for the speciation of *Corynebacterium* spp. (e.g., API Coryne, API(RAPID) Coryne, and RapID CB Plus, Biolog Identification System) (167-173). These identification panels can usually be completed in 24-48 hrs., although rapid enzyme methods are more often becoming a major part of the updated systems. Although these systems may be challenged when assessed with a diverse and reference group of species, they perform generally well in clinical circumstances where the number of different species found is limited for the majority of specimens. Since all systems are unable to accurately speciate all isolates, supplementary tests must often be used to augment the kits; 15-30% of clinical isolates will require such additional tests. In addition to *Corynebacterium* spp., some of these kits also speciate or at least indicate the genus of other diphtheroids. Again, the issue of supplemental tests arises.

Chromatographic methods are useful for distinguishing *Corynebacterium* spp. from other Gram positive rods especially those that are partially acid-fast (see Chapter 14). Cellular fatty acid analysis in particular is of value in this regard, but there are clearly limitations in differentiating within the genus (174).

Skin scales from patients with erythrasma fluoresce red when exposed to Wood's lamp. There is often some confusion in differentiating this bacterium from *C. jeikeium* by biochemical means alone. Skin scales or scrapings from erythrasma characteristically show multiple bacilli when stained with a variety of vital stains [e.g., cotton blue (175)].

Although *C. urealyticum* will grow well on conventional media that are used for urine specimens such as blood agar, a selective medium has been devised (176).

Both ribotyping (177) and 16S rRNA sequencing (151) have been used to attempt speciation. Molecular approaches along this theme will undoubtedly continue to be developed, but at the present time, the databases need frequent additions in order to keep pace with the change in nomenclature and the acquisition of new species.

There are limited roles for typing among the non-diphtheria corynebacteria. Pulse field gel methods are likely to be applicable to all however, although study in this area is minimal.

B. *L. monocytogenes*

Although the morphology on Gram stain is that of a regularly-shaped bacillus when the bacterium is obtained freshly from culture (smaller than most *Bacillus* spp.), the morphology may vary and include coccoid and coccobacillary forms when stained directly in clinical specimens such as cerebrospinal fluid or abscess. The cerebrospinal fluid cell count during meningitis is potentially variable as well; although polymorphonuclear cell predominance is common, the spectrum may include mononuclear cell predominance and any combination in between. The presence of predominant mononuclear cells in the context of newborn meningitis and a positive Gram stain for Gram positive bacteria should strongly raise concern for listeriosis until otherwise proven.

The bacterium may initially be confused with others unless the catalase reaction is performed. The bacterium is possibly identified throught the use of assessments which include catalase (+), oxidase (-), hemolysis (small zone on routine blood agar), salt tolerance, and esculin (+). A GenProbe chemiluminescent probe is available for species confirmation (178), but given the infrequency of *Listeria* isolates in most laboratories, it is unlikely to be commonly available for prospective use. Likewise, identification with API Listeria could be of value, but again most clinical laboratories will not have common use for such a product especially when the bacterium can be reasonably identified by the simple traits as detailed above; identification to the genus level is also possible in the API Coryne system (179) and as well with the API Strep system. Identification methods are more likely to be used in the food and animal industry.

L. monocytogenes is usually obtained in pure culture from previously sterile sites of infection. Difficulty in isolation may be apparent, however, when the bacterium is mixed with normal vaginal flora (where it may be disregarded in light growth or mistaken phenotypically for enterococci) or when epidemiological studies of stool carriage are undertaken. The bacterium will grow well on routine bacteriological media after 24 hrs. when obtained from usually sterile sites. Nevertheless, the use of cold enrichment may be of value since the bacterium, like some pathogenic yersiniae, is capable of growing in refrigeration temperatures. Both cold enrichment and selective media are not usually required for most clinical specimens. Indeed, selective media are more likely to be used for enteric prevalence studies or for screening products in the food industry (180). For the purposes of clinical bacteriology, selective media, when indicated, may include colistin and nalidixic acid, broad-spectrum cephalosporins, and amphotericin B. Dyes have been used to inhibit enterococci. In the food industry, it is apparent that maximal selection can be achieved with the use of more than one selective medium.

Rapid detection with antigen detection methods or genetic amplification with PCR (181) have a limited role in clinical microbiology. Such assays would not enjoy much use, and the ad hoc use and associated complicating features of the same are unlikely to provide information that is more timely than that which is obtained from the timely and knowledgeable selection of clinical specimens.

Typing methods for listeriae have been studied considerably due to the impact on the food industry, although some of these methods have also now been applied to clinical isolates including those from outbreaks of infection. It is evident that serotyping provides only a first line of differentiation among isolates, and it is somewhat problematic that most clinical isolates belong to less than a handful of serotypes. Intraserotype discrimination, however, can be achieved with PFGE or PCR typing methods; these methods are generally equivalent in their discriminatory power. Otherwise, methods for typing have included phage typing, MLEE, ribotyping, PCR-REA, rep-PCR, and AP-PCR (182-188). The RiboPrinter Microbial Characterization System has also been used to rapidly and accurately characterize isolates (189).

C. Bacillus spp.

1. B. anthracis

This bacterium is readily cultured from blood when present, but bacteremia is an indicator of a very serious infection and is associated with a very high mortality rate. Thus, a positive blood culture will not often be of value in managing a patient. The bacterium can also be cultured from cutaneous lesions although not consistently. The potential for *B. anthracis* to act as a biohazard is real, and thus, due care should be exercised in dealing with a suspect isolate. Work should be performed in an appropriate cabinet, and the work surfaces should be thoroughly decontaminated. It is preferable to handle *B. anthracis* as a level 3 pathogen.

As previously detailed, *B. anthracis* grows readily, and selective media, although described, are not generally required. The identification of the bacterium is relatively straight-forward once it is recognized that one is dealing with a *Bacillus* spp. of some sort (190). Colonies are grey-white and hold on to the agar when moved. The bacterium is non-hemolytic, non-motile, and penicillin susceptible. Rare reports of penicillin resistance have been published (191). The identification of capsule will also be helpful. Identification can also be facilitated with the use of API or Biolog biochemical methods (192,193). PCR techniques can be used to identify toxin or capsule genes, although these will obviously not be readily available to most.

2. Other Bacillus spp.

Although some colony morphologies may be typical of *Bacillus* spp. and although experience in judging such morphologies accrues over time, there is nevertheless considerable potential variation. Spores may swell some bacilli and may be suggestive of some species. Spores can be difficult to appreciate after fresh subculture from a clinical specimen and are uncommon when these bacteria are seen in clinical specimens. If the subculture is left at room temperature for 1-2 days, the spores may become more prominent. Spores may be selected by heat treatment (65°C for 15 min.) or by ethanol treatment (50% ethanol for 1 hr.) Stain variability is common either in smears from positive blood cultures or in smears from clinical specimens.

Bacillus spp. all grow readily on common media. Growth in positive blood cultures from true infections is most often readily appreciated by 24 hrs. When contaminating blood cultures, growth may be delayed by 24-48 hrs. in addition since the contaminanting form of the bacterium will often be the spore which requires conversion to the vegetative bacterium. Selective media for these bacteria are not required when clinical samples are cultured, although *B. cereus* selective media have been used for the purposes of culturing food and some clinical samples (194); there are a variety of selective media for such work (e.g., mannitol-egg yolk-polymyxin B agar), and spore selection by the aforementioned methods may also be useful in this regard.

Bacillus spp. are catalase-positive and largely motile. Differentiation may in part depend on whether they are oxidative or fermentative. Differentiation of common species can be achieved with the determination of lecithinase activity, casein hydrolysis, starch hydrolysis, gelatin hydrolysis, arginase dehydrolase activity, indole production, nitrate reduction, and the production of acid from a battery of sugars. A detailed table for such reactions has been provided (195). Again, the combination of API 20E and API 50CHB have been useful for identifying the major species (192,196). The suitability of the latter approach is seemingly dependent on achieving timely updates in the database due to changing nomenclature and new species. Despite these possibilities, the greater issue is simply that of defining whether any such speciation is required. For most isolates where there is a good likelihood of finding a *Bacillus* spp. as a contaminant, speciation should not be encouraged, e.g., a single positive blood culture bottle from an otherwise uncomplicated outpatient. Even for those circumstances where infection is probable, designation to the 'Bacillus spp.' level is usually adequate, e.g., an isolated true bacteremia in an immunocompromised patient with the central venous access device as the likely focus. In the latter case, the provision of some estimate of bacterial susceptibility is probably more critical. Speciation may then be reserved for complicated or rare infections, or for the event of a potential outbreak.

In circumstances of suspect food poisoning, the absolute detection of a *Bacillus* spp., especially *B. cereus*, may be insufficient to define the cause. Quantitation of *B. cereus* in food is often of value (often present $>10^5$/gm. of food), and it should be demonstrated that isolates from both food and patient are the same since these bacteria may normally be present in the bowel as a consequence of acquisition from various foods.

The presence of parasporal crystals is of importance for differentiating *B. cereus* (-) from *B. thuringiensis* (+). Furthermore, differentiation of these very similar species has been accomplished with the use of molecular techniques (197,198). It is of interest that some molecular techniques may not be able to distinguish these species (199) and that *B. thuringiensis* isolates have been found that may produce a *B. cereus*-like enterotoxin (200).

D. *Propionibacterium* spp.

These bacteria are frequent contaminants, and thus the definitive speciation is usually uncalled for when it is evident that an isolate is unlikely to be of clinical relevance. Propionibacteria not uncommonly signal positive in blood cultures at about 5-7 days and essentially always in the anaerobic bottle. If blood cultures are maintained for 5 days only, as has been the trend in many laboratories given the state-of-the-art in blood culture automation, propionibacteria may be missed. Likewise, if the anaerobic bottles are deleted from sets, again a trend in some laboratories, then propionibacteria are unlikely to be found. It must be recognized, however, that most of such isolates do represent contaminants.

P. *acnes* has been encountered by most laboratories. It usually has delayed growth on blood agar and must be incubated for 48-72 hrs. to achieve reasonable colonies especially when obtained from clinical specimens. The bacterium will favour anaerobic growth although microaerophilic atmospheres may suffice after subculture. The bacterium is catalase-positive and indole-positive and typically diphtheroidal in Gram stains.

Other propionibacteria are more difficult to readily speciate. It is fortunate that most clinical isolates prove to be *P. acnes*. RapID ANA performs well for designation to the genus level.

E. *Arcanobacterium* spp.

A. haemolyticum is often easily dismissed as a small colony non-Group A beta-hemolytic streptococcus (i.e., nongroupable) since it is most likely to be cultured from throat swabs. It is catalase-negative and pits the agar. Beta-hemolysis is usually delayed and growth is enhanced in CO_2 (201). The API Coryne system identifies this bacterium. Selective media have been described and these were used to find the bacterium in prospective studies (202,203). The latter are unlikely to be of much practical use given the rarity of this bacterium in acute pharyngitis.

Hemolysis from *A. pyogenes* is enhanced with increased CO_2. The bacterium hydrolyzes gelatin, produces acid from xylose, and produces beta-glucuronidase (204). Some commercial methods have had difficulty with the differentiation of *A. haemolyticum* and *A. pyogenes* (205). *A. pyogenes* is identified with the API Coryne system as is *A. bernardiae*.

F. *E. rhusiopathiae*

This bacterium will grow on routine blood agar and will appear as a diphtheroid. Among clinical samples, it is most likely to be found in blood cultures. Since it is catalase-negative, it is important to ensure that suspect but unusual putative streptococcal colonies are Gram-stained so that *E. rhusiopathiae* is not discarded. It may also be at times mistaken for *Gardnerella*. It is negative for the reactions of indole, VP, esculin, and urease; H_2S production in the butt of a TSI slope is a hallmark. API Coryne identifies this bacterium. PCR techniques for use in veterinary medicine have been defined (206). Also in the latter context, molecular methods have been applied to study heterogeneity within the species for typing purposes.

G. *G. vaginalis*

Good colonial growth may require 48-72 hrs. of incubation. The bacterium is initially suspected on the basis of a negative test for catalase and non-motility. It is positive for alpha-glucosidase, hydrolyzes starch, and is usually hippurate-positive (~90%) (13). It is susceptible to inhibition by SDS and metronidazole (50 μg. disc). *G. vaginalis* is identified in the API Coryne battery, although newer *Actinomyces* spp. are identified as *G. vaginalis* as well. Isolates can be biotyped on the basis of lipase, beta-galactosidase, and hippurate reactions.

Beta-hemolysis is demonstrable on rabbit or human blood agar but not with sheep blood. This trait was exploited for the production of a differential medium when the bacterium was more commonly sought at a time that it was believed to be the etiological agent of bacterial vaginosis (13). Selective media have included colistin-nalidixic agar with human blood base, human blood agar with gentamicin, nalidixic acid, and amphotericin B, and human blood agar bilayer (for better demonstration of hemolysis) with Tween 80, colistin, nalidixic acid, and amphotericin B.

The laboratory diagnosis of bacterial vaginosis currently depends very little on the isolation of *G. vaginalis*. Rather, the vaginal fluid of a symptomatic patient may be subjected to two main assessments: a) production of an amine odour after alkalinization of the fluid on a microscope slide with KOH, and b) Gram stain of a smear with an observation for clue cells, depletion of normal lactobacilli (i.e., Gram positive rod predominance), and relative abundance of Gram negative rods, especially those that are slender, small, and curved. The Gram-stained smear reading is obviously fraught with variable interpretation. Scoring schemata have therefore been proposed in order to provide some measure of standardization (207,208).

H. Miscellaneous Gram positive rods

As for the non-diphtheria *Corynebacterium* spp., it is beneficial to ensure that work which is invested in identifying these bacteria be prefaced by an adequate clinical assessment of whether the isolate is likely to have been causing disease. Much energy and resource can be exhausted in this area, and accurate speciation may be an exercise in futility if the primary laboratory and diagnosticians have not made the effort to ensure that a contaminant has been ruled out.

As detailed by von Graevenitz and Funke (166), there are several preliminary measures that may serve to reasonably categorize these various species. These include oxidation or fermentation status, catalase, assessment of acid-fastness, motility, hemolysis including synergistic hemolysis (CAMP test), nitrate, urease, esculin, and acid production from several sugar substrates. It does not make sense to have smaller inexperienced laboratories overly dwell on such characterization, and the use of reference laboratories for this purpose should be considered. Commercial systems such as API Coryne and Biolog have success in identifying several of the genera and species (166,169,170); these will likely improve as the manufacturers are able to catch up with new designations and new species profiles. Reference laboratories will likely also utilize cellular fatty acid analyses and other assessments of the cell wall constitution. As the databases improve, it is also likely that 16S rRNA sequencing will become useful. At this time, no one method or approach will necessarily identify all such bacteria, but rapid gains are being made.

VII. SUSCEPTIBILITY TESTING

The methods which are used for susceptibility testing of the bacteria that are described in this chapter are open to debate since well-accepted and standardized methods are not clearly identified. For several of these bacteria, clinical experience in the treatment of infection may be altogether limited or perhaps limited to few antibiotics. Nevertheless, on a practical basis, susceptibility testing may be desirable for some circumstances, especially in the context of serious infections. Turnidge and Bell have given some suggestions regarding what methods and criteria may be used for members of this group (see Chapter 8), e.g., using staphylococcal, enterococcal, or streptococcal breakpoints depending on the bacterium. In general, methods such as agar dilution, broth microdilution, and Etest appear satisfactory; in some circumstances, disc diffusion may give a reasonable estimate of susceptibility. Media may include 5%-sheep blood agar with a Mueller-Hinton base; a Columbia base may provide better growth for some lipophilic isolates. For some isolates, incubation may require extension to 48 hrs. rather than 18-24 hrs., and 5% CO_2 supplementation may benefit growth.

Whereas many of these bacteria have predictable susceptibility, it may be prudent to test them when serious infections arise, since the potential to acquire resistance in this era of multi-resistant bacteria is of concern. Traditional resistances when common for a given bacterium should be respected, e.g., cephalosporins for *L. monocytogenes*, regardless of the test results; it is the usual susceptible ones that merit some further consideration. The spectrum of testing should be tempered by knowledge of the site of infection, possible complications and the intensity of infection, published evidence of benefit from the use of antibiotics, and routes of administration that are feasible as well as antibiotics that are practical. Circumstances of infection with these bacteria should be of primary concern to the laboratory and should merit proactive consultation with the patient's physician.

Perhaps it is best to take a pragmatic approach in this regard. Antibiotics that have little or no activity (e.g., no zone by disc diffusion) should be avoided. Antibiotics that have tremendous activity (e.g., zones by disc diffusion > 30 mm. or MICs <0.125 mg./L.) should be considered. The choice may then ultimately depend on the historical data, ease and cost of administration, and pharmacodynamics. Bacteria with intermediate susceptibility, and for which the choice of an evidence-based antibiotic is difficult, should be the subject of discussion.

Generalizing, most of the bacteria that are discussed in this chapter are reasonably susceptible to vancomycin with the few exceptions of *Erysipelothrix* and some lactobacilli; other exceptions have been documented but are rare. Indeed, many are quite exquisitely susceptible to beta-lactam agents such as penicillin which should be preferred for various reasons. One can also generalize that these bacteria are uniformly resistant to nalidixic acid, polymyxins, and mecillinam. Since the applied systematics have been changing, a review of the former literature on susceptibility testing in this area should bear in mind the changes in nomenclature or for that matter, possible mistaken identities, e.g., former *C. xerosis* now recognized to likely have been *C. amycolatum*.

A.   *Corynebacterium* spp.

1.   *C. diphtheriae*

In the context of highly suspect diphtheria, antibiotics and even antitoxin should be administered prior to the actual bacteriological confirmation. The use of antibiotics is associated with a shortening of the pharyngeal illness and will also eliminate pharyngeal shedding which is of benefit to prevent spread. Antibiotics are also advocated for contacts of a case. Nevertheless, it is recognized that pharyngeal carriage may persist after a course of antibiotics for either asymptomatic colonization or active illness, and thus, a test of cure should be considered (209).

Clinical isolates are most often susceptible to penicillin, erythromycin, clindamycin, tetracycline, chloramphenicol, aminoglycosides, advanced spectrum cephalosporins, and rifampin. Penicillin and erythromycin are used for active disease, whereas erythromycin has a better outcome for eradicating the carrier state. Penicillin MICs are usually in the range of 0.025-0.4 mg./L.(210). Erythromycin and ciprofloxacin MICs are usually 0.025-0.4 and 0.12-0.5 mg./L. respectively. The new macrolides have MICs that are similar to those of erythromycin. The contemporary outbreak in Russia was not associated with resistant bacteria, and it appears that the degree of susceptibility is essentially unchanged for most antibiotics when compared to historic data (211). Resistance to erythromycin has been documented, but it is extremely uncommon; it is speculated that such resistance has been acquired from skin corynebacteria (212).

Serious non-toxigenic *C. diphtheriae* infections such as endocarditis have been treated with a combination of a beta-lactam and an aminoglycoside.

2.   Other Corynebacterium spp.

Particular study has been directed to the use of susceptibility testing methods for this group of bacteria (213-215). Etest and agar dilution methods have a good correlation with each other. For erythromycin and vancomycin especially, there is also a good correlation between disc diffusion and broth microdilution; this is less apparent for penicillin susceptibility. Vancomycin is the most active of antibiotics against all *Corynebacterium* spp. (165), and teichoplanin susceptibility is also the norm (164). Most are also susceptible to doxycycline and fusidic acid. *C. jeikeium, C. urealyticum,* and *C. amycolatum* are not uncommonly multiresistant and especially resistant to penicillin. It is highly probable that resistance among *C. jeikeium* is hospital-acquired (216). Given the potential variation in this group of bacteria, it is important to exercise care with the acceptance that penicillin resistance or susceptibility in themselves should absolutely correlate with speciation.

The following generalizations detail patterns of susceptibility or resistance among *Corynebacterium* spp. (always vancomycin susceptible) (164,165,213-222):

> *C. accolens* – susceptible to penicillin and erythromycin
>
> *C. afermentans* – susceptible to penicillin
>
> *C. amycolatum* – susceptible to tetracycline; variable susceptibility to beta-lactams, erythromycin, clindamycin, aminoglycosides, rifampin, ciprofloxacin
>
> *C. auris* – resistant to penicillin; susceptible to gentamicin, ciprofloxacin, tetracycline, and rifampin; variable susceptibility to erythromycin and clindamycin
>
> *C. bovis* – susceptible to erythromycin and rifampin
>
> *C. glucuronolyticum* – susceptible to penicillin, gentamicin, and rifampin; resistant to erythromycin, clindamycin, tetracycline, and ciprofloxacin
>
> *C. jeikeium* – resistant to penicillin and co-trimoxazole; generally multi-resistant to many others (although not always); susceptibility variable to erythromycin, tetracycline, doxycycline, fusidic acid, and ciprofloxacin
>
> *C. minutissimum* – some strains multi-resistant
>
> *C. pseudodiphtheriticum* – susceptible to penicillin, aminoglycosides, tetracycline, rifampin, ciprofloxacin; variable susceptibility to erythromycin and clindamycin
>
> *C. pseudotuberculosis* – susceptible to penicillin, erythromycin, tetracycline, chloramphenicol, and rifampin
>
> *C. striatum* – susceptible to penicillin; resistant to erythromycin, clindamycin, tetracycline, and ciprofloxacin; variably susceptible to aminoglycosides and rifampin
>
> *C. ulcerans* – susceptible to penicillin and erythromycin
>
> *C. urealyticum* – resistant to penicillin and aminoglycosides; variably susceptible to erythromycin, tetracycline, ciprofloxacin, and rifampin
>
> *C. xerosis* – penicillin susceptible

B. *L. monocytogenes*

This bacterium is susceptible to penicillin and ampicillin which are favoured as primary agents in therapy. Serious infections may benefit from the addition of gentamicin which creates a synergistic effect with penicillin (223). The bacterium is also generally susceptible to cotrimoxazole, vancomycin, tetracyclines, erythromycin, and chloramphenicol. It is routinely resistant to all cephalosporins and variably so to quinolones. The robust growth of this bacterium allows the application of breakpoints that are used for enterococci.

The treatment of infection must take into account the need to penetrate cells that harbour intracellular bacterium (224). It is recommended that treatment be prolonged (~3-4 weeks) since there is a possibility of relapse (225).

There are increasing reports of resistance which appear to have emerged mainly since the 1980s. These include plasmid- and transposon-associated resistance to erythromycin, tetracycline, and chloramphenicol (226). Resistance has been transferable from enterococci and streptococci to *Listeria*, and from *Listeria* to enterococci, streptococci, and staphylococci (226).

C. *Bacillus* spp.

B. anthracis is susceptible to penicillin, erythromycin, tetracycline, and chloramphenicol (227). Rare citations of penicillin resistance have been made (191).

   B. cereus commonly possesses beta-lactamases and among these are potentially very potent ones that are capable of cleaving a broad spectrum of beta-lactam agents. These bacteria are not uncommonly susceptible to aminoglycosides, erythromycin, clindamycin, chloramphenicol, and vancomycin (228). Among non-*B. cereus* species, however, the profile may be much different, and indeed they may be susceptible to penicillin and lack beta-lactamases (228). It is suggested, therefore, that such isolates be tested individually when serious infections arise. Since these species grow very well in the laboratory, they may be assessed with breakpoint criteria that are used for staphylococci for example.

D. *Propionibacterium* spp.

These are susceptible to penicillin and vancomycin. There is usually susceptibility to most other antibiotics except metronidazole and aminoglycosides (229).

E. *Arcanobacterium* spp.

A. haemolyticum is often susceptible to penicillin, erythromycin, clindamycin, chloramphenicol, tetracycline, and vancomycin, and variably susceptible to aminoglycosides and ciprofloxacin (230,231). It is resistant to cotrimoxazole. Despite in vitro susceptibility to penicillin, clinical failure has been reported, and erythromycin remains the drug of choice to treat pharyngitis (232).

   A. pyogenes is susceptible to penicillin, tetracycline, chloramphenicol, aminoglycosides, and ciprofloxacin. *A. bernardiae* is susceptible to penicillin, erythromycin, clindamycin, and vancomycin.

F. *E. rhusiopathiae*

As previously indicated, this bacterium is one of the rare Gram positive bacilli that are vancomycin-resistant. Resistance is also common to cotrimoxazole and aminoglycosides. Susceptibility to penicillin is exquisite (MICs range ~0.002-0.06 mg./L.), and susceptibility to erythromycin, clindamycin, tetracycline, chloramphenicol, and ciprofloxacin are also recognized (91).

G. *G. vaginalis*

This bacterium is susceptible to penicillin, ampicillin, and most beta-lactam agents (13). It is also susceptible to metronidazole, erythromycin, and clindamycin.

   Bacterial vaginosis responds very well to treatment with metronidazole, but such an impact is likely due to an effect on vaginal anaerobes in addition to *G. vaginalis*. Metronidazole does not affect lactobacilli which are needed to replenish the normal flora during bacterial vaginosis.

H. Other Gram positive bacilli

Isolates from these genera are vancomycin-susceptible except for some lactobacilli. Generalizations regarding susceptibility include:

   Actinomyces neuii – susceptible to penicillin
   Arthrobacter – susceptible penicillin
   Bifidobacterium – susceptible to penicillin
   Brevibacterium – susceptible to aminoglycosides, tetracycline, and rifampin; variable susceptibility to penicillin, erythromycin, clindamycin, and ciprofloxacin
   Cellulomonas – susceptible to tetracycline and rifampin
   Dermabacter – susceptible to rifampin; variable susceptibility to penicillin, erythromycin, clindamycin, aminoglycosides, tetracycline, and ciprofloxacin

Lactobacillus – susceptible to penicillin; resistant to metronidazole

Microbacterium – susceptible to erythromycin; resistant to aminoglycosides; variable susceptibility to penicillin (former *Aureobacterium* spp. – susceptible to beta-lactams but resistant to clindamycin, aminoglycosides, and ciprofloxacin)

Turicella – susceptible to penicillin; variable susceptibility to erythromycin and clindamycin

REFERENCES

1. Eskola J, Lumio J, Vuopio-Varkila J. Resurgent diphtheria – are we safe? Brit Med Bull 1998; 54:635-645.
2. Vitek CR, Wharton M. Diphtheria in the former Soviet Union; re-emergence of a pandemic disease. Emerg Infect Dis 1998; 4:539-550.
3. van der Lelie H, Leverstein-Van Hall M, Mertens M, van Zaanen HC, van Oers RH, Thomas BL, von dem Borne AE, Kuijper EJ. *Corynebacterium* CDC group JK (*Corynebacterium jeikeium*) sepsis in haematological patients: a report of three cases and a systematic literature review. Scand J Infect Dis 1995; 27:581-584.
4. Jones D. Foodborne listeriosis. Lancet 1990; 336:1171-1174.
5. Bryce EA, Smith JA, Tweeddale M, Andruschak BJ, Maxwell MR. Dissemination of *Bacillus cereus* in an intensive care unit. Infect Cont Hosp Epidemiol 1993; 14:459-462.
6. Thuler LC, Velasco E, de Souza Martins CA, de Faria LM, da Fonseca NP, Dias LM. An outbreak of *Bacillus* species in a cancer hospital. Infect Cont Hosp Epidemiol 1998; 19:856-858.
7. Gray J, George RH, Durbin GM, Ewer AK, Hocking MD, Morgan ME. An outbreak of *Bacillus cereus* respiratory tract infections on a neonatal unit due to contaminated ventilator circuits. J Hosp Infect 1999; 41:19-22.
8. Drobniewski FA. *Bacillus cereus* and related species. Clin Microbiol Rev 1993; 6:324-338.
9. Schnept E, Crickmore N, Van Rie J, Lereclus D, Baum J, Feitelson J, Zeigler DR, Dean DH. *Bacillus thuringiensis* and its pecticidal crystal proteins. Microbiol Mole Biol Rev 1998; 62:775-806.
10. Logan NA. *Bacillus* species of medical and veterinary importance. J Med Microbiol 1988; 25:157-165.
11. Ibrahim KH, Brown G, Wright DH, Rotschafer JC. *Bacillus anthracis*: medical issues of biologic warfare. Phamacotherapy 1999; 19:690-701.
12. Dixon TC, Meselson M, Guillemin J, Hanna PC. Anthrax. N Engl J Med 1999; 341:815-826.
13. Catlin WB. *Gardnerella vaginalis*: characteristics, clinical considerations, and controversies. Clin Microbiol Rev 1992; 5:213-237.
14. Kalapothaki V, Sapounas T, Xirouchaki E, Papoutsakis G, Trichopoulos D. Prevalence of diphtheria carriers in a population with disappearing clinical diphtheria. Infection 1984; 12:387-389.
15. Hoeprich PD. Diphtheria. In: Hoeprich PD, Jordan MC, Ronald AR, eds. Infectious Diseases: A Treatise of Infectious Processes. Philadelphia, PA:JB Lippincott Co., 1994:373-380.
16. Tiley SM, Kociuba KR, Heron LG, Munro R. Infective endocarditis due to nontoxigenic *Corynebacterium diphtheriae*: report of seven cases and review. Clin Infect Dis 1993; 16:271-275.
17. Funke G, von Graevenitz A, Clarridge JE, Bernard K. Clinical microbiology of coryneform bacteria. Clin Microbiol Rev 1997; 10:125-159.
18. Funke G, Lawson PA, Bernard KA, Collins MD. Most *Corynebacterium xerosis* strains identified in the routine clinical laboratory correspond to *Corynebacterium amycolatum*. J Clin Microbiol 1996; 34:1124-1128.
19. Esteban J, Nieto E, Calvo R, Fernandez-Robals R, Valero-Guillen PL, Soriano F. Microbiological characterization and clinical significance of *Corynebacterium amycolatum* strains. Eur J Clin Micrbiol Infect Dis 1999; 18:518-521.
20. Grove DI, Der-Haroutian V, Ratcliff RM. *Aureobacterium* masquerading as 'Corynebcterium aquaticum' infection: case report and review of the literature. J Med Microbiol 1999; 48:965-970.
21. Renaud FN, Gregory A, Barreau C, Aubel D, Freney J. Identification of *Turicella otitidis* isolated from a patient with otorrhea associated with surgery: differentiation from *Corynebacterium afermentans* and *Corynebacterium auris*. J Clin Microbiol 1996; 34:2625-2627.
22. Riegel P, Ruimy R, De Briel D, Prevost G, Jehl F, Bimet F, Christen R, Monteil H. *Corynebacterium argentoratense* sp. nov. from the human throat. Int J Syst Bacteriol 1995; 45:533-537.
23. Riegel P, Heller R, Provost G, Jehl F, Monteil H. *Corynebacterium durum* sp. nov., from human clinical specimens. Int J Syst Bacteriol 1997; 47:1107-1111.
24. von Graevenitz A, Punter-Streit V, Riegel P, Funke G. Coryneform bacteria in throat cultures of healthy individuals. J Clin Microbiol 1998; 36:2087-2088.

25. Funke G, Efstratiou A, Kuklinska D, Hutson RA, De Zoysa A, Engler KH, Collins MD. *Corynebacterium imitans* sp. nov. isolated from patients with suspected diphtheria. J Clin Microbiol 1997; 35:1978-1983.

26. Collins MD, Falsen E, Akervall E, Sjoden B, Alvarez A. *Corynebacterium kroppenstedtii* sp. nov., a novel corynebacterium that does not contain mycolic acids. Int J Syst Bacteriol 1998; 48:1449-1454.

27. Funke G, Hutson RA, Hilleringmann M, Heizmann WR, Collins MD. *Corynebacterium lipophiloflavum* sp. nov. isolated from a patient with bacterial vaginosis. FEMS Microbiol Lett 1997; 150:219-224.

28. Golledge CL, Phillips G. *Corynebacterium minutissimum* infection. J Infect 1991; 23:73-76.

29. Claeys G, Vanhouteghem H, Riegel P, Wauters G, Hamerlynck R, Dierick J, de Witte J, Verschraegen G, Vaneechoutte M. Endocarditis of native aortic and mitral valves due to *Corynebacterium accolens*: report of a case and application of phenotypic and genotypic techniques for identification. J Clin Microbiol 1996; 34:1290-1292.

30. Riegel P, de Briel D, Prevost G, Jehl F, Monteil H, Minck R. Taxonomic study of *Corynebacterium* Group ANF-1 strains: proposal of *Corynebacterium afermentans* sp. nov. containing the subspecies *C. afermentans* subsp. afermentans subsp. nov. and *C. afermentans* subsp. lipophilum subsp. nov. Int J Syst Bacteriol 1993; 43:287-292.

31. Dykhuizen RS, Douglas G, Weir J, Gould IM. *Corynebacterium afermentans* subsp. lipophilum: multiple abscess formation in brain and liver. Scand J Infect Dis 1995; 27:637-639.

32. Funke G, Lawson PA, Collins MD. Heterogeneity within human-derived Centres for Disease Control and Prevention (CDC) coryneform group ANF-1-like bacteria and description of *Corynebacterium auris* sp. nov. Int J Syst Bacteriol 1995; 45:735-739.

33. Funke G, Osorio CR, Frei R, Riegel P, Collins MD. *Corynebacterium confusum* sp. nov., isolated from human clinical specimens. Int J Syst Bacteriol 1998; 48:1291-1296.

34. Funke G, Ramos CP, Collins MD. *Corynebacterium coyleae* sp. nov., isolated from human clinical specimens. Int J Syst Bacteriol 1997; 47:92-96.

35. Sjoden B, Funke G, Izquierdo A, Akervall E, Collins MD. Description of some coryneform bacteria isolated from human clinical specimens as *Corynebacterium falsenii* sp. nov. Int J Syst Bacteriol 1998; 48:69-74.

36. van der Lelie H, Leverstein-Van Hall M, Mertens M, van Zaanen HC, van Oers RH, Thomas BL, von dem Borne AE, Kuijper EJ. *Corynebacterium* CDC group JK (*Corynebacterium jeikeium*) sepsis in haematological patients: a report of three cases and a systematic literature review. Scand J Infect Dis 1995; 27:581-584.

37. Riegel P, Ruimy R, de Briel D, Prevost G, Jehl F, Christen R, Monteil H. Genomic diversity and phylogenetic relationships among lipid-requiring diphtheroids from humans and characterization of *Corynebacterium macginleyi* sp. nov. Int J Syst Bacteriol 1995; 45:128-133.

38. Funke G, Pagano-Niederer M, Bernauer W. *Corynebacterium macginleyi* has to date been isolated exclusively from conjunctival swabs. J Clin Microbiol 1998; 36:3670-3673.

39. Rupp ME, Stiles KG, Tarantolo S, Goering RV. Central venous catheter-related *Corynebacterium minutissimum* bacteremia. Infect Control Hosp Epidemiol 1998; 19:786-789.

40. Funke G, Lawson PA, Collins MD. *Corynebacterium mucifaciens* sp. nov., an unusual species from human clinical material. Int J Syst Bacteriol 1997; 47:952-957.

41. Petit PL, Bok JW, Thompson J, Buiting AG, Coyle MB. Native-valve endocarditis due to CDC coryneform group ANF-3: report of a case and review of corynebacterial endocarditis. Clin Infect Dis 1994; 19:897-901.

42. Morris A, Guild I. Endocarditis due to *Corynebacterium pseudodiphtheriticum*: five case reports, review, and antibiotic susceptibilities of nine strains. Rev Infect Dis 1991; 13:887-892.

43. Cimolai N, Rogers P, Seear M. *Corynebacterium pseudodiphtheriticum* pneumonitis in a leukaemic child. Thorax 1992; 47:838-839.

44. Manzella JP, Kellogg JA, Parsey KS. *Corynebacterium pseudodiphtheriticum*: a respiratory tract pathogen in adults. Clin Infect Dis 1995; 20:37-40.

45. Burke GJ, Malouf MA, Glanville AR. Opportunistic lung infection with *Corynebacterium pseudodiphtheriticum* after lung and heart transplantation. Med J Aust 1997; 166:362-364.

46. Izurieta HS, Strebel PM, Youngblood T, Hollis DG, Popovic T. Exudative pharyngitis possibly due to *Corynebacterium pseudodiphtheriticum*, a new challenge in the differential diagnosis of diphtheria. Emerg Infect Dis 1997; 3:65-68.

47. Gutierrez-Rodero F, Ortiz de la Table V, Martinez C, Masia MM, Mora A, Escolano C, Gonzalez E, Martin-Hidalgo A. *Corynebacterium pseudodiphtheriticum*: an easily missed respiratory pathogen in HIV-infected patients. Diagn Microbiol Infect Dis 1999; 33:209-216.

48. Mills A, Mitchell RD, Lim EK. *Corynebacterium pseudotuberculosis* is a cause of human necrotising granulomatous lymphadenitis. Pathology 1997; 29:231-233.

49. Peel MM, Palmer GG, Stacpoole AM, Kerr TG. Human lymphadenitis due to *Corynebacterium pseudotuberculosis*: report of ten cases from Australia and review. Clin Infect Dis 1997; 24:185-191.
50. Funke G, Lawson PA, Collins MD. *Corynebacterium riegelii* sp. nov., an unusual species isolated from female patients with urinary tract infections. J Clin Microbiol 1998; 36:624-627.
51. Wattiau P, Janssens M, Wauters G. *Corynebacterium simulans* sp. nov., a non-lipophilic, fermentative *Corynebacterium*. Int J Syst Bacteriol Evol Microbiol 2000; 50:347-353.
52. Riegel P, Ruimy R, Renaud FN, Freney J, Prevost G, Jehl F, Christen R, Monteil H. *Corynebacterium singulare* sp. nov., a new species for urease-positive strains related to *Corynebacterium minutissimum*. Int J Syst Bacteriol 1997; 47:1092-1096.
53. Watkins DA, Chahine A, Creger RJ, Jacobs MR, Lazarus HM. *Corynebacterium striatum*: a diphtheroid with pathogenic potential. Clin Infect Dis 1993; 17:21-25.
54. Brandenburg AH, van Belkum A, van Pelt C, Bruining HA, Mouton JW, Verbrugh HA. Patient-to-patient spread of a single strain of *Corynebacterium striatum* causing infections in a surgical intensive care unit. J Clin Microbiol 1996; 34:2089-2094.
55. Collins MD, Bernard KA, Hutson RA, Sjoden B, Nyberg A, Falsen E. *Corynebacterium sundsvallense* sp. nov., from human clinical specimens. Int J Syst Bacteriol 1999; 49:361-366.
56. Anonymous. Respiratory diphtheria caused by *Corynebacterium ulcerans* – Terre Haute, Indiana, 1996. MMWR Morb Mort Weekly Rep 1997; 46:330-332.
57. Dessau RB, Brandt-Christensen M, Jensen OJ, Tonnesen P. Pulmonary nodules due to *Corynebacterium ulcerans*. Eur Respir J 1995; 8:651-653.
58. De Carpentier JP, Flanagan PM, Singh IP, Timms MS, Nassar WY. Nasopharyngeal *Corynebacterium ulcerans*: a different diphtheria. J Laryngol Otol 1992; 106:824-826.
59. Pers C. Infection due to "Corynebacterium ulcerans", producing toxin – a case report from Denmark. APMIS [B] 1987; 95:361-362.
60. Morales JM, Aguado JM, Diaz-Gonzalez R, Salto E, Andres A, Campo C, Praga M, Martinez MA, Leiva O, Rodriguez-Noriega A, Rodicio JL. Alkaline-encrusted pyelitis/cystitis and urinary tract infection due to *Corynebacterium urealyticum*: a new severe complication after renal transplantation. Transplant Proc 1992; 24:81-82.
61. Soriano F, Ponte C, Ruiz P, Zapardiel J. Non-urinary tract infections caused by multiply antibiotic-resistant *Corynebacterium urealyticum*. Clin Infect Dis 1993; 17:890-891.
62. Ryan M, Murray PR. Prevalence of *Corynebacterium urealyticum* in urine specimens collected at a university-affiliated medical center. J Clin Microbiol 1994; 32:1395-1396.
63. Nebreda-Mayoral T, Munoz-Bellido JL, Garcia-Rodriguez JA. Incidence and characteristics of urinary tract infections caused by *Corynebacterium urealyticum* (*Corynebacterium* group D2). Eur J Clin Microbiol Infect Dis 1994; 13:600-604.
64. Porschen RK, Goodman Z, Rafai B. Isolation of *Corynebacterium xerosis* from clinical specimens: infection and colonization. Am J Clin Pathol 1977; 68:290-293.
65. Austin GE, Hill EO. Endocarditis due to *Corynebacterium* CDC group G2. J Infect Dis 1983; 147:1106.
66. Lamont RJ, Postlethwaite R, MacGowan AP. *Listeria monocytogenes* and its role in human infection. J Infect 1988; 17:7-28.
67. Albritton WL, Cochi SL, Feeley JC. Overview of neonatal listeriosis. Clin Invest Med 1984; 7:311-314.
68. MacGowan AP, Cartlidge PH, MacLoed F, McLaughlin J. Maternal listeriosis in pregnancy without fetal or neonatal infection. J Infect 1991; 22:53-57.
69. Silver HM. Listeriosis during pregnancy. Obstet Gynecol Surv 1998; 53:737-740.
70. Limaye AP, Perkins JD, Kowdley KV. *Listeria* infection after liver transplantation: report of a case and review of the literature. Am J Gastroenterol 1998; 93:1942-1944.
71. Decker CF, Simon GL, DiGoia RA, Tuazon CU. *Listeria monocytogenes* infections in patients with AIDS: report of five cases and review. Rev Infect Dis 1991; 13:413-417.
72. Mylonakis E, Hohmann EL, Calderwood SB. Central nervous system infection with *Listeria monocytogenes*: 33 years' experience at a general hospital and review of 776 episodes from the literature. Medicine 1998; 77:313-336.
73. Spyrou N, Anderson M, Foale R. *Listeria* endocarditis: current management and patient outcome – world literature review. Heart 1997; 77:380-383.
74. Ellis LC, Segreti J, Gitelis S, Huber JF. Joint infections due to *Listeria monocytogenes*: case report and review. Clin Infect Dis 1995; 20:1548-1550.

75. Lunde NM, Messana JM, Swartz RD. Unusual caused of peritonitis in patients undergoing continuous peritoneal dialysis with emphasis on *Listeria monocytogenes*. J Am Soc Nephrol 1992; 3:1092-1097.

76. Gauto AR, Cone LA, Woodard DR, Mahler RJ, Lynch RD, Stoltzman DH. Arterial infections due to *Listeria monocytogenes*: report of four cases and review of world literature. Clin Infect Dis 1992; 14:23-28.

77. Braun TI, Travis D, Dee RR, Nieman RE. Liver abscess due to *Listeria monocytogenes*: case report and review. Clin Infect Dis 1993; 17:267-269.

78. LaForce FM. Anthrax. Clin Microbiol Infect 1994; 19:1009-1013.

79. Granum PE, Lund T. *Bacillus cereus* and its food poisoning toxins. FEMS Microbiol Lett 1997; 157:223-228.

80. Crane JK. Preformed bacterial toxins. Clin Lab Med 1999; 19:583-599.

81. Tuazon CU, Murray HW, Levy C, Solny MN, Curtin JA, Sheagren JN. Serious infections from *Bacillus* spp. JAMA 1979; 241:1137-1140.

82. Christenson JC, Byington C, Korgenski EK, Adderson EE, Bruggers C, Adams RH, Jenkins E, Hohmann S, Carroll K, Daly JA, Pavia AT. *Bacillus cereus* infections among oncology patients at a children's hospital. Am J Infect Cont 1999; 27:543-546.

83. David DB, Kirkby GR, Noble BA. *Bacillus cereus* endophthalmitis. Br J Ophthalmol 1994; 78:577-580.

84. Damgaard PH, Granum PE, Bresciani J, Torregrossa MV, Eilenberg J, Valentino L. Characterization of *Bacillus thuringiensis* isolated from infections in burn wounds. FEMS Immunol Med Microbiol 1997; 18:47-53.

85. Brook I, Frazier EH. Infections caused by *Propionibacterium* species. Rev Infect Dis 1991; 13:819-822.

86. Everett ED, Eickhoff TC, Simon RH. Cerebrospinal fluid shunt infections with anaerobic diphtheroids (*Propionibacterium* species). J Neurosurg 1976; 44:580-584.

87. Tunney MM, Ptrick S, Curran MD, Ramage G, Hanna D, Nixon JR, Gorman SP, Davis RI, Anderson N. Detection of prothetic hip infection at revision arthroplasty by immunofluorescence microscopy and PCR amplification of the bacterial 16S rRNA gene. J Clin Microbiol 1999; 37:3281-3290.

88. Gaston DA, Zurowski SM. *Arcanobacterium haemolyticum* pharyngitis and exanthem – three case reports and literature review. Arch Dermatol 1996; 132:61-64.

89. Pacual Ramos C, Foster G, Collins MD. Phylogenetic analysis of the genus *Actinomyces* based on 16S rRNA gene sequences: description of *Arcanobacterium phocae* sp. nov., *Arcanobacterium bernardiae* comb. nov., and *Arcanobacterium pyogenes* comb. nov. Int J Syst Bacteriol 1997; 47:46-53.

90. Funke G, Pascual Ramos C, Fernandez-Garayzabal J, Weiss N, Collins MD. Description of human-derived Centers for Disease Control coryneform group 2 bacteria as *Actinomyces bernardiae* sp. nov. Int J Syst Bacteriol 1995; 45:57-60.

91. Reboli AC, Farrar WE. *Erysipelothrix rhusiopathiae*: an occupational pathogen. Clin Microbiol Rev 1989; 2:354-359.

92. Lawson PA, Falsen E, Akervall E, Vandamme P, Collins MD. Characterization of some *Actinomyces*-like isolates from human clinical specimens: reclassification of *Actinomyces suis* (Soltys and Spratling) as *Actinobaculum suis* comb. nov. and description of *Actinobaculum shaalii* sp nov. Int J Syst Bacteriol 1997; 47:899-903.

93. Funke G, von Graevenitz A. Infections due to *Actinomyces neuii* (former CDC coryneform group 1 bacteria). Infection 1995; 23:73-75.

94. Wust J, Stubbs S, Weiss N, Funke G, Collins MD. Assignment of *Actinomyces pyogenes*-like (CDC coryneform group E) bacteria to the genus *Actinomyces* as *Actinomyces radingae* sp. nov. and *Actinomyces turicensis* sp. nov. Lett Appl Microbiol 1995; 20:76-81.

95. Sabbe LJ, Van De Merwe D, Schouls L, Bergmans A, Vaneechoutte M, Vandamme P. Clinical spectrum of infections due to the newly described *Actinomyces* species *A. turicensis*, *A. radingae*, and *A. europaeus*. J Clin Microbiol 1999; 37:8-13.

96. Vandamme P, Falsen E, Vancanneyt M, Van Esbroeck M, Van de Merwe D, Bergmans A, Schouls L, Sabbe L. Characterization of *Actinomyces turicensis* and *Actinomyces radingae* strains from human clinical samples. Int J Syst Bacteriol 1998; 48:503-510.

97. Funke G, Hutson RA, Bernard K, Pfyffer GE, Wauters G, Collins MD. Isolation of *Arthrobacter* spp. from clinical specimens and description of *Arthrobacter cumminsii* sp. nov. and *Arthrobacter woluwensis* sp. nov. J Clin Microbiol 1996; 34:2356-2363.

98. Wauters G, Charlier J, Janssens M, Delmee M. Identification of *Arthrobacter oxydans*, *Arthrobacter luteolus* sp. nov., and *Arthrobacter albus* sp. nov., isolated from human clinical specimens. J Clin Microbiol 2000; 38:2412-2415.

99. Funke G, von Graevenitz A, Weiss N. Primary identification of *Aureobacterium* spp. isolated from clinical specimens as 'Corynebacterium aquaticum'. J Clin Microbiol 1994; 32:2686-2691.

100. Brook I, Frazier EH. Significant recovery of nonsporulating anaerobic rods from clinical specimens. Clin Infect Dis 1993; 16:476-480.
101. Funke G, Carlotti A. Differentiation of *Brevibacterium* spp. encountered in clinical specimens. J Clin Microbiol 1994; 32:1729-1732.
102. Gruner E, Steigerwalt AG, Hollis DG, Weyant RS, Weaver RE, Moss CW, Daneshvar M, Brown JM, Brenner DJ. Human infections caused by *Brevibacterium casei*, formerly CDC grops B-1 and B-3. J Clin Microbiol 1994; 32:1511-1518.
103. Funke G, Pascual Ramos C, Collins MD. Identification of some clinical strains of CDC coryneform group A-3 and group A-4 bacteria as *Cellulomonas* species and proposal of *Cellulomonas hominis* sp. nov. for some group A-3 strains. J Clin Microbiol 1995; 33:2091-2097.
104. Jones D, Collins MD. Taxonomic studies on some human cutaneous coryneform bacteria: description of *Dermabacter hominis* gen. nov, sp. nov. FEMS Microbiol Lett 1988; 51:51-56.
105. Hollis DG, Weaver RE. Gram-Positive Organisms: A Guide to Identification. Atlanta:Centers for Disease Control, 1981.
106. Husni RN, Gordon SM, Washington JA, Longworth DL. *Lactobacillus* bacteremia and endocarditis: review of 45 cases. Clin Infect Dis 1997; 25:1048-1055.
107. Schlegel L, Lemerle S, Geslin P. *Lactobacillus* species as opportunistic pathogens in immunocompromised patients. Eur J Clin Microbiol Infect Dis 1998; 17:887-888.
108. Cooper CD, Vincent A, Greene JN, Sandin RL, Cobian L. *Lactobacillus* bacteremia in febrile neutropenic patients in a cancer hospital. Clin Infect Dis 1998; 26:1247-1248.
109. Evtushenko LI, Dorofeeva LV, Subbotin SA, Cole JR, Tiedje JM. *Leifsonia poae* gen. nov., sp. nov., isolated from nematode galls on *Poa annua*, and reclassification of 'Corynebacterium aquaticum' Leifson 1962 as *Leifsonia aquatica* (ex Leifson 1962) gen. nov., nom. rev., comb. nov. and *Clavibacter xyli* Davis et al. 1984 with two subspecies as *Leifsonia xyli* (Davis et al. 1984) gen nov., comb. nov. Int J Syst Bacteriol Evol Microbiol 2000; 50:371-380.
110. Takeuchi M, Hatano K. Union of the genera *Microbacterium* Orla-Jensen and *Aureobacterium* Collins et al. in a redefined genus *Microbacterium*. Int J Syst Bacteriol 1998; 48:739-747.
111. Funke G, Falsen E, Barreau C. Primary identification of *Microbacterium* spp. encountered in clinical specimens as CDC coryneform group A-4 and A-5 bacteria. J Clin Microbiol 1995; 33:188-192.
112. Rihs JD, McNeil MM, Brown JM, Yu VL. *Oerskovia xanthineolytica* implicated in peritonitis associated with peritoneal dialysis: case report and review of *Oerskovia* infections in humans. J Clin Microbiol 1990; 28:1934-1937.
113. Simonet M, de Briel D, Boucot I, Minck R, Veron M. Coryneform bacteria from the middle ear. J Clin Microbiol 1993; 31:1667-1668.
114. Howe RA, Brown NM, Spencer RC. The new threats of Gram positive pathogens: re-emergence of things past. J Clin Pathol 1996; 49:444-449.
115. Galazka AM, robertson SE, Oblapenko GP. Resurgence of diphtheria. Eur J Epidemiol 1995; 11:95-105.
116. Pearson LJ, Marth EH. *Listeria monocytogenes* – threat to a safe food supply: a review. J Dairy Science 1990; 73:912-928.
117. McGinley KJ, Webster GF, Leyden JJ. Regional variations of cutaneous propionibacteria. Appl Environ Microbiol 1978; 35:62-66.
118. Antonio MA, Hawes SE, Hillier SL. The identification of vaginal *Lactobacillus* species and the demographic and microbiologic characteristics of women colonized by these species. J Infect Dis 1999; 180:1950-1956.
119. Dembele T, Obdrzalek V, Votava M. Inhibition of bacterial pathogens by lactobacilli. Zentrabl Bakteriol 1998; 288:395-401.
120. Kailasapathy K, Chin J. Survival and therapeutic potential of probiotic organisms with reference to *Lactobacillus acidophilus* and *Bifidobacterium* spp. Immunol Cell Biol 2000; 78:80-88.
121. Uchida T. Diphtheria toxin. Pharmacol Ther 1983; 19:107-122.
122. Pallen MJ, Hay AJ, Puckey LH, Efstratiou A. Polymerase chain reaction for screening clinical isolates of corynebacteria for the production of diphtheria toxin. J Clin Pathol 1994; 47:353-356.
123. Pascual C, Lawson PA, Farrow JAE, Navarro Gimenez M, Collins MD. Phylogenetic analysis of the genus *Corynebacterium* based on 16S rRNA gene sequences. Int J Syst Bacteriol 1995; 45:724-728.
124. Riegel P, de Briel D, Prevost G, Jehl F, Monteil H. Genomic diversity among *Corynebacterium jeikeium* strains and comparison with biochemical characteristics and antimicrobial susceptibilities. J Clin Microbiol 1994; 32:1860-1865.

125. Ellis JA, Lairmore MD, O'Toole DT, Campos M. Differential induction of tumour necrosis factor alpha in ovine pulmonary alveolar macrophages following infection with *Corynebacterium pseudotuberculosis*, *Pasteurella haemolytica*, and lentiviruses. Infect Immun 1991; 59:3254-3260.

126. Wong TP, Groman N. Production of diphtheria toxin by selected isolates of *Corynebacterium ulcerans* and *Corynebacterium pseudotuberculosis*. Infect Immun 1984; 43:1114-1116.

127. Soriano F, Ponte C, Galiano MJ. Adherence of *Corynebacterium urealyticum* (CDC group D2) and *Corynebacterium jeikeium* to intravascular and urinary catheters. Eur J Clin Microbiol Infect Dis 1993; 12:453-456.

128. McKellar RC. Use of the CAMP test for identification of *Listeria monocytogenes*. Appl Environ Microbiol 1994; 60:4219-4225.

129. Hiltbold EM, Ziegler HK. Mechanisms of processing and presentation of the antigens of *Listeria monocytogenes*. Infect Agents Dis 1993; 2:314-323.

130. Kuhn M, Pfeuffer T, Greiffenberg L, Goebel W. Host cell transduction during *Listeria monocytogenes* infection. Arch Biochem Biophys 1999; 372:166-172.

131. Chakraborty T. Molecular and cell biological aspects of infection by *Listeria monocytogenes*. Immunobiology 1999; 201:155-163.

132. Rouquette C, Berche P. The pathogenesis of infection by *Listeria monocytogenes*. Microbiologia 1996; 12:245-258.

133. Schwarzkopf A. *Listeria monocytogenes* – aspects of pathogenicity. Pathol Biol 1996; 44:769-774.

134. Hanna P. Anthrax pathogenesis and host response. Curr Top Microbiol Immunol 1998; 225:13-35.

135. Ash C, Farrow JAE, Wallbanks S, Collins MD. Phylogenetic heterogeneity of the genus *Bacillus* revealed by comparative analysis of small-subunit-ribosomal RNA sequences. Lett Appl Microbiol 1991; 13:202-206.

136. Rossler D, Ludwig W, Schleifer KH, Lin C, McGill TJ, Wisotzkey JD, Jurtshuk P, Fox GE. Phylogenetic diversity in the genus *Bacillus* as seen by 16S rRNA sequencing studies. Syst Appl Microbiol 1991; 14:266-269.

137. Leonard C, Zekri O, Mahillon J. Integrated physical and genetic mapping of *Bacillus cereus* and other grampositive bacteria based on the IS231A transposition vectors. Infect Immun 1998; 66:2163-2169.

138. Ash C, Farrow JE, Dorsch M, Stackebrandt E, Collins MD. Comparative analysis of *Bacillus anthracis*, *B. cereus*, and related species on the basis of reverse transcriptase sequencing of the 16S rRNA. Int J Syst Bacteriol 1991; 41:343-346.

139. Iriarte J, Bel Y, Ferrandis MD, Andrew R, Murillo J, Ferre J, Caballero P. Environmental distribution and diversity of *Bacillus thuringiensis* in Spain. Syst Appl Microbiol 1998; 21:97-106.

140. McNamara PJ, Cuevas WA, Songer JG. Toxic phospholipases D of *Corynebacterium pseudotuberculosis*, *C. ulcerans*, and *Arcanobacterium haemolyticum*: cloning and seuqence homology. Gene 1995; 156:113-118.

141. Billington SJ, Jost BH, Cuevas WA, Bright KR, Songer JG. The *Arcanobacterium* (*Actinomyces*) *pyogenes* hemolysin, pyolysin, is a novel member of the thiol-activated cytolysin family. J Bacteriol 1997; 179:6100-6106.

142. Hudak AP, Lee SH, Issekutz AC, Bortolussi R. Comparison of three serological methods – enzyme-linked immunosorbent assay, complement fixation and microagglutination – in the diagnosis of human perinatal *Listeria monocytogenes* infection. Clin Invest Med 1984; 7:349-354.

143. Campbell PA. Macrophage-*Listeria* interactions. Immunol Ser 1994; 60:313-328.

144. Harty JT, Lenz LL, Bevan MJ. Primary and secondary immune responses to *Listeria monocytogenes*. Curr Opin Immunol 1996; 8:526-530.

145. Busch DH, Kerksiek K, Pamer EG. Processing of *Listeria monocytogenes* antigens and the in vivo T-cell response to bacterial infection. Immunol Rev 1999; 172:163-169.

146. Turnbull PC, Doganay M, Lindeque PM, Aygen B, McLaughlin J. Serology and anthrax in humans, livestock and Etosha National Park wildlife. Epidemiol Infect 1992; 108:299-313.

147. Turnbull PC. Anthrax vaccines: past, present, and future. Vaccine 1991; 9:533-539.

148. Nass M. Anthrax vaccine: model of a response to the biologic warfare threat. Infect Dis Clin North Am 1999; 13:187-208.

149. Nyman M, Alugupalli KR, Stromberg S, Forsgren A. Antibody response to *Arcanobacterium haemolyticum* infection. J Infect Dis 1997; 175:1515-1518.

150. Easmon CSF, Clark L, Crane JP, Green R. Phagocytosis and killing of *Gardnerella vaginalis* by human neutrophils. J Clin Pathol 1985; 38:747-749.

151. Tang YW, von Graevenitz A, Waddington MG, Hopkins MK, Smith DH, Li H, Kolbert CP, Montgomery SO, Persing DH. Identification of coryneform bacterial isolates by ribosomal DNA sequence analysis. J Clin Microbiol 2000; 38:1676-1678.

152. Engler KH, Glushkevich T, Mazurova IK, George RC, Efstratiou A. A modified Elek test for detection of toxigenic corynebacteria in the diagnostic laboratory. J Clin Microbiol 1997; 35:495-498.
153. Snell JJS, Demello JV, Gardner PS, Wantes WK, Brooks R. Detection of toxin production by *Corynebacterium diphtheriae*: results of a trial organized as part of the United Kingdom National External Microbiological Quality Assessment Scheme. J Clin Pathol 1984; 37:796-799.
154. Engler KH, Efstratiou A. Rapid enzyme immunoassay for determination of toxigenicity among clinical isolates of corynebacteria. J Clin Microbiol 2000; 38:1385-1389.
155. Hallas G, Harrison TG, Samuel D, Colman G. Detection of diphtheria toxin in culture supernates of *Corynebacterium diphtheriae* and *C. ulcerans* by immunoassay with monoclonal antibody. J Med Microbiol 1990; 32:247-253.
156. Nielsen PB, Koch C, Friss H, Heron I, Prag J, Schmidt J. Double-sandwich enzyme-linked immunosorbent assay for rapid detection of toxin-producing *Corynebacterium diphtheriae*. J Clin Microbiol 1987; 25:1280-1284.
157. Pietrzak J, Muehlestein S, Gasser M. Sandwich-dot immunobinding assay (sandwich-DIA), a new immunological method for the detection of diphtheria toxin. Zentralbl Bakteriol 1990; 274:61-69.
158. Efstratiou A, Engler KH, Dawes CS, Sesardic D. Comparison of phenotypic and genotypic methods for detection of diphtheria toxin among isolates of pathogenic corynebacteria. J Clin Microbiol 1998; 36:3173-3177.
159. Krech T, de Chastonay J, Falsen E. Epidemiology of diphtheria: polypeptide and restriction enzyme analysis in comparison with conventional phage typing. Eur J Clin Microbiol Infect Dis 1988; 7:232-237.
160. Riegel P, Freitas FI, Prevost G, Andronescu C, Bimet F, Kiredjian M, Estrangin E, Emond JP, Dellion S, Halioua B, Monteil, Patey O. Comparison of traditional and molecular methods for typing nontoxigenic strains of *Corynebacterium diphtheriae*. Eur J Clin Microbiol Infect Dis 1997; 16:610-614.
161. Popovic T, Kim C, Reiss J, Reeves M, Nakao H, Golaz A. Use of molecular subtyping to document long-term persistence of *Corynebacterium diphtheriae* in South Dakota. J Clin Microbiol 1999; 37:1092-1099.
162. De Zoysa AS, Efstratiou A. PCR typing of *Corynebacterium diphtheriae* by random amplification of polymorphic DNA. J Med Microbiol 1999; 48:335-340.
163. Gilbert L. Infections with *Corynebacterium diphtheriae* – changing epidemiology and clinical manifestations. Commun Dis Intell 1997; 21:161-164.
164. Lagrou K, Verhaegen J, Janssens M, Wauters G, Verbist L. Prospective study of catalase-positive coryneform organisms in clinical specimens: identification, clinical relevance, and antibiotic susceptibility. Diagn Microbiol Infect Dis 1998; 30:7-15.
165. Williams DY, Selepak ST, Gill VJ. Identification of clinical isolates of nondiphtherial *Corynebacterium* species and their antibiotic susceptibility patterns. Diagn Microbiol Infect Dis 1993; 17:23-28.
166. von Graevenitz A, Funke G. An identification scheme for rapidly and aerobically growing Gram-positive rods. Zentralbl Bakteriol 1996; 284:246-254.
167. Funke G, Renaud FN, Freney J, Riegel P. Multicenter evaluation of the updated and extended API (RAPID) Coryne database 2.0. J Clin Microbiol 1997; 35:3122-3126.
168. Freney J, Duperron MT, Courtier C, Hansen W, Allard F, Boeufgras JM, Monget D, Fleurette J. Evaluation of API Coryne in comparison with conventional methods for identifying coryneform bacteria. J Clin Microbiol 1991; 29:38-41.
169. Soto A, Zapardiel J, Soriano F. Evaluation of API Coryne system for identifying coryneform bacteria. J Clin Pathol 1994; 47:756-759.
170. von Graevenitz A, Punter V, Gruner E, Pfyffer GE, Funke G. Identification of coryneform and other gram-positive rods with several methods. APMIS 1994; 102:381-389.
171. Hudspeth MK, Gerardo SH, Citron DM, Goldstein EJ. Evaluation of the RapID CB Plus system for identification of *Corynebacterium* species and other gram-positive rods. J Clin Microbiol 1998; 36:543-547.
172. Funke G, Peters K, Aravena-Roman M. Evaluation of the RapID CB Plus system for identification of coryneform bacteria and *Listeria* spp. J Clin Microbiol 1998; 36:2439-2442.
173. Lindenmann K, von Graevenitz A, Funke G. Evaluation of the Biolog System for the identification of asporogenous aerobic gram-positive bacilli. Med Microbiol Lett 1995; 4:287-296.
174. Bernard KA, Bellefeuille M, Ewan EP. Cellular fatty acid composition as an adjunct to the identification of asporogenous, aerobic Gram-positive rods. J Clin Microbiol 1991; 29:83-89.
175. Padilha-Goncalves A. A single method to stain *Malassezia furfur* and *Corynebacterium minutissimum* in scales. Rev Inst Med Trop Sao Paulo 1996; 38:299-302.
176. Zapardiel J, Nieto E, Soriano F. Evaluation of a new selective medium for the isolation of *Corynebacterium urealyticum*. J Med Microbiol 1998; 47:79-83.

177. Bjorkroth J, Korkeala H, Funke G. rRNA gene RFLP as an identification tool for *Corynebacterium* spp. Int J Syst Bacteriol 1999; 49:983-989.

178. Ninet B, Bannerman E, Bille J. Assessment of the Accuprobe *Listeria monocytogenes* culture identification reagent kit for rapid colony confirmation and it application in various enrichment broths. Appl Environ Microbiol 1992; 58:4055-4059.

179. Kerr KG, Hawkey PM, Lacey RW. Evaluation of the API Coryne system for identification of *Listeria* species. J Clin Microbiol 1993; 31:749-750.

180. Curtis GD, Lee WH. Culture media and methods for the isolation of *Listeria monocytogenes*. Int J Food Microbiol 1995; 26:1-13.

181. Jaton K, Sahli R, Bille J. Development of polymerase chain reaction assays for detection of *Listeria monocytogenes* in clinical cerebrospinal fluid samples. J Clin Microbiol 1992; 30:1931-1936.

182. Jacquet C, Thierry D, Veit P, Guesdon JL, Rocourt J. Evaluation of an rDNA *Listeria* probe for *Listeria monocytogenes* typing. APMIS 1999; 107:624-630.

183. Jersek B, Gilot P, Gubina M, Klun N, Mehle J, Tcherneva E, Rijpens N, Merman L. Typing of *Listeria monocytogenes* strains by repetitive element sequence-based PCR. J Clin Microbiol 1999; 37:103-109.

184. Kerouanton A, Brisabois A, Denoyers E, Dilasser F, Grout J, Salvat G, Picard B. Comparison of five typing methods for the epidemiological study of *Listeria monocytogenes*. Int J Food Microbiol 1998; 43:61-71.

185. Van der Mee-Marquet N, Loessner M, Audurier A. Evaluation of seven experimental phages for inclusion in the international phage set for the epidemiological typing of *Listeria monocytogenes*. Appl Environ Microbiol 1997; 63:3374-3377.

186. Boerlin P, Boerlin-Petzold F, Bannerman E, Bille J, Jemmi T. Typing *Listeria monocytogenes* isolates from fish products and human listeriosis cases. Appl Environ Microbiol 1997; 63:1338-1343.

187. Schonberg A, Bannerman E, Courtieu AL, Kiss R, McLauchlin J, Shah S, Wilhelms D. Serotyping of 80 strains from the WHO multicentre international typing study of *Listeria monocytogenes*. Int J Food Microbiol 1996; 32:279-287.

188. Harvey J, Gilmour A. Application of multilocus enzyme electrophoresis and restriction fragment length polymorphism analysis to the typing of *Listeria monocytogenes* strains isolated from raw milk, nondairy foods, and clinical and veterinary sources. Appl Environ Microbiol 1994; 60:1547-1553.

189. Allerberger F, Fritschel SJ. Use of automated ribotyping of Austrian *Listeria monocytogenes* isolates to support epidemiological typing. J Microbiol Meth 1999; 35:237-244.

190. Turnbull PCB. Definitive identification of *Bacillus anthracis* – a review. J Appl Microbiol 1999; 87:237-240.

191. Lalitha MK, Thomas MK. Penicillin resistance in *Bacillus anthracis*. Lancet 1997; 349:1522.

192. Logan NA, Carman JA, Melling J, Berkeley RCW. Identification of *Bacillus anthracis* by API tests. J Med Microbiol 1985; 20:75-85.

193. Baillie LW, Jones MN, Turnbull PC, Manchee RJ. Evaluation of the Biolog system for the identification of *Bacillus anthracis*. Lett Appl Microbiol 1995; 20:209-211.

194. van Netten P, Kramer JM. Media for the detection and enumeration of *Bacillus cereus* in foods: a review. Int J Food Microbiol 1992; 17:85-99.

195. Logan NA, Turnbull PCB. *Bacillus* and recently derived genera. Chapter 23. In: Murray PR, Baron EJ, Pfaller MA, Tenover FC, Yolken RH, eds. Manual of Clinical Microbiology. Washington, DC:ASM Press, 1999:357-369.

196. Logan NA, Berkeley RCW. Identification of *Bacillus* strains using the API system. J Gen Microbiol 1984; 130:1871-1882.

197. te Giffel MC, Beumer RR, Klijn N, Wagendorp A, Rombouts FM. Discrimination between *Bacillus cereus* and *Bacillus thuringiensis* using specific DNA probes based on variable regions of 16S rRNA. FEMS Microbiol Lett 1997; 146:47-51.

198. Brousseau R, Saint-Onge A, Prefontaine G, Masson L, Cabana J. Arbitrary primer polymerase chain reaction, a powerful method to identify *Bacillus thuringiensis* serovars and strains. Appl Environ Microbiol 1993; 59:114-119.

199. Carlson CR, Caugant DA, Kolsto AB. Genotypic diversity among *Bacillus cereus* and *Bacillus thuringiensis* strains. Appl Environ Microbiol 1994; 60:1719-1725.

200. Jackson SG, Goodbrand RB, Ahmed R, Kasatiya S. *Bacillus cereus* and *Bacillus thuringiensis* isolated in a gastroenteritis outbreak investigation. Lett Appl Microbiol 1995; 21:103-105.

201. Cummings LA, Wu WK, Larson AM, Gavin SE, Fine JS, Coyle MB. Effects of media, atmosphere, and incubation time on colonial morphology of *Arcanobacterium haemolyticum*. J Clin Microbiol 1993; 31:3223-3226.

202. Wat LL, Fleming CA, Hodge DS, Krishnan C. Selective medium for isolation of *Arcanobacterium haemolyticum* and *Streptococcus pyogenes*. Eur J Clin Microbiol Infect Dis 1991; 10:443-446.

203. Mackenzie A, Fuite LA, Chan FT, King J, Allen U, MacDonald N, Diaz-Mitoma F. Incidence and pathogenicity of *Arcanobacterium haemolyticum* during a 2-year study in Ottawa. Clin Infect Dis 1995; 21:177-181.

204. Gahrn-Hansen B, Frederiksen W. Human infections with *Actinomyces pyogenes* (*Corynebacterium pyogenes*). Diagn Microbiol Infect Dis 1992; 15:349-354.

205. Brander MA, Jousimies-Somer HR. Evaluation of the RapID ANAII and API ZYM systems for identification of *Actinomyces* species from clinical specimens. J Clin Microbiol 1992; 30:3112-3116.

206. Makino SL, Okada Y, Maruyama T, Ishikawa K, Takahashi T, Nakamura M, Ezaki T, Morita. Direct and rapid detection of *Erysipelothrix rhusiopathiae* DNA in animals by PCR. J Clin Microbiol 1994; 32:1526-1531.

207. Spiegel CA. Diagnosis of bacterial vaginosis by direct Gram stain of vaginal fluid. J Clin Microbiol 1983; 18:170-177.

208. Nugent RP, Krohn MA, Hillier SL. Reliability of diagnosing bacterial vaginosis is improved by a standardized method of Gram stain interpretation. J Clin Microbiol 1991; 29:297-301.

209. Miller LW, Bickham S, Jones WL, Heather CD, Morris RH. Diphtheria carriers and the effect of erythromycin therapy. Antimicrob Agents Chemother 1974; 6:166-169.

210. Zamiri I, McEntegart MG. The sensitivity of diphtheria bacilli to eight antibiotics. J Clin Pathol 1972; 25:716-717.

211. Maple PA, Efstratiou A, Tseneva G, Rikushin Y, Dshevoi S, Jahkola M, Vuopio-Varkila J, George RC. The in vitro susceptibilities of toxigenic *Corynebacterium diphtheriae* isolated in northwestern Russia and surrounding areas to ten antibiotics. J Antimicrob Chemother 1994; 34:1037-1400.

212. Serwold-David TM, Groman NB. Mapping and cloning of *Corynebacterium diphtheriae* plasmid pNG2 and characterization of its relatedness to plasmids from skin coryneforms. Antimicrob Agents Chemother 1986; 30:69-72.

213. Zapardiel J, Nieto E, Gegundez MI, Gadea I, Soriano F. Problems in minimum inhibitory concentration determinations in coryneform organisms: comparison of an agar dilution and the Etest. Diagn Microbiol Infect Dis 1994; 19:171-173.

214. Weiss K, Laverdiere M, Rivest R. Comparison of antimicrobial susceptibilities for *Corynebacterium* species by broth microdilution and disk diffusion methods. Antimicrob Agents Chemother 1996; 40:930-933.

215. Traub WH, Geipel U, Leonhard B, Bauer D. Antibiotic susceptibility testing (agar disk diffusion and agar dilution) of clinical isolates of *Corynebacterium jeikeium*. Chemotherapy 1998; 44:230-237.

216. Garcia-Bravo M, Aguado JM, Morales JM, Noriega AR. Influence of external factors in resistance of *Corynebacterium urealyticum* to antimicrobial agents. Antimicrob Agents Chemother 1996; 40:497-499.

217. Martinez-Martinez L, Suarez AI, Winstanley J, Ortega MC, Bernard K. Phenotypic characteristics of 31 strains of *Corynebacterium striatum* isolated from clinical samples. J Clin Microbiol 1995; 33:2458-2461.

218. Martinez-Martinez L, Pascual A, Bernard K, Suarez AI. Antimicrobial susceptibility pattern of *Corynebacterium striatum*. Antimicrob Agents Chemother 1996; 40:2671-2672.

219. Soriano F, Zapardiel J, Nieto E. Antimicrobial susceptibilities of *Corynebacterium* species and other non-spore-forming gram-positive bacilli to 18 antimicrobial agents. Antimicrob Agents Chemother 1995; 39:208-214.

220. Funke G, Punter V, von Graevenitz A. Antimicrobial susceptibility patterns of some recently defined coryneform bacteria. Antimicrob Agents Chemother 1996; 40:2874-2878.

221. Judson R, Songer JG. *Corynebacterium pseudotuberculosis*: in vitro susceptibility of 39 antimicrobial agents. Vet Microbiol 1991; 27:145-150.

222. Garcia-Rodriguez JA, Garcia-Sanchez J, Munoz-Bellido JL, Nebreda-Mayoral T, Garcia-Sanchez E, Garcia-Garcia M. In vitro activity of 79 antimicrobial agents against *Corynebacterium* group D2. Antimicrob Agents Chemother 1991; 35:2140-2143.

223. Jones EM, MacGowan AP. Antimicrobial chemotherapy of human infection due to *Listeria monocytogenes*. Eur J Clin Microbiol Infect Dis 1995; 14:165-175.

224. Hof H, Nichterlein T, Kretschmar M. Management of listeriosis. Clin Microbiol Rev 1997; 10:345-357.

225. McLauchlin J, Audurier A, Taylor AG. Treatment failure and recurrent human listeriosis. J Antimicrob Chemother 1991; 27:851-857.

226. Charpentier E, Courvalin P. Antibiotic resistance in *Listeria* spp. Antimicrob Agents Chemother 1999; 43:2103-2108.

227. Doganay M, Aydin N. Antimicrobial susceptibility of *Bacillus anthracis*. Scand J Infect Dis 1991; 23:333-335.

228. Weber DJ, Saviteer SM, Rutala WA, Thomann CA. In vitro susceptibility of *Bacillus* spp. to selected antimicrobial agents. Antimicrob Agents Chemother 1988; 32:642-645.

229. Denys GA, Jerris RC, Swenson JM, Thornsberry C. Susceptibility of *Propionibacterium acnes* clinical isolates to 22 antimicrobial agents. Antimicro Agents Chemother 1983; 23:335-337.

230. Carlson P, Kontainen S, Renkonen OV. Antimicrobial susceptibility of *Arcanobacterium haemolyticum*. Antimicrob Agents Chemother 1994; 38:142-143.

231. Carlson P, Korpela J, Walder M, Nyman M. Antimicrobial susceptibilities and biotypes of *Arcanobacterium haemolyticum* blood isolates. Eur J Clin Microbiol Infect Dis 1999; 18:915-917.

232. Osterlund A. Are penicillin treatment failures in *Arcanobacterium haemolyticum* pharyngotonsillitis caused by intracellularly residing bacteria? Scand J Infect Dis 1995; 27:131-134.

14

Mycobacteria and Actinomycetes

Nevio Cimolai
Children's and Women's Health Centre of British Columbia, Vancouver, British Columbia, Canada

William A. Black
Department of Pathology and Laboratory Medicine, University of British Columbia, Vancouver, British Columbia, Canada

Adalbert Laszlo
IUATLD/WHO Consultant on Tuberculosis Bacteriology, Nepean, Ontario, Canada

I. HISTORICAL BACKGROUND

Tuberculosis and leprosy are the most important illnesses that are associated with this group of organisms. The human impact of these has been significant throughout recorded history (1-7), and the classical descriptions of these diseases preceded the recognition of their bacterial etiology by centuries. Unique clinical presentations led to classic descriptions of disease (e.g., consumption) well before the time that the actual bacterial causes were defined by laboratory methods.

Although the majority of historical descriptions will undoubtedly focus on *Mycobacterium tuberculosis* among this large group of micro-organisms, there are several commonalities which broadly apply. With few exceptions, the clinical illnesses that are associated with these bacteria are subacute or chronic. Along with the slow process of disease progression, the immune responses are relatively unique in that there is more often a striking dominance of cell-mediated immune activation and thereafter some histopathological similarity in the affected tissue. Although the number of existing or chronic tuberculosis and leprosy infections are many on a world-wide basis, the absolute number of newly-acquired illnesses is considerably less when compared to other common infectious diseases such as respiratory viral infections. Nevertheless, tuberculosis is among the major infectious causes of mortality. Both the chronicity of illness and the lesser frequency of disease have often resulted in an inadequate level of awareness when clinical differential diagnoses are made. Technically, both mycobacteria and actinomycetes have been regarded as difficult bacteria to work with, in large part as a consequence of slow growth, specialized medium requirements, lack of experience in dealing with these bacteria by most laboratories, unique physical attributes, and unique antimicrobial susceptibility.

Whereas one must consider that the relevant history for this group of bacteria spans centuries, an accentuated recent history has led to a considerable renaissance of interest. This more recent enthusiasm has occurred essentially over the last two decades and is mostly attributable to two factors. Firstly, the degree of compromised immunity for patients has considerably increased despite gains in pharmacology. In particular, the "AIDS era" and the number of patients who become immune compromised as a consequence of transplantation and immunosupressive therapy has increased. Therefore, we have a new and increasing pool of susceptible patients, and the potential to deal with a patient who suffers from an active infection has increased proportionately. Secondly, scientific advances, especially in the field of molecular biology, have given us tools that have the potential to overcome the limitations that could not previously be approached.

Among the actinomycetes, most recent significant gains focus on the application of microbial genetics and speciation. The accurate differentiation of these slower growing bacteria can be accomplished by molecular techniques that may require less time than traditional methods which are otherwise phenotypically based. A case in point must certainly be that of *Tropheryma whippelii* (the cause of Whipple's disease), genetically an actinomycete whose detection was accomplished with new molecular diagnostic techniques in a context where the bacterium cannot yet be reliably cultivated (8).

Among mycobacteria other than *M. tuberculosis* (non-tuberculous mycobacteria; NTM), much of the important history relates to events in recent times that will prove to have revolutionized the field. In recent years, new diseases have become apparent which are related to the increasing number of immunocompromised hosts if not the enhanced intensity of medical interventions. Several new mycobacterial species have been defined; many of these were recognized to be closely related by conventional identification methods. Automation and the trend towards rapid diagnosis has increased the potential to find these bacteria in clinical samples including blood. Again, new genetic technologies have increased the potential to speciate and fingerprint NTM where cumbersome or no such technology previously existed.

Given the frequency and severity of tuberculosis, considerable effort has focused on diagnosis and epidemiology, and the timely gains in this area are unprecedented. Table 1 details some key items of historical importance in these regards.

Just as the recent history has witnessed major changes in the field, the imminent future will feel the impact of these very useful technologies. Predictably, new diagnostic assays will be focused on enhancing the sensitivity and reliability of diagnosis and will benefit patient care by providing a diagnosis

Table 1 Key events in the recent history of tuberculosis.

A.	WHO declares tuberculosis a global emergency.
B.	The AIDS epidemic complicates tuberculosis control.
C.	Short course antituberculous therapy is a viable option for many patients.
D.	Automation for diagnosis is developed (especially with the liquid culture) and decreases culture time.
E.	Direct probe technologies facilitate rapid speciation of automated or other growths, both for *M. tuberculosis* and some NTM.
F.	Multi-resistant *M. tuberculosis* becomes a more prominent menace.
G.	Rapid diagnosis is facilitated with the advent of genetic amplification techniques (e.g., PCR, LCR).
H.	Molecular typing methods enhance epidemiological studies.
I.	Automation for susceptibility testing of mycobacteria becomes available.
J.	Molecular methods become available to determine mycobacterial drug resistance but implementation awaits further study.
K.	CDC/Dept of Health and Human Services' Advisory Committee for Elimination of Tuberculosis state intent to eradicate tuberculosis in the U.S. by 2010.
L.	WHO and IUATLD adopt DOTS strategem for tuberculosis control.

in a reasonably short period of time. As competition in the commercialization of advanced technologies proceeds, cost will likely be altered, and paradigms of cost-effective performance and utilization will emerge. Nevertheless, the availability of such laboratory supports will only be of value to the extent that they may be rationally used in a context where awareness and public health containment are equally fostered. For many western countries, the incidence of tuberculosis continued to decline until the 1980s when a resurgence emerged. A decline in control programs, coupled with the presence of patients (e.g., with AIDS) who failed to respond more typically, led to a resurgence in the subsequent years (9). Our ability to cope with this resurgence and with the international tuberculosis crises can only be a function of our ingenuity or lack thereof given the advanced resources which have and are to evolve.

II. CLINICAL ASPECTS

A. Tuberculosis

Tuberculosis is predominantly an infection of the lower respiratory system, but the potential for systemic complications is considerable. Essentially every body system or organ may directly suffer from disease. From a general perspective, tuberculosis must be viewed as the potential 'great pretender' (analogous to the clinical diagnostic difficulty which was historically seen with syphilis) in that the clinical presentation often mimics other illnesses whether infectious or not. Concern for infection must therefore be maintained in contexts where the illness is cryptic and even more so in areas where tuberculosis is endemic. The inapparent onset of infection along with the chronicity of disease are in a large part responsible for the latter. As well, it is possible for the causative agent to remain relatively dormant and to be contained by the immune system until a later date. Tuberculosis may present in classical fashion within the respiratory tract, but a vast literature exists to detail the many atypical clinical forms. Although systemic illness will often be accompanied by evidence of disease in the lungs, it must also be acknowledged that isolated foci of extra-pulmonary infection do occur and may pose as the first evidence that a patient has tuberculosis. Disease of the lung may be primary or secondary. The latter, classically attributed almost exclusively to reactivation of primary disease, has been recently recognized as due to exogenous reinfection in a proportion of cases, particularly in HIV/AIDS patients or high prevalence areas.

1. Primary pulmonary tuberculosis

Primary tuberculosis can occur at all ages. Primary disease may lead to clinical manifestations as early as two weeks after contact, but the recognition of primary disease most often will vary over four to twelve weeks. Apart from the clinical manifestations that will arise as a consequence of the direct lung disease, constitutional symptoms may include fever, weight loss, and a number of non-specific symptoms.

The initial focus for infection is most often solitary although several areas of the lung may be simultaneously infected. Any area of the lung may be involved as the initial site of infection but certain findings may be more common at different ages. In children, it is not uncommon to see a pulmonary parenchymal infiltrate of the mid- or lower lung along with enlarged lymph nodes of the pulmonary hila. The enlarged lymph nodes in the chest are those directly draining the lung tissue that is involved. As age of the patient increases, hilar node involvement is less likely, and the upper lobes of the lung are more often involved. In the elderly, lower lobe involvement again becomes more common. The diseased lung may progress to cavitation and appear as a pulmonary nodule. As the disease is either healed or continues, other events take place that lead to the clinical manifestations. For example, healing and organization of the active infection may leave a residual pulmonary nodule with or without calcification. In the circumstance when infection extends beyond the original boundaries, the pleural space may become involved. Symptoms can arise as the infectious process spills into an airway or causes parenchymal collapse and/or airway compromise. Sputum production, its character, and its association with blood are variable. Spontaneous resolution may occur, or the disease may continue to spread locally or via the blood route to other organs. Spread within the lung can occur secondarily while the initial focus continues or resolves. Unfortunately, any such disease may occur in the absence of patient complaints. Rapidity of progression is variable but is favoured in young children, patients with compromised immunity (especially those with HIV infection), and those with complicating medical circumstances otherwise. Varied degrees of healing can occur either spontaneously or after the use of antituberculous chemotherapy, and viable tuberculous bacilli may remain although the disease is seemingly quiescent.

Outside of the lung parenchyma and pleural space, disease may occur in the endobronchial tissue and larynx.

2.   Secondary pulmonary tuberculosis

The reactivation of tuberculosis many years after the primary infection can occur in all parts of the lung, but the classical area for this to occur is the upper lobes, usually unilaterally. A local area of pneumonitis initiates this process and the time for reactivation is quite variable. Local parenchymal disease, partial healing and scarring, and cavitation are all possible. Reactivation may then lead to further spread to other areas with primary disease occurring as a consequence. This progression can occur in a matter of weeks to months. The occurrence of a reactivation is influenced by a number of variables, but underlying medical illnesses, especially those which modify host cell-mediated immunity, are particularly influential. Again, it is now recognized that a sizeable proportion of presumed reactivations are actually re-infections.

3.   Tuberculosis and AIDS

Both primary and secondary pulmonary tuberculosis can occur in this specific patient group. The manifestations of either form are greatly affected by the degree of immunosuppression. When disease is advanced, however, there is a high probabilility that secondary disease will occur elsewhere in the body. As well, tuberculosis can progress quickly and is less likely to become dormant; this has tremendous public health implications since spread is facilitated, and it serves as a reminder that improved timeliness for diagnosis is a necessity rather than a luxury. Whereas secondary tuberculosis occurs in about 10% of patients over a lifetime, there is a 10% per annum frequency among untreated HIV-infected patients.

4.   Extra-pulmonary tuberculosis

The potential for spread outside of the pulmonary system is facilitated by the presence of nearby vital anatomic structures and by the possibilities that the bacterium may be mobilized by a variety of routes. Spread to contiguous organs such as pericardium or pleural space can occur by direct extension since the organ boundaries do not provide sufficient barrier to the disease process. Migration of the bacterium within the lung via respiratory airways to the mouth and gastrointestinal tract provide opportunity for other foci of direct infection. Blood-borne transfer to any other organ system will result in renal, central nervous system, and bone infections among others. Spread may also occur along lymphatic channels.

Miliary tuberculosis refers to progressive bloodborne spread to varied organs. Of interest, such spread, and subsequent disease, may return to the lung where the pattern of involvement is now much more diffuse rather than focal.

Table 2 outlines potential sites of systemic tuberculosis. The clinical manifestations are quite variable and have at times mimicked tumours, other infections, benign growths, and other systemic diseases. Clinical suspicion is critical when other evidence of tuberculosis, especially co-existent in the respiratory tract, is not apparent. Indeed the clinical manifestations may be protean.

Table 2   Extra-pulmonary sites for tuberculosis.

Central Nervous System
  cortical
  meningeal
  ophthalmic
	Cutaneous
	
	Gastrointestinal
	  esophageal
	  small intestinal

Genitourinary
  renal
  male genital (e.g., prostatic)
  female genital (e.g., ovarian, endometrial)
  cervical
	large intestinal
	  biliary
	
	Lymphatic
	  mesenteric

Skeletal
  discitis
  skull
  joint
  vertebral (Pott's disease)
  peripheral bone
	supraclavicular
	  retroperitoneal
	
	Thoracic
	  pericardial
	  pleural space

Upper Respiratory
  otitic
	thoracic fistulae
	  mediastinal

Vascular	**Visceral**
	  hepatic
	  splenic
	  pancreatic
	  adrenal
	  peritoneal
	  paravertebral

B. Leprosy

Leprosy has been historically regarded as a disfiguring and unrelenting illness, but the advent of effective antimicrobial treatment has significantly changed the outlook for patients and has also contributed to a better understanding of disease.

The manifestations of clinical disease span a spectrum between two poles. On one hand, patients may have a limited and well-defined involvement of skin. The skin changes may be hypopigmented and are often associated with reduced sensation. These lesions occur directly as a result of the local infection by *M. leprae*. Nerve involvement and thereafter dysfunction may occur. At the other extreme, which is more infectious, the leprosy bacilli are widespread and in large numbers in the skin, and lead to a prominent papular thickening and nodule formation. Areas of the skin that have lower temperature, such as the earlobes, are more likely to be diseased, and ultimately the degree of skin involvement may appear grotesque in its worst form. As a consequence of local invasion and as a function also of peripheral nerve tropism, superficial and deep nerves are progressively affected, and may therefore markedly affect limb function and subsequent appearance. The combination of skin and neural affliction is responsible for the clinical outcome of 'Hansen's Disease'. The nasal passages may also be affected, and shedding of bacilli from this site is important for secondary transmission. These extremes of disease are respectively known as tuberculoid leprosy and lepromatous leprosy, and their manifestations are a function of the form of immune response and its balance with the nature of microbial invasion. Whereas an understanding of these extremes is useful to clarify pathogenesis, in reality most patients have an illness that is somewhat intermediate (borderline leprosy) and again, this will change as the balance between infection and immune response shifts.

Apart from the involvement of large peripheral nerves, most patients will not have any overt evidence of any major organ involvement although bloodborne spread is quite possible in lepromatous disease.

C. NTM

There are many mycobacteria other than *M. tuberculosis* and *M. leprae* which are capable of causing human infection. Many of these bacteria have been described only within the last two decades and indeed some only within the last few years. Table 3 lists a representative number of these and their associated illnesses. As many of the listed illnesses and subsequent mycobacterial isolations are somewhat uncommon, a few relevant examples are highlighted.

Given the complexity among this broad bacterial group, there proves to be a wide variety of clinical illnesses that are possible. These have become even more so varied due to the increasing complexity of medical illnesses and their treatments. Indeed some mycobacteria have been newly identified in large part as a consequence of the contemporary AIDS epidemic. It is likely that more NTM will be identified within the next decade, and these will likely be obtained from illnesses of immunocompromised hosts. New molecular technologies have expanded our understanding of the heterogeneity among the NTM. Where close relationships between current species were likely to have been present, differentiation was historically limited by the reliance on phenotypic assays, many of which were difficult to implement. Current genetic techniques are much more likely to define species although this application should be viewed with some temporary reservation as gold standards are re-established. Hence, it is conceivable that many newly described species (and the description of their associated clinical illnesses) would have been unavoidably merged into the more common species that were known at the time. Whereas the individual NTM may be categorized on the basis of laboratory criteria, the commonalities among the clinical illnesses cross any such division. The more common of clinical illnesses include respiratory infections, cervical lymphadenitis, cutaneous infections, widespread systemic disease, and infection after surgical procedures.

Several mycobacteria other than *M. tuberculosis* are capable of causing a respiratory illness that is clinically indistinguishable from classical tuberculosis, e.g., *M. bovis* (12), *M. africanum* (14), and *M. kansasii*. This is perhaps not surprising for *M. bovis* and *M. africanum* since they closely resemble *M. tuberculosis* and have been categorized as members of the '*M. tuberculosis* complex' and not NTM. More common, however, is the association of varied NTM with chronic infection of the previously diseased lung (37). Essentially in the latter context, these mycobacteria prove to be opportunists. The disease presentations are variable, and there is not uncommonly some difficulty in definitively proving a cause-and-effect relationship. Patients with chronic illness such a cystic fibrosis, cancer of the lung, chronic obstructive pulmonary disease otherwise, and other mechanical problems within the airways are especially at risk. Impaired immunity is another major factor which facilitates such chronic infection of lung. As detailed in Table 3, a majority of NTM have at some time been associated with chronic pulmonary disease, but *M. avium*, *M. intracellulare*, *M. fortuitum*, *M. kansasii*, *M. malmoense*, and *M. xenopi* are among the most common.

Chronic lymphadenitis, particularly of the neck and among children, has historically been associated with varied NTM although *M. tuberculosis* may be the major cause among some populations in particular geographic regions, e.g., aboriginal people in British Columbia, Canada. Usually these lesions are unilateral and may be accompanied by pain and swelling, although patients are less commonly febrile or unwell otherwise. Although most of these are self-limiting, very large swellings or those which do not resolve over many weeks may be directed for further investigation. *M. avium*, *M. intracellulare*, *M. kansasii*, *M. malmoense*, and *M. scrofulaceum* are common among the mycobacteria from these lesions.

Cutaneous infection usually occurs by direct inoculation. A variation of ulcers and nodules are usually found at a well confined site. *M. marinum*, *M. haemophilum*, *M. ulcerans*, and *M. kansasii* are high on the list of mycobacterial causes. It is less common to have cutaneous invasion as a consequence of a systemic illness.

Systemic illnesses (i.e., bloodborne with or without dissemination to limited or multiple organs) with NTM have been documented for many decades, but the last twenty years has particularly been a time when such infections have increased in numbers. The AIDS era, greater medical intervention with

Table 3   NTM that are associated with human disease.

Mycobacterium	Illnesses	Special features	Reference
M. abscessus	pulmonary, cutaneous, post-surgical, systemic	rapid grower, more acute illness, potential contaminant	10
M. asiaticum	pulmonary		11
M. avium	pulmonary, systemic in immunocompromised, lymphadenitis, cutaneous, many other rare	especially in AIDS	13
M. branderi	pulmonary	newly described	15
M. celatum	respiratory, infections in immunocompromised	newly described	16
M. chelonae	pulmonary, cutaneous, post-surgical, systemic	rapid grower, more acute illness, potential contaminant	10
M. conspicuum	infection in immunocompromised	newly described	17
M. fortuitum	pulmonary, cutaneous, post-surgical, systemic	rapid grower, more acute illness, potential contaminant	10
M. gastri	varied		
M. genavense	systemic in immunocompromised	requires prolonged incubation in liquid media	18
M. gordonae	pulmonary, rarely systemic	usually non-pathogen, often contaminant	19
M. haemophilum	mainly lymphocutaneous, rarely systemic	unique hemin	20
M. heidelbergense	lymphadenitis	newly described	36
M. interjectum	lymphadenitis, pulmonary	newly described	21
M. intracellulare	pulmonary, systemic, lymphadenitis, cutaneous	especiallly in AIDS	13
M. kansasii	chronic lung, lymphadenitis , cutaneous, systemic in immunocompromised	rare in children	22
M. lentiflavum	respiratory	newly described	23
M. malmoense	pulmonary, lymphadenitis, cutaneous	occasionally systemic, especially from Europe	24
M. marinum	lymphocutaneous, arthropathy	water-associated, "swimming pool" granuloma	25
M. mucogenicum	post-trauma or surgical	rapid grower, most likely contaminant	26
M. scrofulaceum	lymphadenitis, pulmonary	rarely disseminated	27
M. shimoidei	pulmonary		28
M. simiae	pulmonary	rare systemic	29
M. smegmatis	soft tissue/bone	usually non-pathogen, often contaminant	30
M. szulgai	pulmonary		31
M. terrae	pulmonary, tenosynovitis	mainly contaminant	32
M. triplex	pulmonary, lymphadenitis	newly described	33

Table 3 cont'd.

Mycobacterium	Illnesses	Special features	Reference
M. ulcerans	cutaneous	chronic skin ulcers, geography dependent	34
M. xenopi	pulmonary	rare systemic	35

the outcome of greater host susceptibility, and newer diagnostic technologies have all contributed to this growth. Symptoms among these patients tend to be non-specific and may include fever, weight loss, night sweats, and cachexia, with or without associated pulmonary disease. The pulmonary component here is more likely to be secondary to bloodborne spread rather than primary lung infection with secondary systemic disease. Progression of the disease will lead to manifestations which are indicative of seeding to liver, spleen, bone marrow, gastrointestinal tract, among most other areas. Given the non-specificity of symptoms and given the variability of tissue involvement, the clinician must retain a high index of suspicion to search for NTM causes of systemic disease, especially among HIV-infected patients and those with severe immunosuppression (38). Many NTM have at some time been found in deep tissue including blood, but *M. avium* and *M. intracellulare* are particularly notable here especially among AIDS patients (39). For the latter, the likelihood of systemic illness is particularly a function of the degree of disease progression; this can be determined with some degree of confidence solely by the examination of CD4 lymphocyte count suppression.

Focal areas of infection can arise as a consequence of medical procedures, especially those that are related to the surgical implantation of foreign objects. Wound infections after surgical procedures must also be considered in those where conventional pyogenic bacteria are not found.

Given the ubiquity of many NTM among environmental sources, especially potable water, it follows that they may be easily found in clinical specimens as a consequence of contamination. The finding of these bacteria must carry with it some reservation about whether the underlying illness is truly mycobacterial. This is particularly true when particular bacteria such as *M. gordonae* and *M. smegmatis* are found, and when the isolation has been made from a specimen that originates from a site where a non-pathogen may reside, e.g., mouth or gastrointestinal tract where the bacterium has been obtained from food or water.

D. Actinomycetes

In general, actinomycetes are slow growing bacteria, and like mycobacteria, are therefore more likely to be associated with subacute or chronic illness (40). Infections are more likely to occur among immuno-compromised hosts, but the ubiquity of these bacteria in the environment also makes it more possible for infections of the skin to occur especially in dependent areas of the body. On a proportionate basis, these bacterial infections are much less common than those of more typical pyogenic organisms. Systemic or cutaneous disease is not uncommonly misconstrued initially for a fungal illness.

1. Nocardiosis

Most human illness is caused by *N. asteroides*, but there are no specific clinical presentations which rule out other species (41). In immunocompetent patients, the disease course is protracted; it may resolve without therapy but is capable of recurring. In the immunocompromised host, there is a greater opportunity for acute widespread dissemination. Transplantation is a major risk factor (42).

Most nocardioses are in the lung (43). The pulmonary disease can be quite variable and in many ways as variable as the presentation of pulmonary tuberculosis. Most often the illness appears as cavitary disease with or without major parenchymal involvement. Varied local complications are possible. The pulmonary illness is most often relatively localized, but may also secondarily seed to blood and hence other organs; the potential for the latter to happen will depend on the status of the host. Cutaneous and soft tissue infection most commonly results as a consequence of direct inoculation. Sinus tracts may form within the latter. Chronic infections of the feet (mycetomas) can occur in dependent areas. Central nervous system disease usually occurs as an apparent brain abscess, and there is usually concomitant pulmonary disease. Many other body sites may be involved after bacteremia (44), and nocardiae must now be considered as important pathogens in AIDS (45).

2.   *Rhodococcus*

Rhodococci mainly cause infection in compromised hosts, and again most infections are relatively subacute (46,47). Infection, especially among HIV-infected individuals (48), is likely to occur in the lung where it typically presents as cavitary disease. Isolation from blood-borne illness has also occurred among those with indwelling intravenous lines and again in the context of immunocompromise.

3.   *Other*

Actinomycetes are very common in the environment, and humans must necessarily encounter a large spectrum of species. Only the following however are of noteworthy consequence:

Actinomadura madurae
Causative of mycetomas of the feet especially in tropical areas (49).

Amycolata spp.
Rarely invasive.

Dermatophilus congolensis
A zoonosis that mainly affects skin (50). Dermatophilosis is rare but acquired during superficial contact with animals who are also infected.

Gordona terrae
Rarely seen as a pathogen of lung or skin.

Rothia spp.
Usually oral commensals, they are not uncommonly isolated from specimens from the upper respiratory tract. Infection may be local and there are rare citations of invasive illness.

Streptomyces spp.
Causes of mycetomas; rarely bloodborne systemic pathogens.

Thermophilic actinomycetes
Not a cause of infection per se, but rather associated with hypersensitivity pneumonitis which occurs after inhalation of the bacteria in dust or other aerosols.

III. EPIDEMIOLOGY OF INFECTION

A. *M. tuberculosis*

Humans are the only major vector for tuberculosis. On a numbers basis, tuberculosis is by far the commonest cause of death that can be attributed to an infectious agent. Many of the deaths, and most of the disease, occur in areas of the world where diagnosis and treatment continue to be a problem.

The bacterium is airborne and much transmission necessarily occurs as a result of respiratory transmission from infected individuals. The frequency of secondary transmission will depend on the intensity of infection (i.e., more infectious with more respiratory disease and bacterial shedding) and the duration of exposure. Whereas highly infectious individuals are those whose respiratory smears are positive for the causative agent, transmission can occur from a smear-negative patient. After contact, there is usually an incubation period of several weeks to months prior to the development of infection as measured by a positive tuberculin skin test which denotes reactive cell-mediated immunity. Clinical disease, however, may require many more weeks or months to present. Latent infection may be reactivated years if not decades later. This silent reservoir is at this time indeterminable for any given individual and remains an important obstacle to overcome in future diagnostic endeavours.

The resurgence of tuberculosis in recent years is in substantial part attributable to the HIV epidemic. HIV-positive status is a major risk factor for flagrant clinical tuberculosis after initial acquisition, and such status is also associated with greater opportunity of reactivation, more rapid decompensation, and greater bacterial burden. Nevertheless, there are several factors which will also continue to promote the infection world-wide. Travel and immigration have facilitated movement of the patient, and hence disease, to a degree unprecedented in the history of the human race. Countries with limited resources to combat spread have high endemicity and little in the way of positive outlook for control; these are the same countries where the risk of explosive HIV outbreaks is high. In westernized countries, there is some complacency due to the availability of antituberculosis chemotherapy and the earlier trend towards control. Large urban centres have promoted homelessness, drug use, overcrowding, and lack of medical care. The reservoir for tuberculosis is therefore likely to continue throughout the world, regardless of how developed any country may pose itself to be. These dilemmae are exceedingly relevant to new diagnostic technologies in that the incredible potential gain in science, and thereafter laboratory medicine, may be greatly impeded in its application to truly impact on the disease in regions where such impact is likely to make considerable difference. On a global basis, the continuation of tuberculosis in major endemic areas is everyone's problem.

The emergence of drug resistance in tuberculosis is of great concern. Antituberculous therapy is complicated by the long duration of required treatment, the higher frequency of toxicity per agent, and the difficulty in achieving effective cure at some difficult sites. Multi-drug resistance must be curtailed if possible. Incomplete treatments, partial compliance, and disease in severely compromised patients all may contribute to both treatment failure and the potential for drug resistance to emerge. It must also be recognized that treatment per se will complicate the utilization of diagnostic testing especially when newer techniques may rely on detection where viability is not appreciable.

B. Leprosy

Humans are a major source for leprosy, but theories of transmission have evolved somewhat. Direct contact with an infected individual was maintained historically as the major if not only mode for transmission. The recognition of major nasal carriage/infection in some patients has led to consideration for aerosol transmission, and a role for the nearby environment cannot be ruled out.

Patients with lepromatous leprosy shed more bacterium as a consequence of the much greater bacterial burden, but overall, the infectiousness of leprosy is not as great as was historically portrayed.

Infection is most common is regions of Africa, Asia, and Latin America; disease predominates in rural rather than urban areas. The incubation period after contact is measured in many years, i.e., 4-7 years. Again, the detection of latent infection during this time continues to pose a challenge for modern diagnostics.

C.   NTM and Actinomycetes

The epidemiology of infection with these two broad groups is quite similar with few exceptions. These bacteria are common in the environment, and they are especially common in soil and water (and hence food). As a consequence of this ubiquity, they are very commonly encountered, and it is surprising that more frequent infection is not diagnosed. Both groups are relative opportunists, and they infect patients whose immunity or anatomy are compromised. Nosocomial acquisition is quite possible given that potable water sources may be easily seeded with NTM. The AIDS epidemic has quickly created a new group of high risk patients during a time when immunosuppression has relatively lessened with advances in transplantation and the availability of cyclosporin and similar agents. Zoonotic potential for transmission is present for some examples.

Although the above generalizations hold for most representatives of these groups, notable exceptions include: animal source – *M. simiae*, occasionally *M. kansasii*, occasionally *M. fortuitum* and *chelonae*, occasionally *M. avium* and *intracellulare*, and *D. congolensis*; waterborne – *M. marinum*; normal mouth flora – *Rothia* spp. and *Tropheryma whippelii*. Whereas infections with either NTM or actinomycetes can occur among animals analogous to humans, these animal infections generally do not serve as common sources for humans apart from the exceptions noted above.

There is considerable geographic variation in the frequency of NTM isolation (e.g., *M. malmoense* in Scandinavia and Scotland, e.g., *M. xenopi* in France and England), but the basis for such variation is not understood.

IV. NATURE OF THE BACTERIUM, PATHOGENESIS, AND CLINICAL FEATURES

A. *M. tuberculosis*

Mycobacteria in general are aerobic, weakly Gram positive bacteria with slow generations times. Their genomes have a high GC content and this in effect makes them somewhat similar to actinomycetes and corynebacteria. The cell walls are rich with complex lipids and in particular mycolic acids which are long branched fatty acids (C_{60}-C_{90}). As a function of these unique fatty acids, the cell wall is difficult to penetrate and thereby gives rise to the properties that in common terms is known as acid-fastness. With either the traditional Ziehl-Neelsen stain or the modified Kinyoun, the tough surface coat may be penetrated by dye stains only through the use of heat and/or chemical mordants. After adequate staining, the fixed dye cannot be easily removed even with the use of acid or acid-alcohol decolorizers; a property described as acid or acid-alcohol fastness respectively. Mycobacteria are among the most acid-fast of bacteria but organisms such as legionellae, nocardiae, rhodococci, and other actinomycetes may also be partially acid-fast, again a reflection of some similar properties within the cell wall. Other bacteria are not capable of retaining these particular dyes due to the permeability of the cell wall to such harsh chemical treatment. 'Cord factor' is somewhat unique to *M. tuberculosis* among mycobacteria (although not entirely specific) in that a serpentine formation of multiple bacteria is apparent in smears either from colonies or from most broth systems; this occurs as a function of the predominance of trehalose-containing mycolic acids, and it serves as a rapid presumptive identification method in the laboratory. Apart form mycolic acids, *M. tuberculosis* has a long lipoarabinomannan structure on its surface which may have a role in virulence. Mycobacteria are relatively resistant to the effects of dilute sodium hydroxide solutions (1%), and this facilitates laboratory diagnosis since chemical treatment of contaminated specimens by these solutions may facilitate eradication of salivary or other contaminants prior to culture. Growth of *M. tuberculosis* can occur on a variety of solid and liquid media (e.g., egg-based such as Lowenstein-Jensen, and artificial but lipid-containing Middlebrook media or Bactec media), but the generation time in any medium nevertheless approaches 12-24 hrs. In contrast to some other myco-bacteria, *M. tuberculosis* is not pigmented.

An understanding of pathogenesis has been greatly facilitated by the overall amount of human tissue that is available from surgery or autopsy, by the presence of good animal models for pulmonary and systemic disease (53), and by advances in molecular biology and immunology (51,54). An under-standing of these processes is critical since insight in this area furthers our knowledge of why there are diagnostic limitations. For primary infection, inhalation leads to deposition of the infectious bacterium in the small airways and alveolar spaces. Pulmonary macrophages encounter these bacteria and ingest them. A majority of such latter encounters is likely associated with eradication of the bacterium and hence no infection. Less commonly, the tuberculous bacilli may resist macrophage digestion and indeed grow within these cells, presumably by resistance of intracellular phagosomal-lysosomal fusion or some such similar mechanism (52). As bacterial multiplication continues, foreign antigen is presented to ef-fector immune cells and further macrophage activity is recruited with the subsequent development of delayed-type hypersensitivity (DTH) (55,56). Macrophage activation as well as activation of other im-mune cells subsequently facilitate the cascade of numerous events due to the enhanced production of varied cytokines which promote inflammation, tissue destruction, healing, among other events. As this activity continues, a central focal area of necrosis may emerge which is surrounded by macrophages of varied configuration. As the central focus expands and continues to degenerate, tissue may acquire a 'cheesy' consistency which is referred to as caseation (58). Small foci of this activity may be referred to as granulomata and may contain epithelioid cells and Langhans' giant cells, both of which are macro-phages that have been altered or fused. The initiation of DTH may be associated with healing, and this is therefore analogous to leprosy. In the presence of DTH and hence cell-mediated immunity, there is a reduction in bacterial load with a tendency to healing and tubercle formation. When DTH is diminished, the bacterial load may increase unchecked, and therefore disease progression may ensue (60,61). From an immunological perspective, tuberculosis is fascinating with the potential for both immune activation and suppression or anergy to co-exist (62).

From these local foci of bacterial growth, organism may enter the small airways and then dis-seminate into other areas of the lung. As well, spread may occur as viable bacterium is carried into the lymphatics or blood. Containment in other areas of the body must necessarily depend on the same im-mune mediators and cells as pulmonary infection. It is not surprising therefore that HIV infection is associated with rapid disease progression (57). The process of reactivation is not well understood, but the disappearance of DTH in late adulthood after a much earlier exposure to the bacterium could allow quiescent infection to re-emerge (59).

These events effectively lead to an understanding of the clinical presentation of tuberculosis. The progression, healing, and re-emergence of infection varies on a sliding scale of DTH and no DTH. Acti-vation of macrophages and the subsequent events that follow are greatly related to the release of im-mune and other activators.

B. *M. leprae*

M. leprae cannot be cultivated in vitro including tissue culture. For experimentation purposes, it has been cultivated in the mouse foot pad. Doubling times are measured in 1-2 weeks. The organism may possibly live outside of the body though perhaps in an inactive state, and this suggestion has given rise to the theory that the presence of environmental bacterium may facilitate spread in addition to the more likely person-to-person route.

The bacterium is acid-fast but not to the same extent as *M. tuberculosis*, and it is preferable to use a modification termed the Fite stain. Acid-fast bacilli are found on smears from skin slits or in biopsies of skin. The intensity of staining correlates with the viability of the bacterium, i.e., strong if viable and of interrupted pattern if non-viable.

Prominent antigens consist of phenolic glycolipids and lipoarabinomannan. It has been debated whether these or other antigens participate in immune complex formation or other pathogenic mechanisms (63,64).

In lepromatous disease, there is generally a lack of granulomata. There are free accumulations of bacteria, and anergy may be evident. Macrophage function may be so ineffectual that the macrophage may contain gross vacuoles of bacterium (foamy macrophage). Essentially this will represent a state where DTH and CMI are of insufficient value in containing the organism. When the latter immune functions are prominent, acid-fast bacilli will be relatively uncommon in areas of involvement. Granulomata will be prominent and in fact may play a large part in nerve destruction (65). It must be recognized that although the clinical illness may vary along a spectrum between these two poles, the progression or resolution of illness may lead to conversions from one form to the other. Indeed, the different histopathological forms may be apparent in the same individual at different sites. Therapy will also have a role in such conversion especially with the facilitation towards healing and then DTH emergence as the bacterium is contained. Overall the macrophage has a major role in the resolution process and its activation will lead to the release of cytokines and like substances which promote various clinical manifestations (66).

C. NTM

As there are a large number of NTM, it is not surprising that comparisons and similarities among members of this group would be sought. Historically, limited phenotypic traits were used to group or differentiate. The Runyon classification scheme was mainly developed on the basis of pigment production or rapidity of growth. Four broad groups included are: photochromogens (light induced pigmentation), scotochromogens (pigment regardless of light exposure), non-chromogens (no pigment), and rapid growers. Despite the past and even present convenience of using these attributes for rapid presumptive categorization which then facilitates the choice of other requisite laboratory work, genetic homology and sequencing of rDNA has shown that bacteria within the same group may be quite unrelated. These genetic studies have also been critical to the further differentiation of seemingly similar subgroups. For example, the former subspecies of *M. chelonae* have now been clearly separated into *M. chelonae* and *M. abscessus*. A large number of laboratory phenotypic tests may be used for differentiation as detailed later herein.

Pathogenesis is well-studied for few NTM, and recent interest has more so been kindled by the high frequency of some NTM infections, particularly *M. avium* (67), in HIV-infected patients. *M. avium* binding to eukaryotic cells has been well studied (70). The latter bacterium can induce apoptosis of macrophages (68). Differential cytokine expression can occur depending on whether the macrophages are from HIV-infected patients or normal individuals (69). Strain variation among *M. avium* isolates appears to correlate with colony appearance and this variation can be associated with differences in virulence.

In general, mycobacteria have the ability to inhibit phagosomal-lysosomal fusion in macrophages. Disease is contained with effective CMI, and therefore infection is more likely to occur in those with compromise of said immunity. In AIDS, disseminated disease is highly correlated with low CD4 lymphocyte counts. Reversal of such immune dysfunction, for example with the use of potent antivirals, is then associated with a much lower risk for disseminated mycobacterial infections. For those NTM that produce lung infection, the histopathology is relatively similar to that of tuberculosis. Again, the macrophage has a dominant role in pathogenesis and control. Some NTM may share cross-reactive antigens with *M. tuberculosis*.

D.   Actinomycetes

Nocardiae are generally hardy bacteria and may flourish on simple laboratory media. There is considerable variation in colony morphology and pigmentation even for the same species. Colonial growth on artificial media usually requires 1-4 weeks. When the Gram stain is applied to infected tissue, the bacteria may appear filamentous, and the staining is beaded. The bacteria are partially acid-fast, and modifications in the Ziehl-Neelsen stain (less harsh decolorization) should be used. Many of the features of pathogenesis are similar to those of mycobacterial infection (71), but yet granulomatous changes in tissue are relatively uncommon. Although the macrophage and other components of CMI have critical roles in infection (72), abscess formation is usually apparent.

Rhodococci also grow well on routine bacteriological media but have much shorter growth times that can be measured in a few days. Although the name implies pigmentation, colony pigment may require many days to evolve. These bacteria may also be partially acid-fast like nocardiae. Most research in pathogenesis comes from animal study where the natural disease is more common (46). It is evident that CMI also has a critical role in rhodococcal infections.

D. congolensis has a characteristic staining pattern whereby branched filaments are seen that are scored with divisions in the tranverse plane. Samples from fresh cultures show motility under the microscope.

V.   IMMUNOLOGY OF INFECTION

A.   *M. tuberculosis*

Whereas DTH and CMI are critical to the pathogenesis of tuberculosis, an expression of such immunity on a practical basis is limited as a resource for diagnostic assays with the exception of the tuberculin test which uses purified protein derivative (PPD). Although the standard tuberculin test is extremely useful, there are several limitations to its application. Some patients may be anergic, others in endemic areas may have reactivity due to exposure but no active disease (i.e., non-specificity), and for those where the disease is cured, the tuberculin response persists for a lengthy period of time. Furthermore, the past use of BCG vaccine will often lead to a positive response. It is not surprising, therefore, that studies of humoral immunity would be pursued for various reasons.

Some generalizations are applicable to human antibody responses in this context. Strong antibody responses are measurable in a sizeable proportion of infected individuals, but it is unclear that this response has much to do with any form of protection. A variety of antigenic components have been used as detailed below, and crude preparations are more prone to more non-specificity. When purified antigens are used, however, it becomes apparent how diverse and how variable the antibody repertoire is for any given patient. Patients with severely compromised immunity, and for whom the diagnosis may not be as obvious, are limited in their antibody response.

There are numerous antigens which have been used for studies of humoral immunity and/or for the purposes of serodiagnosis or follow-up of therapy: antigens of 10 kD, 16 kD, 17 kD, 19 kD, 24 kD, 30 kD, 35 kD, 38 kD (antigen 5), and 45/47 kD, Kp 90 antigen, antigen 60 (complex of BCG antigens), antigen 85, acylated trehaloses (of *M. fortuitum*), PPD, autoclaved antigen, polymerized old tuberculin (OT), lipoarabinomannan, glycolipid antigen, and chimeric proteins (73-89). The designations of these antigens are from many different sources, and therefore, it would not be surprising that some of them do prove to be slight inadvertent molecular weight variants (i.e., M_r varying due to methodological differences). In primary tuberculosis, the antibody levels are generally low and are directed especially to cytoplasmic antigens whereas in post-primary disease, antibody is directed mainly to secreted antigens. IgM reponses are much less consistent than IgG. Several antigens cross-react with antigens of other mycobacteria (90) and a few even with other non-mycobacteria (e.g., histoplasmosis). The trend therefore has been to favour component immunogens for antibody detection alone or in combination.

Antibody responses tend to be poor in children. More antibody is generated during active pulmonary tuberculosis rather than in those with merely apparent pleural disease, extra-pulmonary infection, or miliary tuberculosis. Antibody status is more likely to be positive for those with smear positive tuberculosis rather than for those with culture-positive, smear-negative tuberculosis (91). Patients with HIV infection and who especially have CD4 lymphocyte counts that are critically low are likely to have a poor antibody response despite widespread disease (92,93). Intrathecal antibody responses are measurable (94,95) but may persist well after a meningeal tuberculosis is treated. It is not apparent that any particular measure of antibody response has a direct and reliable correlate with severity of illness or outcome.

Overall, the application of humoral response assessment to laboratory diagnosis has been of limited value. Interest in this area remains the focus for commercial tests. Perhaps the hope that any one test or antigen will give a definitive answer is far gone. Rather, it may be more prudent to focus on the use of specific antigens to which a sensitive response is generated and which may be able to give the clinician a sense of probability for illness (96). For example, smear-negative but suspect illness might be one scenario where a diagnostic test, especially in a non-endemic area, could shift the likelihood of active disease and hence affect interventions.

B. *M. leprae*

The role of CMI in leprosy cannot be overstated. Genetic variation (especially at HLA loci) has a role in facilitating the diversity of clinical presentations. A skin test has been assessed (analogous to the tuberculin test but with *M. leprae* antigen) but unfortunately is of insufficient reliability. The lepromin skin test is negative in lepromatous leprosy and more likely, although not absolutely, positive in tuberculoid leprosy. It is not uncommon to have anergy during lepromatous leprosy. It is unlikely that diagnostic tests which rely on measurements of CMI, however configured, will be sufficiently applicable.

Antibody development during leprosy has been studied, and accentuated responses have been noted in lepromatous leprosy. Antibody production will vary depending on the spectrum of disease; more antibody evident in multi-bacillary disease versus less frequent in pauci-bacillary disease. For example, it may be very common to have antibody directed to the PGL-1 antigen in lepromatous disease but significantly less in tuberculoid disease (95% versus 60%). IgG subclasses are recruited differently during the varied forms of the disease (63,97). In general, there is a significant problem with positive serology among undiseased but close contacts of leprosy, e.g., household (98,99). The latter contacts presumably encounter the bacterium in high frequency but do not actively develop an illness. This phenomenon would be analogous to the sensitization of individuals to *M. tuberculosis* during exposure. Antigens that have been used for the detection of immune responses include PGL-1, 29 kD, 35 kD, and 65 kD antigens, crude antigen preparations (e.g., sonicated) and recombinant 35 kD antigen (100-105). Levels of IgM antibodies to PGL-1 and the 65 kD antigen correlate with the presence of circulating immune complexes (64). Antibody to PGL-1 correlates with the 'bacterial index' (quantitative measure of bacteria in skin slits or biopsies). Overall, there is a low predictive value for any such antibody determination in areas where the disease is not endemic (106,107). Furthermore, there may also be problems relating to mycobacterial cross-reactivity in areas where tuberculosis is common. Indeed, immunoblotting studies have defined such cross-reactive antigens (108). Anti-*M. leprae* antibody studies may then find a niche in circumstances where clinical diagnosis is uncertain or where histopathological examination is either impossible or confusing. Similar to tuberculosis, therefore, the serological assessment may alter the probability of diagnosis in a given context where the probability based on other grounds is somewhat indeterminate.

C. NTM

The cell-mediated immune responses as previously discussed are of seemingly greater importance for NTM infections than the humoral arm of immunity. Skin testing with varied NTM have been used in the past mainly for epidemiological studies. The ubiquity of most NTM in the environment and hence the high probability that an encounter of the human immune system with the organism has taken place both ensure that CMI of some sort will exist for many to some NTM. Cross-reactivity of skin testing with that for *M. tuberculosis* has long been acknowledged.

The study of antibody responses to mycobacterial crude or defined antigen has not received the same attention as for *M. tuberculosis* and *M. leprae*. Given the role of *M. avium* and like bacteria in AIDS, some assessment has been made of antibody response for diagnostic purposes (109). The use of antibody status in severely immunocompromised patients is limited.

D. Actinomycetes

The actinomycetes are considerably diverse, and a need for serological diagnosis is limited given the overall infrequency of related illnesses. In general, one can anticipate that there will be problems with cross-reactive antigens between species, strain variability for any given species, and variable host response to infection given that infection is likely to occur among those who are compromised in their ability to produce antibody.

Despite the above, nocardiosis is one illness for which antibody responses have been studied (114). Initial preparations for antibody determination used whole or crude culture filtrate antigens. Subsequent study has focussed on specific antigens of 24/26 kD, 31 kD, 55 kD, and 62 kD; the 55 kD antigen has especially been of interest due to its presence in varied *Nocardia* species (110-113). Patients with rhodococcal infection apparently may have antibody that recognizes the latter. The application of *Nocardia* serology is limited, and the potential for normal individuals to encounter these bacteria is high.

Studies of immune response to infection with rhodococci has been obtained mainly from studies with infected horses. CMI is critical to infection and explains why these infections have emerged in those with HIV infection. Crude antigen preparations have been used to assess humoral responses, and apparently negligible antibody development occurs in horses.

Serology has been of value in determining exposure to thermophilic actinomycetes (115-117). Pulmonary hypersensitivity occurs in the absence of actual infection, but there is sufficient antigenic exposure to facilitate antibody production. This is somewhat remarkable given that only tiny quantities of antigen are usually required to induce an allergic response.

VI. LABORATORY DIAGNOSIS

A. General concepts

Time-honoured methods for the diagnosis of mycobacterial and actinomycete infections will continue to be of value and will of necessity be utilized in areas of the world where resources are limited. The future challenge for diagnosticians will be to develop methods or find resources that will be applicable to those endemic areas where much of the tuberculosis resides.

In regions with sufficient resources and where expectations for state-of-the-art technologies exist, there will undoubtedly be a continuing trend towards greater sophistication and applicability. Not only will the laboratory techniques be enhanced, but the operations and impact of networking should be felt (118). In particular, there will be a continuing emphasis on molecular methods which are timely and cost-effective. These gains will facilitate better liaison with public health authorities for timely control of disease. Molecular techniques will continue to increase our understanding of the complexity and diversity of mycobacteria and actinomycetes; they will also contribute to the better understanding of epidemiology. Given the emergence of resistant bacteria, this enhanced sophistication will also necessarily help define treatment complications early. The provision of a good service can only occur within the context of internal improvements; continuous quality improvement is critical.

The precise definition of how any particular laboratory will offer services is dependent on many factors, but the number of specimens received and the frequency with which positive identifications are made bears highly on these considerations. Algorithms for effective service are not likely to be the same for every provider.

B. Nature of the specimen

The collection of samples for diagnostic procedures, whether for mycobacteria or actinomycetes, merits special consideration as detailed below, but the first critical factor is an appropriate concern for the etiological agents. Whether due to the chronicity of disease or the lack of florid clinical symptoms and signs, there are many clinical presentations of infection which may not necessarily trigger immediate concern. Analogous to the need to collect many cerebrospinal fluids in order to ensure an adequate determination of all of the few bacterial meningitides that actually exist among patients, concerns for tuberculosis should be investigated with the same vigour; an infection not determined has great ramifications to both patient and society.

An adequate amount of specimen must be obtained, and consideration should be given to multiple site sampling where appropriate, e.g., among the elderly or children who may not be able to produce sputum. For children, gastric aspirates may yield useful material as may blood cultures from HIV-infected patients. Critical volumes are especially important for the collection of cerebrospinal fluids and urines.

Maintenance of samples should prevent bacterial overgrowth where the potential exists, e.g., respiratory samples, urines, gastric aspirates, stool. Prompt refrigeration at 4°C will suffice for all specimens, and transfer to the mycobacteriology laboratory should preferably takes place within twenty-four hours. Transport media per se are not required but extremes of pH should be prevented, e.g., gastric aspirates may often benefit from neutralization upon receipt in order to counteract the usual acidity. Nevertheless, most mycobacteria are relatively hardy.

In the case of pulmonary tuberculosis, three consecutive early morning samples of sputum are usully sufficient for diagnosis provided the specimen has sufficient organisms to yield a positive culture. Approximately 15% of infections will not be cultivable, however, and in these situations, it is better to consider alternative approaches such as sputum induction with hypertonic saline (5-10%), gastric washings, and endoscopic bronchial samplings rather than merely increase the number of sputum specimens examined. If timing is of less concern, the opportunity exists to wait for the results of the first collected if it is anticipated that the diagnostic yield will be high prior to further collection. The collection of multiple specimens, when genetic amplification techniques are to be used, has also been studied.

Rejection criteria are somewhat difficult to establish. The rejection criteria that might be used for example with sputa that are submitted for routine bacteriology are not as applicable since the purity of a specimen may not be of great concern as long as the etiological agent is defined. Quantitation of the bacterium is not critical in the vast majority of circumstances. Delayed transport times, acidic pH, or small volumes are not necessarily limitations to successful culture on an all-or-none basis. Any such problem must be viewed in the context of the specimen that is submitted. For example, some specimens may be difficult to re-obtain. Critical information that accompanies any specimen may modify the approach. Cerebrospinal fluids for tuberculosis should be of minimum 5 ml. volumes since it is recognized that a limited quantity of organism may be present. Gastric washes and urines should preferably be acquired in the early morning when neither food ingestion or micturition respectively have taken place so that maximal organism will be residual. Stools are not generally of value for establishing the diagnosis of tuberculosis. In circumstances of suspect mycobacteremia, minimum volumes of blood for culture are approximately 5-10 ml. (119). Pleural effusions may yield the bacterium in tuberculosis, but they are also not uncommonly culture-negative (120). The latter may be supplemented with pleural biopsy which may yield cultivable organism or which may have granulomata that are seen on histopathology. Table 4 outlines some special considerations for specimen acquisition in the context of suspect tuberculosis.

For the diagnosis of leprosy, specimens of choice include skin slits, nasal smears or biopsies, and skin or other special site biopsies.

Several special considerations are to be had for varied NTM. In disseminated *M. avium* infection among HIV-infected individuals, the bacterium may be found in stool. Blood cultures will be of value in suspect mycobacteremia especially when immunosuppression is advanced. Given the ubiquity of NTM in the environment, care must be taken to avoid contamination of specimens. For example, potable water may not uncommonly harbour NTM and thus contamination from the oropharynx is quite possible. Mere presence of the bacteria in a clinical specimen should not be taken as definitively indicative of infection. Repeat specimen collection becomes much more important here especially when the specimens are of a site where mycobacterial contamination is more likely.

Actinomyetes are relatively hardy, although some believe that refrigeration temperature may have some relative detriment to nocardiae, and the same general concerns are had as for mycobacterial specimens. Nevertheless, infection is much more common of lung, skin, and sterile tissue. Routine bacterial cultures of sputum may not yield *Nocardia* spp. as some strains require an extended incubation period. It is critical therefore that there be some due notice given to the laboratory when these bacteria are to be considered. *Nocardia* spp. may occasionally be found in the mouth, but more importantly, they

Table 4 Special considerations for clinical specimens that are acquired for the laboratory diagnosis of tuberculosis.

Site	Volume	Collection time	Number of samples	Added concern
blood	5-10 ml.	random	1-2	Isolator[R] tube sediments may contain inhibitors to growth in BACTEC bottles
CSF	minimum 5 ml.	random	NA	
gastric aspirate	as possible	fasting	3 consecutive early mornings	pH buffering with sodium carbonate or phosphate; especially for pediatrics
pleural fluid	5-10 ml.		NA	pleural biopsy concomitantly obtained
sputum	as possible	random	2-3 samples	avoid NTM contaminant sources; saline induction if needed
other respiratory	5-10 ml.	random	NA	potential value of bronchial biopsy
sterile sites	as possible	random	NA	e.g., liver, brain, lymph node, bone marrow (marrow may be entered into BACTEC bottles)
urine	5-10 ml.	prior to	3 consecutive early mornings	value of repetitive urine cultures should be tempered by review of local experience

may also be colonizers of the respiratory tract. Hence, mere isolation of *Nocardia* spp. from the respiratory tract is not an absolute indication of infection, and a smear should always be examined for the presence of characteristic Gram positive branching filaments.

C. Conventional microscopy

1. *Mycobacteria*

Despite rapid progression in the area of molecular diagnostics, direct staining for mycobacteria, especially in suspect tuberculosis, continues to be an important part of specimen evaluation. In the underdeveloped countries, where 95% of the infections occur and where culture is usually not available, microscopy underpins all tuberculosis control initiatives. In areas where resources are less available, reliance on microscopy will continue for the foreseeable future. The cost of direct staining is proportionately low, and given an appropriate infrastructure, the results can be acquired on a timely basis. A positive smear for acid-fast bacilli in a sputum sample has good specificity for the diagnosis of tuberculosis. In populations where NTM are more common, it might be anticipated that a positive smear should suffer in its predictive value, but this is much less than anticipated. For example, although disseminated *M. avium* infection would be a major concern among patients with AIDS, a positive smear from the respiratory tract in fact has a very good likelihood of indicating the presence of *M. tuberculosis* in many regions.

The diagnostic impact of the Ziehl-Neelsen (ZN) stain or equivalent continues. The test is a rapid one and is unrivaled in potential turn-around time. Only the development of exceedingly rapid genetic amplification assays will likely rival this status. From the perspective of public health, the timeliness of the ZN stain provides impactful information which may diminish subsequent spread. Even in hospitals, the ZN will facilitate appropriate quarantine. Sputum smears which are deplete of acid-fast bacilli or have low numbers correlate with less infectivity in contrast to the specimen which has high bacterial load.

Despite its availability for many decades, the ZN stain is not well understood from a molecular and biochemical perspective. The differential staining ability is essentially attributed to mycolic acid structures of the cell wall. Typical acid-fast bacilli in tuberculosis appear relatively slender and pencil-like. The staining may be beaded. Some variation may exist for specific NTM, and indeed rapid-growing NTM may be easily over-decolourized as the cell wall structures are less taut. The use of fluorochromes (auramine-rhodamine) is a matter of preference over the conventional ZN stain, but it is believed that the fundamental mechanisms of stain penetration and retention are the same.

Quantitatively, the sensitivity of the ZN stain is approximately 10^3-10^5 bacteria/ml. The lower pole of this sensitivity is favoured when the observer is more experienced, when more time is given to viewing of the smear, and when a fluorescence technique is favoured over the traditional light microscopic variations. Experience has a large part to play in the view of how smears should be read. The individual may consume five to fifteen minutes in such an exercise and scan up to 200-400 fields under oil immersion. Fluorochromes are used for screening of smears at lower power (e.g., 400X), and hence there is an improvement in timeliness; 30-50 fields may be screened in two to five minutes. Whichever method is chosen can be compared to culture results as the arbiter in order to better appreciate the relevancy of work so performed. Some have found that the fluorescence screening approach is more susceptible to error due to non-specific fluorescence and its potential interpretation as positive. In order to circumvent such error, it may be possible to have all positive assays from the first method re-read by another interpreter or to have all positive assays from this screening method confirmed by the traditional ZN stain. Both staining approaches lend themselves to semi-quantitation which is based on the number of positive bacilli per microscopic field. Whereas a positive smear is incriminative for tuberculosis regardless of the quantitation of bacilli, quantitation may have some usefulness. Low quantitations, when culture proves to be negative, may support a retrospective concern for contamination. Quantitation will

reflect on infectivity and diminished numbers may be sought as a consequence of commencing antituberculous therapy. If there is a need for direct susceptibility testing from the specimen, smear quantitation may also facilitate the preparation of the inoculum for such assessment. The presence of ten acid-
fast bacilli per high power field is taken to be a 4+ quantitation. The finding of less than four acid-fast
bacilli in 100 light microscopic high-power fields does not generally correlate well with culture positivity.

Table 5 details examples of the comparison of smear to culture. In general, the smear, regardless
of technique, is considerably less sensitive than culture which remains the gold standard for the laboratory diagnosis of tuberculosis. The sensitivity of smears will be influenced by the patient population,
frequency of endemic disease, and culture method. There is also a good correlation with rapid diagnostic techniques which are based on genetic amplification; smear-positive samples are much more often
positive by these new techniques in contrast to smear-negative samples. If comparisons are made only
for those specimens that yield *M. tuberculosis*, the smear-positive rate is higher in contrast to the smear-
positive rate for all specimens that yield mycobacteria by culture. For cerebrospinal fluids, the limitations of direct smears have long been recognized (121). Usually there are few bacilli in tuberculous
meningitis. Therefore, it is preferential to collect a minimum of fluid (approximately 5 ml.) and to either
concentrate it by centrifugation or to layer the fluid by drying in stepwise progression. Concentration of
specimens by centrifugation is preferable when the nature of the specimen will allow it, and smears
should be made from such concentrates rather than from the original specimen. For those with suspect
mycobacteremia, smears of the blood or buffy coat are generally unreliable. Morphology may be affected by the implementation of antituberculous therapy.

The ZN smear has obvious use otherwise in the laboratory. It will be of some benefit to determine
the presence of cording for rapid presumptive identification of *M. tuberculosis* and for the confirmation
that colonies of growth are indeed acid-fast organisms. In addition, analogous methods, whether of the

Table 5 Examples for calculated sensitivity (sens.) and specificity (spec.) of mycobacterial smears
when compared to culture of the same clinical specimen.

Stain	Comparison	Sens.(%)	Spec.(%)	No.	Specimen	Reference
ZN or A-R	L-J	42.7	99.9	6199	all	122
A-R	not stated	32 (all) 46 (TB)	99	10468	all	123
A-R	L-J and Middlebrook	33 (all) 65 (TB)	98.3	3207	all	124
A-R+ ZN	L-J and Middlebrook	48.7 (all) 55.3 (TB)	99.9	2347	all	125
A-R+ ZN	L-J and Middlebrook	41.4	99.9	6550	all	126
ZN	L-J	53.1	99.8	2560	sputa	127

A-R = auramine-rhodamine stain; ZN = Ziehl-Neelsen; L-J = Lowenstein-Jensen; TB = for specimens with *M.
tuberculosis*

conventional ZN stain or the fluorescence counterparts, may be used in histopathological assessment of tissue sections.

Successful use of staining techniques must take the following issues into consideration:

a) performance of smears by less experienced personnel (thereby the need to have positive smears rechecked),
b) diminished sensitivity if the specimen is not concentrated,
c) potential contamination of smears from the positive control when the control is examined initially,
d) carry-over of acid-fast bacilli from other positive smears if the microscope lens is not properly cleaned,
e) lack of differentiation of acid-fast bacilli to indicate *M. tuberculosis* versus NTM,
f) cross-contamination at the time of the staining procedure,
g) contamination of the specimen as the result of using water that has a high burden of naturally present NTM (detected with the negative control),
h) performance of smears in an area with low volume and perhaps low prevalence of infection in the population so served, and
i) insufficient volume of sample, e.g., CSF.

2. Leprosy

As previously detailed, the diagnosis of leprosy is critically related to the use of ZN staining or modifications thereof on skin or biopsy samples. Apart from the mere presence of bacteria as a diagnostic indicator, the appearance of the bacteria on a qualitative basis (Morphological Index) may indicate viability, i.e., less well staining bacteria are less viable. Such indication has some usefulness in determining response to therapy.

3. Actinomycetes

The search for these bacteria by staining techniques will benefit from the application of both the Gram stain and the modified ZN stain. It must be recognized that structures in vivo may differ from their appearance after the bacteria are cultured. In tissue or sputum, nocardiae are branching and have a beaded Gram stain appearance. The filaments tend to be long and may be confused at times with those that are seen in actinomycosis which is caused by very different and anaerobic bacteria. A modified acid-fast stain will differentiate the two. For nocardiae, the traditional ZN stain is modified so that the decolorization steps are less harsh given the lesser tenacity of the nocardial cell wall.

Apart from the Gram stain and the modified ZN stain, these bacteria may also be visualized after silver, methylene blue, or Giemsa stains. The filaments are easily differentiated from fungal elements by the calibre and by the pattern of branching.

In varied actinomycete infections, granules may be present at the site of drainage. These may prove to yield the bacteria better than the drainage otherwise. The granules should be stained and cultured.

Rhodococci are more likely to appear as coccoid or coccobacillary forms after Gram staining. It is unlikely that they will be singled out in a sputum smear where many normal oral flora bacteria may have similar morphological appearance. These bacteria are more likely to be considered when the morphotypes are apparent from otherwise sterile tissue, e.g., open biopsy. Rhodococci may be weakly acid-fast when modified ZN staining is applied.

D. congolensis has a particular staining pattern that is quite characteristic; simples stains such as methylene blue or Giemsa are able to demonstrate a pattern of transverse markings along the length of the bacterial filament.

D. Laboratory isolation

1. Specimen processing and pre-treatment

The receipt of small specimen volumes does not necessarily invalidate the use for diagnostic purposes. When such small volumes are received, all of the tissue should be processed. Specimens from sterile sites usually do not require pre-treatment of any sort apart from centrifugation of fluids. Centrifugation will increase the yield of mycobacteria. Whole tissue may be ground prior to smear and culture. Processing of samples should take place in a Level II safety cabinet which has been so designated for this work.

Specimens from sites which normally contain bacterial flora may benefit from tissue processing. Prolonged transport time for sputa may further increase the likelihood that excessive contamination exists. Whereas the need for decontamination of specimens may significantly vary from specimen to specimen, a routine application to fluids such as sputa, gastric aspirates, urines, and stools is relevant. The routine bacterial culture of specimens to determine the degree of such contamination prior to mycobacterial processing seems at first appealing, but will be cumbersome to most laboratories especially when the focus is mainly diagnostic mycobacteriology. Decontamination efforts make use of the fact that mycobacteria, by virtue of their tough cell walls, are relatively resistant to a variety of chemicals which are otherwise able to inhibit bacteria of other sorts. In addition to decontamination, several specimens, especially sputa, may benefit from chemical homogenization in order to liberate bacteria from mucous and other debris in the clinical specimen. Liquefaction of sputa is achieved with a reducing agent such as dithiothreitol or n-acetyl-cysteine. Decontamination may be achieved by agents such as sodium hydroxide, sodium dodecyl sulphate, and Zephiran (128,129). Sodium hydroxide has the added benefit of acting as a mucolytic as well. The combination of sodium hydroxide (1%) and a reducing agent is popular, but there are several other methods, e.g., sodium hydroxide and sodium dodecyl sulphate, and Zephiran and trisodium phosphate. These agents, however, are nevertheless capable of inhibiting mycobacteria if the concentrations of the agents are high and if the exposure time is prolonged. Many NTM and actinomycetes will be more susceptible to these agents than *M. tuberculosis*. The concentration of sodium hydroxide can be varied in order to alter the frequency of contamination. The clinical specimen can be admixed with the decontamination/mucolytic solution, neutralized, and then centrifuged. Alternatively, the treated suspension may be centrifuged first, and then the centrifugate may be resuspended in a buffered saline. Regardless of approach, the overall contact time with the decontaminating agents must be viewed carefully (130).

Another form of processing includes the use of a lytic agent for blood samples prior to culture. The Isolator[R] tube contains varied agents which lyse red and white blood cells. The resulting pellet is cultured on standard media. It has been recognized, however, that lysing agents in the residual pellet may antagonize mycobacterial growth in liquid culture whereas the same lysing agents may be absorbed or neutralized by solid medium components (131).

2. Mycobacterial culture

The isolation of *M. tuberculosis* from any sample or site is essentially indicative of active tuberculosis.

There has been a considerable number of changes in the area of laboratory isolation for mycobacteria. These changes have mainly related to more consistent and complete culture, increased speed of detection, and automation of culture methodology.

What are the benefits of more timely culture? Epidemiology of infection and its association with control is ever more so important today as a resurgence of tuberculosis must be met with containment. More timely determination of infection will impact on the prevention of secondary cases. In addition, increasing presence of drug resistance among isolates of *M. tuberculosis* necessitates better control. An increasing awareness of systemic illness, especially bacteremia, among immunocompromised patients also warrants more timely intervention.

In general, it is preferable to use a culture system that includes both selective and non-selective media. For the many specimen types, this will be unnecessary since they are obtained from sterile tissue. Unfortunately, many specimens will be acquired from the respiratory tract where the odds of contamination are high. The mechanism for selection is commonly achieved with the use of antibiotics or dyes. Malachite green is a time-honoured inhibitor, but the effects are critically concentration related; excess concentrations will inhibit all mycobacteria. Antibiotics are most commonly used, and the particular selection is varied and may include penicillin, nalidixic acid, lincomycin, carbenicillin, polymyxin B, and trimethoprim; cycloheximide and amphotericin B have been used as antifungals. Again, some of these antibiotics may have anti-mycobacterial properties given sufficient concentration.

Although the potential value for liquid media in mycobacteriology has long been recognized, it is clear from more recent versions of this approach that broth enrichment has a significant role to play in maximizing yield. It is accepted by most that the current standard for mycobacterial culture should include both solid and liquid media; there may still be considerable debate as to which of the specific solid and liquid media (including automated) are best, and part of the debate here continues to be in a state of flux as new automated methods increasingly become available. Certainly the standard for comparison of any new method should include both solid and liquid media. The newer formats for broth culture have undoubtedly decreased the time for detection, and in comparison to traditional solid media alone, the interval to detection of any mycobacterial growth has decreased by 7-10 days. One must acknowledge, however, that increased detection of mycobacteria from specimens will include both true pathogens and mycobacterial contaminants. Broth media alone, especially in an automated format, would seem potentially feasible as a stand-alone method but there are nevertheless some isolates, and importantly including *M. tuberculosis*, which prefer the nutrients from solid media. Broth media nevertheless require subculture, and indeed mixtures of mycobacteria will be difficult to determine from broth cultures. Furthermore, the isolation of colonies may help in preliminary classification since the phenotype (e.g., pigmentation) can provide clues.

Regardless of the culture schema, it must be anticipated that some smear-positive samples will be culture-negative. Firstly, there will obviously be those that are simply false-positive smears; this is likely to be more so when the number of acid-fast bacilli are very few. In addition, however, some of these smears may be truly positive but have the following explanations: a) the patient is on active antimycobacterial therapy, b) a fastidious mycobacterium is encountered which requires longer than the usual incubation time, c) presence of some NTM which may need the addition of special growth factors, and d) persistent non-viable *M. tuberculosis* in some successfully treated culture-negative patients (190).

The use of 'cording', as previously detailed, has reasonable positive predictive value for determining the identification of *M. tuberculosis* or another member of the *M. tuberculosis* complex. This appearance after acid-fast staining was identified historically from conventional media, but it is also present among isolates from broth culture (132). With the realization that this phenotypic feature is not definitively indicative of the *M. tuberculosis* complex and with the recent availability of accurate molecular tools for rapid presumptive identification, there will be less of a reliance on the determination of cording.

Mycobacterial media, whether solid or liquid, are best cultured at 35-37 °C; growth on some solid media such as Middlebrook 7H10 and 7H11 is enhanced with increased carbon dioxide in the atmosphere. Some mycobacteria, especially those which are isolated from skin and superficial soft tissue such as *M. marinum*, *M. ulcerans*, and *M. haemophilum*, grow better at lower temperature, e.g., 30-33 °C. Cultures should be held for 6 to 8 weeks in general although the particulars for any medium must depend on what other media have been included in the overall culture protocol. Positive smears should warrant prolonged incubation when cultures are negative during a six week protocol especially if the patient was not on antituberculous agents before the specimen was collected. Some mycobacteria, e.g., *M. genavense* and *M. ulcerans*, may require prolonged incubation. Some mycobacteria benefit from the addition of supplements, e.g., the best example being the need for *M. haemophilum* to have hemoglobin, heme, or ferric ion added in order to achieve growth. The reading of cultures also depends on the complexity of media that are used overall. Solid media should be observed within the first week for contamination and thereafter, weekly. Liquid media should be examined as regularly if the Bactec bottle culture mechanism is used; newer automated methods will provide continuous or near-continuous monitoring. When several media are being used, the laboratory must determine an efficient method which will provide the most timely of results but which will facilitate the rational use of people and other resources – only each laboratory will be able to determine this balance.

Table 6 provides some attributes for the solid and liquid media and the systems that are currently used or near to be used.

Traditional agar-based media alone are now recognized to have had limitations in detecting mycobacteria as compared to the current standard. Nevertheless, agar media continue to be used in conjunction with the enrichment broths. For the purposes of being more encompassing, different agar media may be used in a bi-plate. Selective solid media incorporate antibiotics into either the traditional egg-based media or Middlebrook-Cohn defined media, e.g., Gruft modification of Lowenstein-Jensen or Mitchinson's modification of 7H11. Regardless of the solid medium variant, colonies of mycobacteria appear in 1-4 weeks. The clear Middlebrook media are more amenable to use for susceptibility testing.

Analogous to the benefit of using enrichment for general bacteriological purposes, enrichment broth has been of benefit for the enhanced detection of mycobacteria. Probably the most contemporary major advance in this area was the advent of the BACTEC 460 and 12B bottle. The automated system detects radioactive CO_2 which is derived from mycobacterial use of labeled palmitic acid. The system improved time to detection by 7-14 days. The 13A bottle is used for blood culture. A pellet of bacterial growth can be used for molecular speciation, and the medium is suitable for use in susceptibility testing. Although of benefit, some detractions in using this system include the repetitive use of needles, a potential for instrument needle contamination and hence bottle contamination during the automated sampling process, and the need for radioactive markers.

The Septi-Chek[R] manufacturers had previously devised a biphasic system for the culture of usual bloodborne bacterial pathogens. The device (see Chapter 9) uses a bottle with broth enrichment and a paddle top which has several forms of solid medium. An inversion of the bottle bathes the agar with broth so that enrichment may lend itself to the isolation of colonies on the solid medium. For mycobacteriology, a similar system was developed with 7H9 broth and a combination of Lowenstein-Jensen, Middlebrook 7H11, and chocolate agar media on the paddle. No special instrumentation is required and the technique was generally comparable to the BACTEC system and slightly better than conventional culture on solid media.

The Mycobacterial Growth Indicator Tube (MGIT) includes broth enrichment but is novel for the detection system. A silicon rubber incorporates a ruthenium compound which acts as an oxygen sensor when viewed with ultraviolet light. Although the system has similar frequencies of culture positives as the original BACTEC system, there is apparently more opportunity for contamination. The detection system however has tremendous potential and has the potential to circumvent problems that are associated with the radiometric BACTEC. This has led to the development of automated systems from BACTEC which use this new detection system: BACTEC 9000 MB (133,134) and BACTEC MGIT 960 (135). These new variations are automated and are contoured to facilitate susceptibility testing. They are also set up in such a way that data management and linkages with existing computer systems are possible. These advances are natural correlates from the progression in blood culture methodology as outlined in Chapter 9. Other automated systems [ESP II (AccuMed)(135) and MB/BacT (Organon Teknika)(137)] have similar general designs although the systems vary in mode of detection. Some of these new detector systems, however, may not function as well when blood is the specimen for culture. Figures 1 and 2 illustrate some example protocols for routine and then for specific blood culture of mycobacteria.

Table 6   Composition of culture media and their attributes.

Medium/Method	Composition	Antibiotics	Characteristics
Lowenstein-Jensen (L-J)	solid egg-based	Malachite green; antibiotics may be added for selection	good growth support; not for susceptibility testing; opaque medium
Petragnani	solid egg-based	Malachite green; antibiotics may be added for selection	similar to L-J but more inhibitory due to more Malachite green; opaque medium
American Thoracic Society	solid egg-based; milk	Malachite green; antibiotics may be added for selection	similar to L-J but less inhibitory due to less Malachite green; opaque medium
Coletsos	egg-based	Malachite green	supplements added
Middlebrook 7H10	solid; defined for salts, co-factors, vitamins, fatty acid	Malachite green; antibiotics may be added for selection	transparent; less Malachite green than egg-based media; used for susceptibility testing; slightly more rapid colonial growth than egg-based media
Middlebrook 7H11	solid; as 7H10 but has added casein hydrolysate	as above	as above
Middlebrook 7H9	broth; defined	as above	
Dubos Tween albumin	broth		
BACTEC 12B (BACTEC 460 model)	broth; defined	added for selection	decreases time to detection compared to solid media; radiometric detection; automated; can be used for susceptibility testing
BACTEC 13A (BACTEC 460 model)	broth; defined		supplement added; for blood and bone marrow; radiometric detection; automated

Table 6 cont'd.

Medium/Method	Composition	Antibiotics	Characteristics
Septi-Chek	biphasic; 7H9 broth and paddle has solid media	added for selection	supplement added; stand-alone and no automation needed; similar sensitivity to BACTEC
Mycobacterial Growth Indicator Tube (MGIT)	broth; 7H9	added for selection	supplement added; stand-alone; oxygen use sensor; need uv; not for use with blood specimens; same sensitivity as BACTEC; more contaminants than BACTEC; amenable to susceptibility testing
BACTEC MGIT 960	broth; 7H9	added for selection	automated version of the MGIT; amenable to susceptibility testing; same sensitivity as BACTEC 12B
BACTEC 9000 MB	broth; 7H9	added for selection	supplements added; automated continuous monitoring; good data management; same detector as MGIT
ESPII	broth; 7H9	added for selection	supplements added; automated continous monitoring; good data management; detection via head space pressure change
MB/BacT	broth; 7H9	added for selection	supplements added; automated continous monitoring; good data management; CO_2 detection based

3.   Culture of actinomycetes

There are many selective media which have been devised for the isolation of actinomycetes from soil, but comparatively few if any selective media have been well studied for the purposes of isolating pathogens from human infection. This may certainly be a function of the rarity of these infections. Growth from sterile tissue usually takes place in several days to several weeks. Actinomycetes are able to grow well on most non-inhibitory routine bacteriological media such as blood agar and chocolate agar; it is critical, however, that the media be incubated for a prolonged period, and hence there is the need to prevent dessication during this time. Perhaps most important is the need for the laboratory to be alerted that

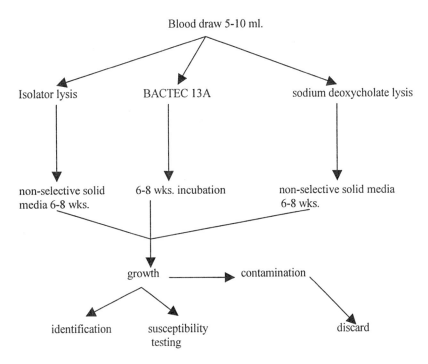

Figure 1 Options for mycobacterial blood culture.

actinomycetes are to be considered so that appropriate considerations can be had. Several actinomycetes may also grow on non-selective fungal and mycobacterial media. When blood is to be cultured for these bacteria, prolonged incubation and blind or terminal subculture should be used. Essentially all pathogenic actinomycetes will grow at 35-37 °C.

Selection for these bacteria is problematic, and no one medium can be necessarily advocated for all actinomycetes. Actinomycetes may be inhibited by the processing that may be used for mycobacteria and by antibiotics that are used for selective mycobacterial and fungal cultures. When the clinical specimen is likely to be contaminated, modified Thayer-Martin or selective buffered charcoal yeast extract (like that used for the detection of legionellae) may be tried for the purposes of finding nocardiae. Otherwise, due diligence in searching for these bacteria and other actinomycetes after prolonged culture on non-selective media may be crucial. Historically, the use of paraffin-baiting has been advocated for nocardiae whereby a glass rod, which is covered with paraffin, acts as the carbon source within a defined balanced salt medium. The bacteria which are able to use this carbon source will attach to the glass rod and may thereafter be subcultured. This approach has had variable results.

E. Laboratory identification

1. Mycobacteria

The identification of mycobacteria can be a laborious task especially when conventional biochemical and other phenotypic methods are used. Fortunately, most of the common isolates cluster within a limited number of species. Furthermore, the recent trends in molecular techniques will facilitate more prompt and accurate determination of speciation.

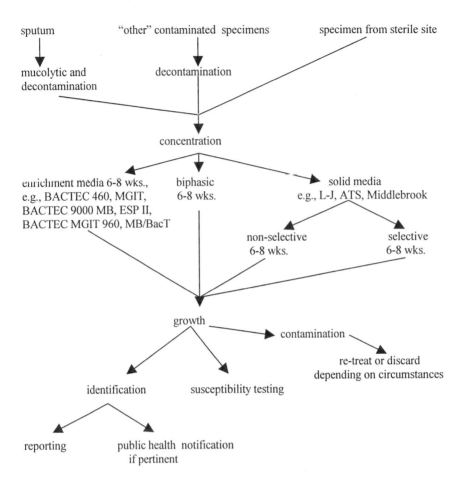

Figure 2   Options for mycobacterial cultures in general.

Traditional methods are relatively well standardized, but despite this, many tests can be of an indeterminate outcome especially when the assessor is less experienced. It is of benefit that mycobacteriology of this nature be confined to few but fairly well experienced laboratories. The traditional methods may require days to complete and thus have the reputation of being slow. When mycobacterial culture mainly relied on the use of solid media, colonies were readily available for the traditional methods to be applied. The current inclusion of enrichment media neccitates that positive broths be subcultured so that colonies will be obtained for these purposes. Thus, the reliance on liquid media for more rapid determination makes it desirable to have non-traditional and new molecular methods for speciation. The latter approach will be susceptible nevertheless perhaps to the issue of mixed cultures. Table 7 outlines some of the more useful traditional phenotypic and biochemical determinations. Details of test performance are provided elsewhere (138-141).

The phenomenon of cording serves as a rapid presumptive method to identify the *M. tuberculosis* complex and, in most circumstances, such isolates will be *M. tuberculosis* proper. Cording is not specific, however, and examples of both false-positive and false-negative are known. *M. tuberculosis* will be positive in tests of niacin accumulation, nitrate reduction, and pyrazinamidase; negative in tests of heat-stable catalase and urease production; and resistant to TCH. Differentiation from *M. bovis* is of

Table 7 Key features of varied biochemical and other assessments which are used in the speciation of mycobacteria.

Arylsulfatase – enzyme assay

BACTEC NAP – chemical analogue of chloramphenicol inhibits protein synthesis; inhibition of *M. tuberculosis* complex; added to BACTEC liquid medium

Catalase – semi-quantitative; assess for heat-stabile or heat-labile forms

Colony morphology – especially facilitated by the use of clear Middlebrook media

Ferric ion utilization (iron uptake) – reduction leads to iron oxide formation

Growth on MacConkey medium – growth or no growth without crystal violet

Growth rate – rapid growers in less than seven days

Inhibition by T2H – thiophene-2-carboxylic acid chemical inhibition

NaCl tolerance – direct growth inhibition in medium

Niacin accumulation – biochemical detection of accumulated nicotinic acid

Nitrate reduction – reduction of nitrate to nitrite

Pigmentation – photoactivated or not; defines Runyon groups

Preferred temperature – growth at room temperature, 30 °C, and 37 °C

Pyrazinamidase – deamination of pyrazinamide (PZA) to pyrazinoic acid

Tellurite reduction – heavy metal reduction

Tween 80 hydrolysis – release of oleic acid alters coloured substrate

Urease activity – colour change after urea utilization and alkalinization

---

value since the vaccine variant BCG has been recently used as an adjunct in human bladder cancer therapy and hence may have a greater probability of being found; the subsequent public health implications are potentially significant when *M. tuberculosis* is falsely identified.

The identification of NTM is obviously more complex due to the variety of species. Traditional methods have obviously not been entirely dependable for such identification since molecular techniques have been able to be more definitive in identifying new species where the traditional methods have been unable to separate them from those previously identified. Further work will be needed to define new standards with the combination of traditional and novel methods. On a preliminary basis, simple features such as colony pigmentation, colony phenotype, rapidity of growth, and preferred temperatures of growth can act to categorize NTM to a point where more specific biochemical assays may be targeted. Runyon's classification based on colony pigmentation is still of some value when mycobacterial colonies are visualized. Colony isolates are categorized as detailed in Table 8 which also gives some examples of the species within these groups. Table 9 illustrates how preliminary knowledge of the Runyon group may bias the choice of other assessments. Again it is evident that the advent of molecular techniques has the potential to help diagnostic mycobacteriology in that the extensive battery of biochemical tests may no longer need to be applied in the future. In the interim, however, an integration of classical and molecular techniques with a practical emphasis on the former may be considered.

There are several possible approaches which could be taken in order to facilitate bacterial identification given the existing laboratory tools. Such approaches could include chromatographic methods, genetic probes, genetic amplification, and direct genetic sequencing to name a few.

Chromatographic analyses can be contoured to provide analysis of metabolites or cellular constitutents, and for the purposes of mycobacterial identification, the variations of thin-layer chromato-

Table 8 Runyon groups of NTM.

Photochromogens (pigment produced with light activation)

M. kansasii	*M. marinum*	*M. simiae*
M. szulgai (@25 °C)	*M. asiaticum*	

Scotochromogens (pigment produced regardless of photoactivation)

M. gordonae	*M. xenopi*	*M. scrofulaceum*
M. szulgai (@37 °C)	*M. vaccae*	*M. flavescens*

Non-chromogenic slow growing (no pigment)

M. avium	*M. intracellulare*	*M. gastri*
M. malmoense	*M. genevense*	*M. terrae*

Rapid growers

M. chelonae	*M. fortuitum*	*M. phlei*
M. abscessus	*M. smegmatis*	*M. mucogenicum*

Table 9 Useful identification tests for various Runyon groups of NTM.

	Photochromogens		Non-chromogens	
		Scotochromogens		Rapid growers
Colony appearance	#	#	#	#
Temp. preference/tolerance	#	#		#
Pigmentation	#	#	#	
Niacin accumulation	#			
Nitrate reduction	#	#	#	#
Catalase	#		#	
Arylsulfatase	#	#	#	#
Pyrazinamidase	#		#	
Urease	#	#	#	
Tween hydrolysis	#	#	#	
NaCl tolerance		#	#	#
Tellurite reduction			#	
Inositol				#
Mannitol				#
Citrate				#
Polymixin B inhibition				#
Iron uptake				#

graphy, gas-liquid chromatography (GLC), and high pressure liquid chromatography (HPLC) have been applied. Essentially, short fatty acids from the bacterium are esterified, and the profile is examined by GLC. A bank of pre-determined profiles is then used for comparison to a given unknown profile for the isolate under study. Such a system has been commercialized (MIDI system) although not widely used; computer software facilitates pattern recognition, but database enhancements for mycobacterial identification are needed. Since the GLC pattern is dependent on fatty acids, which may vary according to the growth substrate that is provided, subcultures must be performed on defined media such as Middlebrook agar. GLC has the potential to obviate the use of several biochemicals, but the level of identification in many circumstances still requires supplementary testing with traditional biochemicals. Due to the need to provide rapid identification for *M. tuberculosis*, GLC is mainly of benefit to facilitate the identification of the more difficult NTM. HPLC provides further advancement and is more likely to replace the need for multiple biochemicals altogether. HPLC is used to create patterns of mycolic acid esters which will be relatively species-specific. As mycolic acids are branched fatty acids with alkyl side chains that possess 60 to 90 carbon lengths, there is considerable potential diversity that can be exploited for diagnostic purposes. A standardized growth of mycobacterial colonies is required, and the time for this growth may be measured in several weeks. It is also desirable to support HPLC with computer-assisted recognition software. Overall, HPLC compares well to the use of traditional biochemicals and genetic probes. There is also the potential to have this technology applied directly to the many enrichment broths that are fashionable. GLC and HPLC will necessarily be confined to reference laboratories as there is a requirement for costly equipment. The material costs thereafter are relatively reasonable. Again, these techniques will be used mainly for the identification of NTM.

The use of DNA probes for bacterial identification became popular in the 1980s and initial methods by necessity incorporated radiolabeled sequences. It was soon determined however that the use of DNA probes was limited when applied directly to clinical samples. Fundamentally, the major problem was the limited amount of bacterium that was available in samples in contrast to the modest sensitivity of the probe, e.g., often lower limit of 10^3-10^5 organisms. Despite this limitation, it was obvious that direct application to colonies or enrichment growths would be possible. Indeed, commercial versions of mycobacterial probes with radiolabel became available. These probes are cDNA that is complementary to a sequence within an rRNA gene. Soon after, the radiolabel was replaced with non-isotopic label which could be detected with chemiluminescence in a luminometer (AccuProbe). The procedural time for these probe assays is measured in a few hours, and therefore, this methodology has much to offer. The combination of enrichment broth culture (e.g., automated) with a rapid probe technology to follow has the potential to shorten an identification time by several weeks and thus to have a marked impact for patient and public health. The need to create species-specific probes, however, has been an impediment, and probes have been limited to a few more common species: *M. tuberculosis* complex, *M. avium* and *intracellulare*, *M. kansasii*, and *M. gordonae*. Despite the long shelf-life of these products (at least 12 months), it is difficult to stock probes for species that might be relatively rare, and thus, it is likely that the selection of products for the more common species will remain. The configuration of these probes and the use of a relatively simple luminometer makes the technology applicable to non-reference laboratories. The probes are certainly of value for quickly identifying members of the *M. tuberculosis* complex (142). The use of probes for provisional classification compares well to other traditional methods. There are nevertheless some problems with both false-positive and false-negative tests; the mere insufficiency of bacterium from a broth culture may in itself be responsible for a false-negative test. There is also the potential problem with mixed cultures.

Given the limitation of commercial probes with respect to the spectrum of NTM that may exist, there continues to be interest in developing to the next level of accurate speciation. In theory, the approaches could include genetic sequencing or genetic amplification which is followed by restriction endonuclease digestion. Both of the latter paths have been explored, published on, and now implemented in some laboratories. DNA sequencing has especially focused on species-specific and stable areas of the 16S rRNA gene (143,144). Although initially demanding for equipment, such sequencing can be easily and rapidly accomplished. This approach has led to the finding of new mycobacterial species and has helped clarify some difficult areas in NTM differentiation. Databanks are available with sequencing data that can be used either manually or via computer to compare with the unknown. Improvements in the area are happening quickly and the opportunity for automation here is evident. This approach detects a wide range of species in contrast to the direct DNA probes. Other methods for speciation are likely. The sequencing of the whole *M. tuberculosis* genome as well as the potential to sequence the genomes of all mycobacteria will provide for a great number of opportunities to find species-specific regions that can be exploited. The use of genetic amplification also has great promise in this area, especially when used in tandem with restriction fragment length polymorphism analysis. As would be anticipated, the latter possibility has already been exploited to some degree. For example, regions of the groEL gene, a heat-shock protein gene (145), and an rRNA gene (146) have been amplified by the polymerase chain reaction, and the products have been subjected to restriction enzyme digests; the patterns which then correlate with particular species. As rapid thermocycling or other rapid amplification processes are fine-tuned, it is quite certain that very timely speciation will be possible with the combination of amplification of early colonies or broth growths. Automation will allow for multiple simultaneous amplifications. Even if only the majority of NTM speciations are capable with these methods, there is likely to be considerable measurable benefit. Use of commercial amplification assays for speciation from BACTEC 12B bottles has already been studied (147).

2. Actinomycetes

The identification of actinomycetes is a highly complex task for rare isolates and should be left to the capability of a referral laboratory that has experience with the same. More complex tests are generally required. Details of such tertiary testing have been published (40,148).

Colonies should be examined for the presence of aerial hyphae. The nature of the colony will, however, depend on the medium that is chosen, and colonies are not uncommonly pigmented. For actinomycetes in general, differentiation can be achieved by a combination of carbohydrate utilization, other substrate utilization, growth in the presence of lyzozyme, arylsulfatase activity, assays for cell wall constituents, and antimicrobial susceptibility. It is anticipated though that molecular techniques will have much impact in the speciation of this group. Techniques such as 16S rRNA sequencing and polymerase chain reaction amplification with (149,150) or without restriction enzyme polymorphism analysis, as for mycobacteria, are likely to replace the aforementioned techniques which are laborious.

F. Antigen detection

Despite many advances in the development of monoclonal antibodies and monospecific antisera, antigen detection through radiometric or ELISA methods has not moved ahead sufficiently to be of practical widespread use. As for other bacteria, the availability of sufficient antigen for detection is a major stumbling block; this is not surprising given the frequency of smear-negative but culture-positive specimens which implies a limited quantity of bacterium in the clinical specimen to begin with. There still remains the possibility though that such technology could be applied to broth enrichments for the purposes of rapid identification.

Due to the limitations of antigen detection through antibody capture, others have pursued the detection of mycobacterial products by biochemical methods, namely chromatography. Tuberculostearic acid is a long-chained, saturated fatty acid from the cell wall that can be assayed by GLC. It is not entirely specific for *M. tuberculosis* but would be of some benefit for the diagnosis of meningeal infection which is unlikely to be caused by other mycobacteria or actinomycetes. The limit for detection, however, is somewhere in the range of 10^3-10^4 bacteria. 2-eicosanol is a long-chained alcohol which is obtained from the hydrolysis of cell wall mycolates and again is detected by a biochemical method. Both of these approaches require sophisticated support and are still limited in scope for the identification of *M. tuberculosis*.

Overall, the genetic amplification technologies have stolen the momentum away, and little ongoing progress in the area of antigen detection has been evident.

G. Direct detection by genetic amplification

1. *Mycobacteria*

Genetic amplification technologies for rapid diagnosis have obviously broad application to diagnostic bacteriology, but ideally they should be applied to those etiological agents which are difficult to grow or which have a prolonged period for finalization of existing diagnostic work-up. Mycobacterial illnesses are certainly among the latter category, and it is not surprising that much work would be focused in this area.

Whereas probe technology will detect the presence of nucleic acids, it is not uncommon to see a grey-zone in the difference between positive signal and background. Nucleic acid amplification technologies are intended to create more positive signal so that this grey-zone is either eliminated or shifted greatly. Several methods for nucleic acid amplification have emerged and mainly for the purposes of diagnosing tuberculosis: polymerase chain reaction (most commonly studied and implemented), rRNA amplification, ligase chain reaction, strand displacement amplification, cycling probe technology, nucleic acid sequence based amplification, and Qbeta replicase amplification (see Chapter 5).

There are numerous variations on PCR-based approaches for detecting *M. tuberculosis*; many of these have focused on the repeat DNA element IS6110 as the target. Optimistically, genetic amplification methods have been able to detect as low as 1-10 mycobacterial cells. All appear reasonably specific (specificity generally >90%). For specimens that are smear-positive (i.e., higher numbers of bacterium), the sensitivity of these assays approaches 90-97%, but among smear-negative specimens, the figures are as low as at 50-70%. Although Roche has commercialized the AMPLICOR MTB Assay (which is based on PCR of rDNA) and GenProbe has made the Mycobacterial Tuberculosis Direct Test available (based on rRNA isothermal amplification), several publications have detailed 'home-brew' methods (151). The reliability of these assays can be markedly biased by the choice for comparison, i.e., high sensitivity when only solid culture media are used. Table 10 gives a representative sampling for studies that have assessed commercial assays.

The nucleic acid amplification tests can be completed in times ranging from several hours to 1-2 days depending on the commercial system that is used and/or number of specimens processed. Specimen preparation is minimal. Unfortunately, the assays cannot differentiate between living and inactivated bacterium and so must be cautiously applied to specimens where the knowledge of positive has relevance. Decontamination procedures for sputa may affect the reliability of nucleic acid amplification, and interference can be variable. Furthermore, the amplification process in itself can be interfered by non-specific inhibitors in the clinical specimen. Nucleic acid extraction can minimize the latter, but it must be realized that a small proportion of specimens may not be amenable to amplification regardless of pre-treatment. The interlaboratory comparison of how these tests perform has provided some interesting discussion (152).

Overall, the limitations of nucleic acid detection impose the need to use culture methods in addition; nucleic acid amplification then becomes an adjunct rather than a replacement. The relevance of false-positive assays cannot be underestimated. If the prevalence of tuberculosis is low in a given population, a false-positive rate of 1-5% can have great impact to the extent that the number of true-positives may be exceeded by false positives. The application of nucleic acid amplification methods is in somewhat of a quandary. It is a subject of debate as to how the rapid methods fit into every day diagnostics, i.e., whether of routine use for every respiratory specimen or simply as an adjunct to confirm positive smears. Cost-containment in an era of escalating laboratory and other medical costs is also certain to have a role in determining the future for these methods.

Widespread use of nucleic acid amplification for all specimens that are submitted is not advocated until reproducible studies verify these applications. For the time being, their use is thus generally restricted to respiratory specimens. Progress for non-respiratory specimens, e.g., CSF, is imminent (153).

Table 10 Efficiencies of commercial methods for the laboratory diagnosis of tuberculosis.

Method	Sens.	Spec.	PPV	NPV	Comparison standard	Reference
AMTDTII	92.8	99.4	98.5	97	BACTEC 12B + L-J or	156
LCx	75.7	98.8	96.4	90.5	MB-Redox + L-J	
LCx	98.5 (smear-pos.)	100	100	98.4	BACTEC 12B + L-J or	157
	41.5 (smear-neg.)	99.9	96.4	98	MB/BacT + L-J	
Amplicor	96.1	100	100	98.1	BACTEC 12B	158
LCx	100	99.3	98.7	100		
AMTDTI	98.6	99.4	98.6	99.4		
AMTDTI	100 (smear-pos.)	77.8	86.7	99.2	BACTEC 12B + Middlebrook biplate	159
	65.2 (smear-neg.)	99.0	60.0	99.2		
LCx	78	100	95	98	L-J + Coletsos agar + BACTEC 12B or MGIT	147
LCx	94.8 (smear-pos.)	90.0	98.2	75.0	BACTEC 12B + Coletsos + Stonebrink or	160
	70.0 (smear-neg.)	97.7	24.1	99.7	BACTEC 12B + L-J + Middlebrook biplate	
Amplicor	83	99	97	95	BACTEC 12B + L-J	161
AMTDTI	83	100	100	96	L-J + Coletsos +	162
AMTDTII	94.7	100	100	98.4	BACTEC 12B	
BDProbe-Tec	94.7				Septi-Chek + Ogawa egg medium	163
Amplicor	89.5					
LCx	93.9	92.3	70.0	98.7	L-J + BACTEC 12B	164
LCx	90.8	100	100	94.7	L-J + Coletsos + BACTEC 12B	165
Amplicor	95.4 (smear-pos.)	90.9	97.7	83.3	BACTEC 12B + L-J + Kirchner + Stonebrink	166
	50.0 (smear-neg.)	99.3	85.7	98.9		

Sens. = sensitivity; Spec. = specificity; PPV = positive predictive value; NPV = negative predictive value; AMTDI or AMTDII = Amplified Mycobacterium Tuberculosis Direct Test (Gen-Probe) version I or version II; LCx = Abbott ligase chain reaction; Amplicor = Cobas Amplicor MTB (Roche); BDProbeTec = strand displacement amplification.

Commercially-available assays have been applied mainly to sputa and they focus on the identification of the *M. tuberculosis* complex. The next wave of nucleic acid amplification diagnostics will likely include multiplex assays which can simultaneously detect several mycobacteria at the same time (154). Genus-specific detection is also a possible starting point (155).

2. Actinomycetes

Acintomycete infections are simply not of sufficient frequency to warrant direct detection methods as detailed above. The methods are more likely to find relevance for the speciation of isolates.

One exception though is the detection of the Whipple's bacillus, *Tropheryma whippelii*. This bacterium is non-cultivable with routine methods but has been detected by genetic methods. Although the histopathology of disease is somewhat characteristic of the disorder, confirmation with direct PCR detection is possible. Indeed such methods have been used by some to propose that *T. whippelii* is a common component of normal body flora.

H. Epidemiological tools

1. Mycobacteria

As the spread of tuberculosis is of great public concern, the availability of means to survey the epidemiology of spread are desirable. Historically, limited approaches were at hand; phage typing was not of much practical benefit. Molecular techniques have now taken hold and have been standardized and widely adopted.

The issue now is not so much whether an acceptable technique for typing is available but rather when it should be implemented, i.e., what role fingerprinting methods have in everyday mycobacteriology. A variety of methods have been detailed, and to name a few, these have included IS6110 typing (see below), PCR typing of the IS6110 sequence, mixed-linker PCR, and spoligotyping (167-169,189). There are a great number of possibilities, but the trend is to develop a method which is reproducible, cost-effective, and timely, and which can be performed on few organisms, i.e., direct from a specimen or from very early growth of the organisms from agar or broth enrichment. Fingerprinting studies have mainly focused on *M. tuberculosis* but it is obvious that analogous methods in principle will be obtained for NTM when the need arises (170,171). For the most part, typing methods will be used to search for epidemic spread. In addition, however, it is possible for such methods to determine whether laboratory contamination has occurred; the latter has been long recognized, but the magnitude of such a problem has not been fully grasped (172,173).

Much of the work in this area for *M. tuberculosis* has focused on the use of the IS6110 repetitive sequence. This genetic element is mobile within the genome of *M. tuberculosis* complex bacteria. Strains of *M. tuberculosis* will have a variable number of such repetitive sequences, and their distribution within the genome will be highly variable (possibly even random). The typing process is laborious but seemingly simple in design. Bacterium must be grown to sufficient quantity, and this may require several weeks. DNA is extracted from the cellular harvest and then subjected to restriction endonuclease digestion which is followed by electrophoresis and Southern blotting with the use of a radiolabeled IS6110 fragment. The Southern blotting process will yield a variable ladder of probe-labeled bands. For those isolates where equivocal discrimination is a problem, other methods may be secondarily applied (174). This method has been standardized and is now used in several reference laboratories thoughout the world. In the future, however, it will likely be replaced by equally reproducible though less labour intensive nucleic acid amplification technologies.

Much interest has been directed to *M. avium* in AIDS, and the pattern of spread among HIV-infected individuals has also garnered attention. Typing methods such as serotyping, pulse field gel electrophoresis, and restriction fragment length polymorphisms of insertion elements IS311 and IS1245 have been used. Various methods have also been devised for furthering the epidemiology of other NTM.

2. Actinomycetes

Fingerprinting for epidemiological purposes is much less often a concern for the actinomycetes especially as they are so infrequently isolated from clinical specimens. Nevertheless, it only requires the translation of approaches from other bacteriological typing tools in order to develop useful methods. For example, methods such as ribotyping, PCR typing with randomly amplified polymorphic DNA, and pulse field gel electrophoresis have been detailed (175,176).

VII. SUSCEPTIBILITY TESTING

A. Mycobacteria

The therapy of tuberculosis and other mycobacterial infections is complicated in part due to the lack of response to many antibiotics that are used for common bacterial infections. Although short and long courses of tuberculosis therapy have been devised, all schemes use multiple antibiotics for several months. Alternate and to some extent strictly anti-mycobacterial agents must be utilized. Table 11 details first- and second-line antibacterials for the treatment of tuberculosis. The site of infection may pose a problem to anti-mycobacterial agents since granulomas and inflammatory tissue must be penetrated; macrophages may exclude antibiotics as ingested mycobacteria are secluded intracellularly. Different antibiotic regimens may therefore be required depending on the specific site of infection. Speciation of the mycobacteria is important in that particular resistance profiles may be more typical for a given species. Most NTM are routinely resistant in vitro to anti-mycobacterial antibiotics. Overall, in vitro results need to be supported by a positive outcome in vivo (177).

Drug resistance among *M. tuberculosis* isolates is recognized, and in the last decade, there has been a trend to increasing resistance especially for antibiotics such as isoniazid and rifampin which are first-line agents. Isolates with multiple resistance have also been encountered. Resistance has emerged on a global basis but has been more prominent among AIDS patients and those whose treatment regimen has been compromised (e.g., lack of completion for a full therapeutic course or inability to obtain more than one drug for therapy). Approximately 10-15% of *M. tuberculosis* isolates will have resistance to at least one drug prior to any therapeutic regimen, and about 2-5% will be resistant to two agents. It is not uncommon for these resistances to include isoniazid or rifampin. Given the problems that have been experienced when drug resistant tuberculosis occurs in epidemic form, *M. tuberculosis* isolates should be tested for susceptibility even though standard therapeutic courses are to be used. Global surveillance of tuberculosis through the WHO/IUATLD program will hopefully yield a more accurate determination of present status and future trends.

Anti-mycobacterial susceptibility among NTM is variable and the mechanisms for susceptibility testing are complicated since the conditions for such assessment may be inconsistent due to the variable

Table 11 First- and second-line anti-tuberculosis agents.

First line	Second line
isoniazid	rifabutin
pyrazinamide	ethionamide
rifampin	para-aminosalicylic acid
streptomycin	cycloserine
ethambutol	capreomycin
	kanamycin
	amikacin
	ciprofloxacin
	ofloxacin
	clofazimine

optimal requirements for bacterial growth among this very diverse group of organisms. Much attention though has been paid to the treatment of *M. avium* and related infections in patients with AIDS. Early after the potential for systemic infections was recognized, it was apparent that treatment of these patients was difficult. Whereas resistance to the antibiotics in themselves was a large part of the problem, it was also acknowledged the that profound immunosuppression which could occur in advanced AIDS might undermine successful antimicrobial therapy. The disastrous consequences of systemic *M. avium* infection among these patients led to the recommendation of anti-mycobacterial prophylaxis with single agents. The new erythromycin analogues, clarithromycin and azithromycin, served this purpose well as did rifabutin. With the advent of combinations of anti-HIV therapies which were associated with a sharp decline in viral load and with a restoration of cell-mediated immunity, less prophylaxis and treatment will be required, but the remaining infections will nevertheless remain difficult tasks to overcome.

Several methods for susceptibility testing have been implemented and these include the proportion method, the absolute concentration technique, the resistance ratio method, and the broth tube critical dilution (e.g., BACTEC enrichment broth variation of the proportion method). The proportion method is time-honoured and continues to be used by most. This technique makes use of clear defined Middlebrook media. Isolates of *M. tuberculosis* are standardized and are spotted onto agar media with and without various predetermined concentrations of anti-mycobacterial agents. Susceptibility is defined as a lack of growth on the antibiotic media which is equivalent to <1% of the total inoculum which has been spotted on the control media without the antibiotic. When the bacterium to be used is that obtained in colony form from primary isolation plates, the method is referred to as indirect. The latter approach may take up to 2-3 weeks to complete, and some *M. tuberculosis* which are antibiotic resistant may be slower to grow. Alternatively, inocula can be estimated by making serial dilutions of smear-positive specimens or their concentrates and subsequent application to antibiotic and control media. The latter approach, the direct method, has been taken in order to expedite the results especially when there is a strong epidemiological concern for drug-resistant *M. tuberculosis*. Problems with inoculum standardization and mixed cultures are recognized, and so the approach must have limited but high priority application. The approach with BACTEC media is relatively simple; essentially, the BACTEC bottles are used with and without a critical concentration of the anti-mycobacterial under study. The bottles are inoculated with standardized bacterium, and again, the inoculum may be direct or indirect. Growth in the bottles is monitored by the automated BACTEC system, and growth suppression is interpreted as susceptibility to that particular agent. Results with the latter technique can be obtained in as little as 1-2 weeks. If the inocula are prepared from other BACTEC bottles that have grown the mycobacterium as a primary isolation medium, it is possible to overlook mixed cultures. The use of this method was confirmed for first-line agents and has been available for several years now. Recent work has shown that the same approach can be applied to second-line agents as well (178). With the arrival of several automated broth enrichment techniques for mycobacterial growth, it is likely that these new systems will also prove to be useful for susceptibility testing analogous to the BACTEC.

Other approaches have also been studied including flow cytometry (179,180) and genetic probes (used to monitor growth rates in broths with and without antibiotics) (181) but are not widely subscribed to.

Whereas the NTM in general pose some difficulty in terms of developing standardized susceptibility testing (182), particular concern occurs when considering rapid growers. These mycobacteria are often resistant to the agents used for tuberculosis whether first- or second-line. Susceptibility and resistance are better assessed by conventional bacterial susceptibility testing methods such as disc diffusion, broth microdilution, or critical agar dilution. (see Chapter 8) (183). Etest has also been evaluated. Rapid growers often multiply sooner after subculture (2-3 days) so that the inoculum standardization and the reading of results are facilitated. Interpretive criteria must be viewed cautiously however.

With the concerns for resistance that have become evident over the last decade, many have studied the molecular basis for the same. It is apparent, however, that resistance to any one agent may be due to several different mutations or mechanisms. The determination of sequences that correlate with resistances have then led to the possibility to detect them with nucleic acid amplification methods (184). Resistance to rifampin and isoniazid have been particularly well-characterized (185). For rifampin resistance, changes in the *rpoB* gene can be determined by a battery of PCR techniques (with or without sequencing). Unfortunately, the many mutations that are possible must be determined, and their numbers may complicate practical application. Nevertheless, automated approaches have the potential to ease the technical difficulties that are posed by the latter, and it is possible to have results completed in 1-2 days in contrast to the time that is required for traditional methods (measured in weeks). Commercial products have already been made available for these purposes (186). Since drug-resistant *M. tuberculosis* most often have rifampin or isoniazid (or streptomycin) resistance, it is possible to at first test for the presence of these and then cascade to the testing of other antibiotics by conventional means if the former resistance is determined. These methods can be applied directly to broth cultures. It is conceivable that the future will see the combination of direct nucleic acid amplification for *M. tuberculosis* and the application of another amplification method(s) for resistance determinants. It is also possible that the use of DNA probe arrays will provide rapid genotypic information that can be exploited for these purposes (187).

B. Actinomycetes

Susceptibility testing for this broad group of organisms must be individualized, but the general approaches should be those which are applicable to routine bacteriology. These bacteria are somewhat more like rapid growing mycobacteria. They will grow quicker after subculture, and the methods which are applicable include disc diffusion, broth dilution, agar dilution, and E test (188). Radiometric methods have also been attempted with some success (188).

Sulphonamides are consistently active against nocardiae in vivo, and hence the need to perform susceptibility testing is less. Its use is more likely to be of benefit in the finding of alternatives when needed.

Given the chronicity of actinomycete infections, it is not uncommon to require prolonged courses of therapy that may last many weeks to possibly months depending on the status of the host. Despite what is seemingly susceptibility to an agent in vitro, a correlation with a positive outcome may not only be a function of the right 'drug-bug' combination; duration of therapy, choice of the particular agent and its pharmacology, as well as resolution of the compromise that has facilitated the infections may all be important. For example, rhodococcal infections in AIDS patients have often relapsed when treatment duration is abbreviated and when the patient has advanced suppression of cell-mediated immunity.

REFERENCES

1. Burke RM. An Historical Chronology of Tuberculosis. 1955.
2. Keers RY. Pulmonary Tuberculosis: A Journey Down the Centuries. London: Bailliere Tindall, 1978.
3. Meachen GN. A Short History of Tuberculosis. New York, NY, USA: AMS Press, 1978.
4. Caldwell M. The Last Crusade: The War on Consumption, 1862-1954. New York: Atheneum, 1988.
5. Daniel TM. Captain of Death: The Story of Tuberculosis. Rochester, NY: Rochester University Press, 1997.
6. Dormandy T. The White Death: A History of Tuberculosis. London: Hambledon Press, 1999.
7. Dubos RJ, Dubos J. The White Plague: Tuberculosis, Man, and Society. Boston, MA: Little and Brown, 1952.
8. Relman DA, Schmidt TM, MacDermott RF, Falkow S. Identification of the uncultured bacillus of Whipple's disease. N Engl J Med 1992; 327:293-301.
9. American Thoracic Society. Control of tuberculosis in the United States. Am Rev Resp Dis 1992; 146: 1623-1633.
10. Wallace RJ, Swenson JM, Silcox V, Good R, Tschen JA, Stone MS. Spectrum of disease due to rapidly growing mycobacteria. Rev Infect Dis 1983; 5:657-679.

11. Blacklock ZM, Dawson DJ, Kane DW, McEvoy D. *Mycobacterium asiaticum* as a potential pulmonary pathogen for humans: a clinical and bacteriologic review of five cases. Am Rev Resp Dis 1983; 127:241-244.
12. Grange JM, Yates MD. Incidence and nature of human tuberculosis due to *Mycobacterium africanum* in South-East England: 1977-87. Epidemiol Infect 1989; 103:127-132.
13. Prince DS, Peterson DD, Steiner RM, Gottlieb JE, Scott R, Israel HL, Figueroa WG, Fish JE. Infection with *Mycobacterium avium* complex in patients without predisposing conditions. N Engl J Med 1989; 321:863-868.
14. Wilkins EG, Griffiths RJ, Roberts C. Pulmonary tuberculosis due to *Mycobacterium bovis*. Thorax 1986; 41:685-687.
15. Koukila-Kahkola P, Springer B, Bottger EC, Paulin L, Jantzen E, Katila ML. *Mycobacterium branderi* sp. nov., a new potential human pathogen. Int J Syst Bacteriol 1995; 45:549-553.
16. Bux-Gewehr I, Hagen HP, Rusch-Gerdes S, Feurle GE. Fatal pulmonary infection with *Mycobacterium celatum* in an apparently immunocompetent patient. J Clin Microbiol 1998; 36:587-588.
17. Springer B, Tortoli E, Richter I, Grunewald R, Rusch-Gerdes S, Uschmann K, Suter F, Collins MD, Kroppenstedt RM, Bottger EC. *Mycobacterium conspicuum* sp. nov., a new species isolated from patients with disseminated infections. J Clin Microbiol 1995; 33:2805-2811.
18. Tortoli E, Brunello F, Cagni AE, Colombrita D, Dionisio D, Grisendi L, Manfrin V, Moroni M, Passerini Tosi C, Pinsi G, Scarparo C, Simonetti MT. *Mycobacterium genavense* in AIDS patients: report of 24 cases in Italy and review of the literature. Eur J Epidemiol 1998; 14:219-224.
19. Douglas JG, Calder MA, Choo-Kang YFJ, Leitch AG. *Mycobacterium gordonae*: a new pathogen? Thorax 1986; 41:152-153.
20. Saubolle MA, Kiehn TE, White MH, Rudinsky MF, Armstrong D. *Mycobacterium haemophilum*: microbiology and expanding clinical and geographic spectra of disease in humans. Clin Microbiol Rev 1996; 9:435-447.
21. Lumb R, Goodwin A, Ratcliff R, Stapleton R, Holland A, Bastian I. Phenotypic and molecular characterization of three clinical isolates of *Mycobacterium interjectum*. J Clin Microbiol 1997; 35:2782-2785.
22. Wolinsky E. Nontuberculous mycobacteria and associated diseases. Am Rev Resp Dis 1979; 119:107-159.
23. Springer B, Wu WK, Bodmer T, Haase G, Pfyffer GE, Kroppenstedt RM, Schroder KH, Emler S, Kilburn JO, Kirschner P, Telenti A, Coyle MB, Bottger C. Isolation and characterization of a unique group of slowly growing mycobacteria: description of *Mycobacterium lentiflavum* sp. nov. J Clin Microbiol 1996; 34:1100-1107.
24. Henriques B, Hoffner SE, Petrini B, Juhlin I, Wahlen P, Kallenius G. Infection with *Mycobacterium malmoense* in Sweden: report of 221 cases. Clin Infect Dis 1994; 18:596-600.
25. Gluckman SJ. *Mycobacterium marinum*. Clin Dermatol 1995; 13:273-276.
26. Springer B, Bottger EC, Kirschner P, Wallace RJ. Phylogeny of the *Mycobacterium chelonae*-like organism based on partial sequencing of the 16S rRNA gene and proposal of *Mycobacterium mucogenicum* sp. nov. Int J Syst Bacteriol 1995; 45:262-267.
27. Hautmann G, Lotti T. Diseases caused by *Mycobacterium scrofulaceum*. Clin Dermatol 1995; 13:277-280.
28. Tortoli E, Simonetti MT. Isolation of *Mycobacterium shimoidei* from a patient with cavitary pulmonary disease. J Clin Microbiol 1991; 29:1754-1756.
29. Valero G, Peters J, Jorgensen JH, Graybill JR. Clinical isolates of *Mycobacterium simiae* in San Antonio, Texas: an 11-year review. Am J Respir Crit Care Med 1995; 152:1555-1557.
30. Newton JA, Weiss PJ, Bowler WA, Oldfield EC. Soft-tissue infection due to *Mycobacterium smegmatis*: report of two cases. Clin Infect Dis 1993; 16:531-533.
31. Maloney JM, Gregg CR, Stephens DS, Manian FA, Rimland D. Infections caused by *Mycobacterium szulgai* in humans. Rev Infect Dis 1987; 9:1120-1126.
32. Tonner JA, Hammond MD. Pulmonary disease caused by *Mycobacterium terrae* complex. South Med J 1989; 82:1279-1282.
33. Floyd MM, Guthertz LS, Silcox VA, Duffey PS, Jang Y, Desmond EP, Crawford JT, Butler WR. Characterization of an SAV organism and proposal of *Mycobacterium triplex* sp. nov. J Clin Microbiol 1996; 34:2963-2967.
34. Van der Werf TS, Van der Graaf WTA, Tappero JW, Asiedu K. *Mycobacterium ulcerans* infection. Lancet 1999; 354:1013-1018.
35. Jiva TM, Jacoby HM, Weymouth LA, Kaminski DA, Portmore AC. *Mycobacterium xenopi*: innocent bystander or emerging pathogen? Clin Infect Dis 1997; 24:226-232.
36. Haas WH, Butler WR, Kirschner P, Plikaytis BB, Coyle MB, Amthor B, Steigerwalt AG, Brenner DJ, Salfinger M, Crawford JT, Bottger EC, Bremer HJ. A new agent of mycobacterial lymphadenitis in children: *Mycobacterium heidelbergense* sp. nov. J Clin Microbiol 1997; 35:3203-3209.

37. Olivier KN. Nontuberculous mycobacterial pulmonary disease. Curr Opin Pulm Med 1998; 4:148-153.

38. Chin DP. *Mycobacterium avium* complex and other nontuberculous mycobacterial infections in patients with HIV. Semin Respir Infect 1993; 8:124-138.

39. Benson C. Disseminated *Mycobacterium avium* complex disease in patients with AIDS. AIDS Res Hum Retroviruses 1994; 10:913-916.

40. McNeil MM, Brown JM. The medically important aerobic actinomycetes: epidemiology and microbiology. Clin Microbiol Rev 1994; 7:357-417.

41. Lerner PI. Nocardiosis. Clin Infect Dis 1996; 22:891-903.

42. Menendez R, Cordero PJ, Santos M, Gobernado M, Marco V. Pulmonary infection with *Nocardia* species: a report of 10 cases and review. Eur Resp J 1997; 10:1542-1546.

43. Wilson JP, Turner HR, Kirchner KA, Chapman SW. Nocardial infections in renal transplant recipients. Medicine 1989; 68:38-57.

44. Kontoyiannis DP, Ruoff K, Hooper DC. *Nocardia* bacteremia: report of 4 cases and review of the literature. Medicine 1998; 77:255-267.

45. Kim J, Minamoto GY, Grieco MH. Nocardial infection as a complication of AIDS: report of six cases and review. Rev Infect Dis 1991; 13:624-629.

46. Prescott JF. *Rhodococcus equi*: an animal and human pathogen. Clin Microbiol Rev 1991; 4:20-34.

47. Cornish N, Washington JA. *Rhodococcus equi* infections: clinical features and labortory diagnosis. Curr Clin Top Infect Dis 1999; 19:198-215.

48. Drancourt M, Bonnet E, Gallais H, Peloux Y, Raoult D. *Rhodococcus equi* infection in patients with AIDS. J Infect 1992; 24:123-131.

49. Venugopal PV, Venugopal TV. *Actinomadura madurae* mycetomas. Austr J Dermatol 1990; 31:33-36.

50. Towersey L, Martins E. Londero AT, Hay RJ, Soares Filho PJ, Takiya CM, Martins CC, Gompertz OF. *Dermatophilus congolensis* human infection. J Am Acad Dermatol 1993; 29:351-354.

51. Lagrange PH, Wargnier A, Herrmann JL. The immune responses in tuberculosis: role for pathogenesis, diagnosis, and prevention. Pediatr Pulmonol 1999; 18:S136-S139.

52. Deretic V, Fratti RA. *Mycobacterium tuberculosis* phagosome. Mol Microbiol 1999; 31:1603-1609.

53. Smith DW, Wiegeshaus EH. What animal models can teach us about the pathogenesis of tuberculosis in humans. Rev Infect Dis 1989; 11:S385-S393.

54. Bloom BR, Flynn J, McDonough K, Kress Y, Chan J. Experimental approaches to mechanisms of protection and pathogenesis in *M. tuberculosis* infection. Immunobiology 1994; 191:526-536.

55. Fenton MJ, Vermeulen MW. Immunopathology of tuberculosis: roles of macrophages and monocytes. Infect Immun 1996; 64:683-690.

56. Schlesinger LS. Role of mononuclear phagocytes in *M. tuberculosis* pathogenesis. J Invest Med 1996; 44:312-323.

57. Daley CL. Current issues in the pathogenesis and management of HIV-related tuberculosis. AIDS Clin Rev 1997-1998; 289-321.

58. Dannenberg AM. Roles of cytotoxic delayed-type hypersensitivity and macrophage-activating cell-mediated immunity in the pathogenesis of tuberculosis. Immunobiology 1994; 191:461-473.

59. Le HQ, Davidson PT. Reactivation and exogenous reinfection: their relative roles in the pathogenesis of tuberculosis. Curr Clin Top Infect Dis 1996; 16:260-276.

60. Dannenberg AM. Delayed-type hypersensitivity and cell-mediated immunity in the pathogenesis of tuberculosis. Immunol Today 1991; 12:228-233.

61. Rook GA. Macrophages and *Mycobacterium tuberculosis*: the key to pathogenesis. Immunol Ser 1994; 60:249-261.

62. Vanham G, Toossi Z, Hirsch CS, Wallis RS, Schwander SK, Rich EA, Ellner JJ. Examining a paradox in the pathogenesis of human pulmonary tuberculosis: immune activation and suppression/anergy. Tuber Lung Dis 1997; 78:145-158.

63. Dhandayuthapani S, Izumi S, Anandan D, Bhatia VN. Specificity of IgG subclass antibodies in different clinical manifestations of leprosy. Clin Exp Immunol 1992; 88:253-257.

64. Rojas RE, Segal-Eiras A. Characterization of circulating immune complexes in leprosy patients and their correlation with specific antibodies against *Mycobacterium leprae*. Clin Exp Dermatol 1997; 22:223-229.

65. Shetty VP, Uplekar MW, Antia NH. Immunohistological localization of mycobacterial antigens within the peripheral nerves of treated leprosy patients and their significance to nerve damage in leprosy. Acta Neuropathol 1994; 88:300-306.

66. Barnes PF, Chatterjee D, Brennan PJ, Rea TH, Modlin RL. Tumor necrosis factor production in patients with leprosy. Infect Immun 1992; 60:1441-1446.
67. Barrow WW. Contributing factors of pathogenesis in the *Mycobacterium avium* complex. Res Microbiol 1991; 142:427-433.
68. Bermudez LE, Parker A, Petrofsky M. Apoptosis of *Mycobacterium avium*-infected macrophages is mediated by both tumour necrosis factor (TNF) and Fas, and involves the activation of caspases. Clin Exp Immunol 1999;116:94-99.
69. Johnson JL, Shiratsuchi H, Toossi Z, Ellner JJ. Altered IL-1 expression and compartmentalization in monocytes from patients with AIDS stimulated with *Mycobacterium avium* complex. J Clin Immunol 1997; 17:387-395.
70. Hayashi T, Rao SP, Catanzaro A. Binding of the 68-kilodalton protein of *Mycobacterium avium* to alpha(v)beta3 on human monocyte-derived macrophages enhances complement receptor type 3 expression. Infect Immun 1997; 65:1211-1216.
71. Beaman BL, Beaman L. *Nocardia* species: host-parasite relationships. Clin Microbiol Rev 1994; 7:213-264.
72. Gupta R, Pancholi V, Vinayak VK, Khuller GK. Immune responses to the protein, carbohydrate and lipid antigens of *Nocardia asteroides* in experimental nocardiosis in mice. J Med Microbiol 1985; 20:255-261.
73. Amicosante M, Barnini S, Corsini V, Paone G, Read CA, Tartoni PL, Singh M, Albera C, Bisetti A, Senesi S. Evaluation of a novel tuberculosis complex-specific 34 kDa protein in the serological diagnosis of tuberculosis. Eur Resp J 1995; 8:2008-2014.
74. Kawamura M, Sueshige N, Imayoshi K, Yano I, Maekura R, Kohno H. Enzyme immunoassay to detect antituberculous glycolipid antigen (anti-TBGL antigen) antibodies in serum for diagnosis of tuberculosis. J Clin Lab Anal 1997; 11:140-145.
75. Arikan S, Tuncer S, Us D, Unal S, Ustacelebi S. Anti-Kp 90 IgA antibodies in the diagnosis of active tuberculosis. Chest 1998; 114:1253-1257.
76. Amicosante M, Richeldi L, Monno L, Cuboni A, Tartoni PL, Angarano G, Orefici G, Saltini C. Serological markers predicting tuberculosis in human immunodeficiency virus-infected patients. Int J Tuberc Lung Dis 1997; 1:435-440.
77. Rosales-Borjas DM, Zambrano-Villa S, Elinos M, Kasem H, Osuna A, Mancilla R, Ortiz-Ortiz L. Rapid screening test for tuberculosis using a 38-kDa antigen from *Mycobacterium tuberculosis*. J Clin Lab Anal 1998; 12:126-129.
78. Gupta S, Bhatia R, Datta KK. Serological diagnosis of childhood tuberculosis by estimation of mycobacterial antigen 60-specific immunoglobulins in the serum. Tuber Lung Dis 1997; 78:21-27.
79. Julian E, Matas L, Ausina V, Luquin M. Detection of lipoarabinomannan antibodies in patients with newly acquired tuberculosis and patients with relapse tuberculosis. J Clin Microbiol 1997; 35:2663-2664.
80. Diagbouga S, Fumoux F, Zoubga A, Sanou PT, Marchal G. Immunoblot analysis for serodiagnosis of tuberculosis using a 45/47-kilodalton antigen complex of *Mycobacterium tuberculosis*. Clin Diagn Lab Immunol 1997; 4:334-338.
81. Bothamley GH. Serological diagnosis of tuberculosis. Eur Resp J 1995; 20:S676-S688.
82. Zheng YJ, Wang RH, Lin YZ, Daniel TM. Clinical evaluation of the diagnostic value of measuring IgG antibody to 3 mycobacterial antigen preparations in the capillary blood of children with tuberculosis and control subjects. Tuber Lung Dis 1994; 75:366-370.
83. Escamilla L, Mancilla R, Glender W, Lopez-Martin LM. *Mycobacterium fortuitum* glycolipids for the serodiagnosis of pulmonary tuberculosis. Am J Resp Crit Care Med 1996; 154:1864-1867.
84. Ma Y, Wang YM, Daniel TM. Enzyme-linked immunosorbent assay using *Mycobacterium tuberculosis* antigen 5 for the diagnosis of pulmonary tuberculosis in China. Am Rev Resp Dis 1986; 134:1273-1275.
85. Alde SL, Pinasco HM, Pelosi FR, Budani HF, Palma-Beltran OH, Gonzalez-Montaner LJ. Evaluation of an enzyme-linked immunosorbent assay using an IgG antibody to *Mycobacterium tuberculosis* antigen 5 in the diagnosis of active tuberculosis in children. Am Rev Resp Dis 1989; 139:748-751.
86. Chau PY, Wan KC, Ng WS, So SY, Lau WY, Fan ST, Lee DK. Enzyme-linked immunosorbent assay of antibodies to purified protein derivative (PPD) in the diagnosis of active tuberculosis: evaluation of its potential and limitation in a high prevalence area. Trop Geogr Med 1987; 39:228-232.
87. Sada E, Ferguson LE, Daniel TM. An ELISA for the serodiagnosis of tuberculosis using a 30,000-Da native antigen of *Mycobacterium tuberculosis*. J Infect Dis 1990; 162:928-931.
88. Sada E, Brennan PJ, Herrera T, Torres M. Evaluation of lipoarabinomannan for the serological diagnosis of tuberculosis. J Clin Microbiol 1990; 28:2587-2590.
89. Hussey G, Kibel M, Dempster W. The serodiagnosis of tuberculosis in children: an evaluation of an ELISA test using IgG antibodies to *M. tuberculosis* strain H37 RV. Ann Trop Pediatr 1991; 11:113-118.

90. Qadri SM, Smith KK. Nonspecificity of the Anda A60-tb ELISA tests for serodiagnosis of mycobacterial disease. Can J Microbiol 1992; 38:804-806.

91. Bothamley GH, Rudd R, Festenstein F, Ivanyi J. Clinical value of the measurement of *Mycobacterium tuberculosis* specific antibody in pulmonary tuberculosis. Thorax 1992; 47:270-275.

92. Thybo S, Richter C, Wachmann H, Maselle SY, Mwakyusa DH, Mtoni I, Andersen AB. Humoral response to *Mycobacterium tuberculosis*-specific antigens in African tuberculosis patients with high prevalence of human immunodeficiency virus infection. Tuber Lung Dis 1995; 76:149-155.

93. Ratansuwan W, Kreiss JK, Nolan CM, Schaeffler BA, Suwanagool S, Tunsupasawasdikul S, Chuchottaworn C, Dejsomritrutai W, Foy HM. Evaluation of the MycoDot test for the diagnosis of tuberculosis in HIV seropositive and seronegative patients. Int J Tuberc Lung Dis 1997; 1:259-264.

94. Sindic CJ, Boucquey D, Van Antwerpen MP, Baelden MC, Laterre C, Cocito C. Intrathecal synthesis of antimycobacterial antibodies in patients with tuberculous meningitis: an immunoblotting study. J Neurol Neurosurg Psychiatry 1990; 53:662-666.

95. Mathai A, Radhakrishnan VV, Shobha S. Diagnosis of tuberculous meningitis confirmed by means of an immunoblot method. J Infect 1994; 29:33-39.

96. Verbon A, Weverling GJ, Kuijper S, Speelman P, Jansen HM, Kolk AH. Evaluation of different tests for the serodiagnosis of tuberculosis and the use of likelihood ratios in serology. Am Rev Resp Dis 1993; 148: 378-384.

97. Sheela R, Shankernarayan NP, Ramu G, Muthukkaruppan VR. IgG subclass antibodies to mycobacterial sonicate and recombinant antigens in leprosy. Lepr Rev 1995; 66:10-18.

98. Chanteau S, Glaziou P, Plichart C, Luquiaud P, Plichart R, Faucher JF, Cartel JL. Low predictive value of PGL-1 serology for the early diagnosis of leprosy in family contacts: results of a 10-year prospective field study in French Polynesia. Int J Lepr Other Mycobact Dis 1993; 61:533-541.

99. Agis F, Schlich P, Cartel JL, Guidi C, Bach MA. Use of anti-*M. leprae* phenolic glycolipid-I antibody detection for early diagnosis and prognosis of leprosy. Int J Lepr Other Mycobact Dis 1988; 56:527-535.

100. Stefani MM, Martelli CM, Morais-Neto OL, Martelli P, Costa MB, De Andrade AL. Assessment of anti-PGL-1 as a prognostic makrer of leprosy. Int J Lepr Other Mycobact Dis 1998; 66:356-364.

101. Triccas JA, Roche PW, Britton WJ. Specific serological diagnosis of leprosy with a recombinant *Mycobacterium leprae* protein purified from a rapidly growing mycobacterial host. J Clin Microbiol 1998; 36:2363-2365.

102. Parkash O, Chaturvedi V, Girdhar BK, Sengupta U. A study on performance of two serological assays for diagnosis of leprosy patients. Lepr Rev 1995; 66:26-30.

103. Escobar-Gutierrez A, Amezcua ME, Pasten S, Pallares F, Cazares JV, Pulido RM, Flores O, Castro E, Rodriguez O. Comparative assessment of the leprosy antibody absorption test, *Mycobacterium leprae* extract enzyme-linked immunosorbent assay, and gelatin particle agglutination test for serodiagnosis of lepromatous leprosy. J Clin Microbiol 1993; 31:1329-1333.

104. Prakash K, Aggarwal R, Sehgal VN. Significance of antibodies to phenolic glycolipid-I in leprosy diagnosis. J Dermatol 1992; 19:953-958.

105. Lefford MJ, Hunegnaw M. Siwik E. The value of IgM antibodies to PGL-1 in the diagnosis of leprosy. Int J Lepr Other Mycobact Dis 1991; 59:432-440.

106. Soares DJ, Failbus S, Chalise Y, Kathet B. The role of IgM antiphenolic glycolipid-1 antibodies in assessing household contacts of leprosy patients in a low endemic area. Lepr Rev 1994; 65:300-304.

107. Kumar B, Sinha R, Sehgal S. High incidence of IgG antibodies to phenolic glycolipid in non-leprosy patients in India. J Dermatol 1998; 25:238-241.

108. Das PK, Rambukkana A, Bass JG, Groothuis DG, Kok A, Halperin M. Identification of mycobacterial antigens for "ELISA" serology in the diagnosis of leprosy and tuberculosis. Acta Leprol 1989; 7:S117-S120.

109. Plum G, Brenden M, Santos P, Schwarz E, Wahnschaffe U, Mauff G, Pulverer G. Serum antibody reactivity to recombinant mig and whole cell antigens in *Mycobacerium avium* infection. Zentralb Bakteriol 1996; 284:348-360.

110. Angeles AM, Sugar AM. Rapid diagnosis of nocardiosis with an enzyme immunoassay. J Infect Dis 1987; 155:292-296.

111. Angeles AM, Sugar AM. Identification of a common immunodominant protein in culture filtrates of three *Nocardia* species and use in etiologic diagnosis of mycetoma. J Clin Microbiol 1987; 25:2278-2280.

112. Boiron P, Provost F. Use of partially purified 54-kilodalton antigen for diagnosis of nocardiosis by Western blot (immunoblot) assay. J Clin Microbiol 1990; 28:328-331.

113. Boiron P, Stynen D. Immunodiagnosis of nocardiosis. Gene 1992; 115:219-222.

114. Salinas-Carmona MC, Welsh O, Casillas SM. Enzyme-linked immunosorbent assay for serological diagnosis of *Nocardia brasiliensis* and clinical correlation with mycetoma infections. J Clin Microbiol 1993; 31:2901-2906.

115. Wenzel FJ, Gray RL, Roberts RC, Emanuel DA. Serologic studies in farmer's lung: precipitins to the thermophilic actinomycetes. Am Rev Resp Dis 1974; 109:464-468.

116. Shen YE, Kurup VP, Fink JN. Circulating antibodies against thermophilic actinomycetes in farmers and mushroom workers. J Hyg Epidemiol Microbiol Immunol 1991; 35:309-316.

117. Van den Bogart HG, Van den Ende G, Van Loon PC, Van Griensven LJ. Mushroom worker's lung: serologic reactions to thermophilic actinomycetes present in the air of compost tunnels. Mycopathologia 1993; 122:21-28.

118. Salfinger M, Hale YM, Driscoll JR. Diagnostic tools in tuberculosis. Respiration 1998; 65:163-170.

119. Stone BL, Cohn DL, Kane MS, Hildred MV, Wilson ML, Reves RR. Utility of paired blood cultures and smears in diagnosis of disseminated *Mycobacterium avium* complex infections in AIDS patients. J Clin Microbiol 1994; 32:841-842.

120. Chan CHS, Arnold M, Chan CY, Mak TW, Hoheisel GB. Clinical and pathological features of tuberculous pleural effusions and its long-term consequences. Respiration 1991; 58:171-175.

121. Kennedy DH, Fallon RJ. Tuberculous meningitis. JAMA 1979; 241:264-268.

122. Burdash NM, Manos JP, Ross D, Bannister ER. Evaluation of the acid-fast smear. J Clin Microbiol 1976; 4:190-191.

123. Murray PR, Elmore C, Krogstad DJ. The acid-fast stain: a specific and predictive test for mycobacterial disease. Ann Intern Med 1980; 92:512-513.

124. Lipsky BJ, Gates J, Tenover FC, Plorde JJ. Factors affecting the clinical value of microscopy for acid-fast bacilli. Rev Infect Dis 1984; 6:214-222.

125. Gordon F, Slutkin G. The validity of acid-fast smears in the diagnosis of pulmonary tuberculosis. Arch Pathol Lab Med 1990; 114:1025-1027.

126. Greenbaum JM, Beyt BE, Murray PR. The accuracy of diagnosing tuberculosis at a large teaching hospital. Am Rev Resp Dis 1980; 121:477-481.

127. Levy H, Feldman C, Sacho H, van den Meulen H, Kellenbach J, Koornhof H. A re-evaluation of sputum microscopy and culture in the diagnosis of pulmonary tuberculosis. Chest 1989; 95:1193-1197.

128. Salfinger M, Kafader FM. Comparison of two pre-treatment methods for the detection of mycobacteria of BACTEC and Loewenstein-Jensen slants. J Microbiol Meth 1987; 6:315-321.

129. Yajko DM, Nassos PS, Sanders CA, Gonzalez PC, Reingold AL, Horsburgh CR, Hopewell PC, Chin DP, Hadley WK. Comparison of four decontamination methods for recovery of *M. avium* complex from stools. J Clin Microbiol 1993; 31:302-306.

130. Krasnow I, Wayne LG. Sputum digestion. I. The mortality rate of tubercle bacilli in various digestion systems. Am J Clin Pathol 1966; 45:352-355.

131. Wasilaukas B, Morrell R. Inhibitory effect of the Isolator blood culture system on growth of *Mycobacterium avium-M. intracellulare* o BACTEC 12B bottles. J Clin Microbiol 1994; 32:654-657.

132. McCarter YS, Ratkiewicz IN, Robinson A. Cord formation in BACTEC medium is a reliable, rapid method for presumptive identification of *Mycobacterium tuberculosis* complex. J Clin Microbiol 1998; 36:2769-2771.

133. Zanetti S, Ardito F, Sechi L, Sanguinetti M, Molicotti P, Delogu G, Pinna MP, Nacci A, Fadda G. Evaluation of a nonradiometric system (BACTEC 9000 MB) for detection of mycobacteria in human clinical samples. J Clin Microbiol 1997; 35:2072-2075.

134. Pfyffer GE, Cieslak C, Welscher HM, Kissling P, Rusch-Gerdes S. Rapid detection of mycobacteria in clinical specimens by using the automated BACTEC 9000 MB system and comparison with radiometric and solid-culture systems. J Clin Microbiol 1997; 35:2229-2234.

135. Hanna BA, Ebrahimzadeh A, Elliott LB, Morgan MA, Novak SM, Rusch-Gerdes S, Acio M, Dunbar DF, Holmes TM, Rexer CH, Savthyakumar C, Vannier AM. Multicenter evaluation of the BACTEC MGIT 960 system for recovery of mycobacteria. J Clin Microbiol 1999; 37:748-752.

136. Tortoli E, Cichero P, Chirillo MG, Gismondo MR, Bono L, Gesu G, Simonetti MT, Volpe G, Nardi G, Marone P. Multicenter comparison of ESP Culture System II with BACTEC 460TB and with Lowenstein-Jensen medium for recovery of mycobacteria from different clinical specimens, including blood. J Clin Microbiol 1998; 36:1378-1381.

137. Rohner P, Ninet B, Metral C, Emler S, Auckenthaler R. Evaluation of the MB/BacT system and comparison to the BACTEC 460 system and solid media for isolation of mycobacteria from clinical specimens. J Clin Microbiol 1997; 35:3127-3131.

genus *Mycobacterium*: tests for pigment, urease, resistance to sodium chloride, hydrolysis of Tween 80, and beta-galactosidase. Int J Syst Bacteriol 1974; 24:412-419.

139. Wayne LG, Engel HWB, Grassi C, Gross W, Hawkins J, Jenkins PA, Kappler W, Kleeberg HH, Krasnow I, Nel EE, Pattyn SR, Richards PA, Showaltar S, Slosarek M, Szabo I, Tarnok I, Tsukamura M, Vergmann B, Wolinsky E. Highly reproducible techniques for use systematic bacteriology in the genus *Mycobacterium*: II. Tests for niacin and catalase and for resistance to isoniazid, thiophene 2-carboxylic acid hydrazide, hydroxylamine, and p-nitrobenzoate. Int J Syst Bacteriol 1976; 26:311-318.

140. Metchock BG, Nolte FS, Wallace RJ. *Mycobacterium*. In: Murray PR, Baron EJ, Pfaller MA, Tenover FC, Yolken RH, eds. Manual of Clinical Microbiology. Washington DC:ASM, 1999:399-437.

141. Heifets L. Mycobacteriology laboratory. Tuberculosis 1997; 18:35-53.

142. Badak FZ, Goksel S, Sertoz R, Nafile B, Ermertcan S, Cavusoglu C, Bilgic A. Use of nucleic acid probes for identification of *Mycobacterium tuberculosis* directly from MB/BacT bottles. J Clin Microbiol 1999; 37:1602-1605.

143. Rogall T, Flohr T, Bottger EC. Differentiation of *Mycobacterium* species by direct sequencing of amplified DNA. J Gen Microbiol 1990; 136:1915-1920.

144. Rogall T, Wolters J, Flohr T, Bottger E. Towards a phylogeny and definition of species at the molecular level within the genus *Mycobacterium*. Int J Syst Bacteriol 1990; 40:323-330.

145. Plikaytis B, Yakrus M, Butler WR, Woodley C, Silcox VA, Shinnick TM. Differentiation of slowly growing *Mycobacterium* species, including *M. tuberculosis*, by gene amplification and restriction fragment length polymorphism analysis. J Clin Microbiol 1992; 30:1815-1822.

146. Vaneechoutte M, de Beenhouwer H, Claeys G, Verschraegen G, de Rouck A, Paepe N, Elaichouni A, Portaels F. Identification of *Mycobacterium* species by using amplified ribosomal DNA restriction analysis. J Clin Microbiol 1993; 31:2061-2065.

147. Garrino MG, Glupczynski Y, Degraux J, Nizet H, Delmee M. Evaluation of the Abbott LCx *Mycobacterium tuberculosis* assay for direct detection of *Mycobacterium tuberculosis* complex in human samples. J Clin Microbiol 1999; 37:229-232.

148. Schaal KP. Laboratory diagnosis of actinomycete diseases. In: Goodfellow M, Mordarski M, Williams ST, eds. The Biology of the Actinomycetes. London:Academic Press, 1984:441-456.

149. Wilson RW, Steingrube VA, Brown BA, Wallace RJ. Clinical application of PCR-restriction enzyme pattern analysis for rapid identification of aerobic actinomycete isolates. J Clin Microbiol 1998; 36:148-152.

150. Laurent FJ, Provost F, Boiron P. Rapid identification of clinically relevant *Nocardia* species to genus level by 16S rRNA gene PCR. J Clin Microbiol 1999; 37:99-102.

151. Sandin RL. Polymerase chain reaction and other amplification techniques in mycobacteriology. Clin Lab Med 1996; 16:617-639.

152. Noordhoek GT, van Embden JDA, Kolk AHJ. Reliability of nucleic acid amplification for detection of *Mycobacterium tuberculosis*: an international collaborative quality control study. J Clin Microbiol 1996; 34:2522-2525.

153. Bonington A, Strang JI, Klapper PE, Hood SV, Rubombora W, Penny M, Willers R, Wilkins EG. Use of Roche AMPLICOR *Mycobacterium tuberculosis* PCR in early diagnosis of tuberculous meningitis. J Clin Microbiol 1998; 36:1251-1254.

154. Kox LF, Jansen HM, Kuijper S, Kolk AH. Multiplex PCR assay for immediate identification of the infecting species in patients with mycobacterial disease. J Clin Microbiol 1997; 35:1492-1498.

155. Stauffer F, Haber H, Rieger A, Mutschlechner R, Hasenberger P, Tevere VJ, Young KK. Genus level identification of mycobacteria fom clinical specimens by using an easy-to-handle *Mycobacterium*-specific PCR assay. J Clin Microbiol 1998; 36:614-617.

156. Piersimoni C, Callegaro A, Scarparo C, Penati V, Nista D, Bornigia S, Lacchini C, Sagnelli M, Santini G, De Sio G. Comparative evaluation of the new Gen-Probe *Mycobacterium tuberculosis* amplified direct test and the semiautomated Abbott LCx *Mycobacterium tuberculosis* assay for direct detection of *Mycobacterium tuberculosis* complex in respiratory and extrapulmonary specimens. J Clin Microbiol 1998; 36:3601-3604.

157. Lumb R, Davies K, Dawson D, Gibb R, Gottlieb T, Kershaw C, Kociuba K, Nimmo G, Sangster N, Worthington M, Bastian I. Multicenter evaluation of the Abbott LCx *Mycobacterium tuberculosis* ligase chain reaction assay. J Clin Microbiol 1999; 37:3102-3107.

158. Wang SX, Tay L. Evaluation of three nucleic acid amplification methods for direct detection of *Mycobacterium tuberculosis* complex in respiratory specimens. J Clin Microbiol 1999; 37:1932-1934.

158. Wang SX, Tay L. Evaluation of three nucleic acid amplification methods for direct detection of *Mycobacterium tuberculosis* complex in respiratory specimens. J Clin Microbiol 1999; 37:1932-1934.
159. Bergmann JS, Yuoh G, Fish G, Woods GL. Clinical evaluation of the enhanced Gen-Probe Amplified Mycobacterium Tuberculosis Direct Test for rapid diagnosis of tuberculosis in prison inmates. J Clin Microbiol 1999; 37:1419-1425.
160. Rohner P, Jahn EI, Ninet B, Ionati C, Weber R, Auckenthaler R, Pfyffer GE. Rapid diagnosis of pulmonary tuberculosis with the LCx *Mycobacterium tuberculosis* assay and comparison with conventional diagnostic techniques. J Clin Microbiol 1998; 36:3046-3047.
161. Rajalahti I, Vuorinen P, Nieminen MM, Miettinen A. Detection of *Mycobacterium tuberculosis* complex in sputum specimens by the automated Roche Cobas Amplicor Mycobacterium Tuberculosis Test. J Clin Microbiol 1998; 36:975-978.
162. Gamboa F, Fernandez G, Padilla E, Manterola JM, Lonca J, Cardona PJ, Matas L, Ausina V. Comparative evaluation of initial and new versions of the Gen-Probe Amplified Mycobacterium Tuberculosis Direct Test for direct detection of *Mycobacterium tuberculosis* in respiratory and nonrespiratory specimens. J Clin Microbiol 1998; 36:684-689.
163. Ichiyama S, Ito Y, Sugiura F, Iinuma Y, Yamori S, Shimojima M, Hasegawa Y, Shimokata K, Nakashima N. Diagnostic value of the strand displacement amplification method compared to those of Roche Amplicor PCR and culture for detecting mycobacteria in sputum samples. J Clin Microbiol 1997; 35:3082-3085.
164. Tortoli E, Lavinia F, Simonetti MT. Evaluation of a commerical ligase chain reaction kit (Abbott LCx) for direct detection of *Mycobacterium tuberculosis* in pulmonary and extrapulmonary specimens. J Clin Microbiol 1997; 35:2424-2426.
165. Ausina V, Gamboa F, Gazapo E, Manterola JM, Lonca J, Matas L, Manzano JR, Rodrigo C, Cardona PJ, Padilla E. Evaluation of the semiautomated Abbott LCx *Mycobacterium tuberculosis* assay for direct detection of *Mycobacterium tuberculosis* in respiratory specimens. J Clin Microbiol 1997; 35:1996-2002.
166. Reischl U, Lehn N, Wolf H, Naumann L. Clinical evaluation of the automated COBAS AMPLICOR MTB assay for testing respiratory and nonrespiratory specimens. J Clin Microbiol 1998; 36:2853-2860.
167. Wilson SM, Goss S, Drobniewski F. Evaluation of strategies for molecular fingerprinting for use in the routine work of a *Mycobacterium* reference unit. J Clin Microbiol 1998; 36:3385-3388.
168. Kremer K, van Soolingen D, Frothingham R, Haas WH, Hermans PW, Martin C, Palittaponarnpim P, Plikaytis BB, Riley LW, Yakrus MA, Musser JM, van Embden JD. Comparison of methods based on different molecular epidemiological markers for typing of *Mycobacterium tuberculosis* complex strains: interlaboratory study of discriminatory power and reproducibility. J Clin Microbiol 1999; 37:2607-2618.
169. Bonora S, Gutierrez MC, Di Perri G, Brunello F, Allegranzi B, Ligozzi M, Fontana R, Concia E, Vincent V. Comparative evaluation of ligation-mediated PCR and spoligotyping as screening methods for genotyping of *Mycobacterium tuberculosis* strains. J Clin Microbiol 1999; 37:3118-3123.
170. Roiz MP, Palenque E, Guerrero C, Garcia MJ. Use of restriction fragment length polymorphism as a genetic marker for typing *Mycobacterium avium* strains. J Clin Microbiol 1995; 33:1389-1391.
171. Picardeau M, Prod'Hom G, Raskine L, LePennec MP, Vincent V. Genotypic characterization of five subspecies of *Mycobacterium kansasii*. J Clin Microbiol 1997; 35:25-32.
172. De Ramos M, Soini H, Roscanni GC, Jaques M, Villares MC, Musser JM. Extensive cross-contamination of specimens with *Mycobacterium tuberculosis* in a reference laboratory. J Clin Microbiol 1999; 37:916-919.
173. Small PM, McClenny NB, Singh SP, Schoolnik GK, Tompkins LS, Mickelsen PA. Molecular strain typing of *Mycobacterium tuberculosis* to confirm cross-contamination in the mycobacteriology laboratory and modification of procedures to minimize occurrence of false-positive cultures. J Clin Microbiol 1993; 31:1677-1682.
174. Yang Z, Barnes PF, Chaves F, Eisenach KD, Weis SE, Bates JH, Cave MD. Diversity of DNA fingerprints of *Mycobacterium tuberculosis* isolates in the United States. J Clin Microbiol 1998; 36:1003-1007.
175. Louie L, Louie M, Simor AE. Investigation of a pseudo-outbreak of *Nocardia asteroides* infection by pulse-field gel electrophoresis and randomly amplified polymorphic RNA PCR. J Clin Microbiol 1997; 35:1582-1584.
176. Exmelin L, Malbruny B, Vergnaud M, Provost F, Boiron P, Morel C. Molecular study of nosocomial nocardiosis outbreak involving heart transplant recipients. J Clin Microbiol 1996; 34:1014-1016.
177. Mitchison DA, Nunn AJ. Influence of initial drug resistance on the response to short-course therapy of pulmonary tuberculosis. Am Rev Respir Dis 1986; 133:423-430.
178. Pfyffer GE, Bonato DA, Ebrahimzadeh A, Gross W, Hotaling J, Kornblum J, Laszlo A, Roberts G, Salfinger M, Wittwer F, Siddiqi S. Multicenter laboratory validation of susceptibility testing of *Mycobacterium tuber-*

culosis against classical second-line and newer antimicrobial drugs by using the radiometric BACTEC 460 technique and the proportion method with solid media. J Clin Microbiol 1999; 37:3179-3186.

179. Moore AV, Kirk SM, Callister SM, Mazurek GH, Schell RF. Safe determination of susceptibility of *Mycobacterium tuberculosis* to antimycobacterial agents by flow cytometry. J Clin Microbiol 1999; 37:479-483.

180. Kirk SM, Schell RF, Moore AV, Callister SM, Mazurek GH. Flow cytometric testing of susceptibilities of *Mycobacterium tuberculosis* isolates to ethambutol, isoniazid, and rifampin in 24 hours. J Clin Microbiol 1998; 36:1568-1573.

181. Martin-Casabona N, Xairo Mimo D, Gonzalez T, Rossello J, Arcalis L. Rapid method for testing susceptibility of *Mycobacterium tuberculosis* by using DNA probes. J Clin Microbiol 1997; 35:2521-2525.

182. Heifets LB. Dilemmas and realities in drug susceptibility testing of *M. avium-intracellulare* and other slowly growing nontuberculous mycobacteria. In: Heifets LB, ed., Drug Susceptibility in the Chemotherapy of Mycobacterial Infections. Boca Raton, FL:CRC Press, 1991:123-140.

183. Woods GL, Bergmann JS, Witebsky FG, Fahle GA, Wanger A, Boulet B, Plaunt M, Brown BA, Wallace RJ. Multisite reproducibility of results obtained by the broth microdilution method for susceptibility testing of *Mycobacterium abscessus*, *Mycobacterium chelonae*, and *Mycobacterium fortuitum*. J Clin Microbiol 1999; 37:1676-1682. 183.

184. Telenti A, Imboden P, Marchesi F, Schmidheini T, Bodmer T. Direct automated detection of rifampin-resistant *Mycobacterium tuberculosis* by polymerase chain reaction and single-strand conformation polymorphism analysis. Antimicrob Agents Chemother 1993; 37:2054-2058.

185. Telenti A, Honore N, Bernasconi C, March J, Ortega A, Heym B, Takiff HE, Cole ST. Genotypic assessment of isoniazid and rifampin resistance in *Mycobacterium tuberculosis*: a blind study at reference laboratory level. J Clin Microbiol 1997; 35:719-723.

186. Watterson SA, Wilson SM, Yates MD, Drobniewski FA. Comparison of three molecular assays for rapid detection of rifampin resistance in *Mycobacterium tuberculosis*. J Clin Microbiol 1998; 36:1969-1973.

187. Troesch A, Nguyen H, Miyada CG, Desvarenne S, Gingeras TR, Kaplan PM, Cros P, Mabiliat C. *Mycobacterium* species identification and rifampin resistance testing with high-density DNA probe arrays. J Clin Microbiol 1999; 37:49-55.

188. Ambaye A, Kohner PC, Wollan PC, Roberts KL, Roberts GD, Cockerill FR. Comparison of agar dilution, broth microdilution, disk diffusion, E test, and BACTEC radiometric methods for antimicrobial susceptibility testing of clinical isolates of the *Nocardia asteroides* complex. J Clin Microbiol 1997; 35:847-852.

189. Haas WH, Butler WR, Woodley CL, Crawford JT. Mixed-linker polymerase chain reaction: a new method for rapid fingerprinting of isolates of the *Mycobacterium tuberculosis* complex. J Clin Microbiol 1993; 31:1293-1298.

190. Al-Moamary MS, Black W, Bessuille E, Elwood RK, Vedal S. The significance of the persistent presence of acid-fast bacilli in sputum smears in pulmonary tuberculosis. Chest 1999; 116:726-731.

15

Enterobacteriaceae and Enteric Infections

Nevio Cimolai
Children's and Women's Health Centre of British Columbia, Vancouver, British Columbia, Canada

G. Balakrish Nair
National Institute of Cholera and Enteric Diseases, Calcutta, India, and Laboratory Sciences Division, International Centre for Diarrhoeal Diseases, Dhaka, Bangladesh

Yoshifumi Takeda
National Institute of Infectious Diseases, Tokyo, Japan

Luiz R. Trabulsi
Laboratorio Especial de Microbiologia, Instituto Butantan, São Paulo, Brazil

I. HISTORICAL BACKGROUND

The history of *Enterobacteriaceae* is captured in a plethora of books and other publications that have been made available over the last century; these are considerably numerous and available for the avid reader. As but one valuable example, the series of manuals published as the "Identification of *Enterobacteriaceae*" by Ewing and Edwards (1) serve to acquaint the uninitiated with the astounding number of changes and contributions to the science and diagnostics in this field. There has been a voluminous literature in this area with the generation of many books and reviews that span not only historical events but also contemporary views of clinical disease, epidemiology, basic microbiology, pathogenesis, immunology, and diagnostics. The importance of these bacteria as a group and individually to medicine and science as a whole has been and will undoubtedly continue to be considerable; the contributions which may be solely attributed to *Escherichia coli*, for example, are monumental in the basic sciences.

Whereas an important subset of the *Enterobacteriaceae* are indeed enteric pathogens for humans, there are several other enteric pathogens which we have considered within this chapter that have very little genetic homology with the former. Our inclusion here is only for convenience since the latter pathogens are often considered in the same breath when a discussion arises in the context of enteric disease.

Enterobacteriaceae is a family designation in the systematics of Gram negative bacteria. There is good reason to refer to pathogens as belonging to this broad group since the name quickly identifies a cluster of pathogens with many common features and with many commonalities among the spectrum of associated infections. Most of these have the capability of residing in the normal human gastrointestinal tract or are gastrointestinal pathogens. The designation of "coliforms" in many ways is synonymous with this group on a practical basis, but in fact is more broad-ranging since the term denotes mainly a morphological appearance as observed from the Gram stain and to a lesser extent may be taken to imply the phenotypic appearance of the bacterial colony from routine culture. Likewise, the term "enteric bacteria" is often taken to be synonymous with this family, although it is well recognized that the true spectrum of enteric, i.e., gastrointestinal, bacteria includes many Gram positive cocci and various anaerobes.

Our intent in this chapter is not to provide copious details about biochemical reactions and identification for the vast number of *Enterobacteriaceae* or non-*Enterobacteriaceae* enteric pathogens. Rather, we provide a microbiological and then clinical background for these human pathogens, and then emphasize practical features of laboratory diagnostics.

Whereas it has been apparent that the *Enterobacteriaceae* and non-*Enterobacteriaceae* enteric pathogens are many, and hence a discussion of the same considerably complex, this diversity has even more so become apparent over the last decade as new genetic technologies define provisional groups and species with a greater degree of certainty (Figures 1 and 2). A relatively new study of the interrelationships, or for that matter differentiation, among species within former genera has provided for an exponential increment of knowledge. As an example of the latter and with relevance to the context overall of this chapter, one need only consider the changes that have taken place in the systematics of *Yersinia enterocolitica* and related bacteria. Almost three decades ago, the genus *Yersinia* was comprised of only three species: *Y. pestis*, *Y. pseudotuberculosis*, and *Y. enterocolitica*. It was recognized, however, that considerable heterogeneity existed among isolates of *Y. enterocolitica*, the more common human pathogen. Several laboratories defined biogroup subsets of *Y. enterocolitica* and ascribed disease causation with some biogroups more than others (2). As work followed in the genetics of these biogroups, it was apparent that several were indeed sufficiently different from *Y. enterocolitica* such that new species were defined by the early 1980s: *Y. intermedia*, *Y. frederiksenii*, and *Y. kristensenii*. The latter nomenclature is of more than academic importance since it defines essentially non-pathogenic species. Despite the latter, there continued to be obvious biogroups that remained among *Y. enterocolitica* (3), but by the end of the same decade, more biogroups were given species designation: *Y. bercovieri* and *Y. mollaretii* (4). With what now remains as *Y. enterocolitica*, there continue to be recognized biotypes, and interspecies heterogeneity remains evident when genetic studies are applied (5). Figure 3 illustrates the genetic relationships among some *Yersinia* species as proposed by Caugant et al. (6).

With the dynamics of the aforementioned change, there have been many new designations of nomenclature for both genera and species. These changes in themselves, let alone other facets of the microbiology and associated diseases, have been at best confusing to both the clinicians who are directly responsible for patient care and to the diagnosticians and microbiologists who deal with these otherwise. Table 1 illustrates only a sample of these changes. As might be anticipated, there has at times been controversy over the choice of species or genus names, and this is inevitable given the number of strong investigators in the field as well as the global history of microbiology. Indeed, as we speak, many such controversies continue to be the subject for healthy academic debate and discussion. The designations so used in this chapter are for the sake of convenience and not in any way intended to pose fully, or in part, as arbiters of these dilemmae. It is for certain that such controversies will not at this time change the pattern of clinical infection or the necessary diagnostic approaches.

In the area of enteric bacteriology, the last two decades have been extremely rewarding, and the definition of common but relatively new enteric pathogens has occurred. For example, the 1970s and early 1980s were times of great excitement in the field as campylobacters were discovered. Although *C. jejuni* and *C. coli* were by far the most common of these, new *Campylobacter* spp. were soon to be found among the enteric specimens of immunocompromised patients and in the blood of others as well. Among the latter bacteria, a group of campylobacters (e.g., *C. fennelliae*, *C. cinaedi*) eventually became

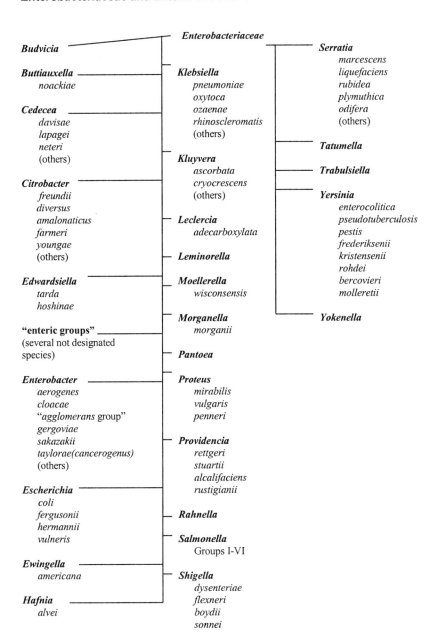

Figure 1 Currently recognized genera and major species of *Enterobacteriaceae* that are found in human clinical specimens.

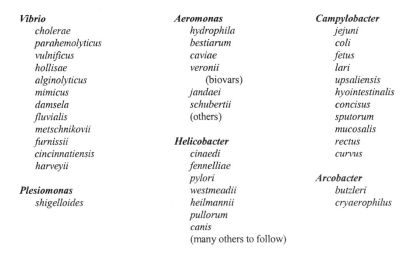

Vibrio
   cholerae
   parahemolyticus
   vulnificus
   hollisae
   alginolyticus
   mimicus
   damsela
   fluvialis
   metschnikovii
   furnissii
   cincinnatiensis
   harveyii

Plesiomonas
   shigelloides

Aeromonas
   hydrophila
   bestiarum
   caviae
   veronii
      (biovars)
   jandaei
   schubertii
      (others)

Helicobacter
   cinaedi
   fennelliae
   pylori
   westmeadii
   heilmannii
   pullorum
   canis
   (many others to follow)

Campylobacter
   jejuni
   coli
   fetus
   lari
   upsaliensis
   hyointestinalis
   concisus
   sputorum
   mucosalis
   rectus
   curvus

Arcobacter
   butzleri
   cryaerophilus

Figure 2   Currently recognized genera and major species of non-*Enterobacteriaceae* enteric pathogens (and their associated species).

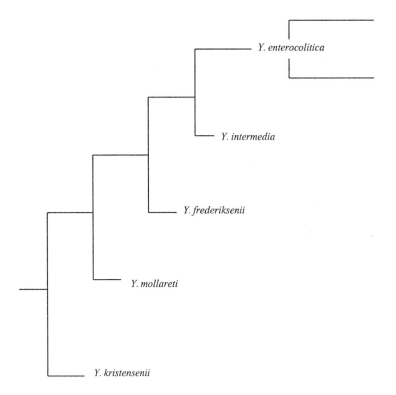

Figure 3   Proposed genetic relationships among five *Yersinia* species based on electrophoretic enzyme typing [adapted from Caugant et al. (6)].

Table 1 Examples of nomenclature changes among members of the *Enterobacteriaceae* and non-*Enterobacteriaceae* enteric pathogens.

Contemporary designation	Former designation
Arcobacter butzleri	*Campylobacter butzleri*
Campylobacter curvus	*Wolinella curva*
Campylobacter gracilis	*Bacteroides gracilis*
Campylobacter rectus	*Wolinella recta*
Hafnia alvei	*Enterobacter hafniae*
Helicobacter cinaedi	*Campylobacter cinaedi*
Helicobacter fenelliae	*Campylobacter fenelliae*
Kluyvera sp.	enteric group 8
Leclercia adecarboxylata	enteric group 41
Leminorella sp.	enteric group 57
Moellerella wisconsensis	enteric group 46
Morganella morganii	*Proteus morganii*
Pantoea agglomerans	*Enterobacter agglomerans*
Photorhabdus luminescens	*Xenorhabdus luminescens*
Providencia rustigianii	*Providencia alcalifaciens* biogroup 3
Tatumella ptyseos	group EF-9
Yokenella sp.	*Koserella trabulsii*/enteric group 45

recognized as *Helicobacter* spp. The latter therefore had more homology to *Helicobacter pylori* (a major gastric pathogen; see Chapter 20) than to *C. jejuni*. Interest in *Aeromonas hydrophila* as an enteric pathogen gained considerable momentum in the 1980s, and such attention led to the realization of heterogeneity among *Aeromonas* spp. Although some degree of heterogeneity was previously acknowledged, there were considerably new views of the systematics, and thereafter disease-associations, once genetic studies were able to further explore and expand on this theme. In the study of diarrheagenic *E. coli*, major gains in the science were also achieved. Enterohemorrhagic (verotoxigenic; Shiga-like toxin producing) *E. coli* were newly discovered and their contributions to disease world-wide soon became apparent. The history of enteropathogenic *E. coli* is a good example of the positive progression that generally took place in this domain and is illustrated below (Figure 4).

Soon after *E. coli* was recognized as a common bacterium of the human gastrointestinal tract, it became suspect that the organism, or at least some versions of it, could be associated with diarrheal illnesses (7). Among these illnesses, there was a common association of *E. coli* with diarrheal outbreaks in pediatric nurseries. Few other bacterial enteric pathogens were known at the time (i.e., outside of *Salmonella* and *Shigella*), and so it may have seemed natural as well that variants of a member of the normal stool flora should be suspect. By the 1940s, a serogrouping (serotyping) scheme had been initiated which was used to classify isolates of *E. coli*; this scheme was quickly adopted world-wide and suspect diarrheagenic *E. coli* were given particular serogroup designations. Once so established, further studies, which were structured along the line of case-control comparisons, confirmed the association of certain *E. coli* serogroups and diarrheal illness, especially that among infants. It was recognized in an episode that a particular *E. coli* serogroup was most commonly found among the aerobic flora of the diarrheal cohort in contrast to controls. Other pathogens were ruled out and many patients seemed to benefit from

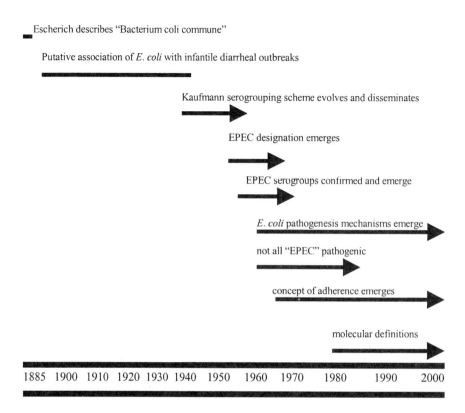

Escherich describes "Bacterium coli commune"

Putative association of *E. coli* with infantile diarrheal outbreaks

Kaufmann serogrouping scheme evolves and disseminates

EPEC designation emerges

EPEC serogroups confirmed and emerge

E. coli pathogenesis mechanisms emerge

not all "EPEC" pathogenic

concept of adherence emerges

molecular definitions

1885 1900 1910 1920 1930 1940 1950 1960 1970 1980 1990 2000

Figure 4   A chronology of events which are related to the emergence of EPEC as pathogens.

an antibiotic treatment. As well, anti-serogroup antibodies developed among patients and among volunteers who often developed a diarrheal illness after experimental inoculation. Further investigations of human disease and animal models continued to provide cause for recognizing these bacteria as distinct pathogens of the gastrointestinal tract. Given the collective experience, these *E. coli* isolates were thus defined as enteropathogenic *E. coli* (EPEC) (8). EPEC were recognized by the 1950s to be inclusive of many different serogroups. Some of these were relatively common in contrast to others which were extremely rare. Nevertheless, the number of EPEC serogroups continued to expand. Soon after the EPEC designation came into use, several mechanisms of pathogenesis were being proposed for diarrheagenic *E. coli*. Initially, these included invasiveness and the production of heat-labile or heat-stable toxins. These were not commonly found among EPEC, however, and attention soon turned to adherence, even though a small subset were also eventually found to produce verotoxins (Shiga-like toxins). It proved that specialized adherence was a common finding among many traditional EPEC, and further work confirmed that a particular form of adherence, termed localized adherence, was particularly identified. Other forms of adherence also became apparent (diffuse adherence and enteroaggregative adherence), but both physiological and molecular investigations during the 1980s and 1990s (and which continue) detailed a very interesting virulence mechanism(s) involving both bacterium and host (9). In summary, it was found that only a subset of traditional EPEC maintained the ability to manifest localized adherence and that several putative EPEC serogroups possessed either no virulence determinant as currently recognized or less commonly possessed a virulence trait that now is recognized among other *E. coli* diarrheagenic groups (Figure 5). In essence, this work has progressed over the course of a century and yet continues to serve as the focus for considerable investigative curiosity.

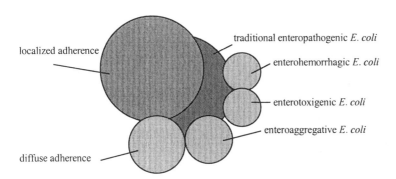

localized adherence

traditional enteropathogenic *E. coli*

enterohemorrhagic *E. coli*

enterotoxigenic *E. coli*

enteroaggregative *E. coli*

diffuse adherence

Figure 5   Traditional EPEC and overlapping subsets of *E. coli*.

Apart from new discoveries, major cycles in the epidemiology of bacterial transmission brought many of the *Enterobacteriaceae* or non-*Enterobacteriaceae* enteric pathogens to the forefront in recent history. Globalization and the massive exchange of food resources has increased the potential for food-borne enteric pathogens to cause large outbreaks, e.g., enterohemorrhagic *E. coli* caused approximately 5-10,000 infections in Japan during closely related epidemics (10,11), e.g., *Salmonella* spp. have caused large international outbreaks of infection as a consequence of dissemination via alfalfa sprouts (12,13). Global climatic changes have apparently had a major influence on the resurgence of cholera in the Americas to the extent that up to a million or more infections may have occurred (14,15). It cannot be under-estimated how such a large epidemic may secondarily be translated into global concerns (16). Increased pressure for antimicrobial resistance to emerge and to be maintained has also been of major concern (Table 2). Whereas significant new antimicrobials have been produced on a semi-regular basis over the last two decades, the development of resistance to these same agents has essentially kept pace in many circumstances. Antibiotic resistance often develops on a focal or regional basis, but the potential for national and international spread has been realized and continues to be of great concern. To maintain stride with these aforementioned changes, health organizations and governments have recognized the need to create timely and communicative surveillance systems.

The great spectrum of infections that are associated with these bacteria continues to be expanded. Given the new age of health care and scientific informatics, there exists a wealth of published international experience to the extent that even less common infections or rare complications can be reviewed within a short time frame. On a numeric basis, these bacteria are commonly associated with community-acquired infections, and they also comprise a significant proportion of the causes for nosocomial infection. Whereas there is some prospect for the control of infection for given examples, it is unlikely that prevention in the form of vaccination will become available for such a broad group of bacteria in general, and thus the cumulative toll of human illness with these bacteria will continue. It should be acknowledged that although the distribution of disease that is associated with these bacteria is worldwide, there is a greater proportion among those in under-developed countries where resources are meager and where conditions are generally unfavourable for rapid progress. If disease was only to occur in the latter circumstances, there would still remain an incredible burden to resolve.

II. CLINICAL ASPECTS

A. *Enterobacteriaceae*

Apart from some enteric pathogens, e.g., *Salmonella*, *Shigella*, and verotoxigenic *E. coli* which cause an acute infection and do not often colonize the normal gastrointestinal tract, most *Enterobacteriaceae* are normal intestinal flora although there is considerable variation in the frequency that individual species inhabit the gastrointestinal tract. In keeping with their common presence in the gut, they are not uncommonly found at other sites temporarily as a consequence of contamination (e.g., vagina, stomach, mouth, and skin), whether from direct anatomic contiguity or from spread via hand contact.

Table 2   Concerning recent trends in the antimicrobial resistance of *Enterobacteriaceae* and non-*Enterobacteriaceae* causes of enteric infection.

Bacterium	Antimicrobial(s)	Issue	Reference
Campylobacter jejuni	quinolones	animal feed-associated; emerging in the 1990s	17,18
Escherichia coli	urinary tract agents	mainly amoxicillin, cotrimoxazole, and quinolones	19,20
Enterobacter spp. *Klebsiella* spp. *Citrobacter* spp. *Serratia marcescens* *Escherichia coli*	advanced cephalosporins	extended spectrum beta-lactamases but also including carbapenemases; spread to *Salmonella* spp. a concern	21-23
Salmonella serotype Typhi	multiple antibiotics	resistance to amoxicillin, cotrimoxazole, chloramphenicol; concerns for resistance emerging for advanced cephalosporins and quinolones	24-26
Salmonella serotype Typhimurium DT104	multiple antibiotics	global spread	27
Shigella dysenteriae	quinolones	quinolone resistance is following the development of widespread resistance to ampicillin and cotrimoxazole	28
Vibrio cholerae	tetracycline	multiple resistance emerging	29

Consequently, they are often present at times when the body is compromised and thus susceptible to the nearest possible pathogen.

The spectrum of illnesses that are associated with these bacteria in general is vast, and there is a large compendium of literature which details the many common and uncommon variations of infections that may include essentially every body system or organ. Very few of these infections, however, are spontaneous among otherwise healthy individuals. For example, enteric infections may arise as a consequence of the first encounter of a non-immune host with the pathogen. *E. coli* urinary tract infections may occur in seemingly normal hosts without any previous or underlying complicating factor. The compromised host, however, is susceptible to almost all *Enterobacteriaceae*, and the risk factors are many: complicated urinary tract with or without indwelling devices, intensive care and its associated procedures, malignancy with or without the use of chemotherapy, surgical intervention, gastrointestinal surgery or catastrophes, burns, neonatal status (especially premature), medical devices, pregnancy and labor and delivery, immunosuppression, inflammatory bowel disease, liver failure, among others. Many of the latter risk factors are most often present among patients who are admitted to hospital, and hence infections with *Enterobacteriaceae* are often nosocomial (30). The occurrence of infections in the hospital environment ensures that both patient and bacteria will be exposed to antimicrobial agents which then increases the chance that resistance will emerge. Furthermore, the commonality of medical interventions as well as the simple fact that susceptible individuals are cared for in close proximity will provide for ample opportunity for outbreaks to occur.

1. *Escherichia*

On a numeric basis, *E. coli* is the most common individual species among the *Enterobacteriaceae* that causes human infection. A wide variety of infections have been reported, but the more frequent include urinary tract infections, gastrointestinal infections, intra-abdominal infections, and bacteremia.

E. coli is by far the most common cause of urinary tract infections. The bacterium is responsible for up to 80-95% of simple cystitides among otherwise normal patients. The frequency is lesser among patients who reside in hospital and whose urinary tract may be compromised by anatomical defects including the placement of a urinary catheter. The bacterium is also the most common cause of pyelonephritis and as a consequence may enter the bloodstream. In addition, *E. coli* has been touted as an uncommon cause of urethritis, but is an important pathogen in acute prostatitis. Urinary tract infections are more common among women perhaps as a simple consequence of the short urethra as well as the proximity of the urethra to fecal sources of the bacterium. Significant asymptomatic bacteriuria is deemed to be present when the organism is present in high numbers (e.g., $\geq 10^8$/L.) in a midstream urine sample and when this finding is reproducible in the context of the asymptomatic state. The latter is a risk factor for symptomatic urinary tract infections whether of the lower or upper pole. Pregnancy also increases the chance for *E. coli* urinary tract infections. In the elderly, asymptomatic colonization of the bladder by bacteria, especially *E. coli*, becomes much more common. The latter poses some risk for symptomatic disease, but is generally so common that treatment is not indicated.

E. coli has the potential to cause diarrhea by a variety of mechanisms and is clearly the most versatile bacterium in this regard (31). Whereas the bacterium is commonly a component of the normal gastrointestinal flora and, as such, is part of a natural defence mechanism which in fact prevents enteric pathogens from causing disease, various strains are capable of maintaining virulence factors which transform them into etiological agents of gastroenteritis. Enterohemorrhagic *E. coli* (EHEC) possess toxins (variably termed verotoxins, Shiga-like toxins, or Shiga-toxins) that are critical to the development of both local bowel pathology and systemic complications. EHEC mainly affect the large bowel. Although advanced disease not uncommonly presents in the form of a dysentery, which includes bloody diarrhea and mucous production (hence the term "enterohemorrhagic"), some patients will have but a mild watery diarrhea, and yet others may be relatively asymptomatic. The diarrheal illness may be accompanied by abdominal pain and emesis, and usually lasts for 2-5 days. Systemic complications mainly include the progression to hemolytic uremic syndrome (HUS) which includes the triad of microangiopathic hemolytic anemia, thrombocytopenia, and renal failure; EHEC-related HUS is among the most common causes of acute kidney failure in children that lead to the need (albeit usually temporary) for dialysis. Various forms of HUS may be incomplete, and some patients may have a greater degree of one manifestation than another, e.g., anemia and thrombocytopenia with little apparent renal disease. HUS occurs in approximately 3-10% of children who suffer from EHEC infections. Enterotoxigenic *E. coli* (ETEC) cause diarrhea that is secondary to the action of one of two toxins on the bowel. These bacteria may produce either a heat-labile or heat-stable enterotoxin, and the resulting disease is mainly a watery (non-bloody) diarrhea. ETEC infections are a major subset of 'turista' or traveller's diarrhea. Enteroinvasive *E. coli* (EIEC) behave similar to invasive shigellae and thus are able to cause a spectrum of illness which varies from watery to bloody diarrhea. Enteroaggregative *E. coli* (EAEC) strains have been found in association with acute and persistent diarrhea, although the number of normal carriers is usually high. The role played by diffuse adhering *E. coli* (DAEC) in diarrheal illnesses is not firmly established. The term enteroadherent *E. coli* has been practically abandoned because it included different diarrheagenic *E. coli* categories. As previously detailed, EPEC have a long history, but it is now acknowledged that this designation had been inclusive of many *E. coli* that were subsequently recognized to be EHEC, ETEC, and EIEC. EPEC generally cause a watery diarrhea.

Intra-abdominal infections with *E. coli* are often of mixed bacterial etiology. Both *E. coli* and these other bacteria arise from the normal intestinal flora. They may enter the abdominal cavity, liver, bowel wall, or bloodstream when the normal barrier is breached through trauma, surgery, or other cause for perforation. In this context, *E. coli* may cause synergistic infections with other gut flora such as anaerobes, enterococci, and streptococci. Spontaneous infections may arise during compromise of the normal intestinal blood flow and host defences, e.g., peritonitis during alcoholic liver disease.

The many other potential infections that *E. coli* may cause is somewhat reflective of the potential for other *Enterobacteriaceae*. The presence of *E. coli* in large quantity in the gastrointestinal tract ensures that it will be present and well- positioned to take advantage of an opportune moment. Accordingly, these other infections will include newborn sepsis (infant acquires the bacterium from a contaminated maternal genital tract), maternal obstetrical and gynecological infections, skin infections (especially around the buttocks and thighs in the form of decubitus ulceration), abscesses of internal organs (that are contiguous to the gastrointestinal tract), pneumonia (especially as a consequence of aspiration of gastric contents that have refluxed), among others.

Bacteremia may arise as a consequence of many of the latter infections.

E. vulneris, fergusonii, and *hermannii* are most often isolated in clinical specimens where they are not etiological agents of infection (32,33). For the few infections that occur, they are often of patients whose host defences are compromised. Citations of infection mostly include wounds (especially after trauma), central venous lines, urinary tract, and bowel-associated pathology.

2. *Salmonelloses*

Salmonellosis is a relatively common human infection. Although most commonly appreciated as a food-borne gastrointestinal illness, human *Salmonella* infection indeed takes various forms, many of which are non-intestinal. On a generic basis, salmonellosis may be divided into two broad groups of clinical entities: a) gastroenteritis-associated including complications, and b) typhoidal or enteric fever.

Gastroenteritis and associated complications

Enteritis occurs with most *Salmonella* infections including those that are more likely to be associated with typhoidal illnesses, but clinical symptomatology is quite variable. For illnesses that are associated with the common causes of salmonellosis, a diarrheal illness occurs. The symptoms often include abdominal pain and fever. The diarrhea may be watery and mild, or prolonged and associated with blood and mucous. The required inoculum for infection is usually >100 bacteria, but greater susceptibility to lower inocula may be associated with compromise in immunity or gastrointestinal function. Disease onset may occur in 1-8 days after ingestion but more typically after 48-72 hrs. Exposure to salmonellae does not consistently lead to infection, since a reasonable proportion will have transient carriage and no actual infection. Yet others may have a clinically silent infection. The duration of the diarrheal illness may range from 2-10 days, and most will be self-limited without any form of medical intervention. Likewise, the intensity of disease may be quite varied, e.g., a transient bloody diarrhea may be apparent for a single day in contrast to others who experience an advanced bloody colitis, i.e., dysentery. After disease resolution, a variable frequency of patients will become carriers of the bacterium for weeks to months. Thereafter, an active infection of the same nature will not occur during this carrier state, but systemic complications may rarely arise; as well, the patient will serve as a reservoir for the spread of infection to others as well as to food sources.

Complications from intestinal salmonellosis are much more likely to occur simultaneous with the acute diarrheal disease or at least within a short time thereafter (34). Most complications arise as a direct extension from the gastrointestinal tract via bloodstream. Most such extensions will simply be manifest with fever and general malaise, and the spread will be documented with a positive blood culture. There will often not be any focal infection as a consequence of the latter. In a small subset of patients, however, and especially those who are compromised (whether of immunity or bowel function), infants under the age of 1 yr., or the elderly, various infections of non-enteric sites will occur. These include almost every body tissue or space, but the more common include soft tissues, bone and joint, hepatobiliary and spleen, pulmonary (usually a secondary pneumonia or empyema), genital, central nervous system (especially meningitis), and vascular (including endocarditis). The urinary tract may be involved with either primary or secondary disease. Apart from increased risk for invasion among the latter groups, invasive complications can occur sporadically in seemingly normal individuals. Given the high frequency of enteric *Salmonella* infection in the general community, such complications are not necessarily a rarity. Apart from complications that involve actual infections of non-enteric sites, a reactive arthritis may occur among some within days to weeks after the enteritis is resolved.

Risk for severity of diarrheal disease and the likelihood of systemic complications are influenced by the particular species or serotype. Even for the same serotype, there may be variation in the occurrence of clinical manifestations among patients from different outbreaks.

Typhoid or enteric fever

Typhoid fever is typically caused by *S.* serotype Typhi or serotype Paratyphi, although there are several other serotypes that have been associated with enteric fever (35). It appears that most enteric fevers worldwide are related to *S.* serotype Typhi. Although the bowel may be involved in typhoid fever, patients often do not have diarrhea in contrast to most other salmonelloses. Typhoid fever is mainly a systemic illness, and the illness is marked by rapid entry of the bacterium into the circulation. Patients will often initially have fever and headache after an incubation period of 5 d. to 3 wks. The required inoculum is relatively less than that which is needed for other salmonelloses. As the disease progresses, patients may develop a cough, bradycardia, and some degree of confusion. Physical findings are limited: patients may have hepatosplenomegaly, and up to one-third may develop Rose spots (a red macular rash) on the skin. Untreated, typhoid fever will often resolve over several weeks, but patients may die during the course of the illness from circulatory collapse. Spread to various tissues can occur and result in complications such as abscesses of liver and spleen, as well as pericarditis. As late complications, bowel hemorrhage and perforation can occur even though a diarrheal illness has never been experienced. Chronic carriage of *S.* serotype Typhi can also arise after acute illnesses.

3. *Shigelloses*

Shigelloses are acquired with a small inoculum which may be as few as several organisms. The incubation period varies from 1-10 days but is most often in the range of 48-96 hrs. The resulting illness is mainly diarrheal and, like salmonelloses, the spectrum of intestinal illness is considerably variable. Nevertheless, it appears that most shigelloses are associated with a more aggressive illness which is often accompanied by fever, abdominal pain, and severe diarrhea. The disease is often categorized as a colitis. Severe diarrhea may be associated with marked dehydration and generalized toxemia. The fever may be sufficiently severe among young children and lead to seizures, although some degree of encephalopathy may be independent of fever. Most disease will be abacteremic, but bacteremia may occur and be associated with a prominent leukocytosis. It is uncommon to see direct consequences of blood-borne spread.

In regions where patients' underlying health status is compromised by malnutrition and lack of medical support, shigelloses are major etiological agents in gastroenteritides that are associated with death. *Shigella dysenteriae* in particular is capable of producing a toxin (Shiga toxin) that leads to the same pattern of systemic illness as enterohemorrhagic *E. coli*, i.e., HUS.

A post-infectious reactive arthritis uncommonly occurs. Chronic carriage is essentially not seen.

4. Yersinioses

The discussion herein relates to *Yersinia* spp. other than *Y. pestis*; the latter is discussed in Chapter 19. Gastrointestinal infection is by far the most common yersiniosis, and both *Y. enterocolitica* and *Y. pseudotuberculosis* are implicated (37,38). Other *Yersinia* spp. have rarely been associated with infection in general, and they are not diarrheal pathogens.

Gastroenteritides caused by *Y. enterocolitica* occur within a period of 2-7 days after initial ingestion, usually through a food-borne mechanism (37). Patients often have prominent abdominal pain with or without fever or emesis. The diarrheal illness itself is quite variable, analogous to the wide spectrum during salmonellosis or shigellosis, but yersiniosis tends to be more prolonged. Although the diarrhea may abate in 3-14 days, the overall illness may last for up to 3 wks. In its severe enteric form, the diarrheal illness is a dysentery. For some patients, disease may be relatively confined to the terminal ileum and hence mimic the regional enteritis of Crohn's disease; the latter is recurrent, however, whereas yersiniosis occurs in a single acute episode. Lymph nodes that drain the ileum or large bowel may be greatly inflamed, thus yielding the entity termed mesenteric adenitis. With either the bowel or mesenteric node involvement, the abdominal pain may be severe and mimic appendicitis (thereby termed pseudoappendicitis). Within days to weeks after the gastroenteritis is clinically resolved, post-infectious immunological sequelae occur among <10% of patients: these may include an arthropathy (especially in HLA-B27 positive individuals), erythema nodosum, and potential involvement of heart, kidney, and thyroid.

During the enteritis or through other mechanisms, *Y. enterocolitica* can become invasive. Most commonly, the latter will take the form of a bacteremia without a specific focus other than gut. Patients who have immune compromise (e.g., malignancies), liver dysfunction, impaired gastrointestinal tracts, and iron overload are especially at risk for these complications. The bacterium has been transmitted through blood transfusions; cold storage does not inhibit the bacterium's growth potential significantly. As a consequence of bacteremic spread, various sites may become involved with secondary infection including large blood vessels (i.e., vascular wall), bone, joint, liver, and central nervous system. Untreated, there is a strong potential for serious morbidity and mortality.

Y. pseudotuberculosis most often causes an intestinal illness as well. This bacterium does not nearly cause as many infections as *Y. enterocolitica*. The enteritis is especially associated with abdominal pain. Post-infectious sequelae as well as extraintestinal infections can occur but are proportionately rare. The species designation of 'pseudotuberculosis' has arisen as a consequence of the appearance of mesenteric lymphadenopathy.

5. Enterobacter

Of the *Enterobacter* spp., *E. cloacae* and to a lesser degree *E. aerogenes* are responsible for most disease (39). All enterobacters are opportunists, and thus are often associated with nosocomial infection. The latter are generally facilitated by the presence of medical devices such as urinary catheters, central venous lines, mechanical ventilation, among other instrumentations. These bacteria are part of the enteric flora, but become enriched when other normal enteric flora is suppressed by antibiotic use. Excess use of cephalosporins especially selects for enterobacters which are often resistant to first generation cephalosporins, and may become resistant to most cephalosporins when broad spectrum beta-lactamases are derepressed. Infections are more common among patients in intensive care, whether adult or neonatal, burn units, and oncology wards. Infections are most common in the urinary tract, lower respiratory tract (especially those who are intubated), wounds, intra-abdominal sites, and central nervous system. These bacteria may contaminate solutions that are used for parenteral nutrition. The "agglomerans" group of enterobacters are especially associated with contamination of infusate or associated administration devices.

6. *Serratia spp.*

S. marcescens accounts for the vast majority of *Serratia* infections (40). Like enterobacters, *S. marcescens* is mainly an opportunist and is an important cause of nosocomial infection. Here too, infection is fostered by medical devices, and antibiotics such as cephalosporins select for this infectious agent as well. *S. marcescens* is particularly resistant to various decontaminant solutions such as detergents and weak dilutions of many others. The spectrum of infections is more diverse than those of enterobacters. These may include urinary tract infections, wound infection, respiratory colonization or infection among those who are chronically ventilated, burns, superficial skin and wound infections, osteomyelitis, endocarditis among intravenous drug users, and blood-borne infections in the absence of a focus.

7. *Citrobacter spp.*

C. freundii causes most citrobacter infections, and although the risk factors for these infections are similar to *Serratia* and enterobacters, the frequency of citrobacter infections is considerably less. Infections occur especially in the urinary tract, respiratory tract (opportunistic), blood, and wounds (41). Infection among newborns in intensive care has been documented in epidemic form, and the latter not uncommonly includes the central nervous system.

Citrobacters with toxins that resemble those of enterohemorrhagic *E. coli* have been described and have been associated with diarrheal illnesses, but the latter are seemingly uncommon.

8. *Proteus group*

P. mirabilis causes most *Proteus* infections, and the vast majority of these are in the urinary tract (42). In otherwise well individuals, especially females, *P. mirabilis* is usually the cause of up to 3-10% of uncomplicated cystitides. As a group, *Proteus* infections are capable of complicating the urinary tract by facilitating stone formation through potent urease production (alkalinizing urine). *P. vulgaris* may be favoured in some urinary tract infections when antibiotics have been used in the presence of a urinary catheter. Infections of wounds, venous lines, and compromised respiratory tracts also occur, as does bacteremia as a consequence.

Morganella morganii behaves very similar to *Proteus* spp. in commonly being associated with urinary tract infections. *M. morganii* not uncommonly has multiple antibiotic resistance so that infection again is favoured by the use of an antibiotic during a time when the urinary tract is compromised, e.g., catheter. Various infections such as those for *Proteus* spp. are also seen but are relatively rare.

Providencia spp. also have a tendency to infect the urinary tract, and they are generally opportunists.

9. *Klebsiellae*

K. oxytoca and *K. pneumoniae* are the most common klebsiellae in human infection. Both of these are essentially opportunists and like many of the other *Enterobacteriaceae*, they are likely to cause nosocomial infection as a consequence of mechanical ventilation, instrumentation, use of other medical devices, and altered gastrointestinal structure and function (43). Both are commonly represented among the normal gut flora. Bacteremias due to the presence of central lines, urinary tract infections, surgical infections, and respiratory infections are most common. *K. pneumoniae* pneumonia is a classically de-scribed entity (Friedlander's pneumonia) which typically occurs among debilitated patients. Both *K. oxytoca* and *K. pneumoniae* are also seen as pathogens among newborns in intensive care. The liberal use of ampicillin in hospital settings selects for these klebsiellae since they are uniformly resistant to this antibiotic. This may explain their importance in neonatal intensive care where ampicillin and gen-tamicin are commonly used as first-line agents in early-onset sepsis.

K. ozaenae is associated with chronic atrophic rhinitis which imparts a putrid odor to the upper respiratory tract (44). The disease if often responsive to antibiotics. *K. rhinoscleromatis* is associated with another upper respiratory tract disease termed rhinoscleroma which is a chronic and deforming illness whereby granulomata form at the site of infection. It too is amenable to antibiotic therapy (45).

10. Edwardsiella

E. tarda is an uncommon cause of bacteremia, wound infections, and meningitis (46). It has been asso-ciated with diarrhea in areas of warm climate; the clinical illness resembles gastrointestinal salmonello-ses.

11. Others

Among the many other species of *Enterobacteriaceae*, clinical infection is quite uncommon, and these bacteria, although present in specimens such as wounds and stools, are often of unknown significance. Some are rare opportunists and uncommon nosocomial pathogens.

An association of *Budvicia*, *Buttiauxella*, *Leminorella*, *Moellerella*, and *Trabulsiella* with disease is most often dubious.

Hafnia alvei is an accepted, albeit uncommon, nosocomial pathogen and has been associated with respiratory, urinary tract, blood-borne, wound, and central nervous system infections. There has been some concern that a variant of *H. alvei* causes diarrhea, but recent work has demonstrated that the strains under study were biochemical variants of *E. coli* (47).

Pantoea spp. have been somewhat newly designated and were formerly of the "*Enterobacter ag-glomerans* group". Studies of genetic relationships indicated that some biogroups among the diverse *E. agglomerans* group had sufficient homology to form these species. They are opportunists and have been associated with urinary tract, wound, and respiratory infections.

Other uncommon species and disease associations include:

Cedecea spp.	bacteremia, respiratory infections
Erwinia spp.	urinary tract infection
Ewingella sp.	bacteremia, respiratory infections, wound infections
Kluyvera spp.	nosocomial infections
Leclercia sp.	bacteremia, respiratory infections
Rahnella sp.	nosocomial infections
Tatumella sp.	bacteremia, respiratory infections, urinary tract infections
Yokenella sp.	respiratory infections, urinary tract infections, wounds

B. Non-*Enterobacteriaceae* enteric pathogens and related bacteria

1. Vibrios

V. cholerae

Different antigenic and bio- types have been etiological agents of diarrhea throughout the world, and their dominance during epidemics over the last century has been variable. The classical O1 serogroup was of major concern on the Indian subcontinent, but subsequent epidemic activity has occurred with the El Tor and O139 'Bengal' variants. Historically, it was observed that the El Tor biotype was associated with milder disease, but recent pandemics have shown that all three of these *V. cholerae* variants are capable of causing severe illnesses.

This species is typically associated with severe watery diarrhea, but indeed there is considerable variability in the gastrointestinal illness (48). In fact, most of the acquisitions will lead to no disease at all or a relatively mild illness. Less than 10-20% will develop classical cholera, and most of these will do well with antibiotic therapy and adequate hydration. Unfortunately, this infrequency will yet necessarily translate into many severe and even lethal infections given that pandemics include many thousands of infections in regions of the world that are over-crowded or are served with inadequate water supplies.

The infectious dose is high (usually $>10^5$ bacteria), although lower quantities may be infectious when the otherwise inhibitory acid of the stomach is neutralized. The incubation period is usually 1-5 days. Patients will often have mild to moderate abdominal cramping with or without emesis. Initial stools will purge the bowel of its contents, and subsequent stools will be mainly watery and pale ('rice-water' stools). The disease does not evolve into a dysentery. In severe illnesses, the amount of fluid loss is dramatic and may include the depletion of several litre equivalents in a few hours. Continuing major fluid loss leads to severe dehydration over hours to a few days. Patients may develop shock due to low circulating blood volume, and electrolyte imbalances may occur as a complication. Rehydration efforts must recreate the balance of fluid and electrolytes. All of these manifestations are due to the cholera toxin's localized effect on the small intestine which is the primary site of infection. Despite the severity for some of these illnesses and despite the high quantity of bacterium in the gut lumen, toxigenic *V. cholerae* does not enter the blood or cause metastatic infection.

Some *V. cholerae* strains do not produce toxin but yet may be associated with a mild diarrheal illness. These bacteria may cause wound infections and subsequent bacteremia as is seen for several of the non-cholera vibrios.

Non-cholera vibrios

There are many non-cholera vibrios which cause human disease, but the absolute number of such illnesses is relatively small (49). In general, and like *V. cholerae*, acquisition is usually linked to contact with saline sea waters or the ingestion of marine sources of food (e.g., raw oysters) that have been inadequately cooked. Most of these have been associated with diarrhea, but the severity of these illnesses does not approach the severe watery diarrhea of cholera. Severity is more likely to be linked with systemic spread. Although outbreaks of these infections can occur, the numbers are very much less than the epidemic and pandemic activity that may be seen with cholera.

V. parahemolyticus causes diarrhea, wound infections, otitis, and superficial ophthalmological infections. In contrast to cholera, fluid loss is not overly problematic, but the diarrheal illness may mimic other forms of colitis with the potential outcome of having blood and mucous in stools. Fever and abdominal pain tend to be more severe. *V. vulnificus* causes sepsis and wound infections. Bacteremia tends to occur in those who have underlying liver dysfunction and has a high fatality rate. Wound infection can rapidly progress to bullous lesions and cellulitis. *V. mimicus*, *V. alginolyticus*, *V. fluvialis*, *V. damsela*, and *V. hollisae* are variably associated with diarrhea, wound infection, otitis externa, and bacteremia. *V. cincinnatiensis* and *V. carchariae* have rarely been associated with infection. It is debatable whether *V. furnissii* is an etiological agent of gastroenteritis.

2. Campylobacter spp.

C. jejuni and to a lesser extent *C. coli* have been associated with community-acquired gastroenteritis. *C. jejuni* usually ranks among the top three diarrheal pathogens in developed countries thoughout the world. Gastroenteritides are often sporadic, but epidemic disease is well-detailed. The bacterium may also be acquired as a form of traveller's diarrhea. Typical *C. jejuni* infections are preceded by fever and abdominal pain; the incubation period is usually 24-72 hrs. (50). Most illnesses are self-limited over 1-7 days. The spectrum of gastroenteritis is somewhat analogous to salmonellosis: the majority are watery diarrheal illnesses, but dysentery is possible. Systemic spread occurs, although the frequency at which this occurs is likely to be underestimated since patients' blood is not often cultured during gastroentertides, and since campylobacters do not grow well in conventional blood culture media. Nevertheless, systemic complications that are due to spread from active gastrointestinal infection appears to occur in less than 1-2%. Bacteremia and central nervous system infection are more likely to occur in those who are immunocompromised. Late non-infectious complications can include reactive arthritis, renal dysfunction (e.g., HUS), and Guillain-Barre disease (ascending neuropathy).

Numerically, *C. coli* infection is not nearly as common as that due to *C. jejuni*, and it appears to be mainly causative of gastroenteritides.

C. fetus is less often a cause of diarrhea, and the clinical illness of gastroenteritis is variable. There are many citations, however, of invasive disease despite the infrequency of intestinal infections (51). These invasive illnesses are more likely to occur among patients whose health is compromised. Bacteremia, septic miscarriages, endocarditis, and meningitis have all been recorded.

Both *C. upsaliensis* and *C. lari* are uncommon causes of diarrhea and are capable of causing bacteremic sepsis (52,53).

3. Helicobacter spp.

Although *H. pylori* (see Chapter 20) is the major pathogen in this genus, there are now several *Helicobacter* spp. that have been identified as minor gastrointestinal pathogens which are capable of becoming blood-borne. These include *H. cinaedi*, *H. fennelliae*, *H. westmeadii*, and *Helicobacter* sp. strain Mainz (54-56). Bacteremia is most often seen among compromised patients and mainly among those who are HIV-infected. *H. pullorum* and *H. canis* have rarely been associated with gastroenteritis. Several of these species have formerly been designated as *Campylobacter* spp., but the advent of more precise molecular definition and the availability of more isolates to use for these studies have facilitated a better understanding of their placement.

4. Arcobacter spp.

This genus is represented by the species *A. butzleri* and *A. cryaerophilus*. Again, both of these bacteria were formerly in the genus *Campylobacter* and indeed share many phenotypic attributes. Both are uncommon diarrheal pathogens and are capable of causing bacteremia. *A. butzleri* has been associated with other systemic illnesses (e.g., peritonitis, endocarditis) in a few patients.

5. Aeromonas spp.

Applied systematics for this genus have been a challenge, and there are several species that have been associated with human disease (57). Fortunately, most of the changes in nomenclature have not applied to the two most common clinical isolates: *A. hydrophila* and *A. caviae*. Both of these species are not uncommonly isolated from stool specimens of individuals with a diarrheal disease. *A. caviae* seems to be relatively non-pathogenic and is likely a fortuitous finding in most circumstances despite some claims that it may be an etiological agent of gastroenteritis. *A. hydrophila* seems to be better justified as a gastrointestinal pathogen, but even so, there are publications of contradictory evidence. *A. hydrophila* can be isolated from asymptomatic individuals, and volunteer studies have not been consistent in demonstrating a cause-and-effect relationship. When *A. hydrophila* is isolated in moderate to large quantities in the context of a diarrheal illness, the clinical course is often relatively benign, and most illnesses consist of a watery diarrhea which is self-limited over the course of a few days.

Both *A. hydrophila* and *A. caviae*, in addition to the other *Aeromonas* spp., are capable of being etiological agents in many other forms of infection. With respect to *A. hydrophila*, these non-intestinal infections do not seem to arise from a preceding or existing gastroenteritis. Non-intestinal infections are more likely to occur among patients who are compromised such as those with liver disease, malignancies, or immunocompromise otherwise. When infection occurs, it is usually somewhat aggressive in its course, and the bacterium can invade blood and lead to bone and joint infection, peritonitis, meningitis, and endocarditis. Superficial skin infections may rapidly progress to cellulitis. Injuries are common reasons for wound and ocular infection. The bacteria can cause respiratory infections and cholecystitis as a consequence of entry from the contiguous areas of mouth or gastrointestinal tract. Invasive *Aeromonas* infections may be associated with considerable morbidity unless attended to promptly.

6. Pleisiomonas

Contact and infection with this bacterium appears to be relatively uncommon in developed countries (58); infection is more often seen in warmer climates. Although uncommon, *P. shigelloides* does seem to be justifiably designated as a gastrointestinal pathogen. Bacteremic illnesses and meningitis are rare but severe.

III. EPIDEMIOLOGY OF INFECTION

A. Enterobacteriaceae

These bacteria are commonly carried in the intestinal tract of humans in high numbers with some exceptions. They are also carried at times on the hands, skin (especially about the pelvis), oropharynx, and genital tract. It is not surprising therefore that direct person-to-person transmission, especially for those species that are components of the normal body flora, should occur and that these bacteria should then serve as major nosocomial pathogens. The latter is on account of both endogenous and exogenous sources. It is not uncommon to find a wider distribution of coliforms on the body among the elderly and especially those in nursing homes.

Several of the *Enterobacteriaceae* also constitute a part of the normal microbial flora of animals; there may be a tendency for some to colonize particular animals more than others. Some also are not uncommonly found on plants and in soil. Thus, there is plenty of opportunity for these bacteria to taint water and food supplies. For those of animal or human source in particular, quantitations in potable water are an indication of the degree of fecal contamination (and hence safety).

The epidemiology of key enteric pathogens is discussed below. In general, however, there is obviously under-recognition and hence under-reporting of diarrheal illnesses. In essentially every major population of the world, these enteric pathogens cause disease. There is often a peak of associated gastroenteritides in the summer months when warmer climate facilitates practices that enhance transmission. Occupational exposure and a role for animal meat processing practices which largely distribute these bacteria are important. Although acquisition of enteric pathogens most often occurs from the food or water itself, some may cause infection after relatively low inocula and thus person-to-person transmission can occur, e.g., for shigellosis and enterohemorrhagic *E. coli*. It is very uncommon to see enteric pathogens cause nosocomial infection especially in developed countries where water and food hygiene is relatively well-guarded.

Typing systems have been devised for all common *Enterobacteriaceae* as discussed later and in Chapter 7. For the purposes of diarrheal pathogens especially, there is a major role for ongoing surveillance of contemporary isolates so that outbreaks, or sporadic but common source infections, may be determined. The vehicles of food and water have the potential to disseminate pathogens to large populations in short order.

1. E. coli

Acquisition of enteric *E. coli* pathogens is most often a function of residence or visitation to areas that are endemic. All of the various *E. coli* that cause diarrhea may be acquired as a form of traveller's diarrhea even though this entity has been traditionally linked with the enterotoxigenic *E. coli*.

Enterohemorrhagic *E. coli* include numerous serotypes although *E. coli* O157:H7 is the most prominent pathogen in developed countries. Infection has been documented throughout the world. Bovine sources are particularly incriminated in transmission (59), but a number of other animals have occasionally carried EHEC, e.g., other farm animals, deer, and horses. Humans do not commonly carry these bacteria chronically, although excretion after acute infection may last for several weeks. Secondary contamination of food products has been linked to massive outbreaks, e.g., via milk, water, processed meat products, sprouts, apple cider, various vegetables, and fruit. There is a summertime peak for both EHEC infection and the associated complication of HUS. Farm families who have livestock are at much greater risk for infection. Person-to-person spread of EHEC can occur from actively infected patients, especially children.

EPEC were traditionally coined on the basis of finding seemingly epidemic strains of *E. coli* among newborns and infants. EPEC infection, however, does occur sporadically, and outbreaks in other populations have been detailed. The epidemiology of EPEC in contemporary times is markedly skewed by changes in the diagnostic laboratory. Decades ago, it was not uncommon for stools from children to be screened for EPEC by serological methods; these methods (as detailed later) were time-consuming. After it was recognized that many presumed EPEC serotype isolates were non-pathogens (i.e., non-specificity of serotyping to find a true EPEC) and since reliable antisera have become less available, most pediatric centres have ceased screening for EPEC by this approach. Requests to search for these pathogens have become a rarity. EPEC are a leading cause of infantile diarrhea in developing countries. The frequency of EPEC infections in developed countries started to fall in the 1960s and is currently relatively rare. The main risk factors for EPEC infection in developing countries are the high endemicity in large unban centres, previous hospital admission, and poverty. Transmission of EPEC is fecal-oral via contaminated hands, weaning foods, and fomites. The reservoir of EPEC is symptomatic or asymptomatic children and asymptomatic adult carriers. Animals are not a source of EPEC since their EPEC-like strains belong to serotypes that are not associated with human infections.

ETEC are the principal agents of traveller's diarrhea, and they are an important cause of childhood diarrhea in the developing world. The most common vehicles for ETEC infections are food and water that have been contaminated by human feces. ETEC infections are rare in developed countries, but several foodborne outbreaks have been recorded. Person-to-person transmission seems not to occur. The infective doses in adult volunteers is high. ST-producing ETEC cause the majority of endemic illnesses.

The epidemiology of EAEC is largely unknown, but it has been demonstrated that these bacteria have the ability to cause endemic diarrhea, mainly persistent diarrhea, among children. Several EAEC diarrheal outbreaks also have been documented. Interestingly enough, it has been suggested that EAEC infection in children may be associated with developmental delay regardless of the presence of diarrheal symptoms.

EIEC is a well-established category of pathogen and is associated with endemic diarrhea and food and waterborne outbreaks. The prevalence of EIEC may be high in people who are living in poor hygienic conditions.

The role played by DAEC in diarrhea is still controversial.

2. Salmonellosis

Human-to-human transmission is much less a problem for salmonellae that cause diarrhea, but it is nevertheless of concern for transmission of typhoid fever bacilli. Food acquisition is the major mechanism, and both poultry and raw eggs are the most important sources (60). Outbreaks are often traced to food from restaurants, but large scale outbreaks in the community have been linked to commonly-consumed items such as dairy products (even seemingly pasteurized milk), sprouts, processed meat, and water. There is less seasonality in the occurrence of salmonellosis. Maternal-newborn transmission at the time of birth has been documented. Asymptomatic human carriage may occur after an acute illness, and such carriage may last for months to years in a small proportion of patients. Both cold-blooded and warm-blooded animals may also serve as reservoirs. Much recent attention has been given to domestic and exotic animals as a reservoir as illustrated in Table 3. The value for serological typing has been evident since ongoing monitoring of these subtypes may allow for recognition of new foci or major changes with existing foci.

    S. serotype Typhi is endemic especially in Africa, Central America, India, and large regions of southeast Asia, although on a historic basis, endemic typhoid fever was found in most parts of the world. Much of the sporadic disease and many outbreaks continue in highly endemic regions as the spread of the bacterium occurs both through food and water sources. *S.* serotype Typhi in the highly developed regions of the world is most often imported. Humans serve as the major reservoir for re-entry of the typhoid bacilli into the water supply and other areas of the environment. Not only does person-to-person spread occur, but *S.* serotype Typhi in particular poses a hazard to patient caregivers and as well to laboratory staff who handle pure cultures. Drug resistance to the most commonly used antibiotics has emerged (26), and this is not surprising given the large burden of disease that continues and which must be treated. Chronic carriage among a small proportion ensures that the bacterium will be available to continue contamination when sanitary conditions are poor. Typhoid vaccines have been produced, but although these may be used for patients from developed countries who travel, they unfortunately have not been available to those in greatest need; as well, break-though inefficacy remains a concern.

3.   Shigellosis

Shigellae are also acquired mainly from contaminated food and water, and travel to endemic areas is a risk factor (62). Human-to-human transmission occurs mostlikely as a consequence of the low inoculum that is required to initiate disease. Long-term human carriage is the exception. Infection is more likely to occur during warmer times of the year.

    In developed countries, *S. sonnei* has become the most common *Shigella* spp. isolate. *S. dysenteriae* (Shiga bacillus) is more common in areas with inadequate resources for water supply and for

Table 3   Salmonella serotypes that have been isolated from salmonelloses which are related to exotic pets in Canada during the period 1991-1996. Data are abstracted from a report of the National Laboratory for Enteric Pathogens, Canada (61). Serotypes are designated as common names rather than in serotype nomenclature for the sake of brevity.

Chameleon	*S. houten*
Frog	*S. ealing*
Hedgehog	*S. tilene, S. typhimurium*
Iguana	*S. abaetetuba, S. anatum, S. cerro, S. chameleon, S. florida, S. fluntern, S. houten, S. javiana, S. kralendyk, S. manhattan, S. marina, S. muenchen, S. newport, S. poona, S. phoenix, S. rubislaw, S. wassenaar*
Lizard	*S. ealing, S. muenchen, S. panama, S. poona, S. wassenaar*
Snake	*S. lome, S. newport, S. panama*
Sugar glider	*S. tilene*
Turtle	*S. ealing, S. java, S. javiana, S. litchfield, S. jangwani, S. miami, S. monschaui, S. muenchen, S. muenster, S. newport, S. panama, S. pomona, S. poona, S. phoenix, S. rubislaw, S. stanley*

other similar hygienic needs; an association with HUS has long been known, and the disease is identical to that which is caused by EHEC.

4. *Yersiniosis*

Pathogenic *Y. enterocolitica* is acquired from animals, especially porcine, who are mainly colonized (2). Although acquisition can be direct from the animal source, transmission more commonly occurs from a tainted food source. Non-pathogenic *Y. enterocolitica* and non-pathogenic *Yersinia* spp. otherwise are commonly found in the environment including water and soil. There is some degree of serogroup specificity among *Y. enterocolitica* for different animals. Serogroups O3, O8, and O9 are the most common among pathogenic isolates from Europe and North America.

Y. pseudotuberculosis is much less common as a pathogen, and there are proportionately fewer outbreaks. Bovine sources are important, as is milk, as the particular vehicles for transmission. A wide variety of animals are capable of carrying the bacterium, including those that are domestic, and birds have also been implicated.

5. *Edwardsiella*

These bacteria have been found among both cold-blooded and warm-blooded animals, particularly fish and reptiles.

B. Non-*Enterobacteriaceae* enteric pathogens and related bacteria

1. *Vibrios*

Vibrios, including *V. cholerae*, are commonly found in the marine environment and especially among ocean waters of warmer climates, e.g., tropical and near-tropical (63). The burden of vibrios is influenced by climate-induced changes and such an influence, e.g., warming of water due to shifting ocean currents as expressed in the recent El Nino phenomenon, has been used to partially explain the recent pandemic of cholera in Central and South America. Water and food, e.g., crustaceans and molluscs, from such marine sources, as well as food that has been contaminated by marine water, are commonly implicated in the transmission of *V. cholerae*. Human asymptomatic carriage, although described, is relatively uncommon, and there are no known animal reservoirs. It is unclear how the bacterium is maintained between epidemic cycles. During epidemic activity, diarrheal stools contain high numbers of bacteria and serve to perpetuate transmission when waters are seeded. A partially protective vaccine is available, but it is not clear that there is a role for major interruption of pandemics. The roles of maintaining a good water and food supply, and of active treatment of cholera illnesses with antibiotics, cannot be underestimated. Changes in the antigenicity of *V. cholerae* isolates from different pandemics has been proposed as the mechanism by which such activity is renewed. For example, it has been proposed that *V. cholerae* O139 has arisen as a consequence of antigenic variation of the O1-El Tor biotype (65).

Non-cholera vibrios are also found in marine waters, but their distribution world-wide is much greater. Apart from ingestion via food and water, contact with these bacteria may occur during recreational events in marine waters. Geographic variation in some infections may be a direct reflection of food habits, e.g., consumption of raw seafood in Japan.

2. *Campylobacters*

The epidemiology of campylobacterioses in many ways parallels that of salmonelloses (64). Food acquisition is common especially from poultry sources; both milk and water are important vehicles as well. Numerous other animals may harbour campylobacters, especially *C. jejuni*, including ovine, porcine, bovine, canine (including domestic), and feline sources. There is a predominance of disease in the summertime as influenced by changes in food preparation. Children are more commonly affected by a

C. jejuni gastroenteritis that requires investigation or treatment. *C. jejuni* is also a common cause of traveller's diarrhea.

C. coli infection is much less common that that from *C. jejuni* (ratios in developed countries are often 1:20-1:50 respectively), and porcine reservoirs are mostly implicated. *C. lari* has been found in birds (including poultry) and domestic cats and dogs. *C. fetus* has been documented among several animal sources.

3. *Helicobacter* spp.

Both *H. cinaedi* and *H. fennelliae* have caused systemic and gastrointestinal infection among patients who have been HIV-infected. It is unclear whether there is any particular tropism to such patients or whether the infections occur as a result simply of more frequently encountering these bacteria though sexual practices of homosexual males. *H. cinaedi* has also been cultured from hamsters.

4. *Arcobacter* spp.

These are generally found among the same animal reservoirs as *C. jejuni*.

5. *Aeromonas* spp.

Aeromonads are ubiquitous. They are found in fresh water sources including potable water. They may also be present in sewage and marine environments. Human and animal gastrointestinal carriage does occur. When asymptomatic carriage is determined among humans, the species most often found is usually *A. caviae*. Therefore, the finding of aeromonads in stool specimens does not incriminate these bacteria in a setting of gastroenteritis.

6. *Pleisiomonas*

P. shigelloides is found in fresh water sources and among numerous animals and fish.

IV. NATURE OF THE BACTERIUM, PATHOGENESIS, AND CLINICAL MANIFESTATIONS

A. *Enterobacteriaceae*

These bacteria are Gram negative rods that maintain the classic coliform morphology when viewed microscopically. They grow well on readily available non-selective laboratory media including MacConkey's medium. They ferment sugars and are oxidase-negative. G+C content is approximately 50%. Members of this family have homology with the type species *E. coli*.

In common with other Gram negative bacteria, these organisms have a double cell membrane (inner and outer membrane) (Figure 5); the periplasmic space between these membranes often maintains critical enzymes such as beta-lactamases. Lipopolysaccharides, porins, and various outer membrane proteins are important constituents that generally factor into the pathogenesis of infection especially when the disease is invasive. The surface of these Gram negative bacteria is highly convoluted and provides for considerable surface area to facilitate exchange with the environment and contact with the host (Figure 6). Motility is variable and is based on the presence of flagellae.

Fimbriae serve to facilitate attachment for many species in this group (Figure 7) (66,67). Some of these adhesins are critical to *E. coli* enteropathogens and serve as "colonization factors" (e.g., CFA I and CFA II for some EPEC). Yet others may contribute to attachment with uroepithelial cells and thus provide a virulence factor for urinary tract infections (P fimbriae). Genetic exchange between organisms within species may be enhanced with pili which morphologically resemble fimbrial attachment proteins.

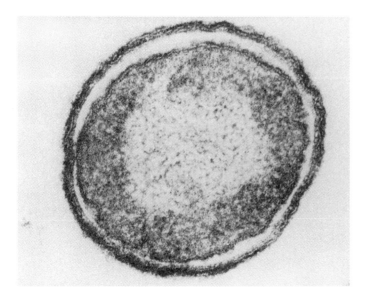

Figure 5 Electronmicrograph of *E. coli* in cross-section which illustrates the presence of inner and outer membranes.

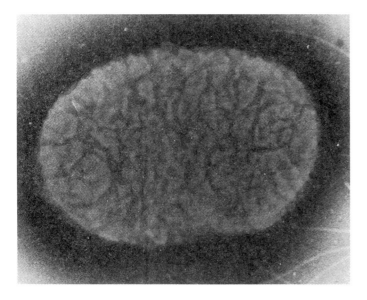

Figure 6 Electronmicrograph of the surface of an *E. coli* isolate demonstrating the highly convoluted bacterial surface.

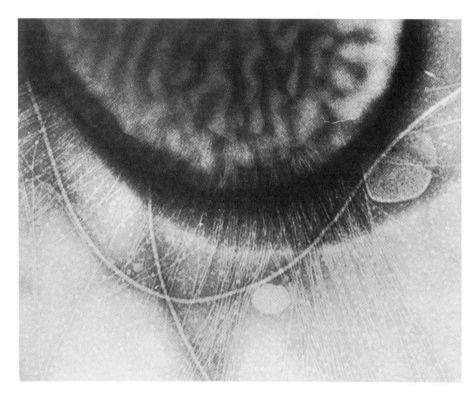

Figure 7   Electronmicrograph of a *Proteus mirabilis* isolate which demonstrates the presence of multiple fimbriae in addition to flagellae.

Lipopolysaccharides (LPS) are in part composed of a lipid A unit and core polysaccharide that may function as endotoxin which has a variety of important physiological effects – these include production and release of various cytokines including tumour necrosis factor, complement activation, activation of kinins, and impact on coagulation and fibrinolysis (68). LPS appears to be pivotal in the initiation of Gram negative shock (also referred to as endotoxic shock), and current work continues to emphasize the role of cytokines as well as nitric oxide and eicosanoids in the molecular pathogenesis (69,70). LPSs may, in addition, have variable long polysaccharide repeat chains. The latter are not uncommonly cross-reactive between species. Variability in these long chains (O side chain) provides for heterogeneity in the subsequent immunological (antibody) responses, and hence provides the basis for typing schemes which indeed have had much historical importance, e.g., *E. coli* and *Salmonella* O typing. Other antigens that have been used for the latter purpose include the flagellar antigens (much less variation than LPS) and capsular (K) antigen (although presumably polysaccharide, these have also included surface proteins and some other structures less commonly).

This group of bacteria has the ability to produce a large number of toxins and extracellular enzymes that either act in large part singly or in concert with various other virulence factors. These can include intracellular toxins, cytotoxins, and hemolysins.

When plasmid analysis has been conducted, most species frequently contain plasmids, and these can potentially carry genes that are critical to pathogenesis, e.g., some EPEC, and especially antimicrobial resistance, e.g., aminoglycoside-modifying genes.

1. Escherichia spp.

The non-*coli* species (*E. hermannii*, *E. fergusonii*, and *E. vulneris*) are not commonly associated with human infection, and hence, they have been barely studied in contrast to *E. coli* which continues to be the focus for many interests. Several virulence factors have been detailed for *E. coli* that are pathogens in many forms of illness. Apart from these particular virulence factors as detailed below, there are many other attributes which may prove to benefit the bacterium in particular circumstances. These include rapid grow rate and response to the environment, motility, variable hemolysis, ubiquity as a component of normal flora, relative resistance to decontaminating agents, possession of endotoxin, ability to evolve antimicrobial resistance, among other factors. In most infections, *E. coli* induces the recruitment of a pyogenic response.

The role of attachment to eukaryotic cells has been highlighted in the study of uropathogenic *E. coli*. In particular, a role for P fimbriae has been accepted, and cellular receptors and their biochemistry have been studied. The designation 'P' for these bacterial attachment factors arises from their ability to bind to P blood group (sialosyl galactosyl globoside) antigens which, apart from their abundance among red blood cells, are present on the surfaces of uroepithelial cells (71,72). Such receptors may explain the differences in likelihood among patients to develop urinary tract infections, especially for those with recurrent disease and in the absence of urinary tract anomalies. Although bacteria with these adhesin capabilities are found more often among isolates from urinary tract infections (UTI), they are nevertheless also common among routine stool isolates. Serotypes of bacteria from both UTI and bowel flora are generally in common. Although adhesion does appear to have a major role in the pathogenesis of urinary tract infections, it has become evident that the disease process is multifactorial and includes an interaction between bacterium and host that is affected by fimbriae, aerobactin, hemolysins, bacterial capsule, and serum resistance. The pattern of UTI may be determined by the complexity of such virulence factors among the offending bacteria (73-75). For *E. coli* isolates from adult males with acute prostatitis, there also appear to be important roles for virulence factors such as adhesins and perhaps even cytotoxins (76).

EIEC invade eukaryotic cells in a mechanism that is quite similar to that of most *Shigella* species. Most EIEC belong to relatively few serotypes. Historically, the definition of invasiveness was in part determined by the ability to induce clinical manifestations in the Sereny test. The molecular basis for invasion has since been explored, and it appears that invasion is dependent on the presence of invasion factors termed *ipa* (invasion plasmid antigens) which are coded for by a 130 Mda plasmid that is common among EIEC (77,78). *IpaH* is copied multiple times and can also exist on the chromosome (79). The invasion plasmid may be lost with in vitro passage of these isolates. Invasion of colonic epithelium is accompanied by a strong polymorphonuclear response, and the histopathology of infection is essentially that of an inflammatory colitis.

ETEC also tend to belong to a few serogroups. Attachment factors play a role in their proclivity to cause intestinal disease; fimbriae [CFA I and CFA II (Colonization Factor Antigen)] are antigenically variable and susceptible to change in vivo (80). Type-specific immunity occurs. ETEC produce one of two enterotoxins (LT and ST) which are critical to pathogenesis. LT is in many ways similar to cholera toxin, and it takes the form of A and B subunits which are responsible for toxin attachment and intracellular derangement respectively. Intracellular events are associated with cAMP modulation and its consequences. ST is comparatively a much smaller molecule, and its stability is a function of considerable cross-linking. The latter acts through cGMP-activated pathways. Both toxins act by affecting fluid excretion at the cellular level with the net outflow of fluid and electrolytes into the intestinal lumen (81). The bowel wall is not infiltrated with inflammatory cells, therefore, in contrast to the illnesses that are attributable to EIEC or EHEC.

EPEC are characterized by their attaching and effacing manner of association with the host cell (31). In this association, the microvilli are disrupted from the apical membrane which then curves around the bacteria to form pedestal structures (9). Along with the bacterial attachment, intracellular events take place with respct to actin aggregation. It has been suggested that the bacterium may be responsible for directing its own attachment by sending a receptor to the eukaryotic membrane. These interactions with the host cell appear to stimulate a number of intracellular signal transduction pathogeways (83). All proteins that are necessary for the A/E phenotype are encoded by genes which are found within a pathogenicity island called LEE (Locus of Enterocyte Effacement) which can be inserted at different sites in the *E. coli* chromosome. The *eae* LEE gene is responsible for the protein called intimin which belongs to a family of proteins that resemble the *Yersinia* invasin protein and which promotes eukaryotic cell attachment and invasion (82). In vitro, attachment and effacement is usually demonstrated with the use of either HeLa or Hep2 cells. Among the several EPEC serotypes, some possess the *eaf* plasmid (typical EPEC) while others do not posses this plasmid (atypical EPEC). In some countries, e.g., England, *eaf*–positive serotypes are rarely isolated. In fact, less than 10% of the EPEC strains in England have the *eaf* plasmid. In Brazil, however, and probably in other developing countries, the *eaf*-psotive serotypes are still more common. The *eaf*-positive EPEC show the localized adherence pattern which is mediated by the BFP fimbriae that are encoded by the EAF plasmid. The adherence pattern that is expressed by the *eaf* negative EPEC is different and has been called LA-like (LAL). This LAL pattern seems to be mediated mainly by intimin (86). At the clinical level, the above interplay between host and bacterium results in altered fluid and electrolyte balance, and hence the production of a watery diarrhea; although bacterial products may invade cells, it is not apparent that invasion occurs to the extent as is seen with EIEC. Two other forms of eukaryotic cell attachment include: enteroaggregative attachment (84) and diffuse adherence that has been found in association with EPEC and other E. coli categories (85,87).

Enteroaggregative *E. coli* have been more strongly linked with diarrheal illnesses especially those that are chronic among children in the developing world (88), but evidence to the contrary has also been published (89,90). The pattern of attachment to eukaryotic cells is unique in that palisade aggregates of the bacterium are seen in contrast to the clustering that is apparent for localized adherence. Enteroaggregative *E. coli* can be asymptomatically carried in the gastrointestinal tract (91). The ability to demonstrate aggregative adherence is susceptible to methodological variation (92). Adherence is a plasmid-associated feature (93) and may be due to a unique outer membrane protein (94). It has been proposed that some enteroaggregative *E. coli* produce a heat-stable toxin; the presence or absence of this toxin may explain why not all enteroaggregative *E. coli* are necessarily etiological agents of diarrhea (90). Of classic EPEC serogroups, up to 10% may have DNA sequences which are associated with the aggregative adherence (87). The pathogenesis is otherwise poorly understood.

Diffuse adherence has been inconsistently associated with gastroenteritis, and the evidence to date which favours a causative role has linked this phenotype with illness in young children (96). Diffuse adherence is identified by the broad pattern of adherence to cultured cells. It is not clear that all putative diffusely adhering *E. coli* are able to attach by a common mechanism. Recent work has indicated that a particular family of adhesins is relevant and that these *E. coli* contain a homologue of the LEE locus that is otherwise seen with EPEC (85). The latter would be consistent with the watery nature of diarrhea that has been seen among some patients.

Cytolethal distending toxin (CLDT) appears to have been first observed in an isolate of *E. coli* O55 (97). It is a heat-labile toxin which is characterized by its ability to cause elongation and distension of susceptible eucaryotic cells (e.g., Chinese hamster ovary, HeLa, or HEp-2) over the first 24 hrs. and then continuing distension and ultimate cell death within the subsequent 24-48 hrs. (98). CLDT has biological properties in common with a family of similar toxins that are found in other bacteria (99). The toxin interrupts the cell cycle at the G2/M phase. The initial in vitro toxin effects on Chinese hamster ovary cells are similar to those which is seen with the *E. coli* heat-labile toxin. Few studies have assessed the relevance of this toxin to diarrheal illnesses, but a study among young children in Bangladesh recently demonstrated the greater frequency of CLDT-bearing *E. coli* in symptomatic patients than among controls (100). Pathogenesis and pathology are not well-characterized.

Cytotoxic necrotizing factor (CNF) was described in the 1980s (101) and exists in two forms: CNF1 and CNF2. These toxins are proteins which activate in mammalian cells to cause actin cytoskeleton reorganization. They deamidate Rho proteins which affect cell cytoskeleton regulation in several ways (102). The presence of CNFs is highly linked to the presence of hemolysins and, to a lesser extent, a novel cytolethal distending factor and an adhesin (103). It is unclear how these virulence traits may or may not work in concert. The role of CNF-producing *E. coli* in acute or chronic diarrhea is still awaiting confirmation. Nevertheless, it is not uncommon to find isolates from extra-intestinal infections that are capable of producing these toxins, and indeed they were found very early on to be present among uropathogenic *E. coli*.

EHEC have been well-studied perhaps due to concerns for the potential consequences of HUS and, in part, due to the numerous outbreaks that have been recorded in the last decade (104-106). A family of toxins, termed verotoxins (VT), Shiga-like toxins, or Shiga toxins, are the major virulence factors. The most important of these for human isolates is VT1 and VT2, and VT2 production in particular has been associated with a somewhat greater risk for progression of the gastroenteritis to HUS. VT1 is essentially identical to the Shiga toxin of *Shigella dysenteriae* which had been recognized well before EHEC were discovered. VT2 is somewhat different from the latter and shares approximately 50% homology with them. EHEC attach to intestinal epithelium and appear to do so most commonly with factors that resemble those of EPEC, i.e., production of intimin from the LEE. Effacement occurs thereafter. A localized enteritis ensues in the large bowel, and it is likely that several factors are responsible for the local response: VTs, attachment and effacement factors, LPS, hemolysins, among others. At the level of the bowel, the histopathology is quite variable. There may be little if no evidence of inflammation, or there may be massive inflammation and necrosis. Transmural necrosis of bowel and bowel perforation may occur in severe infections, and the appendix may also become involved. The response to inflammation is mainly from polymorphonuclear cells, and fecal leucocytosis can be found in a significant proportion. Epithelial erosion and microangiopathy may result in localized bleeding. For most patients, it is unclear why there may be considerable variation in the degree of colitis, but it is apparent that the use of antimotility antidiarrheal agents may make the disease worse. The bacterium does not enter the bloodstream, but its toxin is absorbed. VTs have cellular receptors that are well defined, e.g., globotriaosylceramide (Gb_3) (107). The toxins have A and B subunits that contribute to intracellular change and cellular binding respectively. Within the cell, the A subunit blocks protein synthesis at a ribosomal level, and in doing so, activates apoptosis. Particular tissues have concentrations of binding sites that may explain the regional effects of HUS, i.e., renal disease and microangiopathy. There are many serotypes of *E. coli* that are capable of producing VTs, but the most reknowned is O157:H7. This serotype has virulence factors in common with other EHEC, but in particular, uniformly has a 60 MDa plasmid. EHEC isolates may possess one or more VTs simultaneously. The majority of North American O157 isolates have both VT1 and VT2. VTs can be detected by cell cytotoxicity and neutralization assays. It is apparent from the latter, especially when directly applied to stool specimens, that high and low level VT-positive isolates can be determined. Low level toxin producers may be found in stool specimens, but they do not necessarily cause diarrhea and HUS. The ability to show an effect of antibiotics on the production of VTs seems to be methodologically variable.

2.   Salmonella

Biochemically, salmonellae have several distinct attributes which help separate this species from other *Enterobacteriaceae*. They produce H_2S in appropriate detection media and are neither early nor late lactose fermenters (some lactose-positive *Salmonella* isolates have been found however). In combination with other biochemical studies, they are not difficult to differentiate from most other coliforms.

The nomenclature of this species is somewhat confusing to the uninitiated. Properly, there are several species and subspecies of *Salmonella*, but for the purposes of human infection, almost all belong to *S. enterica* subsp. enterica (subspecies I). Most clinicians are familiar with the common designations for *Salmonella* serotypes which are generally expressed as if they are a species, e.g., 'S. infantis' or 'S. newport'. Although of practical value in the general medical community, the latter names are actually abbreviations for serotypes. Serotypes are based on the serological demonstration of antigenic diversity among the complex carbohydrates of LPS-associated O side chains and then furthermore on the antigenic (protein) diversity of flagellar (H) structures (108). The implementation of such a typing scheme must be viewed historically for the benefit that differentiation of serotypes has held in epidemiological analyses. There was also an important role, and there continues to be, for this serology as a mechanism to confirm, especially presumptively, the speciation of salmonellae. Serotype nomenclature is at first expressed by a numerical and alphabetical series which defines O antigen type and then the H type. O antigen groups are broadly classified by capital letters, and most human isolates are in the groups ranging A-E; within each group, the actual antigen(s) are then expressed as numbers for the purposes of serotyping. H antigens may have more than one serological phenotype in a given isolate, and thus more than one H antigen type may be designated. H antigen shifts in vitro can be induced under laboratory conditions in order to ensure that H antigen diversity is exposed. A serotype can be defined by – O type:H type (phase 1):H type (phase 2), e.g., 9,12:i:1,3. Since this alphanumerical designation, although technically precise, is somewhat cumbersome to employ, the serotype is summarily described with a name that is most often based on the geographical site of origin unless historically otherwise defined. It must be acknowledged that the latter name defines a serotype and not a species proper. Thus, the common epithet 'Salmonella hadar' is more correctly denoted as *Salmonella* serotype Hadar. Whereas there are over 2400 serotypes that have been defined for all *Salmonella* species, only more than one-half have been isolated from human illnesses. Furthermore, very few of the latter are of any great frequency, and the predominant serotypes are influenced by geographical determinants. Serotyping is often accomplished at the O antigen level by local laboratories, but the art of complex O and H serotyping is best left with referral centres. Serotypes can be further differentiated on the basis of phage typing or other epidemiological tools as discussed later.

There are several important exceptions to note in speciation and serotyping. *Salmonella* serotype Typhi has a prominent capsular antigen known as Vi, and the expression of Vi is capable of masking the O antigen. Boiling of the isolates will usually allow for the O antigen to be demonstrated. *S.* serotype Paratyphi often lacks H_2S production, but the biochemicals are otherwise consistent with *Salmonella* spp. *Arizona* spp. of old are now included in the *Salmonella* groups.

Salmonellae must compete with the normal enteric flora in order to establish infection, and thereafter these bacteria are capable of being maintained in a chronic carriage state. They are resistant to bile, and hence, may actually be maintained in the gallbladder during such carriage. A variable infectious dose is required for infection, but in most patients, this quantity is usually high. Various host factors such as age (especially very young and very old), altered gastric function (and decreased acidity), cellular immune suppression (e.g., HIV infection), and antibiotic use among others increase the risk for *Salmonella* infection and decrease the infectious dose that may be required to initiate the process.

Salmonellae often bear multiple plasmids, and some of these carry virulence factor determinants, but key elements for disease causation are also chromosomal in origin (107). Salmonellae induce their own internalization into non-phagocytic intestinal epithelial cells and are able to cross from apical to basolateral surfaces in the form of membrane-bound vesicles (110). Both membrane and cytoskeleton changes are induced by type III (contact-dependent) protein secretion systems. The export and translocation of signaling proteins is encoded by genetic elements from at least two pathogenicity islands (SPI-1 and SPI-2) (111).

These bacteria also invade and persist within phagocytic immune cells of the macrophage series, although they are generally susceptible to polymorphonuclear cell phagocytosis. In particular, they invade M cells of the gastrointestinal tract. As the bacteria migrate through either the intestinal epithelium or M cells, they are then met by macrophages in the Peyer's patches of the intestines. Again, they are often able to escape degradation and may then enter blood via lymphatics by virtue of being carried as internalized pathogens within the circulating mononuclear cell. Spread, and to some extent sequestration, may occur throughout the reticuloendothelial system. Such interactions activate cytokines and induce physiological effects that are of both benefit and detriment to the host.

The diarrheal state is most likely a function of the effects of signal induction on intestinal epithelial cells. The bowel is infiltrated with polymorphonuclear cells. Variation in the intensity and nature of diarrhea and bowel pathology are apparent. Due to their persistence in mononuclear cells, and indeed the use of these cells for transport throughout the body, infection can occur among any organ system. The issue of sequestration is crucial to the understanding of why some of these extraintestinal infections may be particularly difficult to treat, e.g., endovascular infections. Some patients will develop a reactive arthritis or Reiter's syndrome after intestinal infection, and it is presumed at this time that immunological derangement, rather than direct infection, is responsible; this is consistent with the higher frequency of such manifestations among those patients who express HLA B27.

S. serotype Typhi is associated with bowel epithelial erosions even though patients uncommonly suffer from diarrhea. This serotype, and those that are more likely to cause enteric fever, are more closely associated with monocytes and particularly are hidden within the reticuloendothelial system. There must clearly exist some major differences in virulence factors for enteric fever salmonellae to differ in their disease course from most other salmonellae that are responsible primarily for diarrheal illnesses.

3. Shigella

Shigellae are non-motile, lactose-negative, and generally less reactive in sugar fermentation than other *Enterobacteriaceae*. A proportion of *S. sonnei* are capable of late lactose fermentation. In general, shigellae are considerably homologous to *E. coli*, and in particular, to the non-motile *E. coli* that have been referred to as 'alkalescens-dispar' (112). The phylogenetic positioning of *Shigella* spp. is spread among the several phylogenetic groups of *E. coli*. Despite the latter and despite common virulence mechanisms between shigellae and EIEC, it appears that the latter two groups of bacteria have been derived from different ancestral paths (113) during the evolution of *E. coli*.

There are four major serogroups of shigellae, and several serotypes exist among them. These correspond to the commonly used names of: *S. dysenteriae* (Group A), *S. flexneri* (Group B), *S. boydii* (Group C), and *S. sonnei* (Group D). Apart from serotypes of each and apart from the single serotype of *S. sonnei*, there are some biochemical differences between the groups with some exceptions. Serology in this regard is of benefit for epidemiological purposes and for presumptive and confirmatory identification. *S. sonnei* is the most common of shigellae in North America; the predominant shigella is geographically determined elsewhere.

A low inoculum is required ($<10^2$) to initiate infection; these bacteria are relatively resistant to gastric acid. Virulence is controlled by several mechanisms which are dependent on many genes and indeed environmental signals (114). After cell contact, the bacteria release invasins (*ipa* proteins) through activation of the type III secretory apparati. A complex signalling then takes place which effectively causes a major cytoskeleton rearrangement including actin repolarization (115-117). The latter facilitates endocytosis into the eucaryotic cell. Intracellularly, the bacteria lyze the phagocytic vacuole and gain entry into the cellular cytoplasm where events continue to cascade. The bacteria also induce apoptosis of macrophages which then triggers inflammatory and immune pathways, including the major recruitment of polymorphonuclear cells. Both virulence plasmid (130 Mda) and chromosomal elements interact in these regards.

S. dysenteriae is also capable of producing the Shiga toxin which is essentially identical to VT1 of EHEC. As a consequence, it is possible to see the complication of HUS arise during or after the bacillary dysentery. Other Shiga toxin variants are not well-defined for this species.

Shigella dysentery is associated with a localized neutrophilic infiltration and often a systemic leukemoid reaction.

4. Yersinia

The changes in the nomenclature for this species have been previously detailed (see I. Historical Background). Only *Y. enterocolitica* and *Y. pseudotuberculosis* are enteropathogens, and even so, only particular serogroups or biotypes of *Y. enterocolitica* are pathogenic (3,118). These two species are lactose-negative although they are often late-lactose fermenters. They produce urease. Several biochemicals will vary depending on whether the bacteria are grown at 25°C versus 37°C. In addition, motility is better demonstrated at the lower temperature. These yersiniae grow in temperatures ranging from refrigeration to body temperature; growth at 4°C may explain why high titres of bacterium may yet grow in blood products despite seemingly adequate maintenance. Overall, the *Yersinia* spp. differentiation is reliably accomplished by existing biochemical schemata.

Both *Y. enterocolitica* and *Y. pseudotuberculosis* have multiple serogroups. For *Y. enterocolitica*, serogroups O3, O8, and O9 are particularly represented among pathogenic types in Europe and North America (118). *Y. enterocolitica* may be biotyped, and biotype 1A is non-pathogenic (3). Non-pathogenic *Y. enterocolitica* are identified on a practical basis by their ability to degrade esculin and by their production of pyrazinamidase.

Both *Y. enterocolitica* and *Y. pseudotuberculosis* have much in common with respect to virulence factors, but more study has been directed to the former. Enteropathogenic yersiniae are serum-resistant and invasive. Virulence is dependent on both plasmid-borne (65-75 kb) and chromosomal elements. Outer membrane proteins are differentially expressed at various temperatures. Once the bacteria reach M cells in the intestinal tract, they attach via plasmid-encoded factors. Products of the *inv* gene (invasins; outer membrane proteins) (119) then initiate cell penetration which is further facilitated by the gene locus *ail* (attachment invasion locus). It appears that the latter gene product also is involved in serum resistance. A number of other *Yersinia* outer membrane proteins (Yops) (120) are secreted, and they have local and intracellular effects which continue to potentiate the pathogenesis. For example, YopH dephosphorylates proteins in phagocytic cells and induces numerous changes in transduction pathways. YopB causes significant changes in macrophage-derived cytokines. Phenotypic tests for virulence that have been proposed include determination of the presence of the virulence plasmid, autoagglutination, Congo red uptake, and calcium dependence. Some practical problems with such determinations include methodological variation and the spontaneous loss of the virulence plasmid in vitro after passage. It must be acknowledged that virulence is a factor of both plasmid- and chromosomally- mediated products. These bacteria have secretion pathways which resemble other enteric pathogens (111).

After invasion of either M cells or intestinal epithelium, the bacteria migrate to intestinal lymphoid tissue where further replication can occur. The pathological events which result include epithelial ulceration, microabscess formation, and inflammation. On a macroscopic basis, the latter is manifest as colitis, terminal ileitis, and mesenteric adenitis.

A large inoculum is usually required for infection. Although the acquisition of iron has been touted as essential for the virulence of several bacteria, it is especially evident that patients with iron overload, or those who are undergoing therapy for such overload, are at risk for *Y. enterocolitica* bacteremia (118). The mechanisms for the latter are unclear. Reactive arthritis, erythema nodosum, and Reiter's syndrome may also occur after *Yersinia* enteritis and, as for other enteric pathogens, especially among patients with HLA B27 (118). In the case of yersiniae, however, it has been postulated that there is some degree of molecular mimicry.

5. Other Enterobacteriaceae

As previously detailed, these bacteria have a wide variety of traits that might serve as virulence factors, but it is perhaps most important to realize that they are often present in contexts where opportunism is likely to occur. In this sense, many infections may not necessarily be a function of highly specialized or sophisticated virulence factors.

We have not detailed tables of biochemical reactions that are relevant to members of the *Enterobacteriaceae*. These details can be acquired from the many individual publications on taxonomy. The Manual of Clinical Microbiology that is published by the American Society for Microbiology has been consistently complete in providing such tables for enteric Gram negative bacteria. A number of the following species have biotypes, and many of them have had serotyping schemes that have been created on the basis of heat-stable antigens such as LPS. Many of the latter typing schemes are of historic value now that advanced fingerprinting methods have arisen.

Outside of the virulence factors that have been well-studied for *E. coli*, salmonellae, shigellae, and yersiniae, most other *Enterobacteriaceae* have not been as extensively studied with few exceptions.

The *Citrobacter* genus has been considerably enlarged within the last decade, and this has in particular arisen as a consequence of realizations that the 'C. freundii complex' was especially heterogeneous (121). The bacteria in this genus have antigens that may cross-react with other *Enterobacteriaceae*. Some have found evidence of intimin-like proteins in a diarrheal model (122). There are citations of verotoxin production among some isolates (123), but a broad surveillance for such toxin production has not confirmed the same (124). Nevertheless, an outbreak of HUS was linked to VT-positive *C. freundii* (125). Some interest has been directed to the ability of some species to cause central nervous system infections, and the presence of CNS-active outer membrane proteins and intracellular invasion has been highlighted in early work (126,127).

Edwardsiella tarda is lactose-negative and H_2S-positive. Some investigations have questioned whether there is an enterotoxin and whether these bacteria are invasive. Others have described the presence of unique 'membrane ruffles' after cell contact (128).

The common klebsiellae are encapsulated. Bacteria have been typed according to O and H antigens. The capsule appears to be relevant as a virulence factor and interacts with some cell types, but independent adhesins are more important for attachment (129). Some have proposed that capsular or other antigens may stimulate immunological reactions that lead to chronic arthropathies such as ankylosing spondylitis (130), but this area is controversial (131), and no such association is yet confirmed. A citation of cytotoxin production by some isolates has been made (132). *K. rhinoscleromatis* induces a chronic granulomatous disease which, on biopsy, shows large foamy macrophages. The associated illness seems too rare to draw much attention. *K. ozaenae* is associated with an atrophy of the nasal mucosa but also has drawn little attention regarding pathogenesis.

Morganella is strongly urease-positive, and as indicated below, this may serve as a major virulence factor for urinary tract infections.

Proteus spp. also produce urease. This enzyme creates an alkaline environment and promotes the formation of struvite stones. Whereas urease activity is seemingly critical, other possible virulence factors include swarming motility, fimbrial attachment proteins, and invasive potential (74,133). It is not apparent that hemolytic activity (134) is as important as initially believed. Yet others have proposed that the ability to cause urinary tract infections may be more so related to the simple presence of *Proteus* spp. in the nearby enteric reservoir (135).

Some *Providencia alcalifaciens* isolates may be enteropathogenic, but there is no clear-cut concensus (136).

Serratia marcescens are quite resistant to decontaminating agents. Few strains have shown cytotoxic activity, but the latter seems to be methodologically variable (137). More recent interest has been focussed on proteases (138).

B. Non-*Enterobacteriaceae* enteric pathogens and related bacteria

1. Vibrios

V. cholerae

Vibrios are glucose-fermenting, oxidase-positive, curved Gram negative rods. The are relatively resistant to bile but susceptible to acidity as may be encountered in the stomach. To the contrary, they are able to survive alkaline conditions in the environment. Different serotypes of *V. cholerae* vary in their ability to survive in various water habitats. Their growth is stimulated by the presence of salt, and they are resistant to high salt concentrations (6-10%). This species is susceptible to the vibriostatic compound 0/129. Several recent reports, however, have described clinical and environmental strains of *V.*

cholerae that are resistant to 0/129 (139). Strains of the O139 serotype which were isolaed in 1992 were also resistant to 0/129. Therefore, caution should be exercised when relying on this test for differentiting *Vibrio* and *Aeromonas* spp.

As Gram negative bacteria, they possess endotoxin. Serotyping of *V. cholerae* is based on O antigens and is of value for epidemiological purposes. There are over 200 different O serotypes, but very few constitute the ones that have been responsible for epidemic activity. The O1 serotype includes both 'classic' and 'El Tor' biotypes which may be differentiated by phenotypic traits. The O1 serotype has been subtyped into Ogawa, Inaba, and Hikojima groups. Serotype O139 (Bengal) is a recent clone which has caused epidemic disease in several countries on the Asian continent and is believed to be the eighth pandemic strain of cholera. The O1 and O139 serotypes maintain bioactive cholera toxin, but most other serotypes do not. Antigenic shift may be induced in vitro and probably occurs in the field as there is a generally continuous genomic alteration (140). It is not entirely clear how the epidemic clones evolve, but there is the potential for phage conversion (141).

The clinical manifestations of cholera are almost entirely due to the production of cholera toxin which is a heat-labile toxin that bears similarity to the heat-labile toxin of ETEC (CT; choleragen). In 1996, Waldor and Mekalanos discovered that the genes encoding CT (the operon ctxAB) are not integral components of the *V. cholerae* genome but are elements of the genome of a filamentous bacteriophage, CTXφ, that specificially infects *V. cholerae* (142). CTXφ DNA is generally integrated site-specifically at either one (El Tor) or two (classical) loci within the *V. cholerae* genome, and the arrangement of the CTX prophage arrays differ between the two biotypes. This enterotoxin is structured in the A/B subunit form. The B unit binds to cellular receptors, and the A unit has ADP-ribosyl transferase activity. Among *V. cholerae* serotypes that lack CT activity, molecular analyses have demonstrated that there is a lack of the CTXφ. Extensive molecular analyses have shown that very few wild-type strains have natural deletions of other genes (*zot*, *ace*, *cep*) of the CTXφ (143). Other virulence factors appear to include pili (144), the flagellum, adhesins (hemagglutinins), El Tor hemolysin, and protease activity. CT elicits a strong humoral immune response, and on this basis the toxin has been used as an adjuvant for oral vaccines.

The pathogenesis has otherwise been extensively investigated. A large inoculum of bacterium is required ($\sim 10^6$-10^8) for initiation of infection. *V. cholerae* penetrates the mucous layer, attaches to the intestinal epithelial cell, and produces toxin. The B subunit of CT binds to a GM1 ganglioside receptor on the apical side of the intestinal cell; bacterial neuraminidase activity serves to increase such receptor structures on the cell surface. The A subunit of CT is internalized and migrates through the cell most likely via endoplasmic reticulum and the Golgi apparatus (145). The A1 subunit of CT is mobilized to the basolateral side of the cell where it interacts with the adenyl cyclase-G protein complex. As it catalyzes ribosylation of protein G_s alpha, adenylyl cyclase is activated, and the intracellular cAMP increases considerably. Protein kinases are mobilized, and chloride channels which affect fluid and electrolyte balance are stimulated. As a consequence, there is a massive exit of fluid, especially in the small intestine, which exceeds the capacity of the bowel later to absorb. CT may also directly interfere with fluid absorption (146), and furthermore it may also interfere with neurotransmitters at the bowel level (144). These events may translate into massive fluid and electrolyte losses. 'Rice water stools' are a description of such massive watery diarrhea that contains flecks of mucous.

Non-cholera vibrios

These vibrios are oxidase-positive with the exception of *V. metschnikovii*. These bacteria will generally grow on routine bacteriological media since there is often sufficient sodium chloride content (~0.5%). They will also grow on MacConkey's medium and appear as non-lactose fermenters with the exception of *V. vulnificus* which is a lactose-fermenter. Apart from some degree of salt requirement, these vibrios are salt-tolerant like *V. cholerae*; *V. mimicus* is the only exception. Growth and no growth in nutrient broths with 0% and 6% sodium chloride respectively may be useful assessments during speciation attempts. In particular, some may be confused with *Aeromonas* species; both *Aeromonas* and

Plesiomonas do not grow in the presence of 6% sodium chloride. Serotyping schemes have been devised for several non-cholera vibrios, but they are of limited value on a practical basis.

V. parahemolyticus is associated with a more invasive illness, and infection may be accompanied by bloody diarrhea. The bacterium has a strong hemolysin, known as the thermostable hemolysin (TDH), that produces beta-hemolysis with human red cells (Kanagawa phenomenon). Both TDH and a urease enzyme appear to be associated with greater virulence. It has been proposed that the hemolysin may have enterotoxin activity (147). Infections that are caused by *V. parahaemolyticus* are usually associated with diverse serovars. A recent interesting trend has, however, been the emergence of a new O3:K6 clone of *V. parahaemolyticus* in 1995 which is spreading pandemically and which has been responsible for increased infections in seven Asian countries and the United States (148,149).

There are several putative virulence factors for *V. vulnificus* (150), but it is not clear that the cytotoxin is important. Some *V. mimicus* strains have CT-like activity (151). *V. hollisae* has a strong hemolysin.

Localized wound infections may be aggressive, and blood-borne infections cause considerable morbidity.

2.   *Campylobacter spp.*

Campylobacters are curved or apparently spiral Gram negative rods. The extended spiral morphology is a function of curved rods growing end-to-end. In vitro, the morphology may be altered. These bacteria are motile and are capable of passing through 0.45 μm. filters. Growth is enhanced by an increased quantity of hydrogen in the atmosphere and also with a reduction of oxygen to 5-10%. Several species are thermotolerant and will grow well at 42°C; these will also grow at 37°C, but the former temperature may help with selection. *C. fetus* will not culture well at 42°C. *Arcobacter* (formerly *C. cryaerophilus* and *C. butzleri*) also does not thrive at the latter temperature. On solid culture media, it is not uncommon to see *Campylobacter* colonies spread as a function of their motility.

Most campylobacters are catalase-positive except for some of the newer species (e.g., *C. curva/recta*, formerly *W. curva/recta*, e.g., *C. gracilis*, formerly *B. gracilis*) which grow anaerobically.

C. jejuni is hippurate-positive, and this reaction in combination with other crude features of a thermophilic campylobacter are usually sufficient to identify this species with a reasonable probability. Susceptibility to nalidixic acid and cephalothin have been used to facilitate speciation; an increasing frequency of nalidixic acid resistance has jeopardized this approach in some locales.

An inoculum of ~10^3 is required for infection which is relatively low compared to vibrios, although both are relatively susceptible to gastric acid. *C. jejuni* causes most campylobacter infections and has been best studied in this group. Infection can extend from the jejunum to the colon. Predominantly regional disease can be confined to the terminal ileum and colon. Infection is associated with a net in-migration of polymorphonuclear cells. Bacteria penetrate the mucous layer by way of their corkscrew motility; non-motile variants are much less virulent. They are able to adhere and then cause some epithelial ulceration. It has been proposed that *C. jejuni* has some invasive potential (152). Whereas there is some belief that a cholera-like toxin is apparent for some strains (153), more recent evidence supports the presence of a cytolethal-distending toxin for many isolates (154,155).

The association of *C. jejuni* with Guillain-Barre syndrome (an ascending polyneuropathy) has been confirmed by several groups; up to 30% of patients with this illness have evidence of a preceding campylobacter infection. It has been shown that the neural ganglioside GM1 cross-reacts with some but not all *C. jejuni* (156). Significantly more isolates from patients with this illness have GM1-like epitopes (157). Patients with the HLA B27 type are more prone to post-infectious reactive arthropathies.

Extensive serotyping schemes, based either on heat-stable or heat-labile antigens, have been devised for both *C. jejuni* and *C. coli.*

C. fetus is resistant to inactivation by serum and is also relatively resistant to phagocytosis. A capsule-like S-layer (surface) protein may have a role in the latter (158).

3. Helicobacter spp.

Non-*pylori* helicobacters stain poorly with the Gram stain and are weakly Gram negative. They are curved or spiral, and morphology may change after passage in vitro. They are oxidase- and catalase-positive; *H. canis* is catalase-negative. These bacteria grow better in an atmosphere with reduced oxygen and increased carbon dioxide. *H. westmeadii* grows best anaerobically. Growth is best at 37°C, but cultures may require incubation for up to 3-5 days. *H. cinaedi* and *H. fennelliae* are the most common among human isolates (159); they do not grow at 42°C. Brucella agar and anaerobic CDC agar support the growth best.

Pathogenesis has not been studied to any large degree.

4. Aeromonas spp.

Although having some similarities to particular non-cholera vibrios and *Plesiomonas*, *Aeromonas* species are phylogenetically distinct; G+C% content is approximately 60%. Nevertheless, there is considerable diversity within this genus, and several 'DNA groups' or genospecies have been defined (57). Several of these groups are not isolated from humans, but among those that are include: *A. hydrophila* (gp. 1), *A. bestiarum* (gp. 2), *A. caviae* (gp. 4), *A. veronii* biovar sobria (gp. 8), *A. veronii* biovar veronii (gp. 10), *A. jandaei* (gp. 9), *A. schubertii* (gp. 12), and *A. trota* (gp. 14). On a practical basis, most human isolates are *A. hydrophila*, *A. caviae*, and *A. veronii* biovar sobria.

Aeromonads are motile, oxidase-positive, fermentative Gram negative rods that grow well on routine bacteriological media including MacConkey's agar. They grow over a wide range of temperatures.

Many produce a potent and broad range of extracellular enzymes which include lipases, proteases, chitinases, nucleases, amylases, and hemolysins (160). Enterotoxin-like activity of *A. hydrophila* is linked to the hemolysin. *A. caviae* is for the most part generally avirulent in contrast to *A. hydrophila*. Pathogenesis is not well-studied, and in part, the uncertainty of disease associations (e.g., gastroenteritis) has hindered interest.

5. Plesiomonas

There is one species in this genus. It is oxidase- and catalase- positive and is fermentative. The G+C% content is 50%. It has been questioned whether *P. shigelloides* possesses a cholera-like toxin (161).

V. IMMUNOLOGY OF INFECTION

With few exceptions, most of the infections that are associated with the bacteria that are discussed in this chapter are relatively acute, and serodiagnosis of such infections is complicated by the short time between initial contact and disease. Both systemic and mucosal responses are applicable depending on the site of infection. Although cell-mediated immunity may have a role in some infections, most infections are associated with a prominent humoral immune response. For many of these bacteria, the assessment of serological responses is complicated due to the large number of antigens that may be targeted. For example, the large number of serotypes or serogroups that are based on LPS responses leads to certain complexity.

On a generic basis, antibody-coated bacterial studies were at one time used for the differentiation of upper and lower pole urinary tract infections, i.e., positive staining of urinary isolates by IFA for the presence of antibody that is bound to the bacterial cell would be indicative of a renal source. There are several methodological problems with such studies, and they have not survived the test of time (162).

Given the frequency of many enteric infections and their global impact as discussed in this chapter, it is not surprising that several have been the focus of intense study for vaccines.

A. *Enterobacteriaceae*

1. *E. coli*

In active cystitides, polymorphonuclear cells enter the bladder by migrating across the epithelial layer, and they may enter via the kidney if upper pole infection occurs. Antibody production to the offending isolate is prominent in pyelonephritides, but it is often negligible among those patients with cystitis or significant asymptomatic bacteriuria (163). Much of this antibody is directed to bacterial LPS and not capsular antigens. Urinary antibody does have the ability to inhibit bacterial attachment.

In the context of EHEC infections, patients generally have a poor humoral response to VT1 and VT2 including those with the systemic complication of HUS (164). Patients do, however, usually amount a strong anti-LPS response which can last for several months (165). In particular, antibodies to the O157 LPS have been documented, although it must be appreciated that this antigen can cross-react with the LPS of other *Enterobacteriaceae* including other *E. coli* serotypes (166). Antibody to intimin has also been detected after infections (167). Sera from controls as well as pooled (therapeutic) immunoglobulin lots contain both anti-VT1 and anti-VT2 antibody, although the anti-VT1 response is greater quantitatively; sera from infected patients are variable (168).

Among those with EPEC or ETEC infections, antibody does form to colonization factors (169,170). For children with EPEC, antibody production is more likely to be directed to *BfpA* and *EspA* products and lesser to intimin and *EspB* product (165).

LT from ETEC serves as a potent stimulator of the immune response and, like CT from *V. cholerae*, is being promoted as a possible adjuvant for vaccine construction.

2. *Salmonelloses*

Again, the acute nature of diarrheal illnesses due to these bacteria does not allow for serodiagnostic assays to be helpful in most circumstances. Nevertheless, chronic carriage is associated with a persistence of high level antibody (172). For patients with post-infectious reactive arthropathies, the likelihood of this complication is greater with a more severe illness and with the presence of a greater antibody response to infection (173).

Antibody responses to *S.* serotype Typhi have been studied especially with the intent of defining protective epitopes for vaccine purposes. Antibodies are developed to the O, Vi, and H antigens of the bacterium. Typhoid fever elicits some protective immunity, and chronic carriers post-infection are generally immune to any further systemic illness. Protective antibodies are directed mainly to the O antigen, and anti-Vi antibody is of lesser benefit in protection. Cell-mediated immune responses develop after infection and may also have some role in protection. The Widal test has historically been used for serodiagnosis and utilizes O and H antigens in an agglutination format; problems of non-specificity have long been recognized, and in large part, these are due to the cross-reacting LPS. A live-attenuated oral *S.* serotype Typhi vaccine is available and is partially protective.

3. *Shigelloses*

Antibody develops within 7-10 days after an acute infection (174), and this includes sIgA in the bowel after enteric infection. High levels of pre-existing IgG subtypes correlate with a decreased chance of infection (175). Homologous immunity develops after dysentery which includes a prominent anti-LPS response (176). The latter anti-LPS antibody may cross-react with other LPSs.

Immunoblotting studies have revealed a strong antibody response to Ipa (invasion plasmid antigen); this is better appreciated among those who have a new primary infection rather than those who live in endemic areas and who may have pre-existing high titres of antibody (177). Strong responses to Shiga toxin are also found in both animal models and human infection (178,179).

4. *Yersinioses*

The data in this regard is mainly from observations during *Y. enterocolitica* enteritis. A general prominent antibody response is seen by about 2-3 weeks after infection; there is particularly an IgG2 response among those with arthritis (180). The antibody has been characterized by immunoblotting and IgG, IgA, and IgM antibodies have been detected after enteric infection, but patients with post-infectious arthropathies have additional reactivity of IgA with antigens of 34.5, 48, and 240 kD (181).

The use of serodiagnostics has been complicated by the many serotypes that may be causative of disease. For purposes of agglutination serology, therefore, only common serogroups (usually 3 or 4) from human disease have been used.

There has been a resurgence in interest for serodiagnostic studies as a mechanism to confirm the association of previous illness with subsequent post-infectious arthropathy, particularly in regards to IgA status.

5. *Proteus*

Urinary isolates of *P. mirabilis* consistently produce a protease which is active in urine and which may cleave urinary immunoglobulins; a role in providing the bacterium with protection is postulated (182).

B. Non-*Enterobacteriaceae* enteric pathogens and related bacteria

1. *V. cholerae*

Circulating antibodies develop after infection to several antigens including O, H, and CT. Vibriocidal antibodies are assessed by exposure of live bacteria to serum in the presence of complement. Such antibody peaks at approximately 7-10 days post-illness but is lost progressively over several months. The vibriocidal antibody correlates better with protection than anti-CT IgG (183). Local mucosal IgA is also important. There is a decreasing incidence of cholera with increasing age, and long-lasting immunity does occur as recurrent cholera is uncommon.

Infection induces antibody to attachment structures such as fimbriae (184) and particularly the mannose-sensitive hemagglutinin (185). Among those patients who are infected with either the O1 or O139 serotypes, some degree of heterologous protection against the alternate serotype occurs (186). Volunteer challenge studies have examined the immune response to *V. cholerae* O1 by immunoblotting (187). There is a good response post-infection as determined by circulating IgG and jejunal sIgA. The antibodies so generated cross-react with heterologous serotypes. Secretory IgA is especially directed to low molecular weight proteins that are less than 25 kD. Consistent responses to outer membrane proteins occur regardless of whether the El Tor or classic O1 biotypes are used for substrate (188). When bacterium is grown in vitro versus in a rabbit ileal loop, the appreciable immune response varies, which thus implies that antigen expression is different in vivo versus in vitro.

2. *Campylobacter*

Campylobacter infections elicit a systemic immune response which includes both IgG and IgM (189), and there is a correlation between antibody and the quantitative excretion of bacterium during the acute illness (190). A maximal response is seen within two weeks of infection; systemic IgG and IgM persist longer than systemic IgA (191), but local sIgA also forms. There is a decreasing incidence with increasing age. Infection protects against homologous re-infection among volunteers.

Anti-flagellin antibody commonly pre-exists, and it is likely that flagellar antigens from other bacteria cross-react (192). The putative cytotoxin does not recruit a prominent response (193). After intestinal *C. jejuni* infections, antigens of 19, 56, and 92 kD are particularly recognized (194). As for *V. cholerae*, it has been shown that some proteins are expressed only in vivo, and these may command potent responses that might otherwise be unrecognized if in vitro sources of antigen are only used (192).

For patients with post-infection Guillain-Barre syndrome, it is postulated that antibody forms as a consequence of cross-reactivity with LPSs that bear the same epitope, but it appears that the development of anti-GM1 antibody may depend on some other factors as well (195).

Cell-mediated immunity has a small role if any (196).

3. Helicobacters

This area has been understudied perhaps due to the infrequency of such infections. *H. cinaedi* infection is associated with the development of antibody to five antigens as assessed by immunoblotting and these range from 41-96 kD (197).

4. Aeromonas and Plesiomonas

The development of a serological response to putative infection is inconsistent, and in large part, this may be due to the inability to define true infection. It may be that the majority of *Aeromonas* isolations from stool specimens are not truly a function of acute infection.

Studies of secretory antibody have been used to add further science to the association of bacterium and disease. Among a group of adults who suffered traveller's diarrhea after visiting Mexico, secretory antibody was found against *A. hydrophila* and *A. veronii* biovar sobria but not against *A. caviae*. This antibody was directed towards LPS (198).

Interestingly, no such antibody in the above study could be shown to be directed to *P. shigelloides* (198).

VI. LABORATORY DIAGNOSIS

A. Specimen collection, transport, and storage

The *Enterobacteriaceae* are generally hardy bacteria and withstand collection on routine swabs and in routine transport media. Rather than being subject to attrition in specimens, they are more likely to overgrow other pathogens when the bacteriology is mixed. Specimens should generally be processed within 2-4 hours for most samples, but maintenance at refrigeration temperature is acceptable for most specimens and for up to 24 hrs. if not longer. Samples for toxin analysis (e.g., VT detection) may also be preserved at refrigeration temperature with little decay in potency. The need for enrichment is dependent on several factors, but especially late timing during an illness, delay between collection and processing, and antibiotic use. When bacteria such as EPEC or enteroaggregative *E. coli* are to be detected among mixed stool flora, which include normal flora wild-type *E. coli*, it has not been evident that the putative pathogens have any growth disadvantage in comparison to other coliforms; such specimens too may be refrigerated if not immediately processed.

The short generation times for most coliforms is cause to rapidly process urines within a 2 hrs. period. Although urines that have been held longer may still be processed, notation should be made in the reporting that a longer transport time was had, especially if the bacterial counts approach a significant level.

Stool specimens are best submitted in the form of feces, rather than rectal swabs or even biopsies when they are obtained, since more specimen will be available to spread over solid selective media. Stool samples that have been sent early during the course of an illness are more likely to yield the enteric pathogen as numbers of the pathogen tend to be reduced over several days. For example, it is not uncommon for *E. coli* O157:H7 to be absent in a stool specimen by the time that HUS is apparent after the diarrheal illness. The number of stools that are required has been the subject of more interest recently given the need to contain health care costs. In acute diarrheal illnesses, one stool specimen will usually suffice; the submission of a second specimen may increase the yield by only 5-15%. The latter increment will depend on the context, i.e., if the study population is represented more with specimens from patients with subacute illnesses, those on antibiotics, and those who are seen well after the initial onset of disease. Historically, the number of specimens obtained was also in part a function of technical or methodological limitations, but some of the error in the latter regard has been reduced over the last 2-3 decades by the advent, trial, and acceptance of several selective media and the recognition of several effective combinations of the latter. In addition, some have proposed that the culture of specimens from hospital in-patients who have been cared for more than 3 days should not be cultured for routine enteric pathogens (199). The latter may be prudent in general terms among hospitals in developed countries where the experience indicates a low yield and where food and water supplies are secure. The latter may not be as acceptable in countries where nosocomial pathogens truly include enteric pathogens. Even in developed nations, changes in health care and the more liberal use of day-pass discharges or transport of food into the hospital from the outside may enhance the opportunity for patients to encounter food that may have been tainted with enteric pathogens. Another recommendation by some is to avoid processing stool samples that are formed rather than those which are diarrheal in nature. The latter approach will no doubt be applicable to a specimen type that has a lower yield of enteric pathogens, but it is not always clear to the laboratory technologist whether a stool is obtained in a non-diarrheal state, and the paucity of information that accompanies a sample prevents the forwarding of details that might be pertinent (199). Patients with typhoid fever may often not have diarrhea. Patients with *Yersinia*-associated abdominal pain may also not have diarrhea. There are other exceptions as well. Likewise, stool samples should not be rejected for the culture of enteric pathogens in any circumstance where blood and mucous are not apparent, e.g., a non-bloody stool does not necessarily rule out the potential for EHEC or *Shigella* (199).

The transport of stool specimens should depend on the anticipated timing between collection and processing. In general, stool specimens that are processed within 2-4 hrs. after collection do not require a transport medium. Likewise, if stool specimens are collected on-site within a hospital, the enteric pathogens will survive if the specimen is collected in the evening and processed on the next working day after refrigeration. Yersiniae survive and even grow during refrigeration. The use of stool transport media has largely been supported by studies in the field where specimens were transported over long distances and in extreme environmental conditions. For example, shigellae were evidently susceptible to delayed transport. In most scenarios where the specimen may be acquired in the home and then transported to the laboratory on the next day, stool transport media are recommended mainly to provide for an adequate buffer. Several media can be used for this purpose, but Cary-Blair (with reduced agar content) appears to serve this need for all enteric pathogens that require culture; Cary-Blair transport is useful for both campylobacters and vibrios. Glycerol-buffered saline is generally suitable for transport except for vibrios, and *Vibrio* transport with other media should be maintained at room temperature rather than refrigeration. Vibrios may also be transported in enrichment culture media such as alkaline peptone water. Both original stool specimens and stools in transport media can be frozen with little loss in viable enteric pathogens, except for vibrios.

B. Microscopy

The Gram stain of tissue or sample from extra-intestinal sources is useful for detecting these Gram negative organisms. Occasionally, the Gram negatives may be masked by an overabundance of negative staining background tissue or debris. The 'coliform' morphology of *Enterobacteriaceae* is relatively distinctive in many specimens, although the Gram stain does not allow for most *Enterobacteriaceae* to be distinguished from each other. Some bacteria may appear encapsulated with the simple Gram stain, e.g., some klebsiellae. Vibrios, campylobacters, and non-*pylori* helicobacters appear as curved or spiral Gram negative bacteria in clinical samples. Campylobacters do not stain very well with the conventional Gram stain and may require a more intense counterstain or an anticipating eye. Flagellar stains for light microscopy have little role in current times.

The use of light microscopy and stains for stool specimens is of limited value. A few early studies demonstrated some benefit for identifying curved rods in stool and for implicating campylobacters (200,201). The latter seems to be of limited practical value, however, as many laboratories will never accumulate sufficient experience, and many physicians are generally unaware that direct staining could have some diagnostic value in assessing an acute campylobacteriosis. The use of the Gram stain otherwise on stool smears is of limited value but may have some minor use in assessing the balance of or lack of enteric flora in unusual circumstances. The use of wet preparations or saline suspensions (with or without dark-field exam) for detecting motile organisms that are consistent with vibrios (especially in cholera) or campylobacters is likely to gain favour only with the experienced, but these two groups cannot be distinguished reliably from each other on the basis of motility in areas where they are both endemic.

Smears for fecal leucocytes may be processed with the Gram stain, methylene blue stain, or other equivalents. The presence of fecal leucocytosis, even for truly large bowel pathogens, is variable, and the absence should not be used to exclude the processing of particular specimens. Even formed stools may have some leucocytes in them, and thus standard criteria should be used to assign the designation of fecal leucocytosis to any given specimen. White blood cells may be congregated and may vary in their morphology. Both the Gram stain and methylene blue stain do not differentiate neutrophils from eosinophils; the latter may be present in allergic enteritides or some parasitic diarrheas. Therefore, the definition of fecal leucocytosis for the purposes of defining an inflammatory infiltrate should include a numeric standard which is aimed at polymorphonuclear cells, e.g., ≥ 5 polymorphonuclear leucocytes per high power field (1000X) in at least four different fields. One must nevertheless accept that some non-infectious inflammatory colitides, e.g., Crohn's disease or ulcerative colitis, may have an appearance on stool smears which is indistinguishable from bacillary dysenteries. An inflammatory response that is measured in this fashion is most likely to be associated with shigellae, salmonellae, EHEC, yersiniae, and campylobacters (202-206). Although shigellosis may be more often accompanied by fecal leucocytosis, there is too much of an overlap with these other infectious gastroenteritides. Generally, the presence of fecal leucocytes is more useful to differentiate colitis (and its causes) from small bowel diarrhea (more likely viruses and *Giardia*).

The use of direct fluorescence antibody detection for enteric pathogens is fraught with technical difficulty but has been assessed especially for cholera (207). In this example, a monoclonal antibody-based DFA was essentially equivalent to culture in a setting mainly of acute secretory diarrhea. It is unclear how well such a method would perform in specimens with lesser numbers of bacteria.

C. Culture

Routine culture media will support the growth of all of the bacteria that are discussed in this chapter including campylobacters if the appropriate atmosphere and other culture conditions are met. Coliforms will grow very well anaerobically. Routine enrichment broths are of value in circumstances where either very small quantitations of bacterium are present or when antimicrobial therapy has been already given. Selective and differential media are often a valuable addition when mixtures of coliforms or other resident flora are encountered. The choice and use of the latter media will be a function of the nature of the specimen. For example, MacConkey medium continues to enjoy common use. CLED, eosin methylene blue, and equivalent media with new chromogenic substrates (e.g., Rainbow agar) are also preferred by some for particular specimens. Selection against Gram positive organisms is often achieved with bile salts or dyes, e.g., crystal violet in MacConkey. In addition, broadly effective antibiotics, e.g., vancomycin, may also be of value for the latter. To the contrary, it may be of use to suppress coliforms when other pathogens are being sought; antibiotics often provide such inhibition, e.g., colistin and other polymyxins, nalidixic acid. Bile salts may also inhibit Gram negative bacteria, and this effect is concentration dependent; even coliforms may have differential susceptibility to bile salts.

The choice of media for routine bacteriology usually provides little for debate, but the selection specifically for enteric pathogens is somewhat more of an art. In regards to the latter, it must be acknowledged that many such individual media exist, and their use can therefore take place in several combinations. The preference for any given laboratory will be a function of experience, cost, local needs and endemic pathogens, prioritization in the laboratory overall, and the incremental benefit for detecting pathogens.

The culture of these bacteria from blood in current blood culture systems is not difficult, although the detection of campylobacters and vibrios by Gram stain and the subculture of campylobacters and helicobacters may prove somewhat elusive. *S.* serotype Typhi and other enteric fever salmonellae should be sought in blood and stool, but may also be found in urine, bone marrow, and other tissue less often.

Several individual coliforms may have attributes that facilitate presumptive identification. Klebsiellae are not uncommonly mucoid even on MacConkey medium. *Proteus* species are often found to swarm on routine media such as blood or chocolate agar. Some isolates will have pigmentation on routine media especially when the culture has been held, e.g., *Serratia*, some 'E. agglomerans complex'.

1. *Enterobacteriaceae*

E. coli

There is a tremendous diversity of biochemical patterns within the *E. coli* species, and thus, differential media which separate it from other coliforms are often very difficult to design; in addition, *E. coli* is generally susceptible to agents that inhibit these other bacteria. One exception to this difficulty is the use of sorbitol-MacConkey medium for the selective isolation of *E. coli* O157:H7 (208). This EHEC serotype typically does not ferment sorbitol, and therefore, the use of sorbitol rather than lactose in the MacConkey base will differentiate it from other more commonly sorbitol-positive *E. coli*. A few sorbitol-positive *E. coli* O157:H7 isolates, however, have been found. Most other EHEC serotypes are sorbitol-positive, and a small percentage ($\leq$5%) of non-pathogenic *E. coli* are sorbitol-negative as well (59). Fortunately, many areas have *E. coli* O157:H7 as the predominant EHEC. Colonies should be well spread on sorbitol-MacConkey medium in order to appreciate the sorbitol-negative phenotype; this medium provides presumptive evidence only however. Some have added cefixime and tellurite to sorbitol-MacConkey agar to increase selection (209). Enrichment broths are not typically used for EHEC, but a small gain (usually <5-10% increase) in *E. coli* O157:H7 isolation may be had if GN broth is used in the same format as for shigellae except with subculture to sorbitol-MacConkey medium. One may restrict the latter enrichment procedure to high risk scenarios, e.g., bloody stool or patients with HUS (210). Chromogenic media have also been created for the purpose of detecting EHEC (211). Some recent work has examined the use of immunomagnetic separation for the purposes of concentrating *E. coli* O157:H7 from clinical samples, and this has translated into a commerical kit for this purpose (Dynabeads) (212). Essentially, the stool specimen is enriched for a few hours in GN broth. Magnetic beads are prelabelled with anti-O157 antiserum; they are mixed with the enriched stool specimens to cause binding of the bacterium to the beads. Magnetic separation is then used to concentrate the bacterium which is thereafter cultured on sorbitol-MacConkey agar.

Other pathogenic *E. coli* such as non-O157 EHEC, EPEC, and ETEC are not detected with selective media. Rather, a low selective medium or non-selective medium is first used to grow the presumptive *E. coli*, and then phenotypic or genotypic methods are applied to isolated colonies. EIEC isolates grow well on some selective media such as Deoxycholate-Citrate and Hektoen agars. Several EIEC strains ferment lactose from these media in 24 hrs. or in a few days (213).

Salmonella

Most enteric selective and differential media were historically devised with the expressed intention of determining the presence of *Salmonella* spp. and *Shigella* spp. The use of some of these media for other purposes has been fortuitous. These media yield isolates which should be considered suspect, if not presumptive, for enteric pathogens; appropriate biochemical and serological confirmation is thereafter sought. These media rank in varying stringencies for selection and are usually used in combinations (e.g., one less selective and one more selective solid medium along with an enrichment broth). Commonly-used media include MacConkey medium, eosin methylene blue, Salmonella-Shigella agar, Deoxycholate-Citrate medium, xylose-lysine-deoxycholate agar, Hektoen medium, brilliant green agar, and bismuth sulfite agar; Tables 4 and 5 detail some characteristics of the latter as well as enrichment broths. In general, salmonellae are initially suspect as non-fermenting colonies (i.e., lactose-negative and/or sucrose-negative). H_2S production imparts a black colour to colonies in addition on some of

Table 4   Attributes of common selective and differential enteric media for some pathogenic *Enterobacteriaceae*. N.A. – not applicable. H_2S – detection in addition to colour indicator changes from substrate fermentation.

Medium	Inhibition mechanisms	Selectivity	Fermentation substrate	H_2S	Colour indicator
Solid					
Hektoen	bile salts	moderate	lactose, sucrose	yes	bromthymol blue
Deoxycholate-Citrate	sodium deoxycholate, citrate	high	lactose	yes	neutral red
MacConkey	bile salts, Crystal violet	low	lactose	no	neutral red
Eosin-Methylene Blue	eosin, methylene blue	low	lactose, sucrose	no	eosin, methylene blue
Xylose-Lysine Deoxycholate	deoxycholate	moderate	xylose, lactose, sucrose	yes	phenol red
Salmonella-Shigella	bile salts, brilliant green, citrate	high	lactose	yes	neutral red, brilliant green
Bismuth Sulfite	bismuth, brilliant green	high	N.A.	no	brilliant green
Brilliant Green	brilliant green	high	lactose, sucrose	no	phenol red, brilliant green
Enrichment broths					
GN	sodium deoxycholate, mannitol				
Selenite F	sodium hydrogen selenite				
Tetrathionate	bile salts, iodine, ±brilliant green, potassium iodide				

Table 5 Appearances of common bacteria on common solid selective media.

Medium	Appearance	Rationale	Examples
MacConkey agar	pink colony	strong lac+	*E. coli*, klebsiellae, enterobacters
	light/late pink	weak lac+ or late fermenters	citrobacters, *Serratia*, *Hafnia*, *Providencia*
	clear	lactose non-fermenter	*Salmonella*, *Shigella*, *Proteus*, *Edwardsiella*
Eosin-methylene blue	green-black, metallic sheen	strong lac+	as above
	purple-red	weak lac+ or late fermenters	as above
	clear	lactose non-fermenter	as above
	(yersiniae may be purple-black due to sucrose fermentation)		
Deoxycholate-Citrate agar	deep red (small)	strong lac+	as above
	light pink	weak lac+ or late fermenters	as above
	clear	lactose non-fermenter	as above
Salmonella-Shigella agar	red	lac+	as above
	clear with black centers	lac-, H_2S+	
Hektoen agar	orange-pink	lac+	as above
	blue-green with black centers	lac-, H_2S+	*Salmonella*
	green	lac-, H_2S-	*Shigella*
xylose-lysine-deoxycholate agar	bright yellow	lac+	as above
	[yellow with black centers for *Citrobacter* (H_2S+)]		
	red with black centers	lac-, suc-, H_2S+	*Salmonella*
	clear	lac-, suc-, H_2S-	*Shigella*
bismuth sulfite	black with metallic sheen	reduction of sulfite	*S.* serotype Typhi
	black, no sheen	as above	enteric salmonellae
	greenish		some salmonellae

these media. Bismuth sulfite agar should be used after relatively fresh preparation, and it is a good medium for *S.* serotype Typhi isolation. Lesser known media include mannitol-lysine-crystal violet-brilliant green agar, xylose-lysine-Tergitol 4 medium, novobiocin-brilliant green-glycerol-lactose agar, and modified semi-solid Rappaport-Vassiliadis medium (214). Some of the latter are comparable or better than some traditional media for usual enteric salmonellae, but particular ones, e.g., xylose-lysine-Tergitol 4 medium and the modified Rappaport-Vassiliadis medium (214), may be inhibitory to *S.* serotype Typhi and *S.* serotype Paratyphi. More recent variations of the above have incorporated chromogenic substrates, e.g., Rambach agar (214), SM-ID medium (214), CHROMagar Salmonella medium (215), and ABC medium (216). The latter are somewhat more costly for initial reagents although some have proposed that enhanced differentiation on these media prevent much extra work that may be had for the assessment of colonies that prove to be non-pathogens.

More commonly-used enrichment broths include GN broth, tetrathionate broth, selenite F, and Mueller-Kaufmann enrichment (217). Care should be takento ensure that these enrichments are subcultured on a timely basis to solid selective media (tetrathionate ~ 12-24 hrs.; selenite F ~ 8-12 hrs.). Timeliness particularly is an issue for GN broth which should be optimally subcultured at 4-6 hrs. GN broth is less inhibitory by virtue of having a reduced concentration of deoxycholate (0.5%); this medium also has mannitol which slows the growth of some *Proteus* spp. Selenite F is inhibitory to *E. coli* and *Shigella*. Tetrathionate broth requires the addition of iodine which necessitates that the broth be used a short time thereafter.

Lactose-positive salmonellae are relatively uncommon but have been associated with outbreaks (218). Rare lactose-positive *S.* serotype Typhi have also been detailed (219). Occasionally these may be found accidentally when coliforms from urine or other sites are evaluated; detection from stool is complicated by the lactose fermentation effect which will confuse screening biochemicals, although they may be found as suspect colonies on xylose-lysine deoxycholate, bismuth sulfite, and Hektoen media.

Shigella

Shigellae are much more susceptible to inhibition on selective media than are salmonellae, but the same media are generally used for enteric cultures, and shigellae appear as non-fermenters of the major base carbohydrate initially (e.g., of lactose). Media such as Salmonella-Shigella, Hektoen, and Deoxycholate-Citrate are particularly selective. Nevertheless, it is in large part due to the potential problems with *Shigella* inhibition that less selective media should be used in tandem, e.g., MacConkey or xylose-lysine deoxycholate. For example, Deoxycholate-Citrate agar has up to three times the active bile acids equivalent when compared to MacConkey agar. Rare shigellae are lactose-positive (<1%), but most *S. sonnei* and about one-third of *S. dysenteriae* are late-lactose fermenters (i.e., ONPG-positive). Enteric enrichment broths may be relatively inhibitory except for GN broth. On solid selective media, there is not uncommonly some inhibition of *S. dysenteriae*, and thus it may appear as smaller colonies than are anticipated.

Yersinia

Y. enterocolitica and *Y. pseudotuberculosis* are late-lactose fermenters and will appear lactose-negative initially on MacConkey agar. They do not grow well, or at all, on Salmonella-Shigella medium, and they ferment sucrose and xylose on Hektoen and xylose-lysine-deoxycholate agars which renders these media not useful for this purpose.

Cefsulodin-irgasan-novobiocin (CIN) medium is the standard for selective isolation of enteric yersiniae, even though several other media have been created for this purpose (220). Colonies develop a 'bulls-eye' appearance with a red center due to mannitol fermentation. This medium has considerable inhibitory properties for other enteric bacteria, and occasionally even some *Y. enterocolitica* and *Y. pseudotuberculosis* strains are inhibited. Incubation is best held at 30°C, and media should be examined for up to 48 hrs. since colonies may appear small over the first day. The growth should be scored on a semi-quantitative basis since pathogenic enteric yersiniae will typically be present in moderate to large numbers during an acute illness, whereas the non-pathogenic yersiniae are more often present in light quantities (221). A modification of CIN was derived in Japan which incorporates esculin (222). Non-pathogenic *Y. enterocolitica* develop dark colonies in the latter due to the positive esculin reaction, whereas pathogenic types are red colonies.

Cold enrichment of stool at 4°C in a phosphate-buffered saline mixture is a time-honoured method to detect small quantities of these bacteria. The sample is usually held for 3-4 weeks and subcultured once weekly onto CIN. For most routine stool specimens, the incremental gain in enteric yersiniae is of little value since most isolates prove to be of the non-pathogenic types. Nevertheless, this approach may be added to usual cultures when the disease has occurred in the distant past, when patients with seemingly post-infectious reactive arthropathies are investigated, and when a regional enteritis is deserving of more intense work-up.

Congo red agar can be used as a mechanism to differentiate pathogenic from non-pathogenic *Y. enterocolitica*, since the pathogenic variety take up the Congo red dye. This approach is not commonly used now that simple biochemicals, as detailed below, can be used in replacement.

2.   *Non-Enterobacteriaceae enteric pathogens and related bacteria*

V. cholerae

This bacterium will grow on simple media and as a non-lactose fermenter on MacConkey's agar. The oxidase test is a critical reaction when colonies are to be assessed directly from such media or after subculture (although oxidase tests from MacConkey medium may be falsely negative).

Thiosulfate-citrate-bile salts (TCBS) medium is highly selective and being sucrose fermenters, *V. cholerae* yields yellow colonies, although some strains may not grow well on this selective agar (223). Few non-cholera vibrios will have yellow colonies as well. Other solid selective media which are not as commonly used for clinical specimens include: tellurite-taurocholate gelatin agar, Vibrio agar, and polymyxin-mannose-tellurite agar.

Selective enrichment broths may be of value in endemic areas, especially since many infections will be relatively mild or even asymptomatic (224). Alkaline peptone water, which has a high pH (8.4-9.0), is useful for this purpose since vibrios in general multiply well in alkaline conditions; others include sodium phosphate-gelatin, alkaline peptone water with tellurite, and tellurite-taurocholate media.

Non-cholera vibrios

These are also oxidase-positive which again will be useful for initial screening from routine media. Many of these are sucrose-negative, and most will have green colonial appearances on TCBS.

Campylobacter

Microaerophilic conditions with reduced oxygen but enhanced carbon dioxide are crucial for adequate culture of campylobacters, although some newer campylobacter species grow well anaerobically. The 42°C temperature for incubation is strictly relevant for thermophilic varieties; others may not grow at this temperature or very poorly so. When suspect campylobacters are being subcultured from blood culture bottles, selective media are not usually required, and indeed these bacteria may grow on blood agar with varying bases. Media for thermophilic and most other campylobacters should be incubated up to 72 hrs.

Enteric cultures for campylobacters require selection. There are many such selective solid media, and all have antibiotics which suppress other enteric bacteria. The selectivity of such antibiotics is variable, and it must be recognized that some campylobacters may be inhibited by the typical antibiotics which are used to select for thermophilic campylobacters, e.g., *C. jejuni* and *C. coli*, that are most common in clinical specimens. Most initial solid media were blood-based, but newer variations over the last 10-15 years have been blood-free although containing charcoal. The selectivity of these media may vary depending on whether incubation takes place at 37°C versus 42°C. Selective media include Skirrow's medium, Butzler's medium, Campy-CVA, and charcoal-cefoperazone-deoxycholate agar. Cephalothin was not uncommonly used as the selective antibiotic in early media, but it has become apparent that some campylobacters and arcobacters are susceptible to this agent. Cefoperazone is less inhibitory (225). Some have shown that a combination of media, rather than one, enhance the recovery of campylobacters.

Given the susceptibility of some campylobacters and arcobacters to antibiotics, several investigators have examined the value of stool filtration. These bacteria are able to pass through filters that have 0.65 μm. (and as small as 0.45 μm.) openings probably by way of their cork-screw motility. A filter paper is placed on a non-selective medium, and drops of stool suspension (saline) are added to the paper. After a short incubation period, the filter is removed, and the solid medium is incubated under usual conditions. The incubation at 37°C rather than 42°C will then further add to the potential to find non-thermophilic campylobacters. The incremental benefit from the filtration approach is variable (226-228); indeed some have found no benefit at all. This approach should be evaluated to determine if it has a role in a given context, and this will obviously depend on the prevalence of these non-typical campylobacters.

Enrichment broths are several and include Preston medium and Campy-thio broth. Again, the benefit from enrichment is variable (229,230).

The methods for enteric culture are quite complex given the variety of pathogens that are now routinely sought, and thus the addition of more selective plates or enrichment broths must be assessed in the context of the existing cost, recovery, and technical burden.

Helicobacter

From blood cultures, non-pylori helicobacters grow on non-selective media with Brucella base, but often require extended incubation (54,55). These bacteria may occasionally be found on conventional selective campylobacter media. In addition to prolonged incubation, cultures should be maintained at 37°C.

Aeromonas

Most human pathogenic species grow well at 37°C, but some environmental or animal pathogens grow better at 20-25°C. They will thrive on routine media and can be initially suspected with the oxidase test. On MacConkey agar, they may initially appear as lactose-negative colonies.

Several variations of selective media have been proposed. Blood agar (any blood source) will often show beta-hemolysis, even double-zoned, for *A. hydrophila* and *A. veronii* biovar sobria. The addition of ampicillin is often sufficiently selective, although some susceptible aeromonads do arise. CIN, which is used for yersiniae, has been touted for *Aeromonas* selection; rather than the original formulation, it is preferable to reduce the concentration of cefsulodin or to replace it entirely with the same concentration of ampicillin that is used for the ampicillin-blood agar. Some aeromonads will also grow on bismuth sulfite or TCBS media.

Enrichment is not routinely used, but when desired, alkaline peptone water has served this purpose.

Plesiomonas

This bacterium can also be detected by the oxidase-positive reaction on colonies from non-selective media such as blood agar. Isolates are also lactose-negative and sucrose-negative which facilitates their isolation from MacConkey and Hektoen media. Inositol-brilliant green-bile salts agar has been used as a selective medium, since these bacteria are commonly inositol-positive.

As for aeromonads, alkaline peptone water can be used for enrichment.

D. Identification

Identification is still largely dependent on phenotypic assessments, and these most commonly include colony appearance, biochemical assays, and serological reactivities.

For most common coliforms on routine media, colonial morphology has little to offer, although a few features may be indicative of a particular species, e.g., pigmentation, e.g. swarming of *Proteus* spp.

Biochemical profiles are the most important indicators overall for speciation among this large group of bacteria. Detailed tables which outline the many biochemical attributes of genera and species are available. For example, all editions of the Manual of Clinical Microbiology, as published by the American Society for Microbiology (231), have excellent tables for the latter purpose as has historically the Edwards and Ewing's manual (1). In considering these or other such tables, it must be acknowledged that they have often been based on well-defined methods ('tube biochemicals') which may not necessarily be used in most laboratories. It is imperative, therefore, that the consideration of frequencies of positive reactions be tempered by the known data for any given system, whether it be modifications of conventional tube biochemicals or commercial systems. One must also temper these considerations by variation in what may be considered as the standard for assessment. Databanks for identification profiles are usually available for most biochemical systems. In general, the identification of lesser known species tends to be problematic for most identification systems, and the use of reference laboratories may be desirable. The referral of isolates should, however, depend on the context, and there must be a balance between practical, logistic, and cost considerations versus the sentiment of needing to know. With some identification systems, it may be beneficial to use a second system which may be able to overcome the initial system's limitations. Consideration of the bacterium's susceptibility profile may also be a useful adjunct to the biochemical profile (see VII. Susceptibility Testing). A number of molecular methods are emerging which have the potential to radically change the way in which bacteria are routinely identified; in the interim, the current standards are still of great value.

Commercial methods for identification now come in many forms. They differ in the number of biochemicals used, whether rapid enzyme substrates are used, need for supplementary tests, incubation times, inoculum preparation, interpretive criteria, among other things. Most methods are excellent for identifying the most common species of *Enterobacteriaceae*, and up to 90-98% of routine clinical isolates are accurately predicted. Relatively simple methods may be used for some specimens such as outpatients' urines, whereas more complete methods may be chosen for secondary and tertiary care medical centres. Databases for these systems continue to be built on. Problems still occur with the identification of rare species, and it is important that inadvertent mixtures of coliforms, or for that matter any other bacteria, are not being assessed; this may particularly be a problem for systems that use rapid enzyme substrates which may not at all depend on predominant growth of one bacterium. The basis for identification is usually a binary system for probability (see Chapter 2) which is useful in expressing the likelihood that a designated species is truly so.

Screening biochemicals for suspect colonies from selective enteric media are still useful endeavours, since a well-utilized system may save considerably on the cost of more detailed investigations for diarrheal pathogens. The particular choice of screening method may include one or a series of conventional tube biochemicals; the more commonly chosen include triple sugar iron (TSI) agar, Kligler's iron agar (KIA), and lysine iron agar (LIA) along with one or more adjuncts. For example, TSI is often used in tandem with a medium for determining lysine, indole, and motility reactions; urease is also a common addition. Motility-indole-ornithine medium has also been used. Suspect colonies from enteric solid media are inoculated directly into screening biochemicals, and the reactions are used to determine suspect pathogens which will then undergo more definitive biochemical assessment as well as possibly serological assays. Table 6 details the anticipated reactions from these screening enteric biochemicals. Essentially, the core biochemical screen (i.e., TSI, KIA) is a method to assess fermentation pattern, gas from fermentation, and H_2S production. In a solid slant medium, reactions are determined for both the agar deep (bottom of tube) and the slant. Acid production and colour indicator change occurs throughout the medium when lactose (and/or sucrose in TSI) is fermented; the base only will be acidic when

Table 6 Anticipated results of conventional enteric screening biochemicals for selected pathogens.

Test	Reaction	Suspect
TSI	K/K	non-fermenter
	K/A, +gas, +H₂S	*Salmonella*
	K/A, ±gas	*Shigella*/EIEC*
	A/A, no gas, +urea supplemental	*Yersinia*
KIA	K/K	non-fermenter
	K/A, +H₂S, ±gas	*Salmonella, Citrobacter, Proteus*
	K/A, ± gas	*Shigella*/EIEC*
LIA	K/K	*Salmonella*
	K/A	*Shigella*
	K/A, +urea supplemental	*Yersinia*

K – alkaline reaction; A – acid production; * - some *S. flexneri* 6 isolates produce gas.

glucose is fermented since amine generation near the slant, which is exposed to air, will help retain the pH to its original in the slant. Hydrogen sulfide production generates a black discoloration. Gas formation as a product of fermentation can be visualized by pockets of gaseous disruption of the agar medium.

1. Enterobacteriaceae

E. coli

The vast majority of *E. coli* are readily speciated with commerical methods. 'Inactive' (and non-motile) *E. coli* may provide some challenge. For the purpose of screening urine samples, some choose to limit the assessment to standard coliform colony morphology, positive spot indole, and positivity for beta-D-glucuronidase. For the assessment of out-patient urines, this limited profile will yield a high probability for determining the species.

EPEC are defined by their pattern of eukaryotic cell attachment in vitro or by molecular methods which define the associated virulence factors (31). The perception of attachment is method dependent, and is also dependent on having sufficient experience given the variations which may exist. Hep-2 cells are preferred for the attachment pattern assessment. Bacteria are incubated with the live cell substrate for 3 hrs., and then the cells (usually on a cover-slip) are stained to determine the presence of bacteria and their organization. Clustered (bundled) bacterial cells in different areas of the eukaryotic cell surface are consistent with localized attachment. Different phenotypic and molecular tests can be used to identify EPEC. The more practical way to identify these bacteria, however, seems to be the simultaneous use of VT and *eae* probes or the respective PCR primers (232-234). EPEC are VT-negative and *eae*-positive. To distinguish between typical and atypical EPEC, the *eaf* probe is an excellent test. With a very few exceptions (e.g., O142:H6 strains), typical EPEC react regularly with this probe. The *bfpA* probe also can be used to demonstrate the presence of the *eaf* plasmid, but one has to be aware that strains of serotypes O119:H2 and O128:H2, which are relatively frequent, react with this probe but do not have a true *eaf* plasmid. They are *eaf*-negative, and the *bfp* operon is practically absent (235). Other tests that can be used to identify EPEC are adhesion asays, probes, and PCR to demonstrate the presence of the LEE region, the FAS test, and immunological tests to demonstrate the presence of bundle-forming pili. Further useful information can be gained by the use of serotyping. Typical EPEC strains of the EPEC O serogroups always belong to well defined O:H serotypes which are regularly *eae*+, *eaf*+, LA+, and FAS+. For identification of non-motile strains, serotyping needs to be combined with RFLP-PCR analysis of the *fliC* gene. More than 90% of the typical EPEC strains possess antigens H2, H6, or H34. Serotyping alone has limited value for atypical EPEC identification because some strains produce VT and therefore would be identified as EHEC.

Enteroaggregative *E. coli* demonstrate a "stacked brick" pattern of adherence in the HEp-2 cell assay (84). A PCR assay for the genetic determinant has also been detailed, but a discrepancy between probe-positive isolates and adherence to Hep-2 cells has been recorded (236).

DNA probes for diffuse adherence have also been reported (237); their application must await confirmation that diffusely adherent *E. coli* are truly pathogens.

The biological assay of guinea pig keratoconjunctivitis (Sereny test) had initially been used to define EIEC. Probe or PCR methods are now available which target the *ipaC* or *ipaH* determinants. Again, such methods can be performed on 5-10 suspect *E. coli* colonies. Biochemical confirmation of positive isolates is necessary since shigellae will also often be positive in this assessment. The virulence plasmid may be lost on subculture, and therefore the detection of the plasmid itself by agarose electrophoresis is not desirable. Another approach is to detect the *ipaC* associated-antigen of *E. coli* by EIA (238). Some difficulty may be apparent in differentiating EIEC and *Shigella* when detecting one or the other purposely with the use of markers for invasion directly from stool samples; a multiplex PCR will likely serve to provide accurate differentiation (239). EIEC can also be recognized in preliminary form with O antisera and be a few biochemical tests. The non-EIEC strains in the EIEC O serogroups usually are motile and lysine-positive. EIEC strains are lysine-negative and non-motile with exception of O124:H34. As some of the EIEC antigens are shared by *Shigella* which also are lysine-negative and non-motile, further biochemical tests should be used to differentiate both groups of pathogens (240).

As previously detailed, ETEC have usually one of either LT or ST. Both of these were historically determined by bioassay; LT was detected by the rounding of Y1 adrenal cells or the elongation of Chinese hamster ovary cells, and ST with a rabbit ligated ileal loop assay or suckling mouse assay. Agglutination and EIA assays have become commercially available to detect these toxins (241,242), and furthermore, they can now be determined by either direct probes or PCR (243). With PCR, multiplex assays have been proposed to detect these two toxin determinants in tandem or combination with other non-ETEC toxins or factors (244).

The detection of EHEC must necessarily take two approaches. The first is the specific detection of *E. coli* O157:H7 with the use of sorbitol-MacConkey agar as previously defined. Sorbitol-negative colonies are confirmed as *E. coli* and then initially reacted with reagents that will detect the O157 LPS; there are now many commercial sources for such reagents including agglutination and EIA formats (245-247). The finding of the O157 serotype is not specific, however, since some O157-positive isolates are not EHEC, and some other *E. coli* may have cross-reacting LPS. Nevertheless, most sorbitol-negative colonies that are presumptive O157 do indeed prove to be verotoxigenic *E. coli* O157:H7. The probability of the latter will in part be determined by the frequency and endemicity of such a diarrheal pathogen in the given community, and the probability will be high when the isolate is from a patient who suffers from hemorrhagic colitis or HUS. Further O157 serological confirmation, as well as determination of the H7 flagellar type, usually thereafter takes place in a reference centre. Presumptive O157 isolates may also be confirmed by determining toxigenicity either with eukaryotic cell culture or by genetic detection (especially PCR). In addition, commercial kits for the detection of O157 antigen directly in stool by EIA have also appeared (248).

The second approach for detecting EHEC is to screen stool specimens for toxin directly. Cell supernatants or filtrates are applied to the Vero cell line (although several other sensitive cells lines are available) with and without anti(VT)toxin (59). The cell line undergoes cytotoxicity over 24 hrs. although the latter will be neutralized in wells with antitoxin. Toxicity may be seen as early as 4-6 hrs. if the potency (i.e., titre) is sufficient. Weak VT producers may require 48-72 hrs. After determining that a stool sample has evidence of VT, an aliquot of the same refrigerated stool can be grown on solid media to isolate *E. coli* colonies with the intent of assessing individual VT-producing capability. A positive colony can then be serotyped for epidemiological purposes. The vast majority of non-O157 EHEC are sorbitol-positive, and neither the use of biochemical identification tests (as in tube biochemicals or complex commercial strips) nor detection of enterohemolysin in themselves are sufficient to delineate these bacteria. VT in stools has also been detected with EIA assays (249). As well, commercial EIA (e.g., Premier EHEC) and agglutination (e.g., VTEC-RPLA, Oxoid) assays can also be applied to detecting VTs from *E. coli* colonies (250,251). Suspect colonies may also be directly tested for VT genes by direct probes or PCR. There remains the theoretical possibility for some isolates to lose VT genes during subculture. Apart from direct stool toxicity assessment, Karmali and others have used a screening technique to assess VT among colonies of coliforms that are grown on a non-selective medium such as blood agar (252). A broad blind sweep of colonies is extracted with polymyxin, and the extract is applied to cells for toxin detection; the addition of cycloheximide increases the sensitivity of the eukaryotic cells to the toxin. After a positive assay, individual colonies of *E. coli* are then assessed directly and serotyped when proven.

VT detection by PCR is capable of differentiating VT variants termed VT1, VT2, and VTe (the latter being more important in animal-associated EHEC). VT2 can also be further differentiated into VT2 variants VT2 and VT2v (253). Although VT2 has been associated with strains that are more likely to be associated with HUS, the actual toxin type determination does not currently have much relevance to the management of an individual patient's disease.

Given the approaches for EHEC detection and their variations, it may seem initially confusing how the laboratory should proceed in these regards. Certainly, the knowledge base of how frequent EHEC are, including specific serotypes, must weigh heavily on such decisions. Where *E. coli* O157:H7 is common and dominant among EHEC, e.g., many North American regions, the use of sorbitol-MacConkey is generally suffient. There yet remains some debate about whether the latter should be a component of the routine enteric media for all stool specimens in areas where the frequency is low. Furthermore, in areas where other serotypes prevail, it is probably best to use stool toxicity testing or polymyxin-extracted sweeps of coliform growth as the initial screening mechanism. The latter approaches, however, may yield very little practically in highly O157 endemic areas, and they may be reserved for stool specimens from outbreaks or from patients with HUS.

Salmonella

Presumptive salmonellae from enteric media are determined as previously detailed. The use of a commercial strip to confirm the suspicion along with a preliminary O serogrouping (usually using broad polyvalent groupings of A, B, C1, C2, D, and E) are usually sufficient to declare the isolate a *Salmonella* sp. Confirmatory biochemicals or serology are then of epidemiological value if the resources allow.

Commercial kits usually work well for *Salmonella* identification. Among the key biochemicals are lactose (-), ONPG (-), H_2S(+), and citrate (+).

S. serotype Typhi is serotyped as 9,12:d:- which is a Group D serotype. In addition, it expresses the Vi antigen which may at times mask the serological detection of the O antigen. In such cases where Vi is detected for a suspect *S.* serotype Typhi, a bacterial suspension may be boiled to unmask the Group D antigens. Occasionally, the Vi antigen may be detected among other salmonellae and other coliforms. In addition to suspecting this serotype on the basis of serology, several biochemicals are distinctively different from routine enteric salmonellae: ornithine (-), citrate (-),and no gas production from glucose.

Genetic probes and PCR detection of salmonellae have been assessed considerably, although the majority of interest has arisen in the food industry (254,255). Some studies have found greater sensitivity with such methods when compared to standard culture (256). Various modifications of this technology include paramagnetic bead separation (257), in situ hybridization (258), multiplex PCR assay for bacterium and drug resistance (259), and application to clinical samples from typhoid fever illnesses (260). A practical role for such methods in routine practice is yet to be defined.

Shigella

Suspect shigellae from enteric screening are also subjected to both biochemical confirmation and serological assessment. These bacteria are identified with reasonable accuracy from commercial systems. Occasionally, the serological studies may require a boiling pre-treatment of the isolate.

Key determinations include non-motility, lactose (-), ONPG (-; although *S. sonnei* may be positive), lysine (-), and no gas production from glucose.

Genetic detection of shigellae has also been evaluated (261-264). Greater sensitivity of PCR when compared to traditional cultures has been touted (261,262). Differentiation of shigellae and EIEC can also be accomplished (264). Again, a practical role for these methods in routine bacteriology is not yet realized.

Yersinia

As previously detailed, yersiniae may be suspected on the basis of screening slants combined with urease determination from selective enteric media. Currently, however, most laboratories use CIN which is reasonably selective. Thus, suspect yersiniae will be chosen on the basis of the classic 'target' colony on CIN and then assessed biochemically. Key biochemicals include urease (+), PPA (-), and lysine (-). *Yersinia* spp. biochemicals are better determined at 25°C rather than 37°C; motility may also be observed only for organism that is grown at 25-30°C.

Biotyping in the traditional schemata for *Y. enterocolitica* does not have as much relevance today, although three particular biochemicals are useful for delineating pathogenic and non-pathogenic biotypes: esculin, salicin, and pyrazinamidase (all + for putative non-pathogenic biotypes). The isolation of *Y. enterocolitica* which is negative for two of these three biochemicals should be reported; the quantitations will usually be in the moderate to heavy quantity on CIN. Non-pathogenic biotypes should either not be reported or should be reported as " [quantitative description] *Y. enterocolitica* isolated; non-pathogenic biotype". Some prefer the latter approach since there have been some rare citations of non-pathogenic biotypes that were associated with outbreaks (265). Commercial systems are able to speciate both *Y. enterocolitica* and *Y. pseudotuberculosis* well.

Non-*enterocolitica* and non-*pseudotuberculosis* species are also reasonably well defined with commercial identification systems. Although some will be biased to reporting these isolates from stool most likely due to the impression left by the genus designation, they probably should not be reported given their non-pathogenic status since such a report is only likely to confuse the clinician.

Given the simplified use of a few biochemicals to reasonably well categorize *Y. enterocolitica* into pathogenic and non-pathogenic isolates, there is generally little if any role for prospective serological serotyping on an individual basis.

2.   *Non-Enterobacteriaceae enteric pathogens and related bacteria*

Vibrio

When using TCBS as the selective medium, most colonies will warrant some investigation. In non-endemic areas where such a medium is not a routine component of enteric screening, the detection of oxidase-positive fermenters may be the initial cause to further assess an isolate. Commercial kits for identification may perform well for common vibrios but may be of lesser value for some of the uncommon species; the latter are likely to require referral. Some commerical kits may be enhanced with the addition of 1% saline to the inoculum for biochemicals so that vibrios will be supported. Given the oxidase positivity, the more likely confusion will exist between vibrios and *Aeromonas* spp. The former are tolerant to 6% NaCl but not the latter. *Aeromonas* and *Plesiomonas* isolates are also arginine-positive. The 'string test', using a suspension of organism in 0.5% deoxycholate, will yield a mucoid string when a bacteriological loop is lifted from such a suspension for vibrios but not aeromonads.

In areas that are endemic for *V. cholerae*, more economic short-cuts may prove to be of value, whereas areas with rare isolates, and perhaps more resources, may depend mainly on biochemical identification. In endemic areas, serological reactions may be applied directly to a suspect colony in order to confirm the presence of an O1 or O139 serotype; commercial agglutination kits for this purpose are useful (266). *V. cholerae* O1 isolates may be differentiated into 'classic' and 'El Tor' variants as follows:

	Sheep RBC hemolysis	VP	Resistance to polymyxin B (50 U)
Classic	no	-	S
El Tor	yes	+	R

It must be noted, however, that there is considerable variation in the hemolysis and the VP test, and at least two or more of the tests should be used to determine biotype. Sensitivity to polymyxin B and to biotype-specific bacteriophages, classical IV and El Tor 5, are the most reliable to biotype isolates of *V. cholerae* O1. Commercial EIA systems for O1 antigen detection directly from stools have become available (Cholera SMART) (267). The latter are likely to be most applicable when the disease is acute, and thus high quantitations of bacterium are present. Not all *V. cholerae* are necessarily toxigenic, especially those that do not belong to the recognized endemic and actively circulating serotype(s). Assays for toxigenicity were historically biological and utilized either Chinese hamster ovary cells or Y1 adrenal cells. Cholera toxin can now be determined with latex agglutination, EIA, or PCR for *ctx* genes

(268,269). It has been suggested that direct toxin testing by these methods for stools might also be applicable.

Campylobacter and *Arcobacter*

Most pathogenic campylobacters and arcobacters are catalase-positive; the recent campylobacters that have been renamed from *Wolinella* or *Bacteroides* genera are catalase-negative and favour an anaerobic environment with increased hydrogen in the growth atmosphere. Pathogenic campylobacters and arcobacters can be initially suspected on the basis of the Gram stain and colony morphology; obviously the majority will be recovered on *Campylobacter* selective media. They will initially be assessed for hippurate hydrolysis and antibiotic disc susceptibility (i.e., cephalothin and nalidixic acid). The ability to grow at 42°C is consistent with most pathogenic campylobacters especially from stool, but a few, especially systemic pathogens like *C. fetus*, will only grow at 37°C.

Thermophilic catalase-positive campylobacters that are hippurate-positive should be considered as *C. jejuni* without further assessment on a practical basis. Hippurate-negative *C. jejuni* do exist, but hippurate negativity should then prompt consideration for other campylobacters, arcobacters, and helicobacters, especially if the bacterium has been initially obtained from culture at 37°C. Supplementary tests may include catalase, H_2S production, antibiotic discs, indoxyl acetate hydrolysis, and nitrate. Commercial methods for identification have been made available (270), but both these and in-house approaches usually have difficulty in identifying lesser common campylobacters, and most enteric campylobacters will in fact prove to be *C. jejuni* which can be identified by a few simple assessments.

Immunological methods for speciation are not far advanced (271,272). Genetic methods, however, are progressing quickly, and it inevitable that a rapid approach, perhaps with PCR or a similar method, will soon emerge (273). Identification methods for campylobacters have been extensively reviewed by Stephen On recently (274).

Helicobacter

These bacteria do not grow at 42°C, and therefore, they will often be considered in the same context as non-thermophilic campylobacters from which they may be difficult to differentiate. Both *H. cinaedi* and *H. fennelliae* are biochemically differentiated. Again, the review paper of On (274) is a useful reference in these regards. As new *Helicobacter* spp. are so to be defined, the identification of these bacteria will undoubtedly become more complicated (see Chapter 20).

Aeromonas

As oxidase-positive fermentative bacteria that grow well and timely on routine media, *Aeromonas* spp. will be considered early after isolation. Some commerical identification systems accurately identify aeromonads to the genus level and thereafter call most isolates *A. hydrophila*. Other systems may accurately separate *A. caviae* and *A. hydrophila*. The three most common species by far prove to be *A. hydrophila*, *A. caviae*, and *A. veronii* var. sobria (especially the first two). Speciation beyond the latter three is rarely needed. The accurate identification of all aeromonads from human sources is somewhat complicated by the overlapping profiles between some species and by the need to use mechanisms that are uncommon to most laboratories. Often, then, the uncommon species may require referral.

Given the complexity of currently acknowledged genomospecies within this group, both PCR (with or without restriction digest analysis) and PFGE are being assessed in order to more easily provide consistent speciation (275-277).

Plesiomonas

P. shigelloides is accurately defined with most advanced commercial systems and is generally distinctive from *Aeromonas* spp.

E. Serodiagnosis

1. *Enterobacteriaceae*

E. coli

Serodiagnosis is not currently of use for *E. coli* infections with the exception of some EHEC. Although immunological responses to VTs do occur as assessed by neutralization or EIA, these reactions are generally not prominent and indeed not of sufficient measure to be used for diagnostic purposes (278,279).

Antibody responses to the homologous EHEC LPS after hemorrhagic colitis or HUS are much more prolific. Most study has been conducted with the O157 LPS (279,280). IgG antibody to O157 develops in more than 90% of patients within weeks after infection, and the antibody may persist for months (166). The LPS cross-reacts with some brucellae, some *Y. enterocolitica*, *V. cholerae* O1, other *E. coli* LPS (e.g., O55), group N salmonellae, some *C. freundii*, and *E. hermannii*. It is believed that such cross-reactivity may be responsible for false-positive serology when the O157 LPS is being used as the antigenic substrate (281). Some have assessed the use of a collection of common EHEC LPSs (O157, O26, O111, O55, and O128) and have shown that a majority of HUS patients develop antibodies when such a cluster of antigens is used (282). Serology for EHEC has a limited role in the overall diagnostic approach, and it is preferable to focus on stool testing for bacterium and/or toxin. Nevertheless, O157 serology may have some value for assessing the impact of an outbreak (283) or for confirming the cause of an episode of HUS. In the latter respect, the vast majority of gastroenteritis-associated HUS in children is caused by EHEC, and thus, EHEC should be suspected even when they are not cultured from stool samples of such patients.

Salmonella

The use of *Salmonella* serology in general is complicated by the O antigen specificity of the immune response (284). A common antigen for this purpose is not yet available.

The Widal test is an agglutination (tube or microtitre) reaction for the diagnosis of *S.* serotype Typhi infection which has been used historically (285). It has been difficult to standardize and is known to have an associated problem with false-positives. In endemic areas, there will be problems with interpretation due to endemic seroprevalence, and thus its value may be greater for those who return to non-typhoidal areas. Given the potential to recover the Typhi serotype from several body samples and given the potential for non-specific serological results, it is probably best to limit use of this test to those highly suspect illnesses, even retrospectively, that are culture-negative.

The use of the Vi antigen for serology (whether hemagglutination or EIA) has been shown to be of some value for detecting the carrier state (286,287). One such assay was shown to have a sensitivity of up to 75% for detecting carriers when a titre $\geq$1:160 was determined (288). Of interest, such an assay has been used to help identify possible carriers in an outbreak setting who may have been integral to food-borne transmission.

Shigella

Serology is not of sufficient value for diagnostic purposes even though the antibody response correlates well with severity of the clinical illness.

As for EHEC toxins, patients have a relatively poor response to Shiga toxin after *S. dysenteriae* infections. An alternative approach to serology for such infections has made use of LPS as the antigen (289).

Yersinia

Agglutination serology with either heat-killed or formalinized whole cells has been used for many years to establish a diagnosis for either *Y. enterocolitica* or *Y. pseudotuberculosis* infections. Reference sera are used to ensure standardization, and generally, titres $\geq$1:128 are significant among those who have been previously well (290). It is preferable to have paired sera for the assessment of seroconversion, especially among children and immunosuppressed patients who may not respond well and who may have titres as low as ≤1:32 despite bonafide infection. Serology must be interpreted with some knowledge of the antigen preparation (including realization of the circulating serogroup), background endemic seroprevalence which may be geographically variable, the underlying illness, active antibiotic therapy, and history of immunosuppression. As with other precipitation assays, prozone phenomena may be seen. Antibody titres persist for several months. Titres that range from 1:80 to >1:10,000 can develop within 5-10 days after onset of infection. In Europe, where serodiagnosis has been more commonly employed for *Y. enterocolitica* infections, the O:3 and O:9 antigens have been used since bacteria with these serogroups have caused the majority of illnesses.

Cross-reactions of *Y. enterocolitica* with other *Enterobacteriaceae* (e.g., some salmonellae, e.g., *Y. pseudotuberculosis*), brucellae, and rickettsiae have been defined. Given the potential for cross-reactivity and hence apparent endemic seroprevalence in some populations, it may be better to restrict the use of such serology to outbreaks where the serogroup is known or to retrospective diagnosis in regions with low seroprevalence (291).

Given the problems with agglutination, EIAs have been developed (even commercially) which will measure IgA, IgG, and IgM antibodies collectively (292,293). Whole cells or LPS have been used as the antigen in the latter. Problems with false-positive tests nevertheless continue to occur. Among patients with post-reactive arthritis, IgA antibodies tend to persist and may serve as a more reliable marker in themselves.

2. Non-Enterobacteriaceae enteric infections

Vibrio
There is a very limited role for serodiagnostic assays in assessing cholera. Paired sera should be collected when serology is to be used since most disease has a very rapid onset, and thus antibodies form well after; also, such serology is more likely, if at all, to be used in an area that is endemic, and hence, where there is some background antibody.

Among volunteers who were infected, seroconversion occurs by about day 10 after onset of the illness. The antibody levels tend to return to normal in the range of 1-6 months for those who reside in non-endemic areas.

Serology, with the measurement of either vibriocidal or anti-CT antibody (294), should restricted for use mainly in circumstances where a retrospective diagnosis will be of value.

Campylobacter
Serology has a limited role in the diagnosis of active disease, although it is recognized that it may provide an adjunct to culture for maximizing the detection of infectious episodes (295). There is some concern for cross-reactivity of *C. jejuni* serology with that for *H. pylori*. Many serological variants of *C. jejuni* exist.

Antigen extracts have been used to detect IgG, IgA, and IgM in the context of *C. jejuni* disease (189). Almost all patients will develop an IgG response, but only about 2/3 and 1/3 respectively will develop individual IgA and IgM responses. Both IgA and IgM rapidly decline. It has been advocated that all three forms of antibody should be sought. Others have found that the detection of these antibodies (with an acid extract antigen) has a sensitivity approaching 80% and a very high specificity (~99%) when appropriate cut-off values for EIA are selected (296). IgG antibodies seem to arise relatively early in the course of an illness, and it has been proposed that this may be occurring as a function of an anamnestic response given the likelihood that previous exposure has been had (297).

Aeromonas
There is no serological test for routine diagnosis. Most infections, when they may truly occur despite isolation of the bacterium from stool, are self-limited. Nevertheless, some form of serological test

might be of value to determine whether the bacterium has caused disease in a situation where there are other complicating factors; this would likely have limited use.

F. Epidemiological typing

The use of epidemiological typing for these groups of bacteria has been considerable given their frequency as community-acquired enteric pathogens (often occurring in outbreak form) and given their role as common and serious nosocomial pathogens. By necessity, the evolution of typing methods has followed the growth of new technologies over the last three decades, but it is apparent at the present time that essentially all *Enterobacteriaceae* and non-*Enterobacteriaceae* enteric pathogens and related bacteria may be typed by one or more of the current methods (see Chapter 7).

Biotyping has limited use for any of these bacteria, although it should be acknowledged that unique biochemicals may yet serve as a marker for a unique isolate. For many species, especially of the *Enterobacteriaceae*, former biotypes were a function of the limitations that were had for defining current species; some of these biotypes indeed proved to be newly designated species once genetic methods were utilized.

In general, antibiograms have limited value with the exception when very unusual patterns are evident, especially of resistance. For example, S. serotype Typhimurium DT104 has a particularly resistant profile (298). If not of sole value for typing, the antibiogram will at least serve as an initial mechanism to determine whether further typing will be necessary.

The diversity of O antigens was exploited for the purposes of typing most *Enterobacteriaceae* of concern as best evidenced by the development of complex O typing schemes for both *E. coli* and *Salmonella* (which still enjoy considerable use). Such systems used either agglutination or passive hemagglutination (PHA) with heat-stable or heat-labile antigens (e.g., Penner systems for PHA typing of *Proteus*). Although typing sera for this purpose continue to be made available for a few limited examples, the availability of O typing schemes for bacteria such as *Serratia* or *Enterobacter* often required the use of a few international reference laboratories. Outside of the limited uses for *Salmonella* and *E. coli*, therefore, most such systems have been replaced by newer molecular techniques. Likewise, the use of capsular antigens for typing is mainly an approach of the past.

Typing with bacteriophages and bacteriocins (or colicins) has also largely been replaced by new methods. Overall, it is somewhat inconvenient to maintain the series of phages that are required for any one common species. Nevertheless, phage typing of *E. coli* and *Salmonella* was shown to be sufficiently discriminatory in most circumstances, and these are still occasionally used by the most tertiary of reference centres.

The introduction to genetic relatedness as the basis for typing came mainly in the form of plasmid profiles with or without restriction enzyme digest. Although many *Enterobacteriaceae* bear plasmids, the limitation in number of plasmids and the potential for plasmidless isolates limited this approach. The subsequent methods included restriction digests of whole chromosomal material (BRENDA) with or without probes, ribotyping, PCR-based typing, and pulse field gel electrophoresis (PFGE or FIGE). The trend has been to develop methods which have a reasonable number of products or bands for comparison (i.e., having enough to facilitate the perception of differences when they exist but not being overly cumbersome), allow for elimination of radioactive labels, are resource-sparing, are timely, and are sufficiently discriminative. In large part, these characteristics are met especially by PCR–based methods, and to a lesser degree, PFGE. In theory, there should be many possible typing systems that are PCR-based given the format of RAPD (randomly amplified polymorphic DNA)-typing.

Mulitlocus enzyme electrophoresis is an effective but time and resource consuming method, and it will in large part be replaced by genetic methods for most purposes.

In the acceptance of any such method, it has at times been difficult to choose one as the absolute standard. Indeed, such a choice must be tempered by the epidemiological data that accompanies an outbreak where a clonal population is most likely. Nevertheless, in large comparisons, especially international, a method must often be chosen as an arbiter. Some methods may serve to discriminate beyond others, e.g., PCR-based methods or PFGE may continue to distinguish among isolates of a particular *Salmonella* serotype; some may not add any further differentiation, e.g., PCR-based methods such as those that are based on ERIC or REP primers generally do not provide much added information once the O157 serotype of *E. coli* is determined. In addition, it may be that some methods may be overly discriminative, e.g., some PFGE, when minor shifts in genome occur as a natural event during the course of an outbreak. When used for a focal setting such as the comparison of several isolates from an infection control investigation in a hospital, generally simple methods such as those which are PCR-based may be used, especially given that this approach will be amenable to the likely availability of thermocyclers in most large-sized laboratories. For the purposes of international comparisons or when a reference set of types (with numeric or other designations) is to be included, it may be more desirable to choose a method that is less open to variability for the given purpose.

For example, two PCR-based approaches are detailed which are broadly applicable to most *Enterobacteriaceae*. Genetic amplification of areas that are intimately related to **R**epetitive **E**xtragenic **P**alindromic (REP) sequences is known as REP-PCR. REP elements are often found in clusters and are dispersed throughout the bacterial genome (299); they have varying distances between them and may comprise up to 1% of the total chromosome. Their distribution is relatively stable, although an exact role in bacterial functions is not absolutely certain. Given the variable distances between elements, amplifications of bacterial genome with appropriate primers leads to a gradient of amplification product size; such variability thus gives rise to the diversity among isolates. Specimen preparation can be minimal and may simply involve proteinase K digestion and boiling of a standard suspension of bacterium that has been acquired from routine solid culture media. Products of amplification can be assessed on conventional ethidium bromide-stained agarose gels and may be visually inspected for similarites among isolate profiles.

Another similar PCR-based technique with somewhat broader application is methodologically related to the above and abbreviated as ERIC-PCR (300). In this approach, primers are designed which bind to **E**nterobacterial **I**ntergenic **R**epetitive **C**onsensus (ERIC) sequences. These too are interspersed throughout the bacterial genome in such a fashion that gradients of genetic amplification product will be obtained. The product is generated, resolved, and interpreted in much the same fashion as that for REP-PCR. Although it is intentional that both ERIC-PCR and REP-PCR be designed with primers that bind to pre-identified areas of the genome, it is also quite likely, given the short primer sequence, that the process is also in part inclusive of random amplification. For both of these methods, there is some overlapping application to Gram positive bacteria (301) and even yeast. In our experience, one set of ERIC primers, termed ERIC2 and ERIC1R complement, can be used to type a large variety of *Enterobacteriaceae* and pseudomonads (302,303).

A good example of the progress that has been achieved in this general area is that relating to the epidemiological study of *E. coli* O157:H7. As previously detailed, this EHEC serotype is the most common among those that cause both sporadic and epidemic infections, and the need for an accurate and applicable typing scheme is obvious. The pre-definition of the serotype already considerably narrows the opportunity to find diversity as it would in defining a particular, especially uncommon, *Salmonella* serotype; the O157 serotype is otherwise generally uncommon among clinical non-enteric isolates. The antibiogram is generally consistent with typical community-acquired *E. coli* whether pathogens or commensals; occasional ampicillin or co-trimoxazole resistance is encountered, but there is insufficient diversity to use the antibiogram for differentiation. The isolate may be assessed for toxin production. Most isolates produce both VT1 and VT2 (up to 80-90% in North America), but the presence of only VT1 or VT2, or the presence of the VT2v variant may lend some uniqueness. Plasmid profiles may also serve to preliminarily indicate difference or commonality (304), but it is possible to have a single common plasmid-bearing epidemic isolate which then limits this approach. Phage typing does discriminate among isolates and can be used for epidemiological purposes (305). Most PCR typing techniques that are applied to *E. coli* or *Enterobacteriaceae* otherwise, such as ERIC-PCR, REP-PCR, or RAPD-PCR, may not show much diversity among *E. coli* O157:H7 even when it exists (306), although some reports to the contrary have been published (307,308). Ribotyping has also not been of much value (309). Probing of DNA digests with lambda phage probes or labeled toxin probes has been proposed (310), but neither have gained widespread use. Sufficient discrimination can be achieved with variations of PFGE, and this method is currently being touted as a reference technique. Indeed, a large American surveillance network has streamlined a PFGE approach to the extent that multiple typing laboratory sites are able to provide reliable data to an epidemiology central (311). It is the latter approach that will give most relevancy to the typing of *E. coli* O157:H7 on a proactive basis, especially when linked to 'smart' computer programs which will facilitate the task of comparisons. It must be acknowledged, however, that outbreaks can occur with more than one strain.

Serotyping of common campylobacters has been achieved with the use of passive hemagglutination and heat-stable (LPS) antigens (312,313). Molecular methods are quickly being assessed nevertheless (314,315).

As previously detailed, *V. cholerae* is serotyped and biotyped. Subtyping within the common O1 serotype, however, may be desirable and is being increasingly used for epidemiological purposes, and various methods have been assessed including ribotyping, multilocus enzyme electrophoresis, rRNA-RFLP, and ctx-gene/flanking sequence-RFLP (316,317). A standardized ribotyping scheme is now available for both of the biotypes of *V. cholerae* O1 and for the O139 serotype (318,319).

The typing of *Aeromonas* spp. has not received much attention for clinical purposes.

VII. SUSCEPTIBILITY TESTING

A. *Enterobacteriaceae*

Given the growth rate of these bacteria, susceptibility testing is readily completed and interpretable in 24 hrs. The methods which may be used include those that are standard for rapidly-growing non-fastidious aerobic bacteria otherwise: these include agar dilution, modified Kirby-Bauer, microbroth dilution, and Etest (and their variations). There is some discrepancy among break-points from different countries, but on whole, these differences tend to be minor. The use of control bacteria where possible is advocated. Chapter 8 details aspects of susceptibility testing.

Although the details of testing procedures and their interpretation are reasonably set for these bacteria, less is certain about which antibiotics should be tested and indeed reported on routinely. Such decisions are influenced by the context, the local pattern of resistance, the need to conserve resource, the need to impact appropriately on infection control, and the knowledge base of the laboratory user. It is prudent to develop cascades of antibiotic susceptibility reporting that cater to the least expensive, equally effective, and more narrow of spectrum.

Common *Enterobacteriaceae* infections have been treated considerably, and in general, the microbiologist and primary clinician have developed an understanding of in vitro/in vivo correlates over time. It must be accepted, however, that not all beneficial predictions of response from in vitro work will be met with cure or even actual benefit. The complications of infection as well as the pharmacodynamics of the antibiotic(s) must be considered, and experience is just as, if not more important than, the in vitro result. For example, enteric salmonellae are not uncommonly susceptible to a wide variety of antimicrobial agents including ampicillin, cephalosporins, cotrimoxazole, aminoglycosides, among others. Few of these, if any, will have an affect on the acute course of an enteric salmonellosis. For *Shigella* diarrhea, discrepancies in outcome have been noted between oral ampicillin and oral amoxycillin; the former, which has less absorption and hence greater intralumenal concentrations, achieves a better outcome than the latter which is better absorbed and thus achieves better blood levels. In general, there is a good correlation between in vitro susceptibility and cure for common *Enterobacteriaceae*. Whereas such a correlation is then routinely extended to uncommon *Enterobacteriaceae* and their infections, the outcome should be more guarded until a sufficient body of knowledge has been accumulated.

Although susceptibility profiles for *Enterobacteriaceae* can be quite variable, there are nevertheless some predictable patterns among several species for selected antibiotics (Table 7). These are worthy of acknowledgement since susceptibility results to the contrary are often in error, and thus should be re-evaluated when encountered. These patterns may also help in the presumptive speciation given that they are so predictable. For example, cephalosporin susceptibility was often in part used to assist with the identification of common klebsiellae in the past.

Overall, there is a trend towards increasing resistance for these Gram negative bacteria. This is most evident for nosocomial pathogens which, by nature of having been acquired in an environment where antibiotic pressure is common, readily acquire resistance genes or enhance the production of innate mechanisms of resistance as a consequence of mutations in regulatory genes. Bacteria such as *Serratia* and *Enterobacter* have particularly adapted to such antibiotic pressure (320,321). These and other bacteria have acquired the capability to be resistant to broad-spectrum cephalosporins, carbapenems, new quinolones, and aminoglycosides (322,323). The potential for common enteric pathogens to acquire resistance genes from these latter bacteria has been realized (324).

The evolution of broad-spectrum beta-lactamases is of major concern. Currently, and in the past, clinicians have often relied on the availability of beta-lactam antibiotics and congeners for treating serious Gram negative infections, occasionally in combination with other agents such as aminoglycosides. With the advent of each new such agent, resistance has emerged shortly thereafter. *E. coli*, for example, have been found that overproduce TEM-1 beta-lactamase (325). Through exposure to cephalosporins especially, other *Enterobacteriaceae* have evolved potent beta-lactamases (especially AmpC [group 1]) (326) that confer resistance to newer generations of cephalosporins. Although commonly carried on the chromosome and actively expressed, the genes for these beta-lactamases may be derepressed through mutations in the related regulatory genes. As well, dozens of derivatives of both the TEM and SHV family of beta-lactamases have arisen through an accumulation of point mutations that affect the active sites of these enzymes (22,327,328). Whereas the existence of these chromosomal genes in themselves

Table 7   Common resistance profiles for selected *Enterobacteriaceae* and *Aeromonas*.

	Ampicillin	Cephalothin	Polymyxin	Ticarcillin	Nitrofurantoin
S. marcescens	R	R		+/- (50%R)	
C. freundii	R	R			R
M. morganii	R	R	R		R
K. pneumoniae	R			R	
K. oxytoca	R			R	
H. alvei	R	R			
E. cloacae	R	R			+/-(75%R)
P. vulgaris	R		R		R
P. mirabilis			R		R
Providencia		R	R		R
Edwardsiella			R		
A. hydrophila	R	R			

is of great concern, more discomforting is the knowledge that equivalent genes have now been found on plasmids with the potential of having them spread to other *Enterobacteriaceae* (329,330); such mobile elements now also include carbapenemases (331,332). Furthermore, the progression of mutations has also facilitated the development of resistance to beta-lactamase inhibitors (333,334). In addition to the threat of such potent beta-lactamases, it is also critical to realize that this activity is but one mechanism in addition to the potential to alter target sites (i.e., pencillin-binding proteins) for beta-lactams and to alter outer membrane permeability (335). Therefore, it is conceivable and indeed postulated that resistance to seemingly advanced antimicrobials may be a combination of such mechanisms, e.g., overproduction of an AmpC enzyme along with a decrease in outer membrane permeability (336). Overall, the development of 'integrons' which contain gene cassettes that are capable of moving to other integrons poses a threat given the ability to collect resistance genes (337). Although the detection of beta-lactam resistance is usually accomplished with traditional susceptibility testing methods, extended spectrum beta-lactamases may not always be sufficiently expressed. The presence of such activity may be better demonstrated by a modification of the Etest (combines both ceftazidime and clavulanic acid) (338) or the use of 'double-disc' diffusion (339). The role for such testing on a routine basis is yet to be determined, and therapeutic options are often available which allow for beta-lactam antibiotics to be reserved when such concerns arise.

The second category of resistance that is also of major concern is that relating to the aminoglycosides which are commonly used as adjuncts to beta-lactam agents in serious infections. For *Enterobacteriaceae*, the enzymatic modification of aminoglycosides has long been recognized in contrast to some other bacteria, e.g. pseudomonads, which may have resistance that is based more on impermeability. The aminoglycoside-modifying enzymes vary in activity, e.g., acetylation, adenylation, or phosphorylation, and the specific modifying enzyme may confer resistance to one aminoglycoside or many at the same time (340). This form of resistance is high-level, and resistance genes are often borne on plasmids. The more common resistances include those to single aminoglycosides or those with impact on gentamicin and tobramycin (but not amikacin). Isolates with combinations of such enzymes may be resistant to all aminoglycosides. There is considerable variation in both the geographical spread of such resistance genes as well as the frequency among hospitals in a given region (341).

Fluoroquinolones have become a welcome new resource for the management of both complicated and uncomplicated Gram negative infections. They may be conveniently administered in the oral form on many occasions. Unfortunately, resistance to them is emerging quickly, and in part, this may simply be a function of their current widespread (perhaps even excessive) use in the community. Mutations in the DNA gyrase active site are often found when resistance emerges.

1. E. coli

Resistance to the first-line agent ampicillin has increased to approximately 30-50% for community-acquired isolates; this resistance is most often due to the TEM-1 beta-lactamase which confers resistance also to carbenicillin and ticarcillin, and to a lesser degree piperacillin. Resistance to cotrimoxazole has also increased and is often cited in the range of at least 25%. Cephalosporin resistance is much less common. First-generation cephalosporin resistance is usually <5-10%, although citations have been made of broad spectrum beta-lactamases in this species.

Antibiotic use for EHEC infection is controversial and understudied. Some have proposed that in vitro exposure to antibiotics is associated with increased liberation of toxin (342), but such findings have been questioned in the context of methodological variation (343). It is unclear whether any such findings have relevance to clinical care.

Treatment of EPEC infections with oral non-absorbable antibiotics (aminoglycosides or polymyxins) is a tactic of old (344), but does not appear to have been validated in recent times given the new understanding of pathogenesis in regards to attachment. It is conceivable that treatment studies of the past were not privileged in truly having understood what constituted pathogenic EPEC.

ETEC resistance is of concern especially in areas of high attack rate where antibiotic use may not be well-controlled (345).

2. Salmonella

Gastroenteritides

Few if any antibiotics change the course of an acute *Salmonella* gastroenteritis, and thus there is a discrepancy here between in vitro effect and in vivo outcome. Thus, antibiotic susceptibility is usually not necessary and indeed should not be generally reported. Some patients who are at higher risk of developing systemic spread along with the intestinal illness (e.g., children less than one year of age or the elderly) have at times been treated with antibiotics in order to reduce the potential for complications. In the latter circumstance, the antibiotics are used for their activity in blood and tissue for which the correlation with in vitro testing is much better. Nevertheless, such antibiotic use is debatable even if for short periods, and the best choice of an antibiotic is of further uncertainty. The treatment of systemic illness such as bacteremias may generally follow the treatment of Gram negative infections otherwise and do not necessarily require the following of a typhoid fever treatment regimen; the antimicrobial and its administration will depend on the actual site.

There has been a progressive increase in resistance especially with respect to agents such as ampicillin, cotrimoxazole, and tetracyclines. The global dissemination of *S.* serotype Typhimurium DT104 is but one example of a strain with multiple resistance (346). The finding of extended spectrum beta-lactamases and aminoglycoside-modifying enzymes among salmonellae is also becoming more common (23).

Treatment of carriers may be desirable on occasion; treatment may be complicated, however, by the seclusion of bacterium in the biliary system in the presence of stones. Treatments currently often include fluoroquinolones for a prolonged period (~4-6 weeks).

S. typhi

Several antibiotics are of proven value for the treatment of typhoid fever when the bacterium is susceptible, and these include cotrimoxazole, ampicillin, chloramphenicol, ciprofloxacin, cefotaxime, ceftriaxone, and cefoperazone. Relapses do occur regardless of in vitro susceptibility; these are likely due to the sequestration of bacterium in immune cells including the reticuloendothelial system. Treatment should be given for a minimum of 10-14 days. Aminoglycosides and first-generation cephalosporins should not be used regardless of apparent in vitro susceptibility.

Multiple drug resistance is emerging in several locales (26), and is often due to plasmid-borne genes which commonly include factors for chloramphenicol resistance. Whereas chloramphenicol was a first-line therapy in most settings, it is becoming less so. Resistance to ampicillin, chloramphenicol, cotrimoxazole, and tetracyclines is now a global concern (347), and it has prompted recommendations that ciprofloxacin be used as the antibiotic of choice at least for oral therapy. Quinolone-resistant isolates have emerged, and these have been associated with treatment failure (348).

The treatment of carriers is much more relevant given the potential impact of *S.* serotype Typhi. Quinolones have been used for this purpose with some beneficial outcome.

3. Shigella

When shigellae are susceptible to ampicillin, cotrimoxazole, nalidixic acid, or fluoroquinolones, the use of these agents is accompanied by a favourable clinical outcome, and they should generally be used to modify the course of an illness when the presentation is moderate to severe. Some agents, such as oral cephalosporins, may show activity in vitro but will not necessarily have any beneficial impact.

Resistance is increasing, and many isolates from endemic areas not uncommonly manifest resistance to ampicillin and cotrimoxazole. Nalidixic acid has been a treatment option for the latter, but resistance is also emerging to this agent. Given the geographic variation in resistance frequencies, it is recommended that susceptibility testing should be performed.

4. *Yersinia*

Y. enterocolitica commonly produces 'type A and B' beta-lactamases which confer resistance to ampicillin, carbenicillin, and first-generation cephalosporins (349), but occasional ampicillin susceptible serotypes are isolated. This species is often susceptible to aminoglycosides, cotrimoxazole, piperacillin, third-generation cephalosporins, tetracycline, and chloramphenicol (350). The bacterium is, however, resistant to cefsulodin which is used in selective media. Although some have recommended the use of either cotrimoxazole or tetracycline for the treatment of *Yersinia* gastroenteritis, placebo-controlled trials of antibiotic efficacy have not been able to demonstrate a benefit at least for cotrimoxazole (351). The latter study must be reconsidered, however, since many patients were recruited late in the disease, and since former studies did not always consider the issue of pathogenic and non-pathogenic subtypes.

Systemic yersinoses usually respond to an extended-spectrum cephalosporin with or without an aminoglycoside. Fluoroquinolones have also been comtemplated as potentially useful agents. Dual therapy should probably be used especially in endovascular infections which may be more refractory to treatment.

Y. pseudotuberculosis is susceptible to ampicillin, tetracycline, cotrimoxazole, chloramphenicol, aminoglycosides, and extended-spectrum cephalosporins.

B. Non-*Enterobacteriaceae* enteric pathogens and related bacteria

1. *Vibrios*

Vibrios in general grow relatively well on plain Mueller-Hinton medium or equivalent, and therefore, standard methods for susceptibility testing may be used. For example, interpretive criteria are detailed for tetracycline, ampicillin, cotrimoxazole, and chloramphenicol.

V. cholerae

Appropriate antibiotics decrease the severity of cholera and shorten the duration of excretion of the organism. Tetracyclines have been the treatment of choice except for pediatric patients who may receive ampicillin, cotrimoxazole, or chloramphenicol. Fluid and electrolyte support are essential, nevertheless, given the rapid changes in physiology that may arise in short order before antibiotics take their effect.

Resistance for this species is emerging, although it is significantly variable depending on location and sometimes serotypes (352-354). Resistance to ampicillin and cotrimoxazole is now common even for the O139 serogroup (up to 80-95%). In some regions, tetracycline resistance is up to approximately 50%. Cotrimoxazole resistance elements may be carried as conjugative transposons (65), thus explaining the potential for rapid shifts in susceptibility between serotypes. Significant variations in susceptibility among isolates of one serogroup have been determined during different periods, and resistance may emerge during a longstanding epidemic (355). The changing patterns of resistance closely follow the continuous emergence of new clones for any given serogroup (356). It is of interest that non-O1 *V. cholerae* that lack the ability to produce toxin may harbour single or multiple resistance genes (357); perhaps these are the reservoir for transferable resistance to pathogenic serogroups.

Non-cholera vibrios

The treatment of diarrheal illnesses due to these pathogens is debatable, including that due to *V. parahemolyticus*. Treatment of systemic disease can be accomplished with a variety of antibiotics and is critical since vibrio bacteremias have considerable associated morbidity. *V. vulnificus* is susceptible to many antibiotics (358).

2. Campylobacter

Methods for susceptibility testing of these bacteria are not well-standardized for clinical purposes although several methods have been used to study susceptibility for comparative purposes. Agar dilution methods with the use of Mueller-Hinton blood (5%) agar and incubation at 37°C have been detailed as has the use of the Etest with the same conditions.

C. jejuni and *C. coli* not uncommonly possess beta-lactamases (359). They are often susceptible to erythromycin, tetracycline, aminoglycosides, chloramphenicol, and fluoroquinolones. Both erythromycin and ciprofloxacin are recommended for the treatment of moderate to severe gastroenteritides when the patients are seen relatively early during the illness. Resistance to erythromycin and tetracycline have been described, and indeed resistance to the former may be increasing. It is thus of some value to test for erythromycin susceptibility if treatment is contemplated. Resistance to fluoroquinolones has also increased significantly in some regions (360), and there is concern that veterinary use of related antibiotics may be having some influence in this regard.

A variety of antimicrobials have been used to treat rare systemic illnesses from enteric campylobacters including aminoglycosides. *C. fetus* is susceptible to aminoglycosides and beta-lactam agents.

3. Helicobacter

Most experience with the treatment of these rare infections relates to *H. cinaedi* infection of immunocompromised patients. *H. cinaedi* is usually susceptible to tetracyclines, aminoglycosides, and fluoroquinolones.

4. Aeromonas

Most data for susceptibility testing have been obtained for the three common human-associated species (361,362). *A. hydrophila* and *A. caviae* are commonly resistant to ampicillin, first-generation cephalosporins, and ticarcillin due to beta-lactamase production. They are usually susceptible to tetracyclines, aminoglycosides, fluoroquinolones, extended-spectrum cephalosporins, and cotrimoxazole. Treatment for diarrheal episodes is not yet scientifically supported; again, it is questionable whether these bacteria are etiological agents even when they are isolated from the stool of a symptomatic patient. Systemic infections and aggressive localized infections will benefit from single or combination therapy that is otherwise guided by susceptibility testing. The methods for the latter are essentially those that are otherwise used for *Enterobacteriaceae*.

Transferable resistance due to plasmids has been identified (363). Nevertheless, beta-lactamases are usually a function of chromosomal elements; these are inducible. Two major beta-lactamases are recognized. The first is a metallo beta-lactamase which has a broad spectrum of activity including carbapenems (364,365). The second is a serine beta-lactamase which behaves like a group 1 cephalosporinase (364).

5. Plesiomonas

P. shigelloides is often beta-lactamase positive and ampicillin resistant (95,362). It is usually susceptible to cotrimoxazole, aminoglycosides, fluoroquinolones, and cephalosporins (95).

REFERENCES

1. Ewing WH. Edwards and Ewing's Identification of *Enterobacteriaceae* (Fourth Edition). New York, NY:Elsevier, 1986.
2. Bottone EJ. *Yersinia enterocolitica*: a panoramic view of a charismatic microorganism. CRC Crit Rev Microbiol 1977; 5:211-214.

3. Wauters G, Kandolo K, Janssens M. Revised biogrouping scheme of *Yersinia enterocolitica*. Contrib Microbiol Immunol 1987; 9:14-21.

4. Wauters G, Janssens M, Steigerwalt AG, Brenner DJ. *Yersinia mollaretii* sp. nov. and *Yersinia bercovieri* sp. nov. formerly called *Yersinia enterocolitica* biogroups 3A and 3B. Int J Syst Bacteriol 1988; 38:424-429.

5. Lobato MJ, Landeras E, Gonzalez-Hevia MA, Mendoza MC. Genetic heterogeneity of clinical strains of *Yersinia enterocolitica* traced by ribotyping and relationships between ribotypes, serotypes, and biotypes. J Clin Microbiol 1998; 36:3297-3302.

6. Caugant DA, Aleksic S, Mollaret HH, Selander RK, Kapperud G. Clonal diversity and relationships among strains of *Yersinia enterocolitica*. J Clin Microbiol 1989; 27:2678-2683.

7. Robins-Browne RM, Traditional enteropathogenic *Escherichia coli* of infantile diarrhea. Rev Infect Dis 1987; 9:28-53.

8. Neter E. Enteritis due to enteropathogenic *Escherichia coli*. Am J Dig Dis 1965; 10:883-886.

9. Law D. Adhesion and its role in the virulence of enteropathogenic *Escherichia coli*. Clin Microbiol Rev 1994; 7:152-173.

10. Watanabe H, Akihito W, Inagaki Y, Itoh K, Tamura K. Outbreaks of enterohaemorrhagic *Escherichia coli* O157:H7 infection by two different genotype strains in Japan, 1996. Lancet 1996; 348:831-832.

11. Yukioka H, Kurita S. *Escherichia coli* O157 infection disaster in Japan, 1996. Eur J Emerg Med 1997; 4:165.

12. Van Beneden CA, Keene WE, Strang RA, Werker RA, King AS, Mahon B, Hedberg K, Bell A, Kelly MT, Balan VK, MacKenzie WR, Fleming D. Multinational outbreak of *Salmonella enterica* serotype Newport infections due to contaminated alfalfa sprouts. JAMA 1999; 281:158-162.

13. Mahon BE, Ponka A, Hall WN, Komatsu K, Dietrich SE, Siitonen A, Cage G, Hayes PS, Lambert-Fair MA, Bean NH, Griffin PM, Slutsker L. An international outbreak of *Salmonella* infections caused by alfalfa sprouts grown from contaminated seeds. J Infect Dis 1997; 175:876-882.

14. Reeves PR, Lan R. Cholera in the 1990s. Brit Med Bull 1998; 54:611-623.

15. Koo D, Traverso H, Libel M, Drasbek C, Tauxe R, Brandling-Bennett D. Epidemic cholera in Latin America, 1991-1993: implications of case definitions used for public health surveillance. Bull Pan Am Health Organ 1996; 30:134-143.

16. Mossel DA, Struijk CB, Jansen JT. Control of the transmission of *Vibrio cholerae* and other enteropathogens by foods originating from endemic areas in South America and elsewhere as a model situation. Int J Food Microbiol 1992; 15:1-11.

17. Piddock LJ. Quinolone resistance and *Campylobacter* spp. J Antimicrob Chemother 1995; 36:891-898.

18. Smith KE, Besser JM, Hedberg CW, Leano FT, Bender JB, Wicklund JH, Johnson BP, Moore KA, Osterholm MT. Quinolone-resistant *Campylobacter jejuni* infections in Minnesota, 1992-1998. N Engl J Med 1999; 340:1525-1532.

19. Perrin M, Donnio PY, Heurtin-Lecorre C, Travert MF, Avril JL. Comparative antimicrobial resistance and genomic diversity of *Escherichia coli* isolated from urinary tract infections in the community and in hospitals. J Hosp Infect 1999; 41:273-279.

20. Ena J, Lopez-Perezagua MM, Martinez-Peinado C, Cia-Barrio MA, Ruiz-Lopez I. Emergence of ciprofloxacin resistance in *Escherichia coli* isolates after widespread use of fluoroquinolones. Diagn Microbiol Infect Dis 1998; 30:103-107.

21. Nordmann P. Trends in beta-lactam resistance among *Enterobacteriaceae*. Clin Infect Dis 1998; 27:S100-S106.

22. Heritage I, M'Zali FH, Gascoyne-Binzi D, Hawkey PM. Evolution and spread of SHV extended-spectrum beta-lactamases in gram-negative bacteria. J Antimicrob Chemother 1999; 44:309-318.

23. Revathi G, Shannon KP, Stapleton PD, Jain BK, French GL. An outbreak of extended-spectrum beta-lactamase-producing *Salmonella senftenberg* in a burns ward. J Hosp Infect 1998; 40:295-302.

24. Wain J, Hoa NT, Chinh NT, Vinh H, Everett MJ, Diep TS, Day NP, Solomon T, White NJ. Quinolone-resistant *Salmonella typhi* in Vietnam: molecular basis of resistance and clinical response to treatment. Clin Infect Dis 1997; 25:1404-1410.

25. Mermin JH, Townes JM, Gerber M, Dolan N, Mintz ED, Tauxe RV. Typhoid fever in the United States, 1985-1994: changing risks of international travel and increasing antimicrobial resistance. Arch Intern Med 1998; 158:633-638.

26. Rowe B, Ward LR, Threlfall EJ. Multidrug-resistant *Salmonella typhi*: a worldwide epidemic. Clin Infect Dis 1997; 24:S106-109.

27. Akkina JE, Hogue AT, Angulo FJ, Johnson R, petersen KE, Saini PK, Fedorka-Cray PJ, Schlosser WD. Epidemiologic aspects, control, and importance of multiple-drug resistant *Salmonella tyhimurium* DT104 in the United States. J Am Vet Med Assoc 1999; 214:790-798.

28. Legros D, Paquet C, Dorlencourt F, Saoult E. Risk factors for death in hospitalized dysentery patients in Rwanda. Trop Med Int Health 1999; 4:428-432.

29. Materu SF, Lema OE, Mukunza HM, Adhiambo CG, Carter JY. Antibiotic resistance pattern of *Vibrio cholerae* and *Shigella* causing diarrhoea outbreaks in the eastern Africa region: 1994-1996. East Afr Med J 1997; 74:193-197.

30. Jones RN. Impact of changing pathogens and antimicrobial susceptibility patterns in the treatment of serious infections in hospitalized patients. Am J Med 1996; 100:S3-S12.

31. Nataro JP, Kaper JB. Diarrheagenic *Escherichia coli*. Clin Microbiol Rev 1998; 11:142-201.

32. Levine WN, Goldberg MJ. *Escherichia vulneris* osteomyelitis of the tibia caused by a wooden foreing body. Ortho Rev 1994; 23:262-265.

33. Farmer JJ, Fanning GR, Davis BR, O'Hara CM, Riddle C, Hickman-Brenner FW, Asbury MA, Lowery VA, Brenner DJ. *Escherichia fergusonii* and *Enterobacter taylorae*, two new species of *Enterobacteriaceae* isolated from clinical specimens. J Clin Microbiol 1985; 21:77 81.

34. Goldberg MB, Rubin RH. The spectrum of *Salmonella* infection. Infect Dis Clin North Am 1988; 2:571-598.

35. Mandal BK. Typhoid and paratyphoid fever. Clin Gastroenterol 1979; 8:715-735.

36. Keusch GT. *Shigella* infections. Clin Gastroenterol 1979; 8:645-662.

37. Cover TL, Aber RC. *Yersinia enterocolitica*. N Engl J Med 1989; 321:16-24.

38. Tertti R, Vuento R, Mikkola P, Granfors K, Makela AL, Toivanen A. Clinical manifestations of *Yersinia pseudotuberculosis* infection in children. Eur J Clin Microbiol Infect Dis 1989; 8:587-591.

39. Chow JW, Yu VL, Shlaes DM. Epidemiologic perspectives on *Enterobacter* for the infection control professional. Am J Infect Cont 1994; 22:195-201.

40. Acar JF. *Serratia marcescens* infections. Infect Cont 1986; 7:273-278.

41. Lipsky BA, Hook EW, Smith AA, Plorde JJ. *Citrobacter* infections in humans: experience at the Seattle Veterans Medical Center and a review of the literature. Rev Infect Dis 1980; 2:746-760.

42. Peerbooms PG, Verweij AM, MacLaren DM. Uropathogenic properties of *Proteus mirabilis* and *Proteus vulgaris*. J Med Microbiol 1985; 19:55-60.

43. Podschun R, Ullmann U. Klebsiella spp. as nosocomial pathogens: epidemiology, taxonomy, typing methods, and pathogenicity factors. Clin Microbiol Rev 1998; 11:589-603.

44. Goldstein EJ, Lewis RP, Martin WJ, Edelstein PH. Infections caused by *Klebsiella ozaenae*: a changing disease spectrum. J Clin Microbiol 1978; 8:413-418.

45. Miller RH, shulman JB, Canalis RF, Ward PH. *Klebsiella rhinoscleromatis*: a clinical and pathogenic enigma. Otolaryngol Head Neck Surg 1979; 87:212-221.

46. Janda JM, Abbott SL. Infections associated with the genus *Edwardsiella*: the role of *Edwardsiella tarda* in human disease. Clin Infect Dis 1993; 17:742-748.

47. Janda JM, Abbott SL, Albert MJ. Prototypal diarrheagenic strains of *Hafnia alvei* are actually members of the genus Escherichia. J Clin Microbiol 1999; 37:2399-2401.

48. Barua D, Greenough WB – eds. Topics in Infectious Disease: Cholera. New York, NY:Plenum Press, 1992.

49. Hughes JM, Hollis DG, Gangarosa EJ, Weaver RE. Non-cholera vibrio infections in the United States: clinical, epidemiologic, and laboratory features. Ann Intern Med 1978; 88:602-606.

50. Cornick NA, Gorbach SL. *Campylobacter*. Infect Dis Clin North Am 1988; 2:643-654.

51. Morrison VA, Lloyd BK, Chia JK, Tuazon CU. Cardiovascular and bacteremic manifestations of *Campylobacter fetus* infection: case report and review. Rev Infect Dis 1990; 12:387-392.

52. Jimenez SG, Heine RG, Ward PB, Robins-Browne RM. *Campylobacter upsaliensis* gastroenteritis in childhood. Pediatr Infect Dis J 1999; 18:988-992.

53. Tauxe RV, Patton CM, Edmonds P, Barrett TJ, Brenner DJ, Blake PA. Illness associated with *Campylobacter laridis*, a newly recognized *Campylobacter* species. J Clin Microbiol 1985; 21:222-225.

54. Totten PA, Fennell CL, Tenover CL, Wezenberg JM, Perine PL, Stamm WE, Holmes KK. *Campylobacter cinaedi* (sp. nov.) and *Campylobacter fennelliae* (sp. nov.): two new *Campylobacter* species associated with enteric disease in homosexual men. J Infect Dis 1985; 151:131-139.

55. Kiehlbauch JA, Brenner DJ, Cameron DN, Steigerwalt AG, Makowski JM, Baker CN, Patton CM, Wachsmuth IK. Genotypic and phenotypic characterization of *Helicobacter cinaedi* and *Helicobacter fennelliae* strains isolated from humans and animals. J Clin Microbiol 1995; 33:2940-2947.

56. Trivett-Moore NL, Rawlinson WD, Yuen M, Gilbert GL. *Helicobacter westmeadii* sp. nov., a new species isolated from blood cultures of two AIDS patients. J Clin Microbiol 1997; 35:1144-1150.

57. Janda JM, Abbott SL. Evolving concepts regarding the genus *Aeromonas*: an expanding panorama of species, disease presentations, and unanswered questions. Clin Infect Dis 1998; 27:332-344.

58. Brenden RA, Miller MA, Janda JM. Clinical disease spectrum and pathogenic factors associated with *Plesiomonas shigelloides* infections in humans. Rev Infect Dis 1988; 10:303-316.

59. Karmali MA. Infection by verocytotoxin-producing *Escherichia coli*. Clin Microbiol Rev 1989; 2:15-38.

60. Turnbull PC. Food poisoning with special reference to *Salmonella* – its epidemiology, pathogenesis and control. Clin Gastroenterol 1979; 8:663-714.

61. Woodward DL, Khakhria R, Johnson WM. Human salmonellosis associated with exotic pets. J Clin Microbiol 1997; 35:2786-2790.

62. Tjoa WS, DuPont HL, Sullivan P, Pickering LK, Holguin AH, Olarte J, Evans DG, Evans DJ. Location of food consumption and traveller's diarrhea. Am J Epidemiol 1977; 106:61-66.

63. Shears P. Cholera. Ann Trop Med Parasitol 1994; 88:109-122.

64. Slutsker L, Altekruse SF, Swerdlow DL. Foodborne diseases: emerging pathogens and trends. Infect Dis Clin North Am 1998; 12:199-216.

65. Waldor MK, Tschape H, Mekalanos JJ. A new type of conjugative transposon encodes resistance to sulfamethoxazole, trimethoprim, and streptomycin in *Vibrio cholerae* O139. J Bacteriol 1996; 178:4157-4165.

66. Hacker J. Role of fimbrial adhesins in the pathogenesis of *Escherichia coli* infections. Can J Microbiol 1992; 38:720-727.

67. Krogfelt KA. Bacterial adhesion: genetics, biogenesis, and role in pathogenesis of fimbrial adhesins of *Escherichia coli*. Rev Infect Dis 1991; 13:721-735.

68. Dunn DL. Gram-negative bacterial sepsis and sepsis syndrome. Surg Clin North Am 1994; 74:621-635.

69. Heumann D, Glauser MP, Calandra T. Molecular basis of host-pathogen interaction in septic shock. Curr Opin Microbiol 1998; 1:49-55.

70. Opal SM, Cohen J. Clinical gram-positive sepsis: does it fundamentally differ from gram-negative bacterial sepsis? Crit Care Med 1999; 27:1608-1616.

71. Stroud MR, Stapleton AE, Levery SB. The P histo-blood group-related glycosphingolipid sialosyl galactosyl globoside as a preferred binding receptor for uropathogenic *Escherichia coli*: isolation and structural characterization from human kidney. Biochemistry 1998; 37:17420-17428.

72. Stapleton AE, Stroud MR, Hakomori SI, Stamm WE. The globoseries glycosphingolipid sialosyl galactosyl globoside is found in urinary tract tissues and is a preferred binding receptor in vitro for uropathogenic *Escherichia coli* expressing pap-enocded adhesins. Infect Immun 1998; 66:3856-3861.

73. Johnson JR. Virulence factors in *Escherichia coli* urinary tract infection. Clin Microbiol Rev 1991; 4:80-128.

74. Mobley HL, Island MD, Massad G. Virulence determinants or uropathogenic *Escherichia coli* and *Proteus mirabilis*. Kidney Int 1994; 47:S129-S136.

75. Svanborg C, Godaly G. Bacterial viruelence in urinary tract infection. Infect Dis Clin North Am 1997; 11:513-529.

76. Mitsumori K, Terai A, Yamamoto S, Ishitoya S, Yoshida O. Virulence characteristics of *Escherichia coli* in acute bacterial prostatitis. J Infect Dis 1999; 180:1378-1381.

77. Pal T, Al-Sweih NA, Herpay M, Chugh TD. Identification of enteroinvasive *Escherichia coli* and *Shigella* strains in pediatric patients by an *ipaC*-specific enzyme-linked immunosorbent assay. J Clin Microbiol 1997; 35:1757-1760.

78. Buysse JM, Hartman AB, Strockbine N, Venkatesan M. Genetic polymorphism of the *ipaH* multicopy antigen gene in *Shigella* spp. and enteroinvasive *Escherichia coli*. Microb Pathog 1995; 19:335-349.

79. Sethabutr O, Echeverria P, Hoge CW, Bodhidatta L, Pitarangsi C. Detection of *Shigella* and enteroinvasive *Escherichia coli* by PCR in the stools of patients with dysentery in Thailand. J Diarrhoeal Dis Res 1994; 12:265-269.

80. Gaastra W, Svennerholm AM. Colonization factors of human enterotoxigenic *Escherichia coli* (ETEC). Trends Microbiol 1996; 4:444-452.

81. Wolf MK. Occurrence, distribution, and associations of O and H serogroups, colonization factor antigens, and toxins of enterotoxigenic *Escherichia coli*. Clin Microbiol Rev 1997; 10:569-584.

82. Frankel G, Phillips AD, Rosenshine I, Dougan G, Kaper JB, Knutton S. Enteropathogenic and enterohemorrhagic *Escherichia coli*: more subversive elements. Mol Microbiol 1998; 30:911-921.

83. Donnenberg MS. Interactions between enteropathogenic *Escherichia coli* and epithelial cells. Clin Infect Dis 1999; 28:451-455.

84. Nataro JP, Steiner T, Guerrant RL. Enteroaggregative *Escherichia coli*. Emerg Infect Dis 1998; 4:251-261.

85. Beinke C, Laarmann S, Wachter C, Karch H, Greune L, Schmidt MA. Diffusely adhering *Escherichia coli* strains induce attaching and effacing phenotypes and secrete homologs of Esp proteins. Infect Immun 1998; 66:528-539.

86. Pelayo JS, Scaletsky IC, Pedroso MZ, Sperandio V, Giron JO, Frankel G, Trabulsi LR. Virulence properties of atypical EPEC strains. J Med Microbiol 1998; 48:41-49.
87. Scotland SM, Smith HR, Cheasty T, Said B, Willshaw GA, Stokes, Rowe B. Use of gene probes and adhesion tests to characterize *Escherichia coli* belonging to enteropathogenic serogroups isolated in the United Kingdom. J Med Microbiol 1996; 44:438-443.
88. Bhan MK, Raj P, Levine MM, Kaper JB, Bhandari N, Srivastava R, Kumar R, Sazawal S. Enteroaggregative *Escherichia coli* associated with persistent diarrhea in a cohort of rural children in India. J Infect Dis 1989; 159:1061-1064.
89. Albert MJ, Faruque AS, Faruque SM, Sack RB, Mahalanabis D. Case-control study of enteropathogens associated with childhood diarrhea in Dhaka, Bangladesh. J Clin Microbiol 1999; 37:3458-3464.
90. Vila J, Gene A, Vargas M, Gascon J, Latorre C, Jimenez de Anta MT. A case-control study of diarrhea in children caused by *Escherichia coli* producing heat-stable enterotoxin. J Med Microbiol 1998; 47:889-891.
91. Kang G, Sheela S, Mathan MM, Mathan VI. Prevalence of enteroaggregative and other Hep-2 cell adherent *Escherichia coli* in asymptomatic rural south Indians by longitudinal sampling. Microbios 1999; 100:57-66.
92. Haider K, Faruque SM, Albert MJ, Nahar S, Neogi PK, Hossain A. Comparison of a modified adherence assay with existing assay methods for identification of enteroaggregative *Escherichia coli*. J Clin Microbiol 1992; 30:1614-1616.
93. Savarino SJ, Fox P, Deng Y, Nataro JP. Identification and characterization of a gene cluster mediating enteroaggregative *Escherichia coli* aggregative adherence fimbria I biogenesis. J Bacteriol 1994; 176:4949-4957.
94. Spencer J, Chart H, Smith HR, Rowe B. Expression of membrance-associated proteins by strains of enteroaggregative *Escherichia coli*. FEMS Microbiol Lett 1998; 161:325-330.
95. Rautelin H, Sivonen A, Kuikka A, Renkonen OV, Valtonen V, Kosunen TU. Enteric *Plesiomonas shigelloides* infections in Finnish patients. Scand J Infect Dis 1995; 27:495-498.
96. Poitrineau P, Forestier C, Meyer M, Jallat C, Rich C, Malpuech G, De Champs C. Retrospective case-control study of diffusely adhering *Escherichia coli* and clinical features in children with diarrhea. J Clin Microbiol 1995; 33:1961-1962.
97. Anderson JD, MacNab AJ, Gransden WR, Damm SM, Johnson WM, Lior H. Gastroenteritis and encephalopathy associated with a strain of *Escherichia coli* O55:K59:H4 that produced a cytolethal distending toxin. Pediatr Infect Dis J 1987; 6:1135-1136.
98. Johnson WM, Lior H. A new heat-labile cytolethal distending toxin (CDLT) produced by *Escherichia coli* isolates form clinical material. Microb Pathogen 1988; 4:103-113.
99. Cmayras C, Tasca C, Peres SY, Ducommun B, Oswald E, De Rycke J. *Escherichia coli* cytolethal distending toxin blocks the HeLa cell cycle at the G2/M transition by preventing cdc2 protein kinase dephosphorylation and activation. Infect Immun 1997; 65:5088-5095.
100. Albert MJ, Faruque SM, Faruque AS, Bettelheim KA, Neogi PK, Bhuiyan NA, Kaper JB. Controlled study of cytolethal distending toxin-producing *Escherichia coli* infections in Bangladeshi children. J Clin Microbiol 1996; 34:717-719.
101. Caprioli A, Falbo V, Ruggeri FM, Baldassarri L, Bisicchia R, Ippolito G, Romoli E, Donelli G. Cytotoxic necrotizing factor production by hemolytic strains of *Escherichia coli* causing extra-intestinal infections. J Clin Microbiol 1987; 25:146-149.
102. Hofman P, Flatau G, Selva E, Gauthier M, Le Negrate G, Fiorentini C, Rossi B, Boquet P. *Escherichia coli* cytotoxic necrotizing factor 1 effaces microvilli and decreases transmigration of polymorphonuclear leukocytes in intestinal T84 epithelial cell monolayers. Infect Immun 1998; 66:2494-2500.
103. De Rycke J, Milon A, Oswald E. Necrotoxic *Escherichia coli* (NTEC): two emerging categories of human and animal pathogens. Vet Res 1999; 30:221-233.
104. Paton JC, Paton AW. Pathogenesis and diagnosis of Shiga toxin-producing *Escherichia coli* infections. Clin Microbiol Rev 1998; 11:450-479.
105. Kaper JB. Enterohemorrhagic *Escherichia coli*. Curr Opin Microbiol 1998; 1:103-108.
106. Noel JM, Boedeker EC. Enterohemorrhagic *Escherichia coli*: a family of emerging pathogens. Dig Dis 1997; 15:67-91.
107. Lingwood CA. Role of verotoxin receptors in pathogenesis. Trends Microbiol 1996; 4:147-153.
108. Popoff MY, Le Minor L. Antigenic Formulae of the *Salmonella* Serovars. Paris:Pasteur Institute, 1997.
109. Collazo CM, Galan JE. The invasion-associated type-III protein secretion system in *Salmonella* – a review. Gene 1997; 192:51-59.
110. Darwin KH, Miller VL. Molecular basis of the interaction of *Salmonella* with the intestinal mucosa. Clin Microbiol Rev 1999; 12:405-428.

111. Lee VT, Schneewind O. Type III secretion machines and the pathogenesis of enteric infections caused by *Yersinia* and *Salmonella* spp. Immunol Rev 1999; 168:241-255.

112. Dodd CE, Jones D. A numerical taxonomic study of the genus *Shigella*. J Gen Microbiol 1982; 128:1933-1957.

113. Rolland K, Lambert-Zechovsky N, Picard B, Denamur E. *Shigella* and enteroinvasive *Escherichia coli* strains are derived from distinct ancestral strains of *E. coli*. Microbiology 1998; 144:2667-2672.

114. Dorman CJ, Porter ME. The *Shigella* virulence gene regulatory cascade: a paradigm of bacterial gene control mechanisms. Mole Microbiol 1998; 29:677-684.

115. Sansonetti PJ, Tran Van Nhieu G, Egile C. Rupture of the intestinal epithelial barrier and mucosal invasion of *Shigella flexneri*. Clin Infect Dis 1999; 28:466-475.

116. Sansonetti PJ. Molecular and cellular mechanisms of invasion of the intestinal barrier by enteric pathogens: the paradigm of *Shigella*. Folia Microbiol 1998; 43:239-246.

117. Sansonetti PJ, Egile C. Molecular bases of epithelial cell invasion by *Shigella flexneri*. Antonie von Leeuwenhoek 1998; 74:191-197.

118. Bottone EJ. *Yersinia enterocolitica*: the charisma continues. Clin Microbiol Rev 1997; 10:257-276.

119. Miller VL, Falkow S. Evidence for two genetic loci in *Yersinia enterocolitica* that can promote invasion of epithelial cells. Infect Immun 1988; 56:1242-1248.

120. Straley SC, Skrzypek E, Plano GV, Bliska JB. Yops of *Yersinia* spp. pathogenic for humans. Infect Immun 1993; 61:3103-3110.

121. Brenner DJ, Grimont PA, Steigerwalt AG, Fanning GR, Ageron E, Riddle CF. Classification of citrobacteria by DNA hybridization: designation of *Citrobacter farmeri* sp. nov., *Citrobacter youngae* sp. nov., *Citrobacter braakii* sp. nov., *Citrobacter werkmanii* sp. nov., *Citrobacter sedlakii* sp. nov., and three unnamed *Citrobacter* genomospecies. Int J Syst Bacteriol 1993; 43:645-658.

122. Frankel G, Candy DC, Everest P, Dougan G. Characterization of the C-terminal domains of intimin-like proteins of enteropathogenic and enterohemorrhagic *Escherichhia coli*, *Citrobacter freundii*, and *Hafnia alvei*. Infect Immun 1994; 62:1835-1842.

123. Schmidt H, Montag M, Bockemuhl J, Heesemann J, Karch H. Shiga-like toxin II-related cytotoxins in *Citrobacter freundii* strains from humans and beef samples. Infect Immun 1993; 61:534-543.

124. Giraldi R, Guth BE, Trabulsi LR. Production of Shiga-like toxin among *Escherichia coli* strains and other bacteria isolated from diarrhea in Sao Paulo, Brazil. J Clin Microbiol 1990; 28:1460-1462.

125. Tschape H, Prager R, Steckel W, Fruth A, Tietze E, Bohme G. Verotoxigenic *Citrobacter freundii* associated with severe gastroenteritis and cases of haemolytic uraemic syndrome in a nursery school: green butter as the infection source. Epidemiol Infect 1995; 114:441-450.

126. Badger JL, Stins MF, Kim KS. *Citrobacter freundii* invades and replicates in human brain microvascular endothelial cells. Infect Immun 1999; 67:4208-4215.

127. Doran TI. The role of *Citrobacter* in clinical disease of children: review. Clin Infect Dis 1999; 28:384-394.

128. Phillips AD, Trabulsi LR, Dougan G, Frankel G. *Edwardsiella tarda* induces plasma membrane ruffles on infectin of HEp-2 cells. FEMS Microbiol Lett 1998; 161:317-323.

129. Favre-Bonte S, Joly B, Forestier C. Consequences of reduction of *Klebsiella pneumoniae* capsule expression on interactions of this bacterium with epithelial cells. Infect Immun 1999; 67:554-561.

130. Maki-Ikola O, Nissila M, Lehtinen K, Granfors K. IgA class serum antibodies against three different *Klebsiella* serotypes in ankylosing spondylitis. Br J Rheumatol 1998; 37:1299-1302.

131. Russell AS, Suarez Almazor ME. Ankylosing spondylitis is not caused by *Klebsiella*. Rheum Dis Clin North Am 1992; 18:95-104.

132. Minami J, Okabe A, Shooide J, Hayashi H. Production of a unique cytotoxin by *Klebsiella oxytoca*. Microb Pathogen 1989; 7:203-211.

133. Latta RK, Schur MJ, Tolson DL, Altman E. The effect of growth conditions on in vitro adherence, invasion, and NAF expression by *Proteus mirabilis*. Can J Microbiol 1998; 44:896-904.

134. Mobley HL, Belas R. Swarming and pathogenicity of *Proteus mirabilis* in the urinary tract. Trends Microbiol 1995; 3:280-284.

135. Peerbooms PG, Verweij AM, Oe PL, MacLaren DM. Urinary pathogenicity of *Proteus mirabilis* strains isolated form faeces or urine. Antonie van Leeuwenhoek 1986; 52:53-62.

136. Albert MJ, Alam K, Ansaruzzaman M, Islam MM, Rahman AS, Haider K, Bhuiyan NA, Nahar S, Ryan N, Montanaro J, Mathan MM. Pathogenesis of *Providencia alcalifaciens*-induced diarrhea. Infect Immun 1992; 60:5017-5024.

137. Carbonell GV, Fonseca BA, Figueiredo LT, Darini AL, Yanaguita RM. Culture conditions affect cytotoxin production by *Serratia marcescens*. FEMS Immunol Med Microbiol 1996; 16:299-307.
138. Molla A, Matsumoto K, Oyamada I, Katsuki T, Maeda H. Degradation of protease inhibitors, immunoglobulins, and other serum proteins by *Serratia* protease and its toxicity to fibroblasts in culture. Infect Immun 1986: 53:522-529.
139. Ramamurthy T, Pal A, Pal SC, Nair GB. Taxonomical implications of emergence of high frequency of occurrence of 2,4-diamino-6,7-diisopropylpteridine-resistant strains of *Vibrio cholerae* from clinical cases of cholera in Calcutta, India. J Clin Microbiol 1992; 30:742-743.
140. Khetawat G, Bhadra RK, Nandi S, Das J. Resurgent *Vibrio cholerae* O139: rearrangement of cholera toxin genetic elements and amplification of rrn operon. Infect Immun 1999; 67:148-154.
141. Faruque SM, Albert MJ, Mekalanos JJ. Epidemiology, genetics, and ecology of toxigenic *Vibrio cholerae*. Microbiol Mol Biol Rev 1998; 62:1301-1314.
142. Waldor MK, Mekalanos JJ. Lysogenic conversioin by a filamentous phage encoding cholera toxin. Science 1996; 272:1910-1914.
143. Kurazano H, Pal A, Bag BK, Nair GB, Karasawa T, Mihara T, Takeda Y. Distribution of genes encoding cholera toxin, zonula occludens toxin, accessory cholera toxin, and El Tor hemolysin in *Vibrio cholerae* of diverse origins. Microb Pathogen 1995; 18:231-235.
144. Herrington DA, Hall RH, Losonsky G, Mekalanos JJ, Taylor RK, Levine MM. Toxin, toxin-coregulated pili, and the toxR regulon are essential for *Vibrio cholerae* pathogenesis in humans. J Exp Med 1988; 168:1487-1492.
145. Lencer WI, Hirst TR, Holmes RK. Membrane traffic and the cellular uptake of cholera toxin. Biochem Biophys Acta 1999; 1450:177-180.
146. Raufman JP. Cholera. Am J Med 1998; 104:386-394.
147. Nishibuchi M, Fasano A, Russell RG, Kaper JB. Enterotoxigenicity of *Vibrio parahemolyticus* with and and without gene encoding thermostable direct hemolysin. Infect Immun 1992; 60:3539-3545.
148. Okuda J, Ishibashi M, Hayakawa E, Nishino T, Takeda Y, Mukhopadhyay AK, Garg S, Bhattacharya SK, Nair GB, Nishibuchi M. Emergence of a unique O3:K6 clone of *Vibrio parahaemolyticus* in Calcutta, India, and isolation of strains from the same clonal group from southeast Asian travellers arriving in Japan. J Clin Microbiol 1997; 35:3150-3155.
149. Matsumoto C, Okuda, Ishibashi M, Iwanaga M, Garg P, Ramamurthy T, Wong H, Depaola A, Kim YB, Albert MJ, Nichibuchi M. Pandemic spread of an O3:K6 clone of *V. parahaemolyticus* and emergence of related strains evidenced by arbitrarily primed PCR and *toxRS* sequence analyses. J Clin Microbiol 2000; 38:578-585.
150. Linkous DA, Oliver JD. Pathogenesis of *Vibrio vulnificus*. FEMS Microbiol Lett 1999; 174:207-214.
151. Shinoda S. Protein toxins produced by pathogenic vibrios. J Nat Toxins 1999; 8:259-269.
152. Ketley JM. Pathogenesis of enteric infections by *Campylobacter*. Microbiology 1997; 143:5-21.
153. Wassenaar TM. Toxin production by *Campylobacter* spp. Clin Microbiol Rev 1997; 10:466-476.
154. Whitehouse CA, Balbo PB, Pesci EC, Cottle DL, Mirabito PM, Pickett CL. *Campylobacter jejuni* cytolethal distending toxin causes a G2-phase cell cycle block. Infect Immun 1998; 66:1934-1940.
155. Eyigor A, Dawson KA, Langlois BE, Pickett CL. Cytolethal distending toxin genes in *Campylobacter jejuni* and *Campylobacter coli* isolates: detection and analysis by PCR. J Clin Microbiol 1999; 37:1646-1650.
156. Oomes PG, Jacobs BC, Hazenberg MP, Banffer JR, van der Meche FG. Anti-GM1 IgG antibodies and *Campylobacter* bacteria in Guillain-Barre syndrome: evidence of molecular mimicry. Ann Neurol 1995; 38:170-175.
157. Nachamkin I, Ung H, Moran AP, Yoo D, Prendergast MM, Nicholson MA, Sheikh K, Ho T, Asbury AK, McKhann GM, Griffin JW. Ganglioside GM1 mimicry in *Campylobacter* strains from sporadic infection in the United States. J Infect Dis 1999; 179:1183-1189.
158. Blaser MJ. *Campylobacter fetus* – emerging infection and model system for bacterial pathogenesis at mucosal surfaces. Clin Infect Dis 1998; 27:256-258.
159. Kiehlbauch JA, Brenner DJ, Cameron DN, Steigerwalt AG, Makowski JM, Baker CN, Patton CM, Wachsmuth KI. Genotypic and phenotypic characterization of *Helicobacter cinaedi* and *Helicobacter fennelliae* strains isolated from humans and animals. J Clin Microbiol 1995; 33:2940-2947.
160. Pemberton JM, Kidd SP, Schmidt R. Secreted enzymes of *Aeromonas*. FEMS Microbiol Lett 1997; 152:1-10.
161. Gardner SE, Fowlston SE, George WL. In vitro production of cholera toxin-like activity by *Plesiomonas shigelloides*. J Infect Dis 1987;156:720-722.
162. Riedasch G, Ritz E, Rauterberg E. Do antibody-coated bacteria reflect local immune response in the urinary tract? Am J Nephrol 1984; 4:361-366.

163. Hanson LA, Ahlstedt S, Fasth A, Jodal U, Kaijser B, Larsson P, Lindberg U, Olling S, Sohl-Akerlund A, Svanborg-Eden C. Antigens of *Escherichia coli*, human immune respne, and the pathogenesis of urinary tract infections. J Infect Dis 1977; 136:S144-S149.

164. Chart H, Law D, Rowe B, Acheson DW. Patients with haemolytic uraemic syndrome caused by *Escherichia coli* O157: absence of antibodies to Vero cytotoxin 1 (VT1) or VT2. J Clin Pathol 1993; 46:1053-1054.

165. Ludwig K, Bitzan M, Zimmermann S, Kloth M, Ruder H, Muller-Wiefel DE. Immune response to non-O157 Vero toxin-producing *Escherichia coli* in patients with hemolytic uremic syndrome. J Infect Dis 1996; 174:1028-1039.

166. Chart H, Jenkins C. The serodiagnosis of infections caused by Verocytotoxin-producing *Escherichia coli*. J Appl Microbiol 1999; 86:731-740.

167. Voss E, Paton AW, Manning PA, Paton JC. Molecular analysis of Shiga toxigenic *Escherichia coli* O111:H-proteins which react with sera from patients with hemolytic-uremic syndrome. Infect Immun 1998; 66:1467-1472.

168. Bitzan M, Klemt M, Steffens R, Muller-Wiefel DE. Differences in verotoxin neutralizing activity of therapeutic immunoglobulins and sera from healthy controls. Infection 1993; 21:140-145.

169. Levine MM, Ristaino P, Marley G, Smyth C, Knutton S, Boedeker E, Black R, Young C, Clements ML, Cheney C, Patnaik R. Coli surface antigens 1 and 3 of colonization factor antigen II-positive enterotoxigenic *Escherichia coli*: morphology, purification, and immune responses in humans. Infect Immun 1984; 44:409-420.

170. Karch H, Heesemann J, Laufs R, Kroll HP, Kaper JB, Levine MM. Serological response to type 1-like somatic fimbriae in diarrheal infection due to classical enteropathogenic *Escherichia coli*. Microb Pathogen 1987; 2:425-434.

171. Martinez MB, Taddei CR, Ruiz-Tagle A, Trabulsi LR, Giron JA. Antibody response of children with enteropathogenic *Escherichia coli* infection to the bundle-forming pilus and locus of enterocyte effacement-encoded virulence determinants. J Infect Dis 1999; 179:269-274.

172. Persson MA, Ekwall E, Hammarstrom L, Lindberg AA, Smith CI. Immunoglobulin G (IgG) and IgA subclass pattern of human antibodies to *Shigella flexneri* and *Salmonella* serogroup B and D lipopolysaccharide O antigens. Infect Immun 1986; 52:834-839.

173. Samuel MP, Zwillich SH, Thomson GT, Alfa M, Orr KB, Brittain DC, Miller JR, Phillips PE. Fast food arthritis – a clinicopathologic study of post-*Salmonella* reactive arthritis. J Rheumatol 1995; 22:1947-1952.

174. Munoz C, Baqar s, van de Verg L, Thupari J, Goldblum S, Olson JG, Taylor DN, Heresi GP, Murphy JR. Characteristics of *Shigella sonnei* infection of volunteers: signs, symptoms, immune responses, changes in selected cytokines and acute-phase substances. Am J Trop Med Hyg 1995; 53:47-54.

175. Robin G, Cohen D, Orr N, Markus I, Slepon R, Ashkenazi S, Keisari Y. Characterization and quantitative analysis of serum IgG class and subclass response to *Shigella sonnei* and *Shigella flexneri* 2a lipopolysaccharide following natural *Shigella* infection. J Infect Dis 1997; 175:1128-1133.

176. Ekwall E, Haeggmann S, Kalin M, Svenungsson B, Lindberg AA. Antibody response to *Shigella sonnei* infection determined by an enzyme-linked immunosorbent assay. Eur J Clin Microbiol 1983; 2:200-205.

177. Oberhelman RA, Kopecko DJ, Salazar-Lindo E, Gotuzzo E, Buysse JM, Venkatesan MM, Yi A, Fernandez-Prada C, Guzman M, Leon-Barua R, Sack RB. Prospective study of systemic and mucosal immune responses in dysenteric patients to specific *Shigella* invasion plasmid antigens and lipopolysaccharides. Infect Immun 1991; 59:2341-2350.

178. Schultsz C, Qadri F, Hossain SA, Ahmed F, Ciznar I. *Shigella*-specific IgA in saliva of children with bacillary dysentery. FEMS Microbiol Immunol 1992; 4:65-72.

179. Keren DF, McDonald RA, Wassef JS, Armstrong LR, Brown JE. The enteric immune response to *Shigella* antigens. Curr Top Microbiol Immunol 1989; 146:213-223.

180. Mattila PS, Valtonen V, Tuori MR, Makela O. Antibody responses in arthritic and uncomplicated *Yersinia enterocolitica* infections. J Clin Immunol 1985; 5:404-411.

181. Gronberg A, Fryden A, Kihlstrom E. Humoral immune response to individual *Yersinia enterocolitica* antigens in patients with and without reactive arthritis. Clin Exp Immunol 1989; 76:361-365.

182. Loomes LM, Kerr MA, Senior BW. The cleavage of immunoglobulin G in vitro and in vivo by a proteinase secreted by the urinary tract pathogen *Proteus mirabilis*. J Med Microbiol 1993; 39:225-232.

183. Glass RI, Svennerholm AM, Khan MR, Huda S, Huq MI, Holmgren J. Seroepidemiological studies of El Tor cholera in Bangladesh: association of serum antibody levels with protection. J Infect Dis 1985; 151:236-242.

184. Ehara M, Ichinose Y, Iwani M, Utsunomiya A, Shimodori S, Kangethe SK, Neves BC, Supawat K, Nakamura S. Immunogenicity of *Vibrio cholerae* O1 fimbriae in animal and human cholera. Microbiol Immunol 1993; 37:679-688.

185. Qadri F, Jonson G, Begum YA, Wenneras C, Albert MJ, Salam MA, Svennerholm AM. Immune response to the mannose-sensitive hemagglutinin in patients with cholera due to *Vibrio cholerae* O1 and O139. Clin Diagn Lab Immunol 1997; 4:429-434.
186. Qadri F, Mohi G, Hossain J, Azim T, Khan AM, Salam MA, Sack RB, Albert MJ, Svennerholm AM. Comparison of the vibriocidal antibody response in cholera due to *Vibrio cholerae* O139 Bengal with the response in cholera due to *Vibrio cholerae* O1. Clin Diagn Lab Immunol 1995; 2:685-686.
187. Richardson K, Kaper JB, Levine MM. Human immune response to *Vibrio cholerae* O1 whole cells and isolated outer membrane antigens. Infect Immun 1989; 57:495-501.
188. Sears SD, Richardson K, Young C, Parker CD, Levine MM. Evaluation of the human immune response to outer membrane proteins of *Vibrio cholerae*. Infect Immun 1984; 44:439-444.
189. Herbrink P, van den Munckhof HA, Bumkens M, Lindeman J, van Dijk WC. Human serum antibody response in *Campylobacter jejuni* enteritis as measured by enzyme-linked immunosorbent assay. Eur J Clin Microbiol Infect Dis 1988; 7:388-393.
190. Taylor DN, Perlman DM, Echeverria PD, Lexomboon U, Blaser MJ. *Campylobacter* immunity and quantitative excretion rates in Thai children. J Infect Dis 1993; 168:754-758.
191. Blaser MJ, Duncan DJ. Human serum antibody response to *Campylobacter jejuni* infection as measured in an enzyme-linked immunosorbent assay. Infect Immun 1984; 44:292-298.
192. Panigrahi P, Losonsky G, DeTolla LJ, Morris JG. Human immune response to *Campylobacter jejuni* proteins expressed in vivo. Infect Immun 1992; 60:4938-4944.
193. Perez-Perez GI, Cohn DL, Guerrant RL, Patton CM, Reller LB, Blaser MJ. Clinical and immunologic significance of cholera-like toxin and cytotoxin production by *Campylobacter* species in patients with acute inflammatory diarrhea in the USA. J Infect Dis 1989; 160:460-468.
194. Mills SD, Bradbury WC. Human antibody response to outer membrane proteins of *Campylobacter jejuni* during infection. Infect Immun 1984; 43:739-743.
195. Gregson NA, Rees JH, Hughes RA. Reactivity of serum IgG anti-GM1 ganglioside antibodies with the lipopolysaccharide fractions of *Campylobacter jejuni* isolates from patients with Guillain-Barre syndrome (GBS). J Neuroimmunol 1997; 73:28-36.
196. Wallis MR. The pathogenesis of *Campylobacter jejuni*. Br J Biomed Sci 1994; 51:57-64.
197. Flores BM, Fennell CL, Stamm WE. Characterization of *Campylobacter cinaedi* and *C. fenelliae* antigens and analysis of the human immune response. J Infect Dis 1989; 159:635-640.
198. Jiang ZD, Nelson AC, Mathewson JJ, Ericsson CD, DuPont HL. Intestinal secretory immune response to infection with *Aeromonas* species and *Plesiomonas shigelloides* among students from the United States in Mexico. J Infect Dis 1991; 164:979-982.
199. Fan K, Morris AJ, Reller LB. Application of rejection criteria for stoll cultures for bacterial enteric pathogens. J Clin Microbiol 1993; 31:2233-2235.
200. Park CH, Hixon DL, Polhemus AS, Ferguson CB, Hall SL, Risheim CC, Cook CB. A rapid diagnosis of *Campylobacter* enteritis by direct smear examination. Am J Clin Pathol 1983; 80:388-390.
201. Sazie ESM, Titus AE. Rapid diagnosis of *Campylobacter* enteritis. Ann Intern Med 1982; 96:62-63.
202. Harris JC, Dupont HL, Hornick RB. Fecal leucocytes in diarrheal illness. Ann Intern Med 1972; 76:697-703.
203. Pickering LK, Dupont HL, Olarte J, Conklin R, Ericcson C. Fecal leucocytes in enteric infections. Am J Clin Path 1977; 68:562-565.
204. Korzienowski OM, Barada FA, Rouse JD, Guerrant RL. Value of examination for fecal leucocytes in the early diagnosis of shigellosis. Am J Trop Med Hyg 1979; 28:1031-1035.
205. Siegel D, Cohen PT, Neighbor M, Larkin H, Newman M, Yajko D, Hadley K. Predictive value of stool examination in acute diarrhea. Arch Pathol Lab Med 1987; 111:715-718.
206. Cimolai N. Fecal leucocytes in *Escherichia coli* O157:H7 enteritis. J Clin Pathol 1990; 43:347.
207. Hasan JAK, Bernstein D, Huq A, Loomis L, Tamplin ML, Colwell RR. Cholera DFA: an improved direct fluorescent-monoclonal antibody staining kit for rapid detection and enumeration of *Vibrio cholerae* O1. FEMS Microbiol Lett 1994; 120:143-148.
208. Gransden WR, Damm MAS, Anderson JD, Carter JE, Lior H. Further evidence associating hemolytic uremic syndrome with infection by verotoxin-producing *Escherichia coli* O157:H7. J Infect Dis 1986; 154:522-524.
209. Zadik PM, Chapman PA, Siddons CA. Use of tellurite for the selection of verocytotoxigenic *Escherichia coli* O157. J Med Microbiol 1993; 39:155-158.
210. Sanderson MW, Gray JM, Hancock DD, Gray CC, Fox LK, Besser TE. Sensitivity of bacteriologic culture for detection of *Escherichia coli* O157:H7 in bovine feces. J Clin Microbiol 1995; 33:2616-2619.

211. Bettelhiem KA. Studies of *Escherichia coli* cultured on Rainbow Agar O157 with particular reference to enterohemorrhagic *Escherichia coli*. Microbiol Immunol 1998; 42:265-269.
212. Wright DJ, Chapman PA, Siddons CA. Immunomagnetic separation as a sensitive method for ioslating *Escherichia coli* O157 from food samples. Epidemiol Infect 1994; 113:31-39.
213. Silva RM, Toledo MR, Trabulsi LR. Biochemical and cultural characteristics of invasive *Escherichia coli*. J Clin Microbiol 1980; 11:441-444.
214. Dusch H, Altwegg M. Evaluation of five new plating media for isolation of *Salmonella* species. J Clin Microbiol 1995; 33:802-804.
215. Gaillot O, Di Camillo P, Berche P, Courcol R, Savage C. Comparison of CHROMagar Salmonella Medium and Hektoen Enteric Agar for isolation of salmonellae from stool samples. J Clin Microbiol 1999; 37:762-765.
216. Perry JD, Ford M, Taylor J, Jones AL, Freeman R, Gould FK. ABC Medium, a new chromogenic agar for selective isolation of *Salmonella* spp. J Clin Microbiol 1999; 37:766-768.
217. Poisson DM, Niocel B, Florence S, Imbault D. Comparison of Hektoen and Salmonella-Shigella agar on 6033 stools of human origin submitted for routine isolation of *Salmonella* sp. and *Shigella* sp. Pathol Biol 1992; 40:21-24.
218. Falcao DP, Trabulsi LR, Hickman FW, Farmer JJ. Unusual *Enterobacteriaceae*: lactose-positive *Salmonella typhimurium* which is endemic in sao Paulo, Brazil. J Clin Microbiol 1975; 2:349-353.
219. Cohen SL, Wylie BA, Sooka A, Koornhof HJ. Bacteremia caused by a lactose-fermenting, multiply resistant *Salmonella typhi* strain in a patients recovering from typhoid fever. J Clin Microbiol 1987; 25:1516-1518.
220. Head CB, Whitty DA, Ratnam S. Comparative study of selective media for recovery of *Yersinia enterocolitica*. J Clin Microbiol 1982; 16:615-621.
221. Cimolai N, Trombley C, Blair GK. Implications of *Yersinia enterocolitica* biotyping. Arch Dis Child 1994; 70:19-21.
222. Fukushima H. New selective medium for isolation of virulent *Yersinia enterocolitica*. J Clin Microbiol 1987; 25:1068-1073.
223. Gangarosa EJ, Dewitt WE, Huq I, Zarifi A. Laboratory methods in cholera: isolation of *Vibrio cholerae* (El Tor and classical) on TCBS medium in minimally equipped laboratories. Trans R Soc Trop Med Hyg 1968; 62:693-699.
224. Kaper JB, Morris JG, Levine MM. Cholera. Clin Microbiol Rev 1995; 8:48-86.
225. Karmali MA, Simor AE, Roscoe M, Fleming PC, Smith SS, Lane J. Evaluation of a blood-free, charcoal-based, selective medium for the isolation of *Campylobacter* organisms from feces. J Clin Microbiol 1986; 23:456-459.
226. Piersimoni C, Bornigia S, Curzi L, De Sio G. Comparison of two selective media and a membrane filter technique for isolation of *Campylobacter* species from diarrhoeal stools. Eur J Clin Microbiol Infect Dis 1995; 14:539-542.
227. Lopez L, Castillo FJ, Clavel A, Rubio MC. Use of a selective medium and a membrane filter method for isolation of *Campylobacter* species from Spanish paediatric patients. Eur J Clin Microbiol Infect Dis 1998; 17:489-492.
228. Engberg J, On SL, Harrington CS, Gerner-Smidt P. Prevalence of *Campylobacter*, *Arcobacter*, *Helicobacter*, and *Sutterella* spp. in human fecal samples as estimated by a re-evaluation of isolation methods for campylobacters. J Clin Microbiol 2000; 38:286-291.
229. Agulla A, Merino FJ, Villasante PA, Saz JV, Diaz A, Velasco AC. Evaluation of four enrichment media for isolation of *Campylobacter jejuni*. J Clin Microbiol 1987; 25:174-175.
230. Ribeiro CD, Fitzgerald TC. Is enrichment culture necessary for isolating *Campylobacter jejuni* from faeces? J Clin Pathol 1988; 41:1135.
231. Murray PR, Baron EJ, Pfaller MT, Tenover FC, Yolken RH. Manual of Clinical Microbiology. 7th Edition. Washington, DC:American Society for Microbiology, 1999.
232. Scotland SM, Smith HR, Cheasty T, Said B, Wilshaw GA, Stokes N, Rowe B. Use of gene probes and adhesion tests to characterize *Escherichia coli* belonging to enteropathogenic serogroups isolated in the United Kingdom. J Med Microbiol 1996; 44:438-443.
233. Cimolai N, Cheong ACH, Trombley C. Markers of virulence among prospectively acquired putative enteropathogenic *Escherichia coli* serogroups. Pediatr Pathol Lab Med 1997; 17:267-274.
234. Rosa AC, Mariano AT, Pereira AM, Tibana A, Gomes TA, Andrade JR. Enteropathogenicity markers in *Escherichia coli* isolated from infants with acute diarrhoea and healthy controls in Rio de Janeiro, Brazil. J Med Microbiol 1998; 47:781-790.

235. Bortolini MF, Trabulsi LR, Keller R, Frankel G, Sperandio V. Lack of expression of bundle-forming pili in some clinical isolates of enteropathogenic *Escherichia coli* (EPEC) is due to a conserved large deletion in the bfp operon. FEMS Microbiol Lett 1999; 179:169-174.

236. Okeke IN, Lamikanra A, Steinruck H, Kaper JB. Characterization of *Escherichia coli* strains from cases of childhood diarrhea in provincial southwestern Nigeria. J Clin Microbiol 2000; 38:7-12.

237. Jallat C, Livrelli V, Darfeuille-Michaud A, Rich C, Joly B. *Escherichia coli* strains involved in diarrhea in France: high prevalence and heterogeneity of diffusely adhering strains. J Clin Microbiol 1993; 312:2031-2037.

238. Pal T, Serichantalerg O, Echeverria P, Scheutz F, Cam PD. The use of an *ipaC*-specific ELISA to identify enteroinvasive *Escherichia coli* strains of unusual serogroups. Diagn Microbiol Infect Dis 1998; 32:255-258.

239. Houng HS, Sethabutr O, Echeverria P. A simple polymerase chain reaction technique to detect and differentiate *Shigella* and enteroinvasive *Escherichia coli* in human feces. Diagn Microbiol Infect Dis 1997; 28:19-25.

240. Toledo MR, Trabulsi LR. Correlation between biochemical and serological characteristics of *Escherichia coli* and results of the Sereny test. J Clin Microbiol 1983; 17:419-421.

241. Scotland SM, Flowman RH, Rowe B. Evaluation of a reversed passive latex agglutination test for detection of *Escherichia coli* heat-labile toxin in culture supernatants. J Clin Microbiol 1989; 27:339-340.

242. Cryan B. Comparison of three assay systems for detection of enterotoxigenic *Escherichia coli* heat-stable enterotoxin. J Clin Microbiol 1990; 28:792-794.

243. Stacy-Phipps S, Mecca JJ, Weiss JB. Multiplex PCR assay and simple preparation method for stool specimens detect enterotoxigenic *Escherichia coli* DNA during the course of infection. J Clin Microbiol 1995; 33:1054-1059.

244. Tsen HY, Jian LZ, Chi WR. Use of a multiplex PCR system for the simultaneous detection of heat labile toxin I and heat stable toxin II genes of enterotoxigenic *Escherichia coli* in skim milk and porcine stool. J Food Protect 1998; 61:141-145.

245. March SB, Ratnam S. Latex agglutination test for detection of *Escherichia coli* serotype O157. J Clin Microbiol 1989; 27:1675-1677.

246. Sowers EG, Wells JG, Strockbine NA. Evaluation of commercial latex reagents for identification of O157 and H7 antigens of *Escherichia coli*. J Clin Microbiol 1996; 34:1286-1287.

247. Borczyk AA, Harnett N, Lombos M, Lior H. False-positive identification of *Escherichia coli* O157 by commercial latex agglutination tests. Lancet 1990; 336:946-947.

248. Dylla BL, Vetter EA, Hughes JG, Cockerill FR. Evaluation of an immunoassay for direct detection of *Escherichia coli* O157 in stool specimens. J Clin Microbiol 1995; 33:222-224.

249. Ball HJ, Finlay D, Zafar A, Wilson T. The detection of verocytotoxins in bacterial cultures from human diarrhoeal samples with monoclonal antibody-based ELISAs. J Med Microbiol 1996; 44:273-276.

250. Acheson DW, DeBreuker S, Donohue-Rolfe A, Kozak K, Yi A, Keusch GT. Development of a clinically useful diagnostic enzyme immunoassay for enterohemorrhagic *Escherichia coli* infection. In: Karmali MA, Goglio AG – eds. Recent Advances in Verocytotoxin-Producing *Escherichia coli* Infections. Amsterdam:Elsevier, 1994:109-112.

251. Beutin L, Zimmerman S, Gleier K. Rapid detection and isolation of Shiga-like toxin (verocytotoxin)-producing *Escherichia coli* by direct testing of individual enterohemolytic colonies from washed sheep blood agar plates in the VTEC-RPLA assay. J Clin Microbiol 1996; 34:499-502.

252. Karmali MA, Petric M, Lim C, Cheung R, Arbus GS. Sensitive method for detecting low numbers of verotoxin-producing *Escherichia coli* in mixed cultures by use of colony sweeps and polymyxin extraction of verotoxin. J Clin Microbiol 1985; 22:614-619.

253. Tyler SD, Johnson WM, Lior H, Wang G, Rozee KR. Identification of verotoxin type 2 variant B subunit genes in *Escherichia coli* by the polymerase chain reaction and restriction fragment length polymorphism analysis. J Clin Microbiol 1991; 29:1339-1343.

254. Baumler AJ, Heffron F, Reissbrodt R. Rapid detection of *Salmonella enterica* with primers specific for *iroB*. J Clin Microbiol 1997; 35:1224-1230.

255. Olsen JE, Aabo S, Nielsen EO, Nielsen BB. Isolation of a *Salmonella*-specific DNA hybridization probe. APMIS 1991; 99:114-120.

256. Chiu CH, Ou JT. Rapid identification of *Salmonella* serovars in feces by specific detection of virulence genes, *invA* and *spvC*, by an enrichment broth culture-multiplex PCR combination assay. J Clin Microbiol 1996; 34:2619-2622.

257. Haedicke W, Wolf H, Ehret W, Reischl U. Specific and sensitive two-step polymerase chain reaction assay for the detection of *Salmonella* species. Eur J Clin Microbiol Infect Dis 1996; 15:603-607.

258. Nordentoft S, Christensen H, Wegener HC. Evaluation of a fluorescence-labelled oligonucleotide probe targeting 23S rRNA for in situ detection of *Salmonella* serovars in paraffin-embedded tissue sections and their rapid identification in bacterial smears. J Clin Microbiol 1997; 35:2642-2648.

259. Khann AA, Nawaz MS, Khan SA, Cerniglia CE. Detection of multidrug-resistant *Salmonella typimurium* DT104 by multiplex polymerase chain reaction. FEMS Microbiol Lett 2000; 182:355-360.

260. Chaudhry R, Laxmi BV, Nisar N, Ray K, Kumar D. Standardisation of polymerase chain reaction for the detection of *Salmonella typhi* in typhoid fever. J Clin Pathol 1997; 50:437-439.

261. Islam MS, Hossain MS, Hasan MK, Rahman MM, Fuchs G, Mahalanabis D, Baqui AH, Albert MJ. Detection of shigellae from stools of dysentery patients by culture and polymerase chain reaction techniques. J Diarrhoeal Dis Res 1998; 16:248-251.

262. Gaudio PA, Sethabur O, Echeverria P, Hoge CW. Utility of a polymerase chain reaction diagnostic system in a study of the epidemiology of shigellosis among dysentery patients, family contacts, and well controls living in a shigellosis-endemic area. J Infect Dis 1997; 176:1013-1018.

263. Oberhelman RA, Kopecko DJ, Venkatesan MM, Salazr-Lindo E, Gotuzzo E, Yi A, Chea-Woo E, Ruiz R, Fernandez-Prada C, Leon-Barua R, Sack RB. Evaluation of alkaline phosphatase-labelled *ipaH* probe for diagnosis of *Shigella* infections. J Clin Microbiol 1993; 31:2101-2104.

264. Houng HS, Sethabur O, Echeverria P. A simple polymerase chain reaction technique to detect and differentiate *Shigella* and enteroinvasive *Escherichia coli* in human feces. Diagn Microbiol Infect Dis 1997; 28:19-25.

265. Bottone EJ. *Yersinia enterocolitica*: a panoramic view of a charismatic microorganism. Crit Rev Microbiol 1977; 5:211-214.

266. Rahman M, Sack DA, Wadood A, Yasmin M, Latif A. Rapid identification of *Vibrio cholerae* serotye O1 from primary isolation plates by a coagglutination test. J Med Microbiol 1989; 28:39-41.

267. Hasan JAK, Huq A, Tamplin ML, Siebeling RJ, Colwell RR. A novel kit for rapid detection of *Vibrio cholerae* O1. J Clin Microbiol 1994; 32:249-252.

268. Ramamurthy T, Pal A, Bag PK, Bhattacharya SK, Nair GB, Kurozano H, Yamasaki S, Shirai H, Takeda T, Uesaka Y, Horigome K, Takeda Y. Detection of cholera toxin gene in stool specimens by polymerase chain reaction: comparison with bead enzyme-linked immunosorbent assay and culture method for laboratory diagnosis of cholera. J Clin Microbiol 1993; 31:3068-3070.

269. Shirai H, Nishibuchih M, Ramamurthy T, Bhattacharya SK, Pal SC, Takeda Y. Polymerase chain reaction for detection of the cholera enterotoxin operon of *Vibrio cholerae*. J Clin Microbiol 1991; 29:2517-2521.

270. Huysmans MB, Turnidge JD, Williams JH. Evaluation of API Campy in comparison withy conventional methods for identification of thermophilic campylobacters. J Clin Microbiol 1995; 33:3345-3346.

271. Hodinka RL, Gilligan PH. Evaluation of the Campyslide agglutination test for confirmatory identification of selected *Campylobacter* species. J Clin Microbiol 1988; 26:47-49.

272. Nachamkin I, Barbagallo S. Culture confirmation of *Campylobacter* species by latex agglutination. J Clin Microbiol 1990; 28:817-818.

273. Al Rashid ST, Dakuna I, Louie H, Ng D, Vandamme P, Johnson W, Chan VL. Identification of *Campylobacter jejuni*, *C. coli*, *C. lari*, *C. upsaliensis*, *Arcobacter butzleri*, and *A. butzleri*-like species based on the *glyA* gene. J Clin Microbiol 2000; 38:1488-1494.

274. On SLW. Identification methods for campylobacters, helicobacters, and related organisms. Clin Microbiol Rev 1996; 405-422.

275. Cascon A, Anguita J, Hernanz C, Sanchez M, Fernandez M, Naharro G. Identification of *Aeromonas hydrophila* hybridization group 1 by PCR assays. Appl Environ Microbiol 1996; 62:1167-1170.

276. Borrell N, Acinas SG, Figueras MJ, Martinez-Murcia AJ. Identification of *Aeromonas* clinical isolates by restriction fragment length polymorphism of PCR-amplified 16S rRNA genes. J Clin Microbiol 1997; 35:1671-1674.

277. Moyer NP, Martinetti G, Luthy-Hottenstein J, Altwegg M. Value of rRNA gene estriction patterns of *Aeromonas* spp. for epidemiological investigations. Curr Microbiol 1992; 24:15-21.

278. Greatorex JS, Thorne GM. Humoral immune responses to Shiga-like toxins and *Escherichia coli* O157 lipopolysaccharide in hemolytic-uremic syndrome patients and healthy subjects. J Clin Microbiol 1994; 32:1172-1178.

279. Barrett TJ, Green JH, Griffin PM, Pavia AT, Ostroff SM, Wachsmuth IK. Enzyme-linked immunosorbent assays for detecting antibodies to Shiga-like toxin I, Shiga-like toxin II, and *Escherichia coli* O157:H7 lipopolysaccharide I human serum. Curr Microbiol 1991; 23:189-195.

280. Chart H, Smith HR, Scotland SM, Rowe B, Milford DV, Taylor CM. Serological identification of *Escherichia coli* O157:H7 infection in haemolytic uraemic syndrome. Lancet 1991; 337:138-140.

281. Chart H, Evans J, Chalmers RM, Salmon RL. *Escherichia coli* O157 serology: false-positive ELISA results caused by human antibodies binding to bovine serum albumin. Lett Appl Microbiol 1998; 27:76-78.

282. Ludwig K, Bitzan M, Zimmermann S, Kloth M, Ruder H, Muller-Wiefel DE. Immune response to non-O157 Vero toxin-producing *Escherichia coli* in patients with hemolytic uremic syndrome. J Infect Dis 1996; 174:1028-1039.

283. Cheasty T, Robertson R, Chart H, Mannion P, Syed Q, Garvey R, Rowe B. The use of serodiagnosis in the retrospective investigation of a nursery outbreak associated with *Escherichia coli* O157:H7. J Clin Pathol 1998; 51:498-501.

284. Smith BP, Dilling GW, House JK, Konrad H, Moore N. Enzyme-linked immunosorbent assay for *Salmonella* serology using lipopolysaccharide antigen. J Vet Diagn Invest 1995; 7:481-487.

285. Shukla S, Patel B, Chitnis DS. 100 years of Widal test & its reappraisal in an endemic area. Ind J Med Res 1997; 105:53-57.

286. Engleberg NC, Barrett TJ, Fisher H, Porter B, Hurtado E, Hughes JM. Identification of a carrier by using Vi enzyme-linked immunosorbent assay serology in an outbreak of typhoid fever on an Indian reservation. J Clin Microbiol 1983; 18:1320-1322.

287. Lanata CF, Tafur C, Benavente L, Gotuzzo E, Carillo C. Detection of *Salmonella typhi* carriers in food handlers by Vi serology in Lima, Peru. Bull Pan Am Health Organ 1990; 24:177-182.

288. Lanata CF, Levine MM, Ristori C, Black RE, Jimenez L, Salcedo M, Garcia J, Sotomayor V. Vi serology in detection of chronic *Salmonella typhi* carriers in an endemic area. Lancet 1983; ii:441-443.

289. de Silva DG, Candy DC, Mendis LN, Chart H, Rowe B. Serological diagnosis of infection by *Shigella dysenteriae*-1 in patients with bacillary dysentery. J Infect 1992; 25:273-278.

290. Bottone EJ, Sheehan DJ. *Yersinia enterocolitica*: guidelines for serologic diagnosis of human infections. Rev Infect Dis 1983; 5:898-906.

291. Lange S, Larsson P. What do serum antibodies to *Yersinia enterocolitica* indicate? Rev Infect Dis 1984; 6:880-881.

292. Paerregaard A, Shand GH, Gaarslev K, Espersen F. Comparison of crossed immunoelectrophoresis, enzyme-linked immunosorbent assays, and tube agglutination for serodiagnosis of *Yersinia enterocolitica* serotype O:3 infection. J Clin Microbiol 1991; 29:302-309.

293. Vesikari T, Granfors K, Maki M, Gronroos P. Evaluation of ELISA in the diagnosis of *Yersinia enterocolitica* diarrhoea in children. Acta Pathol Microbiol Scand 1980; 88:139-142.

294. Clements ML, Levine MM, Young CR, Black RE, Lim YL, Robins-Browne RM, Craig JP. Magnitude, kinetics, and duration of vibriocidal antibody responses in North Americans after ingestion of *Vibrio cholerae*. J Infect Dis 1982; 145:465-473.

295. Figueroa G, Galeno H, Troncosco M, Toledo S, Soto V. Prospective study of *Campylobacter jejuni* infection in Chilean infants evaluated by culture and serology. J Clin Microbiol 1989; 27:1040-1044.

296. Rautelin H, Kosunen TU. Single and multiple acid extract antigens in *Campylobacter* serology. Acta Pathol Microbiol Immunol Scand [B] 1987; 95:277-281.

297. Walder M, Forsgren A. Enzyme-linked immunosorbent assay (ELISA) for antibodies against *Campylobacter jejuni*, and its clinical application. Acta Pathol Microbiol Immunol Scand [B] 1982; 90:423-433.

298. Akkina JE, Hogue AT, Angulo EJ, Johnson R, Petersen KE, Saini PK, Fedorka-Cray PJ, Schlosser WD. Epidemiologic aspects, control, and importance of multiple-drug resistant *Salmonella* Typhimurium DT104 in the United States. J Am Vet Med Assoc 1999; 214:790-798.

299. Stern MJ, Ames GF, Smith NH, Robinson EC, Higgins CF. Repetitive extragenic palindromic sequences: a major component of the bacterial genome. Cell 1984; 37:1015-1026.

300. Versalovic J, Koeuth T, Lupski JR. Deistribution of repetitive DNA sequences in eubacteria and application to fingerprinting of bacterial genomes. Nucleic Acids Res 1991; 19:6823-6831.

301. Cimolai N, Cogswell A, Hunter R. Nosocomial transmission of penicillin-resistant *Streptococcus pneumoniae*. Pediatr Pulmonol 1999; 27:432-434.

302. Cimolai N, Trombley C. Verification of a PCR-based typing method for *Acinetobacter baumannii* in a pseudo-outbreak investigation. Diagn Microbiol Infect Dis 1997; 28:61-64.

303. Cimolai N, Trombley C, Wensley D, LeBlanc J. Heterogeneous *Serratia marcescens* genotypes from a nosocomial pediatric outbreak. Chest 1997; 111:194-197.

304. Cimolai N, Basalyga S, Mah DG, Morrison BJ, Carter JE. A continuing assessment of risk factors for the development of *Escherichia coli* O157:H7-associated hemolytic uremic syndrome. Clin Nephrol 1994; 42:85-89.

305. Frost JA, Smith HR, Willshaw GA, Scotland SM, Gross RJ, Rowe B. Phage-typing of Vero-cytotoxin (VT) producing *Escherichia coli* O157 isolated in the United Kingdom. Epidemiol Infect 1989; 103:73-81.

306. Grif K, Karch H, Schneider C, Daschner FD, Beutin L, Cheasty T, Smith H, Rowe B, Dierich MP, Allerberger F. Comparative study of five differeent techniques for epidemiologicl typing of *Escherichia coli* O157. Diagn Microbiol Infect Dis 1998; 32:165-176.
307. Madico G, Akopyants NS, Berg DE. Arbitrarily primed PCR DNA fingerprinting of *Escherichia coli* O157:H7 strains by using templates from boiled cultures. J Clin Microbiol 1995; 33:1534-1536.
308. Birch M, Denning DW, Law D. Rapid genotyping of *Escherichia coli* O157 isolates by randomo amplification of polymorphic DNA. Eur J Clin Microbiol Infect Dis 1996; 15:297-302.
309. Martin IE, Tyler SD, Tyler KD, Khakria R, Johnson WM. Evaluation of ribotyping as epidemiological tool for typing *Escherichia coli* serogroup O157 isolates. J Clin Microbiol 1996; 34:720-723.
310. Paros M, Tarr PI, Kim H, Besser TE, Hancock DD. A comparison of human and bovine *Escherichia coli* O157:H7 isolates by toxin genotype, plasmid profile, and bacteriophage lambda-restriction fragment length polymorphism profile. J Infect Dis 1993; 168:1300-1303.
311. Stephenson S. New approaches for detecting and curtailing foodborne microbial infections. JAMA 1997; 277:1337-1340.
312. Hebert GA, Penner JL, Hennessy JN, McKinney RM. Correlation of an expanded direct fluorescent-antibody system with an established passive hemagglutination system for serogrouping strains of *Campylobacter jejuni* and *Campylobacter coli*. J Clin Microbiol 1983; 18:1064-1069.
313. Wong KH, Skelton SK, Patton CM, Feeley JC, Morris G. Typing of heat-stable and heat-labile antigens of *Campylobacter jejuni* and *Campylobacter coli* by coagglutination. J Clin Microbiol 1985; 21:702-707.
314. Duim B, Wassenaar TM, Rigter A, Wagenaar J. High-resolution genotyping of *Campylobacter* strains isolated from poultry and humans with amplified fragment length polymorphism fingerprinting. Appl Environ Microbiol 1999; 65:2369-2375.
315. Hanninen ML, Pajarre S, Klossner ML, Rautelin H. Typing of human *Campylobacter jejuni* isolates in Finland by pulsed-field gel electrophoresis. J Clin Microbiol 1998; 36:1787-1789.
316. Koblavi S, Grimont F, Grimont PAD. Clonal diversity of *Vibrio cholerae* O1 evidenced by rRNA gene restriction patterns. Res Microbiol 1990; 141:645-657.
317. Wachsmuth IK, Evans GM, Fields PI, Olsvik O, Popovic T, Bopp CA, Wells JG, Carrillo C, Blake PA. The molecular epidemiology of cholera in Latin America. J Infect Dis 1993; 167:621-626.
318. Popovic T, Bopp CA, Olsvik O, Wachsmuth IK. Epidemiologic application of a standardized ribotype scheme for *Vibrio cholerae* O1. J Clin Microbiol 1993; 31:2474-2482.
319. Faruque SM, Saha MN, Asadulghani J, Bag PK, Bhadra RK, Bhattacharya SK, Sack RB, Takeda Y, Nair GB. Genomic diversity among *Vibrio cholerae* O139 strains isolated in Bangladesh and India between 1992 and 1998. FEMS Microbiol Lett 2000; 15:279-284.
320. Hejazi A, Falkiner FR. *Serratia marcescens*. J Med Microbiol 1997; 46:903-912.
321. Sanders WE Jr., Sanders CC. *Enterobacter* spp.: pathogens posed to flourish at the turn of the century. Clin Microbiol Rev 1997; 10:220-241.
322. Sirot J, Chanal C, Petit A, Sirot D, Labia R, Gerbaud G. *Klebsiella penumoniae* and other *Enterobacteriaceae* producing novel plasmid-mediated beta-lactamases markedly active against thrid-generation cephalosporins: epidemiologic studies. Rev Infect Dis 1988; 10:850-859.
323. Tessier F, Arpin C, Allery A, Quentin C. Molecular characterization of a TEM-21 beta-lactamase in a clinical isolate of *Morganella morganii*. Antimicrob Agents Chemother 1998; 42:2125-2127.
324. Barnaud G, Arlet G, Verdet C, Gaillot O, Lagrange PH, Philippon A. *Salmonella enteritidis: AmpC* plasmid-mediated inducible beta-lactamase (DHA-1) with an *ampR* gene from *Morganella morganii*. Antimicrob Agents Chemother 1998; 42:2352-2358.
325. Thornsberry C. Trends in antimicrobial resistance among today's bacterial pathogens. Pharmacotherapy 1995; 15:S3-S8.
326. Hanson ND, Sanders CC. Regulation of inducible *AmpC* beta-lactamase expression among *Enterobacteriaceae*. Curr Pharm Design 1999; 5:881-894.
327. Petrosino J, Cantu C, Palzkill T. Beta-lactamases: protein evolution in real time. Trends Microbiol 1998; 6:323-327.
328. Moosdeen F. The evolution of resistance to cephalosporins. Clin Infect Dis 1997; 24:487-493.
329. Tzouvelekis LS, Bonomo RA. SHV-type beta-lactamases. Curr Pharm Design 1999; 5:847-864.
330. Jones RN. Important and emerging beta-lactamase-mediated resistances in hsopital-based pathogens: the *AmpC* enzymes. Diagn Microbiol Infect Dis 1998; 31:461-466.
331. Bush K. Metallo-beta-lactamases: a class apart. Clin Infect Dis 1998; 27:S48-S53.

332. Rasmussen BA, Bush K. Carbapenem-hydrolyzing beta-lactamases. Antimicrob Agents Chemother 1997; 41:223-232.
333. Bonomo RA, Rice LB. Inhibitor resistant class A beta-lactamases. Front Biosciences 1999; 4:34-41.
334. Chaibi EB, Sirot D, Paul G, Labia R. Inhibitor-resistant TEM beta-lactamases: phenotypic, genetic and biochemical characteristics. J Antimicrob Chemother 1999; 43:447-458.
335. Pitout JD, Sanders CC, Sanders WE. Antimicrobial resistance with focus on beta-lactam resistance in gram-negative bacilli. Am J Med 1997; 103:51-59.
336. Jacoby GA. Extended-spectrum beta-lactamases and other enzymes providing resistance to oxyimino-beta-lactams. Infect Dis Clin North Am 1997; 11:875-887.
337. Fluit AC, Schmitz FJ. Class 1 integrons, gene cassettes, mobility, and epidemiology. Eur J Clin Microbiol Infect Dis 1999; 18:761-770.
338. Cormican MG, Marshall SA, Jones RN. Detection of extended-spectrum beta-lactamase (ESBL)-producing strains by the Etest ESBL screen. J Clin Microbiol 1996; 34:1880-1884.
339. Schumacher H, Bengtsson B, Bjerregaard-Andersen H, Jensen TG. Detection of extended-spectrum beta-lactamases: the reliability of methods for susceptibility testing as used in Denmark. APMIS 1998; 106:979-986.
340. Anonymous. The most frequently occurring aminoglycoside resistance mechanisms – combined results of surveys in eight regions of the world. J Chemother 1995; 7(Suppl. 2):17-30.
341. Miller GH, Sabatelli FJ, Hare RS, Glupczynski Y, Mackey P, Shlaes D, Shimizu K, Shaw KJ. The most frequent aminoglycoside resistance mechanisms – changes with time and geographic area: a reflection of aminoglycoside usage patterns? Clin Infect Dis 1997; 24:S46-S62.
342. Walterspiel JN, Ashkenazi S, Morrow AL, Cleary TG. Effect of subinhibitory concentrations of antibiotics on extracellular Shiga-like toxin I. Infection 1992; 20:25-29.
343. Grif K, Dierich MP, Karch H, Allerberger F. Strain-specific differences in the amount of Shiga toxin released from enterohemorrhagic *Escherichia coli* O157 following exposure to subinhibitory concentrations of antimicrobial agents. Eur J Clin Microbiol Infect Dis 1998; 17:761-766.
344. Kauffman F, Dupont A. *Escherichia coli* from infantile epidemic gastroenteritis. Acta Pathol Micro Scand 1950; 27:552-564.
345. Sack RB, Rahman M, Yunus M, Khan EH. Antimicrobial resistance in organisms causing diarrheal disease. Clin Infect Dis 1997; 24:S102-S105.
346. Poppe C, Smart N, Khakria R, Johnson W, Spika J, Prescott J. *Salmonella typhimurium* DT104: a virulent and drug-resistant pathogen. Can Vet J 1998; 39:559-565.
347. Hampton MD, Ward LR, Rowe B, Threlfall EJ. Molecular fingerprinting of multidrug-resistant *Salmonella enterica* serotype Typhi. Emerg Infect Dis 1998; 4:317-320.
348. Threlfall EJ, Ward LR, Skinner JA, Smith HR, Lacey S. Ciprofloxacin-resistant *Salmonella typhi* and treatment failure. Lancet 1999; 353:1590-1591.
349. Cornelis G. Distribution of beta-lactamases A and B in some groups of *Yersinia enterocolitica* and their role in resistance. J Gen Microbiol 1975; 91:391-402.
350. Stolk-Engelaar V, Meis J, Mulder J, Loeffen F, Hoogkamp-Korstanje J. Activity of 24 antimicrobials against *Yersinia enterocolitica*. Contrib Microbiol Immunol 1995; 13:172-174.
351. Pai CH, Gillis F, Tuomanen E, Marks MI. Placebo-controlled double-blind evaluation of trimethoprim-sulfamethoxazole treatment of *Yersinia enterocolitica* gastroenteritis. J Pediatr 1994; 104:308-311.
352. Vijayalakshmi N, Rao RS, Badrinath S. Minimum inhibitory concentration (MIC) of some antibiotics against *Vibrio cholerae* O139 isolates from Pondicherry. Epidemiol Infect 1997; 119:25-28.
353. Yamamoto T, Nair GB, Albert MJ, Parodi CC, Takeda Y. Survey of in vitro susceptibilities of *Vibrio cholerae* O1 and O139 to antimicrobial agents. Antimicrob Agents Chemother 1995; 39:241-244.
354. Dhar U, Bennish ML, Khan WA, Seas C, Huq Khan E, Albert MJ, Abdus Salam M. Clinical features, antimicrobial susceptibility and toxin production in *Vibrio cholerae* O139 infection: comprison with *V. cholerae* O1 infection. Trans R Soc Trop Med Hyg 1996; 90:402-405.
355. Mukhopadhyay AK, Garg S, Nair GB, Kar S, Ghosh RK, Pajni S, Ghosh A, Shimada T, Takeda T, Takeda Y. Biotype traits and antibiotic susceptibility of *Vibrio cholerae* serogroup O1 before, during and after the emergence of the O139 serogroup. Epidemiol Infect 1995; 115:427-434.
356. Basu A, Garg P, Datta S, Chakraborty S, Bhattacharya T, Yamasaki S, Takeda Y, Nair GB. *Vibrio cholerae* O139 in Calcutta, 1992-1998: incidence, antibiograms, and genotypes. Emerg Infect Dis 2000; 6:139-147.
357. Dalsgaard A, Serichantalergs O, Pitarangsi C, Echeverria P. Molecular characterization and antibiotic susceptibility of *Vibrio cholerae* non-O1. Epidemiol Infect 1995; 114:51-63.

358. Dalsgaard A, Frimodt-Moller N, Bruun B, Hoi L, larsen JL. Clinical manifestations and molecular epidemiology of *Vibrio vulnificus* infections in Denmark. Eur J Clin Microbiol Infect Dis 1996; 15:227-232.
359. Taylor DE, Courvalin P. Mechanisms of antibiotic resistance in *Campylobacter* species. Antimicrob Agents Chemother 1988; 32:1107-1112.
360. Piddock LJ. Quinolone resistance and *Campylobacter* spp. J Antimicrob Chemother 1995; 36:891-898.
361. Morita K, Watanabe N, Kurata S, Kanamori M. Beta-lactam resistance of motile *Aeromonas* isolates form clinical and environmental sources. Antimicrob Agents Chemother 1994; 38:353-355.
362. Reinhardt JF, George WL. Comparative in vitro activities of selected antimicrobial agents against *Aeromonas* species and *Plesiomonas shigelloides*. Antimicrob Agents Chemother 1985; 27:643-645.
363. Chaudhury A, Nath G, Shukla BN, Sanyal SC. Biochemical characterisation, enteropathogenicity and antimicrobial resistance plasmids of clinical and environemental *Aeromonas* isolates. J med Microbiol 1996; 44:434-437.
364. Jones BL, Wilcox MH. *Aeromonas* infections and their treatment. J Antimicrob Chemother 1995; 35:453-461.
365. Stunt RA, Amyes AK, Thomson CJ, Payne DJ, Amyes SG. The production of a novel carbapenem-hydrolysing beta-lactamase in *Aeromonas veronii* biovar sobria, and its association with imipenem resistance. J Antimicrob Chemother 1998; 42:835-836.

16

Gram Negative Cocci and Moraxellae

Nevio Cimolai

Children's and Women's Health Centre of British Columbia, Vancouver, British Columbia, Canada

Dominique A. Caugant

WHO Collaborating Centre for Reference and Research on Meningococci, National Institute of Public Health, Oslo, Norway

I. HISTORICAL BACKGROUND

Neisseriae and moraxellae are a small group of medically-important bacteria. The neisseriae are Gram negative cocci, while the moraxellae comprise both Gram negative cocci and coccobacilli. The family *Neisseriaceae* includes several other genera that are not considered as neisseriae per se, i.e., *Acineto-bacter*, *Alysiella*, *Eikenella*, *Kingella*, and *Simonsiella*. Whereas phylogenetic studies indicate that these latter genera are indeed more closely related to the neisseriae than the moraxellae are (1) (Figure 1), we included the discussion of the neisseriae and moraxellae together for historical reasons and given the practical similarities that exist in the laboratory. The other genera of *Neisseriaceae* are mentioned in Chapters 17 and 18. Our discussion therefore highlights the major human pathogens (*Neisseria gonor-rhoeae*, *Neisseria meningitidis*, and *Moraxella catarrhalis*) and other medically relevant species, most of which belong to the commensal flora.

N. gonorrhoeae (the 'gonococcus') has historically been a prominent human pathogen and at one time the most commonly recognized bacterium that was associated with sexually transmitted diseases. Many decades of work have focussed on obtaining simple methods for identification and on the critical needs of specimen transport. Shortly after antibiotics became available to treat gonococcal infections, antibiotic resistance emerged, and in particular, penicillin-resistant gonococci spread throughout all continents (3). This translated into work that determined appropriate short course therapy with the use of new antibiotics as detailed later. The notoriety of N. gonorrhoeae lessened as it became apparent that *Chlamydia trachomatis* (see Chapter 27) was a much more common cause of sexually transmitted dis-eases (STDs); the numbers of documented C. trachomatis infections increased exponentially when bet-ter diagnostic methods became available for this organism to replace the traditional culture techniques. The recognition that both N. gonorrhoeae and C. trachomatis could, and often did, cause disease to-gether led to the use of treatment regimens that would cover both organisms and hence that would im-prove control for these infections. The latter progress, as well as the onset of the AIDS epidemic (with its associated emphasis on the prevention of STDs), have had a tremendous impact on the decline of gonorrhea.

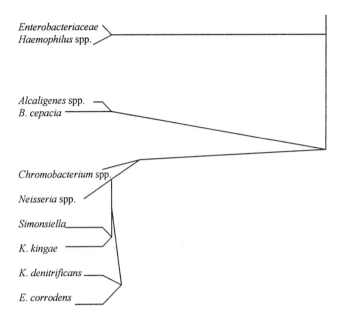

Figure 1   Dendrogram of the phylogeny of beta group *Proteobacteria* including the placement of *Neisseria* spp. based on 16S rRNA sequences [adapted from (1) and (2)].

Neisseria meningitidis (the 'meningococcus') causes sporadic meningitis throughout most of the developed world, but foci of epidemic activity continue to exist (4). On a historic basis, the disease burden has been considerable due to large epidemics sometimes encompassing several continents. While the bacterium caused infection at an alarming frequency among military recruits during the last century's wars, large epidemics are currently occurring periodically in parts of Africa and China. The advent of antibiotic therapy and, perhaps more important than the latter, antibiotic prophylaxis were critical to control the disease although antibiotic resistance to prophylaxis agents (e.g., sulphonamides) quickly emerged. There is much activity in the vaccination field (5), but no preparation is conferring protection against all of the common meningococcal strains.

Moraxella catarrhalis (formerly known as *Neisseria catarrhalis* and *Branhamella catarrhalis*) became recognized as an important respiratory pathogen in the last three decades (6). Prior to that, it was mainly viewed as a relatively non-pathogenic *Neisseria* species that colonized the upper respiratory tract of humans (7). Although invasive disease beyond the respiratory tract is a rarity, the bacterium continues to be a relatively common cause of infection, in part because of its presence in high frequency within the human oropharynx. The taxonomic status (and hence nomenclature) of this bacterium remains a subject for debate (8,9).

Other *Neisseria* spp. and other moraxellae are uncommon causes of infection and mainly present as opportunists in the compromised patient. Since most of the *Neisseria* spp. are highly competent in genetic transformation, there have been some concerns that this group of commensal bacteria might serve as a reservoir for antibiotic resistance to be transferred to *N. meningitidis* as well as to other bacteria (10).

II. CLINICAL ASPECTS

A. *N. gonorrhoeae*

N. gonorrhoeae is mainly acquired through sexual transmission, although newborns may become infected as they descend through an infected maternal genital tract. Both males and females may develop an infection of the genital tract that is asymptomatic. The latter is much more common among females. This silent reservoir is crucial for transmission. It is believed that particular strains are more likely to be associated with asymptomatic disease than others. In males, an incubation period of approximately 2-4 days occurs before the onset of symptoms; this timing may be longer in females and again contributes to the under-recognition of the infection during a time period that may be crucial for secondary transmission. Whether symptomatic or not, gonorrhea may spontaneously resolve over a 2-3 week period although some patients may have a very protracted course if untreated.

Males often first present with symptomatic urethritis which is most commonly manifest by discharge and dysuria. Systemic features such as fever are quite uncommon at this stage. The bacterium will not cause cystitis but rather has a proclivity to ascend the genital system. Epididymitis, prostatitis, and orchitis are all possible complications. Nevertheless, proportionately few males will have disease that ascends beyond the urethra. The manifestations in females vary considerably (11). Apart from asymptomatic disease, many will develop a mild to moderate discharge which emanates from the endocervix. Others may present with urethritis with or without discharge; again, cystitis per se does not occur. The bacterium may ascend the genital tract and infect the fallopian tubes. Thereafter, the infection may extend to the tubo-ovarian area and potentially spill over into the abdomen to cause peritonitis either locally or diffusely. This progression may reach the liver capsule, i.e., perihepatitis, and may be accompanied by fever and varying forms of abdominal pain, but it also has the potential to remain relatively silent. When clinically apparent, the intra-abdominal illness is commonly referred to as pelvic inflammatory disease. Untreated, the involvement of the tubo-ovarian area can progress to create permanent damage and scarring which may lead to infertility or ectopic pregnancy. Although these illnesses may occur with *N. gonorrhoeae* as the sole etiological agent, it is not uncommon for *C. trachomatis* to be a co-pathogen. In chronic tubal infection, vaginal-source anaerobes not uncommonly participate in the disease process as well. The latter complications, in addition to those that are detailed in the following paragraphs, emphasize the fact that *N. gonorrhoeae* is much more than a simple urethral pathogen.

Other forms of relatively superficial infection may occur at alternate mucosal sites. Depending on sexual practices, both pharyngeal and anal areas may be involved. Pharyngeal infection may occasionally include symptomatic pharyngitis. In the anal region, the infection may ascend to the lower rectum, thus causing a proctocolitis. Both of the latter sites may also be asymptomatically infected. The newborn may first become infected at the ocular site which may present as purulent conjunctivitis; adults too, however, are susceptible to superficial ocular disease.

Whereas most infections are confined to the genital tract, *N. gonorrhoeae* has the potential to be a systemic pathogen. Newborns may develop early-onset sepsis following invasion into the bloodstream from the superficial mucosal sites. Other age groups also are susceptible to bloodborne infection. The latter may manifest itself initially as a febrile illness where the bacterium may not have extended to areas outside of the bloodstream. In other cases, the infection may spread to joint, skin, bone, heart, and meninges. Among young sexually active adults, *N. gonorrhoeae* is not an uncommon cause of septic arthritis (12). Some individuals may have direct infection of the skin which presents as a vesicular lesion(s). The simultaneous occurrence in joint and skin has been translated into an "arthritis-dermatitis" syndrome. Disseminated gonococcal infections occur in less than 3% of those patients who have symptomatic or asymptomatic genital infection (12). Infection with certain strains is more likely to progress to systemic disease.

B. N. meningitidis

N. meningitidis is commonly carried in the normal flora of the nasopharynx and may be present in about 5-20% of the healthy population in the absence of disease outbreaks. In some closed populations, e.g., military recruits, carriage may reach 100%. Both encapsulated and unencapsulated strains are represented in the carrier state. During episodes of viral upper respiratory infections, relative overgrowth of this bacterium may be found in comparison to other typical organisms of the normal flora, i.e., analogous to that occurring with *S. pneumoniae* and *H. influenzae* in the same context. Systemic infection occurs nearly exclusively with encapsulated strains. All age groups may be affected, but most of the sporadic illnesses occur among children who are under the age of five. Invasive disease is less common among the elderly. Risk factors for repeated episodes of invasive disease include various complement deficiencies (13) which are due to defective serum bactericidal activity and/or phagocytosis. Meningococcal disease recurs in up to one-third of the individuals who have late component deficiency and nearly one-tenth of those who are properdin deficient (14).

Invasive meningococcal disease can take several forms. Most concerning, however, is advanced bacteremic disease with complications or meningeal infection. The bacterium presumably gains access to the circulation by penetrating through the mucosal membrane. Many patients who develop invasive disease probably have acquired the bacterium only a short while prior. Progression to severe meningococcal infection is rapid, and death may occur within hours. The bacteremia is often accompanied by acute fever, the onset of chills, and general malaise. Sepsis may progress to severe hypotension, shock state, pulmonary edema, and disseminated intravascular coagulation. A petechial or hemorrhagic rash is one of few manifestations that are relatively characteristic of the systemic illness. Some patients, especially children, may present with sepsis and no apparent focus; their initial blood cultures may be positive, and they may otherwise be well even during the next day despite a lack of therapy. The latter form of illness mimics "walking" pneumococcal bacteremia. A chronic form of bacteremia has also been described which is somewhat analogous to gonococcal bacteremia whereby the illness may have an associated rash and arthropathy. Central nervous system infection is not uncommonly associated with evidence of sepsis otherwise, although purely meningitis without evidence of bloodborne infection is also frequently seen. Meningococcal meningitis is the second most common form of bacterial meningitis among children and adults in developed countries (after pneumococcal meningitis). As with bacteremic illness, the mortality rate is high if left untreated. Primary pneumonia is also a direct manifestation of invasive disease, but occurs much less often than either meningococcemia or meningitis. Although penicillin has been and continues to be an effective antimeningococcal agent, some patients will have their illness progress despite the initiation of appropriate therapy. This probably occurs as a direct result of massive outgrowth of meningococci and response to residual bacterial products such as endotoxin. Even in countries where appropriate therapy is available, the case-fatality rate for systemic meningococcal disease is approximately 10%. The hemorrhagic rash may be followed by gangrene of the extremities. Some patients will develop post-infectious arthritis, pericarditis, or central nervous system sequelae.

Less severe illnesses can also occur such as conjuctivitis, urethritis, arthritis, and secondary respiratory infection. The respiratory infections, which may include pneumonia, bacterial tracheitis, and acute-on-chronic bronchitis, occur among individuals who may be compromised, e.g., chronic lung disease or post-viral illness. Patients with chronic intubation and artificial ventilation frequently develop some form of bacterial overgrowth in the trachea; *N. meningitidis* may be one of the bacteria that takes advantage of this situation even though symptomatic disease is not necessarily seen.

C. M. catarrhalis

M. catarrhalis has been recognized as a component of the normal respiratory bacterial flora for decades, but the significance of this bacterium as a pathogen was lacking. Eventually, it was confirmed mainly as a pathogen of the respiratory tract, and it has been implicated in otitis media, sinusitis, and mid- to lower respiratory infections (15). Acute respiratory illnesses may include acute-on-chronic bronchitis and bacterial tracheitis. Most instances of disease will occur after a viral infection or in patients who have some form of chronic respiratory compromise. Thus, *M. catarrhalis* appears to be mainly an opportunistic pathogen which creates infection in areas that are proximal to the oropharynx. Damage of the mucosa by viruses will lead to mucous trapping and airway blockade that will facilitate the sequestration of bacteria in a closed space (16). *M. catarrhalis* is often present in greater numbers in the respiratory tract when intercurrent viral infections exist. These infections are thus similar to those that are caused by *H. influenzae* and *S. pneumoniae* in the upper respiratory system (17).

Systemic disease with this bacterium is extremely rare (16), but may include meningitis, bacteremia, endocarditis, and septic arthritis. Most of these illnesses are likely to occur during compromise of the upper airways (facilitating the transgression of bacterium across the mucosal barrier) or in states of immune compromise. For example, oncology patients may have systemic spread as a consequence of immunocompromise and mucosal disruption (e.g., mucositis) from antineoplastic chemotherapy. Most of these infections respond promptly to antibiotics, and the mortality rate is low.

D. Other *Neisseria* spp.

Neisseria spp. (not *N. gonorrhoeae* and *N. meningitidis*) are mainly commensals of the upper respiratory tract and may be found in the proximal small intestine. Low numbers of these bacteria may also be present in the vagina. *N. cinerea* can potentially be misidentified as *N. gonorrhoeae*, but it generally does not cause disease. *N. polysaccharea* can be confused with *N. meningitidis*, but it too is not associated with infection on a practical basis. *N. lactamica* very frequently colonizes the nasopharynx of children.

These *Neisseria* spp. rarely cause invasive disease, and when they are found in blood cultures, their presence most often indicates salivary contamination. Nevertheless, rare infections have included bacteremia, meningitis, peritonitis during ambulatory peritoneal dialysis, conjunctivitis (although mostly found as a commensal at the conjunctival site), endocarditis, and septic arthritis. When found in the context of a complicated respiratory infection, e.g., empyema, these bacteria are most commonly only one component of a mixture of infecting microbes.

E. Other moraxellae

Moraxellae are also most commonly found in the normal upper respiratory tract and sometimes in the bowel and female genital tract. Most infections are superficial, e.g., conjunctivitis, but rare severe or invasive infections may include lower respiratory infection, bacteremia, septic arthritis, meningitis, and post-surgical ocular infections (18). *Oligella urethralis* (formerly *M. urethralis*) is especially found in the urinary tract but is not commonly encountered. *M. osloensis* is mainly found in the female genital tract. *M. lacunata* has been historically associated with chronic external eye infections (19). As a group, these bacteria are very rare causes of significant infection.

III. EPIDEMIOLOGY OF INFECTION

A. *N. gonorrhoeae*

Humans are the only reservoir for this bacterium, and thus human-to-human spread and the mechanisms by which it occurs, mainly sexual, are readily apparent. The risk of acquiring a gonococcal infection is influenced by many variables (11), but the major ones include: low socioeconomic status, unmarried status, number of sexual partners, sex trade work, lack of use of barrier protection, race, ethnicity, urban locale, difficult access to health care supports, lack of proper diagnostic facilities, and drug abuse. The potential for transmission seems to be greatest from infected male to uninfected female rather than the opposite, but asymptomatic patients of either gender may serve as reservoirs for ongoing spread. Given the degree of asymptomatic carriage in the community, it is of value to screen populations who may be at high risk. Knowledge of infected patients should prompt the determination of contacts who will also be screened and treated if necessary.

In Europe and North America, the incidence of gonorrhea peaked in the late 1970s and early 1980s (20), and a sharp reduction in the number of cases then occurred. It is likely that the AIDS epidemic and related factors have significantly contributed to effect this change. Some countries have been extremely efficient at control, e.g., Sweden. This downward trend is continuing into the new millenium although a minor increase has recently been recorded in the United States.

The frequency of penicillinase-producing *N. gonorrhoeae* (PPNG) is quite variable among different geographic locales (21,22). Some countries have had rates as high as 50% over the last decade whereas others continue to have frequencies <5%. The frequencies of other antibiotic resistances are variable, but they are commonly associated with penicillin resistance. Although penicillin resistance through beta-lactamase production was initially the primary concern, beta-lactamase-independent penicillin resistance has also emerged over the last two decades.

B. *N. meningitidis*

N. meningitidis is also strictly associated with humans. Transmission by direct contact or through large particle aerosols is critical to the spread of meningococci. These bacteria are normal components of respiratory flora. Meningococcal infections are seen sporadically throughout the world (23,24). Outbreaks and epidemics are relatively continuous in some regions, e.g., sub-Saharan Africa which is called the "meningitis belt" (25,26). Although the infection can affect all age groups, sporadic infections occur mainly in children. In all ages, crowding is a major risk factor. The relationship between the frequency of invasive disease and the frequency of carriage in a population has been the subject of numerous studies. As many strains from healthy carriers have a low pathogenic potential, overall carriage rates do not correlate, however, with the frequency of disease. Historically, it has been well-recognized that newly-acquired carriage was very important, and the potential for invasive disease correlated with a lack of circulating bactericidal antibody. It is believed that chronic carriage imparts increased immunity to meningococci. When invasive infection does occur, there is a very high fatality rate (up to 5-20%).

When a virulent meningococcal strain begins to spread in a susceptible population, the frequency of disease will exceed a particular threshold, and epidemic activity is defined (25). The recognition of epidemic activity in its beginnings therefore depends on accurate surveillance so that the attack rates can be used with some certainty when attempting to define the incidence of disease above a particular threshold. A change towards older patient age groups will generally occur, and epidemic disease will involve a larger proportion of teenagers and young adults in contrast to sporadic disease.

The availability of antibiotics has markedly changed the magnitude of epidemic infection in developed countries. This impact is due both to effective treatment and effective prophylaxis (of contacts). Almost as soon as antibiotics were used for prophylaxis, resistance emerged. Such was the case for sulphonamides, but resistance probably was in part a function of the use of this antibiotic for other infections. Prophylactic rifampin, in its current pattern of use, does not appear to pose the same problem, although secondary cases caused by rifampin-resistant strains in contacts who received prophylactic rifampin have been reported. Chloramphenicol is a cheap and simple treatment that is used extensively for the treatment of patients during epidemics in the meningitis belt of Africa. The development of resistance to that drug is feared especially given the finding of chloramphenicol-resistant meningococci in Vietnam.

Meningococci can be serogrouped on the basis of the structure of their capsular carbohydrates, and this system has over 10 such serogroups which are labeled with upper case alphabets (e.g., A, B, C, 29E, H, I, J, K, L, X, Y, Z, and W-135). The most commonly isolated serogroups are A, B, and C; X, Y, and W-135 are next common but nevertheless relatively rare overall from infections. The serogroup B polysaccharide has been shown to cross-react with some human tissue. Serogroup Y appears to have a greater tendency towards association with primary pneumonia. In developed countries, serogroup B is the main cause of sporadic disease. Recent outbreaks and epidemics throughout the world are especially represented by serogroups A and C. The biochemistry of the common capsule carbohydrates is well studied. Some capsular carbohydrates cross-react with other pathogens, e.g., some invasive *E. coli.*

Non-encapsulated (non-groupable) meningococci exist within the pool of normal flora, but these are only exceptionally associated with disease. Polysaccharide vaccines that were developed in the 1960s have been used particularly to control serogroup A and C disease. At present, a tetravalent preparation which contains serogroups A, C, W135, and Y is available, but unconjugated vaccines do not confer protection in children under the age of two years, and they do not provide long-term immunity. A serogroup B vaccine is not available because the serogroup B polysaccharide is a poor immunogen, and there is a risk for induction of autoimmunity.

Typing systems which examine strain variation within serogroups are discussed in detail later, and these have been of tremendous value in determining trends in epidemic and global spread (4).

C. *M. catarrhalis*

Carriage rates for *M. catarrhalis* vary from 5-50%. Human-to-human transmission occurs. Nosocomial transmission has been frequently documented among patients in intensive care units who are intubated and artificially ventilated (27).

IV. NATURE OF THE BACTERIUM, PATHOGENESIS, AND CLINICAL MANIFESTATIONS

The *Neisseria* spp. and *Moraxella catarrhalis* maintain the classical bean-shaped diplococcoid morphology when Gram stained. These bacteria grow well aerobically on enriched media (e.g., enriched chocolate agar) at 35-37°C, and colonies are visible after 24 hrs. in most circumstances; growth is enhanced by, and on occasion dependent on, CO_2 enrichment. These bacteria are non-motile, and oxidase-positive, and catalase-positive. *N. elongata* is an exception in having a short rod or coccobacillary morphology and lacks catalase. Bacteria within this group, including other moraxellae, have the characteristic Gram negative double membrane which includes lipopolysaccharide extending from the outer membrane (analogous for example to that of *Enterobacteriaceae*; see Chapter 15). Moraxellae other than *M. catarrhalis* may have short rod shapes which may vary to coccoid; they are also non-motile.

Moraxellae do not produce acid from carbohydrates when assessed by conventional laboratory methods. *Neisseria* spp., in contrast, are oxidative but produce small amounts of acid by-products. These small amounts can be detected by the use of methods to ensure that peptone alkaline products do not interfere in the appreciation of the acid-induced colour indicator changes, e.g., CTA (cystine trypticase agar) sugars.

The G+C% content of *Neisseria* spp. varies around 49-54%. They are quite clearly separated phylogenetically from *Moraxella* spp. Figure 2 illustrates the relationships of *Neisseria* spp. (2). The species *N. gonorrhoeae, N. meningitidis, N. lactamica,* and *N. polysaccharea* form one genospecies, although they can be differentiated by phenotypic traits. The two major human pathogens, *N. gonorrhoeae* and *N. meningitidis,* are especially related more to each other than to other *Neisseria* spp., and it has been suggested that *N. gonorrhoeae* is in fact a lineage of *N. meningitidis* that has adapted to a different ecological niche (28). Figure 3 demonstrates the inter-relationships of moraxellae (8).

The pathogenesis of pathogenic *Neisseria* infections has been extensively reviewed (29-31).

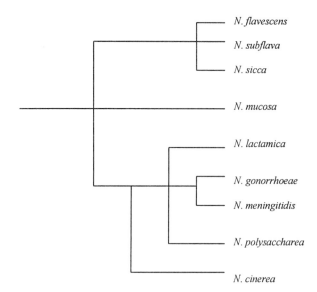

Figure 2 Dendrogram illustrating the relationships among *Neisseria* spp. based on 16S rRNA sequences [adapted from (2)].

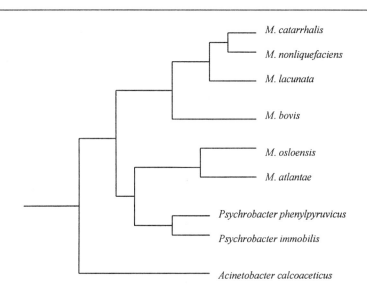

Figure 3 Dendrogram illustrating relationships among moraxellae and other bacteria based on 16S rRNA sequences [adapted from (8)].

A. *N. gonorrhoeae*

N. gonorrhoeae isolates are generally fastidious, and enriched media that have added amino acids, purines, and pyrimidines serve best to support growth. Enriched chocolate agar is most commonly used. Various nutritional auxotrophs, e.g., arginine, proline, xanthine, and uracil dependent, have been recognized (32); the diversity of these facilitates the division of isolates by their auxotype status. This species is unable to grow at temperatures below $33^{\circ}C$, requires CO_2, and is susceptible to drying. The bacterium is also susceptible to some fatty acids. Bacterial cells may autolyze when cultures are maintained for prolonged periods, and thus, fresh subcultures should be maintained when working with this pathogen. Plasmids are often carried, and these are especially critical for antimicrobial resistance.

This bacterium has been considerably studied for virulence factors, and there are several key features (33). Pili facilitate bacterial attachment, and piliated strains are more virulent. Pili are antiphagocytic and facilitate genetic transformation. Pili vary antigenically among isolates (34), but despite this potential, they have been targeted as vaccine candidates. *N. gonorrhoeae* produces an IgA protease that may protect the organism at mucosal sites of colonization and infection. The bacterial outer membrane possesses a porin [an outer membrane protein, designated protein I (PI)] which is also antigenically variable. PI participates in reducing serum bactericidal activity and promotes intracellular invasion. Variation in PI has been the basis for an array of serovars (Por serotyping) that can be used for discrimination of strains for epidemiological purposes. The lipopolysaccharide (LPS) is relatively weak for inducing cytokine and other cascades when compared, for example, to the LPS of *N. meningitidis*. The *N. gonorrhoeae* LPS lacks complex O side chains.

N. gonorrhoeae is selective in binding to cervical and urethral cells that are cuboidal, and does not adhere to squamous vaginal cells. After the initial attachment, the bacterium may become intracellular or penetrate between cell junctions. The bacterium will not only invade cells but also multiplies within them. A strong neutrophilic response ensues, and localized infections are therefore commonly associated with pus formation. Some strains, as defined by auxotroph typing or Por serotyping, are more likely to invade. Those that are more commonly associated with asymptomatic illness attract less of an inflammatory response. It is surprising how this bacterium is able to persist despite the development of a local immune response during chronic infection (35).

B. *N. meningitidis*

Growth of this bacterium occurs on simple media in contrast to *N. gonorrhoeae*, and medium supplements are not as important. *N. meningitidis* also has autolysins which may interrupt in vitro growth. Susceptibility to some detergents such as sodium polyanethol sulphonate (SPS) in blood culture media may also inhibit growth.

The study of virulence factors has received considerable attention. In addition to the capsular polysaccharide which protects the bacterium against complement-mediated bacteriolysis and phagocytosis, a number of other structures may be involved in the pathogenic process. As for *N. gonorrhoeae*, an IgA protease is produced by all strains. The role of iron-binding proteins and iron acquisition has received considerable interest and has been of some interest to those who are attempting to define novel vaccine antigens. Pili play a key role in attachment to mucosal cells, and some outer membrane proteins bind receptors on phagocytic and endothelial cells and stimulate endocytosis. The outer membrane proteins are not specific to the pathogenic serogroups, and their diversity has been exploited for the purposes of serotyping. Two porins, PorA and PorB, are used to respectively serosubtype and serotype meningococci. Numerous monoclonal antibodies have been developed for strain characterization. LPS has a critical role in pathogenesis and is implicated in the induction of many adverse events. Like other potent Gram negative LPSs, it influences complement activation, kinin interactions, coagulation factors, fibrinolytic mediators, and cytokines. The massive induction of these factors in disseminated infection may result in profound hypotension, leaky capillaries, respiratory distress, disseminated intravascular coagulation, among other features of shock. A reversal of this cascade of events is difficult when the disease is advanced. Variation in the LPS has been recognized, and is used as the basis of an immunotyping scheme. Certain immunotypes tend to be more commonly associated with strains that cause invasive disease.

Purulent responses with a predominance of polymorphonuclear cells typically occur during infection.

C. *M. catarrhalis*

Apart from being non-saccharolytic, *M. catarrhalis* is also characterized on the basis of grey-coloured colonies and the production of DNAase. *M. catarrhalis* is piliated, but attachment is complex and is dependent on several factors in addition to pili (27,36). Despite the high frequency of this bacterium in the upper respiratory tract and despite its modest frequency in infection of the sinuses, middle ear, and compromised respiratory tract, it is a very infrequent systemic pathogen (37).

The choice of the genus designations *Moraxella* or *Branhamella* continues to be a subject for healthy debate. It has become obvious with the renaming of several former *Moraxella* spp. that the systematics of these organisms is more complex than historically realized.

D. Other

The pathogenesis of other *Neisseria* spp. infections has not gained much attention as these bacteria rarely cause serious disease. Nevertheless, these other neisseriae have cross-reactive epitopes with both *N. gonorrhoeae* and *N. meningitidis*, especially the latter (38,39). It is believed that these cross-reactions allow for development of some protection against *N. meningitidis* as the commensal *Neisseria* spp. stimulate local mucosal immune responses over a long period of time.

Apart from *M. catarrhalis*, pathogenesis of other *Moraxella* spp. human infections is essentially unstudied. These bacteria are not fastidious but may pose a problem to the laboratory for identification due to the rarity of associated infections.

Lautropia mirabilis is a pleomorphic motile Gram negative coccus with some unique structural features, but its role in human disease is not apparent despite its presence in the normal flora of the mouth (40,41). It appears to be more closely related to the genera of *Burkholderia* and *Alcaligenes* rather than those of the more common Gram negative cocci. This bacterium is not discussed further herein.

Morococcus cerebrosus is an aerobic Gram negative coccus whose individual cells measure less than 1 μm., but mulberry-like aggregates of 10-20 cells are visualized when stained. It is non-motile and produces both oxidase and catalase. Clinical isolates are a rarity, but this organism has been isolated on one occasion from a brain abscess (42).

V. IMMUNOLOGY OF INFECTION

A. *N. gonorrhoeae*

Both the local (mucosal) and systemic immune responses after gonococcal infections are modest (43), and there is a discordance between the two (44). IgA mucosal responses do develop as a consequence of infection, but it is not clear how much these contribute to protection (45). Judging from the presence of both systemic and mucosal antibody among those who have been previously infected, it does not appear that humoral immunity is highly protective of genital infection. By a variety of serological techniques, it has been shown that acute infection is accompanied by a variable IgM response; IgG develops over 1-2 weeks after the initial infection.

Immunoblotting has been used to assess the antibody level in patients with active disease, and some quantitative differences between patients and controls have been found (46). Unfortunately, these differences are not consistent enough to allow for a dichotomy of infected and uninfected individuals. Systemic antibodies often recognize antigens such as pili, protein II (PII), a family of hypervariable outer membrane proteins of 23-33 kD, and LPS. At the mucosal site (vaginal), antibody is especially directed to PI, PII, and pili (47). Other outer membrane proteins have especially been assessed for their role in immunity, but several of these are not apparently accessible at the cell surface and thus may be hidden from the humoral response (48). Anti-PI antibody enhances serum bactericidal activity and experimentally induces a mucosal response (49). Serovar specific immunity does not seem to occur however (50). Both PI and LPS confer resistance to killing by human sera and changes in the LPS modify the latter (51). Gonococcal outer membrane proteins have some degree of immunological homology to those of meningococci. Gonococcal LPS cross-reacts with some *H. influenzae* LPSs (52).

A role for cell-mediated immunity is uncertain in either pathogenesis or protection.

B. *N. meningitidis*

Clinical illness with meningococci leads to a measurable acute immune response. The common presence of meningococci in the pharyngeal flora may, however, complicate the serological differentiation of asymptomatic and diseased individuals.

Carriage of meningococci is an immunizing process in itself, and antibodies develop within a few weeks after new colonization. Both the capsule and other antigens provoke this response; some degree of cross-reactivity between the meningococcal capsule and that of enteric bacteria may also provide for protective immunity. The likelihood of invasion is increased when specific serum bactericidal antibody against a new colonizing strain is lacking. At birth, maternal bactericidal antibody is often in existence from transplacental migration. This bactericidal antibody in serum then increases with age, and indeed in adulthood, the presence of bactericidal antibody to meningococci that express common serogroups is often in the range of 60-90%. Bactericidal antibody that accrues after colonization is relatively serotype-specific (53). Children who convalesce from a meningococcal infection develop bactericidal antibody. There may be a link between human genotype and the quality of anti-meningococcal capsular antigen response (54).

Natural infection induces an antibody response to several antigens including LPS (55), outer membrane proteins (56), IgA protease (57), and serogroup carbohydrates (58). The anticapsular response to serogroups A, C, Y, and W-135 are considerable. Antibody presence, though, does not always indicate protection.

C. *M. catarrhalis*

The study of immunology for *M. catarrhalis* infections is somewhat complicated by the lack of an adequate animal model. As for the pathogenic neisseriae, the outer membrane proteins have been studied in this regard, and antibodies to these structures have been found (59). In particular, there is a common response to outer membrane protein B1 (84 kD) (60). Antibody in the middle ear fluid of those with otitis media does react with outer membrane proteins (61,62). This local production of antibody though is not necessarily matched by a systemic response. An immune response to iron-binding proteins has also been detailed (63).

VI. LABORATORY DIAGNOSIS

A. Staining

Staining of clinical specimens for rapid presumptive diagnosis of infection due to gonococci, meningococci, and *M. catarrhalis* has been of practical relevance for many decades. The predictive values for identifying these bacteria, however, is subject to considerable variation and is dependent on the nature of the underlying illness, gender, the site of specimen acquisition, the quality of the stain, and the experience of the observer among other things.

Apart from the Gram reaction itself, the morphology of these bacteria is often distinctive to the extent that other staining methods have been used simply to identify the bean-shaped diplococcoid forms, e.g., methylene blue staining of genital specimens for the presumptive identification of gonococci from genital sites. In the case of the methylene blue stain, the predictive value for finding these morphotypes from the urethral samples of males is relatively high. The predictive value in the latter example is further increased when many polymorphonuclear cells are present and the bean-shaped diplococci are seemingly intracellular. The demonstration of bacterial morphotypes and cellularity can be captured by several other stains in addition to methylene blue.

The Gram stain is nevertheless more likely to be used for direct staining because of the added value of Gram differentiation and of its use in the general bacteriology laboratory. Among males, the predictive value for gonococcal infection is high (~85-95%); only exceptionally will such bacterial morphotypes be due to other Gram negative diplococci, e.g., *N. meningitidis*. The same findings from a urethral swab of a symptomatic female will also be indicative with a high predictive value, but this is not so for a specimen from the cervix. In many cases, the swab from the female cervix will be contaminated by bacteria from the vaginal pool of normal flora. The latter adds morphotypes which closely resemble cocci and indeed may include non-pathogenic *Neisseria* spp., moraxellae, and acinetobacters. In addition, the presence of an abundant normal flora may obscure the finding of Gram negative diplococci, especially when these are few. It is of benefit when large numbers of Gram negative diplococci are found and when these are apparently intracellular bacteria (sensitivity ~50-70%). In asymptomatic individuals, especially females, the predictive value for the finding of Gram negative diplococci suffers considerably and possibly to the extent where the staining of the clinical specimen for the diagnosis of asymptomatic infection is irrelevant. Such inaccuracy is important given the stigma of infection when misdiagnosed. The application of the Gram stain to other sites, e.g., rectal or oropharygeal, is even more fraught with difficulty regardless of whether the patient is asymptomatic or symptomatic again due to abundance of similar morphotypes (especially in the throat where non-pathogenic *Neisseria* spp. are in abundance). Gonococci are extremely rare causes of meningitis, and thus the finding of Gram negative cocci in the cerebrospinal fluid should not practically raise concern for this species. As well, they are generally uncommon in blood cultures and should not be considered of high probability among young children, the elderly, and immunocompromised hosts. In contrast, the finding of these morphotypes in a joint fluid which has been obtained from a symptomatic arthropathy of a sexually active young adult has a very high predictive value for gonococci.

Meningococci are most often encountered in cerebrospinal fluids, blood cultures, sputa, and skin lesions of meningococcemia. In cerebrospinal fluid, the predictive value for indicating that these bacteria are present when Gram negative diplococci are seen is very high; most often there will be a very prominent polymorphonuclear response. It is much more likely that the bacterium is sparse in the cerebrospinal fluid, however, and hence it is often difficult to find the bacterium in this context. Occasionally, overly decolourized pneumococci may resemble meningococci. The value of Gram stains for petechial skin lesions during active meningococcemia has historically been underestimated. Superficial layers of epidermis should be gently scraped away, and a deep epidermal scraping will often show the bacterium. Assessment of meningococcal presence needs to be made early in the course of the illness, e.g., at initial presentation, since antibiotic therapy lyses bacteria, and the finding of these morphotypes is less certain after 24-48 hrs. of antibiotic therapy. In the context of a septic child without a clinical infectious focus or in the midst of an active respiratory illness, a positive blood culture with Gram negative diplococci is highly likely to indicate meningococcal disease. Such a positive culture in the context of clinical meningococcemia or meningitis is also likely to reflect the same. The finding of Gram negative diplococci from a sputum, middle ear fluid, sinus aspirate, or clinical bacterial tracheitis is more complicated due to the potential for both meningococci and *M. catarrhalis* to cause illness at these sites and due to the higher likelihood of encountering non-pathogenic *Neisseria* spp. in these sites.

Gram stain morphology does not distinguish pathogenic neisseriae and *M. catarrhalis*, but other moraxellae not uncommonly have more of a coccobacillary or bacillary shape. The latter are relatively uncommon systemic humans pathogens, and thus, they are often not initially considered when positive blood cultures are stained. Gram negative anaerobic cocci are generally smaller, are very uncommonly seen in clinical specimens, and are generally not present in specimens that are otherwise used to find pathogenic neisseriae.

B. Culture

Prior to the acquisition of specimens, it must be acknowledged that *N. gonorrhoeae* is capable of infecting several sites simultaneously, and thus the collection of multiple specimens should be contemplated depending on the pattern of sexual practices.

The transport of specimens with potential gonococci and meningococci has been the subject of much study. The problem of maintaining viable gonococci and meningococci in specimens that are transported over long distances led in large part to the development of microbial transport media and their modifications. Potential gonococcal-bearing specimens that are sent in difficult transport circumstances would benefit from the simultaneous submission of an unstained smear (microscope slide). The collection swab itself has the potential to be inhibitory. For example, both the swab material and the applicator stick in untreated cotton swabs has been recognized to be capable of inhibition. It is prudent, therefore, to ensure that the collection kit is of proven value for maintaining gonococci and meningococci (64). The use of a charcoal-based minimal medium or salt solution are the time-honoured transport mechanisms, and these are available in several forms, e.g., modified Amies' and Stuart's transport media (65). The specimen is best kept at room temperature for a short period of time before processing. Apart from swab collection, the use of urine centrifugates has been advocated for gonococcal culture, but the latter is likely to be more complicated by transport issues (66).

Despite the use of an appropriate collection kit and transport mechanism, however, gonococci may yet succumb to other factors that may hinder the laboratory isolation of gonococci (66). Given the latter, it is not surprising that many clinicians and investigators have studied the value of directly applying the clinical specimen to solid growth media at the 'bedside' (65). If culture in the appropriate atmosphere is to follow shortly after such set-up, the solid medium may be sent directly to the laboratory for culture. If transport is to be delayed, it may be preferable to incubate the solid media at the site of acquisition for 24 hrs. before they are forwarded to the laboratory (65). Conditions for maintaining humidity and an appropriate growth atmosphere have been provided commercially from several sources (65). The recipient laboratory is left to further incubate, if necessary, and then to perform the actual bacteriology work. Limitations of this approach include poor technique in application to the solid media (e.g., all of the swab is spread over a narrow area) and inappropriate processing at the site of collection and initial incubation. Meningococci and *M. catarrhalis* are somewhat more resilient, however, to extremes of collection and transport, as are the other Gram negative cocci and moraxellae that we discuss in this chapter.

Culture should include an environment with a temperature of 35-37°C, added humidity, and CO_2 supplementation (65). The latter can be provided by commercial or conventional methods. The use of a plain candle (non-toxic) jar may still suffice, although most medium-to-large laboratories make use of large incubation chambers which provide all of the essential atmospheric components.

Both non-selective and selective media should be used when specimens are collected from sites that may contain normal body flora (65). Selective media are not required of course when a sterile site, e.g., knee fluid, is being sampled. Non-selective media for gonococci require enrichment beyond the usual components of a traditional chocolate medium. This enrichment should include various amino acids, co-factors, and other ingredients that are included in additives such as Isovitalex or equivalent (65). These supplements are needed to ensure that potential fastidious auxotrophs are not missed. Selective media usually include the latter solid medium base, but they are further supplemented with antibiotics that will reduce or eliminate the undesirable normal flora of anterior urethra, vagina and cervix, anorectal area, and pharynx. These antibiotics often include vancomycin, colistin, trimethoprim, and an antifungal agent. The selective media in most common use include Martin-Lewis, modified Thayer-Martin, and New York City media. These media are often held for up to 72 hrs. and should be incubated for no less than 48 hrs. Some gonococci (especially particular auxotrophs) are susceptible to vancomycin, and thus non-selective media should always be used in addition to a selective one. There does not appear to be any major benefit for using more than one selective medium. Occasionally, other *Neisseria* spp., e.g., especially *N. lactamica*, may be found on selective media in addition to a few other bacteria that are resistant to the incorporated antibiotics. Despite the latter, however, it is of value that most clinical specimens are relatively depleted of contaminating bacteria by the aforementioned selective mechanisms.

By way of their restricted metabolic pathways, some *N. gonorrhoeae* auxotrophs may form small colonies after several days. Meningococcal colonies may occasionally appear mucoid, and these will be encapsulated strains. Non-gonococcal neisseriae and moraxellae grow reasonably well on routine blood and chocolate agars. The colonial characteristics for particular isolates of the latter species may be somewhat distinctive, e.g., agar pitting of *M. lacunata*, e.g., pigmentation of some non-pathogenic *Neisseria* spp.

For blood culture, the potential inhibition of gonococci and meningococci by SPS [a component of the blood culture medium which may serve as an anticoagulant and in part as a lytic agent for eucaryotic cells (67)] may explain why a modest proportion of patients with meningococcemia fail to have associated positive blood cultures even when antibiotics have not been used. It has been suggested that the addition of gelatin to the blood culture medium may neutralize SPS and enhance the possibility that these bacteria will be cultured (68). There are inherent problems with this approach: a) these bacteria may be present when there is insufficient clinical evidence in a suspect infection that these microorganisms should be considered, b) the separate introduction of an agent into the blood culture bottle introduces in itself the potential for contamination which may obscure the presence of meningococci, c) the gelatin must be available on an ad hoc basis, and d) the frequency of both gonococcemia and meningococcemia in most laboratories is so small as to make the addition of gelatin impractical. In addition, two studies have not been able to confirm a benefit for this approach (69,70). The addition of gelatin is best left for circumstances of clinical meningococcemia which may have more predictive tell-tale signs. The use of lysis-centrifugation may obviate the need for gelatin (71). One must bear in mind the possibility that even in the latter case, patients are likely to have received an appropriate antibiotic regardless of whether the patient's blood culture is positive or not.

C. Identification

Neisseriae and moraxellae are oxidase-positive, and this initial knowledge is a valuable screening method for the purposes of presumptively identifying gonococci and meningococci from non-selective media on which a few colonies may be obscured amidst colonies of the normal flora. The oxidase test may be performed separately on a filter paper or other support, or directly on the solid agar medium; in the latter circumstance, a subculture should be made of the bacterium after the oxidase reagent has given a positive reaction to the colony, since the organism may be inhibited after prolonged exposure.

1.   N. gonorrhoeae

Whether based on the oxidase test or suspicious colonial morphology from selective media, the time-honoured methods for confirmation of species initially include the demonstration of growth or no growth on simple media and at room temperature (see Table 1). The mere growth on selective media should raise concern for gonococci. The production of acid from CTA sugars (fructose, glucose, lactose, maltose, and sucrose) is then a standard for identification. Rapid methods for the latter sugar utilization have been commercialized, e.g., QuadFerm (72,73), but are variably used (74,75). A rapid chromogenic substrate has also been devised for the latter purposes (Gonochek II) (76); pre-formed enzymes are assessed withsubstrates that are cleaved to form coloured end-products as an indicator of activity.

The implications of a definitive diagnosis of gonorrhea weigh on clinical outcome, control of spread, and psychosocial factors. Thus, an accurate diagnosis is imperative, and it is critical to have a definitive confirmation of *N. gonorrhoeae*. The latter is best accomplished by increasing the probability of confirmation by the use of an alternate method to culture; these may include immunofluorescence (with species-specific monoclonal or polyclonal antibodies) (77,78), agglutination with antibacterial antibody that is adherent to particles which are amenable to the interpretation of an agglutination reac-

Table 1   Differentiation of *Neisseria* spp. and *M. catarrhalis*.

	1	2	3	4	5	6	7	8	9	10	11
Acid from (CTA):											
fructose	-	-	-	-	-	-	-	+	-	+	+/-
glucose	-	-	-	-	+	+	+	+	+	+	+
lactose	-	-	-	-	-	+	-	-	-	-	-
maltose	-	-	-	-	-	+	+	+	+	+	+
sucrose	-	-	-	-	-	-	-	+	-	+	+/-
NO$_3$ reduction	+	-	-	-	-	-	-	+	-	-	-
Growth on nutrient agar (35°C)	+	+	+	+	-	+	+/-	+	+	+	+
DNAase	+	-	-	-	-	-	-	-	-	-	-
Tributyrin hydrolysis	+	-	-	-	-	-	-	-	-	-	-
Coccobacilli/bacilli	-	-	+	-	-	-	-	-	-	-	-

(1 – *M. catarrhalis*; 2 – *N. cinerea*; 3 – *N. elongata*; 4 – *N. flavescens*; 5 – *N. gonorrhoeae*; 6 – *N. lactamica*; 7 – *N. meningitidis*; 8 – *N. mucosa*; 9 – *N. polysaccharea*; 10 – *N. sicca*; 11 – *N. subflava*)

tion (e.g., Phadebact, GonoGen I, GonoGen II) (79-82), and DNA probing (Accuprobe) (83). Each of the latter is susceptible to false-positive or false-negative reactions, and thus, it is preferable overall to use two different methods for confirmation. These methods should include two entirely different approaches, e.g., not the use of CTA sugars and a rapid sugar method, e.g., not two antibody agglutination methods. Figure 4 outlines an approach for gonococcal isolation and identification.

2.   N. meningitidis, M. catarrhalis, and others

N. meningitidis has a pattern of acid production that is somewhat unique, and it will grow variably on simple media at 35°C. It is differentiated from *N. polysaccharea* by the inability to produce a mucoid appearance in the presence of sucrose. Several other species of non-pathogenic *Neisseria* also produce a capsule but have much different acid production profiles. Gamma-glutamyl transferase is present in all meningococci, while other species that grow on media that are selective for neisseriae do not produce this enzyme. The identification of meningococcal serogroup antigens (for encapsulated isolates) will also be of supportive value.

M. catarrhalis manifests DNAase activity and is among the few Gram negative cocci that are capable of reducing nitrate (84). Some investigators have proposed the use of tributyrin hydrolysis or of 4-methyl umbelliferyl butyrate (MUB; rapid chromogenic enzyme substrate) (85,86) as a rapid presumptive method for identification.

The differentiation of other *Neisseria* spp. and moraxellae rests mainly with the biochemical and other criteria as detailed in Tables 1 and Figure 5. *N. cinerea* is not a common clinical isolate, but care must be taken not to confuse it with *N. gonorrhoeae*. *N. cinerea* may be found on selective media, especially from sources such as pharynx and rectum (87). It will grow on simple media at 35°C, but it may weakly produce acid from glucose or provide a rapid chromogenic substrate profile that is very similar to *N. gonorrhoeae* (81). In general, moraxellae and related bacteria are relatively inert, and care must be take to avoid confusion with brucellae. Several moraxellae and *Neisseria* spp. are nevertheless identified by commercial kits (73).

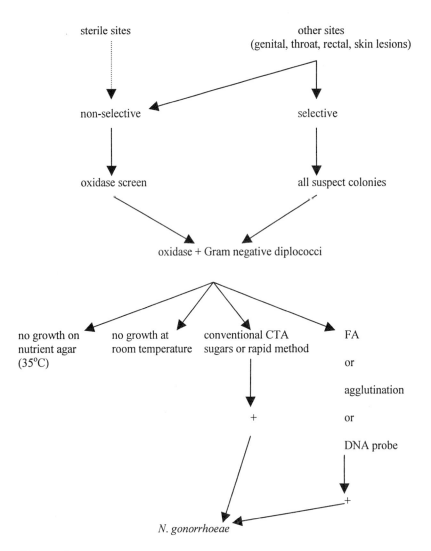

Figure 4   An approach to the culture and identification of *N. gonorrhoeae* from clinical specimens.

D.   Antigen detection

Antigen detection of *N. gonorrhoeae* by enzyme immunoassay has been commercialized (Gonozyme) (88). The application of this method alongside a similar such assay for *C. trachomatis* has appeal. The sensitivity of the assay is limited by the amount of bacterium that is available. Due to the colorimetric (indirect) mechanism for result determination, this format is susceptible to false positive tests. The application of this technology to assessments of gonococcal infection as an indicator for sexual abuse must be guarded. The positive predictive value in such a setting is compromised by the low pre-test probability for true infection. Likewise, such an assay is more likely to be accurate in a symptomatic population of high risk where the amount of organism is considerable and where the frequency of disease is higher. Screening asymptomatic populations is likely also to be compromised for the aforementioned reasons (89).

Agglutination tests for meningococcal antigen detection have several potential uses. For positive blood cultures, the detection of meningococcal serogroups will serve as rapid presumptive identification. The detection of such antigen in a culture-negative cerebrospinal fluid will also be of value (90). For both of these purposes, agglutination of serogroups A, C, Y, and W-135 antigen is possible. The serogroup B reagent cross-reacts with *Escherichia coli* K1 capsule. Thus, the result of the reaction must be interpreted with care; in newborns, a positive reaction likely indicates *E. coli* K1, while in older patients the presence of serogroup B *N. meningitidis* is more probable.

E.   Genetic detection

Given the worldwide problem with gonorrhea, the recent emergence and assessment of new molecular techniques for detection of the bacterium were very welcome. The first of these methods for direct genetic detection was DNA probing. Apart from investigative probes, commercial DNA probes are now

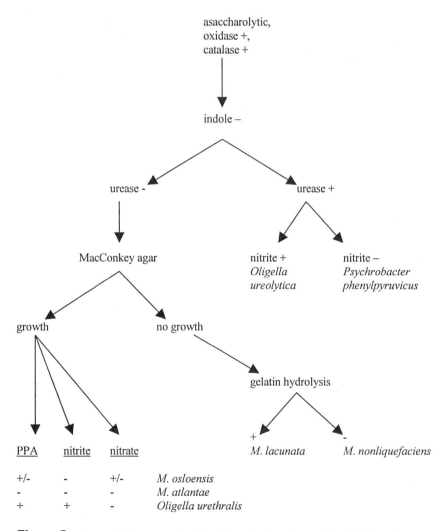

Figure 5   A simplified approach or the differentiation of moraxellae (additional assays may be required).

available (Pace II, GenProbe). A detection kit which could determine the presence of *N. gonorrhoeae* in a few hours has been developed. As with other direct probe assays, the test is limited by the absolute quantity of organism that is present in the specimen. The value of such technology to samples from asymptomatic individuals is thus reduced. The detection of organism by this approach also prevents availability of the bacterium for susceptibility testing when it is desirable.

Genetic amplification technologies thereafter assumed priority, and at least three versions have become commercially available: a) polymerase chain reaction (Roche) (91-93), b) ligase chain reaction (Abbott) (94,95), and c) transcription-mediated amplification (GenProbe) (95,96). New such technologies are emerging continuously. When run alongside *Chlamydia trachomatis* genetic amplification assays (i.e., multiplex amplifications), there is the potential for a very powerful approach to detecting and and thus improving control of these sexually transmitted infections. Amplification also allows for the detection of small quantities of genetic material and may potentially be applied to urine sediments (97). Non-genital specimens may also be assessed with these methods (98). The limitation of not having bacterium available for susceptibility testing along with the inability to use these assays predictably for test of cure in the short term (residual bacterial DNA despite non-viability) provide some uncertainty. It must be recognized, however, that current short course treatment for urethral and female genital infections is highly effective and is often based on the use of potent antibiotics that most gonococci are very susceptible to. Thus, susceptibility testing may not often be required. In the history of contemporary bacteriology, however, resistance of gonococci to several antibiotics has emerged, and some form of antibiotic surveillance must be maintained.

Numerous genetic amplification methods have been described to detect meningococcal DNA in blood and cerebrospinal fluid using a variety of target DNA sequences, but none is commercially available. For example, these targets have included an insertion sequence, the capsule gene, and the *porA* gene (which is species-specific and determines the serosubtype of the strain). A method which is based on 16S rRNA facilitates the differentiation of meningococcal meningitis from meningitis that is due to other pathogens (99).

F. Typing

1. N. gonorrhoeae

Auxotyping was historically used for typing and was of benefit in at least defining some strains that were more likely associated with invasive disease (100). Plasmid profiles and restriction enzyme digests of plasmids has been applied, but limitations due to plasmidless bacteria became evident. Pulsed-field gel electrophoresis has been applied as it has for most other bacteria (101).

Diversity in the outer membrance proteins of *N. gonorrhoeae* was determined with the use of monoclonal antibodies especially to PI. These antibodies could then be used for typing purposes (102). An evolution of porin proteins during infection in a community has been recognized, thus limiting the value of Por serotyping (103).

The discriminatory power of numerous typing methods has been compared (104).

2. N. meningitidis

Serogroup determination for invasive isolates is an obvious first step in characterizing meningococcal isolates since the vast majority of such isolates are encapsulated, and the results are essential if vaccination of groups of the population is to be considered. There is usually very little in the way of practical value for typing non-invasive unencapsulated isolates outside of the research context.

As monoclonal antibody technology was exploited to investigate surface proteins of meningococci, it became apparent that surface protein (especially outer membrane proteins) variability was considerable such that pools of monoclonal antibodies could be used to demonstrate differences among porin (PorA and PorB) proteins. The PorB (class 2 or 3 outer membrane protein) molecule diversity was thus used to define the serotype status, and the PorA (class 1 outer membrane protein) molecule diversity was used to define the serosubtype. Serosubtype designations are determined on the basis of two surface-exposed variable regions within PorA (105). An immunotype designation is based on the variation among bacterial lipopolysaccharides. A serological type has been defined by description of the following in order – serogroup:serotype:serosubtype:immunotype (4). For example, a particular serogroup A strain that was of concern in China was designated A:21:P1.7,10. Despite the success in the use of monoclonal antibodies for typing, it must be acknowledged that horizontal genetic exchange and the human immune response drive ongoing changes in the variable regions of these surface structures that are targets for typing, and thus, some antigenic shifts among highly related strains are readily occurring.

Multilocus enzyme electrophoresis (MLEE) has been applied to the study of population genetics for meningococci (4,106) and it is a useful adjunct to the other typing methods defined above. MLEE establishes phylogenetic relationships by detecting allelic variation in housekeeping genes that are not under selective pressure. Thus, the variation in these genes is accumulating much more slowly. Since recombinational events are so frequent in meningococci, the clonal structure of the populations may be disrupted over a relatively short period of time. Most epidemic clones of meningococci have been reasonably stable over decades, however, and MLEE has proven valuable for the global molecular epidemiological study of *N. meningitidis*.

DNA-based typing methods are now numerous and include restriction enzyme analysis, pulsed-field gel electrophoresis, Rep-PCR, ribotyping, random amplification of polymorphic DNA, insertion sequence analyses, virulence gene sequencing, restriction length polymorphism of PCR products, and multilocus sequence typing (MLST) (107-109). These approaches have their merits and limitations; some are more applicable to population genetics rather than typing of localized outbreaks. MLST, an adaptation of MLEE which is based on the sequencing of fragments of multiple housekeeping genes, is emerging as an international standard, especially as automation facilitates interpretation and record keeping. A central database that is accessible via the Internet is now allowing for the exchange of typing results between all laboratories.

VII. SUSCEPTIBILITY TESTING

A. *N. gonorrhoeae*

Methods for susceptibility testing of these bacteria are well detailed. Critical agar dilution, disc diffusion, and Etest are acceptable alternatives. The recommended medium for use is GC agar which has a defined 'XV-like' supplement (110). This medium should not have added cysteine since the latter has the potential to inactivate some beta-lactams (110).

The major concern is not so much how to test for susceptibility but rather when to test (111). In countries where resources are limited, traditional antibiotics such as penicillin, amoxycillin, and tetracyclines continue to enjoy use, but high rates of resistance in these same areas necessitate the performance of some susceptibility testing. In many developed countries, treatment has been modified over the last decade to favour shorter treatment courses, e.g., single doses, and the use of more broad spectrum antibiotics which are essentially very potent antigonococcal agents, e.g., cefixime, ceftriaxone, and ciprofloxacin. The pre-treatment likelihood of resistance with the latter approach is minimal. Thus, some would argue that susceptibility testing is not warranted if a standard form of potent therapy is to be given regardless (111). In addition, such potent therapies make it much less desirable to have tests of cure since the success rates of therapy are so high. The bacterial isolates from patients with treatment failures should be assessed for susceptibility. Whereas it may not be desirable to test all isolates, it is useful periodically to assess susceptibility in order to ensure that emerging resistance does not make these potent antibiotics quickly irrelevant. An assessment of beta-lactamase status is easily done, and other antibiotics that may be tested should reflect antibiotics in use or those which are referred to as secondary options. Regardless of gonococcal treatment, it is recommended that an anti-*Chlamydia trachomatis* therapy also be administered given the high frequency of co-infections.

Penicillin resistance due to beta-lactamase was the first major resistance that became apparent by on a large scale; by the 1970s, such resistance emerged and quickly spread through all continents. In some regions, this resistance has been present in as many as 50% of isolates. Beta-lactamase production is plasmid-mediated and several different plasmids have been shown to carry the relevant gene (112). Beta-lactamase activity is reliably identified by several methods, including the chromogenic cephalosporin (e.g., nitrocefin) assays (113). Penicillin resistance may also be conferred by chromosomal genes, but this level of resistance tends to be low level and not associated with penicillinase activity (3). Rather, decreased binding of penicillin at the active site due to altered penicillin-binding proteins is responsible. The latter resistance confers some increased resistance to other beta-lactam agents but in a relative fashion (3). This low-level non-beta-lactamase form of resistance is associated with a slight increase in treatment failure when beta-lactam agents are used; the potency of short course advanced cephalosporins diminishes the chance for treatment failure.

Tetracycline resistance is also plasmid-mediated, and the major resistance gene, *tetM*, has been well characterized (112,114). Resistance has been documented to most other antigonococcal agents (e.g., spectinomycin, cotrimoxazole, and erythromycin) although the frequencies are low (3). Of particular concern, quinolone resistance emerged and has been associated with treatment failures; this has occurred within a very short period after these agents were introduced for the treatment of gonorrhea (115,116). The basis for this resistance includes mutations in the *gyrA* gene and reduced drug accumulation into bacterial cells (117). It is not uncommon to see linked resistances, especially in regions where gonorrhea continues to be highly endemic and where bacterial exposure to antibiotics is therefore considerable. For example, linkages of beta-lactamase and tetracycline resistance have historically been observed (118). In many developed countries, the frequency of gonococcal infections has diminished, but as the number of isolates declined, the frequency of resistance increased. Thus, the proportion of resistance has increased even though the absolute numbers of resistant isolates may have reached a plateau. Some have projected that the use of more potent short-course agents might be met with new and more concerning trends in bacterial resistance. While the potential for the latter resistance to emerge is certainly a threat, it must be recognized that gonococcal infections are decreasing in numbers, and thus, the need for antibiotic use is declining and may continue to decline if these short-term potent therapies maintain a high degree of treatment success. This balance will require careful attention over the next decade.

Although resistance genes among gonococci may be mobilized by plasmids (112), it has been observed that the genes are often situated in genetic arrays that are highly mobile (i.e., transposons). It is likely therefore that the issue of resistance among gonococci with respect to existing and new therapies will continue.

B. *N. meningitidis*

Penicillin still remains the antibiotic of choice for meningococcal infections, and resistance to this agent is uncommon on a world-wide basis. This is somewhat surprising given the extent of horizontal transfer that is thought to occur between *N. meningitidis* and other *Neisseria* spp. in the oropharynx (119). It is also surprising given that meningococci have developed resistance to other antibiotics quickly on some occasions when widespread prophylaxis was being advocated after sulphonamides became available many decades ago.

Penicillin resistance does occur, albeit uncommon. Rare isolates have been identified which have either chromosomal- or plasmid-mediated resistance due to beta-lactamase (120), and these are anticipated to be resistant from a clinical perspective. A low level of penicillin resistance due to alterations of penicillin-binding proteins is a more common form of resistance (121). The latter form has emerged over the last decade and represents an incremental resistance in comparison to the generally exquisite susceptibility that was witnessed previously. It is not clear that this low level resistance has any clinical impact when treating either meningococcemia or meningococcal meningitis. Concerns have been extended that this may be the first step towards a higher level of resistance, perhaps analogous to the progressive change that occurred for penicillin resistance among *Streptococcus pneumoniae*. Recent work has shown that such resistance can be predicted by genetic methods (122). Isolates with low-level resistance show some degree of cross-resistance to beta-lactam agents, but advanced-level cephalosporins, e.g., cefotaxime, are nevertheless quite active (123). High rates of this intermediate resistance have especially been found in Spain (up to 40%) (124,125). In contrast, frequencies <10% have been reported from the U.S. (126).

Chloramphenicol and second- or third-generation cephalosporins are active against meningococci in the cerebrospinal fluid, although chloramphenicol resistance was recently reported in some isolates. First-generation cephalosporins are not recommended regardless of apparent in vitro susceptibility.

Sulphonamides were first used for prophylaxis, and eventually, agents such as rifampin, minocycline, and fluoroquinolones were deemed to be appropriate for such purposes. The introduction of sulphonamides was quickly followed by a high frequency of resistance. Rifampin is now commonly used for this purpose. This antibiotic remains highly effective, but resistance following widespread use has occurred (127). These agents must penetrate the nasopharyngeal reservoirs in order for prophylaxis to be effective, but even for these agents, oral ingestion translates into nasopharyngeal concentrations that may sufficiently test the ability for resistance to emerge. Despite the history of sulphonamide resistance, many contemporary isolates (often particular serogroups more than others) are indeed quite susceptible to these agents, e.g., cotrimoxazole, and should be tested during outbreaks (128).

Susceptibility testing of meningococci may be accomplished with disc diffusion, agar dilution, microbroth dilution, and Etest (128-132).

C. *M. catarrhalis*

The luxuriant growth of *M. catarrhalis* on simple media facilitates susceptibility testing. This bacterium was frequently penicillin-susceptible until the last 2-3 decades (133). Now, the frequency of beta-lactamase positivity reaches 70-90% in most surveys (133). The latter are penicillin and amoxycillin resistant. Variations in the spectrum of beta-lactamase activity have been determined; the most common versions are produced by chromosomal genes and include BRO-1 and BRO-2 beta-lactamases (134).

Despite this high frequency of beta-lactamase positivity in the current era, the bacterium has retained susceptibility to a number of alternatives including advanced level cephalosporins, amoxycillin/clavulanic acid, tetracyclines, cotrimoxazole, quinolones, erythromycin, chloramphenicol, and aminoglycosides (113,134,135).

D. Other *Neisseria* spp.

Most of these species are usually penicillin susceptible, but reports of beta-lactamase positivity have been published. It is prudent then to formally test these bacteria for beta-lactamase status when serious infections are to be treated. Low level chromosomal resistance which is analogous to that of *N. meningitidis* has also been found (124).

Some isolates have shown evidence for *tetM* which mediates tetracycline resistance. It is also prudent to test for susceptibility when alternative, non-penicillin agents, are used.

E. Moraxellae

Most of these bacteria grow well and thus are amenable to susceptibility testing with conventional methods (136). Criteria for susceptibility and resistance are not clearly defined, but the majority are very susceptible to penicillin (18). Beta-lactamase activity is uncommon, but should be assessed in the context of serious infections. *M. liquefaciens* isolates have been identified which possess BRO-1 and BRO-2 beta-lactamases which are similar to those of *M. catarrhalis* (137).

REFERENCES

1. Dewhirst FE, Paster BJ, Bright PL. *Chromobacterium, Eikenella, Kingella, Neisseria, Simonsiella,* and *Vitreoscilla* species comprise a major branch of the beta group *Proteobacteria* by 16S ribosomal ribonucleic acid sequence comparison: transfer of *Eikenella* and *Simonsiella* to the family *Neisseriaceae* (emend.). Int J Syst Bacteriol 1989; 39:258-266.
2. Rossau R, Vandenbussche G, Thielemans, Segers P, Grosch H, Gothe E, Mannheim W, De Ley J. Ribosomal ribonucleic acid cistron similarities and deoxyribonucleic acid homologies of *Neisseria, Kingella, Eikenella, Simonsiella, Alysiella,* and Centers for Disease Control Groups EF-4 and M-5 in the emeneded family *Neisseriaceae.* Int J Syst Bacteriol 1989; 39:185-198.
3. Ison CA. Antimicrobial agents and gonorrhea: therapeutic choice, resistance, and susceptibility testing. Genitourin Med 1996; 72:253-257.
4. Caugant DA. Population genetics and molecular epidemiology of *Neisseria meningitidis.* APMIS 1998; 106:505-525.
5. Peltola H. Meningococcal vaccines. Current status and future possibilities. Drugs 1998; 55:347-366.
6. Murphy TF. Lung infections. 2. *Branhamella catarrhalis*: epidemiological and clinical aspects of a human respiratory tract pathogen. Thorax 1998; 53:124-128.
7. Henriksen SD. *Moraxella, Neisseria, Branhamella,* and *Acinetobacter.* Ann Rev Microbiol 1976; 30:63-83.
8. Pettersson B, Kodjo A, Ronaghi M, Uhlen M, Tonjum T. Phylogeny of the family *Moraxellaceae* by 16S rDNA sequence analysis, with special emphasis on differentiation of *Moraxella* species. Int J Syst Bacteriol 1998; 48:75-78.
9. Tonjum T, Bukholm G, Bovre K. Differentiation of some species of *Neisseriaceae* and other bacterial groups by DNA-DNA hybridization. APMIS 1989; 97:395-405.
10. Cimolai N, Bryce E. Beta-lactamase antibiotic resistance in *Neisseria* species. Lancet 1990; 335:1404.
11. McNeeley SG Jr. Gonococcal infections in women. Obstet Gynecol Clin North Am 1989; 16:467-478.
12. Eisenstein BI, Masi AT. Disseminated gonococcal infection and gonococcal arthritis: I. Bacteriology, epidemiology, host factors, pathogen factors, and pathology. Semin Arthritis Rheum 1981; 110:155-172.
13. Ross SC, Densen P. Complement deficiency states and infection: epidemiology, pathogenesis and consequences of neisserial and other infections in an immune deficiency. Medicine 1984; 63:243-273.
14. Figueroa J, Andreoni J, Densen P. Complement deficiency states and meningococcal disease. Immunol Res 1993; 12:295-311.
15. Hager H, Verghese A, Alvarez S, Berk SL. *Branhamella catarrhalis* respiratory infections. Rev Infect Dis 1987; 9:1140-1149.
16. Marchant CD. Spectrum of disease due to *Branhamella catarrhalis* in children with particular reference to acute otitis media. Am J Med 1990; 88:S15-S19.
17. Christensen JJ. *Moraxella (Branhamella) catarrhalis*: clinical, microbiological and immunological features in lower respiratory tract infections. APMIS 1999; 88:S1-S36.
18. Graham DR, Band JD, Thornberry C, Hollis DG, Weaver RE. Infections caused by *Moraxella, Moraxella urethralis, Moraxella*-like groups M-5 and M-6, and *Kingella kingae* in the United States, 1953-1980. Rev Infect Dis 1990; 12:423-431.
19. Ringvold A, Vik E, Bevanger LS. *Moraxella lacunata* isolated from epidemic conjunctivitis among teen-aged females. Acta Ophthalmol 1985; 63:427-431.
20. Barnes RC, Holmes KK. Epidemiology of gonorrhea: current perspectives. Epidemiol Rev 1984; 6:1-30.
21. Lind I. Epidemiology of antibiotic resistant *Neisseria gonorrhoeae* in industrialized and developing countries. Scand J Infect Dis 1990; 69:S77-S82.
22. Ison CA, Dillon JA, Tapsall JW. The epidemiology of global antibiotic resistance among *Neisseria gonorrhoeae* and *Haemophilus ducreyi.* Lancet 1998; 351:S8-S11.
23. Voss L, Lennon D. Epidemiology, management, and prevention of meningococcal infections. Curr Opin Pediatr 1994; 6:23-28.
24. Riedo FX, Plikaytis BD, Broome CV. Epidemiology and prevention of meningococcal disease. Pediatr Infect Dis J 1995; 14:643-657.
25. Moore PS. Meningococcal meningitis in sub-Saharan Africa: a model for the epidemic process. Clin Infect Dis 1992; 14:515-525.
26. Hart CA, Cuevas LE. Meningococcal disease in Africa. Ann Trop Med Parasitol 1997; 91:777-785.

27. Murphy TF. *Branhamella catarrhalis*: epidemiology, surface antigenic structure, and immune response. Microbiol Rev 1996; 60:267-279.

28. Vasquez JA, de la Fuente L, Berron S, O'Rourke M, Smith NH, Zhou J, Spratt BG. Ecological separation and genetic isolation of *Neisseria gonorrhoeae* and *Neisseria meningitidis*. Curr Biol 1993; 3:567-572.

29. Meyer TF. Pathogenic neisseriae – a model of bacterial virulence and genetic flexibility. Zentralb Bakteriol 1990; 274:135-154.

30. Nassif X, Pujol C, Morand P, Eugene E. Interactions of pathogenic *Neisseria* with host cells. Is it possible to assemble the puzzle? Mol Microbiol 1999; 32:1124-1132.

31. Meyer TF. Pathogenic neisseriae: complexity of pathogen-host cell interplay. Clin Infect Dis 1999; 28:433-441.

32. Chen CY, Genco CA, Rock JP, Morse SA. Physiology and metabolism of *Neisseria gonorrhoeae* and *Neisseria meningitidis*: implications for pathogenesis. Clin Microbiol Rev 1989; 2:S35-S40.

33. Britigan BE, Cohen MS, Sparling PF. Gonococcal infection: a model of molecular pathogenesis. N Engl J Med 1985; 312:1683-1694.

34. Cannon JG, Sparling PF. The genetics of the gonococcus. Ann Rev Microbiol 1984; 38:111-133.

35. Sparling PF, Tsai J, Cornelissen CN. Gonococci are survivors. Scand J Infect Dis 1990; 69:S125-S136.

36. Catlin BW. *Branhamella catarrhalis*: an organism gaining respect as a pathogen. Clin Microbiol Rev 1990; 3:293-320.

37. Enright MC, McKenzie H. *Moraxella* (*Branhamella*) *catarrhalis* – clinical and molecular aspects of a rediscovered pathogen. J Med Microbiol 1997; 46:360-371.

38. Kim JJ, Mandrell RE, Griffiss JM. *Neisseria lactamica* and *Neisseria meningitidis* share lipo-oligosaccharide epitopes but lack common capsular and class 1, 2, and 3 protein epitopes. Infect Immun 1989; 57:602-608.

39. Cann KJ, Rogers TR. Detection of antibodies to common antigens of pathogenic and commensal *Neisseria* species. J Med Microbiol 1989; 30:23-31.

40. Gerner-Smidt P, Keiser-Nielsen H, Dorsch M, Stackebrandt E, Ursing J, Blom J, Christensen AC, Christensen JJ, Frederiksen W, Hoffman S, Holten-Andersen W, Ying YT. *Lautropia mirabilis* gen. nov., sp. nov., a Gram-negative motile coccus with unusual morphology isolated from the human mouth. Microbiology 1994; 140:1787-1797.

41. Rossmann SN, Wilson PH, Hicks J, Carter B, Cron SG, Simon C, Flaitz CM, Demmler GJ, Shearer WT, Kline MW. Isolation of *Lautropia mirabilis* from oral cavities of human immunodeficiency virus-infected children. J Clin Microbiol 1998; 36:1756-1760.

42. Long PA, Sly LI, Pham AV, Davis GHG. Characterization of *Morococcus cerebrosus* gen. nov., sp. nov. and comparison with *Neisseria mucosa*. Int J Syst Bacteriol 1981; 31:294-301.

43. Hedges SR, Mayo MS, Mestecky J, Hook EW, Russell MW. Limited local and systemic antibody responses to *Neisseria gonorrhoeae* during uncomplicated genital infections. Infect Immun 1999; 67:3937-3946.

44. Tapchaisri P, Sirisinha S. Serum and secretory antibody responses to *Neisseria gonorrhoeae* in patients with gonococcal infections. Br J Vener Dis 1976; 52:374-380.

45. Russell MW, Hedges SR, Wu HY, Hook EW, Mestecky J. Mucosal immunity in the genital tract: prospects for vaccines against sexually transmitted diseases – a review. Am J Reprod Immunol 1999; 42:58-63.

46. Ison CA, Hadfield SG, Bellinger CM, Dawson SG, Glynn AA. The specificity of serum and local antibodies in female gonorrhea. Clin Exp Immunol 1986; 65:198-205.

47. Lammel CJ, Swet RL, Rice PA, Knapp JS, Schoolnik GK, Heilbron DC, Brooks GF. Antibody-antigen specificity in the immune response to infection with *Neisseria gonorrhoeae*. J Infect Dis 1985; 152:990-1001.

48. Swanson J, Barrera O. Immunological characteristics of gonococcal outer membrane protein II assessed by immunoprecipitation, immunoblotting, and coagglutination. J Exp Med 1983; 157:1405-1420.

49. Jeurissen SH, Sminia T, Beuvery EC. Induction of mucosal immunoglobulin A immune response by preparations of *Neisseria gonorrhoeae* porin proteins. Infect Immun 1987; 55:253-257.

50. Ross JD, Moyes A, Young H. Serovar specific immunity to *Neisseria gonorrhoeae*: does it exist? Genitourin Med 1995; 71:367-369.

51. Hook EW, Olsen DA, Buchanan TM. Analysis of the antigen specificity of the human serum immunoglobulin G immune response to complicated gonococcal infection. Infect Immun 1984; 43:706-709.

52. Virji M, Weiser JN, Lindberg AA, Moxon ER. Antigenic similarities in lipopolysaccharides of *Haemophilus* and *Neisseria* and expression of a digalactoside structure also present on human cells. Microb Pathog 1990; 9:441-450.

53. Jones GR, Christodoulides M, Brooks JL, Miller AR, Cartwright KA, Heckels JE. Dynamics of carriage of *Neisseria meningitidis* in a group of military recruits: subtype stability and specificity of the immune response following colonization. J Infect Dis 1998; 178:451-459.

54. Pandey JP, Ambrosch F, Fudenberg HH, Stanek G, Wiedermann G. Immunoglobuliin allotypes and immune response to meningococcal polysaccharides A and C. J Immunogenet 1982; 9:25-29.
55. Estabrook MM, Baker CJ, Griffiss JM. The immune response of children to meningococcal lipo-oligosaccharides during disseminated disease is directed primarily against two monoclonal antibody-defined epitopes. J Infect Dis 1993; 167:966-970.
56. Mandrell RE, Zollinger WD. Human immune response to meningococcal outer membrane protein epitopes after natural infection or vaccination. Infect Immun 1989; 57:1590-1598.
57. Brooks GF, Lammel CJ, Blake MS, Kusecek B, Achtman M. Antibodies against IgA1 protease are stimulated both by clinical disease and asymptomatic carriage of serogroup A *Neisseria meningitidis*. J Infect Dis 1992; 166:1316-1321.
58. Griffiss JM, Brandt BL, Broud DD, Goroff DK, Baker CJ. Immune response of infants and children to disseminated infections with *Neisseria meningitidis*. J Infect Dis 1984; 150:71-79.
59. Helminen ME, Beach R, Maciver I, Jarosik G, Hansen EJ, Leinonen M. Human immune response against outer membrane proteins of *Moraxella* (*Branhamella*) *catarrhalis* determined by immunoblotting and enzyme immunoassay. Clin Diagn Lab Immunol 1995; 2:35-39.
60. Sethi S, Hill SL, Murphy TF. Serum antibodies to outer membrane proteins (OMPs) of *Moraxella* (*Branhamella*) *catarrhalis* in patients with bronchiectasis; identification of OMP B1 as an important antigen. Infect Immun 1995; 63:1516-1520.
61. Faden H, Hong J, Murphy T. Immune response to outer membrane antigens of *Moraxella catarrhalis* in children with otitis media. Infect Immun 1992; 60:3824-3829.
62. Mathers K, Leinonen M, Goldblatt D. Antibody response to outer membrane proteins of *Moraxella catarrhalis* in children with otitis media. Pediatr Infect Dis J 1999; 18:982-988.
63. Yu RH, Bonnah RA, Ainsworth S, Schryvers AB. Analysis of the immunological responses to transferrin and lactoferrin receptor proteins from *Moraxella catarrhalis*. Infect Immun 1999; 67:3793-3799.
64. Hosty TS, Freear MA, Baker C, Holston J. Comparison of transportation media for the culturing of *N. gonorrhoeae*. Am J Clin Pathol 1974; 62:435-437.
65. Evangelista AT, Beilstein HR, Abramson C. Laboratory Diagnosis of Gonorrhea. Cumitech 4A. Washington, DC:American Society for Microbiology, 1993.
66. Sng EH, Rajan VS, Yeo KL, Goh AJ. The recovery of *Neisseria gonorrhoeae* from clinical specimens: effects of different temperatures, transport times, and media. Sex Transm Dis 1982; 9:74-78.
67. Rintala L, Pollock HM. Effects of two blood culture anticoagulants on growth of *Neisseria meningitidis*. J Clin Microbiol 1978; 7:332-336.
68. Eng J, Holten E. Gelatin neutralization of the inhibitory effect of sodium polyanethol sulfonate on *Neisseria meningitidis* in blood culture media. J Clin Microbiol 1977; 6:1-3.
69. McDonald JC, Knowles K, Sorger S. Assessment of gelatin supplementation of PEDS Plus BACTEC blood culture medium. Diagn Microbiol Infect Dis 1993; 17:193-196.
70. McDonald JC, Knowles K, Sorger S, Richards GK. Assessment of gelatin-supplemented BACTEC blood culture medium in a pediatric hospital. Diagn Microbiol Infect Dis 1992; 15:277-280.
71. Scribner RK, Welch DF. Neutralization of the inhibitory effect of sodium polyanetholsulfonate on *Neisseria meningitidis* in blood cultures processed with the Du Pont Isolator System. J Clin Microbiol 1984; 20:40-42.
72. Gradus MS, Ng CM, Silver KJ. Comparison of the QuadFERM+ 2-hr identification system with conventional carbohydrate degradation tests for confirmatory identification of *Neisseria gonorrhoeae*. Sex Transm Dis 1989; 16:57-59.
73. Janda WM, Zigler KL, Bradna JJ. API QuadFERM+ with rapid DNAase for identification of *Neisseria* spp. and *Branhamella catarrhalis*. J Clin Microbiol 1987; 25:203-206.
74. Durussel C, Siegrist HH. Evaluation of three commercial systems for the identification of pathogenic *Neisseria* and *Branhamella* species against the conventional method. Zentralb Bakteriol Mikrobiol Hyg [A] 1988; 268:318-324.
75. Dolter J, Bryant L, Janda JM. Evaluation of five rapid systems for the identification of *Neisseria gonorrhoeae*. Diagn Microbiol Infect Dis 1990; 13:265-267.
76. Welborn PP, Uyeda CT, Ellison-Birang N. Evaluation of Gonochek-II as a rapid identification system for pathogenic *Neisseria* species. J Clin Microbiol 1984; 20:680-683.
77. Laughon BE, Ehret JM, Tanino TT, Van der Pol B, Handsfield HH, Jones RB, Judson FN, Hook EW. Fluorescent monoclonal antibody for confirmation of *Neisseria gonorrhoeae* cultures. J Clin Microbiol 1987; 25:2388-2390.

78. Welch WD, Cartwright G. Fluorescent monoclonal antibody compared with carbohydrate utilization for rapid identification of *Neisseria gonorrhoeae*. J Clin Microbiol 1988; 26:293-296.

79. Janda WM, Ulanday MG, Bohnhoff M, LeBeau LJ. Evaluation of the RIM-N, Gonochek II, and Phadebact systems for the identification of pathogenic *Neisseria* spp. and *Branhamella catarrhalis*. J Clin Microbiol 1985; 21:734-737.

80. Dillon JR, Carballo M, Pauze M. Evaluation of eight methods for identification of pathogenic *Neisseria* species: Neisseria-Kwik, RIM-N, Gonobio-Test, Minitek, Gonochek II, GonoGen, Phadebact Monoclonal GC OMNI Test, and Syva Micro Trak Test. J Clin Microbiol 1988; 26:493-497.

81. Boyce JM, Mitchell EB Jr. Difficulties in differentiating *Neisseria cinerea* from *Neisseria gonorrhoeae* in rapid systems used for identifying pathogenic *Neisseria* species. J Clin Microbiol 1985; 22:731-734.

82. Philip A, Garton GC. Compartive evaluation of five commercial systems for the rapid identification of pathogenic *Neisseria* species. J Clin Microbiol 1985; 22:101-104.

83. Young H, Moyes A. Comparative evaluation of AccuProbe culture identification test for *Neisseria gonorrhoeae* and other rapid methods. J Clin Microbiol 1993; 31:1996-1999.

84. Doern GV. *Branhamella catarrhalis*: phenotypic characteristics. Am J Med 1990; 88:S33-S35.

85. Singh S, Cisera KM, Turnidge JD, Russell EG. Selection of optimum laboratory tests for the identification of *Moraxella catarrhalis*. Pathology 1997; 29:206-208.

86. Speeleveld E, Fossepre JM, Gordts B, Van Landuyt HW. Comparison of three rapid methods, tributyrine, 4-methylumbelliferyl butyrate, and indoxyl acetate, for rapid identification of *Moraxella catarrhalis*. J Clin Microbiol 1994; 32:1362-1363.

87. Knapp JS, Totten PA, Mulks MH, Minshew BH. Characterization of *Neisseria cinerea*, a nonpathogenic species isolated on Martin-Lewis medium selective for pathogenic *Neisseria* spp. J Clin Microbiol 1984; 19:63-67.

88. Thomas JG, Dul MJ, Badger S, Grecco A, Immerman RS, Jackson N, Jacob CV. Multicenter clinical trial and laboratory utilization of an enzymatic detection method for gonococcal antigens. Am J Clin Pathol 1986; 86:71-78.

89. Thomason JL, Gelbart SM, Sobieski VJ, anderson RJ, Schulien MB, Hamilton PR. Effectiveness of Gonozyme for detection of gonorrhea in low-risk pregnant and gynecologic populations. Sex Transm Dis 1989; 16:28-31.

90. Tilton RC, Dias F, Ryan RW. Comparative evaluation of three commercial products and counterimmunoelectrophoresis for the detection of antigens in cerebrospinal fluid. J Clin Microbiol 1984; 20:231-234.

91. Farrell DJ. Evaluation of AMPLICOR *Neisseria gonorrhoeae* PCR using *cppB* nested PCR and 16S rRNA PCR. J Clin Microbiol 1999; 37:386-390.

92. Palladino S, Pearman JW, Kay ID, Smith DW, Harnett GB, Woods M, Marshall L, McCloskey J. Diagnosis of *Chlamydia trachomatis* and *Neisseria gonorrhoeae* genitourinary infections in males by the Amplicor PCR assay of urine. Diagn Microbiol Infect Dis 1999; 33:141-146.

93. Jungkind D, Direnzo S, Beavis KG, Silverman NS. Evaluation of automated COBAS AMPLICOR PCR system for detection of several infectious agents and its impact on laboratory management. J Clin Microbiol 1996; 34:2778-2783.

94. Carroll KC, Aldeen WE, Morrison M, Anderson R, Lee D, Mottice S. Evaluation of the Abbott LCx ligase chain reaction assay for detection of *Chlamydia trachomatis* and *Neisseria gonorrhoeae* in urine and genital swab specimens from a sexually transmitted disease clinic population. J Clin Microbiol 1998; 36:1630-1633.

95. Koumans EH, Johnson RE, Knapp JS, St Louis ME. Laboratory testing for *Neisseria gonorhoeae* by recently introduced nonculture tests: a performance review with clinical and public health considerations. Clin Infect Dis 1998; 27:1171-1180.

96. Modarress KJ, Cullen AP, Jaffurs WJ Sr., Troutman GL, Mousavi N, Hubbard RA, Henderson S, Lorincz AT. Detection of *Chlamydia trachomatis* and *Neisseria gonorrhoeae* in swab specimens by the Hybrid Capture II and PACE 2 nucleic acid probe tests. Sex Transm Dis 1999; 26:303-308.

97. Xu K, Glanton V, Johnson SR, Beck-Sague C, Bhullar V, Candal DH, Pettus KS, Farshy CE, Black CM. Detection of *Neisseria gonorrhoeae* infection by ligase chain reaction testing of urine among adolescent women with and without *Chlamydia trachomatis* infection. Sex Transm Dis 1998; 25:533-538.

98. Stary A, Ching SF, Teodorowicz L, Lee H. Comparison of ligase chain reaction and culture for detection of *Neisseria gonorrhoeae* in genital and extragenital specimens. J Clin Microbiol 1997; 35:239-242.

99. Radstrom P, Backman A, Qian N, Kragsbjerg P, Pahlson C, Olcen P. Detection of bacterial DNA in cerebrospinal fluid by an assay for simultaneous detection of *Neisseria meningitidis*, *Haemophilus influenzae*, and streptococci using a seminested PCR strategy. J Clin Microbiol 1994; 32:2738-2744.

100. Backman M, Ruden AK, Bygdeman SM, Falk ES, Jonsson A, Kallings I, Ringertz O, Sandstrom EG. Comparison between serological classification and auxotyping in the analysis of *Neisseria gonorrhoeae* infections. Acta Pathol Microbiol Scand [B] 1987; 95:181-188.

101. Xia M, Whittington WL, Holmes KK, Plummer FA, Roberts MC. Pulsed-field gel electrophoresis for genomic analysis of *Neisseria gonorrhoeae*. J Infect Dis 1995; 171:455-458.

102. Kohl PK, Ison CA, Danielsson D, Knapp JS, Petzoldt D. Current status of serotyping of *Neisseria gonorrhoeae*. Eur J Epidemiol 1990; 6:91-95.

103. Hobbs MM, Alcorn TM, Davis RH, Fischer W, Thomas JC, Martin I, Ison C, Sparling PF, Cohen MS. Molecular typing of *Neisseria gonorrhoeae* causing repeated infections: evolution of porin during passage within a community. J Infect Dis 1999; 179:371-381.

104. Van Looveren M, Ison CA, Ieven M, Vandamme P, Martin IM, Vermeulen K, Renton A, Goosens H. Evaluation of the discriminatory power of typing methods for *Neisseria gonorrhoeae*. J Clin Microbiol 1999; 37:2183-2188.

105. Sacchi CT, Lemos AP, Brandt ME, Whitney AM, Melles CE, Solari CA, Frasch CE, Mayer LW. Proposed standardization of *Neisseria meningitidis* PorA variable-region typing nomenclature. Clin Diagn Lab Immunol 1998; 5:845-855.

106. Enright MC, Spratt BG. Multilocus sequence typing. Trends Microbiol 1999; 7:482-487.

107. Verdu ME, Coll P, Fontanals D, March F, Pons I, Van Esso D, Prats G. Comparison of conventional ribotyping and PCR-RFLP ribotyping for the analysis of endemic strains of *Neisseria meningitidis* isolated in a local community over 7 years. FEMS Microbiol Lett 1999; 179:247-253.

108. Woods CR, Koeuth T, Estabrook MM, Lupski JR. Rapid determination of outbreak-related strains of *Neisseria meningitidis* by repetitive element-based polymerase chain reaction genotyping. J Infect Dis 1996; 174:760-767.

109. Yakuau DE, Abadi FJ, Pennington TH. Molecular typing methods for *Neisseria meningitidis*. J Med Microbiol 1999; 48:1055-1064.

110. Jones RN, Gavan TL, Thornsberry C, Fuchs PC, Gerlach EH, Knapp JS, Murray P. Standardization of disk diffusion and agar dilution susceptibility tests for *Neisseria gonorrhoeae*: interpretive criteria and quality control guidelines for ceftriaxone, penicillin, spectinomycin, and tetracycline. J Clin Microbiol 1989; 27:2758-2766.

111. Fekete T. Antimicrobial susceptibility testing of *Neisseria gonorrhoeae* and implications for epidemiology and therapy. Clin Microbiol Rev 1993; 6:22-33.

112. Johnson SR, Morse SA. Antibiotic resistance in *Neisseria gonorrhoeae*: genetics and mechanisms of resistance. Sex Transm Dis 1988; 15:217-224.

113. Doern GV, Jones RN. Antimicrobial susceptibility testing of *Haemophilus influenzae*, *Branhamella catarrhalis*, and *Neisseria gonorrhoeae*. Antimicrob Ag Chemother 1988; 32:1747-1753.

114. Turner A, Gough KR, Leeming JP. Molecular epidemiology of *tetM* genes in *Neisseria gonorrhoeae*. Sex Transm Infect 1999; 75:60-66.

115. Ison CA, Woodford PJ, Madders H, Claydon E. Drift in susceptibility of *Neisseria gonorrhoeae* to ciprofloxacin and emergence of therapeutic failure. Antimicrob Ag Chemother 1998; 42:2919-2922.

116. Ehret JM, Judson FN. Quinolone-resistant *Neisseria gonorrhoeae*: the beginning of the end? Report of quinolone-resistant isolates and surveillance in the southwestern United States, 1989 to 1997. Sex Transm Dis 1998; 25:522-526.

117. Trees DL, Sandul AL, Peto-Mesola V, Aplasca MR, Leng HB, Whittington WL, Knapp JS. Alterations within the quinolone resistance-determining regions of *GyrA* and *ParC* of *Neisseria gonorrhoeae* isolated in the Far East and the United States. Int J Antimicrob Agents 1999; 12:325-332.

118. Ison CA, Gedney J, Easmon CS. Chromosomal resistance of gonococci to antibiotics. Genitourin Med 1987; 63:239-243.

119. Bowler LD, Zhang QY, Riou JY, Spratt BG. Interspecies recombination between the penA genes of *Neisseria meningitidis* and commensal *Neisseria* species during the emergence of penicillin resistance in *N. meningitidis*: natural events and laboratory simulation. J Bacteriol 1994; 176:333-337.

120. Fontanals D, Pineda V, Pons I, Rojo JC. Penicillin-resistant beta-lactamase producing *Neisseria meningitidis* in Spain. Eur J Clin Microbiol Infect Dis 1989; 8:90-91.

121. Woods CR, Smith AL, Wasilaukas BL, Campos J, Givner LB. Invasive disease caused by *Neisseria meningitidis* relatively resistant to penicillin in North Carolina. J Infect Dis 1994; 170:453-456.

122. Maggs AF, Logan JM, Carter PE, Pennington TH. The detection of penicillin insensitivity in *Neisseria meningitidis* by polymerase chain reaction. J Antimicrob Chemother 1998; 42:303-307.

123. Perez Trallero E, Garcia Arenzana JM, Ayestaran I, Munoz Baroja I. Comparative activity in vitro of 16 antimicrobial agents against penicillin-susceptible meningococci and meningococci with diminished susceptibility to penicillin. Antimicrob Ag Chemother 1989; 33:1622-1623.

124. Saez-Nieto JA, Vazquez JA. Moderate resistance to penicillin in *Neisseria meningitidis*. Microbiologia 1997; 13:337-342.

125. Saez-Nieto JA, Lujan R, Berron S, Campos J, Vinas M, Fuste C, Vazquez JA, Zhang QY, Bowler LD, Martinez-Suarez JV, Spratt BG. Epidemiology and molecular basis of penicillin-resistant *Neisseria meningitidis* in Spain: a 5-year history. Clin Infect Dis 1992; 14:394-402.

126. Jackson LA, Tenover FC, Baker C, Plikaytis BD, Reeves MW, Stocker SA, Weaver RE, Wenger JD. Prevalence of *Neisseria meningitidis* relatively resistant to penicillin in the United States, 1991. Meningococcal Disease Study Group. J Infect Dis 1994; 169:438-441.

127. Cooper ER, Ellison RT, Smith GS, Blaser MJ, Reller LB, Paisley JW. Rifampin-resistant meningococcal disease in a contact patient given prophylactic rifampin. J Pediatr 1986; 108:93-96.

128. Abadi FJ, Yakubu DE, Pennington TH. In vitro activities of meropenem and other antimicrobial agents against British meningococcal strains. Chemotherapy 1999; 45:253-257.

129. Abadi FJ, Yakubu DE, Pennington TH. Antimicrobial susceptibility of penicillin-sensitive and penicillin-resistant meningococci. J Antimicrob Chemother 1995; 35:687-690.

130. Campos J, Trujillo G, Seuba T, Rodriguez A. Discriminative criteria for *Neisseria meningitidis* isolates that are moderately susceptible to penicillin and ampicillin. Antimicrob Ag Chemother 1992; 36:1028-1031.

131. Gomez-Herruz P, Gonzalez-Palacios R, Romanyk J, Cuadros JA, Ena J. Evaluation of the Etest for penicillin susceptibility testing of *Neisseria meningitidis*. Diagn Microbiol Infect Dis 1995; 21:115-117.

132. Campos J, Mendelman PM, Sako MU, Chaffin DO, Smith AL, Saez-Nieto JA. Detection of relatively penicillin G-resistant *Neisseria meningitidis* by disk susceptibility testing. Antimicrob Ag Chemother 1987; 31:1478-1482.

133. Wallace RJ Jr., Nash DR, Steingrube VA. Antibiotic susceptibilities and drug resistance in *Moraxella* (*Branhamella*) *catarrhalis*. Am J Med 1990; 88:S46-S50.

134. McGregor K, Chang BJ, Mee BJ, Riley TV. *Moraxella catarrhalis*: clinical significance, antimicrobial susceptibility and BRO beta-lactamases. Eur J Clin Microbiol Infect Dis 1998; 17:219-234.

135. Davies BI, Maesen FP. Treatment of *Branhamella catarrhalis* infections. J Antimicrob Chemother 1990; 25:1-4.

136. Rosenthal SL, Freundlich LF, Gilardi GL, Clodomar FY. In vitro antibiotic susceptibility of *Moraxella* species. Chemotherapy 1978; 24:360-363.

137. Eliasson I, Kamme C, Vang M, Waley SG. Characterization of cell-bound papain-soluble beta-lactamases in BRO-1 and BRO-2 producing strains of *Moraxella* (*Branhamella*) *catarrhalis* and *Moraxella nonliquefaciens*. Eur J Clin Microbiol Infect Dis 1992; 11:313-321.

17

Gram Negative Infections: Pseudomonads and Other Gram Negative Non-Fermentative Bacteria

Kathryn Bernard

Special Bacteriology Laboratory, Canadian Science Centre for Human and Animal Disease, Winnipeg, Manitoba, Canada

I. HISTORICAL BACKGROUND

Gram negative non-fermentative bacteria constitute a complex group of taxonomically unrelated genera and species or provisionally designated taxa. They share the fundamental characteristic that, when tested using classic microbiological methods such as by Triple Sugar Iron (TSI) or Kligler's agar, they lack the ability to ferment carbohydrates. Glucose non-fermenting Gram negative bacteria (GNFGNB) may either utilize substrates via oxidative pathways or are inherently unable to either ferment or oxidize carbohydrates (1). Certain GNFGNB are serious pathogens which can be associated with both epidemics or sporadic infections. They include risk level 3 bacteria (e.g., *Burkholderia pseudomallei*, *B. mallei*) as well as risk level 2 pathogens (e.g., *Pseudomonas aeruginosa*, *B. cepacia*, *Acinetobacter* spp., and *Stenotrophomonas maltophilia*), all of which may be resistant to multiple antibiotics and disinfectants (2) and may cause serious, debilitating disease that can be associated with significant mortality. Most GNFGNB, however, are uncommon opportunistic pathogens which, when isolated, must be carefully evaluated for clinical relevancy in order to assess if full identification to genus and species or taxon group is justified. Such relevancy should include considerations for underlying patient disease, immune status, and recovery of the pathogen from normally sterile body sites or in highly significant numbers from other clinical sources. The taxonomy, risk factors for infection, and virulence markers of GNFGNB have been the subject of intense study in recent years. This work has resulted in greater precision for defining virulence factors as well as a dramatic increase in the number of genera and species and provisional taxa with which the microbiologist must contend. The pathogens described in this chapter have all been associated with disease in humans (rather than being recovered solely from animals, plants, or the environment). (Table 1) Using that criterion, *B. mallei*, which is derived from equine disease, is not further discussed here.

Table 1   Glucose non-fermenting Gram negative bacteria which have been associated with human disease.

Taxon, current designation	Recent taxonomic changes or comment	References or review
Achromobacter spp.	some formerly *Alcaligenes*	50,157
(provisional) 'Achromobacter groups B, E, F'	data suggestive of new genus, species	158,159
Acidovorax spp.	formerly *Pseudomonas*	3,155
Acinetobacter spp.		206-208, Table 2
Afipia spp.		93,216
Agrobacterium spp.		50
Alcaligenes spp.	some formerly *Achromobacter* spp.	50,157
Balneatrix alpica		66
Bergeyella zoohelcum	*Weeksella zoohelcum*	122
Brevundimonas spp.	formerly *Pseudomonas*, relationship with *Caulobacter, Maricaulis*, and *Sphingomonas*	3,63-65
Burkholderia cepacia genomovars I, III	remaining members of the *B. cepacia* complex	3,141,151
B. multivorans	formerly *B. cepacia* genomovar II	141
B. stabilis	formerly *B. cepacia* genomovar IV	151
B. vietnamiensis	formerly *B. cepacia* genomovar V	150
other *Burkholderia* spp.	formerly *Pseudomonas*	3
Caulobacter, Maricaulis genera	with respect to relationship to *Brevundimonas, Sphingomonas*	64,65
(provisional) CDC groups O-1, O-2,)-3, OFBA-1, EO-4, EO-5, WO-1		1,50,83,132, 134,219,220
(provisional) CDC groups EO-2, EO-3	discussed with respect to relationship with *Paracoccus, Rhodobacter*	1,50, unpublished
Chryseobacterium spp.	formerly *Flavobacterium* spp.	122
Comamonas spp.		3,81
Deftia acidovorans	formerly *Comamonas acidovorans*	81
Empedobacter breve	formerly *Flavobacterium* spp.	122
Flavobacterium spp.	see *Bergeyella, Chryseobacterium, Empedobacter, Myroides, Sphingobacterium, Weeksella*	122

Table 1 cont'd.

Taxon, current designation	Recent taxonomic changes or comment	References or review
(provisional) *Flavobacterium* species CDC groups IIb, IIc, IIe, IIh, IIi		1,162,163
(provisional) Gilardi rod group 1	discussed with respect to 'Schineria spp.'	221,unpublished
Methylobacterium spp.		50,87
Myroides spp.	formerly *Flavobacterium* spp.	129
Ochrobactrum spp.		50,113
Oligella spp.		50
Pandoraea spp.	new genus housing outliers most like *R. pickettii*, *R. paucula*, and *B. cepacia*	15
Paracoccus, Rhodobacter	discussed with respect to CDC groups EO-2, EO-3	unpublished
Pseudomonas aeruginosa, other named species or taxon groups		7,24,25
P. luteola	formerly *Chryseomonas luteola*	24
P. oryzihabitans	formerly *Flavimonas oryzihabitans*	24
Psychrobacter spp., including *Psy. phenylpyruvicus*	formerly *Moraxella phenylpyruvica*	116
Ralstonia pickettii, solanacearum	formerly *Burkholderia (Pseudomonas) pickettii, B. solanacearum*	3,42
R. eutropha	formerly *Alcaligenes eutropha*	42
R. gilardii	formerly *Alcaligenes faecalis*-like	43
R. paucula	formerly CDC group IVc-2	44-46
Roseomonas spp. genospecies	formerly part of Gram negative Pink cocci	84
Shewanella spp.		50
Schineria spp.	compared with Gilardii rod group 1	unpublished
Sphingobacterium spp.	formerly *Flavobacterium*	50
Sphingomonas spp.	also compared with *Caulobacter, Maricaulis, Brevundimonas*	50
Stenotrophomonas spp.	formerly *Pseudomonas, Xanthomonas*	3,76,153,154
unknown (novel) Gram negative non-fermenter associated with cystic fibrosis		16
Weeksella virosa		50

II. CLINICAL ASPECTS

A. Role of GNFGNB in Cystic Fibrosis (CF)

B. cepacia, P. aeruginosa, other *Burkholderia* species or genomospecies, *Alcaligenes xylosoxidans*, and *Stenotrophomonas maltophilia* play critical but as yet not completely understood roles in the pulmonary disease of CF.

1. B. cepacia and CF

When infected with *B. cepacia*, some CF patients may exhibit a rapid decline in lung function or an acute illness (3). Other CF patients are colonized with no apparent clinical deterioration or demonstrate a slower decline of lung function (4).

Colonization with drug-resistant organisms, including *B. cepacia*, had been considered a contra-indication to lung transplantation; that assumption is controversial (5). CF patients with *B. cepacia* infection or colonization have increased costs for medical care when compared to *B. cepacia*-negative CF patients (6). Therefore, rapid and correct identification of this organism for these patients is deemed crucial by many.

2. P. aeruginosa and CF

The association of *P. aeruginosa* and severe disease among CF patients is thought to be a function of colonization of the respiratory tree by microcolonies of (primarily) the mucoid form of *P. aeruginosa* that are surrounded by alginate. The microcolonies together create an enhanced immune response with elastin formation which results in long-term damage, compromised lung function, and subsequently death (7). The mucoid form of *P. aeruginosa* is difficult to eradicate, and it is recognized to infect 70-80% of adult CF patients (8). Pulmonary outcome for CF patients is detrimentally influenced by the presence of the mucoid form and by the specific patient immune status rather than strain genotype (9). Small-colony variants of *P. aeruginosa* have been recovered from a significant percentage of CF patients and were found to be associated with multiresistance, poor lung function, and daily inhalation of tobramycin or colistin (10). Presence of *P. aeruginosa* is consequently associated with higher costs for CF patient care (6).

3. CF-associated pathogens other than Burkholderia spp. and P. aeruginosa

S. maltophilia is widespread in the environment, and independent studies suggest that infection in CF patients occurs by multiple independent acquisitions from a variety of sites, within or outside hospitals, rather than from a small number of nosocomially-derived clones (11-13). This agent may cause severe disease that is associated with high mortality, and it exhibits a high degree (up to 84%) of multiple antibiotic resistance, although persistence of *S. maltophilia* in CF patients varies markedly when compared to *P. aeruginosa* (14).

Acinetobacter spp., particularly *A. baumannii*, and like *S. maltophilia*, are becoming of increasing concern for CF patients because of the high prevalence of multiple antibiotic resistant strains (2).

Strains that are recovered primarily from the sputa of CF patients have been assigned to a newly described genus *Pandoraea*, which was proposed after careful polyphasic examination of isolates which were originally identified as being most like one of *B. cepacia, Ralstonia pickettii*, or *R. paucula*. Clinical data suggests that at least some *Pandoraea* isolates were derived from chronic infection in and transmitted among CF patients (15).

Novel agents may cause severe disease in CF patients. In one instance, a bacterium described as a 'very mucoid Gram negative rod' was recovered from a CF patient after double lung transplantation. It has been described as a novel agent of the alpha-*Proteobacteria* with no close or specific relative identified (16).

B. Clinical disease other than cystic fibrosis.

1. *Pseudomonas*

P. aeruginosa is the most significant pathogen among species in this genus and arguably among all GNFGNB described here. It is associated with a broad range of illnesses ranging from superficial skin infections such as folliculitis to fulminant sepsis (7). This bacterium is well-documented to cause serious nosocomial infections, particularly pneumonia among intubated intensive care unit patients (2,7,17) or among patients in intensive care in general (18,19). It is a cause of nosocomial urinary tract infections, peritonitis in patients on continuous ambulatory peritoneal dialysis, and wound infections, especially among burn patients (7). Bacteremia caused by this organism is associated with increased mortality and morbidity, particularly among the immunocompromised (20,21). Infections are often device-associated (17,22). *P. aeruginosa* is known to be a cause of various community-acquired infections including post-puncture osteomyelitis of the foot, invasive external otitis among diabetics (2), and endocarditis among intravenous drug users (7). *P. aeruginosa* bacteremias and pneumonia are associated with severe mortality and morbidity among HIV-1 infected patients (23).

Other *Pseudomonas* species which occasionally cause human disease include (species nova described after 1996 are cited specifically) *P. alcaligenes*, *P. fluorescens*, *P. luteola* formerly *Chryseomonas luteola* (24), *P. mendocina*, *P. monteilii* (25), *P. oryzihabitans* formerly *Flavimonas oryzihabitans* (24), *P. pseudoalcaligenes*, *P. putida* and *P. stutzeri*. Provisionally-named *Pseudomonas* spp. CDC group 1 and group 2 have occasionally been associated with disease (1). *P. oryzihabitans* has been found to be an opportunistic pathogen among immunosuppressed hosts including patients with HIV and leukemia causing community-acquired pneumonia and bacteremia (26). Among such a population, this bacterium is thought to be nosocomially-acquired and may also cause biliary tract infection with peritonitis as well as subdural empyema, in addition to pneumonia and bacteremia (27). *P. luteola* strains have been associated with facial cellulitis and bacteremia in an immunocompetent patient (28). Device-associated illnesses have been attributed to both *P. oryzihabitans* and *P. luteola* (29). Newly-described species *P. monteilii* has been recovered from a variety of specimens, including placenta, stool, bile, bronchial aspirate, urine and pleural fluid, but clinical relevancy is often poorly understood (25).

2. *Burkholderia species (not associated with CF)*

B. pseudomallei is the causative agent of melioidosis, which clinically ranges from an asymptomatic disease as inferred by high seropositivity rates among healthy people (30) to fulminant sepsis that is associated with high mortality rates (3,30). It is thought to be markedly underdiagnosed and under-reported. Disease may include fever of unknown origin and a tuberculosis-like illness among patients who are from or have travelled to areas that are endemic for this bacterium, including Thailand, other South East Asian countries, Northern Australia (particularly during the rainy season), and other tropical and subtropical countries (3,30). An outbreak, traced to a contaminated water treatment plant, has been reported during the dry season in Western Australia (31). It has also been reported as occurring in the Americas, particularly in Puerto Rico (32). Risk factors include being adult or elderly (30), chronic granulomatous disease (32), non-Hodgkin's lymphoma (33), diabetes, and chronic renal disease (31). It has been observed as well as in otherwise healthy individuals (34). *B. pseudomallei* has been implicated in spinal cord disease (35), neonatal meningitis and septicemia (36), brain abscess (37), and multiple abscesses in organs of the reticuloendothelial and other systems (3). Relapse occurs in about 5% of treated cases (3).

B. cepacia, being ubiquitous in the environment, is associated with nosocomial disease among non-CF patient populations, but otherwise it is considered a rare cause of invasive disease among other patients (38,39). *B. cepacia* bacteremias have been linked to underlying malignancies (39), stays in an ICU, invasive procedures, and the use of devices such as catheters (38). This agent has been the cause of an outbreak in a cardiology ward having been disseminated by contaminated heparin (40). It has been linked to respiratory tract infections, particularly if nebulizers were used, as well as peritonitis, and septic arthritis (3). *B. gladioli* is a very rare pathogen among non-CF patients. In one report, severely compromised patients had bacteremia, pneumonia, and cervical adenitis which were caused by this bacterium, but correct identification using commercial systems was difficult (41).

3. Ralstonia

The genus *Ralstonia* was first described in 1995 (42), and the species that have been reported to cause human disease include *R. pickettii* (formerly *P. pickettii* and *B. pickettii*), *R. gilardii* (43) and *R. paucula* (formerly CDC group IVC-2, 44-47). To date, newly re-assigned *Ralstonia* species, *R. solanacearum* and *R. eutropha*, have only been recovered from the environment (42). *R. pickettii* has been described as causing sporadic opportunistic disease (1), but it has also been the cause of to outbreaks. Geographically widespread or localized outbreaks have been associated with a contaminated saline solution that was used during endotracheal suction (48) or for the flushing of intravenous devices. *R. gilardii* has been recovered from cerebrospinal fluid, skin infections, and bone marrow. It has been obtained environmentally from whirlpool water (43). *R. paucula* (CDC group IV-C2) has been recovered from sporadic disease (1,44,46,47) including the indwelling catheter of an AIDS patient (49).

4. Pandoraea

This genus is closely related to *Burkholderia* and *Ralstonia*, and it comprises the four species *P. apista*, *P. norimbergensis*, *P. pulmonicola*, and *P. pnomenusa*. As described earlier, these bacteria have been recovered from the sputa of CF patients, other respiratory specimens (not CF-associated), and the environment (15).

5. Acinetobacter

Named species and genomic *Acinetobacter* taxa are widely distributed in nature and hospital environments, and they are the second most common GNFGNB after *P. aeruginosa* that are recovered from human clinical specimens (50). Acinetobacters are considered as having low pathogenic potential among healthy people, but they cause infections among seriously debilitated patients. This is due to their ability to acquire multiresistance to antibiotics and to survive on environmental surfaces, on dry surfaces, and in the presence of some common disinfectants (50-52). Nosocomial *Acinetobacter* infections may involve the respiratory tract (related to the use of intubation devices, endotracheal tubes, and tracheostomies), urinary tract, wounds, and ambulatory peritoneal dialysis, and they may progress to septicemia, meningitis, osteomyelitis, or arthritis (51). *A. baumannii* is the most prominent pathogen of this genus. Infections by this agent that are associated with malignancies, surgical procedures, severe thermal injury, catheter use, or the initial use of an inappropriate antibiotic leading to multiresistance, are well-described (51,53-59). *A. baumannii* has been reported as a cause of thyroiditis with bacteremic pneumonia (60). Infection by other species such a *A. junii* have been reported (61). *Acinetobacter* genomic species 13TU have been associated with an outbreak; these bacteria were originally identified as *A. junii* when a rapid identification strip was used (62).

6. Brevundimonas, Caulobacter, and Balneatrix

The genus *Brevundimonas* was first described in 1994 to house reassigned former *Pseudomonas* species, *B. diminuta* and *B. vesicularis* (63). Like other GNFGNB, they have been associated with sporadic disease (1). Polyphasic studies have revealed that environmentally-derived *Caulobacter* spp. are closely related to and difficult to distinguish from members of the genus *Brevundimonas*, and so it remains to be seen whether *Caulobacter* spp. (64,65) have been recovered from human disease but misidentified as *Brevundimonas* or other closely related taxa.

Balneatrix alpica was originally described as a cause of an outbreak of pneumonia and meningitis in a spa (66).

7. *Stenotrophomonas maltophilia and Stenotrophomonas species.*

S. maltophilia is well-recognized as a nosocomial pathogen, particularly among elderly, debilitated, and immunosuppressed patients, and it has been associated with numerous infections including meningitis, pneumonia, conjunctivitis, soft tissue infections, endocarditis, and urinary tract infections (7,11,67,68). *S. maltophilia* is the fourth most common non-mycobacterial pathogen causing bacteremia among HIV-infected patients (69). It had been found to colonize and then cause infections in preterm infants in a neonatal intensive care unit (70). *S. maltophilia* has caused prosthetic valve endocarditis in a compromised patient (71) and in a healthy person following dental work (72). This bacterium was thought to cause nosocomial pneumonia for two patients with polymyositis (73). It is recognized as an opportunistic pathogen among acute leukemic patients (74), and it has been reported as a cause of necrotizing pancreatitis (67). It has been an etiological agent of infection in outbreak fashion among allogenic bone marrow transplant patients for whom the infection was enhanced by severe neutropenia and mucositis (75). *S. maltophilia* (formerly *P. maltophilia, Xanthomonas maltophilia*) was the sole species in the genus *Stenotrophomonas* until recently when additional taxa consistent with the genus have been described. *S. africana* was recovered from the CSF of an HIV seropositive patient with meningoencephalitis (76).

8. *Shewanella species*

Members of the genus *Shewanella* are widely distributed in the environment, and natural habits especially include water and soil. Disease in humans has only infrequently been described. For a number of years, *S. putrefaciens* (formerly *P. putrefaciens, Achromobacter putrefaciens, Alteromonas putrefaciens*) was the sole species in the genus. It has been associated with a variety of infections such as cellulitis, otitis media, ocular infections, abscesses, osteomyelitis, peritonitis, and septicemia (1,50). Recent studies of these bacteria have indicated that the genus was heterogeneous, and that it consists of multiple taxa. A second human pathogen, *S. alga*, has been described (77) and recovered from bacteremias arising from leg ulcers (78) as well as from a septic hemodialysis patient concomitant with the recovery of *E. coli* (79). *Shewanella* species has been recovered from a patient with endocarditis (80).

9. *Acidovorax, Comamonas, Delftia, and CDC group weak oxidizer (WO)-1*

These taxa are extremely rare opportunistic human pathogens. *D. acidovorans* has been associated with sporadic infections (1,81), and multiresistant strains have been reported to cause ocular infections (82). CDC group WO-1 and WO-1-like bacteria have been recovered from a variety of human specimens including blood cultures after causing bacteremias (1,83).

10. *Methylobacterium extorquens and Roseomonas species, the 'pink' GNFGNB*

Members of both genera have been recovered from a variety of infections (1,84,85). *M. extorquens* infection occurred in association with a central venous catheter among patients with acute leukemia (86). *M. zatmanii* has been found to cause bacteremia and fever in an immunocompromised host (87). The genus *Roseomonas* is comprised of four named species and four unnamed species. The most clinically relevant appears to be *R. gilardii* (88). This agent has been implicated in catheter-related bacteremia (89), vertebral osteomyelitis (90), and peritonitis in a CAPD patient (91). *R. fauriae* has been implicated in a case of CAPD peritonitis (92).

11. Afipia species

The genus *Afipia* is comprised of three names species, *A. felis*, *A. clevelandensis*, and *A. broomeae*, as well as three unnamed genomospecies (93). *Afipia felis* had been initially called the 'cat scratch fever (CSF) bacillus' and was thought to be the causative agent of cat scratch disease (CSD) (93). It has now been shown that in fact *Bartonella henselae* (see Chapter 22) is the primary causative agent of CSD, and that *A. felis* and other *Bartonella* spp. are very rare causes of this infection (94). Otherwise, *Afipia* spp. have been recovered from a variety of clinical specimens which are largely from sterile sites (1,93).

12. Achromobacter sensu stricto, Alcaligenes, "Achromobacter-like groups B, E, F", Agrobacterium, Ochrobactrum, Oligella, Psychrobacter, Sphingomonas

Achromobacter

Like other GNFGNB described here, these taxa are rare human pathogens whose native habitat is the environment. The most serious pathogen in this genus is *A. xylosoxidans* subsp. xylosoxidans (subspecies designation is not always apparent among reports in the literature). As briefly alluded to above, this agent may play a significant and emerging role in CF disease (95). This bacterium has caused serious disease among HIV-positive patients including bacteremia and/or respiratory disease (96). A multiresistant intraocular isolate which caused endophthalmitis has been reported (97). *A. piechaudii* has only occasionally been isolated from clinical infections (1), but *A. ruhlandii* has not been associated with disease. The genus *Alcaligenes* is now restricted to those species that are consistent with the rare pathogen *A. faecalis* as well as the two species that are not found to cause human disease: *A. defragrans* and *A. latus* (1,50,98,157).

"Achromobacter-like groups B, E, F"

Members of these taxa have been isolated from blood cultures of patients with septicemia (99,100). It has been found that agents which are consistent with "*Achromobacter*-like groups B and E" had caused an outbreak with bacteremia among four patients in western Canada (K. Bernard, unpublished data).

Agrobacterium

The genus *Agrobacterium* is noted primarily as a phytopathogen although at least one of the species, *A. radiobacter* (synonym *A. tumefaciens*), has long been documented as a rare human pathogen (1,101). This agent has been recovered from venous catheter infections, peritonitis, bacteremias or endocarditis among CAPD patients, and urinary tract infections (102) as well as bacteremia in patients with chronic obstructive pulmonary disease (103). This bacterium was recovered from blood cultures of a pregnant woman and that of her premature stillborn (104). *A. radiobacter* has been recovered from the blood of HIV-infected patients (105).

Ochrobactrum

Ochrobactrum anthropi has been recovered from a variety of clinical sources (1,50,106) including bacteremias among seriously debilitated patients who have indwelling venous catheters (101,107) and nosocomial bacteremias in a renal and pancreatic transplant unit where this agent was found to be a contaminant of rabbit anti-thymocyte globulin (108). *O. anthropi* bacteremia has been documented in a pediatric population (109) and among HIV-positive patients (110). Meningitis with this pathogen has been reported after the implantation of an allograft tissue during craniotomy (111) and endophthalmitis after vitreous surgery (112). *O. intermedium* has been associated with bacteremia and concomitant liver abscesses (113,114).

Oligella

The genus *Oligella* includes two clinically relevant species: *O. urethralis* and *O. ureolyticus*. Both species are rare pathogens, and more typically are commensals of the genitourinary tract (1). *O. ure-*

thralis has been recovered from CAPD-associated peritonitis; ciprofloxin resistance was selected after extensive usage (115).

Psychrobacter

The genus *Psychrobacter* has been revised to include *P. immobilis, P. phenylpyruvicus*, and two psychrophilic environmental species that are not found in human disease (116). *P. immobilis* has caused infection in HIV-positive patients (117) and ocular infection in a neonate (118), and otherwise has been occasionally recovered from a variety of other clinical specimens (1,119).

Sphingomonas

The *Sphingomonas* genus currently has at least sixteen species, but only *S. paucimobilis* (formerly *P. paucimobilis*) has been recovered from human clinical specimens, including blood cultures, CSF, urine, wounds, female genital tract, and peritoneal fluid (50). It can be a cause of nosocomial infections (120). *S. parapaucimobilis* and other species in the genus are described (1), but they have not been definitively recovered to date from human disease. A bacterium that is consistent with CDC group O-1 has been described to have caused pneumonia with bronchopulmonary fistulae and bacteremia (121).

13. Flavobacteriaceae/Flavobacterium-Cytophaga complex bacteria

Flavobacterium species sensu stricto (122) have not been associated with human disease, and so they are not discussed further. *Chryseobacterium meningosepticum* has been well-described as being associated with meningitis among neonates (1,123,124). This agent can also cause sepsis, pneumonia, endocarditis, cellulitis, peritoneal disease, eye infections, epididymitis, and sinusitis (123). It has also been associated with bacteremia from central intravenous line-related infection (125). *C. meningosepticum* may play a significant pathogenic role among patients with advanced AIDS (126). Other *Chryseobacterium* spp. only occasionally cause human disease. *C. indologenes* has been reported to have caused bacteremias (127) and infections that are associated with the use of indwelling devices (128). Even though recovered from clinical material, it is thought to be rarely significant (50). *C. gleum* has been recovered from a variety of sources and may be difficult to phenotypically discern from *C. indologenes* (50). Other species in this genus (*C. indotheticum, C. balustinum*, and *C. scophthalum*) have not been associated with human disease (122).

The genus *Myroides* includes *M. odoratus* (formerly *F. odoratum*) and *M. odoratimimus* (129). *M. odoratus* has been associated with recurrent cellulitis and bacteremia in a patient with chronic obstructive pulmonary disease (130), and these species have been recovered from other sources, including urine, wounds, sputum, and ear specimens (50). *M. odoratus* has been recovered from patients with advanced AIDS (126). *Empedobacter breve* (formerly *F. brevis*) has been recovered from a variety of clinical specimens and has a unique CFA composition profile (1). *Bergeyella zoohelcum* (formerly *Weeksella zoohelcum*) has been recovered from human wounds after bites from dogs or after close contact with cats. Some of these superficial infections have led to meningitis or sepsis (50). A case of community-acquired pneumonia with subsequent residual disease due to *B. zoohelcum* has been reported (131). *Sphingobacterium mizutae, S. multivorum, S. spiritivorum*, and *S. thalpophilum* are rare pathogens that have been recovered from various clinical sources (1).

14. Provisional Taxa: CDC Oxidizer group (O)-1, O-2, O-3, OFBA-1, Eugonic Oxidizer (EO)-2, EO3, EO-4, EO-5, Non-Oxidizer (NO)-1, and Gilardii rod group 1

Yellow-pigmented CDC group O-1 has been recovered from a wide variety of sources including the infected lung (121). CDC group O-3 may be recovered from sites that are associated with invasive disease including the duodenum (132). CDC group OFBA was originally recovered from a CAPD patient (133). CDC group NO-1 has been recovered from infections following dog or cat bites (134).

CDC group EO-3 is a Gram negative bacillus that is usually found to exhibit a yellow pigment (1). CDC group EO-3 has been recovered from a variety of clinical specimens and has been found to cause peritonitis (135).

III. EPIDEMIOLOGY OF INFECTION

GNFGNB may be recovered from wide variety of environmental sources such as plants (3), soil, and water (7,136). Environmentally-derived isolates of *P. aeruginosa, B. cepacia*, and *S. maltophilia* have been directly linked with community-acquired and nosocomial disease in adults or pediatric patients (17,20,22,137,138). The other rare opportunistic GNFGNB pathogens which are described herein are primarily derived from the environment.

B. cepacia colonization of a CF patient has prompted patient segregation which is an approach that is thought to limit person-to-person spread of this pathogen (139). Epidemic strains of *B. cepacia* which are derived from a single dominant clone have been transmitted between CF and non-CF patients in a single institution with the result of having previously *B. cepacia*-negative CF patients develop an increased risk of morbidity (140). *Burkholderia* spp. which are not members of the *B. cepacia* cluster, such as *B. gladioli*, have occasionally been recovered from CF patients (140-142) including nosocomial acquisition (143).

Multi-resistant *P. aeruginosa* strains are often thought to be polyclonal in origin (144,145), and resistance is driven more by the continuous admittance of colonized patients to intensive care units in particular and selection pressure from antibiotics, rather than by cross-acquisition among patients (145). Nevertheless, epidemic nosocomial infection has been described especially in association with devices.

Acinetobacter infections appear to occur with some seasonal variation; there is a greater frequency that is observed from July to October than November to June (146). Acquisition of *Acinetobacter* infections are associated with increased mortality and increased length of stays in hospital (147). Some *Acinetobacter* species (*A. lwoffii, A. johnsonii, A. radioresistens*, and *Acinetobacter* genomic species 3) can be recovered from the skin of healthy or hospitalized people; however, the agents considered as the most important pathogens, *A. baumannii* and *Acinetobacter* genomic species 13TU, are only rarely recovered from skin, and their habitat remains unknown (148).

IV. NATURE OF THE BACTERIUM, PATHOGENESIS, CLINICAL MANIFESTATIONS

Precise identification of CF-related pathogens from the genus *Burkholderia* can be difficult, no matter if conventional, manual, or automated kits, or molecular means are employed (149). The process of identification became more complicated when, in 1997, the phrase 'B. cepacia complex' was introduced whereby precise genotypic, phenotypic, and chemotaxonomic characterization of *B. cepacia* isolates that were obtained from CF patients gave rise to at least four discernable genomospecies. All members of this cluster have been associated with disease in CF patients (141). The *B. cepacia* cluster therefore is comprised of: a) *B. cepacia* genomospecies I (which includes the *B. cepacia* type strain (derived from an onion) and the type strain of *B. pyrrocina*, b) genomospecies II, now assigned to the new species *B. multivorans*, c) genomospecies III which is thought to be the one that is most frequently associated with CF-related disease, d) *B. stabilis*, formerly *B. cepacia* genomovar IV, and e) *B. vietnamensis*, first proposed in 1995, has also been described as genomovar V (141,150,151). A descriptive panel that consists of representative strains for each genomovar in order to facilitate further studies of the *B. cepacia* complex has been proposed (152) .

The genus *Stenotrophomonas* was a monophyletic genus that consisted only of *S. maltophilia* until the recent description of *S. africana* (76). The validity of species level distinction for that taxon, however, has been questioned (153). Additional *Stenotrophomonas*-like taxa, which are distinguishable from *S. maltophilia* and *S. africana* by CFA composition and by 16S rRNA sequence analysis, have been reported (153,154).

Acidovorax, Comamonas, Delftia, and CDC group weak oxidizer (WO)-1 are consistent with the "acidovorans" rRNA complex in rRNA superfamily III, and so in recent years, they have been assigned to new genera and species within the family *Comamonadaceae* (81). They exhibit qualitatively similar CFA compositions (1). *Acidovorax delafieldii, A. facilis*, and *A. temperans* were first described in 1990 (155), of which *A. facilis* has only been recovered from soil. The genus *Comamonas* was recently redefined when the new genus *Delftia*, with a single species *D. acidovorans*, formerly *C. acidovorans*, was described (81). The genus *Comamonas*, now consisting of *C. terragena* and *C. testosteroni*, were recovered from hay or soil and not conclusively from human clinical material (1). CDC group WO-1, a temporary designation described by Hollis in 1992, is included in this discussion because it has a number of features in common with members of the *Comamonadaceae*, including biochemical characteristics and similarity by CFA analysis (83). This group has not been analyzed genotypically, and so it may include bacteria that are better assigned to *Acidovorax* species or *D. acidovorans* (1).

Methylobacterium spp. and *Roseomonas* spp. were first designated as 'Gram-Negative Pink Cocci' whose colonies were observed to be various shades of pink when grown from clinical material (1,156), but they are not closely related phylogenetically.

Phylogenetic studies have revealed that *Achromobacter* sensu stricto and *Alcaligenes* are closely related to *Bordetella* species (*Bordetella* are described in Chapter 23) (157) and have qualitatively similar CFA composition profiles (1). *Achromobacter* species, sensu stricto (to differentiate these from *Alcaligenes* species formerly classified as *Achromobacter* or those taxa called '*Achromobacter*-like groups B, E, and F') currently include *Achromobacter xylosoxidans* subsp. xylosoxidans, *A. xylosoxidans* subsp. denitrificans, *A. ruhlandii*, and *A. piechaudii* (98,157).

Achromobacter-like groups B, E, and F were first described by Holmes while studying GNFGNB strains that are related to what was later described as the genus *Ochrobactrum* (158,159). "*Achromobacter*-like groups B and E" are thought to be biotypes of the same as yet to be described genus and species, while 'group F' is thought to be genetically distinct from B and E and other described taxa. They have a unique CFA composition which is similar to but distinct from true *Achromobacter* species, *Alcaligenes, Bordetella, Ochrobactrum*, and *Agrobacterium* (1,160). They have unique protein profiles (159). These strains were identical by biochemical, CFA composition, and by 16S rRNA sequence analysis, when compared with reference strains of *Achromobacter*-like group B and E (Laboratoire Microbiologie de Ghent 5410, LMG 5411, LMG 5430 and LMG 5431). Unpublished phylogenetic analyses for these taxa suggests that they represent a new genus and species which are related to but distinguishable from *Ochrobactrum, Rhizobium, Agrobacterium*, and other closely related alpha-*Proteobacteria* genera (K. Bernard, unpublished data), thus corroborating the conclusions of Holmes (158).

The genera *Agrobacterium* and *Ochrobactrum* are phylogenetically related to each other and often compared phenotypically, but *Ochrobactrum* species are phylogenetically most closely related to *Brucella* species (113). The CFA composition of these three genera in particular may be qualitatively similar (1). The genus *Ochrobactrum* includes two species, *O. anthropi* and *O. intermedium*, which are described as having caused human disease.

Members of the family *Flavobacteriaceae* and other closely-related genera share a number of commonalities. These include: a) being of environmental origin, b) if motile, being so by 'gliding', c) are (often) yellow-pigmented, d) have similar respiratory quinones, e) qualitatively similar CFA compositions (which are very different from most other GNFGNB), and f) have undergone considerable taxonomic changes in recent years (122,161). The genus *Flavobacterium*, which formerly housed most of the taxa that are described here, has been amended to include only those species which are closely related and phenotypically similar to the environmental bacterium *F. aquatile*. Taxa that were formerly assigned to the genus *Flavobacterium* include *Chryseobacterium* species, which have menaquinone 6 as the major respiratory quinone, and *Chryseobacterium gleum* as the type species of the genus (122). C.

gleum and *C. indologenes* (which may share attributes with CDC group IIb) are phylogenetically closely related (122,161). Some *Flavobacterium* CDC groups have characteristics that are consistent with the genus *Chryseobacterium*. CDC group IIc (associated with blood culture isolates) and CDC groups IIe and IIh have menaquinone 6 as the major respiratory quinone and qualitatively similar CFAs to *Chryseobacterium* species, but may be differentiated from named species and each other by phenotypic means (1,162,163). Genotypic studies of provisionally-named groups have not been fully completed.

There is only a limited amount of information available concerning the various provisional CDC groups which are clustered on the basis of similar phenotypic and, in some instances, chemotaxonomic characteristics. Genotypic studies have not been completed as yet.

V. IMMUNOLOGY OF INFECTION

There has been much work in recent years which has elucidated the complex immunological response to infection by GNFGNB particularly with respect to those agents that are associated with CF-related diseases. A dramatic and chronic immunological response to *P. aeruginosa* infection in CF patients, with activation of large numbers of neutrophils, a profound antibody response in serum, saliva, and pulmonary secretions such as sputum, and a high level of circulating immune complexes, is often found. There is a strong correlation between the severity of lung disease and the titre of anti-pseudomonal antibodies (164). It has been suggested that the damage from chronic inflammatory processes to both the epithelium and the structural proteins of the lung is thought to be more serious than the damage which is caused by the bacterium itself (164,165). CF patients may eventually succumb to progressive *P. aeruginosa* infection which is characterized by massive neutrophilic infiltration without bacterial destruction (166). Virulence factors from these bacteria play crucial roles (164). Elastase produced by *P. aeruginosa* plays a mitigating role in CF disease by preventing or delaying airway repair that is being attempted by the host immune system (167). Lipid A of *P. aeruginosa* isolates that are derived from CF patients is thought to affect pathogenesis in two ways: by promoting the colonization and survival of the organism, and by generating increased or unique inflammatory responses (166). Pili are important adhesins for *P. aeruginosa*. Other virulence factors include flagellar biosynthesis protein, exotoxin A, LPS, phospholipase C, rhamnolipid, lipase, histamines, leukocidin, exoenzyme S, and alginate (164).

Burn patients who are experimentally vaccinated with several of the outer membrane proteins (OMP) of *P. aeruginosa* were found to have anti-OMP antibodies which provide some protection from infection, thus suggesting a promising approach for the prevention of nosocomial transmission in this population (168).

B. cepacia has been found to survive intracellularly within phagocytic cells which is then followed by a period of cellular activation where elements such as the tumour necrosis factor were stimulated. A deleterious inflammatory response due to phagocytosis and cellular activation without bacterial killing occurs; it causes chronic tissue destruction and decay of lung function (169). Virulence may be associated with the LPS chemotypes of *B. cepacia* complex bacteria (170).

Much work has been directed to the discovery of how some strains aggrevate disease among CF patients. A highly transmissible strain of *B. cepacia*, thought to be the major strain that is associated with fatal 'cepacia syndrome' (the Edinburgh-Toronto strain), has been especially scrutinized. This strain has been characterized as RAPD type 2/*B. cepacia* genomovar III which harbours the DNA fragment called the *B. cepacia* epidemic strain marker [BCESM] (a hybrid of two insertion sequences – IS1356 and IS402). It possesses surface cable pili (*cbl*A gene) which specifically bind to cytokeratin 13 of patient epithelial cells, thus suggesting a biological target in the respiratory tract for the bacterium (171,171a). This latter marker is thought to be the most specific marker of the 'epidemic strain', and so it is recommended that *B. cepacia* that are derived from CF patients be screened for the presence of this gene (171a).

Levels of circulating markers of inflammation among CF patients, whether clinically stable or exacerbated disease, were found to be increased when compared to a population of colonized, non-CF patients; colonization with *B. cepacia*, however, was not associated with a heightened inflammatory response when compared with *P. aeruginosa* colonization (165,172).

Strains of *B. pseudomallei* produce a cytolethal toxin, the amount of which is thought to correlate with the severity of melioidosis (173). This bacterium survives intracellular killing within a phagosome after phagocytosis (174). Flagellin proteins and O-polysaccharide endotoxin have been touted as promising candidates for use in the development of a melioidosis vaccine (175).

Little is known about factors and immunological responses that are associated with *Stenotrophomonas*-related infections, and indeed some argue that this organism is usually not the definitive cause of infections, but rather that it acts synergistically with other pathogens (176). Protease and elastase production and an ability to adhere to glass, teflon, and plastic materials have been described for clinically-derived *S. maltophilia* isolates (176).

The immunological dynamics of *Acinetobacter* disease are poorly understood. Strain level virulence is thought to be enhanced by the presence of a polysaccharide capsule, the ability to adhere to human epithelial cells, the ability to produce enzymes which damage host tissue, the toxic effect of LPS on host cell walls, and the presence of lipid A (51,147). Endotoxin production in vivo is probably responsible for symptoms that are observed during *Acinetobacter* septicemia (51).

VI. LABORATORY DIAGNOSIS

GNFGNB share some phenotypic characteristics. In contrast to enteric bacteria, they may be oxidase-positive, and nearly all are catalase-positive, non-motile, or exhibit polar or peritrichous flagella. They are often strict aerobes or to a lesser extent facultative anaerobes. Some grow readily and luxuriantly on commonly-used microbiological media over 24 hrs. at mesophilic temperatures, but many grow slowly or poorly in comparison to enteric pathogens (1,50). If bacillary, they are often similar in appearance when assessed with the Gram stain: 1-5 μm. in length to 0.5-1 μm in width (3-5); some taxa, e.g., CDC group EO-2, are more coccobacillary or coccoidal (1). Should identification to genus and species or taxon group be required, many laboratories use commercial kits with or without electronically-based identification schemes (50,177-180) rather than conventional methods (1). Complex taxonomic schemes which are based on phenotypic and some chemotaxonomic criteria have been described (1,3,7,50), and so they are not reproduced here. Some Gram negative bacilli may be poorly reactive or nonreactive towards most or all substrates whether associated with a commercial kit or assessed by traditional means. Automated identification systems have been found to perform reasonably well but require supplemental testing to obtain a >90% accuracy level (177-179,181). Automated blood culture systems have been reported to fail detection of certain GNFGNB after 7 days, and so care must be taken to avoid false-negatives by these methods (182).

A polyphasic approach, which includes both phenotypic and genotypic technologies, is therefore recommended for reference centre-level identification and for characterizing new, rare, or difficult taxa (183,184). One component of a polyphasic approach, that of cellular fatty acid (CFA) composition analysis using computer-assisted gas-liquid chromatography, is widely used. This technique is very useful for characterizing Gram negative nonfermentative bacilli, particularly for those taxa which are not well-discerned or nonreactive with respect to biochemical tests (1,185,186). Many of the taxa described in this chapter have sufficiently unique CFA composition patterns so that such a method can provide a substantive preliminary identification. Genotypic methods such as universal 16S rDNA (141) or *gyr*B (187) gene sequence analysis are now widely used to establish phylogenetic relationships among novel or described taxa. In some instances, genotypic methods provide the sole means of definitive bacterial identification (184).

Selective agars which are directed towards the isolation of these agents from CF patient specimens have been described, and they include oxidation-fermentation polymyxin-bacitracin-lactose agar

(OFPBL), *Pseudomonas cepacia* agar (PCA), and *Burkholderia cepacia* selective agar (BCSA) (188,189). The use of selective media with an enrichment broth is debatable (190). *P. aeruginosa* and other GNFGNB grow more rapidly than *B. cepacia*, and so they may competitively overgrow the latter if present (189). Much work has been directed towards enabling microbiologists to rapidly and specifically identify CF isolates as members of the *B. cepacia* complex with the apparent potential for severe disease, or as another *Burkholderia* species or genomovar that is not part of the *B. cepacia* complex (such as *B. gladioli* or other species less frequently associated with severe CF disease and morbidity). Vandamme et al. proposed phenotypic means used to differentiate *B. cepacia* genomovars I and III from *B. multivorans* and *B. vietnamiensis*, in addition to definitive genotypic methods (141,151). Metabolically inert or poorly-reactive strains of those genomospecies, however, are not well-identified using only biochemical means (4). Additional methods which characterize the *B. cepacia* complex taxa include highly specific PCR-based procedures (4,191), 16S rRNA gene sequence analysis (184), and capillary electrophoresis-single-strand conformation polymorphism analysis (CE-SSCP, 192). CFA composition analysis provides a good presumptive identification of an isolate as a member of the genus *Burkholderia*, but it is not sufficiently specific for species identification (1,141,186). Rapid systems such as the Vitek 2 or Crystal systems are promising, but accuracy problems still exist, nor have these systems been specifically evaluated with respect to detecting individual taxa within the *B. cepacia* cluster (178,179). Misidentification of *B. gladioli* by several commercial systems as *B. cepacia* has been reported (149). The proposed species *B. cocovenenans* was found to be a junior synonym of *B. gladiolii* (193). Species-specific probes for *B. gladioli* have been described (194).

Careful microbiological and epidemiological studies in areas of Thailand which had low prevalence of melioidosis yielded environmentally-derived bacteria which are most like *B. pseudomallei*, but which express a specific phenotype including the fermentation of arabinose (195). Microbiological examination of environmental and clinical specimens provided evidence that the environmental bacterium represented a new arabinose-positive species, *B. thailandensis*, which otherwise phenotypically and closely resembles the arabinose-negative species *B. pseudomallei* (196,197). Melioidosis occurred almost exclusively where arabinose-negative strains were recovered from the nearby environment (198). Only one verified clinically-relevant strain of arabinose-positive *B. pseudomallei* has been reported (199). Some researchers have questioned the validity of describing arabinose-positive and rarely pathogenic strains as a new and separate species, and they have suggested that they likely represent biovars of *B. pseudomallei*; this discussion continues to prove controversial (199). *B. pseudomallei* is considered a risk level 3 agent in many countries, and so it is recommended that manipulations should be done where possible in a risk level 3 suite (200-202). Misidentification of *B. pseudomallei* as *Chromobacterium violaceum* has been reported when using an API 20NE strip (203). Rapid identification methods, including monoclonal antibody assays (204, 205), are under development.

Pandoraea spp. that are obtained from CF patient sputa or other sources must be carefully differentiated from *Ralstonia pickettii*, *R. paucula*, and *B. cepacia* complex isolates with the use of one or more biochemical studies, CFA composition, whole cell protein profiles, and genotypic analyses until rapid identification systems include these taxa in their databases (15).

Acinetobacter spp. are Gram negative coccobacilli or cocci which by phenotypic testing are nearly homogenous (50). The taxonomy of *Acinetobacter* became more complex when 12 genospecies were described based on DNA-DNA hybridization of which 5 were assigned to named species (206). This was later augmented by studies in Sweden and France, which further described genomic species 13-17 (207,208,Table 2). *Acinetobacter* genomic species are highly related to each other by 16S rDNA sequence analysis, and genomic species that are separated by that method may not related well to DNA-DNA hybridization groups (209,210). *Gyr*B sequence analysis may be a useful tool to demonstrate phylogenetic relationships (187). Identification of the 16S-23S intergenic spacer sequences using restriction analysis has been described (211). Since it is difficult to correctly differentiate acinetobacters by phenotypic means alone, it is recommended that the method which is used and the phrase 'presumptive identification' be provided in a report except if genetically-based identification methods are used

Table 2 *Acinetobacter* taxonomic designations.

Species or genomic species	DNA homology group	Other
A. calcoaceticus	1	part of 'A. calcoaceticus and A. baumannii complex'
A. baumannii	2	part of 'A. calcoaceticus and A. baumannii complex'
Acinetobacter genomic species 3	3	
A. haemolyticus	4	beta-hemolytic
A. junii	5	
Acinetobacter genomic species 6	6	
A. johnsonii	7	no growth or poor growth at 37°C
A. lwoffii	8	8 and 9 cannot be differentiated phenotypically
Acinetobacter genomic species 9	9	as above
Acinetobacter genomic species 10	10	
Acinetobacter genomic species 11	11	
A. radioresistans	12	
Acinetobacter genomic	BJ 13; TU 13	BJ 13 = TU 14, but differs from TU species 13 which utilizes substrates
Acinetobacter genomic species 14	BJ 14; TU 14	BJ 14 differs from TU 14; TU 14 = BJ 13
Acinetobacter genomic species 15	BJ 15	unique to ref. 207
Acinetobacter genomic species	TU 15	unique to ref. 208
Acinetobacter genomic species 16	BJ 16	unique to ref. 207
Acinetobacter genomic species 17	BJ 17	unique to ref. 207
Acinetobacter CTTU13, Strain 36527, DNA group 1-3		from ref. 209; 3 taxa given separate accession #s. in Genebank based on ability to separate using 16S rDNA gene sequence analyses

(BJ – Bouvet and Jeanjean (207); TU – Tjerning and Ursing (208). *A. radioresistans* is described in ref. 50 and 251.)

(51). Members of the 'A. calcoaceticus-A. baumannii complex' oxidize glucose (50,206). This characteristic has prompted the creation of a blood agar medium that is enriched with glucose, whereby glucose-utilizing species are observed to produce a browning effect on the agar that is not observed among other glucose non-utilizing *Acinetobacter* taxa (212). CFA composition is a useful tool for the identification of *Acinetobacter* to the genus level, but it cannot be used to differentiate among genomic species (1).

Rapid identification methods based on phenotypic criteria do not readily distinguish *S. putrefaciens* and *S. alga* (79); in fact, it has been proposed, after using precise genotypic methods, that infection in humans may very well be primarily caused by *S. alga* and not *S. putrefaciens* (213).

Balneatrix has a CFA composition like those of *P. aeruginosa* and closely related taxa (1); by 16S rRNA sequence analysis, *B. alpica* is most closely related to, but well-separated from, the genus *Pseudomonas* (66).

Genotypic typing methods have been applied to some of these species, such as *P. stutzeri,* and they have revealed great genetic diversity among clinically- and environmentally-derived strains (214). *P. fluorescens* was implicated in an outbreak of bacteremia among oncology patients; correct identification of the outbreak bacterium was delayed until a polyphasic approach, which included both biochemicals and CFA composition analysis, was used (215).

Methylobacterium and *Roseomonas* may or may not grow well at 35°C on common laboratory media which contain blood, but they may grow better on media that lack blood such as BCYE media which is normally used for the growth of *Legionella* spp. (1). Means to differentiate *Methylobacterium* spp. from *Roseomonas* spp. and genospecies have been described (1,50). *M. extorquens* generally have dry coral-pigmented colonies and appear as distinctive vacuolated Gram negative coccobacilli in the Gram stain, whereas *Roseomonas* has more mucoid pink colonies which are observed to be Gram negative plump cocci or coccobacilli. The two genera may be separated by CFA composition analysis due to significant qualitative differences of CFAs that are present (1,84,156). Differentiation of those species may be accomplished by using biochemical tests and to some extent on the basis of CFA composition analysis (1,50,84). Interestingly, the CFA composition for several of these taxa (*R. gilardii, R. cervicalis,* and *Roseomonas* genomospecies 4 and 5) can qualitatively resemble those that are found for some *Brucella* species (1). A clinically relevant isolate of *M. zatmanii* was found to grow only on BCYE, and definitive identification was achieved using molecular means (87).

Afipia-named species and genomospecies are somewhat fastidious growers in the laboratory, but are considerably less so than *Bartonella* species. They may be recovered on standard laboratory media such as sheep blood agar or BCYE (216). Optimal growth may occur at 30°C rather than 35°C (1,216). *Afipia* spp. are motile and are poorly reactive using standard biochemical tests, but differential characteristics may include the use of catalase, oxidase, xylose, mannitol, urea, and nitrate reactions (1). Genomospecies 2 and *A. broomae* are phenotypically indistinguishable, and so they must be differentiated using molecular methods (1). CFA composition analysis is particularly useful to distinguish *Afipia* species and genomospecies from nearly all other GNFGNB as the profile contains significant volumes of a unique CFA which is found at Equivalent Chain length (ECL) 18.081 (11 methyl 18:1w7c) (217).

Psychrobacter immobilis was once thought to be related with, but distinguished from, provisional taxa CDC groups EO-2 and EO3 (50,119). This proved to be unfounded, however, as described below. *P. phenylpyruvicus*, formerly *Moraxella phenylpyruvica,* has rarely caused infection (1,119). It has been reported that certain *Brucella* species have been misidentified as *P. phenylpyruvicus* if rapid identification methods were used (218). These taxa can be differentiated by careful review of the Gram stain (*Brucella* species are observed to be tiny Gram negative coccobacilli), phenylalamine (PPA)-negative and xylose-positive reactions, whereas *P. phenylpyruvicus* is generally PPA-positive and xylose-negative. They also may be easily differentiated by CFA composition analysis since those taxa have qualitatively different CFAs (1,119).

The CFA composition of *Sphingomonas* spp. and *Caulobacter* spp. are qualitatively somewhat unique and are of the branched-chained type so that this method of characterization can be useful for these bacteria (1,64). The provisional taxon group, CDC group O-1, which has been recovered from a wide variety of clinical sources, has a CFA composition that is consistent with the *Sphingomonas* genus but may be differentiated from *S. paucimobilis* by phenotypic means (1). Provisional taxon 'Agrobacterium yellow group' has been compared phenotypically with *Sphingomonas* species, but CFA composition or genotypic data have not been determined (1).

It is difficult to distinguish *Myroides* species solely by standard phenotypic tests, but they do have some quantitative differences in key CFAs with *M. odoratimimus* having a significant quantity of CFA i-13:0 (129).

CDC group O-2 is observed to have a CFA composition that is consistent with *Sphingomonas* species (1,50). CDC group O-2 is yellow-pigmented, but it is otherwise heterogenous with respect to CFA composition (1,50). CDC group O-3 is observed to be a curved Gram negative rod with a single polar flagellum. CDC group OFBA is highly reactive in conventional substrates and has a unique CFA composition (1,133). Although CDC group NO-1 is phenotypically similar to biochemically nonreactive *Acinetobacter* species or genomospecies, it may be distinguished from members of that genus by CFA composition analysis (1,134). CDC group EO-2 has been described as a Gram negative coccus which is biochemically saccharolytic, has nonpigmented and often mucoid colonies, and has a unique CFA composition profile that is qualitatively similar to *Roseomonas* species and EO-3 (1). Recent studies using 16S rRNA sequence analysis of seven strains that are consistent with CDC group EO-2 description (1) indicate that they represent a novel taxon group in the genus *Paracoccus*, a genus previously not associated with human clinical disease (K. Bernard, unpublished data). Three strains of EO-3 have been studied with the use of 16S rRNA sequence analysis, and they were found to represent a novel *Paracoccus* species which differed from other named species in that genus and from those described above as a novel EO-2 taxon group (K. Bernard, unpublished data). Additional EO-3 strains were found by that method to be single representatives of novel *Paracoccus* or (next closest phylogenetic genus) *Rhodobacter* species. These have not been ascribed to causing or being associated with human infection (K. Bernard, unpublished data). CDC groups EO-4 and EO-5 have been recently described and may be differentiated from CDC groups EO-2 and EO-3 by phenotypic means (219,220). Gilardi rod group 1, recovered from a variety of clinical specimens, is characteristically and strongly phenylalanine deaminase-positive (221). Three strains studied with the use of 16S rRNA sequence analysis indicate a close relationship with a new taxon group with the proposed designation 'Schineria' (K. Bernard, unpublished data).

B. cepacia strains, which have been recovered from CF and non-CF patients, have been analyzed by a variety of subtyping methods including outer-membrane protein profiling (222), electrophoretic (ET) types, PCR restriction fragment length polymorphism (RFLP), and PFGE analysis (140,223,224). Typing methods, in addition to those that are described for the typing CF strains, include randomly amplified polymorphic DNA (RAPD) assays (225).

As for *B. cepacia* isolates that are derived from CF patients, ET typing (223) and CE-SSCP (192) have been successfully used to subtype CF-associated *P. aeruginosa*. PFGE for typing *P. aeruginosa* strains has been described (226).

P. oryzihabitans outbreaks have been successfully typed using PFGE and enterobacterial repetitive intergenic consensus (ERIC)-PCR (227).

PFGE appears to provide greater discrimination for strain typing than ribotyping or biotyping (228) for *Ralstonia*.

A variety of typing methods have been employed to study acinetobacters. The specificity of serotyping has become questionable given the recent taxonomic developments (51). A proposed phage typing scheme generated a large percentage of non-typeable isolates, and its usage is restricted essentially to one reference centre (51). Other typing methods include antibiogram analysis, protein profiling, MLEE, plasmid profiling, ribotyping, PFGE, ALFP, ARDRA, RAPD, ERIC, and infrequent restriction site-PCR (51,229–232).

When a number of different methods were used to type *S. maltophilia* strains from clinical sources or from the environment, PFGE was found to provide the greatest discrimination. It was also found that *S. maltophilia* revealed high intraspecies diversity (233). Three methods (arbitrarily-primed PCR, PFGE, and ERIC-PCR) were used to provide evidence that cross-transmission of this agent had occurred and had caused infections among babies in a neonatal unit (234).

As for other GNFGNB, PFGE provided satisfactory discrimination when performing epidemiological typing for *Alcaligenes* (235,236). Among CF patients, neither cross-infection nor common exposure source of *A. xylosoxidans* subsp. xylosoxidans could be found when genotypic typing methods were used to study clinically significant CF-associated strains (13).

Ribotyping has been used to study epidemiological relationships among unrelated reference, wild-type, and outbreak strains of *Chryseobacterium meningosepticum* (124).

VII. SUSCEPTIBILITY TESTING

Methods to perform and interpret antibiotic susceptibilities, using internationally recognized standards such as those maintained by the NCCLS, are not specifically described for many GNFGNB, except for the most clinically relevant taxa which are also prone to multiresistance to antibiotics (237-239). Appropriate antimicrobial agents and interpretative standards for *P. aeruginosa* are applicable to the susceptibility testing of non-fastidious, glucose nonfermenting Gram negative bacilli with the caveats that the MIC method, not disk diffusion method, is used and that the clinician be provided with the information that the method and interpretive breakpoints are not specific for any GNFGNB other than *P. aeruginosa* (237). As well, it is noted that *P. aeruginosa* may develop resistance during prolonged therapy with all antibiotics, and so strains that are initially found to be susceptible may become resistant within three to four days of therapy thus warranting testing of subsequent isolates (237). *P. aeruginosa* CF isolates and non-CF associated infections alike are prone to the development of multiresistance to antipseudomonal antibiotics (240).

Multi-resistant *P. aeruginosa* strains may be induced in a stepwise fashion after exposure to antipseudomonal antibiotics, and resistance is associated with adverse outcomes (241). Multi-resistance is not necessarily a factor that is associated with an increased risk of death (20). High level resistance to imipenem and meropenem has been recognized in several outbreaks involving VIM-1 carbapenemase-producing *P. aeruginosa* (242). The Etest (AB BioDisk North America Inc., Piscataway, New Jersey) has been shown to provide excellent correlation to reference MIC methods for the mucoid morphotype of CF-derived *P. aeruginosa* strains (morphotypes are described further below), but it is expensive and so is not a recommended choice for routine testing (243). Disk diffusion methods may be more difficult to interpret for the mucoid morphotype (244). The NCCLS guidelines suggest that ticarcillin/clavulanic acid may be useful for some *Pseudomonas* species that are not *P. aeruginosa* (237).

The incidence of endemic infection by *Acinetobacter* spp., particularly *A. baumannii*, is influenced by selective pressures of antibiotic use (58), and so susceptibility testing of clinical isolates must be carefully monitored (245). The use of the Etest MIC method has been described (246). Resistance to amikacin has been reported (247). Imipenem resistance is being increasingly reported (55,248,249), and the mechanism of resistance is being elucidated. Imipenem resistance is verified on the observance of carbapenem-hydrolyzing activity and detection of the carbapenemase gene bla_{imp} which, when transferred, confers resistance to imipenem, meropenem, cefotaxime, ampicillin, and piperacillin (248,249). Multi-drug resistance may also occur among *A. calcoaceticus* and *A. haemolyticus* isolates (50). Consistent use of barrier infection control measures and compliance with handwashing protocols are effective in minimizing outbreaks (53,54).

As discussed previously, the management of *Stenotrophomonas* infection is problematic because of multiple antibiotic resistance and the lack of formal guidelines for in vitro antibiotic susceptibility testing that are specifically directed towards *Stenotrophomonas*, although specific recommendations such as the inclusion of antibiotics ticarcillin/clavulanic acid and moxalactam exist (11,237).

Documented cases of *Afipia* infections are few, and so it is difficult to corroborate antimicrobial susceptibilities to clinical efficacy. In one study, *A. felis* was found to be multiresistant to antibiotics but nevertheless was susceptible to aminoglycosides, imipenem, and rifampin (216). *Oligella urethralis* infection in a CAPD patient was complicated by quinolone resistance (115). Antimicrobial susceptibility testing of flavobacteria has been described (250). Etest methods have been shown not to correlate well with conventional MIC methods for some of the more rare GNFGNB pathogens such as *Chryseobacterium* spp., and so they are not currently recommended (50).

REFERENCES

1. Weyant RS, Moss CW, Weaver RE, Hollis DE, Jordan JE, Cook EC, Daneshvar MI. Identification of Unusual Pathogenic Gram-Negative Aerobic and Facultatively Anaerobic Bacteria. Washington, DC: Williams & Wilkins, 1996.
2. Quinn JP. Clinical problems posed by multiresistant nonfermenting gram-negative pathogens. Clin Infect Dis 1998; 27:S117-S124.
3. Gilligan PH, Whittier S. *Burkholderia, Stenotrophomonas, Ralstonia, Brevundimonas, Comamonas* and *Acidovorax*. In: Murray PR, Baron EJ, Pfaller MA, Tenover FC, Yolken RH, eds. Manual of Clinical Microbiology. Washington, DC:ASM Press, 1999:526-538.
4. Bauernfeind A, Schneider I, Jungwirth R, Roller C. Discrimination of *Burkholderia multivorans* and *Burkholderia vietnamiensis* from *Burkholderia cepacia* genomovars I, III, and IV by PCR. J Clin Microbiol 1999; 37:1335-1339.
5. Kanj SS, Tapson V, Davis RD, Madden J, Browning I. Infections in patients with cystic fibrosis following lung transplantation. Chest 1997; 112:924-930.
6. Johnson JA, Connolly MA, Jacobs P, Montgomery M, Brown NE, Zuberbuhler P. Cost of care for individuals with cystic fibrosis: a regression approach to determining the impact of recombinant human DNase. Pharmacotherapy 1999; 19:1159-1166.
7. Kiska DL, Gilligan PH. *Pseudomonas* In: Murray PR, Baron EJ, Pfaller MA, Tenover FC, Yolken RH, eds. Manual of Clinical Microbiology. Washington, DC:ASM Press, 1999:517-525.
8. Gilligan PH. Microbiology of airway disease in patients with cystic fibrosis. Clin Microbiol Rev 1991; 4:35-51.
9. Parad RB, Gerard CJ, Zurakowski D, Nichols DP, Pier GB. Pulmonary outcome in cystic fibrosis is influenced primarily by mucoid *Pseudomonas aeruginosa* infection and immune status and only modestly by genotype. Infect Immun 1999; 67:4744-4750.
10. Haussler S, Tummler B, Weissbrodt H, Rohde M, Steinmetz I. Small-colony variants of *Pseudomonas aeruginosa* in cystic fibrosis. Clin Infect Dis 1999; 29:621-625.
11. Denton M, Todd NJ, Kerr KG, Hawkey PM, Littlewood JM. Molecular epidemiology of *Stenotrophomonas maltophilia* isolated from clinical specimens from patients with cystic fibrosis and associated environmental samples. J Clin Microbiol 1998; 36:1953-1958.
12. Denton M, Kerr KG. Microbiological and clinical aspects of infection associated with *Stenotrophomonas maltophilia*. Clin Microbiol Rev 1998; 11:57-80.
13. Vu-Thien H, Moissenet D, Valcin M, Dulot C, Tournier G, Garbarg-Chenon A. Molecular epidemiology of *Burkholderia cepacia, Stenotrophomonas maltophilia*, and *Alcaligenes xylosoxidans* in a cystic fibrosis center. Eur J Clin Microbiol Infect Dis 1996; 15:876-879.
14. Demko CA, Stern RC, Doershuk CF. *Stenotrophomonas maltophilia* in cystic fibrosis: incidence and prevalence. Pediatr Pulmonol 1998; 25:304-308.
15. Coenye T, Falsen E, Hoste B, Ohlen M, Goris J, Govan JR, Gillis M, Vandamme P. Description of *Pandoraea* gen. nov. with *Pandoraea apista* sp. nov., *Pandoraea pulmonicola* sp. nov., *Pandoraea pnomenusa* sp. nov., *Pandoraea sputorum* sp. nov., and *Pandoraea norimbergensis* comb. Nov. Int J Syst Bacteriol 2000; 50:887-899.
16. Pitulle C, Citron DM, Bochner B, Barbers R, Appleman MD. Novel bacterium isolated from a lung transplant patient with cystic fibrosis. J Clin Microbiol 1999; 37:3851-3855.
17. Richards MJ, Edwards JR, Culver DH, Gaynes RP. Nosocomial infections in medical intensive care units in the United States. National Nosocomial Infections Surveillance System. Crit Care Med 1999; 27:887-92.
18. Hanberger H, Garcia-Rodriguez JA, Gobernado M, Goossens H, Nilsson LE, Struelens MJ. Antibiotic susceptibility among aerobic gram-negative bacilli in intensive care units in five European countries. French and Portuguese ICU Study Groups. JAMA 1999; 281:67-71.
19. Krause R, Mittermayer H, Feierl G, Allergerger F, Wendelin I, Hirschl A, Reisinger EC. In vitro activity of newer broad spectrum beta-lactam antibiotics against *Enterobacteriaceae* and non-fermenters: a report from Austrian intensive care units. Austrian Carbapenem Susceptibility Surveillance Group. Wien Klin Wochenschr 1999; 111:549-554.
20. Harbarth S, Rohner P, Auckenthaler R, Safran E, Sudre P, Pittet D. Impact and pattern of gram-negative bacteraemia during six years at a large university hospital. Scand J Infect Dis 1999; 31:163-168.

21. Martino R, Santamaria A, Munoz L, Pericas R, Altes A, Prats G, Sierra J. Bacteremia by Gram-negative bacilli in patients with hematologic malignancies: comparison of the clinical presentation and outcome of infections by enterobacteria and non-glucose-fermenting gram-negative bacilli. Acta Haematol 1999; 102:7-11.

22. Edgeworth, JD, Treacher DF, Eykyn SJ. A 25-year study of nosocomial bacteremia in an adult intensive care unit. Crit Care Med 1999; 27:1421-1428.

23. Vidal F, Mensa J, Martinez JA, Almela M, Marco F, Gatell JM, Richart C, Soriano E, Jimenez de Anta MT. *Pseudomonas aeruginosa* bacteremia in patients infected with human immunodeficiency virus type 1. Eur J Clin Microbiol Infect Dis 1999; 18:473-477.

24. Anzai Y, Kudo Y, Oyaizu H. The phylogeny of the genera *Chryseomonas, Flavimonas,* and *Pseudomonas* supports synonymy of these three genera. Int J Syst Bacteriol 1997; 47:249-251.

25. Elomari M, Coroler L, Verhille S, Izard D, Leclerc H. *Pseudomonas monteilii* sp. nov., isolated from clinical specimens Int J Syst Bacteriol 1997; 47:846-852.

26. Giacometti A, Cirioni O, Quarta M, Schimizzi AM, Del Prete MS, Scalise G. Unusual clinical presentation of infection due to *Flavimonas oryzihabitans*. Eur J Clin Microbiol Infect Dis 1998; 17:645-648.

27. Lin RD, Hsueh PR, Chang JC, Teng LJ, Chang SC, Ho SW, Hsieh WC, Luh KT. *Flavimonas oryzihabitans* bacteremia: clinical features and microbiological characteristics of isolates. Clin Infect Dis 1997; 24:867-873.

28. Rastogi S, Sperber SJ. Facial cellulitis and *Pseudomonas luteola* bacteremia in an otherwise healthy patient. Diagn Microbiol Infect Dis 1998; 32:303-305.

29. Rahav G, Simhon A, Mattan Y, Moses AE, Sacks T. Infections with *Chryseomonas luteola* (CDC group Ve-1) and *Flavimonas oryzihabitans* (CDC group Ve-2). Medicine (Baltimore) 1995; 74:83-88.

30. Leelarasamee A. *Burkholderia pseudomallei*: the unbeatable foe? Southeast Asian J Trop Med Public Health 1998; 29:410-415.

31. Inglis TJJ, Garrow SC, Henderson M, Clair A, Sampson J, O'Reilly L, Cameron B. *Burkholderia pseudomallei* traced to water treatment plant in Australia. Emerg Infect Dis 2000; 6:56-59.

32. Dorman SE, Gill VJ, Gallin JI, Holland SM. *Burkholderia pseudomallei* infection in a Puerto Rican patient with chronic granulomatous disease: case report and review of occurrences in the Americas. Clin Infect Dis 1998; 26:889-894.

33. Beeker A, Van de Stadt KD, Bakker K. Melioidosis. Neth J Med 1999; 54:76-79.

34. Thummakul T, Wilde H, Tantawichien T. Melioidosis, an environmental and occupational hazard in Thailand. Mil Med 1999; 164:658-662.

35. Bartley PP, Pender MP, Woods ML, Walker D, Douglas JA, Allworth AM, Eisen DP, Currie BJ. Spinal cord disease due to melioidosis. Trans R Soc Trop Med Hyg 1999; 93:175-176.

36. Halder D, Zainal N, Wah CM, Haq JA. Neonatal meningitis and septicaemia caused by *Burkholderia pseudomallei*. Ann Trop Paediatr 1998; 18:161-164.

37. Padiglione A, Ferris N, Fuller A, Spelman D. Brain abscesses caused by *Burkholderia pseudomallei*. J Infect 1998; 36:335-337.

38. Lu DC, Chang SC, Chen YC, Luh KT, Lee CY, Hsieh WC. *Burkholderia cepacia* bacteremia: a retrospective analysis of 70 episodes. J Formos Med Assoc 1997; 96:972-978.

39. Yu WL, Wang DY, Lin CW, Tsou MF. Endemic *Burkholderia cepacia* bacteraemia: clinical features and antimicrobial susceptibilities of isolates. Scand J Infect Dis 1999; 31:293-298.

40. van Laer F, Raes D, Vandamme P, Lammens C, Sion JP, Vrints C, Snoeck J, Goossens H. An outbreak of *Burkholderia cepacia* with septicemia on a cardiology ward. Infect Control Hosp Epidemiol 1998; 19:112-113.

41. Graves M, Robin T, Chipman AM, Wong J, Khashe S, Janda JM. Four additional cases of *Burkholderia gladioli* infection with microbiological correlates and review. Clin Infect Dis 1997; 25:838-842.

42. Yabuuchi E, Kosako Y, Yano I, Hotta H, Nishiuchi Y. Transfer of two *Burkholderia* and an *Alcaligenes* species to *Ralstonia* gen. Nov.: Proposal of *Ralstonia pickettii* (Ralston, Palleroni and Doudoroff 1973) comb. Nov., *Ralstonia solanacearum* (Smith 1896) comb. Nov. and *Ralstonia eutropha* (Davis 1969) comb. Nov. Microbiol Immunol 1995; 39:897-904.

43. Coenye T, Falsen E, Vancanneyt M, Hoste B, Govan JR, Kersters K, Vandamme P. Classification of *Alcaligenes faecalis*-like isolates from the environment and human clinical samples as *Ralstonia gilardii* sp. nov. Int J Syst Bacteriol 1999; 49:405-413.

44. Moissenet D, Goujon CP, Garbarg-Chenon A, Vu-Thien H. CDC group IV C-2: a new *Ralstonia* species close to *Ralstonia eutropha*. J Clin Microbiol 1999; 37:241-244.

45. Vandamme P, Goris J, Coenye T, Hoste B, Janssens D, Kersters K, De Vos P, Falsen E. Assignment of Centers for Disease Control group IVc-2 to the genus *Ralstonia* as *Ralstonia paucula* sp. nov. Int J Syst Bacteriol 1999; 49:663-669.

46. Osterhout GJ, Valentine JL, Dick JD. Phenotypic and genotypic characterization of clinical strains of CDC group IVc-2. J Clin Microbiol 1998; 36:2618-2622.

47. Noyola DE, Edwards MS. Bacteremia with CDC Group IV c-2 in an immunocompetent infant. Clin Infect Dis 1999; 29:1572.

48. Labarca JA, Trick WE, Peterson CL, Carson LA, Holt SC, Arduino MJ, Meylan M, Mascola L, Jarvis WR. A multistate nosocomial outbreak of *Ralstonia pickettii* colonization associated with an intrinsically contaminated respiratory care solution. Clin Infect Dis 1999; 29:1281-1286.

49. Anderson RR, Warnick P, Schreckenberger PC. Recurrent CDC group IVc-2 bacteremia in a human with AIDS. J Clin Microbiol 1997; 35:780-782.

50. Schreckenberger PC, von Graevenitz A. *Acinetobacter, Achromobacter, Alcaligenes, Moraxella, Methylobacterium* and other nonfermentative Gram-negative rods. In: Murray PR, Baron EJ, Pfaller MA, Tenover FC, Yolken RH, eds. Manual of Clinical Microbiology. Washington, DC: ASM Press, 1999:539-560.

51. Bergogne-Berezin E, Towner KJ. *Acinetobacter* spp. as nosocomial pathogens: microbiological, clinical, and epidemiological features. Clin Microbiol Rev 1996; 9:148-165.

52. Jawad A, Seifert H, Snelling AM, Heritage J, Hawkey PM. Survival of *Acinetobacter baumannii* on dry surfaces: comparison of outbreak and sporadic isolates. J Clin Microbiol 1998; 36:1938-1941.

53. Dy ME, Nord JA, LaBombardi VJ, Kislak JW. The emergence of resistant strains of *Acinetobacter baumannii*: clinical and infection control populations. Infect Cont Hosp Epidemiol 1999; 20:565-567.

54. Husni RN, Goldstein LS, Arroliga AC, Hall GS, Fatica C, Stoller JK, Gordon SM. Risk factors for an outbreak of multi-drug resistant *Acinetobacter* nosocomial pneumonia among intubated patients. Chest 1999; 115:1378-1382.

55. Lai SW, Ng KC, Yu WL, Liu CS, Lai MM, Lin CC. *Acinetobacter baumannii* bloodstream infection: clinical features and antimicrobial susceptibilities of isolates. Kao Hsiung I Hsueh Tsa Chih 1999; 15:406-413.

56. Traub WH, Geipel U, Schwarze I, Bauer D. A cluster of nosocomial cross-infection due to multiple antibiotic-resistant *Acinetobacter baumannii*: characterization of the strain and antibiotic susceptibility studies. Chemotherapy 1999; 45:349-359.

57. Vila J, Ruiz J, Navia M, Becerril B, Garcia I, Perea S, Lopez-Hernandez I, Alamo I, Ballester F, Planes AM, Martinez-Beltran J, de Anta TJ. Spread of amikacin resistance in *Acinetobacter baumannii* strains isolated in Spain due to an epidemic strain. J Clin Microbiol 1999; 37:758-761.

58. Villers D, Espaze E, Coste-Burel M, Giauffret F, Ninin E, Nicholas F, Richet H. Nosocomial *Acinetobacter baumannii* infections: microbiological and clinical epidemiology. Ann Intern Med 1998; 129:182-189.

59. Wisplinghoff H, Perbix W, Seifert H. Risk factors for nosocomial bloodstream infections due to *Acinetobacter baumannii*: a case-control study of adult burn patients. Clin Infect Dis 1999; 28:59-66.

60. Yu EH, Ko WC, Chuang YC, Wu TJ. Suppurative *Acinetobacter baumannii* thyroiditis with bacteremic pneumonia: case report and review. Clin Infect Dis 1998; 27:1286-1290.

61. de Beaufort AJ, Bernards AT, Dijkshoorn L, van Boven CP. *Acinetobacter junii* causes life-threatening sepsis in preterm infants. Acta Paediatr 1999; 88:772-775.

62. McDonald A, Amyes SG, Paton R. The persistence and clonal spread of a single strain of *Acinetobacter* 13TU in a large Spanish teaching hospital. J Chemother 1999; 11:338-344.

63. Segers P, Vancanneyt M, Pot B, Torck U, Hoste B, Dewettinck D, Falsen E, Kersters K, De Vos P. Classification of *Pseudomonas diminuta* Leifson and Hugh 1954 and *Pseudomonas vesicularis* Busing, Doll, and Freytag 1953 in *Brevundimonas* gen. nov. as *Brevundimonas diminuta* comb. nov. and *Brevundimonas vesicularis* comb. nov., respectively. Int J Syst Bacteriol 1994; 44:499-510.

64. Abraham WR, Strompl C, Meyer H, Lindholst S, Moore ER, Christ R, Vancanneyt M, Tindall J, Bennasar A, Smit J, Tesar M. Phylogeny and polyphasic taxonomy of *Caulobacter* species: proposal of *Maricaulis* gen. nov. with *Maricaulis maris* (Poindexter) comb. nov. as the type species, and emended description of the genera *Brevundimonas* and *Caulobacter*. Int J Syst Bacteriol 1999; 49:1053-1073.

65. Sly LI, Cox TL, Beckenham TB. The phylogenetic relationships of *Caulobacter, Asticcacaulis* and *Brevundimonas* species and their taxonomic implications. Int J Syst Bacteriol 1999; 49:483-488.

66. Dauga C, Gillis M, Vandamme P, Ageron E, Grimont F, Kersters K, de Mahenge C, Peloux Y, Grimont PA. *Balneatrix alpica* gen. nov., sp. nov., a bacterium associated with pneumonia and meningitis in a spa therapy center. Res Microbiol 1993; 144:35-46.

67. Monkemuller KE, Morgan DE, Baron TH. *Stenotrophomonas* (*Xanthomonas*) *maltophilia* infection in necrotizing pancreatitis. Int J Pancreatol 1999; 25:59-63.

68. Gopalakrishnan R, Hawley HB, Czachor JS, Markert RJ, Bernstein JM. *Stenotrophomonas maltophilia* infection and colonization in the intensive care units of two community hospitals: a study of 143 patients. Heart Lung 1999; 28:134-141.

69. Manfredi R, Nanetti A, Ferri M, Chiodo F. *Xanthomonas maltophilia*: an emerging pathogen in patients with HIV disease. Int J STD AIDS 1998; 9:201-207.

70. Verweij PE, Meis JF, Christmann V, Van der Bor M, Melchers WJ, Hilderink BG, Voss A. Nosocomial outbreak of colonization and infection with *Stenotrophomonas maltophilia* in preterm infants associated with contaminated tap water. Epidemiol Infect 1998; 120:251-256.

71. Munter RG, Yinnon AM, Schlesinger Y, Hershko C. Infective endocarditis due to *Stenotrophomonas* (*Xanthomonas*) *maltophilia*. Eur J Clin Microbiol Infect Dis 1998; 17:353-356.

72. Shimoni S, Abend Y, Shimon A, Landau Z, Caspi A. *Stenotrophomonas maltophilia* endocarditis following dental treatment in a previously healthy patient. J Infect 1998; 37:305-306.

73. Amano K, Maruyama H, Takeuchi T. Nosocomial pneumonia likely caused by *Stenotrophomonas maltophilia* in two patients with polymyositis. Intern Med 1999; 38:910-916.

74. Sefcick A, Tait RC, Wood B. *Stenotrophomonas maltophilia*: an increasing problem in patients with acute leukaemia. Leuk Lymphoma 1999; 35:207-211.

75. Labarca JA, Leber AL, Kern VL, Territo MC, Brankovic LE, Bruckner DA, Pegues DA. Outbreak of *Stenotrophomonas maltophilia* bacteremia in allogenic bone marrow transplant patients: role of severe neutropenia and mucositis. Clin Infect Dis 2000; 30:195-197.

76. Drancourt M, Bollet C, Raoult D. *Stenotrophomonas africana* sp. nov., an opportunistic human pathogen in Africa. Int J Syst Bacteriol 1997; 47:160-163.

77. Nozue H, Hayashi T, Hashimoto Y, Ezaki T, Hamasaki K, Ohwada K, Terawaki Y. Isolation and characterization of *Shewanella alga* from human clinical specimens and emendation of the description of *S. alga* Simidu et al., 1990, 335. Int J Syst Bacteriol 1992; 42:628-634.

78. Dominguez H, Vogel BF, Gram L, Hoffmann S, Schaebel S. *Shewanella alga* bacteremia in two patients with lower leg ulcers. Clin Infect Dis 1996; 22:1036-1039.

79. Iwata M, Tateda K, Matsumoto T, Furuya N, Mizuiri S, Yamaguchi K. Primary *Shewanella alga* septicemia in a patient on hemodialysis. J Clin Microbiol 1999; 37:2104-2105.

80. Dhawan B, Chaudhry R, Mishra BM, Agarwal R. Isolation of *Shewanella putrefaciens* from a rheumatic heart disease patient with infective endocarditis. J Clin Microbiol 1998; 36:2394.

81. Wen A, Fegan M, Hayward C, Chakraborty S, Sly LI. Phylogenetic relationships among members of the *Comamonadaceae*, and description of *Delftia acidovorans* (den Dooren de Jong 1926 and Tamaoka et al. 1987) gen. nov., comb. nov. Int J Syst Bacteriol 1999; 49:567-576.

82. Stonecipher KG, Jensen HG, Kastl PR, Faulkner A, Rowsey JJ. Ocular infections associated with *Comamonas acidovorans*. Am J Ophthalmol 1991; 112:46-49.

83. Hollis DG, Weaver RE, Moss CW, Daneshvar MI, Wallace PL. Chemical and cultural characterization of CDC group WO-1, a weakly oxidative gram-negative group of organisms isolated from clinical sources. J Clin Microbiol 1992; 30:291-295.

84. Rihs JD, Brenner DJ, Weaver RE, Steigerwalt AG, Hollis DG, Yu VL. *Roseomonas*, a new genus associated with bacteremia and other human infections. J Clin Microbiol 1993; 31:3275-3283.

85. Struthers M, Wong J, Janda JM. An initial appraisal of the clinical significance of *Roseomonas* species associated with human infections. Clin Infect Dis 1996; 23:729-733.

86. Kaye KM, Macone A, Kazanjian PH. Catheter infection caused by *Methylobacterium* in immunocompromised hosts: report of three cases and review of the literature. Clin Infect Dis 1992; 14:1010-1014.

87. Hornei B, Luneberg E, Schmidt-Rotte H, Maass M, Weber K, Heits F, Frosch M, Solbach W. Systemic infection of an immunocompromised patient with *Methylobacterium zatmanii*. J Clin Microbiol 1999; 37:248-250.

88. Lewis L, Stock F, Williams D, Weir S, Gill VJ. Infections with *Roseomonas gilardii* and review of characteristics used for biochemical identification and molecular typing. Am J Clin Pathol 1997; 108:210-216.

89. Alcala L, Vasallo FJ, Cercenado E, Garcia-Garrote F, Rodriguez-Creixems M, Bouza E. Catheter-related bacteremia due to *Roseomonas gilardii* sp. nov. J Clin Microbiol 1997; 35:2712.

90. Nahass RG, Wisneski R, Herman DJ, Hirsh E, Goldblatt K. Vertebral osteomyelitis due to *Roseomonas* species: case report and review of the evaluation of vertebral osteomyelitis. Clin Infect Dis 1995; 21:1474-1476.

91. Sandoe JA, Malnick H, Loudon KW. A case of peritonitis caused by *Roseomonas gilardii* in a patient undergoing continuous ambulatory peritoneal dialysis. J Clin Microbiol 1997; 35:2150-2152.

92. Bibashi E, Sofianou D, Kontopoulou K, Mitsopoulos E, Kokolina E. Peritonitis due to *Roseomonas fauriae* in a patient undergoing continuous ambulatory peritoneal dialysis. J Clin Microbiol 2000; 38:456-457.

93. Brenner DJ, Hollis DG, Moss CW, English CK, Hall GS, Vincent J, Radosevic J, Birkness KA, Bibb WF, Quinn FD, Swaminathan B, Weaver RE, Reeves MW, O'Connor SP, Hayes PS, Tenover FC, Steigerwalt AG, Perkins BA, Daneshvar MI, Hill BC, Washington JA, Woods TC, Hunter SB, Hadfield TL, Ajello GW, Kaufmann AF, Wear DJ, Wenger JD. Proposal of *Afipia* gen. nov., with *Afipia felis* sp. nov. (formerly the cat scratch disease bacillus), *Afipia clevelandensis* sp. nov. (formerly the Cleveland Clinic Foundation strain), *Afipia broomeae* sp. nov., and three unnamed genospecies. J Clin Microbiol 1991; 29:2450-2460.

94. Giladi M, Avidor B, Kletter Y, Abulfia S, Slater LN, Welch DR, Brenner DJ, Steigerwalt AG, Whitney AM, Ephros M. Cat scratch disease: the rare role of *Afipia felis*. J Clin Microbiol 1998; 36:2499-2502.

95. Moissenet D, Baculard A, Valcin M, Marchand V, Tournier G, Garbarg-Chenon A, Vu-Thien H. Colonization by *Alcaligenes xylosoxidans* in children with cystic fibrosis: a retrospective clinical study conducted by means of molecular epidemiological investigation. Clin Infect Dis 1997; 24:274-275.

96. Manfredi R, Nanetti A, Ferri M, Chiodo F. Bacteremia and respiratory involvement by *Alcaligenes xylosoxidans* in patients infected with the human immunodeficiency virus. Eur J Clin Microbiol Infect Dis 1997; 16:933-938.

97. Swart J, Volker-Dieben HJ, Reichert-Thoen JW. *Alcaligenes xylosoxidans* endophthalmitis eight months after cataract extraction. Am J Ophthalmol 1999; 127:345-346.

98. Euzeby JP. List of Bacterial Names with Standing in Nomenclature. 2000. URL http://www-sv.cict.fr/bacteriol/

99. Holmes B, Lewis R, Trevett A. Septicemia due to *Achromobacter* group B: a report of two cases. Med Microbiol Lett 1992; 1:177-184.

100. Jenks PJ, Shaw EJ. Recurrent septicemia due to '*Achromobacter* group B' J Infect 1997; 34:143-145.

101. Alnor D, Frimodt-Moller N, Espersen F, Frederiksen W. Infections with the unusual human pathogens *Agrobacterium* species and *Ochrobactrum anthropi*. Clin Infect Dis 1994; 18:914-920.

102. Hulse M, Johnson S, Ferrieri P. *Agrobacterium* infections in humans: experience at one hospital and review. Clin Infect Dis 1993; 16:112-117.

103. Yu WL, Wang DY, Lin CW. *Agrobacterium radiobacter* bacteremia in a patient with chronic obstructive pulmonary disease. J Formos Med Assoc 1997; 96:664-666.

104. Southern PM Jr. Bacteremia due to *Agrobacterium tumefaciens* (*radiobacter*): report of infection in a pregnant women and her stillborn fetus. Diagn Microbiol Infect Dis 1996; 24:43-45.

105. Manfredi R, Nanetti A, Ferri M, Mastroianni A, Coronado OV, Chiodo F. Emerging gram-negative pathogens in the immunocompromised host: *Agrobacterium radiobacter* septicemia during HIV disease. New Microbiol 1999; 22:375-382.

106. Cieslak TJ, Drabick CJ, Robb ML. Pyogenic infections due to *Ochrobactrum anthropi*. Clin Infect Dis 1997; 25:225-229.

107. Yu WL, Lin CW, Wang DY. Clinical and microbiologic characteristics of *Ochrobactrum anthropi* bacteremia. J Formos Med Assoc 1998; 97:106-112.

108. Ezzedine H, Mourad M, Van Ossel C, Logghe C, Squifflet JP, Renault F, Wauters G, Gigi J, Wilmotte L, Haxhe JJ. An outbreak of *Ochrobactrum anthropi* bacteraemia in five organ transplant patients. J Hosp Infect 1994; 27:35-42.

109. Saavedra J, Garrido C, Folgueira D, Torres MJ, Ramos JT. *Ochrobactrum anthropi* bacteremia associated with a catheter in an immunocompromised child and review of the pediatric literature. Pediatr Infect Dis J 1999; 18:658-660.

110. Manfredi R, Nanetti A, Ferri M, Calza L, Tadolini M, Chiodo F. *Ochrobactrum anthropi* as an agent of nosocomial septicemia in the setting of AIDS. Clin Infect Dis 1999; 28:692-694.

111. Christenson JC, Pavia AT, Seskin K, Brockmeyer D, Korgenski EK, Jenkins E, Pierce J, Daly JA. Meningitis due to *Ochrobactrum anthropi*: an emerging nosocomial pathogen: a report of three cases. Pediatr Neurosurg 1997; 27:218-221.

112. Inoue K, Numaga J, Nagata Y, Sakurai M, Aso N, Fujino Y. *Ochrobactrum anthropi* endophthalmitis after vitreous surgery. Br J Ophthalmol 1999; 83:502.

113. Velasco J, Romero C, Lopez-Goni I, Leiva J, Diaz R, Moriyon I. Evaluation of the relatedness of *Brucella* spp. and *Ochrobactrum anthropi* and description of *Ochrobactrum intermedium* sp. nov., a new species with a closer relationship to *Brucella* spp. Int J Syst Bacteriol 1998; 48:759-768.

114. Moller LVM, Arends JP, Harmsen HJM, Talens A, Terpstra P, Slooff MJH. *Ochrobactrum intermedium* infection after liver transplantation. J Clin Microbiol 1999; 37:241-244.

115. Riley UB, Bignardi G, Goldberg L, Johnson AP, Holmes B. Quinolone resistance in *Oligella urethralis*-associated chronic ambulatory peritoneal dialysis peritonitis. J Infect 1996; 32:155-156.

116. Bowman JP, Cavanagh J, Austin JJ, Sanderson K. Novel *Psychrobacter* species from Antarctic ornithogenic soils. Int J Syst Bacteriol 1996; 46:841-848.

117. Lozano F, Florez C, Recio FJ, Gamboa F, Gomez-Mateas JM, Martin E. Fatal *Psychrobacter immobilis* infection in a patient with AIDS. AIDS 1994; 8:1189-1190.

118. Gini GA. Ocular infection caused by *Psychrobacter immobilis*. J Clin Microbiol 1990; 28:400-401.

119. Moss CW, Wallace PL, Hollis DG, Weaver RE. Cultural and chemical characterization of CDC groups EO-2, M-5, and M-6, *Moraxella (Moraxella)* species, *Oligella urethralis*, *Acinetobacter* species, and *Psychrobacter immobilis*. J Clin Microbiol 1988; 26:484-492.

120. Hsueh PR, Teng LJ, Yang PC, Chen YC, Pan HJ, Ho SW, Luh KT. Nosocomial infections caused by *Sphingomonas paucimobilis*: clinical features and microbiological characteristics. Clin Infect Dis 1998; 26:676-681.

121. Purcell BK, Dooley DP. Centers for Disease Control and Prevention group O1 bacterium-associated pneumonia complicated by bronchopulmonary fistula and bacteremia. Clin Infect Dis 1999; 29:945-946.

122. Vandamme P, Bernardet J-F, Segers P, Kersters K, Holmes B. New perspectives in the classification of the flavobacteria: description of *Chryseobacterium* gen. Nov., *Bergeyella* gen. Nov., and *Empedobacter* nom. rev. Int J Syst Bacteriol 1994; 44:827-831.

123. Bloch KC, Nadarajah R, Jacobs R. *Chryseobacterium meningosepticum*: an emerging pathogen among immunocompromised adults: report of six cases and literature review. Medicine (Baltimore) 1997; 76:30-41.

124. Quilici ML, Bizet C. Ribotyping of *Chryseobacterium meningosepticum*: its use as an epidemiological tool and its correlation with serovars. Res Microbiol 1996; 147:415-25.

125. Yannelli B, Koj IG, Cunha BA. *Chryseobacterium meningosepticum* bacteremia secondary to central intravenous line-related infection. Am J Infect Control 1999; 27:533-535.

126. Manfredi R, Nanetti A, Ferri M, Mastroianni A, Coronado OV, Chiodo F. *Flavobacterium* spp. organisms as opportunistic bacterial pathogens during advanced HIV disease. J Infect 1999; 39:146-152.

127. Hsueh PR, Hsiue TR, Wu JJ, Teng LJ, Ho SW, Hsieh WC, Luh KT. *Flavobacterium indologenes* bacteremia: clinical and microbiological characteristics. Clin Infect Dis 1996; 23:550-555.

128. Hsueh PR, Teng LJ, Ho SW, Hsieh WC, Luh KT. Clinical and microbiological characteristics of *Flavobacterium indologenes* infections associated with indwelling devices. J Clin Microbiol 1996; 34:1908-1913.

129. Vancanneyt M, Segers P, Torck U, Hoste B, Bernardet J-F, Vandamme P, Kersters K. Reclassification of *Flavobacterium odoratum* (Stutzer 1929) strains to a new genus *Myroides*, as *Myroides odoratus* comb. nov. and *Myroides odoratimimus* sp. nov. Int J Syst Bacteriol 1996; 46:926-932.

130. Bachman KH, Sewell DL, Strausbaugh LJ. Recurrent cellulitis and bacteremia caused by *Flavobacterium odoratum*. Clin Infect Dis 1996; 22:1112-1113.

131. Grimault E, Glerant JC, Aubry P, Laurans G, Poinsot JP, Jounieaux V. Uncommon site of *Bergeyella zoohelcum*. Apropos of a case. Rev Pneumol Clin 1996; 52:387-389.

132. Daneshvar MI, Hill B, Hollis DG, Moss CW, Jordan JG, Macgregor JP, Tenover F, Weyant RS. CDC group O-3: phenotypic characteristics, fatty acid composition, isoprenoid quinone content, and in vitro antimicrobic susceptibilities of an unusual gram-negative bacterium isolated from clinical specimens. J Clin Microbiol 1998; 36:1674-1678.

133. von Graevenitz A, Pfyffer G E, Pickett M J, Weaver R E, Wust J. Isolation of am unclassified nonfermentative gram-negative rod from a patient on continuous ambulatory peritoneal dialysis. Eur J Clin Microbiol Infect Dis1993; 12:568-570.

134. Hollis DG, Moss CW, Daneshvar MI, Meadows L, Jordan J, Hill B. Characterization of Centers for Disease Control group NO-1, a fastidious, nonoxidative, gram-negative organism associated with dog and cat bites. J Clin Microbiol 1993;31:746-748.

135. Daley D, Neville S, Kociuba K. Peritonitis associated with a CDC group EO-3 organism. J Clin Microbiol 1997; 35:3338-3339.

136. Rusin PA, Rose JB, Haas CN, Gerba CP. Risk assessment of opportunistic bacterial pathogens in drinking water. Rev Environ Contam Toxicol 1997; 152:57-83.

137. Vegelin, AL, Bissumbhar P, Joore JC, Lammers JW, Hoepelman IM. Guidelines for severe community-acquired pneumonia in the western world. Neth J Med 1999; 55:110-117.

138. Jang TN, Kuo BI, Shen SH, Fung CP, Lee SH, Yang TL, Huang CS. Nosocomial gram-negative bacteremia in critically ill patients: epidemiologic characteristics and prognostic factors in 147 episodes. J Formos Med Assoc 1999; 98:465-473.

139. Ensor E, Humphrey HH, Peckham D, Webster C, Knox, AJ. Is *Burkholderia* (*Pseudomonas*) *cepacia* disseminated from cystic fibrosis patients during physiotherapy? J Hosp Infect 1996; 32:9-25.

140. Holmes A, Nolan R, Taylor R, Finley R, Riley M, Jiang RZ, Steinbach S, Goldstein R. An epidemic of *Burkholderia cepacia* transmitted between patients with and without cystic fibrosis. J Infect Dis 1999; 179:1197-205.

141. Vandamme P, Holmes B, Vancanneyt M, Coenye T, Hoste B, Coopman R, Revets H, Lauwers S, Gillis M, Kersters K, Govan JR. Occurrence of multiple genomovars of *Burkholderia cepacia* in cystic fibrosis patients and proposal of *Burkholderia multivorans* sp. nov. Int J Syst Bacteriol 1997; 47:1188-1200.

142. Christenson JC, Welch DF, Mukwaya G, Muszynski MJ, Weaver RE, Brenner DJ. Recovery of *Pseudomonas gladioli* from respiratory tract specimens of patients with cystic fibrosis J Clin Microbiol 1989; 35:1398-1403.

143. Clode FE, Metherell LA, Pitt TL. Nosocomial acquisition of *Burkholderia gladioli* in patients with cystic fibrosis. Am J Respir Crit Care Med 1999; 160:374-375.

144. Arruda EA, Marinho IS, Boulos M, Sinto SI, Caiaffa HH, Mendes CM, Oplustil CP, Sader H, Levy CE, Levin AS. Nosocomial infections caused by multiresistant *Pseudomonas aeruginosa*. Infect Control Hosp Epidemiol 1999; 20:620-623.

145. Bonten MJ, Bergmans DC, Speijer H, Stobberingh EE. Characteristics of polyclonal endemicity of *Pseudomonas aeruginosa* colonization in intensive care units. Implications for infection control. Am J Respir Crit Care Med 1999; 160:1212-1219.

146. McDonald LC, Banerjee SM, Jarvis WR. Seasonal variation of *Acinetobacter* infections: 1987-1996. Clin Infect Dis 1999; 29:1133-1137.

147. Garcia-Garmendia JL, Ortiz-Leyba C, Garnacho-Montero J, Jimenez-Jimenez FJ, Monterrubio-Villar J, Gili-Miner M. Mortality and the increase in length of stay attributable to the acquisition of *Acinetobacter* in critically ill patients. Crit Care Med 1999; 27:1794-1799.

148. Seifert H, Dijkshoorn L, Gerner-Smidt P, Pelzer N, Tjernberg I, Vaneechoutte M. Distribution of *Acinetobacter* species on human skin: comparison of phenotypic and genotypic identification methods. J Clin Microbiol 1997; 35:2819-2925.

149. Van Pelt C, verduin CM, Goessens WH, Vos MC, Tummler B, Segonds C, Rebsaet F, Verbrugh H, van Belkum A. Identification of *Burkholderia* spp. in the clinical microbiology laboratory: comparison of conventional and molecular methods. J Clin Microbiol 1999; 37:2158-2164.

150. Gillis M, Van Van T, Bardin R, Goor M, Hebbar P, Willems A, Segers P, Kersters K, Heulin T, Fernandez MP. Polyphasic taxonomy in the genus *Burkholderia* leading to an amended description of the genus and proposition of *Burkholderia vietnamensis* sp. nov. for N2-fixing isolates from rice in Vietnam. Int J Syst Bacteriol 1995; 45:274-289.

151. Vandamme P, Mahenthiralingam E, Holmes B, Coenye T, Hoste B, De Vos P, Henry D, Speert DP. Identification and population structure of *Burkholderia stabilis* sp. nov. (formerly *Burkholderia cepacia* genomovar IV) J Clin Microbiol 2000; 38:1042-1047.

152. Mahenthiralingam E, Coeyne T, Chung JW, Govan JR, Taylor P, Vandamme P. Diagnostically and experimentally useful panel of strains from *Burkholderia cepacia* complex. J Clin Microbiol 2000; 38:910-913.

153. Hauben L, Vauterin L, Moore ERB, Hoste B, Swings J. Genomic diversity of the genus *Stenotrophomonas*. Int J Syst Bacteriol 1999; 49:1749-1760.

154. Bernard K, Tessier S, Munro C, Oughton M, Tyler S. Characterization of two clusters of previously undescribed gram-negative bacteria, possibly genus *Stenotrophomonas* species nova. Abstr. C407. In: Abstracts of the 96th General Meeting of the American Society for Microbiology. Washington, DC:American Society for Microbiology, 1996:73.

155. Willems A, Falsen E, Pot B, Jantzen E, Hoste B, Vandamme P, Gillis M, Kersters K, De Ley J. *Acidovorax*, a new genus for *Pseudomonas facilis*, *Pseudomonas delafieldii*, E. Falsen (EF) group 13, EF group 16, and several clinical isolates, with the species *Acidovorax facilis* comb. nov., *Acidovorax delafieldii* comb. nov., and *Acidovorax temperans* sp. nov. Int J Syst Bacteriol 1990; 40:384-398.

156. Wallace PL, Hollis DG, Weaver RE, Moss CW. Biochemical and chemical characterization of pink-pigmented oxidative bacteria. J Clin Microbiol 1990; 28:689-693.

157. Yabuuchi E, Kawamura Y, Kosako Y, Ezaki T. Emendation of genus *Achromobacter* and *Achromobacter xylosoxidans* (Yabuuchi and Yano) and proposal of *Achromobacter ruhlandii* (Packer and Vishniac) comb. nov., *Achromobacter piechaudii* (Kiredjian et al.) comb. nov., and *Achromobacter xylosoxidans* subsp. denitrificans (Ruger and Tan) comb. nov. Microbiol Immunol 1998; 42:429-438.

158. Holmes B, Costas M, Wood AC, Owen RJ, Morgan DD. Differentiation of *Achromobacter*-like strains from human blood by DNA restriction endonuclease digest and ribosomal RNA gene probe patterns. Epidemiol Infect 1990; 105:541-551.

159. Holmes B, Costas M, Wood AC, Kersters K. Numerical analysis of electrophoretic protein patterns of '*Achromobacter*' group B, E and F strains from human blood. J Appl Bacteriol 1990; 68:495-504.

160. Holmes B, Moss CW, Daneshvar MI Cellular fatty acid compositions of "*Achromobacter* groups B and E". J Clin Microbiol 1993; 31:1007-1008.

161. Bernardet J-F, Segers P, Vancanneyt M, Berthe F, Kersters K, Vandamme P. Cutting a Gordian knot: amended classification and description of the genus *Flavobacterium*, emended description of the family *Flavobacteriaceae*, and proposal of *Flavobacterium hydatis*, nom. nov. (basonym, *Cytophaga aquatilis* Strohl and Tait 1978). Int J Syst Bacteriol 1996; 46:128-148.

162. Hollis DG, Moss CW, Daneshvar MI, Wallace-Shewmaker PL. CDC group IIc: phenotypic characteristics, fatty acid composition, and isoprenoid quinone content. J Clin Microbiol 1996; 34:2322-2324

163. Hollis DG, Daneshvar MI, Moss CW, Baker CN. Phenotypic characteristics, fatty acid composition, and isoprenoid quinone content of CDC group IIg bacteria. J Clin Microbiol 1995; 33:762-764.

164. Wilson R, Dowling RB. *Pseudomonas aeruginosa* and other related species. Thorax 1998; 53:213-219.

165. Hendry J, Elborn JS, Nixon L, Shale DJ, Webb AK. Cystic fibrosis: inflammatory response to infection with *Burkholderia cepacia* and *Pseudomonas aeruginosa*. Eur Respir J 1999; 14:435-438.

166. Ernst RK, Yi EC, Guo L, Lim KB, Burns JL, Hackett M, Miller SI. Specific lipopolysaccharide found in cystic fibrosis airway *Pseudomonas aeruginosa*. Science 1999; 286:1561-1565.

167. de Bentzmann S, Polette M, Zahm JM, Hinrasky J, Kilezky C, Bajolet O, Klossek JM, Filloux A, Lazdunski A, Puchelle E. *Pseudomonas aeruginosa* virulence factors delay airway epithelial wound repair by altering the actin cytoskeleton and inducing overactivation of epithelial matrix metalloproteinase-2. Lab Invest 2000; 80:209-219.

168. Lee N, Jung SB, Ahn BY, Kim YH, Kim J, Kim D, Kim I, Yoon SM, Nam SW, Kim H, Park WJ. Immunization of burn patients with a *Pseudomonas aeruginosa* outer membrane protein vaccine elicits antibodies with protective efficacy. Vaccine 2000; 18:1952-1961.

169. Saini LS, Galsworthy SB, John MA, Valvano MA. Intracellular survival of *Burkholderia cepacia* complex isolates in the presence of macrophage cell activation. Microbiology 1999; 145:3465-3475.

170. Evans E, Poxton IR, Govan JR. Lipopolysaccharide chemotypes of *Burkholderia cepacia*. J Med Microbiol 1999; 48:825-832.

171. Sajjan US, Sylvester FA, Forstner JF. Cable-piliated *Burkholderia cepacia* binds to cytokeratin 13 of epithelial cells. Infect Immun 2000; 68:1787-1795.

171a. Clode FE, Kaufmann ME, Malnick H, Pitt TL. Distribution of genes encoding putative transmissibility factors among epidemic and nonepidemic strains of *Burkholderia cepacia* from cystic fibrosis patients in the United Kingdom. J Clin Microbiol 2000; 38:1763-1766.

172. Hendry J, Nixon L, Dodd M, Elborn JS, Govan J, Shale DJ, Webb AK. Pulmonary function, serum markers of inflammation, and IgG antibodies to core lipopolysaccharide of *Burkholderia cepacia* in adults with cystic fibrosis, following colonization with *Burkholderia cepacia*. Pediatr Pulmonol 2000; 29:8-10.

173. Haase A, Janzen J, Barrett S, Currie B. Toxin production by *Burkholderia pseudomallei* strains and correlation with severity of melioidosis. J Med Microbiol 1997; 46:557-563.

174. Harley VS, Dance DA, Tovey G, McCrossan MV, Drasar BS. An ultrastructural study of the phagocytosis of *Burkholderia pseudomallei*. Microbios 1998; 94:35-45.

175. Brett PJ, Woods DE. Pathogenesis of and immunity to melioidosis. Acta Trop 2000; 74:201-210.

176. Denton M, Kerr KG. Microbiological and clinical aspects of infection associated with *Stenotrophomonas maltophilia*. Clin Microbiol Rev 1998; 11:57-80.

177. Wauters G, Boel A, Voorn GP, Verhaegen J, Meunier F, Janssens M, Verbist L. Evaluation of a new identification system, Crystal Enteric/Non-Fermenter, for gram-negative bacilli. J Clin Microbiol 1995; 33:845-849.

178. Funke G, Monnet D, deBernardis C, von Graevenitz A, Freney J. Evaluation of the VITEK 2 system for rapid identification of medically relevant gram-negative rods. J Clin Microbiol 1998; 36:1948-1952.

179. O'Hara CM, Westbrook GL, Miller JM. Evaluation of Vitek GNI+ and Becton Dickinson Microbiology Systems Crystal E/NF identification systems for identification of members of the family *Enterobacteriaceae* and other gram-negative, glucose-fermenting and non-glucose-fermenting bacilli. J Clin Microbiol 1997; 35:3269-3273.

180. Miller J, O'Hare CM. Manual and automated systems for microbial identification. In: Murray PR, Baron EJ, Pfaller MA, Tenover FC, Yolken RH, eds. Manual of Clinical Microbiology. Washington, DC:ASM Press, 1999:193-201.

181. Sung LL, Yang DI, Hung CC, Ho HT. Evaluation of autoSCAN-W/A and the Vitek GNI+AutoMicrobic system for identification of non-glucose-fermenting gram-negative bacilli. J Clin Microbiol 2000; 38:1127-1130.

182. Klaerner H, Eschenbach U, Kamereck K, Lehn N, Wagner H, Miethke T. Failure of an automated blood culture system to detect nonfermentative gram-negative bacteria. J Clin Microbiol 2000; 38:1036-1041.

183. Vandamme P, Pot B, Gillis M, de Vos P, Kersters K, Swings J. Polyphasic taxonomy, a consensus approach to bacterial systematics. Microbiol Rev 1996; 60:407-438.

184. Tang YW, Ellis NM, Hopkins MK, Smith DH, Dodge DE, Persing DH. Comparison of phenotypic and genotypic techniques for identification of unusual aerobic pathogenic gram-negative bacilli. J Clin Microbiol 1998; 36:3674-3679.

185. Welch DF. Applications of cellular fatty acid analysis. Clin Microbiol Rev 1991; 4:422-438.

186. Kellogg JA, Bankert DA, Brenneman TM, Grove MA, Wetzel SL, Young KS. Identification of clinical isolates of non-*Enterobacteriaceae* gram-negative rods by computer-assisted gas-liquid chromatography. J Clin Microbiol 1996; 34:1003-1006.

187. Yamamoto S, Bouvet PJ, Harayama S. Phylogenetic structures of the genus *Acinetobacter* based on *gyr*B sequences: comparison with the grouping by DNA-DNA hybridization. Int J Syst Bacteriol 1999; 49:87-95.

188. Henry DA, Campbell ME, LiPuma JJ. Identification of *Burkholderia cepacia* isolates from patients with cystic fibrosis and use of a simple new selective medium. J Clin Microbiol 1997; 35:614-619.

189. Henry D, Campbell M, McGimpsey C, Clarke A, Louden L, Burns JL, Roe MH, Vandamme P, Speert D. Comparison of isolation media for recovery of *Burkholderia cepacia* complex from respiratory secretions of patients with cystic fibrosis. J Clin Microbiol 1999; 37:1004-1007.

190. Flanagan PG, Paull A. Isolation of *Burkholderia* cepacia by enrichment. J Clin Pathol 1998; 51:557-558.

191. LiPuma JJ, Dulaney BJ, McMenamin JD, Whitby PW, Stull TL, Coenye T, Vandamme P. Development of rRNA-based PCR assays for identification of *Burkholderia cepacia* complex isolates recovered from cystic fibrosis patients. J Clin Microbiol 1999; 37:3167-3170.

192. Ghozzi R, Morand P, Ferroni A, Beretti JL, Bingen E, Segonds C, Husson MO, Izard D, Berche P, Gaillard JL. Capillary electrophoresis-single-strand conformation polymorphism analysis for rapid identification of *Pseudomonas aeruginosa* and other gram-negative nonfermenting bacilli recovered from patients with cystic fibrosis. J Clin Microbiol 1999; 37:3374-3379.

193. Coenye T, Holmes B, Kersters K, Govan JR, Vandamme P. *Burkholderia cocovenenans* (van Damme et al. 1960) Gillis et al. 1995 and *Burkholderia vandii* Urakami et al. 1994 are junior synonyms of *Burkholderia gladioli* (Severini 1913) Yabuuchi et al. 1993 and *Burkholderia plantarii* (Azegami et al. 1987) Urakami et al. 1994, respectively. Int J Syst Bacteriol 1999; 49:37-42.

194. Whitby PW, Pope LC, Carter KB, LiPuma JJ, Stull TL. Species-specific PCR as a tool for the identification of *Burkholderia gladioli*. J Clin Microbiol 2000; 38:282-285.

195. Wuthiekanun V, Smith MD, Dance DA, Walsh AL, Pitt TL, White NJ. Biochemical characteristics of clinical and environmental isolates of *Burkholderia pseudomallei*. J Med Microbiol 1996; 45:408-412.

196. Brett PJ, Deshazer D, Woods DE. Characterization of *Burkholderia pseudomallei* and *Burkholderia pseudomallei*-like strains. Epidemiol Infect 1997; 118:137-148.

197. Brett PJ, DeShazer D, Woods DE. *Burkholderia thailandensis* sp. nov., a *Burkholderia pseudomallei*-like species. Int J Syst Bacteriol 1998; 48:317-320.

198. Parry CM, Wuthiekanun V, Hoa NT, Diep TS, Thao LT, Loc PV, Wills BA, Wain J, Hien TT, White NJ, Farrar JJ. Melioidosis in Southern Vietnam: clinical surveillance and environmental sampling. Clin Infect Dis 1999; 29:1323-1326.

199. Woods DE. Species versus biotype status. J Clin Microbiol 1999; 37:3786-3787.

200. Centers for Disease Control and Prevention. Office of Health and Safety. BMBL Section VII Agent Summary Statements. Section VII-A: Bacterial Agents. 2000.
URL:http://www.cdc.gov/od/ohs/biosfty/bmbl4/bmbl4s7a.htm

201. Euzeby JP. Risk group classification (bacteria): European Community classification. 2000.
URL:http://www-sv.cict.fr/bacterio/hazard.html#group3

202. Health Canada. Risk Group 3 Agents: requiring containment Level 3 2000.
URL:http://www.hc-sc.gc.ca/hpb/lcdc/biosafty/docs/lbg4_e.html#4.6.3

203. Inglis TJ, Chiang D, Lee GS, Chor-Kiang L. Potential misidentification of *Burkholderia pseudomallei* by API 20NE. Pathology 1998; 30:62-64.

204. Pongsunk S, Thirawattanasuk N, Piyasangthong N, Ekpo P. Rapid identification of *Burkholderia pseudomallei* in blood cultures by a monoclonal antibody assay. J Clin Microbiol 1999; 37:3662-3667.

205. Dharakul T, Songsivilai S, Smithikarn S, Thepthai C, Leelaporn A. Rapid identification of *Burkholderia pseudomallei* in blood cultures by latex agglutination using lipopolysaccharide-specific monoclonal antibody. Am J Trop Med Hyg 1999; 61:658-662.

206. Bouvet PJ, Grimont PA. Identification and biotyping of clinical isolates of *Acinetobacter*. Ann Inst Pasteur Microbiol 1987; 138:569-578.

207. Bouvet PJ, Jeanjean S. Delineation of new proteolytic genomic species in the genus *Acinetobacter*. Res Microbiol 1989; 140:291-299.

208. Tjernberg I, Ursing J. Clinical strains of *Acinetobacter* classified by DNA-DNA hybridization. APMIS 1989; 97:595-605.

209. Ibrahim A, Gerner-Smidt P, Liesack W. Phlyogenetic relationship of the twenty-one DNA groups of the genus *Acinetobacter* as revealed by 16S ribosomal DNA sequence analysis. Int J Syst Bacteriol 1997; 47:837-841.

210. Rainey FA, Lang E, Stackebrandt E. The phylogenetic structure of the genus *Acinetobacter*. FEMS Microbiol Lett 1994; 124:349-353.

211. Dolzani L, Tonin E, Lagatolla C, Prandin L, Monti-Bragadin C. Identification of *Acinetobacter* isolates in the *A. calcoaceticus-A. baumannii* complex by restriction analysis of the 16S-23S rRNA intergenic-spacer sequences. J Clin Microbiol 1995; 33:1108-1113.

212. Siau H, Yuen KY, Ho PL, Luk WK, Wong SS, Woo PC, Lee RA, Hui WT. Identification of acinetobacters on blood agar in presence of D-glucose by unique browning effect. J Clin Microbiol 1998; 36:1404-1407.

213. Khashe S, Janda JM. Biochemical and pathogenic properties of *Shewanella alga* and *Shewanella putrefaciens*. J Clin Microbiol 1998; 36:783-787.

214. Sikorski J, Rossello-Mora R, Lorenz MG. Analysis of genotypic diversity and relationships among *Pseudomonas stutzeri* strains by PCR-based genomic fingerprinting and multilocus enzyme electrophoresis. Syst Appl Microbiol 1999; 22:393-402.

215. Hsueh PR, Teng LJ, Pan HJ, Chen YC, Sun CC, Ho SW, Luh KT. Outbreak of *Pseudomonas fluorescens* bacteremia among oncology patients. J Clin Microbiol 1998; 36:2914-2917.

216. Welch DF, Slater LN. *Bartonella* and *Afipia*. In: Murray PR, Baron EJ, Pfaller MA, Tenover FC, Yolken RH, eds. Manual of Clinical Microbiology. Washington, DC:ASM Press, 1999:638-646.

217. Moss CW, Holzer G, Wallace PL, Hollis DG. Cellular fatty acid compositions of an unidentified organism and a bacterium associated with cat scratch disease. J Clin Microbiol 1990; 28:1071-1074.

218. Barham WB, Church P, Brown JE, Paparello S. Misidentification of *Brucella* species with use of rapid bacterial identification systems. Clin Infect Dis 1993; 18:1068-1069.

219. Weyant RS, Daneshvar MI, Jordan JG, Macgregor JP, Hollis DG. Eugonic oxidizer group 4: an unusual Gram-negative bacterium isolated from clinical specimens. Abstr. C196. In: Abstracts of the 99th General Meeting of the American Society for Microbiology. Washington, DC: American Society for Microbiology, 1999:144.

220. Daneshvar MI, Hollis DG, Moss CW, Jordan JG, Macgregor JP, Weyant RS. Eugonic oxidizer group 5: an unusual Gram-negative nonfermenter isolated from clinical specimens. Abstr. C204. In: Abstracts of the 98th General Meeting of the American Society for Microbiology. Washington, DC:American Society for Microbiology, 1998:165.

221. Moss CW, Daneshvar MI, Hollis DG. Biochemical characteristics and fatty acid composition of Gilardi rod group 1 bacteria. J Clin Microbiol 1993; 31:689-691.

222. Livesley MA, Baxter IA, Lambert PA, Govan JR, Weller PH, Lacey DE, Allison DG, Giwercman B, Hoiby N. Subspecific differentiation of *Burkholderia cepacia* isolates in cystic fibrosis. J Med Microbiol 1998; 47:999-1006.

223. Martin C, Boyd EF, Quentin, R., Massicot P, Selander RK. Enzyme polymorphism in *Pseudomonas aeruginosa* strains recovered from cystic fibrosis patients in France. Microbiology 1999; 145:2587-2594.

224. Segonds C, Heulin T, Marty N, Chabanon G. Differentiation of *Burkholderia* species by PCR-restriction fragment length polymorphism analysis of the 16S rRNA gene and application to cystic fibrosis isolates. J Clin Microbiol 1999; 37:2201-2208.

225. Okazaki M, Watanabe T, Morita K, Higurashi Y, Araki K, Shukuya N, Baba S, Watanabe N, Egami T, Furuya N, Kanamori M, Shimazaki S, Uchimura H. Molecular epidemiological investigation using a randomly amplified polymorphic DNA assay of *Burkholderia cepacia* isolates from nosocomial outbreaks. J Clin Microbiol 1999; 37:3809-3814.

226. Romling U, Tummler B. Achieving 100% typeability of *Pseudomonas aeruginosa* by pulsed-field gel electrophoresis. J Clin Microbiol 2000; 38:464-465.

227. Liu PY, Shi ZY, Lau YJ, Hu BS, Shyr JM, Tsai WS, Lin YH, Tseng CY. Epidemiological typing of *Flavimonas oryzihabitans* by PCR and pulsed-field gel electrophoresis. J Clin Microbiol 1996; 34:68-70.
228. Chetoui H, Melin P, Struelens MJ, Delhalle E, Nigo MM, De Ryck R, De Mol P. Comparison of biotyping, ribotyping, and pulsed-field gel electrophoresis for investigation of a common-source outbreak of *Burkholderia pickettii* bacteremia. J Clin Microbiol 1997; 35:1398-1403.
229. Biendo M, Laurans G, Lefebvre JF, Daoudi F, Eb F. Epidemiological study of an *Acinetobacter baumannii* outbreak by using a combination of antibiotyping and ribotyping. J Clin Microbiol 1999; 37:2170-2175.
230. Dijkshoorn L, Van harsselaar B, Tjernberg I, Bouvet PJ, Vaneechoutte M. Evaluation of amplified ribosomal DNA restriction analysis for idenfication of *Acinetobacter* genomic species. Syst Appl Microbiol 1998; 21:33-39.
231. Koeleman JG, Stoof J, Biesmans DJ, Savelkoul PH, Vandenbroucke-Grauls CM. Comparison of amplified ribosomal DNA restriction analysis, random amplified polymorphic DNA analysis, and amplified fragment length polymorphism fingerprinting for identification of *Acinetobacter* genomic species and typing of *Acinetobacter baumannii*. J Clin Microbiol 1998; 36:2522-2529.
232. Yoo JH, Choi JH, Shin WS, Huh DH, Cho YK, Kim KM, Kim MY, Kang MW. Application of infrequent-restriction site PCR to clinical isolates of *Acinetobacter baumannii* and *Serratia marcescens*. J Clin Microbiol 1999; 37:3594-3600.
233. Berg G, Roskot N, Smalla K. Genotypic and phenotypic relationships between clinical and environmental isolates of *Stenotrophomonas maltophilia*. J Clin Microbiol 1999; 37:3594-3600.
234. Garcia de Viedma D, Marin M, Cercenado E, Alonso R, Rodriguez-Creixems M, Bouza E. Evidence of nosocomial *Stenotrophomonas maltophilia* cross-infection in a neonatology unit analyzed by three molecular typing methods. Infect Control Hosp Epidemiol 1999; 20:816-820.
235. Lin YH, Liu PY, Shi ZY, Lau YJ, Hu BS. Comparison of polymerase chain reaction and pulsed-field gel electrophoresis for the epidemiological typing of *Alcaligenes xylosoxidans* subsp. xylosoxidans in a burn unit. Diagn Microbiol Infect Dis 1997; 28:173-178.
236. Knippschild M, Ansorg R. Epidemiological typing of *Alcaligenes xylosoxidans* subsp. xylosoxidans by antibacterial susceptibility testing, fatty acid analysis, PAGE of whole-cell protein and pulsed-field gel electrophoresis. Int J Med Microbiol Virol Parasitol Infect Dis 1998; 288:145-157.
237. National Committee for Clinical Laboratory Standards. Performance standards for antimicrobial susceptibility testing. Supplement M100-S10. Wayne, PA.:National Committee for Clinical Laboratory Standards, 2000.
238. National Committee for Clinical Laboratory Standards. Performance standards for antimicrobial disk susceptibility tests. Approved standard M2-A7. Wayne, PA.:National Committee for Clinical Laboratory Standards, 2000.
239. National Committee for Clinical Laboratory Standards. Methods for dilution antimicrobial susceptibility tests for bacteria that grow aerobically. Approved standard M7-A5. Wayne, PA.:National Committee for Clinical Laboratory Standards, 2000.
240. Saiman L, Burns JL, Whittier S, Krzewinski J, Marshall SA, Jones RN. Evaluation of reference dilution test methods for antimicrobial susceptibility testing of *Pseudomonas aeruginosa* strains isolated from patients with cystic fibrosis. J Clin Microbiol 1999; 37:2987-2991.
241. Harris A, Torres-Viera C, Venkataraman L, DeGirolami P, Samore M, Carmeli Y. Epidemiology and clinical outcomes of patients with multiresistant *Pseudomonas aeruginosa*. Clin Infect Dis 1999; 28:1128-1133.
242. Tsakris A, Pournaras S, Woodford N, Palepou MF, Babini GS, Douboyas J, Livermore DM. Outbreak of infections caused by *Pseudomonas aeruginosa* producing VIM-1 carbapenemase in Greece. J Clin Microbiol 2000; 38:1290-1292.
243. Gilligan PH. Report on the consensus document for microbiology and infectious diseases in cystic fibrosis. Clin Microbiol Newsl 1996; 18:83-87.6.
244. Burns JL, Saiman L, Whittier S, Larone D, Krzewinski J, Liu Z, Marshall SA, Jones RN. Comparison of agar diffusion methodologies for antimicrobial susceptibility testing of *Pseudomonas aeruginosa* isolates from cystic fibrosis patients. J Clin Microbiol 2000; 38:1818-1822.
245. Ruiz J, Nunez ML, Perez J, Simarro E, Martinez-Campos L, Gomez J. Evaluation of resistance among clinical isolates of *Acinetobacter* over a 6-year period. Eur J Clin Microbiol Infect Dis 1999; 18:292-295.
246. Visalli MA, Jacobs MR, Moore TD, Renzi FA, Appelbaum PC. Activities of beta-lactams against *Acinetobacter* genospecies as determined by agar dilution and Etest MIC methods. Antimicrob Agents Chemother 1997; 41:767-770.

247. Vila J, Ruiz J, Navia M, Becerril B, Garcia I, Perea S, Lopez-Hernandez I, Alamo I, Ballester F, Planes AM, Martinez-Beltran J, deAnta TJ. Spread of amikacin resistance in *Acinetobacter baumannii* strains isolated in Spain due to an epidemic strain. J Clin Microbiol 1999; 37:758-761.
248. Da Silva GJ, Leitao GJ, Peixe L. Emergence of carbapenem-hydrolyzing enzymes in *Acinetobacer baumannii* clinical isolates. J Clin Microbiol 1999; 37:2109-2110.
249. Takahashi A, Yomoda S, Kobayashi I, Okubo T. Detection of carbapenemase-producing *Acinetobacter baumannii* in a hospital. J Clin Microbiol 2000; 38:526-529.
250. Chang JC, Hsueh PR, Wu JJ, Ho SW, Hsieh WC, Luh KT. Antimicrobial susceptibility of flavobacteria as determined by agar dilution and disk diffusion methods. Antimicrob Agents Chemother 1997; 41:1301-1306.
251. Nishimura Y, Ino T, Iizuka H. *Acinetobacter radioresistans* sp. nov. isolated from cotton and soil. Int J Syst Bacteriol 1988; 38:209-211.

18

Gram Negative Infections: *Haemophilus* and Other Clinically Relevant Gram Negative Coccobacilli

José Campos and Juan A. Saez-Nieto
Centro Nacional de Microbiología, Instituto de Salud Carlos III, Madrid, Spain

I.   HISTORICAL BACKGROUND

A.   *Haemophilus* spp.

Pfeiffer first reported *Haemophilus influenzae* in 1892 as the primary agent of epidemic influenza. In the 1930s, based on the capsular polysaccharide composition, Pittman identified six *H. influenzae* serotypes (a to f) (1). In 1988, conjugate vaccines which prevent *H. influenzae* type b infection were first licensed; since then, most western countries have included this vaccine into their national vaccination programs with the subsequent result of a drastic reduction in the number of infections. According to the World Health Organization, however, the prevalence of *H. influenzae* type b invasive infections worldwide continues to be elevated as the vaccine has not been introduced in the majority of underdeveloped countries (2).

The most pathogenic member of the genus *Haemophilus* for humans is *H. influenzae*, followed by *H. parainfluenzae*, *H. ducreyi*, and *H. aphrophilus*; other less common species are *H. segnis*, *H. paraphrophilus*, *H. haemolyticus* and *H. parahaemolyticus*. The genus status of *H. ducreyi* and *H. aphrophilus* is questionable; *H. aegyptius* is very similar to *H. influenzae* biotype III; *H. parahaemolyticus* appears to be also very similar to *H. parainfluenzae* biotype III, and *H. segnis* is closely related to *H. parainfluenzae* biotype IV (3,4).

B.   Non-*Haemophilus* spp.

The bacteria in this group, as we discuss herein, are commonly referred to as "fastidious bacteria"; the term in this context has been applied to micro-organisms that grow poorly or not at all on conventional media and that require prolonged incubation in microaerophilic or capnophilic atmospheres before growth is detected (4,5). The micro-organisms within this group can vary in size from small coccobacilli (e.g., *Kingella*) to fusiform and with curved shapes (e.g., *Capnocytophaga*). The inclusion of non-coccobacilli in this chapter relates to historic issues as well as common concerns that arise within the laboratory. Some of them are included in the "HACEK group" (*Haemophilus aphrophilus/H. paraphrophilus, Actinobacillus actinomycetemcomitans, Cardiobacterium hominis, Eikenella corrodens, Kingella* spp.) which is a historic term used to designate this collection of somewhat similar and fastidious bacteria (6).

The genera *Actinobacillus, Pasteurella*, and *Haemophilus* are closely related: similar % G+C, phenotypic features, and in having animal reservoirs for human disease (*Actinobacillus, Pasteurella*). These three groups present problems of differentiation at the genus level (3) and several changes of nomenclature have been proposed (3). The genus *Actinobacillus* includes ten species. It has been proposed that some of them should be transferred to *Haemophilus*, e.g., *H.* (*A.*) *actinomycetemcomitans* (7) or to *Actinobacillus* from *Haemophilus*, e.g., *A.* (*H.*) *pleuropneumoniae* (8) or from *Pasteurella* to *Actinobacillus*, e.g., *A.* (*P.*) *ureae* (9). The species of *Actinobacillus* included in this chapter are: *A.* (*H.*) *actinomycetemcomitans, A. equuli, A. hominis, A. lignieresii, A. suis, A. ureae, A. minor, A. muris,* and *A. capsulatus*.

Slotnick and Dougherty proposed the name *Cardiobacterium hominis* in 1964 (10) for a *Pasteurella*-like bacterium that was isolated previously from the blood of patients with endocarditis.

Suttonella indologenes was previously named *Kingella indologenes* and is included now in the Family *Cardiobacteriaceae* together with the genera *Cardiobacterium* and *Dichelobacter* (11).

Eiken in 1958 (12) found that most of the strains previously described as "corroding bacillus" and named *Bacteroides corrodens* were microaerophilic or facultatively anaerobic; they were renamed *E. corrodens* by Jackson and Goodman in 1972 (13).

Henriksen and Bovre in 1976 transferred the species *Moraxella kingii* to the new genus *Kingella* (14). These organisms are non-motile, non-spore forming, Gram negative rods, and are included in the family *Neisseriaceae*. The species included in the genus *Kingella* are: *K. denitrificans, K. kingae,* and the recently described *K. orale* (previously *K. oralis*) which was isolated from human dental plaque (15).

The genus *Chromobacterium* includes two species: *C. violaceum* and *C. fluviale* (3). Only the first species has been implicated in human disease.

Calymmatobacterium granulomatis (formerly *Donovania granulomatis*) was named by Aragao and Vianna in 1913 (16) and renamed as *Donovania* by Anderson et al. (17).

Williams et al. gave the historical background of *Capnocytophaga* in 1979 (18). After several author descriptions of species such as *Ristella ochracea, Bacteroides oralis, Bacteroides ochraceus,* and CDC group DF-1, Leadbetter et al. isolated strains from dental plaque that were capnophilic and showed gliding motility, and incorporated these into in a new genus *Capnocytophaga* (19). The species included in this genus are: *C. gingivalis, C. ochracea, C. sputigena, C. granulosa,* and *C. haemolytica* from human oral flora; and *C. canimorsus* and *C. cynodegmi* that colonize the oral cavity of dogs.

II. CLINICAL ASPECTS

A. *H. influenzae*

This organism causes two major types of infection: a) *invasive* (meningitis, septicemia, bacteremia, epiglottitis, pneumonia, arthritis, cellulitis, osteomyelitis, and pericarditis), often acute and life-threatening, caused by encapsulated (typeable) strains, generally b, although other types have also been described particularly e and f (20), and b) *non-invasive*, mostly due to unencapsulated (non-typeable) strains, less serious but more common, that generally involve the respiratory tract (otitis, sinusitis, conjunctivitis, and bronchial infections) and other mucosal infections. Many exceptions do exist, however, as unencapsulated strains are well-recognized invasive pathogens in patients with impaired immune response such as neonatal sepsis and pneumonia and other infections in the elderly. Outbreaks of a new syndrome,

Brazilian Purpuric Fever, were described in young children who presented with a clinical picture similar to meningococcemia but which were caused by unencapsulated *H. influenzae* biotype aegyptius (21,22).

1. Clinical manifestations caused by H. influenzae type b strains

Meningitis is the most serious of the systemic infections that are caused by the organism. It is usually a disease of young children; adult cases are rare, often appearing as a result of head trauma, CSF leak, neurosurgery, sinusitis, otitis, and deterioration of the immune system. No clinical features distinguish *H. influenzae* type b meningitis from other types of purulent meningitis. The most common signs are fever and altered central nervous system function. Previous upper respiratory infection including otitis media are common but the onset can also be fulminating with death occurring in a few hours, particularly in children younger than one year old. Before effective vaccines were available, mortality from meningitis caused by *H. influenzae* type b was about 5% in developed countries and much higher in the developing world. Permanent neurological damage occurred in 15-20% of survivors. Antibiotic resistance to ampicillin and/or chloramphenicol also compromised effective treatment before third generation cephalosporins became available (23).

Epiglottitis is a potentially lethal disease of acute onset causing acute respiratory obstruction due to cellulitis and local edema of the supraglottis in children aged two to five years. Initial symptoms include sore throat, fever, and dyspnea which may progress rapidly to airway obstruction within a few hours. Blood cultures are usually positive for *H. influenzae* type b.

Cellulitis usually occurs in young children who present with fever and a reddish-blue tender area that is most often located on one cheek or in the periorbital region and that progresses rapidly to soft tissue involvement. Accompanying bacteremia is very common and other localized infections, like meningitis, may be present.

The true frequency of pneumonia due to *H. influenzae* is unknown as only bacteremic cases with positive blood cultures are usually recognized. Patient age is usually four months to four years. Primary pneumonia can be accompanied by other infections like meningitis, epiglottitis, and otitis. In adults, *H. influenzae* pneumonia is increasingly recognized as a consequence of previous lung diseases and alcoholism.

In children of two years or younger, *H. influenzae* used to be the most common cause of arthritis which involves a single large weight-bearing joint without co-existent osteomyelitis. Cultures of blood and joint fluid are normally positive. The child presents with decreased mobility, pain, and swelling. Response to treatment with systemic antibiotics is excellent although long-term follow-up is necessary because of residual joint dysfunction.

2. Diseases caused by non-typeable H. influenzae

These organisms are important causes of pneumonia in children and adults, particularly among the elderly and among patients with chronic lung diseases. Usually, only bacteremic cases are diagnosed. Clinical symptoms are similar to that of other bacterial pneumonias. In poor countries, acute pneumonia in infants due to non-typeable *H. influenzae* is an important cause of morbidity and mortality. The organism can be recovered in high colony counts, alone or with other micro-organisms, from the sputum of patients with exacerbations of chronic bronchitis and cystic fibrosis (24).

Non-typeable *H. influenzae* is a well-documented cause of tubo-ovarian abscess, salpingitis, amnionitis, and endometritis, especially after premature rupture of membranes. In this context, they may occasionally be associated with septicemia. Infants who are born to such mothers may develop life-threatening neonatal septicemia, meningitis, and acute respiratory distress syndrome which is clinically indistinguishable from early-onset Group B streptococcal disease.

The micro-organisms are important causes of purulent conjunctivitis that can occur in outbreaks during cold months. The most frequent causative strains are *H. influenzae* biotype aegyptius although other biotypes can also be involved. In 1984, a new disease was described in Brazil among children who developed life-threatening infections caused by biotype aegyptius, known as Brazilian Purpuric Fever, and which were characterized by purulent conjunctivitis, high fever, purpura, vascular collapse, and high mortality. In most cases, blood cultures, but not CSF, are positive for biotype aegyptius (21,22).

Acute otitis media is a common illness in children of five months to five years. It is estimated that 20 to 30% of cases of acute bacterial otitis are caused by non-typeable *H. influenzae*. It is also a common cause of sinusitis in both children and adults.

It is well established that non-typeable *H. influenzae* can cause invasive infections both in children and adults (25). Predisposing underlying conditions include alcoholism, malignancy, chronic obstructive pulmonary disease, and human immunodeficiency virus (HIV) infection (26,27).

B. Other *Haemophilus* spp.

H. parainfluenzae is the most frequently isolated pathogen among the *Haemophilus* spp. group. Reported infections include otitis, conjunctivitis, dental abscess, pneumonia, empyema, septicemia, endocarditis, septic arthritis, osteomyelitis, peritonitis, hepatobiliary infection, meningitis, brain abscess, urinary tract, and genital (prostatic and urethral) infection (28-31). *H. aphrophilus* has been described as a cause of sinusitis, otitis, pneumonia, osteomyelitis, and soft tissue abscesses. *H. paraphrophilus* causes endocarditis, brain abscess, hepatobiliary infection, osteomyelitis, and others (32). *H. parainfluenzae*, *H. aphrophilus*, and *H. paraphrophilus* may be the etiological agents in 5% of cases of endocarditis which are secondary to dental procedures or oral trauma. Other predisposing factors include respiratory tract infections, intravenous drug abuse and underlying valvular heart disease (33). Secondary embolization in *Haemophilus* spp. endocarditis can occur in the 50-60% of cases. Polymicrobial endocarditis caused by *H. parainfluenzae* and Gram positive cocci has been described among intravenous drug abusers.

Soft chancre or 'Chancroid' is a sexually transmitted disease that is caused by *H. ducreyi*. The median incubation period is 5-7 days. Lesions are generally confined to the genitalia and perianal areas, and usually begin as tender papules with erythema which become pustular and, later on, form an ulcer that is painful and non-indurated. Ulcers may be single or multiple. Inguinal lymphadenopathy, usually unilateral and painful, occurs in half of the patients. Only 10% of cases are reported in women probably due to an asymptomatic state and/or under-recognized lesions. Infected prostitutes can serve as reservoirs for outbreaks, both among the military and civilians (34).

C. Non-*Haemophilus* spp.

Although these bacteria are recognized as relevant causes of endocarditis (35,36), they can also cause of a broad range of serious infections such as bacteremias, abscesses, and periodontal infections. In the other hand, several of these species are isolated from animal bite wounds particularly some actinobacilli and others (4,37). The most relevant species of Gram negative coccobacilli that are isolated in human infections are included in part in this chapter and listed in Table 1.

1. *Actinobacillus spp.*

Actinobacillus spp. are inhabitants of the upper respiratory and genitourinary tracts of humans and animals. These micro-organisms produce several infections when introduced into healthy tissues by means of trauma or localized injury (e.g., animal bite). These infections are more common in immunocompromised patients.

In humans, *A. hominis*, *A. ureae*, and *A. actinomycetemcomitans* are primarily associated with disease. Other species colonize animals such as horses, pigs, cattle, and others, and these sources may serve as reservoirs for opportunistic infections usually after animal bites. *A. ureae* and *A. hominis* are isolated from sputum and tracheal secretions from patients with chronic respiratory diseases. Occasionally, episodes of bacteremia and meningitis have been reported (38). *A. lignieresii* and *A. equuli* are involved in animal bites and can be isolated from wound and blood samples (39).

A. actinomycetemcomitans is a small Gram negative coccobacillus that is associated with juvenile periodontal disease, bacteremia, endocarditis, and abcesses (40-43). The principal predisposing factors for the development of native or prosthetic valve endocarditis due to this micro-organism include poor dentition and recent dental manipulations. Complications include septic emboli, congestive heart failure, hematogenous dissemination, and death (41,43). Other infections caused by *A. actinomycetemcomitans* result either by spread of the organism from its habitat in the mouth or from hematogenous spread during bacteremia. Cervical and submaxillary lymphadenitis, cellulitis, septic arthritis, urinary tract infections, pericarditis, and other localized infections have been reported (41). The organism is specifically associated with a distinct clinical entity called localized juvenile periodontitis (44) but a cause-and-effect relationship is not certain.

Table 1   Relevant genera and species included in the Gram negative coccobacilli group (as discussed within) according to the source of isolation (4). (* - URT: upper respiratory tract and/or dental plaque; ** - including wound and/or animal bites; + - majority of strains from genitourinary infections. Note: for *Pasteurella*, see Chapter 19)

Species	Source of Human Infection				Common Host
	URT*	Wound**	Blood	Other	
A. actinomycetemcomitans	X	X	X	X	human
A. equuli		X			equine, porcine, others
A. hominis	X				human
A. lignieresii		X			bovine, canine, rat, ovine
A. suis	X	X	X		bovine, equine, porcine
A. ureae	X		X	X	human
P. aerogenes		X			porcine
P. bettyae			X	X+	human
P. canis	X	X		X	canine, human
P. dagmatis	X	X	X	X	canine, feline
P. haemolytica	X	X			bovine, ovine, others
P. multocida	X	X	X	X	canine, feline, human
P. pneumotropica	X	X			canine, feline, rabbit, others
P. stomatis	X	X	X		feline
E. corrodens	X	X	X	X	human
C. hominis			X	X	human
S. indologenes			X	X	human
C. violaceum		X	X	X	human, water
K. denitrificans	X			X	human
K. kingae	X		X	X	human
K. oralis	X				
C. gingivalis	X		X	X	human
C. ochracea	X		X	X	human
C. sputigena	X		X	X	human
C. haemolytica	X				human
C. canimorsus		X	X	X	canine
C. cynodegni		X		X	canine
C. granulosa	X				human

Potential virulence factors for *A. actinomycetemcomitans* include the production of leukotoxin, collagenase, a bone-resorption inducing toxin, alkaline phosphatase and other (44-46).

2. C. hominis

Infection follows a subacute course with an insidious onset and vague symptoms, and can affect either natural or prosthetic heart valves (47). Several complications include septic emboli, mycotic aneurysm, and congestive heart failure. *C. hominis* is rarely associated with infections other than endocarditis, meningitis (48), or abdominal abscess (49).

3. S. indologenes

S. indologenes has been implicated in endocarditis (50) and human eye infections (51).

4. E. corrodens

This bacterium is part of the normal flora of the human upper respiratory tract, and it is associated both with dental and periodontal infections (52) (e.g., periapical abscess, gingivitis, root canal infections), ocular infections, and head and neck infections, and various others (53,54). Bacteremia and endocarditis are also among the more serious infections caused by *E. corrodens* (55-58).

5. Kingella and EF-4

K. kingae appears to have a specific tropism for joint, skeletal, and cardiac tissues, being an opportunistic pathogen that is responsible for endocarditis, osteomyelitis, and septicemia (59,60). These infections are most often seen in young children (61). *K. denitrificans* is a rare cause of septicemia and endocarditis (62,63). *K. oralis* has not been associated with any infection. EF-4 strains (EF4a and EF4b) are part of the normal oral flora of dogs (EF4a) and cats (EF4b), and produce disease in humans following animal bites and scratches (4).

6. C. violaceum

C. violaceum is an uncommon cause of serious pyogenic or septicemic infections in humans and other animals (64,65).

7. C. granulomatis

Growing bacteria form the characteristic "Donovan bodies". *C. granulomatis* is the presumed causative agent of granuloma inguinale, a rare but important cause of genital ulceration that occurs in small endemic foci with a worldwide distribution (66). The lesions of granuloma inguinale reveal: macrophages, neutrophils, lymphocytes, dendritic cells, and multinucleated giant cells. The primary lesion usually occurs in the urogenital area but the throat and/or mouth, neck, and nasopharynx can become infected after orogenital contact. Hematogenous spread to bones, liver, and other organs has been described (67,68).

8. Capnocytophaga spp.

Localized and systemic infections have been described among both immunocompromised and immunocompetent patients (69-71). *C. canimorsus* and *C. cynodegmi* are responsible for some infectious complications of dog bites (72,73).

III. EPIDEMIOLOGY OF INFECTION

A. *H. influenzae*

Whether encapsulated or not, humans are the natural and exclusive hosts for *Haemophilus influenzae*. The bacterium spreads from the upper respiratory tract, particularly pharynx, by airborne droplets. Up to 80% of healthy persons are naso-pharyngeal carriers. Usually, carriage of one or several strains is common but the vast majority of people are colonized with unencapsulated strains; in the general population only 1 to 5% of persons carry encapsulated strains, most commonly serotype b. In close contacts of cases of *H. influenzae* type b invasive infections, however, e.g., children in day care centers, up to 40% can be carriers of encapsulated strains (74).

Before the *H. influenzae* type b vaccine became available, the most serious clinical situation posed by *H. influenzae* was an acute illness in young children which was usually in the form of meningitis, epiglotittis, and pneumonia with or without septicemia. *H. influenzae* type b, which produces capsular polysaccharide made up of repeating units of ribosyl-ribitol phosphate (polyribose phosphate, PRP), accounted for almost 95% of the systemic *H. influenzae* infections in children (mostly aged <3 years and with a peak attack rate of 7-14 months). In the United States, about 8,000 cases of meningitis per year were diagnosed. It was estimated that about 1 in 200 children developed invasive *H. influenzae* type b disease before the age of five years. Alaskan Inuit, Navajo, and Apache Indians had attack rates higher than the general populations with a peak incidence of infection in much younger children. Epiglottitis occurred in older children of two to four years. The incidence was 20-50/100,000 cases in children of less of five years and much higher in developing regions (75). After massive immunization, the incidence in the United States declined by 96%, from 41/100,000 among children below five years to 1.6/100,000 cases in 1995 (76).

B. Other *Haemophilus* spp.

Haemophilus spp. that are described as human pathogens include *H. parainfluenzae*, *H. paraphrophilus*, and *H. ducreyi*. All *Haemophilus* spp. are members of the normal flora of the oral cavity and pharynx. *H. aphrophilus* and *H. segnis* are often found in dental plaque. *H. ducreyi* is a pathogen of the genital site. The infection is of worldwide distribution and typically is associated with low socioeconomic status and poor hygienic conditions. Major outbreaks have been reported. *H. parainfluenzae* can also be isolated from both the urethra and vagina.

C. Non-*Haemophilus* spp.

A common characteristic of several members of this group as we consider herein is that they are accepted as normal flora of the upper respiratory tract and dental plaque. After disturbance of the mucosal integrity, however, they can become invasive and pathogenic. Also, many of them are inhabitants of the respiratory tract of animals. The fact that these organisms are considered as uncommon pathogens may be due in part to the difficulties that are involved in their isolation as a consequence of their growth requirements and that may then complicate their identification in clinical samples. The natural habitat of *C. hominis* is the nose or throat (up to ¾) of healthy human subjects (10). *Kingella* spp. are part of the normal upper respiratory and genitourinary tract flora of humans. *C. violaceum* is common in tropics and is found in the soil and water.

IV. NATURE OF THE BACTERIUM, PATHOGENESIS, AND CLINICAL MANIFESTATIONS

A. *Haemophilus* spp.

Haemophilus spp. are Gram negative, occurring as a short rods or as coccobacilli which are variable in length with marked pleomorphism, non-motile, and aerobic or facultatively anaerobic. These bacteria require preformed growth factors, particularly X factor (protoporphyrin IX or protoheme) and/or V factor (nicotinamide adenine dinucleotide (NAD) or NAD phosphate (NADP) (3). The requirement for these factors, however, is not a definitive proof for *Haemophilus* spp. since some species of *Actinobacillus* and *Pasteurella* do need NAD (4). Other growth factors have been described like pantothenic acid, thiamine, and uracil; some strains also require a purine or cysteine. Complex media are generally required for growth such as chocolate agar. Optimum temperature for growth is 35-37°C. Usually, most species of the genus *Haemophilus* reduce nitrates to nitrites and are positive for alkaline phosphatase. Oxidase and catalase reactions vary among strains. All species have both a respiratory and fermentative type of metabolism. All occur as obligate parasites or commensals on the mucous membranes of humans and some animals. The mol % G+C of the DNA is 37-44. The cell walls resemble those of other Gram negative bacteria in structure, composition, and endotoxic activity. Fimbriae have been detected in hemagglutinating strains of *H. influenzae* and *H. aegyptius* (3).

1. H. influenzae

Non-typeable strains of *H. influenzae* are not micro-organisms that no longer express capsule, but rather are phylogenetically distinct from typeable strains; in contrast with non-typeable strains, encapsulated strains, particularly type b, express little genetic diversity (77). Variations of virulence in nontypeable strains have been correlated with lipopolysaccharide (LPS) composition (78). There are a number of important surface-exposed antigens in *H. influenzae* including proteins (P1, P2, P4, P5, P6 and others which have a variety of functions like adhesins, porins, pili, and proteases), capsules, and lipooligosaccharides (LPS). Most of these antigens undergo antigenic diversity and can therefore be used as epidemiological markers (79). The whole genome of *H. influenzae* strain Rd has been sequenced (80).

H. influenzae colonizes the human nasopharynx over an extended period of time despite specific mucosal antibodies. Explanations for prolonged carriage include intracellular persistence and surface antigenic variation among colonizing strains (81). *H. influenzae* also chronically infects patients with underlying respiratory tract disease such as cystic fibrosis or chronic obstructive pulmonary disease. In these patients, changes in the surface antigens of the organism result in the development of new epitopes which are not recognized by antibodies that are specific for the original infecting strain (82). The process of upper respiratory tract colonization and bloodstream invasion is not well understood. Microbial factors include surface adhesins such as fimbriae (pili), secretion of IgA1 proteases, and inhibition of human epithelial cells by lipopolysaccharide and heat-stable glycopeptide. The importance of type b capsule in the pathogenesis of invasive diseases is well established by genetic techniques and in the rat model of meningitis (83-85). After intranasal inoculation, *H. influenzae* type b invades the submucosa of the nasopharynx and enters the blood stream within minutes. Meningitis occurs secondarily to hematogenous spread. Duration and intensity of bacteremia correlates with meningitis. In the animal model, depletion of complement or splenectomy increases the incidence of meningitis. In contrast, immune stimulation with the administration of specific serum antibodies or other procedures decreases the severity of bacteremia and incidence of meningitis (84-86).

2. *Other Haemophilus spp.*

Pathogenicity of these species is low as compared with *H. influenzae*, and clinical infection is the consequence of local or bloodstream invasion from upper respiratory flora; they may cause local (head and respiratory tract) infection or systemic disease .

B. Non-*Haemophilus* spp.

Actinobacillus spp. are non-motile, gram negative, oval, spherical, or rod-shaped cells of 0.4 x 1 µm. They grow both aerobically and anaerobically at 37°C. Colonies in chocolate agar or sheep blood agar are small (1 to 2 mm.) and are very sticky from primary isolation on solid media.

C. *hominis* appears as pleomorphic rods that may form rosettes and clusters and with variable retention of the Gram stain. It is a facultative anaerobe which grows best on enriched media under microaerophilic conditions with CO_2 supplementation. After incubation for 48-72 hrs., colonies are yellowish to white and are approximately 1-2 mm. in diameter. Although the virulence of *C. hominis* appears to be extremely low, it is occasionally isolated from blood, usually from cases of endocarditis (87,88).

Cells of *S. indologenes* appear as Gram negative rods of 3 µm. length. As with *C. hominis* and *Kingella*, it resists decolorization with the Gram stain. Its colonies are small (1 mm.) and pitting of agar or spreading edges may occur. *S. indologenes* grows in a microaerophilic atmosphere.

E. *corrodens* are Gram negative, slender straight rods that characteristically form depressed or pitting colonies on the surface of agar media.

Kingella spp. are coccobacillary, 0.6-1 µm. in diameter and 2-3 µm. in length, and occur in pairs and short chains. EF-4 bacteria also have coccobacillary forms but appear singly.

C. *violaceum* is usually a rod-shaped Gram negative bacterium, 1.5 to 3.5 µm. in length, usually straight, and arranged singly, in pairs, or in short chains. Characteristic violet colonies are formed on simple media. Unpigmented variants may occur (4).

C. *granulomatis* is an intracellular Gram negative bacterium. The micro-organism has been linked to *Klebsiella* spp. by antigenic cross-reactions and due to the similarity of associated lesions with rhinoscleroma (*K. rhinoscleromatis*). Genetic and phylogenetic studies of *C. granulomatis* have found that it is closely related to the genus *Klebsiella* and it has been proposed that *C. granulomatis* should be reclassified as *Klebsiella granulomatis* comb. nov. (89,90).

Capnocytophaga spp. are short to elongate, flexible Gram negative rods or filaments of 2-5.7 µm. in length. They have gliding motility. Growth occurs with CO_2 supplementation (5%). The colonies are yellow-orange. The species *C. ochracea*, *C. gingivalis* and *C. sputigena* are opportunistic pathogens and have been implicated in adult and juvenile periodontitis (91).

V. IMMUNOLOGY

A. *H. influenzae*

Blood from young children generally lacks bactericidal activity against *H. influenzae* type b strains in contrast to the serum of neonates, older children, and adults (85). When antiserum that contains high levels of antibodies to the type b capsule were administrated as a treatment for meningitis, a dramatic increase in the phagocytic activity was observed thus suggesting that PRP had an antiphagocytic activity. Phagocytosis was increased by opsonization with type-specific antibodies (84). Anti-PRP serum antibodies are a major determinant in protective immunity as they activate complement-mediated bactericidal and opsonic (85) activity, and mediate protective immunity against systemic infections in humans (74). The antigenic stimulus for antibody development could be both the carriage of type b strains and exposure to commensals that have cross-reactive epitopes (86).

At the time of infection with *H. influenzae* type b, serum anti-PRP antibodies are low or absent, and in convalescence levels remain low in young infants. Failure to produce anti-PRP antibodies even after infection is related to the poor immune response of humans to polysaccharides and other T-cell independent antigens (86). The protective minimum serum antibody concentration is about 1.0 µg./ml. (135). Other factors, like the functional avidity of anti-PRP antibody subclasses and responses to other antigens such as LPS and membrane proteins, could also be important for protection (85).

The first generation of vaccines against *H. influenzae* type b consisted of the purified high molecular weight type b polysaccharide (PRP), but clinical trials showed that vaccine was effective in toddlers but did not protect infants of less than 18 months (135). In the second generation, conjugate vaccines were developed through covalent linkage of PRP to a carrier protein which thereby confers T-cell dependent memory and increased immunogenicity. *H. influenzae* type b conjugate vaccines have been shown to be safe, immunogenic, and protective (92,93). Proteins which are used as a carriers include tetanus toxoid, diphtheria toxoid, and outer membrane protein from *Neisseria meningitidis* serogroup B. Four conjugate vaccines have undergone clinical evaluation: PRP-D (Connaught Laboratories), PRP-T (Pasteur-Merieux), PRP-OMC (Merck Sharp and Dohme), and HbOC (Praxis Biologicals). Each of these vaccines is distinguished by its carrier molecule, the size of the hapten saccharide, the type of linkage between hapten and carrier, and the ratio of polysaccharide to protein. All are well-tolerated and result in a high degree of protection, although there are differences in the immunogenicity for the different conjugates (94,95). Conjugate vaccines can be administered at the same time and mixed with diphtheria-pertussis-tetanus (DPT) and polio immunizations as part of the routine program of childhood immunization. The inclusion of the *H. influenzae* type b conjugate vaccines in the routine immunization schedule has resulted in the virtual disappearance of invasive *H. influenzae* type b disease in young children (96). Conjugate vaccines also reduce colonization of the upper respiratory tract with type b strains (97). Although the efficacy of conjugate vaccines is >90%, vaccine failures have been described (98).

VI. LABORATORY DIAGNOSIS

A. *H. influenzae*

Clinical symptoms may suggest a diagnosis of meningitis or other invasive disease but confirmation requires microbiological studies. Positive cultures of CSF, blood, and other sterile fluids such as pleural, subdural, pericardial, or joint fluids, can be diagnostic, even if antibiotic therapy has already been started. Given the fastidious nature of the organism, samples for culture need to be processed without delay in appropriate rich culture media like chocolate agar or other rich media bases to which X and V factors have been added. Selective use of invasive procedures such as tympanocentesis, transtracheal aspirates, bronchoscopy, lung aspirate, and lung needle aspiration may be necessary in selected patients to overcome upper respiratory flora. When possible, samples for culture should also be Gram stained in search of typical Gram negative cocobacilli; in up to 80% of cases of *H. influenzae* meningitis, direct CSF smears reveal typical micro-organisms after centrifugation (99). Positive Gram stains can be reconfirmed by direct detection of type b capsular antigen in CSF by latex agglutination or other immunological techniques. The latter technique can be carried out with CSF in most cases of meningitis including those previously treated. False positive results can occur as a consequence of cross-reactivity between shared antigens of different bacterial species.

The presence of *Haemophilus* in cultured sputa from cystic fibrosis patients should not be overlooked due to mixed flora. Either anaerobic incubation of chocolate agar which is supplemented with 300 mg./L. of bacitracin, use of the NAG medium (blood agar base, *N*-acetyl-D-glucosamine, hemin, NAD, and bacitracin), or use of monoclonal antibodies, increases the detection of *Haemophilus* (100).

Serotyping by slide agglutination or co-agglutination are the most commonly used methods in clinical laboratories for identifying the capsular type of *H. influenzae* isolates. Both methods are commercially available. These methods may give both false positive results due to cross-reactivity with other antigens like outer membrane proteins and LPS, and false negative results due to poor sensitivity (101); to overcome these draw-backs, a PCR-based method for the molecular capsular typing has been described (102).

Differentiation of species from the genus *Haemophilus* are given in Table 2 and differentiation of biotypes in Table 3. There are commercial kits available which identify and biotype *Haemophilus* as well as a commercial DNA probe for the identification of *H. influenzae* in culture. Several biochemical tests and outer membrane protein profiles have been proposed to distinguish between *H. influenzae* biotype III and *H. aegyptius* (103). The easiest way to determine X and V factor requirement is the traditional application of commercial paper disks which are impregnated with X and V factors after swabbing the surface of a culture medium without these factors, e.g., Mueller-Hinton agar. Care must be taken to avoid the carry-over of factors from the primary growth medium. The most reliable means of determining X-factor requirement in *Haemophilus* is the test for porphyrin synthesis (104). When supplied with δ-aminolevulinic acid, X-factor negative or independent strains (typically hemin-independent *H. parainfluenzae*) produce and excrete porphobilinogen and porphyrins which can be detected either by Kovacs's reagent or positive fluorescence at 360 nm. In contrast, X-factor dependent (typically, *H. influenzae*) bacteria lack the enzymes which are needed for the synthesis of these compounds. The substrate for the porphyrin test is 2mM δ-aminolevulinic acid, 2 mM $MgSO_4$ in 0.1 M phosphate buffer (pH 6.9) which is distributed in small tubes with 0.3 to 0.5 ml., being inoculated with a heavy loopful of bacteria. After incubation for a minimum of 4 hrs. at 37°C, the test result can be read in a dark room with Wood's light at 360 nm.; a red fluorescence is indicative of porphyrin production (the strain is X factor or hemin-independent). A practical and alternative method of reading is by adding two drops of Kovacs' reagent; development of a red color in the lower water phase is a positive test. When the strain is also indole positive, a reddish color can develop in the upper phase in the presence of the Kovacs' reagent.

B. Other *Haemophilus* species

All *Haemophilus* spp. other than *H. influenzae* are small pleomorphic Gram negative coccobacilli with fastidious growth requirements and require the presence of X factor (hemin), V factor (nicotinamide adenine dinucleotide, NAD), or both. Organisms with the "para-" designation require V factor only for growth whereas the others require X factor or both X and V factors (Table 2). Initial isolation from specimens other than blood should be on chocolate agar that is incubated with added CO_2 (e.g., 5-10%). Solid media which are effective for the isolation of *H. ducreyi* include enriched chocolate agar that contains Isovitalex and vancomycin, and gonococcal agar base which is supplemented with 5% fetal calf serum, 1% bovine hemoglobin, 1% cofactors-vitamins-amino acid enrichment, and 3 mg./L. of vancomycin; plates should be incubated in a water-saturated atmosphere with 5% of CO_2 at 33°C for 72 hrs. (105).

The clinical diagnosis of chancroid is difficult and often inaccurate because other genital diseases due to other pathogens may be similar. Culture of material that is obtained from the purulent ulcer base should be performed. The Gram stain may show Gram negative coccobacilli, sometimes forming the so-called "school-of-fish" pattern. Non-culture methods used to detect *H. ducreyi* in suspected cases include immunofluorescence (106), enzyme immunoassay (107), and PCR-based probe assay (108). It is essential to exclude syphilis and HIV in all cases of suspected chancroid.

Table 2   Biochemical identification tests of the genus *Haemophilus*.

	H. influenzae	H. haemolyticus	H. ducreyi	H. parainfluenzae	H. aphrophilus*	H. parahaemolyticus	H. paraphrophilus
V factor requirement	+	+	+	-	-	+	+
X factor requirement	+	+	-	+	-	-	-
porphyrin	-	-	+	-	w	+	+
beta-galactosidase ONPG test	-	-	+	-	+	v	+
catalase	+	+	v	-	-	v	-
hemolysis	+	-	-	-	-	+	-
acid from							
D-glucose	+	+	+	v	+	+	+
sucrose	-	-	+	-	+	+	+
lactose	-	-	-	-	+	-	+
D-xylose	v	+	-	-	-	-	-
D-ribose	+	+	-	-	+	-	+
D-mannose	-	-	+	-	+	-	+
D-mannitol	-	-	-	-	-	-	-
maltose	+	+	+	-	+	+	+
raffinose	-	-	-	-	+	-	-

Symbols: + = 90% or more of isolates are positive; - = 90% or more isolates are negative; v = variable results; w = positive weak results; * = genus status is questionable, 100% positive for acid TSI (slant and butt).

C. Non-*Haemophilus* spp.

1.   *Actinobacillus spp.*

Samples that are submitted for bacteriology and for which *Actinobacillus* spp. may be isolated include tracheal secretions, bronchial washings, wound aspirates, blood, and others less common.

Isolation of these bacteria requires blood agar (5% sheep blood) or chocolate agar that is supplemented with vitamins or NAD for V-dependent strains (*A. pleuropneumoniae, A. minor*). The incubation should be in a humid atmosphere with 5% CO_2 for 24-72 hrs. Colonies have a diameter of 0.5 to 3 mm. after incubation for two to three days, and appear round, smooth, and strongly adherent to the agar. Gram stained cells revealed small, oval, and coccobacillary rods.

The identification of species can be accomplished with several tests that are employed otherwise for the differentiation of *Pasteurella* spp. and *Haemophilus* spp.: oxidase, catalase, urease, mannitol, mannose, V-factor dependence, ornithine decarboxylase, esculin hydrolysis, and acid production from several carbohydrates (Table 4) (5).

Tests which differentiate *A. actinomycetemcomitans* from others in the "HACEK group" are found in Figure 1.

Table 3   Differentiation of *H. influenzae* and *H. parainfluenzae* biotypes.

	indole production	urease	ornithine decarboxylase	D-xylose
H. influenzae biotypes				
I	+	+	+	+
II	+	+	-	+
III	-	+	-	+
aegyptius	-	+	-	-
IV	-	+	+	+
V	+	-	+	+
VI	-	-	+	+
VII	+	-	-	+
VIII	-	-	-	+
H. parainfluenzae biotypes				
I	-	-	+	-
II	-	+	+	-
III	-	+	-	-
IV	+	+	+	-
V	+	-	+	-
VI	+	+	-	-

Symbols: + = 90% or more isolates are positive; - = 90% or more isolates are negative; v = variable results.

Table 4   Differential tests for *Actinobacillus* spp. (4,5).

	Test				acid from:		
Species	urease	ONPG	esculin hydrolysis	V-factor need	manl	man	xyl
A. actinomycetemcomitans	-	-	-	-	+L	V	+
A. hominis	+	+	V	-	+	-	+
A. ureae	+	-	-	-	+L	V	-
A. equuli	+	+	-	-	+	+	+
A. lignieresii	+	-	-	-	+	+	+L
A. suis	+	+	+	-	-	+	+
A. muris	+	-	+	-	+	+	-
A. minor	+	+	-	+	-	+	ND

L – delayed reaction; V – variable reaction; ND – not determined; manl – mannitol; man – mannose; xyl – xylose.

2.   C. hominis

Differential characteristics that are useful for the identification of *C. hominis*, and the very similar species *Suttonella indologenes*, are summarized in Table 5. The differentiation into the "HACEK group" is shown in Figure 1.

3.   E. corrodens

The identification of *E. corrodens* is based on the presence of characteristically pitting pale yellow pigmented colonies and on several phenotypic tests as shown in Figure 2. Most of the strains have an odour that is suggestive of chlorine bleach when grown on chocolate or blood agar (6). *E. corrodens* is fastidious and its growth is enhanced by CO_2.

4.   Kingella and EF-4

The differential phenotypic characteristics of *Kingella* and EF-4 strains are summarized in Figure 2. All of the *Kingella* spp. grow aerobically on chocolate and blood agar when incubated at 35-37°C for two or more days. Growth is enhanced in a 5% CO_2 atmosphere. Only *K. kingae* colonies are β-hemolytic on blood agar. Colonies are smooth and convex although spreading, and some strains of EF-4 are weakly pigmented with pale yellow colonies.

5.   C. violaceum

C. violaceum grows on simple peptone agar or MacConkey agar. Some strains are slightly hemolytic on blood agar. After the isolation of typical colonies, further identification requires positive reactions to catalase, nitrate reductase, and arginine dihydrolase. Acid is produced from glucose. Several tests show variable reactions such as oxidase, urease, and indole production.

6.   C. granulomatis

C. granulomatis cannot be grown on conventional bacteriological media but can be isolated in egg yolk sacs and in several cell lines such as Hep-2 or peripheral blood mononuclear cells (109,110). The bacterium is a pleomorphic rod and measures 0.5-1.5 μm. wide by 1-2 μm. in length with rounded ends. Staining may be complete or bipolar. When stained by Wright-Giemsa method, the exudate from infected tissues demonstrates intracellular organisms in the cytoplasm of large mononuclear phagocytes.

Table 5   Phenotypic characteristics of *Cardiobacteriaceae* (*C. hominis* and *S. indologenes*).

Test	C. hominis	S. indologenes
oxidase	+	+
catalase	-	-
nitrate reduction	-	-
indole	+	+
Tween 20 hydrolysis	-	+
Tween 40 hydrolysis	-	+
alkaline phosphatase	-	+
acid from:		
glucose	+	+
maltose	+	V
mannitol	+	-
sorbitol	+	-

V – variable.

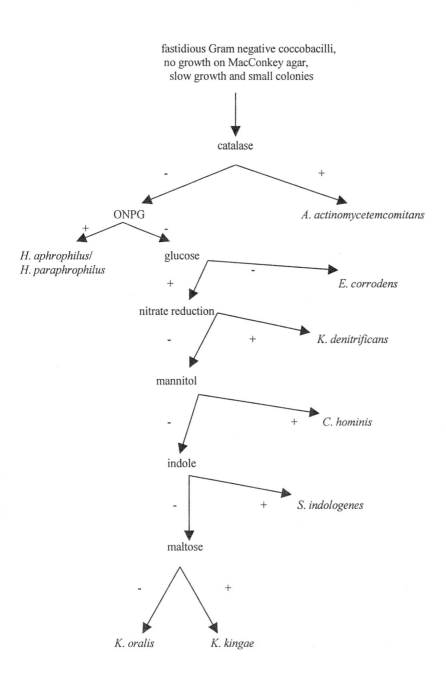

Figure 1   An algorithm for differentiation of "HACEK group" bacteria.

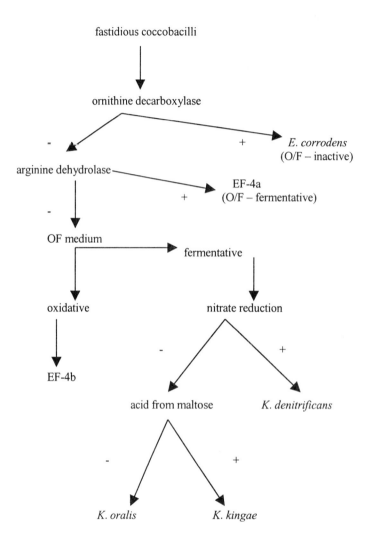

Figure 2 Differential characteristics of *E. corrodens*, *Kingella* spp., and EF-4 strains. O/F – oxidation/fermentation medium.

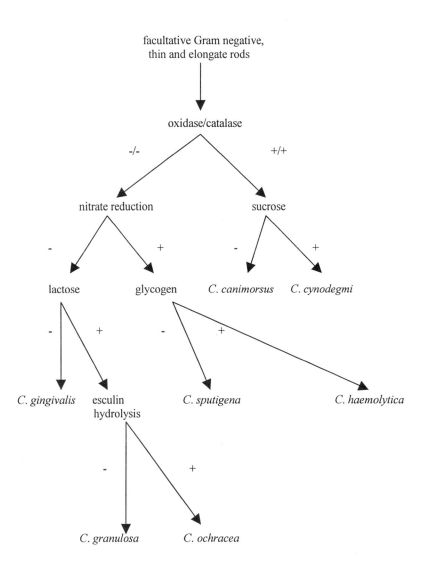

Figure 3 Differential characteristics of *Capnocytophaga* spp.

7. *Capnocytophaga spp.*

The differentiation between *C. ochracea*, *C. gingivalis*, and *C. sputigena* is difficult because most phenotypic tests have variable reactions. Figure 3 shows a simple differential scheme for the presumptive identification of *Capnocytophaga* spp. Recently, several alternative techniques for the detection and identification of *Capnocytophaga* spp. have been described including DNA homology analysis, restriction fragment length polymorphism of 16S rRNA, and protein profiles (111,112).

VII. SUSCEPTIBILITY TESTING

A. *H. influenzae*

Since ampicillin resistance was first reported in the 1970s, resistance to other antibiotics alone or in combination, has been reported for other beta-lactams, chloramphenciol, tetracycline, aminoglycosides, trimethoprim-sulphamethoxazole, rifampin, and fluoroquinolones. Epidemiology of resistance shows variation at continental, national, and local levels. As a general rule, encapsulated strains are usually more antibiotic resistant than non-typeable ones, strains that are isolated from childhood infections are more resistant than those which are isolated from adults, and isolates from chronic infections tend to be more resistant than those isolated from acute infections. Ampicillin resistance is generally due to the production of plasmid-mediated beta-lactamase (113). A comparatively rare mechanism for ampicillin resistance is decreased affinity of penicillin-binding proteins (114). The most common mechanism of chloramphenicol resistance is the production of plasmid-mediated chloramphenicol acetyltransferase (115). Resistance to trimethroprim is due to to mutations in the gene that codes for dihydrofolate reductase (116). Resistance to a ciprofloxacin is consequence of point mutations and amino acid changes in the proteins Gyr A and ParC (117). Simultaneous resistance to several antibiotics is due to a combination of resistance mechanisms, both plasmid and chromosomally mediated, in the same isolate (118).

Both beta-lactamase and chloramphenicol acetyltransferase can be determined by rapid methods (119,120).

Historically, numerous approaches using different methods for *Haemophilus* susceptibility testing were used (121). Haemophilus Test Medium (HTM) was proposed in an attempt to overcome several drawacks of previous media (122). HTM has been adopted by the NCCLS as a recommended medium for *Haemophilus influenzae* susceptibility testing. Zone diameter interpretative criteria and minimal inhibitory concentrations (MICs) have been proposed for disk diffusion and microdilution methods respectively (123,124).

B. Other *Haemophilus* spp.

Chocolate agar and Haemophilus Test Medium can be used to study antibiotic susceptibility for these pathogens (125).

Among *H. ducreyi*, most strains are resistant to ampicillin and amoxicillin due to plasmid mediated beta-lactamase production. Resistance to trimethoprim-sulphamethoxazole is also common. Due to poor patient compliance, single-dose treatment has been attempted with ceftriaxone, spectinomycin, and ciprofloxacin. It is important to identify sexual partners and treat them with effective antibiotics (126).

C. Non-*Haemophilus* spp.

Actinobacilli are susceptible to many antibiotics. Cephalosporins, carbapenems, penicillins, aminoglycosides and quinolones have good activity against *Actinobacillus* infections (127). Only *A. actinomycetemcomitans* is resistant to penicillin. Tetracycline and metronidazole in combination as well as aminoglycosides and beta-lactam antibiotics have been effective in the treatment of infections (128).

C. hominis is susceptible to most antimicrobial agents including penicillins, aminoglycosides, tetracyclines, and others. Sporadic resistance to erythromycin (129) or penicillin (130) has been described.

Like *C. hominis*, *S. indologenes* is susceptible to most antibiotics.

Most *E. corrodens* strains are susceptible to penicillins, cephalosporins, carbapenems, quinolones, and tetracycline; rare β-lactamase positive strains have been reported (131).

Kingella and EF-4 strains are uniformly susceptible to most antibiotics (132).

C. violaceum is susceptible to aminoglycosides, chloramphenicol, and tetracyclines, but is resistant to β-lactam antibiotics (5).

The treatment of donovanosis has included a wide range of antibiotics: tetracycline, chloramphenicol, macrolides, cotrimoxazole, aminoglycosides, and ampicillin.

Capnocytophaga spp. is usually susceptible to extended spectrum cephalosporins, carbapenems, quinolones, macrolides, and chloramphenicol, but are resistant to aminoglycosides, trimethoprim, and aztreonam (133). Although most strains are susceptible to penicillin, β-lactamase production has been described (134).

Standardization of susceptibility testing methods for some of these organisms (HACEK group) has not been defined. In this group, E-Test was found to be a good method because it is not compromised by media, incubation, or inoculum size requirements as required for most types of antimicrobial susceptibility testing (132); interpretive criteria provided by NCCLS guidelines are usually followed (124). In several cases, however, other authors have employed specific media for growth and susceptibility tests according to the species studied, i.e., BY agar for *E. corrodens* or Wilkins-Chalgren agar for *Capnocytophaga* spp (127,131,133).

REFERENCES

1. Pittman M. Variation and type specificity in the bacterial species *Haemophilus influenzae*. J Exp Med 1931; 53:471-492.
2. Global Program for Vaccines and Immunization. The WHO position paper on *Haemophilus influenzae* type b conjugate vaccines. Wkly Epidemiol Rec 1998; 73:64-68.
3. Holt JG, Krieg NR, Sneath PHA, Staley JT, Williams ST. In: Hensyl WR, ed. Bergey's Manual of Determinative Bacteriology, 9th Edn. Baltimore MD:Williams and Wilkins, 1994:195.
4. Weyant RS, Moss CW, Weaver RE, Hollis DG, Jordan JG, Cook EC, Daneshvar MI . Identification of unusual pathogenic Gram negative aerobic and facultatively anaerobic bacteria, 2nd Edn. Baltimore MD:Williams and Wilkins, 1996.
5. Mutters R. *Actinobacillus*, *Capnocytophaga*, *Eikenella*, and other fastidious or rarely encountered gram negative rods. In: Murray PR, Baron, EJ, Pfaller MA, Tenover FC, Yolken RH, eds. Manual of Clinical Microbiology. Washington, DC:American Society for Microbiology, 1999:561-571.
6. Janda WM. The "HACEK group" enigmatic fastidious gram negative bacilli. Rev Med Microbiol 1999; 10:37-50.
7. Potts TV, Zambon JJ, Genco RJ. Reassignment of *A. actinomycetemcomitans* to the genus *Haemophilus* as *H. actinomycetemcomitans* comb. nov. Int J Syst Bacteriol 1985; 35:337-341.
8. Pohl S, Bertschinger HV, Frederiksen W, Mannheim W. Transfer of *Haemophilus pleuropneumoniae* and the *Pasteurella haemolytica*-like organism causing porcine necrotic pleuropneumonia to the genus *Actinobacillus* (*A. pleuroneumoniae* comb. nov.) on the basis of phenotypic and deoxyribonucleic acid relatedness. Int J Syst Bacteriol 1983; 33:510-514.
9. Mutter R, Pohl S, Mannheim W. Transfer of *Pasteurella ureae* Jones 1962 to the genus *Actinobacillus* Brunnpt 1910: *A. ureae* comb. nov. Int J Syst Bacteriol 1986; 36:343-344.
10. Slotnick IJ, Dougherty M. Further characterization of an unclassified group of bacteria causing endocarditis in man: *Cardiobacterium hominis* gen. et sp. nov. Antonie Van Leeuwenhoek J Microbiol Serol 1964; 30:261-272.
11. Dewhirst FE, Poster BJ, La Fontaine S. Transfer of *Kingella indologenes* (Snell and Lapage 1976) to the genus *Suttonella* gen. nov. as *Suttonella indologenes* comb. nov.; transfer of *Bacteroides nudosus* (Beneridge 1941) to the genus *Dichelobacter* gen. nov. and *Dichelobacter nudosus* comb. nov.; and assignments of the genera *Cardiobacterium*, *Dichelobacter* and *Suttonella* to *Cardiobacteriaceae* fam. nov. in the gamma division of *Proteobacteria* on the basis of 16s rRNA sequence comparisons. Int J Syst Bacteriol 1990; 40:426-433.
12. Eiken M. Studies on an anaerobic rod shaped gram negative microorganism: *Bacteroides corrodens* N *sp*. Acta Path Microbiol Scand 1958; 43:404-416.
13. Jackson FL, Goodman YE. Transfer of the facultatively anaerobic organism *Bacteroides corrodens* Eiken to a new genus *Eikenella*. Int J Syst Bacteriol 1972; 22:73-77.
14. Henriksen SD, Boivre K. Transfer of *Moraxella kingae* Henriksen and Bovre to the genus *Kingella* gen. nov. in the family *Neisseriaceae*. Int J Syst Bacteriol 1976; 26:447-450.

15. Dewhirst FE, Casey Chen CK, Paster BJ, Zambon JJ. Phylogeny of species in the family *Neisseriaceae* isolated from human dental plaque and description of *Kingella orale* sp. nov. Int J Syst Bacteriol 1993; 43:490-499.

16. Aragao H, Vianna G. Pesquisas sobre o granuloma venereo. Mem Oswaldo Cruz 1913; 5:211-238.

17. Anderson K, De Monbrem WA, Goodpasture EW. An etiologic consideration of *Donovania granulomatis* cultivated from granuloma inguinale (three cases) in embryonic yolk. J Exp Med 1945; 81:25-39.

18. Williams BL, Hollis D, Holdeman LV. Synonymy of strains of Center for Disease Control group DF-1 with species of *Capnocytophaga*. J Clin Microbiol 1979; 10:550-562.

19. Leadbetter ER, Holt SC, Socransky SS. *Capnocytophaga:* new genus of gram negative gliding bacteria. I. General characteristic, taxonomic considerations and significance. Arch Microbiol 1979; 122:9-16.

20. Waggoner-Fountain LA, Hendley JO, Cody EJ, Perriello VA, Donowitz LG. The emergence of *Haemophilus influenzae* types e and f as significant pathogens. Clin Infect Dis 1995; 21:1322-1324.

21. Brazilian Purpuric Fever Study Group. Brazilian Purpuric Fever: epidemic purpura fulminans associated with antecedent purulent conjunctivitis. Lancet 1987; 2:757-761.

22. Brazilian Purpuric Fever Study Group. *Haemophilus aegyptius* bacteremia in Brazilian purpuric fever. Lancet 1987; 2:761-763.

23. Campos J, Garcia-Tornel S, Gairi JM, Fabregues I. Multiply resistant *Haemophilus influenzae* type b causing meningitis: comparative clinical and laboratory study. J Pediatr 1986; 108:897-902.

24. Regelink AG, Dahan D, Moller LVM, Coulton JW, Eijk P, Ulsen PV, Dankert J, Van Alphen L. Variation in the composition and pore function of major outer membrane pore protein P2 of *Haemophilus influenzae* from cystic fibrosis patients. Antimicro Agents Chemother 1999; 43:226-232.

25. Farley MM, Stephens DS, Brachman PS, Harvey C, Smith JD, Wenger JD, CDC Meningitis Surveillance Group. Invasive *Haemophilus influenzae* disease in adults: a prospective population-based surveillance. Ann Intern Med 1992; 116:806-812.

26. Strausbaugh LJ. *Haemophilus influenzae* infections in adults: a pathogen in search of respect. Postgrad Med 1997; 101:191-196.

27. Murphy TF, Apicella MA. Nontypeable *Haemophilus influenzae*: a review of clinical aspects, surface antigens, and the human immune response to infection. Rev Infect Dis 1987; 9:1-15.

28. Oil PA, Chow AW, Guze LB. Adult bacteremic *Haemophilus parainfluenzae* infections. Arch Intern Med 1979; 139:985-988.

29. Blaylock BL, Baber S. Urinary tract infections caused by *Haemophilus parainfluenzae*. Am J Clin Pathol 1980; 71:285-287.

30. Sturm AW. *Haemophilus influenzae* and *Haemophilus parainfluenzae* in non-gonococcal urethritis. J Infect Dis 1986; 153:165-167.

31. Julander I, Lindberg AA, Svanbom M. *Haemophilus parainfluenzae*: an uncommon cause of septicemia and endocarditis. Scand J Infect Dis 1980; 12:85-89.

32. Bieger RC, Brewer NS, Washington JA. *Haemophilus aphrophilus*: a microbiologic and clinical review and report of 42 cases. Medicine 1978; 57:345-355.

33. Lynn DJ, Kane JG, Parker RH. *Haemophilus parainfluenzae* and *influenzae* endocarditis: a review of forty cases. Medicine 1977; 56:115-128.

34. Trees DL, Morse SA. Chancroid and *Haemophilus ducreyi*: an update. Clin Microbiol Rev 1995; 8:357-375.

35. Geraci JE, Wilson WR. Endocarditis due to gram negative bacteria. Report of 56 cases. Mayo Clin Proc 1982; 57:145-148.

36. Berbari EF, Cockerill III FR, Stecklelberg JM. Infective endocarditis due to unusual or fastidious microorganisms. Mayo Clin Proc 1997; 72:532-542.

37. Brook I. Microbiology of human and animal bite wounds in children. Pediatr Infect Dis 1987; 6:29-32.

38. Verhaegen J, Verbraeken H, Cauby A, Vandenen J, Van Depitte J. *Actinobacillus* (formerly *Pasteurella*) *ureae* meningitis and bacteremia: report a case and review of the literature. J Infect 1988; 17:249-253.

39. Peel MM, Hornidge KA, Luppino M, Stacpoole AM, Weaver RE. *Actinobacillus* spp. and related bacteria in infected wounds of human bitten by horses and sheeps. J Clin Microbiol 1991; 29:2535-2538.

40. El Khizzi N, Lasab SA, Osoba AO. HACEK group endocarditis at the Riyadh Armed Forces Hospital. J Infect 1997; 34:69-74.

41. Kaplan AH, Weber DJ, Oddone EZ, Perfect JR. Infection due to *A. actinomycetemcomitans*: 15 cases and review. Rev Infect Dis 1989; 11:46-63.

42. Müller HP, Flores de Jacoby L. The composition of the subgingival microflora of young adults suffering from juvenile periodontitis. J Clin Periodontol 1985; 12:113-123.

43. Wilson ME. Prosthetic valve endocarditis and paravalvular abscess by *A. actinomycetemcomitans*. Rev Infect Dis 1989; 11:665-667.
44. Bouly KJ, Ashkenazi M. Juvenile periodontitis: a review of pathogenesis, diagnosis, and treatment. J Clin Pediatr Dent 1992; 16:73-78.
45. Robertson PB, Lantz M, Marucha PT, Kornman KS, Trummel CL, Holt SC. Collagenolytic activity associated with *Bacteroides* spp. and *A. actinomycetemcomitans*. J Periodont Res 1982; 17:275-283.
46. Zambon JJ, DeLuca C, Slots J, Genco RJ. Studies of leukotoxin from *A. actinomycetemcomitans* using the promyelocytic HL-60 cell line. Infect Immun 1983; 40:205-212.
47. Pritchard TM, Foust RT, Cantey RT, Cantey JR, Lennan RB. Prosthetic valve endocarditis due to *Cardiobacterium hominis* occuring after upper gastrointestinal endoscopy. Am J Med 1991; 90:516-518.
48. Francioli PB, Foussianos D, Glauser MP. *Cardiobacterium hominis* endocarditis manifesting as bacterial meningitis. Arch Intern Med 1983; 143:1483-1484.
49. Rechtman DJ, Madler JP. Abdominal abscess due to *Cardiobacterium hominis* and *Clostridium bifermentans*. Rev Infect Dis 1991; 13:418-419.
50. Jenny DB, Lenendre PW, Iverson G. Endocarditis caused by *Kingella indologenes*. Rev Infect Dis 1987; 9:787-788.
51. Sutton RGA, O'Keeffe MF, Budock MA, Jeboult J, Tester MP. Isolation of a new *Moraxella* from corneal abscess. J Med Microbiol 1972; 5:148-150.
52. Soder PO, Jin LJ, Soder B. DNA probe detection of periodontopathogens in advanced periodontitis. Scand J Dent Res 1993; 101:363-370.
53. Chen CK, Wilson ME. *Eikenella corrodens* in human oral and non-oral infections: a review. J Periodont 1992; 63:941-953.
54. Flesher SA, Bottone EJ. *Eikenella corrodens* cellulitis and arthritis of the knee. J Clin Microbiol 1989; 27:2606-2608.
55. Joshi N, O'Bryan T, Appelbaum PC. Pleuropulmonary infections caused by *Eikenella corrodens*. Rev Infect Dis 1991; 13:1207-1212.
56. Stoloff AL, Gillies ML. Infections with *Eikenella corrodens* in a general hospital: a report of 33 cases. Rev Infect Dis 1986; 8:50-53.
57. Decker MD, Graham BS, Hunter EB, Liebowitz SM. Endocarditis and infections of intravascular devices due to *Eikenella corrodens*. Am J Med Sci 1986; 292:209-212.
58. Angus BJ, Green ST, Mc Kinley JJ, Goldberg DJ, Frisher M. *Eikenella corrodens* septicaemia among drug injectors: a possible association with "licking wounds". J Infect 1994; 28:102-103.
59. Adachi R, Hammerberg O, Richardson H. Infective endocarditis caused by *Kingella kingae*. Can Med Assoc J 1983; 128:1087-1089.
60. Morrison VA, Wagner KF. Clinical manifestations of *Kingella kingae* infections: case report and review. Rev Infect Dis 1989; 11:776-782.
61. Yagupsky P, Dagan R. *Kingella kingae*: an emerging cause of invasive infections in young children. Clin Infect Dis 1997; 24:860-866.
62. Swann RA, Holmes B. Infective endocarditis caused by *Kingella denitrificans*. J Clin Pathol 1984; 37:1384-1387.
63. Hassan IJ, Hayek L. Endocarditis caused by *Kingella denitrificans*. J Infect 1993; 27:291-295.
64. Georghiou PR, O'Kane GM, Sin S, Kemp RJ. Near fatal septicemia with *Chromobacterium violaceum*. Med J Aust 1989; 150:720-721.
65. Sorensen RV, Jacobs MR, Shurin SB. *Chromobacterium violaceum* adenitis acquired in the northern United States as a complication of chronic granulomatous disease. Pediatr Infect Dis 1985; 4:701-702.
66. Richens J. Donovaniosis – a review. Papua New Guinea Med J 1985; 28:67-74.
67. Paterson DL. Disseminated donovanosis (granuloma inguinale) causing spinal cord compression: case report and review of donovanosis involving bone. Clin Infect Dis 1998; 26:379-383.
68. Rajam RV, Rangiah PN, Arguli VC. Systemic donovaniosis. Brit J Vener Dis 1954; 30:73-80.
69. Bun-Hol AY, Joundy S, Acar JF. Endocarditis caused by *Capnocytophaga ochracea*. J Clin Microbiol 1988; 26:1061-1062.
70. Font R, Jay V, Misra R, Jones D, Wilhelmus K. *Capnocytophaga* keratitis: a clinicopathologic study of three patients including electron microscopic observations. Ophthalmology 1994; 101:1929-1934.
71. Seger R, Kloeti J, von Graevenitz A, Wüst J, Briner J, Willi V, Siegrist H. Cervical abscess due to *Capnocytophaga ochracea*. Pediatr Infect Dis 1982; 1:170-172.

72. Pers C, Gahrn-Hansen B, Frederiksen W. *Capnocytophaga canimorsus* septicemia in Denmark, 1982-1995 a review of 39 cases. Clin Infect Dis 1996; 23:71-75.

73. Brenner DJ, Hollis DG, Fanning GR, Weaver RE. *Capnocytophaga canimorsus* sp. nov. (formerly CDC group DF-2) a cause of septicemia following dog bite and *Capnocytophaga cynodegmi* sp. nov. a cause of localized wound infection following dog bite. J Clin Microbiol 1989; 27:231-235.

74. Campos J, Garcia-Tornel S, Musser J, Selander RK, Smith AL. Molecular epidemiology of multiply resistant *Haemophilus influenzae* type b in day care centers. J Clin Microbiol 1987; 156:483-489.

75. Jordens JZ, Slack MPE. *Haemophilus influenzae*: then and now. Eur J Clin Microbiol Infect Dis 1995; 14:935-948.

76. Centres for Disease Control. Progress toward elimination of *Haemophilus influenzae* type b disease among infants and children – United States, 1987-1995. MMWR 1996; 45:901-906.

77. Musser JM, Kroll JS, Moxon ER, Selander RK. Clonal population of encapsulated *Haemophilus influenzae*. Infect Immun 1988; 56.1837-1845.

78. Melhus A, Hermansson A, Forsgren A, Prellner K. Intra- and inter-strain differences of virulence among nontypeable *Haemophilus influenzae* strains. APMIS 1998; 106:858-868.

79. Gilsdorf JR. Antigenic diversity and gene polymorphisms in *Haemophilus*. Infect Immun 1998; 66:5053-5059.

80. Fleischmann RD, Adams MD, White O, Clayton RA, Kirkness EF, Kerlavage AR, Bult CJ, Tomb JF, Dougherty BA, Merrick JM, McKenney K, Sutton G, FitzHugh W, Fields C, Gocayne JD, Scott J, Shirley R, Liu LI, Glodek A, Kelley JM, Weidman JF, Phillips CA, Spriggs T, Hedblom E, Cotton MD, Utterback TR, Hanna MC, Nguyen DT, Saudek DM, Brandon RC, Fine LD, Fritchman JL, Fuhrmann JL, Geohagen NSM, Gnehm CL, McDonald LA, Small KV, Fraser CM, Smith HO, Venter JC. Whole genome random sequencing and assembly of *Haemophilus influenzae* Rd. Science 1995; 269:496-512.

81. Moxon ER, Gewurz BE, Richards JC, Inzana T, Jennings MP, Hood DW. Phenotypic switching of *Haemophilus influenzae*. Mol Microbiol 1996; 19: 1149-1150.

82. Regelink AG, Dahan D, Moller LVM, Coulton JW, Eijk P, Van Ulsen P, Dankert J, Van Alphen L. Variation in the composition and pore function of major outer membrane pore protein P2 of *Haemophilus influenzae* from cystic fibrosis patients. Antimicrob Agents Chemother 1999; 43:226-232.

83. Halsey NA, Johansen TL, Browman LC, Glode MP. Evaluation of the protective efficacy of *Haemophilus influenzae* type vaccines in an animal model. Infect Immun 1983; 39:1196-1200.

84. Granoff DM, Rockwell R. Experimental *Haemophilus influenzae* type meningitis: immuologic investigation of the infant rat model. Infect Immun 1978; 20:705-713.

85. Schreiber JR, Barrus V, Cates KL, Siber GR. Functional characterization of human IgG, IgM, and IgA antibody directed to the capsule of Haemophilus influenzae type b. J Infect Dis 1986; 153:8-16.

86. Kayhty H, Karanko V, Peltola H, Makela PH. Serum antibodies after vaccination with *Haemophilus influenzae* type b capsular polysaccharide and response to reimmunization: no evidence of immunologic tolerance of memory. Pediatrics 1984; 74:857-865.

87. Wormser GP, Bottone EJ. *Cardiobacterium hominis*: review of microbiologic and clinical features. Rev Infect Dis 1983; 5:680-691.

88. Geraci JE, Greipp PR, Wilkowske CJ, Wilson WR, Washington III JA. *Cardiobacterium hominis* endocarditis four cases with clinical and laboratory observations. Mayo Clin Proc 1978; 53:49-53.

89. Carter JS, Bowden FJ, Bastian I, Myers GM, Sriprakash KS, Kemp DJ. Phylogenetic evidence for reclassification of *Calymmatobacterium granulomatis* as *Klebsiella granulomatis* comb. nov. Int J Syst Bacteriol 1999; 49:1695-1700.

90. Kharsay ABM, Hoosen AA, Kiepiela P, Kirby R, Sturm AW. Phylogenetic analysis of *Calymmatobacterium granulomatis* based on 16S rRNA gene sequences. J Med Microbiol 1999; 48:841-847.

91. Conrads G, Mutters R, Fisher J, Branner A, Lütticken R, Lampert F. PCR reaction and dot-blot hybridization to monitor the distribution of oral pathogens within plaque sample of periodontally healthy individuals. J Periodontol 1996; 67:994-1003.

92. Eskola J, Peltola H, Takala AK, Kayhty H, Hakulinen M, Karanko V, Kela E, Rekola P, Ronnberg PR, Samuelson JS, Gordon LK, Makela PH. Efficacy of *Haemophilus influenzae* type b polysaccharide-diphtheria toxoid conjugate vaccine in infancy. N Engl J Med 1987; 317:712-722.

93. Peltola H, Kilpi T, Anttila M. Rapid disappearance of *Haemophilus infuenzae* type b meningitis after routine childhood immunization with conjugate vaccines. Lancet 1992; 340:592-594.

94. Bisgard KM, Kao A, Leake J, Strebel PM, Perkins BA, Wharton M. *Haemophilus influenzae* invasive disease in the United States, 1994-1995: near disappearance of a child vaccine preventable disease. Emerg Infect Dis 1998; 4:229-237.

95. Centers for Disease Control. Progress toward eliminating *Haemophilus influenzae* type b disease among infants and children – United States, 1987-1997. MMWR 1998; 47:993-998.

96. Eskola J, Kayhty H. Ten years' experience with *Haemophilus influenzae* type b conjugate vaccines in Finland. Rev Med Microbiol 1996; 7:231-241.

97. Barbour ML, Phil D. Conjugate vaccines and carriage of *Haemophilus influenzae* type b. Emerg Infect Dis 1996; 2:176-182.

98. Booy R, Heath PT, Slack MPE, Bewgg N, Moxon ER. Vaccine failures after immunization with *Haemophilus influenzae* type b vaccines. Lancet 1997; 349:1197-1202.

99. Greenlee JL. Approach to diagnosis of meningitis. Cerebrospinal fluid evaluation. Infect Dis Clin NA 1990; 4:583-597.

100. Moller LV, Ruijs GJ, Heijerman GM, Dankert J, Van Alphen L. *Haemophilus influenzae* is frequently detected with monoclonal antibody 8BD9 in sputum samples from patients with cystic fibrosis. J Clin Microbiol 1992; 30:2495-2497.

101. Shrively RG, Shigei JYT, Peterson EM, de la Maza LM. Typing of *Haemophilus influenzae* by coagglutination and conventional slide agglutination. J Clin Microbiol 1985; 18:1-16.

102. Falla TJ, Crook DWM, Brophy LN, Maskell D, Moxon ER. PCR for capsular typing of *Haemphilus influenzae*. J Clin Microbiol 1994; 32:2382-2386.

103. Carlone GM, Sottnek FO, Plikaytis BD. Comparison of outer membrane protein and biochemical profiles of *Haemophilus influenzae* biotype III. J Clin Microbiol 1985; 22:708-713.

104. Kilian M. A rapid method for the differentiation of *Haemophilus* strains – the porphyrin test. Acta Path Micro Scand [B] 1974; 82:835-842.

105. Hannah P, Greenwood JR. Isolation and rapid identification of *Haemophilus ducreyi*. J Clin Microbiol 1982; 16:861-864.

106. Karim QN, Finn G, Easmon CSF, Dangor Y, Dance DAB, Ngeow YF, Ballard RC. Rapid detection of *Haemophilus ducreyi* in clinical and experimental infections using monoclonal antibody: a preliminary evaluation. Genitourin Med 1989; 65:361-365.

107. Roggen EI, Pansaerts R, Van Dyck E, Piot P. Antigen detection and immunological typing of *Haemophilus ducreyi* with a specific rabbit polyclonal serum. J Clin Microbiol 1993; 31:1820-1825.

108. Orle KA, Gates CA, Martin DH, Body BA, Weiss JB. Simultaneous PCR detection of *Haemophilus ducreyi*, *Treponema pallidum*, and herpes simplex virus types 1 and 2 from genital ulcers. J Clin Microbiol 1996; 34:49-54.

109. Kharsany ABM, Hoosen AA, Kiepiela P, Naicker J, Sturm AW. Growth and cultural characteristics of *Calymmatobacterium granulomatis*: the etiological agent of granuloma inguinale (Donovanosis). J Med Microbiol 1997; 46:579-585.

110. Carter J, Hutton S, Sriprakash KS, Kemp DJ, Lum G, Savage J, Bowden FJ. Culture of the causative organism of donovanosis (*Calymmatobacterium granulomatis*) in Hep-2 cells. J Clin Microbiol 1997; 35:2915-2917.

111. Wilson MJ, Wade WG, Weightman AJ. Restriction fragment length polymorphism analysis of PCR-amplified 16S ribosomal DNA of human *Capnocytophaga*. J Appl Bacteriol 1995; 78:394-401.

112. Kwhaja KJ, Parish P, Aldred MJ, Wade WG. Protein profiles of *Capnocytophaga* species. J Appl Bacteriol 1990; 68:385-390.

113. Sykes RB, Matthew M, O'Callaghan CH. R factor mediated beta-lactamase production by *Haemophilus influenzae*. J Med Microbiol 1975; 8:437-441.

114. Mendelman PM, Chaffin DO, Stull TL, Rubens CE, Mack KD, Smith AL. Characterization of non-beta-lactamase mediated ampicillin resistance in *Haemophilus influenzae*. Antimicrob Agents Chemother 1984; 26:235-244.

115. van Kingeren BJ, van Embden JDA, Dessens-Kroon M. Plasmid mediated chloramphenicol resistance in *Haemophilus influenzae*. Antimicrob Agents Chemother 1977; 11:383-387.

116. De Groot R, Sluijter M, Bruyn A, Campos J, Goessens WHF, Smith AL, Hermans PWM. Genetic characterization of trimethoprim resistance in *Haemophilus influenzae*. Antimicrob Agents Chemother 1996; 40:2131-2136.

117. Georgiou M, Munoz R, Roman F, Canton R, Gomez-Lus R, Campos J, De la Campa A. Ciprofloxacin resistant *Haemophilus influenzae* strains possess mutations in analogous positions of GyrA and ParC. Antimicrob Agents Chemother 1996; 40:1741-1744.

118. Campos J, Chanyangam M, de Groot R, Smith AL, Tenover F, Reig R. Genetic relatedness of antibiotic resistance determinants in multiply resistant *Haemophilus influenzae*. J Infect Dis 1989; 160:810-817.

119. O'Callaghan CH, Morris A, Kirby SM, Shingler AH. Novel method for detection of beta-lactamases by using a chromogenic cephalosporin substrate. Antimicrob Agents Chemother 1972; 1:283-288.
120. Azemun P, Stull T, Roberts M, Smith AL. Rapid detection of chloramphenicol resistance in *Haemophilus influenzae*. Antimicrob Agents Chemother 1981; 20:168-170.
121. Needham CA. *Haemophilus influenzae*: antibiotic susceptibility. Clin Microbiol Rev 1988; 1:218-227.
122. Jorgensen JH, Redding JS, Maher LA, Howell AW. Improved medium for antimicrobial susceptibility testing of *Haemophilus influenzae*. J Clin Microbiol 1987; 25:2105-2113.
123. National Committee for Clinical Laboratory Standards. Performance standards for antimicrobial disc susceptibility tests – approved standard. NCCLS Document M2-A6. Wayne, PA:NCCLS, 1997.
124. National Committee for Clinical Laboratory Standards. Methods for dilution antimicrobial susceptibility tests for bacteria that grow aerobically – approved standard. NCCLS Document M7-A4. Wayne, PA:NCCLS, 1997.
125. Jorgensen JH, Howell AW, Maher LA. Antimicrobial susceptibility testing of less commonly isolated *Haemophilus* species using Haemophilus Test Medium. J Clin Microbiol 1990; 28:985-988.
126. Schmid GP. Treatment of chancroid. Rev Infect Dis 1990; 12:S580-S589.
127. Pavivic MJ, van Winkelhoff AJ, de Graaff J. In vitro susceptibilities of *A. actinomycetemcomitans* to a number of antimicrobial combinations. Antimicrob Agents Chemother 1992; 36:2634-2638.
128. Noyan U, Yilmaz S, Kuru B, Kadir T, Acar O, Buget E. A clinical and microbiological evaluation of systemic and local metronidazole delivery in adult periodontitis patients. J Clin Periodontol 1997; 24:158-165.
129. Prior RB, Spagna VA, Perkins RL. Endocarditis due to strain of *Cardiobacterium hominis* resistant to erythromycin and vancomycin. Chest 1979; 75:85-86.
130. Le Quellec A, Bessis D, Perec C, Ciurana AJ. Endocarditis due to a β-lactamase-producing *Cardiobacterium hominis*. Clin Infect Dis 1994; 19:994-995.
131. Lacroix JM, Walker C. Characterization of a beta-lactamase found in *Eikenella corrodens*. Antimicrob Agents Chemother 1991; 35:886-891.
132. Kluger KC, Biedenbach DJ, Jones RN. Determination of the antimicrobial activity of 29 clinical important compounds tested against fastidious HACEK group organisms. Diagn Microbiol Infect Dis 1999; 34:73-76.
133. Roscoe DL, Zemcov SJV, Thorber D, Wise R, Clarke AM. Antimicrobial susceptibilities and β-lactamase characterization of *Capnocytophaga* species. Antimicrob Agents Chemother 1992; 36:2197-2200.
134. Roscoe D, Clarke A. Resistance of *Capnocytophaga* species to β-lactam antibiotics. Clin Infect Dis 1993; 17:284-285.
135. Shapiro ED, Murphy TV, Wald ER, Brady CA, Phil M. The protective efficacy of *Haemophilus* b polysaccharide vaccine. JAMA 1988; 260:1419-1428.

19

Gram Negative Infections: Gram Negative Zoonoses

C. Anthony Hart and Malcolm Bennett
Centre for Comparative Infectious Diseases, University of Liverpool, Liverpool, England

I. HISTORICAL BACKGROUND

The term zoonosis was coined by Virchov in 1901, but it was not formally adopted until 1959 when a Joint Expert Committee of the WHO and FAO produced its deliberations (1). In the latter, zoonoses were defined as "those diseases and infections naturally transmitted between vertebrate animals and man". It is clear, however, that man has long been afflicted with zoonotic infections. Possibly the earliest reference is from Deuteronomy (14:8): "The swine also because it divideth the hoof but cheweth not the cud shall be unclean to you, ye shall not eat of their flesh nor touch their dead carcasses, ye shall not eat anything that dieth of itself". On further reading of this text, it is clear that godliness does not extend to neighbourliness: "thou shalt give it to the stranger that is in thy gates that he may eat it, or thou mayest sell it unto an alien" (14:21).

Although it is estimated that up to two-thirds of the infections newly described over the last 30 years are zoonotic, we have few accurate estimates of their impact. This is, in part, because we have no simple classification scheme which would direct the clinician to include a zoonosis in the differential diagnosis of a particular infection (2,3). In many cases, the specific diagnosis is delayed while the pathogen is isolated and identified. In this chapter, we will consider some of the Gram negative zoonotic pathogens, namely *Brucella* spp., *Francisella* spp., *Pasteurella* spp., *Streptobacillus moniliformis* and *Yersinia pestis*.

A. *Brucella* spp.

Brucellosis was first described clinically by Marston who was an assistant surgeon in the British Army in 1859. It has been referred to as undulant fever, Mediterranean fever, Malta fever, and Bang's disease. The organism was first isolated in 1886 by Bruce, another British army doctor (after whom the genus is named) (14), from splenic tissue that was obtained from soldiers who had died from Malta fever. This organism was eventually named *Brucella melitensis* (after the Roman name for Malta, Melita, the honey island). A Royal Commission was established to examine epidemics of *B. melitensis* that were causing such problems for the garrison in Malta (5). This described the epidemiology of the infection, and demonstrated that goats were persistently infected with *B. melitensis* and that ingestion of unpasteurized goat's milk was the major mode of transmission.

B. abortus was isolated in 1895 from aborted material of cattle by Bang in Denmark, but it was not until the 1920s that human infections were recognized. *B. suis* was isolated from aborted material of pigs by Traum in the U.S. in 1914. Finally, *B. canis* was isolated from dogs who suffered from contagious abortions by Carmichael in the U.S. in 1966. The other major figure in the history of brucellosis is the famous microbiologist from St. Mary's Hospital, London, Sir Almroth Wright who, in 1897, developed an agglutination test to diagnose brucellosis by measuring specific serum antibody titres.

B.   *Franciscella* spp.

The genus is named after the American bacteriologist Edward Francis who contributed greatly to the understanding the bacterium and its pathogenesis. The species name is derived from its place of isolation, Tulare County, California. Tularemia was first described in Japan in 1837 (6), in the U.S. in 1911 (7), and in Sweden in 1931 (8). The disease tularemia has also been called rabbit fever, deerfly fever, market men's disease, wild hare disease, Ohara's disease, and water-rat trapper's disease.

C.   *Pasteurella* spp.

The genus is named in honour of Louis Pasteur who described the bacterial cause of fowl cholera (9). It is only in recent years that it has been recognized as a cause of human infections (10), mostly associated with animal bite wounds.

D.   *Streptobacillus moniliformis*

This almost forgotten bacterium is a cause of rat-bite fever and Haverhill fever in man. Rat-bite fever has been described for over 2000 years, although in Asia, infection is usually with *Spirillum minus*. An infection was described in the U.S. in 1839 (11). The bacterium was originally isolated in 1916 and named *Streptothrix muris* (12). In 1926, a similar bacterium was isolated from an epidemic illness which resembled rat-bit fever in Haverhill, MA and thus named *Haverhillia multiformis* (13). The two bacteria were subsequently shown to be the same and named *Streptobacillus moniliformis* because of the necklace-like morphology on Gram staining.

E.   *Yersinia pestis*

Yersinia pestis causes plague (derived from the Latin plaga: 'a blow that wounds'). It is transmitted by fleas from its reservoir of wild rodent hosts, and it is largely a disease of antiquity. There have been three pandemics of plague or the pestilence as it was known previously. The first pandemic (Justinian) began in 542 AD (14). It probably escaped from its homeland in the Himalayan borderlands of India and China perhaps by the opening of trade routes to the Eastern Roman Empire. At this time, Justinian the Eastern Emperor was trying to re-unite Constantinople with Rome, and this facilitated the plague's westward spread. It is estimated to have killed 10,000 people in Constantinople in one day. Justinian himself became infected but survived. It swept westward through Italy to Southern France and along the North African coast. It is thought to have arrived in Britain in 544 AD. Overall, it is estimated to have killed 100 million people and to have heralded the advent of the Dark Ages. Plague apparently vanished from Europe in 767 AD and did not return for another 600 years.

The Black Death was the next pandemic. It began in 1348 having spread to Europe across the Asian steppes and along the southern Muslim trade routes (15). It was estimated to have killed between one quarter and one third of the population of Europe. It became an early example of bioterrorism when commanders of the Tartar army lobbed plague corpses into the city of Kaffa to which they were laying siege. It returned in a series of epidemics, the last of which was in 1720 in Marseille. Quarantine, meaning isolation for 40 days, was introduced originally in Dubrovnik, Croatia, and in its initial form prevented the entry of anyone into the city in contrast to the current usage of the term which is to isolate the infected individual. It is unclear why this pandemic disappeared.

The third and current pandemic began in Yunan Province, China, in 1860 and reached Hong Kong in 1894 (16). It then spread via black rats (*Rattus rattus*) on ships around the world thus becoming established in the endogenous sylvatic rodents throughout the world. Alexandre Yersin and Shibasaburo Kitasato both went to Hong Kong to isolate the causative organism. Both succeeded, but it is clear that Yersin made the first isolation and described the role of rats. The genus *Yersinia* is named in his honour.

II.   CLINICAL ASPECTS

A.   Brucellosis

Brucellosis is a systemic illness with a multitude of presentations (Table 1). The onset may be acute or insidious. There are no absolute clinical diagnostic signs or symptoms, but fever and lymphadenopathy occur in 80-90% of cases. The fever can wax and wane (hence undulant fever) especially in well-established, untreated cases. Often there are surprisingly few physical signs to match the patients' description of their illness. Chronic brucellosis has been defined as symptoms persisting for more than twelve months, but this can be difficult to establish especially when the onset is insidious. Infection may become localized especially to those organs that are rich in reticulo-endothelial cells.

1.   Gastrointestinal tract

Up to 70% of patients report anorexia, abdominal pain, weight loss, nausea, or vomiting. It may also cause acute cholecystitis, acute pancreatitis, and mesenteric adenitis. The liver is involved in most cases, but disease is not always clinically expressed. It can cause acute or chronic hepatitis and abscess formation.

2.   Respiratory tract

Inhalation of aerosolized bacteria is a well-recognised route of infection but rarely causes respiratory signs; up to 15% have cough and dyspnea.

3.   Bones and joints

Infection here is manifest in 20-60% of patients (17). Sacro-iliitis, usually unilateral, is the most common manifestation followed by arthritis of large peripheral joints and spondylitis in approximately 6% of infections.

4.   Nervous system

Neurobrucellosis occurs in about 5% of patients. It can present at any time in the illness, and meningitis is the most common form. Other syndromes such as myelitis, peripheral neuropathy, central nervous system abscesses, or neuropsychiatric problems can occur.

5.   Cardiovascular system

Endocarditis is the most common infection (only 2-3% of cases) and is the most common cause of death during active brucellosis. Mycotic aneurysms and thrombophlebitis are very rare but do occur.

6.   Genito-urinary system

Acute orchitis or epididymo-orchitis can be presenting illnesses or later complications. Renal abscesses are rare complications. Brucellae can be excreted in urine asymptomatically.

Table 1   Symptoms and signs of brucellosis.

Symptoms	
abdominal pain	joint pain
aches and pains	lethargy
back pain	loss of appetite
chills	rashes
constipation	sleep disturbances
cough	sweating
diarrhea	testicular pain
fever	weight loss
headache	

Signs	
arthritis	pallor
cardiac murmur	pneumonia
CNS abnormalities	psychiatric problems
epididymo-orchitis	rashes
hepatomegaly	spinal tenderness
jaundice	splenomegaly
looks ill	weight loss
lymphadenopathy	

7. Skin

Approximately 5% of patients have cutaneous manifestations including erythema nodosum, ulcers, maculopapular rashes, and petechial purpuric rashes.

B. Tularemia

The clinical features vary from asymptomatic infection (probably the most common) to acute fatal septicemia depending on the virulence of the bacterium, the portal of entry, and state of host immunity. Although there is considerable overlap, the major presentations of tularemia (Table 2) are ulceroglandular, glandular, oculoglandular, pharyngeal, typhoidal, and pneumonic (6,8,18).

Table 2   Major presentations of tularemia.

Ulceroglandular	45-85% of cases	skin ulcers (hands especially) with draining lymphadenopathy
Glandular	10-25% of cases	regional lymphadenopathy with no apparent skin focus
Oculo-glandular	<5% of cases	conjunctivitis; discrete ulcers; periauricular, parotid, or submandibular lymphadenopathy; blepharitis and eyelid edema
Oropharyngeal	<5% of cases	exudative pharyngitis (may be mistaken for diphtheria); cervical lymphadenopathy
Typhoidal	<5% of cases	fever; rigors
Pneumonic	<5% of cases	bronchopneumonia; pleurisy; hilar lymphadenopathy

The onset is sudden with fever and all or some of aches, chills, rigors, cough, and chest pain. Without effective antimicrobial therapy, this can persist for weeks, and at any time, the bacteria can emerge from their focus of infection to cause septicaemia, pneumonia, or meningitis. In the latter case, the mortality can be as high as 60%, but overall without antibiotic therapy, the mortality used to be 5-10%.

The ulceroglandular form of disease begins with a papule at the site of inoculation and a few days after onset of generalized symptoms and signs. The papule evolves through pustule to ulcer which may be covered by an eschar. The nodes draining the area will be enlarged by the time the ulcer develops. Oculoglandular tuleremia is similar except that the ulcer is on the conjunctiva, and the surrounding tissue may become inflamed and edematous. In glandular tularemia, there is no cutaneous or mucosal lesion, but groups of regional nodes are enlarged.

Oropharyngeal tularemia is acquired by ingestion, and the patient usually presents with exudative pharyngitis or tonsillitis (which may be mistaken for diphtheria) occasionally with ulcers. There will often be cervical lymphadenopathy. Typhoidal or septicemic tularemia presents suddenly as a fulminant sepsis syndrome, often with no localizing signs. Up to 50% will develop pneumonia with a dry unproductive cough and occasionally pleurisy and hemoptysis.

C. Pasteurellosis

There are three major clinical manifestations: infection of bite wounds, pneumonia, and bacteremia/septicemia with or without focal lesions (9,10,19). Pasteurellae, principally *P. multocida*, are part of the normal oral flora of dogs and cats, and infection is associated with biting, licking, or scratching by those species (others such as lion, oppossum, and rat are implicated rarely). Local inflammation with local or regional lymphadenitis develops in 1-2 days. Other localized complications include arthritis, tenosynovitis, or osteomyelitis depending on the site and severity of the bite. Pasteurellae can rarely colonize the human upper airways and may thus cause pneumonia especially in those with compromised lung function such as in chronic obstructive airways disease or post-influenza. Bacteremic spread can occur from any infected site leading to septicemia and metastatic disease such as meningitis. Single deep abscesses in many sites are described usually as single case reports.

D. Streptobacillosis

The two modes of transmission (ingestion or rat bite) produce similar clinical syndromes. Haverhill fever follows ingestion of water, foodstuffs, or milk that is contaminated by rats, whereas the mode of transmission for rat-bite fever is obvious (but may occur by close contact and no bite!). The only major difference between the two is that pharyngitis occurs frequently in Haverhill fever. It is characterized by an acute onset of irregularly relapsing fever, chills, headache, vomiting, myalgia, arthralgia, and an erythematous rash (20). The rash may be maculopapular, morbilliform, or even petechial/purpuric. Regional lymphadenopathy is not a feature of streptobacillary rat-bite fever in contrast to that due to *Spirillum minus*. Untreated, the mortality is over 10%. Complications include endocarditis, myocarditis, pericarditis, meningitis, and pneumonia. Abscess formation in almost each of the internal organs has been described.

E. Plague

The three major clinical forms of illness are bubonic, septicemic, and pneumonic plague (21).

1. Bubonic

A bubo (βουβων is 'groin' in Greek) is a lump consisting of an enlarged lymph node and edema of the surrounding tissue. Illness begins with a sudden onset of fever, rigors, and severe headache. The bubo usually begins within 24-36 hours of this. The bubo is usually painful and tender, and the overlying skin is often red and inflamed. Initially, it is hard and rubbery, but as the illness progresses it becomes fluctuant and may rupture. There is usually a solitary bubo, but a minority of patients will have several. The patient becomes more septic as the disease progresses, often with mood changes, insomnia, or slurred speech. By day two or three, the patient will be severely ill, and some may develop a petechial/purpuric rash. In some, the purpuric areas become necrotic with cutaneous gangrene of the extremities in particular. This is probably the origin of the term the Black Death. Occasionally, skin ulcers can occur at the site of the flea bite. The diagnostic lesion, however, is the bubo. Most deaths occur between the third and sixth day, and 30-50% will die if untreated.

2. Septicemic

Although all patients with plague will be septicemic, the term is reserved for those who get overwhelming infection and die, most often, without bubo formation.

3. Pneumonia

In a proportion of patients during bubonic or septicemic plague, *Y. pestis* reaches the lungs via the bloodstream and causes a patchy secondary bronchopneumonia along with cavities or major pulmonary consolidation. Such a patient is highly infectious to others by the airborne route as the sputum contains large numbers of bacteria. On inhalation, patients develop primary pneumonia of rapid onset with tachypnea that may progress to severe respiratory distress, shock, and death. Such patients are highly infectious since their sputa are teeming with *Y. pestis*.

Other manifestations include meningitis, which may occur at presentation or after the bubo has developed, and tonsillar or pharyngeal plague. The latter occurs by inhalation from a case of pneumonic plague, but cases have occurred when fleas are crushed between the teeth (21).

III. EPIDEMIOLOGY OF INFECTION

A. Brucellosis

Brucellosis has a world-wide distribution in domestic and wild animals. It is found especially in countries that border the Mediterranean, the Arabian Peninsula, the Indian subcontinent, and parts of South and Central America. The U.K., U.S., Canada, Australia, and New Zealand have been declared "*Brucella*-free", and there are only rare citations in most of western Europe. *B. abortus* is principally associated with cattle but may be found in buffalo, yaks, and camels. *B. melitensis* is primarily found in sheep and goats, although camels may occasionally be affected. *B. suis* biovars 1-3 are found in swine, domestic, or wild, but biovar 4 is restricted to reindeer, caribou, and their predators. *B. canis* occurs in dogs, but it is usually a laboratory-acquired infection in humans.

Brucellae set up chronic infection in their animal host which tends to excrete them principally in urine, faeces, milk, and products of conception throughout a lifetime. Human infections are acquired by direct contact with the shed brucellae through abrasions, cuts, or mucus membranes, by ingestion of unpasteurized milk or dairy products, and as an occupational hazard in microbiology laboratories. A number of infections have occurred among veterinary surgeons who have inoculated themselves with the live 'attenuated' *B. abortus* strain 19 vaccine. Person-to-person transmission is very rare, but *B. melitensis* has been isolated from human semen which thus raises the possibility of sexual spread (27).

B. Tularemia

Tularemia is primarily a disease of the Northern Hemisphere (Figure 1) and most frequently from latitudes 30° to 71° north. Its absence from the U.K., Africa, South and Central America, and Australia is noteworthy. It is a rare infection, e.g., the highest incidence in the U.S. is 0.15/100,000. Infection can be either sporadic or occur in epidemic foci as has occurred in Spain recently (22). In general, tularemia in

North America is due to *F. tularensis* biovar tularensis (biotype A) and that in Europe due to *F. tularensis* biovar palaearctica (type B). The biovar designation, however, does not necessarily fit with genomic taxonomy (23), and *F. tularensis* biovar tularensis has been isolated from fleas and mites which feed on small mammals in Slovakia (24). *F. philomiragia* has been isolated from both Europe and the U.S.

1. Reservoirs

A large range of vertebrates and invertebrates are able to maintain *F. tularensis*, but a smaller number, however, are involved in transmission to man. In North America, these include lagomorphs, principally *Sylvilagus* (rabbit) and *Lepus* (hare) species, and rodents such as squirrels, rats, voles, mice, muskrats, and beavers. In Europe, the most important reservoirs are hares, voles, hamsters, mice, and even birds. Occasionally, domestic pets such as cats are implicated in transmission of tularemia usually as a consequence of their claws having caught an infected rodent (25) or via bites (26).

2. Transmission and vectors

Infection can be acquired from arthropod vectors, by direct contact with infected animals (skinning, dressing, or eating them), by transmission from the environment (water, dust, hay), or percutaneous inoculation by carnivorous animals that have eaten an infected lagomorph or rodent. Human-to-human transmission has not been described, but infections do occur in laboratory workers with over 200 cases in the U.S. alone (21).

The most important anthropod vectors are ticks, tabanid flies such as the deer-fly (*Chrysops discalis*), fleas, and mosquitoes, although there is some doubt over the role of the latter (28). Tabanids are important in the U.S., and ticks are important in both U.S. and Europe. The ticks most frequently involved are *Ixodes* and *Dermacentor* spp., including *D. andersoni* (wood tick), *D. variabilis* (dog tick), *Amblyomma americanum* (the Lone Star tick), and *I. ricinus* in Europe. Trans-stadial (across the feeding stages of development: larva, nymph, adult) and trans-ovarial (down the generations) is possible. The bacteria are present in the tick gut, tissues, and haemolymph so they may be transmitted by biting, by contamination of broken skin with tick feces, or by crushing them between the teeth or fingernails.

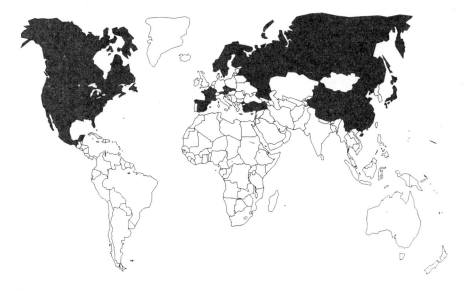

Figure 1   The geographic distribution of tularemia by country over the last 40 years.

C.   Pasteurellosis

P. multocida has a world-wide distribution and has been found wherever it has been sought. It is the cause of fowl cholera in chickens, turkeys, and game birds. It appears to be maintained in flocks by chronically infected but asymptomatic birds that have been infected in previous outbreaks. It is unclear how pathogenic for humans these are. It is a cause of hemorrhagic septicemia and enzootic pneumonia in cattle, pneumonia in sheep, and together with *Bordetella bronchiseptica* atophic rhinitis in pigs. Again whether these can be sources of human infection is unknown. It is found in the oropharynx of cats (50-90%), dogs (50-70%), and rats (14%), and the most frequent zoonotic transfer occurs with bites from these species. Pasteurellae are the most frequent isolates from dog (50%) and cat (75%) bite wounds (29). *P. canis* was most often associated with dog bites and *P. multocida subsp multocida* or *septica* with cat bites, but in most cases other potential pathogens were also present.

P. multocida can be detected in the throats of veterinary students (2.5%), animal handlers (2%), and farm-workers (5%), but not in hospital out-patients (19), thus indicating that animal contact might result in a carrier state. There is a possibility of person-to-person transmission for respiratory tract infection between patients with chronic lung disease (30).

D.   Streptobacillosis

Human streptobacillosis has been described in the U.S., Canada, Brazil, Mexico, Paraguay, Europe (Denmark, Finland, France, Germany, Greece, Holland, Italy, Norway, Spain, Sweden, U.K.), Australia, and India, mostly as case reports but with some outbreaks (e.g., 13,31,32). Although the rat appears to be the natural reservoir of *S. moniliformis*, it has been isolated from other species including mice, guinea-pigs, gerbils, turkeys, squirrels, koala bears, and spinifex hopping mice (20,33,34). Rats carry the bacterium in the upper airway, and it has even been isolated from the middle ear and conjunctivae (35,36). It can cause disease in the rat, but this is exceptional. Most cases of human infection are related to a rat-bite, but one has been related to a dog bite (37). The other major mode of transmission (Haverhill fever) is by ingestion of foodstuffs or water that are contaminated by rat excreta.

E.   Plague

Plague has a world-wide distribution but it is currently absent from many countries (Figure 2). Although its prevalence had been decreasing in previous decades, there has been an increase in reports to the WHO in the 1990s with a yearly average of 2025 cases (38). Those countries reporting the greatest number of cases include Tanzania, Vietnam, Zaire, and Madagascar (39). A recent epidemic in north-west India led to over fifty deaths (40). A few infections occur each year in the U.S. (38).

1.   Reservoir

The predominant reservoirs are urban and sylvatic rats, *R. rattus* (the black rat) and *R. norvegicus* (brown or sewer rat). The former is most important in human infection since it likes to live in houses and travel by ship. Plague normally kills its rat host and 'rat-fall' is a typical precursor of human epidemics. *Y. pestis* has been isolated, however, from more than 230 rodent species, and some of these undoubtedly act as reservoir hosts for infection of other rodents and occasionally for man. These include the multimammate rat (*Mastomys natalensis*) and gerbils in Africa, *R. exulans* in Asia, and ground squirrels (*Spermophilus richardsoni*), rock squirrels (*S. variegatus*) and prairie dogs (*Cynomys spp.*) in the U.S. Companion animals such as dogs and cats can get plague, most often by ingestion of *Y. pestis* infected prey, but these are rarely sources of human infection.

2.   Vectors and transmission

Over 1500 flea species have been found to carry *Y. pestis*, but plague is most likely to be transmitted by fleas whose hypopharynx (proventiculus) becomes blocked by masses of bacteria. This occurs very

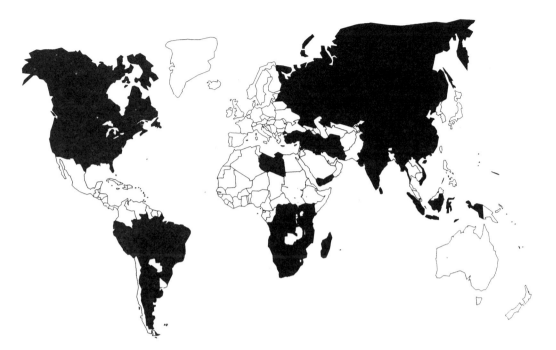

Figure 2 The geographic distribution of plague by country over the last 40 years.

readily in the oriental rat flea (*Xenopsylla cheopis*) which is a very efficient transmitter. Blockage of the hypopharynx causes the flea to bite more often in order to relieve hunger and thirst. The human flea (*Pulex irritans*) is a less efficient vector but is important especially when there is heavy human infestation. The flea ingests blood plus bacteria from a bacteremic host. The bacteria multiply in the clotted blood, and the flea regurgitates some bacteria into the patient's skin when it next feeds. Fleas harbour *Y. pestis* for up to a year, and rodent burrows maintain the plague ecosystems as they provide a humid environment for flea reproduction and a constant traffic of potential hosts. Most human infections are acquired via fleas, but person-to-person spread can occur in pneumonic plague via the respiratory route. Finally, there are cases of plague that are reported following the handling of or the inhalation of aerosols from infected animal tissues.

IV. NATURE OF THE BACTERIA, PATHOGENESIS, AND CLINICAL MANIFESTATIONS

A. *Brucella* spp.

Based on 5S and 16S rRNA sequencing, *Brucella* is taxonomically placed among the α-2 group of the *Proteobacteria* along with *Bartonella henselae* and *Agrobacterium tumefaciens* (41,42). They are small Gram negative coccobacilli with no flagellae, endospores, capsule, or plasmids. They are facultatively intracellular pathogens that can grow aerobically although growth is improved with additional (10%) CO_2 (Table 3). The latter is essential for the initial isolation of *B. ovis* and *B. abortus*. *B. melitensis* has a 2.27×10^3 MDa genome with a G+C ratio of 58-59 mol% and possesses two independent replicons (43). Most of the other species have two replicons except *B. suis* biovar 3 (44). Although they are subdivided into separate species and biovars, 5S and 16S rRNA gene studies indicate they comprise a sin-

Table 3 Characteristics of the genus *Brucella*.

Table 3   Characteristics of the genus *Brucella*.

Species	Host	Human pathogenicity	CO₂ needs	H₂S production	Urease production	Growth on thionine	fuchsin
B. melitensis							
biovar 1	goats,sheep	3	-	-	variable	+	+
biovar 2	goats,sheep	3	-	-	variable	+	+
biovar 3	goats,sheep	3	-	-	variable	+	+
B. abortus							
biovar 1	cattle	2	[+]	+	slow	-	-
biovar 2	cattle	2	[+]	+	slow	-	-
biovar 3	cattle	2	[+]	+	slow	+	+
biovar 4	cattle	2	[+]	+	slow	-	[+]
biovar 5	cattle	2	-	-	slow	+	+
biovar 6	cattle	2	-	[+]	slow	-	+
biovar 9	cattle	2	-	+	slow	+	+
B. suis							
biovar 1	porcines	3	-	+	rapid	+	[-]
biovar 2	porcines	1	-	-	rapid	+	-
biovar 3	porcines	3	-	-	rapid	+	+
biovar 4	reindeer,caribou	2	-	-	rapid	+	[-]
biovar 5	rodents	3	-	-	rapid	+	-
B. canis	canine	1	-	-	rapid	+	-
B. ovis	sheep	0	+	-	-	+	[-]
B. neotomae	rats	0	-	+	rapid	-	-

Human pathogenicity: 0 = none, 1 = low potential, 2 = moderate potential, 3 = high potential. Key: + = positive, - = negative, [+] = most strains positive, [-] = most strains negative.

gle species (*B. melitensis*). Since the original subdivisions are useful for epidemiological purposes, however, they have been maintained (Table 3).

All will grow on peptone-based media that are enriched with blood or serum, but prolonged incubation may be necessary for primary isolation. *Brucella* spp. are catalase-positive but variable in oxidase, urease, and H₂S production (Table 3). Speciation and biovar designation is based on the above, the ability to grow on media that contain thionine or fuchsin, agglutination by monospecific antisera, lysis by phages, and the ability to oxidize various amino acids and sugars. Such assessment is normally the province of a reference laboratory. Use of automated biochemical identification systems can produce misleading results (45). *B. canis* and *B. ovis* are naturally rough whereas primary isolates of the rest are smooth (but may produce rough mutants on subculture). The major surface or O antigen is carried on lipopolysaccharide molecules (or endotoxin). There are cross-reactions between these and O antigens of *Enterobacteriaceae*, e.g., between *Y. enterocolitica* 0:9 and *B. abortus*. The lipid A (or toxic moiety of endotoxin) differs from that of other Gram negative bacteria in being more hydrophobic (more saturated long chain fatty acids with few hydroxylated molecules). This, for example, renders it less active in stimulating IL-1 and TNF-α release from monocytes (46).

Brucellae gain entry directly through skin abrasions and mucosal surfaces (e.g., conjunctivae, bronchial tree) and by ingestion. Ingestion via fatty foods such as dairy products will give some protection against gastric acid, and *B. melitensis* appears more resistant to low pH than other *Brucellae*. The incubation period is usually two to three weeks. During this time the bacteria enter the local lymphatics, grow in the draining lymph nodes, and then spread through the bloodstream. The smooth strains are able to resist the bactericidal activity of serum. Strains of *B. melitensis*, in particular, have a greater ability to resist the killing effect of neutrophils (47). The major site of replication, however, is within the macrophages of the reticulo-endothelial system. It is unclear how the bacteria survive inside phagocytes. Some strains of *B. abortus*, however, produce superoxide dismutase (48), and GMP and adenine production by *B. abortus* has been linked to inhibition of hypohalite production (49). *B. suis* expresses a type IV secretion system and loss of the latter resulted in poor intramacrophage growth (50). It has also recently been shown that *B. suis* prevents apoptosis in monocytes which might prolong their survival (51). The affinity of *B. abortus* for the placenta might be related to enhancement of its growth by erythritol (52).

B. *F. tularensis*

Francisellae are small non-motile, aerobic Gram negative coccobacilli. In early culture, they are encapsulated and show considerable pleomorphism. The capsule is rich in lipid. Optimum growth occurs aerobically at 37°C on media that are supplemented with cysteine or cystine and erythrocytes (human or rabbit). There are two species, *F. tularensis* and *F. philomiragia* (23,53), and they are in the gamma subclass of *Proteobacteria*. They are closely related to endosymbionts of ticks, such as *Wolbachia persica* (23,54), which might cause difficulties in DNA-based surveys of *F. tularensis* in ticks. There are three biovars of *F. tularensis* namely tularensis (old Jellison type A), palearctica (old type B), and novicida which are differentiated by virulence, geographic location, and biochemical reactions (Table 4). There are antigenic differences between biovars tularensis and novicida but not the others. These biovar differences, however, are not always apparent on analysis of 16S rRNA genes (23).

The infective dose is 10-50 colony-forming units by intradermal inoculation but as high as 10^8 by ingestion. The infective dose by aerosol is also very low, but what underlies the differing virulence of *F. tularensis* biotype tularensis and palaearctica is unknown. In the first days after intradermal inoculation, bacteriamultiply to produce the local lesions. They drain to the local lymph nodes and may disseminate to produce bacteremia. They then localize in various lymphoid organs throughout the body. There, they produce necrotic foci, abscesses, and even granulomas which may rarely show caseation. Virulent

Table 4   Characteristics of the genus *Francisella*.

| | | *F. tularensis* | | |
	biovar tularensis	biovar palaeartica	biovar novicida	*F. philomiragia*
requires cystine	+	+	-	-
growth in saline broth	-	-	+	-
oxidase	-	-	-	+
acid from:				
glucose	+	+	+	+
glycerol	+	-	+	n.a.
geographic location	North America	Eurasia	worldwide	worldwide
virulence for:				
humans	high	moderate	low	low
rabbit	high	low	low	low

(n.a. = not applicable)

strains are able to resist the bactericidal action of serum by virtue of their capsule and long O-polysaccharide LPS chains (55). They are also able to survive in neutrophils and even multiply within macrophages. The former property might be related to inhibition of the respiratory burst by bacterial acid phosphatase (56). Growth within macrophages is regulated by mglA and mglB (macrophage growth loci), but the precise mechanism is unclear (57) and apparently does not involve the bacterial acid phosphatase (58). Interestingly, *F. tularensis* shows phase variation in which an antigenically distinct LPS is produced (59). The LPS and lipid A of one variant does not induce nitric oxide (NO) in macrophages thus permitting intramacrophage growth. It is possible for reverse phase shift to occur so perhaps the bacterium is altering macrophage NO production for its survival either during acute infection or in establishing a carrier state. There is also evidence that, in order to survive in macrophages, *F. tularensis* remain in acidified endosomes perhaps to aid the iron uptake that is necessary for growth (60).

C.   *Pasteurella* spp.

Pasteurellae are small non-motile unencapsulated Gram negative bacilli except for *P. multocida* which is coccoid and encapsulated. All grow optimally at 35-37°C on blood-enriched media. They are in the gamma subclass of the Proteobacteria. There are 11 species and three subspecies of *Pasteurella* (Table 5). *P. testudinis, P. haemolytica, P. aerogenes, P. ureae, P. piscidida*, and *P. pneumotropica* (biovars Jawetz and Heyl) are all excluded from the genus and some have been re-assigned to the genus *Actinobacillus*. *P. multocida* is the most important human pathogen. Presence or absence of capsule is not always related to the ability to cause disease, but the amount of capsular material is. *P. multocida* produces neuraminidase and hyaluronidase, but their role in pathogenesis is unknown. In general, infection is apparent more rapidly after a cat (median 23 hrs.) than a dog (median 35 hrs.) bite (29). It is unclear how tissue damage is produced.

D.   *S. moniliformis*

S. moniliformis is a pheomorphic non-motile Gram negative bacillus. In serum supplemented liquid media, it produces typical 'puff-ball' colonies. Growth on solid media requires blood or serum supplements and optimal conditions are 35-37°C with a microaerophilic atmosphere. Two colonial forms occur on subculture, the normal bacillary form and an L-form. *S. moniliformis* is characterized by its negative oxidase, catalase, indole production, and nitrate reduction tests. Its genome has a mol% G+C content of 24-25 (24-26% for the L-form) which is significantly lower than for other Gram negative bacilli (20). In fact, the closest to this value are the *Mycoplasmatales*, but analysis of l6S rRNA genes does not confirm such a relationship (20). *S. moniliformis* has been shown to have two subspecies, however, that cluster with *Sebaldella termitidis* and *Fusobacterium* spp. (20). Recently, a bacterium causing disease in farmed Atlantic salmon has been shown to be related to *S. moniliformis* (61), and presumptive *S. moniliformis* have been isolated from human female genital abscesses (62). The incubation period of *S. moniliformis* rat bite fever is 2-10 days (range 1-22 days) and that of Haverhill fever is similar. It is not known how *S. moniliformis* causes disease and what virulence traits it carries.

E.   *Y. pestis*

Y. pestis is a Gram negative, encapsulated bacillus that exhibits bipolar staining. It is a member of the *Enterobacteriaceae* with a G+C molar content of 46-50%. There are ten species in the genus, but *Y. pseudotuberculosis* is the closest to *Y. pestis* (90% DNA relatedness). It appears that *Y. pestis* is a clone of *Y. pseudotuberculosis* that diverged some 1,500 to 20,000 years ago (63). It will grow on most media albeit slowly with a growth optimum of 25-29°C, but can grow over a range of 2-42°C. On blood agar, it is non-hemolytic but produces characteristic colonies with a 'hammered copper' or 'fried egg' appearance after 48 hrs. at 37°C. It differs from other *Yersinia* in being non-motile at all temperatures, ur-

Table 5   Characteristics of the genus *Pasteurella*.

Species	Pathogenic for humans	Animal reservoir
P. multocida subsp. multocida	+	mammals, birds
P. multocida subsp. septica	+	mammals, birds
P. multocida subsp. gallicida	+	birds
P. dagmatis	+	dogs, cats
P. gallinarum	-	chickens
P. volantium	+	chickens
P. canis	+	dogs
P. stomatis	+	dogs, cats
P. avium	-	chickens
P. langaa	-	chickens
P. anatis	-	ducks
Pasteurella A	-	fowl
Pasteurella B	+	dogs, cats

ease negative, and non-fermentative for melibiose or rhamnose. Three different variants, Antiqua, Medievalis, and Orientalis, (corresponding to the Justinian plague, Black Death, and current plague respectively) are described and are based on glycerol fermentation and nitrate reduction. They do not differ in virulence, but are distinguisable by ribotyping (64) and other techniques (63). In vivo, it produces a capsule, a component of which is the fraction 1 antigen (F1). In culture, it releases cytoplasmic antigens V and W which appear to be involved in growth regulation.

   Y. pestis is a facultative intracellular pathogen. Following inoculation by a flea bite, *Y. pestis*, which at this stage possesses very little capsular F1 antigen, is readily taken up by neutrophils and macrophages. It is able to survive and multiply within macrophages, and during this process capsule production is switched on. Thus, the next generation of bacteria are able to resist phagocytes. The bacteria are released from macrophages by the induction of apoptosis. Some appear to persist by dividing slowly in macrophages perhaps by elaboration of V and W antigens which are related to a growth requirement for calcium. Calcium levels in the macrophage cytoplasm are low. How these activities occur and how they are co-ordinated is gradually being unraveled.

   Both plasmid and chromosomally encoded genes are important in pathogenesis. Some genes and mechanisms are common to several *Yersinia* spp. and others are unique to *Y. pestis*. *Y. pestis* possesses two plasmids that are not found in other species (65). The 100 kb *Tox* plasmid encodes the synthesis of the F1 antigen (*caf* 1) and a toxin that is lethal for rats and mice; the latter is a phospholipase D superfamily member (66) and might thus be responsible for tissue damage. The 9.5 kb *Pst* plasmid encodes a plasminogen activator which is involved in the binding of these bacteria to cell surface glycolipids (67) and in post-translational modification of Yops (outer membrane proteins). Another 70 kb *Lcr* (low calcium response) plasmid is found in all pathogenic *Yersinia* spp. The latter encodes the V and W antigens and regulates vegetative growth in the absence of Ca^{2+} at 37°C, perhaps slowing intramacrophage bacterial growth. Its effect is reversed by addition of Ca^{2+} or by incubation at 26°C (perhaps flea temperature). This plasmid encodes a type III secretion system (composed of YopB, YopD and *LcrV*) which is assembled and dismantled according to environmental conditions. Through this, it secretes a number of intracellular effector proteins (Yop E, Yop H, YpkA/Yopo, Yop P/ Yop J, Yop M and Yop T) (68). The function of some Yops are gradually being understood, e.g., Yop E is a cytotoxin and causes actin depolymerization, Yop H has tyrosine phosphatase activity, and Yop M is anti-inflammatory (69). In addition, the V antigen inhibits neutrophil chemotaxis (70) and suppresses TNF-α production via activated T cells (71). On the chromosome, *Y. pestis* has an unstable 102 kb region which includes a high pathogenicity island (HP1) of 68 kb and an iron acquisition and colony pigmentation locus of 35 kb (72). Interestingly, the HPI sequence is also found in enteroaggregative *Escherichia coli* and among *E. coli* blood culture isolates (73). Loss of colony pigmentation occurs spontaneously, and this is associated with decreased murine virulence. This occurs due to mutations or deletions in the 35 kb region which encodes, among other things, the siderophore which is termed yersiniabactin (71). Within this locus, there are also a fimbriae gene cluster and a regulatory system that is similar to BvgAS of *Bordetella pertussis* (74). A second smaller pathogenicity island that encodes the iron uptake genes has recently been described (75).

V.   IMMUNOLOGY OF INFECTION

A.   *Brucella* spp.

Serum antibodies to *Brucella* spp. appear at about one week post-infection. They are predominantly of the IgM class and are directed against the LPS O antigens. By week two, class switching has occurred, and levels of IgG begin to rise. Both classes continue to rise, but the IgG quantitation soon exceeds IgM. Following the recovery from infection, IgG levels decline over several months, but low levels of IgM can persist for years (76). Antibodies play a role in protection against infection (77), but it is the onset of a cell-mediated immune response that initiates the killing of brucellae which are residing in macrophages (77,78,79) perhaps via interferon-γ NO, and a Th-1 response (79). It appears, however, that the T cell cytotoxic effect may play a more important role than NO at least in murine brucellosis (80). Although live attenuated *B. abortus* (B19) and *B. melitensis* (Rev-1) vaccines are available for the prevention of brucellosis in cattle and sheep and goats respectively, neither are suitable for use in humans. Indeed, accidental inoculation of humans with the vaccine has resulted in brucellosis. Nevertheless, such vaccines do have an effect indirectly on human brucellosis by decreasing the extent of brucellosis in animals.

B.   *F. tularensis*

Infection with *F. tularensis* does confer protection against re-infection. Second attacks of tularemia have not been described. Antibodies that are directed against LPS and other carbohydrate antigens, and agglutinating IgG, IgM, and IgA antibodies appear during the second and third weeks of infection (81). These persist for at least eight years (82), but are present in only a minority (4%) after 25 years (83). Antibodies do not appear to play a major role in defense against infection, but B cells themselves play an as yet unknown role (84). In the initial phase of the infection, neutrophils are critical in the defense against primary infection and help in defense against re-infection (85). In addition, there is evidence of nitric oxide-independent killing of *F. tularensis* in macrophages stimulated by interferon-γ (86). Cell-mediated immunity that is directed principally against protein antigens is required to limit and then cure the infection (81); this appears to persist for at least 25 years (83). Although athymic nu/nu mice (no mature T cells) succumb to a normally sublethal *F. tularensis* infection, this is not the case in mice depleted of either CD4(+) or CD8(+) T-lymphocytes (87). Nevertheless, soon after infection of mice with *F. tulerensis*, there is growth of bacteria in the liver with an expression of Th-1 cytokines (TNF-α, IFN-γ, and IL-12) but not Th-2 cytokines (IL-3, IL-4). No such expression occurred if heat-killed bacteria were inoculated (88). Protection against infection is provided by a live attenuated vaccine (LVS) but not by killed bacteria or subunits (89). In contrast, protection in mice was induced by immunization with LPS from LVS but not with an outer membrane protein (90). Interestingly, although LVS does produce protective immunity, it induces only a minor expansion of γ-δ-T cells compared to natural infection (91). This difference was related to the expression of phosphoantigens by the virulent *F. tularensis* (91).

C. Pasteurellosis

Although it is known that agglutinating, anti-LPS, and anticapsular antibodies can be detected after infection (19), little is known of their role in immunity. Infection via bites or other routes are more likely to be disseminated in those with impaired immunity (e.g., neonates, cirrhosis, malignancy, CSF shunts, diabetes). Formalin-killed whole bacterial cell vaccines have been used successfully to prevent pasteurellosis in fowl, cattle, and pigs (9). There seems little need for such a vaccine for humans.

D. *S. moniliformis*

Although it is known that agglutinating antibodies develop after infection (13), little is known of immune responses and immunity to *S. moniliformis*. There is no vaccine.

E. Plague

Subclinical or asymptomatic infection with *Y. pestis* does occur in the course of epidemics (92), but most often there is an overwhelming infection that proceeds despite immune defenses. In mice that have recovered from a *Y. pestis* infection, the major epitopes that are recognized in convalescent sera were F1, V-antigen, Yop H, Yop M, Yop D, and plasminogen activator protease (93). The various cell-mediated immune responses are poorly understood. The suppression of TNF-α production by *Y. pestis* V antigen occurs not by direct action on macrophages but appears to require a soluble factor that is released by activated T cells (71).

There is a formalin-killed whole cell vaccine that has been used since 1946 for immunization against plague. There is epidemiological evidence that it is effective (94). There is also a live attenuated vaccine (EV76) which is a non-pigmented variant of a wild strain. It also appears effective (94). There is a great deal of interest, however, in subunit vaccines. In mouse models, IgG1 responses to F1 and V antigens correlate with protection against plague (95), and an F1-V fusion protein provided best protection against experimental bubonic or pneumonic plague (96).

VI. LABORATORY DIAGNOSIS

A. *Brucella* spp.

Specific diagnosis is based on the detection of the bacterium by culture, detection of its genome, or by detection of a serological response. Brucellae can be grown in most good quality peptone-based media, and their growth is greatly enhanced by the addition of whole blood or serum. Bone marrow cultures have a higher detection rate than blood cultures (97). In either case, prolonged incubation (up to 30 days) is necessary. Automated culture systems such as BACTEC or BacT/Alert do, however, speed up detection rates (98,99). Bacteria should be subcultured onto blood agar-based media preferably in a 10% CO_2 atmosphere to ensure growth of *B. ovis* and some biovars of *B. abortus*. Identification can be problematic especially if automated or biochemical strip tests are used (45). Brucellae are ACDP category 3 pathogens and should be sent to appropriate reference laboratories for final identification. Brucellae can be detected and identified in clinical material by using genome amplification. Targets that have been utilized include 16S and 23S rRNA genes and spacer region, a major outer membrane, and 31kD antigen gene sequences (100-103).

Since brucellosis is indolent, and often not suspected until late into the disease, serological tests are often utilized. The serum agglutination test (SAT) is still the gold standard but must employ standardized reagents. The test uses *B. abortus* 19 as antigen and detects both IgM and IgG agglutinating antibody. To differentiate the two classes of antibody, an aliquot of serum is treated with 2-mercaptoethanol or dithiothreitol (which reduce disulphide bridges) in order to destroy IgM as a pentamer. It has no effect on IgG (104). Most patients with active brucellosis have a titre of greater than 1/160 with only a portion being IgG. *B. canis,* which is rough, is not detected by this test and low level cross-reactions occur with antibodies to *Y. enterocolitica* 0:9, *Vibrio cholerae*, and *F. tularensis*. Thus, care must be taken in the interpretation of serological results, and they should be used as part of the diagnostic screen together with clinical and epidemiological data. Enzyme-linked immunosorbent assays are commercially available but must always be confirmed by SAT.

B.   *F. tularensis*

The diagnosis requires an awareness of the epidemiology and clinical features of tularemia including a history of possible exposure. Gram staining of tissues is rarely of value for rapid diagnosis, but immunofluorescence may be useful. *F. tularensis* can be cultured from skin ulcers, lymph nodes, sputum, gastric aspirates, pleural fluid, or blood at 37°C in media supplemented with cystine or cysteine. For sites with a normal flora (e.g., skin or sputum), antibiotic-containing media such as Thayer-Martin chocolate agar can be used. Great care must be taken with this high risk pathogen and identification should be done in a reference laboratory. Genome detection by PCR is increasingly used for diagnosis and identification using 16S rRNA, T cell epitope, or FopA genes (105,106,107).

   Antibody detection is the most frequent method for obtaining a specific diagnosis. For this, tube agglutination, micro-agglutination, and ELISA are the most commonly-used techniques (82,108). The latter two assays are the most sensitive and can provide early diagnosis, but for a definitive diagnosis, a rising (4-fold) titre must be demonstrated. Heterophile antibodies, and low level cross-reaction with *Brucella* spp., *Yersinia* spp. or *Proteus* 0X19 do occur but can be eliminated by treatment of the serum with dithiothreitol.

C.   *Pasteurella* **spp.**

Culture of bite wound, blood, CSF, or other infected sites is done on blood or chocolate agar. In many cases, however, bite wounds contain a number of other potential pathogens so that samples should be cultured for aerobes and anaerobes. Selective media have been devised for the isolation of pasteurellae from sites with a normal flora, such as from animals (109), but these are not often used in the diagnosis of human disease.

   Isolates can be confused with *Haemophilus influenzae*, and thus it is of importance for the laboratory to be informed of a possible diagnosis of pasteurellosis (110). Genomic and serological diagnosis are not often used in human medicine.

D.   *S. moniliformis*

S. moniliformis can be isolated from bite wounds or blood, but again, clinical suspicion of infection is needed to alert the laboratory (20). The incorporation of liquoid (sodium polyanethol sulphonate) in blood culture media slows bacterial growth (111). It forms characteristic colonies on, for example, blood agar, and it can be identified by the APIZYM system (112), fatty acid profiles, or 16S rRNA gene sequencing (20). Serological tests are not available.

E.   *Y. pestis*

Diagnosis depends on the suspicion of possible plague which is based on travel and exposure histories. Aspiration of a bubo, which may require prior saline instillation, will provide material for microscopy and culture. The aspirate should be stained using Gram, Wayson, and/or Giemsa techniques. Gram staining will demonstrate intraphagocytic Gram negative bacilli, and the other two stains are useful for demonstrating bipolar staining. Immunofluorescence can also be of value in rapid diagnosis (113). For culture, samples (bubo, blood, CSF, or sputum) should be inoculated onto on blood and MacConkey agar and placed in blood culture bottles. It can take two days for colonies to appear (69). For identification, the API 20E has proved less specific than the BBL Crystal System (114). This is a high risk pathogen, and specific identification should be performed under ACDP category 3 containment in an appropriate reference laboratory. *Y. pestis* can be detected in clinical samples or even fleas using PCR amplification with or without probes (115,116). The latter have a sensitivity as low as 10-100 colony-forming units.

Serological diagnosis is possible by antigen or antibody detection. Detection of F1 antigen in clinical samples has proved useful in the acute diagnosis of plague (39,117). Retrospective diagnosis can be made by demonstrating a four-fold rise or fall in titre to the F1 antigen by passive haemagglutination (118) or ELISA (69). A single titre of greater than 1/10 in a previously unexposed or vaccinated patient provides a presumptive diagnosis.

VII. ANTIMICROBIAL SUSCEPTIBILITY AND TREATMENT

A. *Brucella* spp.

In vitro, *Brucella* spp. are susceptible to a wide range of antimicrobials when tested by disc susceptibility, breakpoint, plate dilution MICs, or E-test (119,120). In such tests, brucellae are susceptible to tetracycline (MICs and MBCs all <1.25 mg./L. except chlortetracycline which has much higher values), aminoglycosides (gentamicin MIC and MBC all <5mg./L.), macrolides (erythromycin MICs and MBCs all <2.5 mg./L.), chloramphenicol (MICs and MBCs <5mg./L.), rifampicin (MICs and MBCs <2.5 mg./L.), and fluoroquinolones (MICs and MBCs <2 mg./L.) (120,121). Of the β-lactams, ampicillin and the carbapenems are active but not the cephalosporins or other penicillins (121,122).

Such in vitro activities, however, are not translated into in vivo efficacy principally because brucellae are facultative intracellular pathogens, and many antimicrobials do not achieve high enough intramacrophage concentrations. Antimicrobials that achieve high concentrations inside macrophages and other cells include the tetracyclines, macrolides, fluoroquinolones and rifampicin. The pH inside the phagocytic vacuole which contains brucellae is low (~ pH 5.0), however, and at this pH, the fluoroquinolones and macrolides such as azithromycin are far less active (123). Even with the tetracyclines (e.g., doxycycline or minocycline) alone, there is a relapse rate such that combinations of antimicrobials, (e.g., doxycycline plus gentamicin or rifampicin) are considered optimal therapy. Even with these, six weeks of therapy is needed. Resistance can develop during therapy, especially with fluoroquinolones. Plasmids are rarely, if ever, found in brucellae (124), and thus plasmid-encoded resistance is not a problem.

B. *F. tularensis*

F. tularensis is sensitive to a wide range of antimicrobials in vitro including the fluoroquinolones (125,126). Exceptions to this include penicillin, cephalexin, cefuroxime, ceftazidime, aztreonam, imipenem, and meropenem with MICs >32 mg./L. (125). The treatment of choice is either streptomycin or gentamicin, and most clinical experience is with streptomycin (127). The fluoroquinolones have proven effective (126), but despite good in vitro activity, ceftriaxone therapy is less successful (128). Little is known of plasmid-encoded resistance in *F. tularensis*.

C. *Pasteurella* spp.

Pasteurella multocida and other species are susceptible to penicillin, ampicillin, cefuroxime, amoxycillin/clavulanic acid, tetracycline, minocycline, cotrimoxazole, and fluoroquinolones at clinically achievable concentrations, (19,129,130). The oral cepholosporins (e.g., cefaclor and cephalexin), erythromycin, and oxacillin are less active (131). Antibiotic resistance plasmids have been detected in fowl and cattle isolates of *P. multocida*, and these encode resistance to tetracycline, streptomycin, and sulphadimidine, but they were small and non-conjugative (109). Recently, a transposon-like element that encodes tetracycline resistance has been found in *P. multocida* (132), and a β-lactamase producing strain was isolated from a lung abscess (133). The optimal therapy of bite wounds is local wound debridement and, because of the above and the mixed nature of the infection, administration of amoxycillin/clavulanic acid (19,29).

D. *S. moniliformis*

In vitro susceptibility testing of *S. moniliformis* by disc diffusion or agar incorporation MICs have produced similar results (20,112). MICs of penicillin (0.015 mg./L.), ampicillin (0.06 mg./L.), tetracycline (0.5 mg./L.), and cefotaxime (0.5 mg./L.) are within clinically achievable levels. In vitro, erythromycin, chloramphenicol, fluoroquinolones, and aminoglycosides are less active but the former has been used successfully in at least one case (134). Penicillin is the treatment of choice and this does not seem to be affected by the bacterium's propensity to produce L-forms during in vitro culture.

E. *Y. pestis*

Y. pestis isolates are usually sensitive in vitro to agents that are active against Gram negative bacteria including ampicillin, tetracyclines, chloramphenicol, streptomycin, gentamicin, sulphonamides, cefotaxime (MIC 0.03 mg./L.), and fluoroquinolones such as ofloxacin and ciprofloxacin (MIC 0.03 mg./L.) (135,136). Prompt and effective antimicrobial chemotherapy can decrease mortality from over 60% to under 15%. Effective regimens include streptomycin or gentamicin by intramuscular injection, doxycycline orally, or chloramphenicol (especially in plague meningitis) orally or intravenously. Although active in vitro, β-lactam antibiotics are not active in experimental models of pneumonic plague, but gentamicin, netilmicin, ciprofloxacin, and ofloxacin were as effective as streptomycin (137). Pneumonic plague is the most difficult therapeutic challenge, and the above agents were effective even when therapy was commenced after forty hours of infection (137), but doxycyline and ciprofloxacin were not effective in a similar model when given 48 hours post-infection (138). In an intraperitoneal challenge model, ciprofloxacin, when commenced 48 hours pre-challenge, was completely effective but less so when given 24 hours post-challenge (139) thus indicating that ciprofloxacin might be of value for prophylaxis, but perhaps less so for therapy.

The view that antimicrobial resistance does not develop in *Y. pestis* has been overturned by the recent isolation of strains in Madagascar that carry a conjugative 150 kb inc6-C plasmid (140). This encoded resistance to ampicillin (TEM-1 β-lactamase; MIC 2048 mg./L.), chloramphenicol (type I chloramphenicol acetyl transferase; MIC 128 mg./L.), streptomycin (3″-9 aminoglycoside adenylyl transferase; MIC >2048 mg./L.), tetracycline (*tet*D; MIC 1024 mg./L.) and sulphonamides (*sul* I; MIC 1024 mg./L.). It was considered that this plasmid could have originated in other enterobacterial species, but it was also able to transfer between *Y. pestis* isolates. Ominously, its appearance could render all the first-line therapies ineffective.

REFERENCES

1. World Health Organization. Zoonoses. Technical Report Series. No. 169. Geneva:WHO, 1959. No. 169.
2. Hart CA, Trees AJ, Duerden BI. Zoonoses. J Med Microbiol 1997; 46:4-33.
3. Hart CA, Bennett M, Begon ME. Zoonoses. J Epidemiol Community Health 1999; 53: 514-515.
4. Evans AC. Further studies on *Bacterium abortus* and related bacteria. II. A comparison of *Bacterium abortus* and *Bacterium bronchisepticum* and with the organism that causes Malta Fever. J Infect Dis 1918; 22:580-587.
5. Mediterranean Fever Commission (1905-1907). Report of the Commissions appointed by the Admiralty, the War Office and the Civil Government of Malta for the investigation of Malta Fever under the supervision of an Advisory Committee of the Royal Society. London: Harrison and Sons.

6. Ohara Y, Sato T, Fujita H, Ueno T, Homma M. Clinical manifestations of tularaemia in Japan: analysis of 1355 cases observed between 1924 and 1987. Infection 1991; 19:14-17.

7. McCoy GW, Chapin CW. *Bacterium tularense*, the cause of plague-like disease of rodents. Publ Hlth Bull 1912; 57:17-23.

8. Tarnvik A, Sandstrom G, Sjostedt A. Infrequent manifestations of tularaemia in Sweden. Scand J Infect Dis 1997; 29:443-446.

9. Adlam C, Rutter JM, eds. *Pasteurella* and Pasteurellosis. London:Academic Press, 1989.

10. Goldstein EJC, Citron DM, Wield B, Blachman U, Sutter VL, Miller TA, Feingold SM. Bacteriology of human and animal bite wounds. J Clin Microbiol 1978; 8:667-672.

11. Wilcox W. Violent symptoms from bite of rat. Am J Med Sci 1839; 26:245.

12. Blake FC. Etiology of rat-bite fever. J Exp Med 1916; 23:39.

13. Parker F, Hudson NP. The etiology of Haverhill fever (erythema arthriticum epidemicum). Am J Pathol 1926; 2:357-359.

14. Kiple KF. The plague of Justinian: an early lesson in the Black Death. In: Kiple KF, ed. Plague, Pox and Pestilence. London:Wiedenfeld and Nicholson, 1997:26-31.

15. Carmichael AG. Bubonic plague: the Black Death. In: Kiple KF, ed. Plague, Pox and Pestilence. London:Wiedenfeld and Nicholson, 1997: 60-67.

16. Christie AB, Corbel MJ. Plague and other yersinial diseases. In: Smith GR, Easmon CSF, eds. London:Edward Arnold, 1990:399-421.

17. Mousa ARM, Muhtaseb SA, Almudallal DS, Khodeir SM, Marafie AA. Osteoarticular complications of brucellosis: a study of 169 cases. Rev Infect Dis 1987; 9:531-543.

18. Evans ME, Gregory DW, Schaffner W, McGee ZA. Tularemia – a 30 year experience with 88 cases. Medicine 1985; 64:251-269.

19. Frederiksen W. Pasteurellosis of man. In: Adlam C, Rutter JM, eds. *Pasteurella* and Pasteurellosis. London:Academic Press, 1989:303-320.

20. Wullenweber M. *Streptobacillus moniliformis* – a zoonotic pathogen. Taxonomic considerations, host species, diagnosis, therapy, geographical distribution. Lab Anim 1995; 29:1-15.

21. Christie A. Plague, tularaemia. In: Christie AB, ed. Infectious Diseases, 3rd Edn. Edinburgh:Churchill Livingstone, 1980:747-774.

22. Lugue PB, Castrillon JLP, Luquero MM, Martin FJM, Lopez-Areal JDL, Pascual PP, Mazon MA, Guilarte VH. Preliminary report of an epidemic tularaemia outbreak in Valladolid. Rev Clin Esp 1998; 198:789-793.

23. Forsman M, Sandstrom G, Sjostedt A. Analysis of 16S ribosomal DNA sequences of *Francisella* strains and utilisation for determination of the phylogeny of the genus and for identification of strains by PCR. Int J Syst Bacteriol 1994; 44:38-46.

24. Gurycova D. First isolation of *Francisella tularensis* subsp tularensis in Europe. Eur J Epidemiol 1998; 14:797-802.

25. Rodon P, Levallois D, Akli J, Leaute E, Friocourt P. Tularemia acquired from a cat-scratch. Medicine et Maladies Infectieuses 1998; 28:223-224.

26. Quezner RW, Mostow SR, Emerson JK. Cat-bite tularemia. J Amer Med Soc 1977; 238:1845-1849.

27. Vandercam B, Zech F, de Cooman S, Bughin C, Gigi J, Wauters C. Isolation of *Brucella melitensis* from human sperm. Eur J Clin Microbiol Infect Dis 1990; 9:303-304.

28. Hubalek Z, Halouzka J. Mosquitoes (*Diptera: Culicidae*) in contrast to ticks (*Acar: Ixodidae*) do not carry *Francisella tularensis* in a natural focus of infection in the Czech Republic. J Med Entomol 1997; 34:660-663.

29. Talan DA, Citron DM, Abrahamian FM, Moran GJ, Goldstein EJC. Bacteriologic analysis of infected dog and cat bites. N Eng J Med 1999; 340:85-92.

30. Itoh M, Tierno PM, Milstoc M, Berger AR. A unique outbreak of *Pasteurella multocida* in a chronic disease hospital. Am J Public Health 1980; 70:1170-1173.

31. Shanson DC, Midgley J, Gazzard BG, Dixey J, Gibson GL, Stevenson J, Finch RG, Cheesbrough J. *Streptobacillus moniliformis* isolated from blood in four cases of Haverhill fever – first outbreak in Britain. Lancet 1983; ii:92-94.

32. McEvoy MB, Noah ND, Pilsworth R. Outbreak of fever caused by *Streptobacillus moniliformis*. Lancet 1987; ii:1361-1363.

33. Hopkinson WI, Lloyd JM. *Streptobacillus moniliformis* septicaemia in spinifex hopping mice (*Notomys alexis*). Austral Vet J 1981; 57:533-534.

34. Glunder G, Hinz KH, Stiburek B. Arthritis in turkeys caused by *Streptobacillus moniliformis* in Germany. Deutsche Tierarzt Wochenschr 1982; 89:367-370.

35. Wullenweber M, Jonas C, Kunstyr I. *Streptobacillus moniliformis* isolated from otitis media of conventionally kept laboratory rats. J Exp Anim Sci 1992; 35:49-57.

36. Al Hadithi HT. Incidence of *Streptobacillus moniliformis* in laboratory rats and mice. Biomed Lett 1997; 55:7-11.

37. Peel MM. Dog-associated bacterial infection in humans – isolates submitted to an Australian reference laboratory, 1981-1992. Pathology 1993; 25:379-384.

38. Anonymous. Human plague in 1994. Wkly Epidemiol Rec 1996; 71:165-168.

39. Ratsitorahina M, Chanteau S, Rahalison L, Ratsifasoamanana L, Boisier P. Epidemiological and diagnostic aspects of the outbreak of pneumonic plague in Madagascar. Lancet 2000; 355:111-113.

40. Mavalankar DV. Indian plague epidemic – unanswered questions and key lessons. J Roy Soc Med 1995; 88:547-551.

41. Moreno E, Stackebrandt E, Dorsch M, Wolters J, Busch M, Mayer H. *Brucella abortus* 16S rRNA and lipid A reveal a phylogenetic relationship with members of the alpha-2 subdivision of the class *Proteobacteria*. J Bacteriol 1990; 172:3569-3576.

42. Minnick MF, Steigler GL. Nucleotide sequence and comparison of the 5S ribosomal RNA genes of *Rochalimea henselae, R. quintana* and *Brucella abortus*. Nucleic Acid Res 1993; 21:2518.

43. Michaux S, Paillisson J, Carles-Nurit MJ, Bourg G, Allardet-Servent A, Ramuz M. Presence of two independent chromosomes in the *Brucella melitensis* 16M genome. J Bacteriol 1993; 175:701-705.

44. Ugalde RA. Intracellular lifestyle of *Brucella* spp. Common genes with other animal pathogens, plant pathogens and endosymbionts. Microbes Infect 1999; 1:1211-1219.

45. Peiris V, Fraser S, Fairhurst M, Weston D, Kaczmarski E. Laboratory diagnosis of brucella infection: some pitfalls. Lancet 1990; 339:1415-1416.

46. Goldstein J, Hoftman T, Frasch C, Lizzio EF, Beining PR, Hochstein D, Lee YL, Angus RD, Golding B. Lipopolysaccharide (LPS) from *Brucella abortus* is less toxic than that from *Escherichia coli* suggesting the possible use of *B. abortus* or LPS from *B. abortus* as a carrier in vaccines. Infect Immun 1992; 60:1385-1389.

47. Young EJ, Borchert M, Kretzer FL, Musher DM. Phagocyosis and killing of *Brucella* by human polymorphonuclear leukocytes. J Infect Dis 1985; 15:682-690.

48. Tatum FM, Detilleux PG, Sacks JM, Halling SM. Construction of Cu-Zn superoxide dismutase deletion mutants of *Brucella abortus*: analysis of survival in vitro in epithelial and phagocytic cells and in vivo in mice. Infect Immun 1992; 60:2863-2869.

49. Canning PC, Roth A, Deyoe BL. Release of guanosine monophosphate and adenine by *Brucella abortus* and their role in the intracellular survival of the bacteria. J Infect Dis 1986; 154:464-470.

50. O'Callaghan D, Cazevieille C, Allardet-Servent A, Boschiroli ML, Bourg G, Foulonge V, Frutos P, Kulakov Y, Ramuz M. A homologue of the *Agrobacterium tumefaciens* VirB and *Bordetella pertussis* Ptl type IV section systems is essential for intracellular survival of *Brucella suis*. Mol Microbiol 1999; 33:1210-1220.

51. Gross A, Terraza A, Ouahrani-Bettache S, Liautard JP, Dornand J. In vitro *Brucella suis* infection prevents the programmed cell death of human monocytic cells. Infect Immun 2000; 68:342-351.

52. Keppie J, Williams AE, Witt K, Smith H. The role of erythritol in the tissue localization of the *Brucellae*. Br J Exp Pathol 1965; 46:104-110.

53. Hollis DG, Weaver RE, Steigerwalt AG, Wenger JD, Moss CW, Brenner DJ. *Francisella philomiragia* comb. nov. (formerly *Yersinia philomiragia*) and *Francisella tularensis* biogroup Novicida (formerly *Francisella novicida*), associated with human disease. J Clin Microbiol 1989; 27:1601-1608.

54. Noda H, Munderloh UG, Kurtti TG. Endosymbionts of ticks and their relationship to *Wolbachia* spp and tick-borne pathogens of humans and animals. Appl Environ Microbiol 1997; 63:3926-3932.

55. Sorokin VM, Pavlovich NV, Prozorova LA. *Francisella tularensis* resistance to bactericidal action of normal human serum. FEMS Immunol Med Microbiol 1996; 13:249-252.

56. Reilly TJ, Baron GS, Nano FE, Kuhlenschmidt MS. Characterization and sequencing of a respiratory burst inhibiting acid phosphatase from *Francisella tularensis*. J Biol Chem 1996; 271:10973-10983.

57. Baron GS, Nano FE. Mgl A and Mgl B are required for the intramacrophage growth of *Francisella novicida*. Mol Microbiol 1998; 29:247-259.

58. Baron GS, Reilly TJ, Nano FE. The respiratory burst inhibiting acid phosphatase AcpA is not essential for the intramacrophage growth or virulence of *Francisella novicida*. FEMS Microbiol Lett 1999; 176:85-90.

59. Cowley SC, Myltseva SV, Nano FE. Phase variation in *Francisella tularensis* affecting intracellular growth, lipopolysaccharide antigenicity and nitric acid production. Mol Microbiol 1996; 20:867-874.

60. Fortier AH, Leiby DA, Narayanan RB, Asafoadjei E, Crawford RM, Nacy CA, Meltzer MS. Growth of *Francisella tularensis* LVS in macrophages – the acidic intracellular compartment provides essential iron required for growth. Infect Immun 1995; 63:1478-1483.

61. Maher M, Palmer R, Gannon F, Smith T. Relationship of a novel bacterial fish pathogen to *Streptobacillus moniliformis* and the fusobacteria group, based on 16S ribosomal RNA analysis. Syst Appl Microbiol 1995; 18:79-84.

62. Pins MR, Holden JVM, Yang JM, Madoff S, Ferraro MJ. Isolation of presumptive *Streptobacillus moniliformis* from abscesses associated with the female genital tract. Clin Infect Dis 1996; 22:471-476.

63. Achtman M, Zurth K, Morelli G, Torren G, Guiyoule A, Carniel A. *Yersinia pestis*, the cause of plague, is a recently emerged clone of *Yersinia pseudotuberculosis*. Proc Natl Acad Sci USA 1999; 96:14043-14048.

64. Guiyoule A, Grimont F, Iteman I, Grimont PAD, Lefevre M, Carniel E. Plague pandemic investigated by ribotyping of *Yersinia pestis* strains. J Clin Microbiol 1994; 32:634-641.

65. Brubaker RR. Factors promoting acute and chronic diseases caused by *Yersiniae*. Clin Microbiol Rev 1991; 4:309-324.

66. Rudolph AE, Stuckley JA, Zhao Y, Matthews HR, Patton WA, Moss J, Dixon JE. Expression, characterization and mutagenesis of the *Yersinia pestis* mutine toxin, a phospholipase D superfamily member. J Biol Chem 1999; 274:11824-11831.

67. Kienle Z, Emody L, Svanborg C, O'Toole PW. Adhesive properties conferred by the plasminogen activator of *Yersinia pestis*. J Gen Microbiol 1994; 38:1679-1687.

68. Cornelis GR, Boland A, Boyd AP, Geuijen C, Iriate M, Neyt C, Sory MP, Stainier I. The virulence plasmid of *Yersinia*, an antihost genome. Microbiol Mol Biol Rev 1998; 62:1315-1352.

69. Perry RD, Fetherston RD. *Yersinia pestis* – etiologic agent of plague. Clin Microbiol Rev 1997; 10:35-66.

70. Welkos S, Friedlander A, McDowell D, Weeks J, Tobery S. V antigen of *Yersinia pestis* inhibits neutrophil chemotaxis. Microb Pathog 1998; 24:185-196.

71. Schmidt A, Rollinghoff M, Beuscher HU. Suppression of TNF by V antigen of *Yersinia* spp. involves activated T-cells. Eur J Immunol 1999; 29:1149-1157.

72. Buchrieser C, Prentice M, Carniel E. The 102-kilobase unstable region of *Yersinia pestis* comprises a high-pathogenicity island linked to a pigmentation segment which undergoes internal rearrangement. J Bacteriol 1998; 180:2321-2329.

73. Schubert S, Rakin A, Karch H, Carniel E, Heesemann J. Prevalence of the "high pathogenicity island" of *Yersinia* species among *Escherichia coli* strains that are pathogenic to humans. Infect Immun 1998; 66:480-485.

74. Buchrieser C, Rusniok C, Frangeul L, Couve E, Billault A, Kunst F, Carniel E, Glaser P. The 102 kilobase *pgm* locus of *Yersinia pestis* : sequence analysis and comparison of selected regions among different *Yersinia pestis and Yersinia pseudotuberculosis* strains. Infect Immun 1999; 67:4851-4861.

75. Hare JM, Wagner AK, McDonough KA. Independent acquisition and insertion into different chromosomal locations of the same pathogenicity island in *Yersinia pestis* and *Yersinia pseudotuberculosis*. Mol Microbiol 1999; 31:291-303.

76. Gazapo E, Gonzalez-Lahoz J, Subiza JL, Baquero M, Gil J, de la Concha EG. Changes in IgM and IgG antibody concentrations in brucellosis over time: importance for diagnosis and follow-up. J Infect Dis 1989; 159:219-225.

77. Young EJ. An overview of human brucellosis. Clin Infect Dis 1995; 21:283-290.

78. Splitter GA, Everlith KM. Collaboration of bovine T-lymphocytes and macrophages in T-lymphocyte response to *Brucella abortus*. Infect Immun 1986; 51:776-783.

79. Jiang X, Baldwin CL. Effects of cytokines on intracellular growth of *Brucella abortus*. Infect Immun 1993; 61:124-129.

80. Eze MO, Yuan L, Crawford RM, Paranavitana CM, Hadfield TL, Bhattacharjee AK, Warren RL, Hoover DL. Effects of opsonization and gamma-interferon on growth of *Brucella melitensis* in mouse peritoneal macrophages in vitro. Infect Immun 2000; 68:257-263.

81. Tarnvik A. Nature of protective immunity to *Francisella tularensis*. Rev Infect Dis 1989; 11:440-450.

82. Bevanger L, Maeland JA, Kvam AI. Comparative analysis of antibodies to *Francisella tularensis* antigens during the acute phase of tularemia and 8 years later. Clin Diagn Lab Immunol 1994; 1:238-240.

83. Ericsson M, Sandstrom G, Sjostedt A, Tarnvik A. Persistence of cell-mediated immunity and decline of humoral immunity to the intracellular bacterium *Francisella tularensis* 25 years after natural infection. J Infect Dis 1994; 170:110-114.

84. Elkins KL, Bosio CM, Rhinehart-Jones TR. Importance of B-cells, but not specific antibodies in primary and secondary protective immunity to the intracellular bacterium *Francisella tularensis* live vaccine strain. Infect Immun 1999; 67:6002-6007.

85. Sjostedt A, Conlan JW, North RJ. Neutrophils are critical for host defenses against primary infection with the facultative intracellular bacterium *Francisella tularensis* in mice and participate in defense against re-infection. Infect Immun 1994; 62:2779-2783.

86. Polsinelli T, Meltzer MS, Fortier AH. Nitric oxide independent killing of *Francisella tularensis* by IFN-gamma stimulated murine alveolar macrophages. J Immunol 1994; 153:1238-1245.

87. Yee D, Rhinehart-Jones TR, Elkins KL. Loss of either CD4(+) or CD8(+) T cells does not affect the magnitude of protective immunity to an intracellular pathogen *Francisella tularensis* strain LVS. J Immunol 1996; 157:5042-5048.

88. Golovliov I, Sandstrom G, Ericsson M, Sjostedt A, Tarnvik A. Cytokine expression in the liver during the early phase of murine tularemia. Infect Immun 1995; 63:534-538.

89. Waag DM, Sandstrom G, England MJ, Williams JC. Immunogenicity of a new lot of *Francisella tularensis* live vaccine strain in human volunteers. FEMS Immunol Med Microbiol 1996; 13:205-209.

90. Fulop M, Manchee R, Titball R. Role of lipopolysaccharide and a major outer membrane protein from *Francisella tularensis* in the induction of immunity against tularemia. Vaccine 1995; 13:1220-1225.

91. Poquet Y, Kroca M, Halary F, Stenmark S, Peyrat MA, Bonneville M, Fournie JJ, Sjostedt A. Expansion of V gamma 9V delta 2 T cells is triggered by *Francisella tularensis* – derived phosphoantigens in tularaemia but not after tularaemia vaccination. Infect Immun 1998; 66:2107-2114.

92. Legsters LJ, Cottingham AJ, Hunter DH. Clinical and epidemiological notes on a defined outbreak of plague in Vietnam. Am J Trop Med Hyg 1970; 19:639-652.

93. Benner GE, Andrews GP, Byrne WR, Strachen SD, Sample AK, Heath DG, Friedlander AM. Immune responses to *Yersinia* outer proteins and other *Yersinia pestis* antigens after experimental plague infection in mice. Infect Immun 1999; 67:1922-1928.

94. Meyer KF. Effectiveness of live or killed plague vaccines in man. Bull WHO 1970; 42:653-666.

95. Williamson ED, Vesey PM, Gillhespy KJ, Eley SM, Green M, Titball RW. An IgG1 titre to the F1 and V antigens correlates with protection against plague in the mouse model. Clin Exp Immunol 1999; 116:107-114.

96. Heath DG, Anderson GW, Mauro JM, Welkos SL, Andrews GP, Adamovic J, Friedlander AM. Protection against experimental bubonic and pneumonic plague by recombinant capsular F1-V antigen fusion protein vaccine. Vaccine 1998; 16:1131-1137.

97. Gotuzzo E, Carillo C, Guerra J, Llosa L. An evaluation of diagnostic methods for brucellosis: the value of bone marrow cultures. J Infect Dis 1986; 153:122-125.

98. Ruiz J, Lorente I, Perez J, Simarro E, Martinez-Campos I. Diagnosis of brucellosis by using blood cultures. J Clin Microbiol 1997; 35:2417-2418.

99. Zimmerman SJ, Gillikin S, Safat N, Bartholomew WR, Amsterdam D. Case report and seeded blood culture study of *Brucella* bacteremia. J Clin Microbiol 1990; 28:2139-2141.

100. Herman L, De Ridder H. Identification of *Brucella* spp by using the polymerase chain reaction. Appl Environ Microbiol 1992; 58:2099-2101.

101. Leal-Klevezas DS, Lopez-Merino A, Martinez-Soriano JP. Molecular detection of *Brucella* spp.: rapid identification of *B. abortus* biovar 1 using PCR. Arch Med Res 1995; 26:263-267.

102. Matar GM, Khneisser IA, Abdelnoor AM. Rapid laboratory confirmation of human brucellosis by PCR analysis of a target sequence of the 31-kilodalton *Brucella* antigen DNA. J Clin Microbiol 1996; 34:477-478.

103. Fox KF, Fox A, Nagpal M, Steinberg P, Heroux K. Identification of *Brucella* by ribosomal-spacer region PCR and differentiation of *Brucella canis* from other *Brucella* spp. pathogenic for humans by carbohydrate profiles. J Clin Microbiol 1998; 36:3217-3222.

104. Buchanan TM, Faber LC. 2-Mercaptoethanol *Brucella* agglutination test: usefulness for predicting recovery from brucellosis. J Clin Microbiol 1980; 11:691-693.

105. Long GW, Oprandy JJ, Narayanan RB, Fortier AH, Porter KR. Detection of *Francisella tularensis* in blood by polymerase chain reaction. J Clin Microbiol 1993; 31:152-154.

106. Fulop M, Leslie D, Titball R. A rapid highly sensitive method for the detection of *Francisella tularensis* in clinical samples using the polymerase chain reaction. Am J Trop Med Hyg 1996; 54:364-366.

107. Zhai JH, Yang RF, Lu JC, Zhang GL, Chen ML, Che FX, Hong C. Detection of *Francisella tularensis* by the polymerase chain reaction. J Med Microbiol 1996; 45:477-482.

108. Bevanger L, Maelund JA, Naess AI. Agglutinins and antibodies to *Francisella tularensis* outer membrane antigens in the early diagnosis of disease during an outbreak of tularemia. J Clin Microbiol 1988; 26:433-437.

109. Rimmler RB, Rhoades KR. *Pasteurella multocida* In: Adlam C, Rutter JM - eds. *Pasteurella* and Pasteurellosis. London:Academic Press, 1989:37-73.

110. Wade T, Booy R, Teare EL, Kroll S. *Pasteurella multocida* meningitis in infancy (a lick may be as bad as a bite). Pediatr Infect Dis J 1999; 158:875-878.

111. Shanson DC, Pratt J, Greene P. Comparison of media with and without panmede for the isolation of *Streptobacillus moniliformis* from blood cultures and observations on the inhibitory effect of sodium polyanethol sulphonate. J Med Microbiol 1985; 19:181-186.

112. Edwards R, Finch R. Characterization and antibiotic susceptibilites of *Streptobacillus moniliformis*. J Med Microbiol 1986; 21:39-92.

113. Winter CC, Moody MD. Rapid identification of *Pasteurella pestis* with fluorescent antibody. II Specific identification of *Pasteurella pestis* in dried smears. J Infect Dis 1959; 104:281-287.

114. Wilmoth BA, Chu MC, Quan TJ. Identification of *Yersinia pestis* by BBL Crystal enteric/non-fermenter identification system. J Clin Microbiol 1996; 34:2829-2830.

115. Trebesius K, Harmsen D, Rakin A, Schmelz J, Heeseman J. Development of rRNA-targeted PCR and in situ hybridization with fluorescently labelled digonucleotides for detection of *Yersinia* species. J Clin Microbiol 1999; 37:1980-1984.

116. Engelthaler DM, Gage KL, Montenieri JA, Chu M, Carter LG. PCR detection of *Yersinia pestis* in fleas: comparison with mouse inoculation. J Clin Microbiol 1999; 37:1980-1984.

117. Cao LK, Anderson GP, Ligler FS, Ezzell J. Detection of *Yersinia pestis* fraction 1 antigen with a fiber optic biosensor. J Clin Microbiol 1995; 33:336-341.

118. Chen TH, Meyer KF. An evaluation of *Pasteurella pestis* fraction-1-specific antibody for the confirmation of plague infections. Bull WHO 1966; 34:911-918.

119. Gur D, Kocagoz S, Akova M, Unal S. Comparison of E-test to microdilution for determining in vitro activities of antibiotics against *Brucella melitensis*. Antimicrob Agents Chemother 1999; 43:2337.

120. Trujillano-Martin I, Garcia-Sanchez E, Martinez IM, Fresnadillo MJ, Garcia-Sanchez JE, Garcia-Rodriguez JA. In vitro activities of six new fluoroquinolones against *Brucella melitensis*. Antimicrob Agents Chemother 1999; 43:194-195.

121. Hall WH, Manion LE. In vitro suceptibility of *Brucella* to various antibiotics. Appl Microbiol 1970; 20:600-604.

122. Kropp W, Gerkens L, Sundelof JG, Kahan FM. Antibacterial activity of imipenem the first thienamycin antibiotic. Rev Infect Dis 1985; 7:S389-S396.

123. Akova M, Gur D, Livermore DM, Kocagoz T, Akalia HE. In vitro activities of antibiotics alone and in combination against *Brucella melitensis* and neutral and acid pHs. Antimicrob Agents Chemother 1999; 43:1298-1300.

124. Moreno E. Genome evolution within the alpha *Proteobacteria*: why do some bacteria not possess plasmids and others exhibit more than one different chromosome? FEMS Microbiol Rev 1998; 22:255-275.

125. Scheel O, Hoel T, Sandvik T, Berdal BP. Susceptibility pattern of Scandinavian *Francisella tularensis* isolates with regard to oral and parenteral antimicrobial agents. APMIS 1993; 101:33-36.

126. Syrjala H, Schildt R, Raisainen S. In vitro suceptibility of *Francisella tularensis* to fluoroquinolones and treatment of tularemia with norfloxacin and ciprofloxacin. Eur J Clin Microbiol Infect Dis 1991; 10:68-70.

127. Enderlin G, Morales L, Jacobs RF, Cross JT. Streptomycin and alternative agents for the treatment of tularemia – review of the literature. Clin Infect Dis 1994; 19:42-47.

128. Cross JT, Jacobs RF. Tularemia treatment failures with outpatient use of ceftriaxone. Clin Infect Dis 1993; 17:976-980.

129. Goldstein EJC, Citron DM. Comparative activities of cefuroxime, amoxicillin/clavulanic acid, ciprofloxacin, enoxacin and ofloxacin against aerobic and anaerobic bacteria isolated from bite wounds. Antimicrob Agents Chemother 1988; 32:1143-1148.

130. Watts JL, Yancey RJ, Salmon SA, Case CA. A four-year survey of antimicrobial susceptibility trends for isolates from cattle with bovine respiratory disease in North America. J Clin Microbiol 1994; 32:725-738.

131. Goldstein EJC, Citron DM, Richwald GA. Lack of in vitro efficacy of oral forms of certain cephalosporins, erythromycin and oxacillin against *Pasteurella multocida*. Antimicrob Agents Chemother 1988; 32:213-215.

132. Kehrenberg C, Werckenthin C, Schwarz S. Tn 5706, a transposon-like element from *Pasteurella multocida* mediating tetracycline resistance. Antimicrob Agents Chemother 1998; 42:2116-2118.

133. Lion C, Lozniewski A, Rosner V, Weber M. Lung abscess due to beta-lactamase-producing *Pasteurella multocida*. Clin Infect Dis 1999; 29:1345-1346.

134. Konstanopoulos K, Skarpos P, Hitjazis F, Georgakopoulos D, Matrangas Y, Andreopoulou M, Koutras E. Rat-bite fever in a Greek child. Scand J Infect Dis 1992; 24:531-533.

135. Smith MD, Vinh D, Hoa NTT, Wain J, Thung D, White NJ. In vitro antimicrobial susceptibilities of strains of *Yersinia pestis*. Antimicrob Agents Chemother 1995; 39:2153-2154.

136. Frean JA, Arntzen L, Capper T, Bryskier A, Klugman KA. In vitro activity of 14 antibiotics against 100 human isolates of *Yersinia pestis* from a Southern African plague focus. Antimicrob Agents Chemother 1996; 40:646-2647.

137. Byrne WR, Welkos SL, Pitt ML, Davis KJ, Brueckner RP, Ezzell JW, Nelson GO, Vaccaro JR, Battersby LC, Friedlander AM. Antibiotic treatment of experimental pnuemonic plague in mice. Antimicrob Agents Chemother 1998; 42:675-681.

138. Russell P, Eley SM, Green M, Stagg AJ, Taylor RR, Nelson M, Beedham RJ, Bell DL, Rogers D, Whittington D, Titball RW. Efficacy of doxycycline and ciprofloxacin against experimental *Yersinia pestis* infection. J Antimicrob Chemother 1998, 41.301-305.

139. Russell P, Eley SM, Bell DL, Manchee RJ, Titball RW. Doxycycline or ciprofloxacin prophylaxis and therapy against experimental *Yersinia pestis* infection in mice. J Antimicrob Chemother 1996; 37:769-774.

140. Galimand M, Guigoule A, Gerbaud G, Rasoamanana B, Chanteau S, Carniel E, Courvalin P. Multidrug resistance in *Yersinia pestis* mediated by a transferable plasmid. N Eng J Med 1997; 337:677-680.

20

Gastric Helicobacters

John Holton
Department of Bacteriology, Royal Free & University College London Medical School, Windeyer Institute of Medical Science, London, England

Dino Vaira
First Medical Clinic, University of Bologna, Bologna, Italy

I. HISTORICAL BACKGROUND

A. *Helicobacter pylori*

Spiral organisms were demonstrated in animal stomach by Rappin as long ago as 1881. In 1938, spiral organisms were also identified in human gastric tissue by Doenges but were considered to be commensal organisms, and therefore interest in them waned. Further confirmation that the human stomach was colonized by spiral-shaped organisms was made in 1975 by Steer who noted for the first time that there was an association with inflammation; a possible link with duodenal ulceration was suggested. It was not until the appropriate culture techniques were available, however, that these organisms were isolated from the human stomach in 1983 by Warren and Marshall (1). Warren again noted that the organisms were associated with gastritis and made the suggestion that they may be related to ulceration. This was met with some widespread skepticism because duodenal ulceration was believed to be caused by excess stomach acid: the "no acid-no ulcer" hypothesis. Gradually, however, with accumulating clinical and scientific evidence, a paradigm shift in medical opinion has occurred, and an increasing number of physicians (although some non-believers still remain) have become convinced that *H. pylori* is causally related to gastro-duodenal disease: the "no *H. pylori*-no ulcer" hypothesis. This paradigm shift has had enormous implications for treatment because ulcers can now be cured by a short eradicative course of antibiotics (instead of continuous acid-suppressive medication only). The 'campylobacter-like organism' (CLO) isolated by Warren has been called at various times, *Campylobacter pylori* or *Campylobacter pyloridis*; only receiving its current name of *H. pylori* in 1989 (2) when it was convincingly demonstrated that it was a novel genus and that it did not belong to the genus *Campylobacter*. The organism's complete genome sequence was first published in the August issue of Nature (3) in 1997 thus testifying to its current perceived importance as a human pathogen.

B. Other *Helicobacter* species

Studies on a wide range of animals (4-17) have demonstrated an increasing number of different *Helicobacter* species which have been isolated from the gastrointestinal tract, and the genus now contains at least 30 species (Table 1). They can broadly be divided into those which are found in the stomach, and those that are found in the lower gastrointestinal tract or the hepatobiliary system (some *Helicobacter* species are associated with malignancies in the liver of mice).

In addition to *H. pylori* causing gastritis in humans, a morphologically distinct organism was noticed (18) in stomach biopsies of patients that were attending endoscopy. This bacterium is larger than *H. pylori* and has a tightly curled spiral protoplasm and bipolar flagellae. It is found principally in the mucous layer rather than being adherent to the gastric epithelial cells and was initially named *Gastrospirillum hominis* on morphological grounds. Analysis of 16S rDNA sequences from two separate isolates established 97% homology to each other; they most closely resemble *H. felis*. *G. hominis* has provisionally been renamed *Helicobacter heilmannii* type 1 and 2 (some choose to retain the designations *Gastrospirillum hominis* type 1 and 2) recognizing that it may represent more than one species. An exact taxonomic position remains unresolved. It could not be cultured axenically but was maintained by in vivo mouse passage. More recently, an organism morphologically indistinguishable from *H. heilmannii* has been isolated from the human stomach, and 16S rDNA sequencing has indicated that it is closely linked to the original two genome sequences of *H. heilmannii* and to *H. felis, H. bizzozeroni,* and *H. salomonis* (19). Morphologically similar organisms have been seen in specimens from dogs, cats, and pigs. For porcine sources, the organism was originally called *Gastrospirillum suis* and was associated with ulceration of the esophagus. Sequence analysis now indicates that it is 99% homologous to *H. heilmannii* type 1 (20). In humans, the organism complex is found in less than 1% of endoscopies and is associated with a focal antral gastritis that is milder than that caused by *H. pylori*. This complex may be

Table 1   Species of *Helicobacter* and their distribution in the gastrointestinal tract. Several other helicobacters have been recorded either without yet validly published names (e.g., H. ulmiensis, H. typhlonicus) or with simple alphanumeric designations (e.g., H. sp. mainz, H. sp. cotton top, H. sp. MZ640285)

Gastric helicobacters	Lower intestinal helicobacters
H. pylori – human	*H. cinaedi* – human
H. heilmanii – human, dog, pig	*H. fennelliae* – human
H. acinonyx – cheetah	*H. westmeadii* – human
H. mustaelae – ferret	*H. canis* – dog
H. felis – cat, dog	*H. pamatensis* – gulls
H. bizzeronii – dog	*H. muridarum* – rodent
H. salomonis – dog	*H. bilis* – rodent
H. nemestrinae – monkey	*H. rodentium* – rodent
H. suncus – shrew	*H. trogontum* – rodent
H. suis – pig	*H. pullorum* – chicken
H. salomonis – dog	*H. cholecystus* – hamster
H. bovis – cattle	*H. rappini* – human, sheep
	H. hepaticus – rodent
	H. mesocrietorum – hamster
	H. canadensis – human

more frequently linked to gastric MALT (**M**ucosal **A**ssociated **L**ymphoid **T**issue) lymphoma (21). Epidemiological evidence suggests that it may be especially a zoonosis that is acquired from dogs.

II. CLINICAL ASPECTS

A. Classification of gastritis: the Sydney system

Individuals who are colonized by *H. pylori* have either an acute or chronic gastritis depending on the stage of the infection (Figure 1). There have been several histopathological systems for classifying gastritis, but in an attempt both to unify them and to provide a common and globally acceptable method of classifying gastritis, the World Congress of Gastroenterologists published the Sydney system. This classification system is a dual one that is based on histological and endoscopic criteria. The histological division of the system consists of data of three sorts: the etiology, the topography of the gastritis, and the histopathology of the inflammation. The endoscopic division of the system records the visual appearance by descriptive terms such as erosion, ulcer, nodularity, etc., and topographical distribution in the stomach. The Sydney system was updated shortly after its publication (22) particularly with respect of the presence or absence of atrophic gastritis.

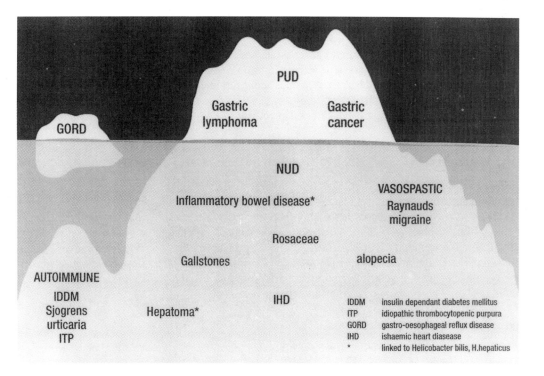

Figure 1 Clinical manifestations that are or may be associated with *H. pylori*.

B. Non-ulcer dyspepsia (NUD)

Despite the fact that probably everyone who is colonized by *H. pylori* has gastritis, relatively few individuals have symptoms of dyspepsia. In fact, the relationship between colonization by *H. pylori* and dyspepsia in the absence of an ulcer, i.e., non-ulcer dyspepsia, is controversial. In studies of patients with NUD, evidence suggests that some may benefit from eradication of *H. pylori*, but no uniquely characteristic profile is at hand to indicate which patient may benefit. Despite a considerable number of studies on the relationship between colonization by *H. pylori* and symptoms, there is still no clear answer. In one study, a beneficial effect of eradication has been demonstrated, but yet in similar studies, no beneficial effect was seen (23,24).

C. Peptic ulcer disease (PUD)

H. pylori is the principle cause of peptic ulcer disease, both gastric and duodenal ulceration (25), although the latter usually occur in different subgroups of patients. The lines of evidence which support this causal role come from six areas: 1) the close statistical correlation between colonization and disease, 2) the use of animal models to mimic disease, 3) the presence of naturally occurring infection in animals where there is presence of both animal-associated helicobacters and stomach ulcers, 4) plausable pathogenic mechanism(s), 5) the correlation between eradication of *H. pylori*, using only antibiotics, and the healing of ulcers, and 6) the correlation between the relapse rate of ulceration and the eradication of *H. pylori*.

D. Pre-cancerous conditions - atrophic gastritis and intestinal metaplasia

Long-term colonization with *H. pylori* may lead to the development of atrophic gastritis and intestinal metaplasia. Atrophic gastritis is characterized by infiltration with inflammatory cells throughout the mucosa and with atrophy of the deep antral glands alongside deposition of fibrous materials. Early chronic atrophic gastritis may be characterized by lymphocytic adherence to antral glands causing focal distortion of the gland. Atrophic gastritis is often a precursor to intestinal metaplasia, and both are considered pre-cancerous lesions.

E. Gastric neoplasms

H. pylori is classified as a Class I carcinogen (26). Colonization by *H. pylori* increases the risk of developing gastric adenocarcinoma six-fold and is linked to the development of gastric MALT lymphomas (27, 28). The evidence for the causal association between *H. pylori* and both gastric adenocarcinoma and B-cell gastric lymphomas is similar. There are geographical correlations in both the prevalence of gastric lymphoma or carcinoma and *H. pylori*. Secondly, patients who have gastric lymphoma or carcinoma also have high colonization rates for *H. pylori*. Further evidence that *H. pylori* is etiologically linked to the development of gastric lymphoma comes from in vitro and therapeutic studies where regression of the lymphoma occurs with eradication of the organism.

F. Extra-gastrointestinal conditions

H. pylori is also associated with a number of extra-gastrointestinal conditions (29) such as rosaceae, urticaria, and vasospastic disorders, the latter which include Raynaud's phenomenon and migraine. In the general population, there is also the potential for *H. pylori* to be a risk factor for the development of vascular disease such as coronary heart disease or for short stature in young girls, although the evidence for both of these is contradictory. There have also appeared associations between colonization by *H. pylori* and various autoimmune diseases such as insulin-dependent diabetes mellitus (IDDM) and thyroiditis; there may be an association with idiopathic thrombocytopenic purpura (ITP). Further work in needed is order to clarify these issues.

III. EPIDEMIOLOGY OF INFECTION

The route of transmission of *H. pylori* is still undecided, although most of the evidence points toward humans as the principal source of infection. Sero-epidemiological studies have identified socio-economic and demographic factors, and indicate that close personal contact is important in the transmission cycle. Some evidence, however, indicates that a poor public health infrastructure may be an important factor, and that the environment may serve as a possible reservoir of infection. Circumstantial evidence also is suggestive that some domestic pets may be potential sources of infection for humans.

A. Demographic and socio-economic factors

The evidence that close personal contact is important for transmission of *H. pylori* is derived from several sero-epidemiological studies which have identified low socio-economic status as being inversely correlated with the prevalence of *H. pylori* (30). These results reflect the childhood living conditions and overcrowding in areas of social deprivation which are correlated with colonization by *H. pylori*. Additional evidence that overcrowding is important in transmission of *H. pylori* is derived from sero-epidemiological studies of institutions such as orphanages, psychiatric institutions, military barracks, submarine crews, and families (31); these all support a role for person-to-person transmission of *H. pylori*.

In industrialized countries, the prevalence of *H. pylori* increases with age. In non-industrialized countries, the prevalence of infection in childhood is high, and there is minimal age-related increase (32). There is therefore a significant correlation between seropositivity and the ethnic origin of the population being assessed. The explanation for this age-related increase in seropositivity among industrialized countries is most readily explained by a cohort effect on patients who, now aged over 60 years, had been exposed to *H. pylori* in childhood. The lower prevalence in younger age groups currently noted reflects some loss of the source or perhaps diminished transmission due to changing social conditions.

B. Source and route of transmission of infection

Epidemiological evidence supports the person-to-person transmission of *H. pylori* with colonization occurring primarily in childhood. Under natural circumstances, transmission might occur by either of two routes: mouth-to-mouth (or gastro-oral by vomit in children) or fecal-oral. In support of these routes, *H. pylori* has been detected in oral secretions, gastric juice, and feces. There is no strong evidence to support either the oral or fecal route as the primary one, and both may be relevant depending on other factors. The oral route is a more direct mode and is consistent with direct person-to-person transmission. The fecal route may, in addition to the direct fecal-oral spread that occurs within a family unit, also allow for indirect spread via fecally-contaminated food or water. Additionally, it may be hypothesized that there are multiple routes for transmission which may vary in importance according to geographic and socio-demographic factors.

1. Fecal route and environmental sources

H. pylori has been isolated from the feces of individuals in Africa (33), but reports of isolation in the U.K. are infrequent. *H. pylori* has also been detected in feces by the polymerase chain reaction (PCR). In addition to the direct fecal-oral transmission that may occur in children or is otherwise associated with poor hygiene, *H. pylori* may also be spread indirectly by the fecal route via food or contaminated water. Sero-epidemiological evidence from Peru and Chile has shown that the prevalence of *H. pylori* in children is strongly correlated both with socio-economic status and the presence of an external water supply or the consumption of raw vegetables, presumably due to irrigation which is inclusive of human sewage. An analysis of potable water samples from Peru by PCR demonstrated the presence of

H. pylori in a sizeable proportion thus suggesting that water is potentially important in transmission (34).

2. *Animals as a source of infection*

Certain occupations have been noted to be risk factors for seropositivity to *H. pylori*: pest-control officers, veterinary surgeons, and meat workers are all more likely to be seropositive when compared to a control population of blood donors. This sero-epidemiological evidence can potentially be dismissed as cross-reaction between *H. pylori* and the known animal helicobacters. *H. pylori* has been detected in laboratory cats thus raising the possibility of a zoonotic transmission from domestic pets. *H. pylori*, however, has not been isolated from feral cats, and it is possible that colonization of cats may have been an anthropnosis. Additionally, there is no serological evidence to support the notion that subjects who own a cat have a higher seroprevalence to *H. pylori* when compared to a general population. It is therefore unlikely that animals are a reservoir of infection for humans although helicobacters other than *H. pylori* (*H. heilmannii*, *H. canis*, and *H. pullorum*) have been shown to have zoonotic spread, and may cause gastritis and gastroenteritis especially among children and immunocompromised individuals. Again, these subjects are the focus of future study.

IV. NATURE OF THE BACTERIUM, PATHOGENESIS, AND CLINICAL MANIFESTATIONS

A. Morphology

H. pylori is a non-spore forming, motile Gram negative bacterium with a helical shape measuring 2.5-4.5 x 0.5-1.0 μm. It has 1-5 unipolar sheathed flagella. In addition to the helical shape, curved forms

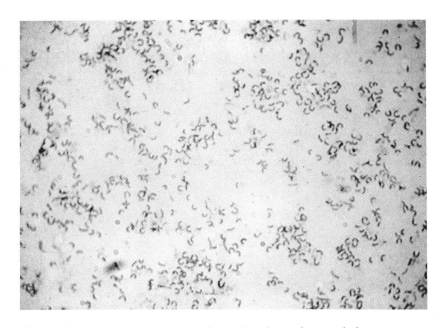

Figure 2   Gram stain appearance of *H. pylori* shown for morphology.

occur (Figure 2), and the bacillus also converts to a coccoid morphology when under environmental stress. Other helicobacters have a similar spiral morphology but may differ in the number and location of flagellae. Some species possess prominent periplasmic fibrils, e.g., *H. felis*, and some are larger than *H. pylori* and have more prominent spirals, e.g., *H. heilmannii*.

B. Cellular constituents

The lipopolysaccharide (LPS) of *H. pylori* is of a generally similar structure to that of other Gram negative bacteria, i.e., lipid A linked to a constant core region and with strain-specific side chains. The lipid A, however, is both underphosphorylated and has fewer fatty acids in comparison to that of *Escherichia coli*, presumably explaining its poor endotoxin activity as contrasted to the endotoxin of *E. coli*. Side chains of the LPS in *H. pylori* carry Lewis blood group antigen-like structures (35) which may be important in the pathogenesis. *H. pylori* maintains a number of enzymes that are commonly found in bacteria, although uniquely, it has prominent urease activity which is the basis for several diagnostic tests and is also important for virulence.

C. Growth and metabolism

H. pylori is a microaerophile and requires up to five days to grow on primary isolation. It produces small (1-2 mm. diameter) colonies on 5% horse blood agar with Columbia agar base. The colonies are domed, glistening, entire, grey, or water-clear, and are sufficiently characteristic to suggest the presence of the organism. *H. pylori* grows at temperatures between 30°C and 37°C in an atmosphere of 5-15% oxygen, 5-12% carbon dioxide, and 70-90% nitrogen. The CampyPak (Oxoid) can be used to provide the appropriate atmospheric culture conditions. The organism is oxidase-positive and demonstrates rapid urease activity which, in combination with a Gram stain and the colonial morphology, are sufficient to identify *H. pylori* on a routine basis.

D. Pathogenesis

Disease is caused by four general mechanisms: a) direct action of surface exposed or secreted toxins, b) indirectly by the modulation of the normal gastric homeostasis as affecting gastrin and pepsinogen levels, and acid secretion, c) as part of a by-stander effect caused by *H. pylori*-induced activation of inflammatory cells with subsequent release of inflammatory mediators, and d) *H. pylori*-stimulated autoimmunity.

1. Direct toxic action

The bacterium must penetrate the viscid mucous layer which covers the gastric epithelial cells before it can adhere to them. Motility is thus an important virulence characteristic as shown by the observation that aflagellate mutants of *H. pylori* lack pathogenicity. Flagellar variants also differentially affect cytokine activation. *H. pylori* possesses a phospholipase which may have a direct effect on the host cell membrane or mucous. Urease activity can release ammonia which has the potential to be directly toxic. Additionally, urease suppresses the bactericidal activity of peroxynitrite by the production of CO_2/HCO_3 which is produced by the hydrolysis of urea. This scavenging of a strong oxidizing/nitriting agent may facilitate the long term survival of *H. pylori* in the midst of an acute inflammatory response (36).

Exposure of gastric cells to *H. pylori* leads to apoptosis (37) and an increased cellular turnover which seems to be facilitated by bacterial lipopolysaccharide. In studies with Mongolian gerbils, a transient increase in apoptosis occurs following colonization by *H. pylori* which is then followed several weeks later by a significant increase in antral cell proliferation that is related to serum gastrin levels (38). Among in vitro studies, chronic exposure of human gastric cells to *H. pylori* induces an apoptosis-resistant phenotype that is associated with a decrease in p27[kip1] expression. Similar reduced levels of this cyclin-dependent kinase inhibitor can be demonstrated in gastric biopsies of patients who are colonized by *H. pylori* (39). By disturbing the balance between normal proliferation and apoptosis, this effect may be highly relevant to the association between *H. pylori* and gastric adenocarcinoma.

Vacuolating cytotoxin

The majority of *H. pylori* strains possess the *vacA* gene (40), but only about 50-60% of strains actively secrete the toxin. Within the gene coding for toxin, there is molecular heterogeneity with four signal sequences (S1a, S1b, S1c, and S2) and two mid-region sequences (M1 and M2). Although most strains possess the *vacA* gene, only those that are also *cagA* positive (see below) are phenotypically toxigenic (Type I strains). Those that are *vacA* positive but *cagA* negative are non-toxigenic (Type II strains). Phenotypic toxigenicity is correlated with molecular genotype with S1/M1 being highly toxigenic and S2/M2 being non-toxigenic when tested on HeLa cells but able to induce vacuolation in gastric epithelial cells. The vacuolating cytotoxin induces vacuolation in cells of the gastric epithelium leading to cytotoxicity.

2. *Disturbed gastric physiology*

Individuals who are colonized with *H. pylori* have hypergastrinemia, due to an inhibition of somatostatin (a negative regulator of gastrin secretion) (41), hyperpepsinogenemia, and elevated meal-stimulated acid secretion. Patients who have duodenal ulcers tend to have a higher nocturnal and meal-stimulated acid output and a larger parietal cell mass than individuals who do not have a duodenal ulcer. The high levels of pepsin and acid in the stomach, as well as the deficient mucous barrier properties that are caused by *H. pylori*, may all contribute to damage of the gastric epithelium and may enhance ulcerogenesis.

3. *Inflammation*

An inflammatory response is mounted by the host in the presence of *H. pylori*. Persistence of the organism leads to the development of a chronic inflammatory response. In addition to polymorphonuclear (PMN) cell infiltration, there is also infiltration of the mucosa and lamina propria by lymphocytes and plasma cells. The severity of gastritis (assessed by the number of PMNs seen) is strongly correlated with the density of colonization by *H. pylori* as shown by several investigators.

Along with adhesion of *H. pylori*, there is up-regulation of NFκB (the chronic inflammatory transcription factor) and an increase in synthesis and release of IL-8, a potent chemo-attractant for inflammatory cells (42). The higher the level of IL-8, the greater the degree of neutrophil infiltration which *H. pylori* may activate to release reactive oxygen metabolites that can damage gastric cells. Additionally, presence of *H. pylori* also stimulates the production of other pro-inflammatory mediators such as IL-1, IL-6, IL-10, IL-12, TNF-alpha, INF-gamma, platelet-activating factor (PAF), Gro-alpha, and leukotriene B4.

CagA pathogenicity island

Fifty to sixty percent of isolates carry the *cagA* (cytotoxin-associated gene) locus (43) which acts as a marker for the *cag* pathogenicity island: an assembly of some 40 genes that are linked to virulence. The significance of *cagA* is that patients who are colonized by *cagA* positive strains have higher levels of IL-8, hence a more intense inflammatory response. They are also more likely to develop ulcer (duodenal or gastric) disease and are more likely to develop gastric adenocarcinoma. The association between *cagA* and PUD and cancer, however, holds only for some geographic areas. Upstream of the *cagA* locus, there are two loci, *picA* and *picB* (*cagE*), which if ablated markedly reduce the induction of IL-8 by epithelial cells.

4. *Auto-immunity*

Antibodies which are directed against *H. pylori* may include those that cross-react with gastric tissue, and high levels of these cross-reacting antibodies can lead to pathological changes in the gastric mucosa. These auto-antibodies are directed against muco-substances in the epithelium. The Lewis antigen is a further target for an autoimmune reaction. Antibodies which are directed against the Lewis epitopes, as expressed on the bacterial LPS, may be involved in the development of gastric atrophy (44) by cross-reacting with Lewis antigen that is expressed on the parietal cell. Some evidence suggests, however, that antibodies to Lewis epitopes may not be relevant to autoimmunity (45) and that antibodies may be directed to some component of the oligosaccharide other than the Lewis carbohydrate. Further, auto-antibodies to gastric tissue may arise by mechanisms other than molecular mimicry to *Helicobacter* epitopes (46).

5. Host factors

In addition to bacterial virulence characteristics, the varying clinical outcome of colonization may be related to host characteristics. A significant finding in this respect is the demonstration that IL-1 polymorphisms are related to an increased risk of hypochlorhydria and the development of gastric cancer (47). Further evidence which supports a role for host components in the disease presentation is the enhanced binding of *H. pylori* to gastric epithelial cells from patients with blood group O and the increased secretion of IL-6 and TNF from leukocytes that are derived from patients with group O blood (48). Animal studies also support the importance of host genetics. Mice that have a reduced or absent inflammatory response to colonization by *H. pylori* produce large amounts of IL-10 compared to mice that have an inflammatory response to the organism (49).

6. Clinical manifestations

The vast majority of individuals who are colonized with *H. pylori* are asymptomatic. The acute manifestations of infection may be minimal or absent, and it is only when the patient complains of dyspepsia or other symptoms of severe gastroduodenal disease, such as ulcers, that colonization by *H. pylori* may be suspected. Both intentional and accidental ingestion of *H. pylori* have been associated with transient upper gastrointestinal symptoms of dyspepsia and vomiting within one week of ingestion. In children, a similar syndrome of upper gastrointestinal symptoms, nausea, and vomiting has been recorded immediately following acquisition of *H. pylori*. Recently, it has been suggested that some strains of *H. pylori* may be "beneficial" to the host. This is based on the findings, in limited studies, that eradication of *H. pylori* in some patients is followed by gastro-esophageal reflux disease (GERD). The evidence for the latter proposal is incomplete.

V. IMMUNOLOGY OF INFECTION

The most complete sequential record of the serological response to *H. pylori* follows intentional ingestion. A small number of sequential sera following natural infection have also been studied. The levels of anti-*H. pylori* IgM rise quickly and return to normal within one week. Thereafter, the levels of IgG and IgA increase and persist indefinitely. A systemic IgE response is also produced. In adults, the host responds to high molecular weight antigens initially, but in children, a response to low molecular weight antigens occurs first (50). There is both a systemic and local response. Gastric and duodenal antibody-secreting cells principally produce IgA and IgM. The antigens that are predominantly recognized include Mrs of 120-125 kD (*cagA*), 87 kD (*vacA*), 74 kD, 66 kD (Ure), 54 kD, 48 kD, 46 kD, 42 kD, 35 kD, 30 kD (*Ure*), and 19.5 kD (51). Several studies, however, have shown detection of antigens with differing molecular weights which probably reflect strain variation. After successful eradication of the organism, the IgG antibody levels begin to fall, and by 6 months, they have usually fallen to a quarter of their original value. As shown by immunoblot analysis, the humoral immune response to antigens of different molecular weight extinguishes at variable rates (52).

The cellular response to *H. pylori* is principally one of an increase in the lamina propria CD4 Th1 cell profile.

VI. DIAGNOSIS

A. General considerations

There are both differences in the perceived role of *H. pylori* in a number of clinical conditions, such as its relationship to NUD, as well as geographic differences in the relationship of virulence markers to distinct disease groups. These differences may affect one's decision to test for *H. pylori* or furthermore, for specific virulence markers. Invariably these concerns prompt the question: "Should I screen for *H. pylori* colonization?"

Additionally, in considering the entire patient population, several well-defined patient groups for whom a diagnosis of colonization by *H. pylori* must be made include: 1) children, 2) pregnant women, 3) elderly, 4) patients presenting for the first time with symptoms, 5) patients who have had previous visits with the same complaint, and 6) patients with known *H. pylori*-related disease.

Subdivisions of these categories can be made according to the venue of consultation (i.e., whether or not the patient visit is taking place in a primary health care setting or a referral gastroenterology clinic), the presence of groups 4-6 (aforementioned) risk factors, and age (i.e., whether or not the patient is over the age of 45 years). Accordingly, such considerations prompt the question: "Which test(s) should I [physician] use?"

If testing is deemed of need, it is necessary to take several factors into account when considering which specific test would be the most appropriate. These factors include ethnicity and the associated regional variance in the prevalence of *H. pylori*; both of which affect the accuracy of some tests.

Although there are many different types of tests for *H. pylori*, not all are appropriate for the various patient groups. Test-specific factors, which must be taken into account when making a decision of which test to use and when, include: 1) the positive/negative predictive values for the test, 2) the cost, and 3) the ease of clinical application.

The various assessments have traditionally been divided into those that require an endoscopy (invasive tests) and those that do not (non-invasive tests).

1. Invasive tests

These are performed with a biopsy of the stomach, a sample of gastric juice, or the use of a swallowed gastric string which facilitates sample collection. They include histology, culture, rapid urease test, polymerase chain reaction, and analysis of gastric juice. It must be acknowledged that diagnostic procedures may suffer from sampling errors given the patchy distribution of bacterium and disease in the stomach.

2. Non-invasive tests

These are performed on samples of blood, serum, saliva, feces, or exhaled breath, and they include serology, urea breath test, fecal antigen test, and PCR amplification of fecally-excreted bacterium.

Comparisons of the tests as listed above have shown that no single test can be relied on to definitively detect colonization by *H. pylori*, but that a combination of culture and histology can predict 99.5% of all infections. The single test with both the highest sensitivity and specificity is the urea breath test. Culture, of course, has by its nature a specificity of 100% for bacterial presence.

B. Histology

Histology provides information both about the presence of *H. pylori* and the presence of inflammation, atrophy, or metaplasia. *H. pylori* can be readily recognized by its characteristic curved or S-shaped morphology, and its location beneath the epithelial cell surface as within the gastric pits or in the mucous overlaying the cell surface (Figure 3). The histological stain that was originally used to detect *H.*

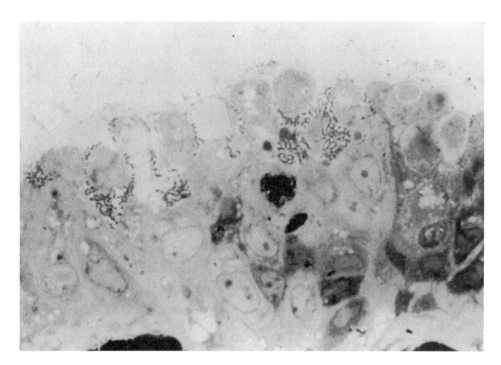

Figure 3 Section of stomach showing *H. pylori*.

pylori was the Warthin-Starry silver stain. This stain, however, is technically difficult and expensive to perform, and it has been replaced by other stains, notably the Giemsa stain, although stains such as the Gimenez, acridine orange, cresyl violet Genta, and carbol fuchsin have also been used. The stain most commonly used for histological analysis is the hematoxylin and eosin stain. Genta's stain has the advantage of demonstrating both the presence of *H. pylori* and the histolopathology simultaneously (53).

The use of stains to detect *H. pylori* in tissue sections relies on the experience of the histopathologist to recognize the typical morphological appearance of the organism. Clearly, small numbers of organisms may be missed, and there is the recognized error of inter-observer variation (54). Also, as the distribution of the organism in the stomach is not uniform, it is recommended that more than one biopsy is taken for examination. Alternatively, "jumbo"-sized biopsies may be acquired.

Compared to culture, the various stains have reported sensitivities of 72% (Gram stain), 67% (Warthin-Starry stain), 79% (Giemsa stain), and 85% (acridine orange stain). Many histopathologists use the Giemsa stain because of its technical ease. The specificity of histology can be increased by immunochemical staining with the use of monoclonal antibodies. Sensitivity can be augmented by fixing the tissue in Carnoy's solution which preserves the surface mucous layer (55). The use of frozen sections which are stained with toluidine blue demonstrates a sensitivity and specificity of 98% as compared to routine histology, and the results can be given to the endoscopist within 20 minutes (56) as opposed to the usual 2-3 days for a histological report.

C. Culture

Culture has had a critical role in establishing *H. pylori* as a causal agent of disease. As mentioned, *H. pylori* has been visualized in stomach specimens for decades, but it was only after the application of culture that it was established as a veritable topic for academic medical interest. Culture continues to have an important role to play in diagnosis, and although it is relatively inexpensive, it is the slowest of the tests currently available since the organism typically requires 3-5 days to grow in primary isolation. An invaluable advantage for culture is the availability of data pertaining to antibiotic susceptibility. In clinical terms, this may be particularly relevant to the treatment of relapsing disease. The second main reason to advocate culture of *H. pylori* is to follow trends in antibiotic resistance which are important when needing to consider empirical treatment. Culture generally has a high sensitivity (70-95%) and specificity (100%). The organism grows very well on 5% horse blood agar with Columbia base that has amphotericin B for selection, but a number of selective culture media are available (57-62). The media are usually, but not exclusively, based on either Columbia or Brain Heart Infusion agar, and containing either blood or blood products, starch, charcoal, cyclodextrin, or bovine serum albumin. The latter additions are thought to act somewhat like serum, and it is intended that they inactivate toxic substances or metabolites in the medium. Table 2 details the constituents of some commonly-used media. Selectivity is provided by the addition of different combinations of antibiotics. Addition of triphenyltetrazolium chloride (TPTZ) to the medium imparts a characteristic golden sheen to the *H. pylori* colonies. It is recommended that more than one culture medium be used, including a non-selective medium, in order to maximize the isolation rate.

    H. pylori soon loses viability when exposed to the environment, and biopsies should be homogenized and cultured quickly to maximize recovery. A number of transport media have been advocated with varying results, although sterile 0.9% saline is probably as good as any if the organism is cultured within a few hours (63). If items are to be transported to a regional laboratory over a prolonged period, cultures can be submitted on chocolate agar slants, and biopsy material can be maintained in selective brain heart infusion broth which is supplemented with horse serum and yeast extract; yields of up to 80% survival by 5 days have been reported.

    H. pylori has also been isolated from oral specimens (e.g., dental plaque) and feces. The overall clinical relevance of these findings is unknown, but isolation from either oral or stool samples does suggest that the organism is also present in the stomach. This is a topic that requires further study since it is easy to collect these specimens. Selective media that are developed to date have been designed for culture of *H. pylori* from stomach specimens where the degree of contamination is comparatively less. Oral and fecal specimens on the other hand have a much more complex microbial flora that may inhibit the isolation of *H. pylori*. Techniques for the isolation of *H. pylori* from feces include the preparation of a fecal slurry in phosphate buffer, separation of fecal material by sieving, concentration of the bacterial pellet by centrifugation, and culture on a selective medium.

    H. pylori has been isolated from blood culture on one occasion as an incidental finding. Isolation

Table 2   Components of some selective media for *H. pylori*. BHIA – brain heart infusion agar.

BHIA	BHIA	BHIA
horse blood 7%	horse serum 10%	sheep blood 10%
Isovitalex 1%	charcoal 0.2%	
	yeast extract 1%	....
	TPTZ 40 mg./ml.	TPTZ 40 mg./ml.
CAB	CAB	CAB
egg yolk emulsion 10%	hemin 10 mg./L.	cyclodextrin 1 gm./L.
Isovitalex 1%	Isovitalex 2%	
	urea 20 gm./L.	
TPTZ 40 mg./ml.	phenol red 1.2 mg./L.	....

CAB – Columbia agar base. Antibiotic combination frequently added is: vancomycin 10 mg./L. + trimethoprim 5 mg./L. + cefsulodin 5 mg./L. + amphotericin 5 mg./L.

of *H. pylori* from blood may be diminished due to its relative inability to grow well in several conventional blood culture media. Brucella broth without bisulphite, biphasic Brain Heart Infusion broth, and supplemented peptone broth have all supported growth of *H. pylori*. Other *Helicobacter* species such as *H. cinaedi*, *H. westmeadii*, *Helicobacter* strain Mainz, and as yet uncharacterized *Helicobacter* species are increasingly being isolated from the blood of immunocompromised patients.

D. Rapid urease test

H. pylori has abundant urease activity; urea is converted to carbon dioxide and ammonia. This chemical reaction is the basis for the detection of the organism in gastric biopsies with the use of the biopsy rapid urease test. The release of ammonia alters the pH of the test medium, and this is detected by a colour change in the pH indicator. Biopsy rapid urease tests (RUT) are used by the clinician in the endoscopy room to establish colonization by *H. pylori* within a short time span, e.g., potentially before the patient leaves the endoscopy department. Compared to culture and histology, urease tests are economical. The sensitivity of the test varies dramatically with the grade of colonization. When large numbers of organisms (grade 4: equivalent to 100 organisms per high power field) are present on the gastric mucosa, the test had a high sensitivity; this may fall to 30% in grade 2 (<29 organisms per hpf). Thus, the urease assay may be less useful in determining colonization after eradication treatment. Furthermore, the sensitivity of the test is reduced by high dose proton pump inhibitor therapy and acid reduction surgery. Overall, the sensitivity and specificity of the RUT are reported as 80-90% and 90-100% respectively. A number of different RUTs are commercially available, e.g., "CLO", "HUT", and "CP" tests, and a reagent strip rapid urease (Pyloritek) determination has also been commercialized; each have slightly different reported sensitivity and specificity (64). The density of microbial colonization can be assessed using a multi-scaled rapid urease test (Hp-Fast) which is graded to give colour reactions varying from yellow to green to light blue and blue. Overall, the sensitivity and specificity of this test when compared to histology is 89% and 88% respectively with the highest positivity of 70% at 30 min. for the highest density of *H. pylori* compared to 62% at 24 hrs. for the lowest density. More recent modifications of the RUT, using a chemiluminescent pH indicator, provide more rapid results and a 50-fold higher sensitivity compared to the routine RUT (65). The rapid urease test, which may require only one minute to complete (66), can also be performed endoscopically with the use of a pH sensitive biosensor; a sensitivity and specificity of 92% and 95% respectively have been reported.

E. Biochemical analysis of gastric aspirate

The measurement of urea and ammonia levels in the gastric juice can be used to detect the presence of *H. pylori*. In uninfected subjects, the ratio of urea to ammonia is high, e.g., 3-4, and in infected subjects as low as < 1.0. The sensitivity and specificity of this test are reported to be 90% to 100%. If performed manually, the technique is rather laborious, but there is the potential for automation. This test is not often used as a routine.

F. Molecular biological methods of detection

1. In-situ hybridization

In-situ hybridization assays have been developed for the detection of *H. pylori* in stomach biopsies with the use of either a biotinylated or ^{32}P-labelled probe which are based on the 16S rRNA sequences. These probes are more sensitive than routine staining and could be particularly useful if low numbers of organisms are present or perhaps for investigating archival paraffin sections. The technique of hybridization is complex and labour intensive when compared to the staining of tissue sections. The biopsy may be inhibitory for the hybridization reaction and false negative reactions may be seen if minor variations in nucleotide sequence occur in the target sequence (67). Thus, in-situ hybridization is not in widespread use as a diagnostic method. A simple hybridization assay, however, has been developed that uses colorimetric detection, and it may be useful for follow-up studies in order to detect eradication of *H. pylori* (68).

2. Polymerase chain reaction

The polymerase chain reaction can used to detect *H. pylori* in gastric biopsies, gastric juice, dental plaque, and feces. It can used diagnostically and as a method for typing; the latter either from cultures or directly from a clinical specimen (69-71). Several different loci have been used as targets for amplification (e.g., 16S rRNA gene, e.g., the urease gene (A and B subunits) and the phosphoglucomutase gene *glmM* (formerly urease C), amongst others (72-77). Due to the clinical significance of the *cagA* and *vacA* loci in their relationship to serious gastroduodenal disease, both of these genes have also been used as targets for PCR (76,78-83); the latter particularly as specific *vacA* alleles have clinical associations with pathology. The majority of the PCR assays have been simple one-step amplifications, although some are nested to increase sensitivity; others have been combined with probes to enhance specificity. Primers for the various loci as targeted are given in Tables 3 and 4. Although most diagnostic PCR amplicons are detected by gel electrophoresis, there is a growing trend to use a colorimetric method for detection, because of the speed for detection and the potential for automation. Three such PCR-enzyme immunoassays assays have been assessed (84). The GEN-ETI-K DEIA (Sorin, Italy) uses streptavidin-coated microwell plates to which a biotinylated specific probe is added. The probe is based on the *glmM* gene. The amplified product is added to the microtitre plate, and the duplex DNA is detected with an enzyme-linked antibody that recognizes double-stranded DNA. PYLORI-PROB (Biocode, Belgium) is a solid-phase sandwich hybridization assay. A specific capture probe (based also on the *glmM* gene) is bound to the microwell plate. The amplified product is added to the well and thereafter detected with a biotinylated probe. PCR-ELISA (Boehringer, Germany) uses a capture probe that is labelled with biotin (*glmM*) which in turn is bound to the solid phase with streptavidin. Thereafter, the digoxigenin-labelled amplified product is added, and the hybridized product is detected with anti-DIG-peroxidase. Assessment of these three kits showed that the colorimetric DNA immunoassays were 100 times more sensitive than standard PCR, and a result could be obtained within 4 hours. The sensitivity and specificity of the three tests were 85% and 88% for GEN-ETI-K DEIA, 87% and 82% for PYLORI-PROB, and 80% and 68% for PCR-ELISA. A further modification of the PCR is the development of LightCycler technology in which the PCR takes place within a sealed glass ampule and in which the accumulation of amplified duplex DNA is measured continuously by fluorophor emission from SybrGreen. The use of a LightCycler can significantly shorten the time for a result to be obtained. Generally, PCR is more technically complex to perform than the RUT, histology, or culture, and may currently offer only a marginal advantage in terms of sensitivity if used only on gastric biopsies. It is perhaps more useful, however, in detecting *H. pylori* in specimens where there is a rich normal flora, where culture is less sensitive, or where there are likely to be small numbers of organisms. PCR may facilitate strain typing which in the future may be valuable for epidemiological studies or to facilitate the rapid detection of antibiotic resistance. PCR can also potentially be used to quantify bacterial load in gastric biopsies through the use of a non-homologous fragment that is linked to specific primers that are being employed to amplify a portion of the *H. pylori* genome. Co-amplification of a known added internal standard (PCR MIMIC) facilitates quantification of the *H. pylori* target. There is, however, no clinical advantage to determining the quantity of *H. pylori* in most contexts, and as the polymerase chain reaction has the ability to detect non-viable forms as well as viable organisms, false positives may occur and thus makes its value doubtful for post-treatment follow-up.

G. Labeled urea tests

Accurate non-invasive tests that indicate current infection with *H. pylori* may be based on the ingestion of labeled urea and the subsequent detection of the breakdown product as evidence for infection.

Table 3 Primers for polymerase chain reaction amplification for *H. pylori*. bp – base-pairs fragment length.

Designation	Forward	Reverse	size (bp)	ref.erence
16S rRNA	GCgACCTgCTggACCATTAC	CgTTAgCTgCATTACTggAgA	139	68
1.9 kD cloned genomic fragment	CATCTTgTTAgAgggATTgg	TAACAAACCgATAATggCgC	203	69
species-specific antigen cistron	TggCgTgTCTATTgACAgCgAgC	CCTgCTgggCATACTTCACCATg	298	70
urease A	GCCAATggTAAATTAgTT	CTCCTTAATTgTTTTTAC	411	71
urease B	TgggATTAgCgAgTATgT	CCCATTTgACTCAATg	132	71
	AATTgCAgAAAATATCAC	ACTTTATTggCTggTTT	115	
glmM	AAgCTTTTAggggTgTTAggggTTT	AAgCTTACTTTCTAACACTAACgC	293	72
(nested)	CTTTCTTCTCAAgCAATTgTC	CAAgCCATCgCCggTTTTAgC	252	73

Table 4 Primers for polymerase chain reaction amplification of *H. pylori* virulence factor genes *cagA* and *vacA*. bp – base-pairs fragment length.

Designation	Forward	Reverse	size (bp)	reference
cagA	TtggACCAACAACCACAAACCgAAg	CTTCCCTTAATTgCgAgATTCC	183	77
	AATACACCAACgCCTCCAAg	TTgTTgCCgCTTTTgCTCTC	396	72
	CCATgAAATTTTgATCCgTTCgg	GATAACAggCAAgCTTTTgAgAgggA	393	74
	1 – ggAATTgTCTgATAAACTTg	3 – CCATTATTgTTATTgTTATTg	612-615 (cag1/3)	76
	2 – ggAACCCTAgTCggTAATg	4 – ATCTTTgAgCTTgTCTATCg	450-558 (cag2/4)	
vacA	(VA1F) ATggAAATACAACAAACACAC	(VA1R) CTgCTTgAATgCgCCAAAC	259 (S1) 286 (S2)	75
	(SS1) gTCAGCATCACACCgCAAC	as above VA1R	190 (S1a)	
	(SS3) AgCgCCATACCgCAAAATgATCC	as above VA1R	187 (S1b)	
	(SS2) gCTAACACgCCAAATgATCC	as above VA1R	199 (S2)	
	(VA3F) ggTCAAAATgCggTCATgg	(VA3R) CCATTggTACCTgTAgAAAC	290 (M1)	
	(VA4F) ggAgCCCCAggAAACATTg	(VA4R) CATAACTAgCgCCTTgCAC	352 (M2)	
	(VAC1F) gAAATACAACAAACACACCgC	(VAC1R) GgCTTgTTTgAgCCCCCAg	201 (S1) 228 (S2)	76
	as above VA3F	(VAC3R) CATCAgTATTTCgCACCACA	388 (M1)	
	(VAC4F) CCAggACCAATTgCCggCAAA	as above VA4R	346 (M2)	

Urea is labelled with ^{14}C, ^{13}C, or ^{15}N and is given as a test meal. Hydrolysis of labeled urea by the urease enzyme releases labeled carbon dioxide which is found in the exhaled breath. Labelled ammonia is excreted in the urine and labelled bicarbonate can be detected in the blood (Figure 4). The routinely-used version of the test, the urea breath test, can be used for epidemiological studies, to screen patients prior to endoscopy, and as a follow-up assessment to determine the effect of treatment in eradication of *H. pylori*. The urea breath test may be unreliable in assessing patients who have had gastric surgery, and in patients who have been on proton pump inhibitors or ranitidine, as false negatives may occur in up to 40% of such patients.

1. ^{14}C-urea breath test

In the ^{14}C-urea breath test, labelled urea is given to the patient with a test meal in order to delay gastric emptying. Various doses of labelled urea have been used which include 0.4 MBq, 0.1 MBq, 110 kBq, and 37 kBq. Breath samples are collected for up to two hours or a single sample can be collected at 40 min. by exhaling into hyamine (a CO_2-trapping agent). The radioactivity of each sample is measured by a scintillation counter. The results are expressed as a percentage of the administered dose as adjusted for endogenous CO_2 directly as counts per minute. Due to the potential adverse effect of radiation, microdose (37 kBq or 1 micro Ci) capsulated formulations (PYtest) have been used. The sensitivity and specificity of the test is recorded as 100% and 97% respectively (85), and although the dose of radiation is no greater than background with the microdose formulation, there is obvious hesitation in using the test among children or pregnant women.

2. ^{13}C-urea breath test

The ^{13}C-urea breath test is identical to the ^{14}C-urea breath test in principle except that ^{13}C is a non-radioactive isotope of ^{12}C, and its measurement requires a mass spectrometer rather than a scintillation counter, thus limiting the availability of this procedure. Several private enterprises offer to analyze ex-

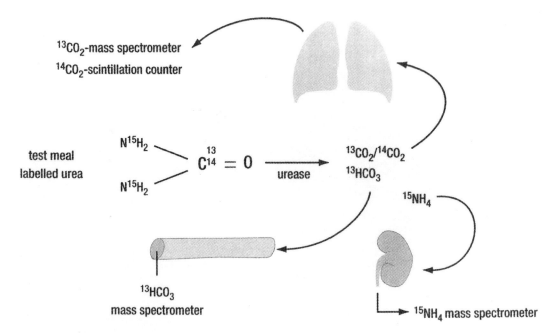

Figure 4   Diagnostic assays which are based on labeled substrate meals.

pired breath samples if sent by mail. The non-radioactive nature of ^{13}C implies that the test can safely be used in children and pregnant females. Since ^{13}C is naturally occurring, it is measured as a ratio of ^{12}C which is the most abundant isotope. Deviations from the naturally occurring ratio of $^{13}C:^{12}C$, defined as zero, are recorded after ingestion of 75-200 mg. ^{13}C-urea. As the ratio is being measured, the volume of expired breath collected is immaterial.

A European protocol for a standard test has been agreed (86) in which a baseline sample is taken prior to the ingestion of 100 mg. of ^{13}C-urea via a test meal. Between 10 and 40 min. after, serial five-minute samples of breath are collected in a bag, and at 40 min., the ratio of $^{13}C:^{12}C$ is measured in a sample of the pooled expired air. The specificity and sensitivity of the ^{13}C-urea breath test are above 98%.

Several possible modifications of the test have been investigated, such as changes to the timing and method of measurement, the dose of labeled urea, the type of test meal, requisite for fasting, and the actual cut-off value. The most limiting factor in the widespread use of the test is the availability of a mass spectrometer given its complexity and cost. The cost of the ^{13}C-UBT has decreased recently, however, owing to the utilization of non-dispersive infrared spectrometry or laser assisted ratio analyzer (LARA) which detects the exhaled CO_2. Both are cheaper than an isotope ratio mass spectrometer (IRMS) that was used in the original tests (87,88). Comparable sensitivity and specificity for the IRMS can also be achieved through gas chromatography with a mass selective detector, and this technology can be found in most biochemistry laboratories. Tests which include either a standard semi-liquid meal or a standard fatty meal have both been used in order to delay gastric emptying. Citric acid has been shown to be effective as a test meal (89) and is marketed in a test kit (Helikit) which also contains 75 mg. labelled urea; its reported use is associated with a sensitivity and specificity of 93% and 97% respectively (90). Data also indicate that 4-hour fasting prior to the meal may not be required (91). In adults, the cut-off is normally taken as a delta value of 5.0, but in children 3.0 appears to be a more appropriate cut-off (92).

3. ^{15}N-urea excretion test

There is one report of urea being labelled with ^{15}N, a naturally occurring non-radioactive isotope of ^{14}N. The excretion of $^{15}NH_4$ is detected by a mass spectrometer, and although urine is an easier specimen to collect than breath, the test is not used routinely. It has a comparable sensitivity and specificity to the ^{13}C breath test.

H. Serology

Serology has frequently been used in epidemiological studies for understanding the population distribution of *H. pylori*, but serology is also used diagnostically as a screening test. Unlike the urea breath test, it is not useful as a follow-up test to establish success of the eradication regimen, because the antibody titres may take up to six months to fall sufficiently in order to ascertain a significant difference. The three main types of commercially-available serological tests are based on a crude or partially purified antigen(s), Western blotting, and recombinant (virulence factor) antigens. The majority of serological tests are laboratory-based although point-of-care assays are increasingly becoming available. Some serological kits are also available for determining anti-*H. pylori* antibody in saliva rather than serum. Recently, a fecal antigen detection test has also become available.

1. Serum antibody assays

The most common antibody assay is that of an ELISA-based format, although latex agglutination and immunochromatographic variations are also available (Table 5). There have been many publications (93-105) which detail the accuracy of these various serological kits, and the reported sensitivity, specificity, and positive and negative predictive values are shown in Tables 6 and 7. Antibody tests are also available for the virulence markers *cagA* and *vacA* by ELISA or immunoblot (e.g., HelicoBlot 2 and

Table 5   Commercial immunoassays for *H. pylori* antibody determination.

Kit name	Test format	Manufacturer
Pylori Elisa II	ELISA	BioWittaker, U.S.
Pyloriset update		Orion, Finland
Helico G2		Shield, U.K.
Premier HP		Meridian, U.S.
Cobas Core		Roche, Switzerland
Hel-p Test II		Amrad, Australia
Malakit		BioLab, Belgium
GAP IgG2		BioRad, U.S.
Roche MTP		Roche, Switzerland
Hp-G screen		Genesis
Microstar EIA		Kenstar, U.K.
SIA Helicobacter		Sigma, U.S.
HM-CAP EIA		Enteric Prod., U.S.
Helisal EIA		Cortecs, U.K.
Helori CTX		Eurospital, Italy
H. pylori IgG		Dako Denmark
Autozyme		Cambridge LS, U.K.
Pyloragen		Hycor, U.S.
Enzygnost HP		Behring, U.K.
Quickvue HP EIA		Quidel, U.S.
Enzywell HP EIA		Dresse Monteriggioni, Italy
Color Vue Pylori		Seradyn, U.S.
Autoplate		Menarini
BioLife		BioLife
Pyloriset Dry	LA	Orion, Finland
Helicoblot 2.0	WB	GeneLab, Singapore
RIBA		Chiron, U.S.
Helisan One step	IMC	Cortecs, U.K.
Helisal RBT		Cortecs, U.K.
FlexSureHPS		SmithKline, U.S.
Genesis Dot		Genesis, U.K.
QuickVueOnestep		Quidel, U.S.
Launch immunocard		Meridian, U.S.
Quadratech HEP		VEDA, France
CLOser		Medical Inst. Corp, Switzerland

Table 6 Sensitivity, specificity, positive predictive value (PPV), and negative predictive value (NPV) for selected immunoassays.

Kit name	Sensitivity	Specificity	PPV	NPV
Pylori Elisa II	100	96	97	100
Helico G 2	85	76	74	87
Premier HP	85-100	80-100	76-100	88-100
Cobas Core	87-98	83-98	87	86
Pyloriset update	100	79	95	100
Hel-p Test	89-100	62-93	65-90	91-100
Malakit	79-87	86-98	96	60
GAP IgG	76-100	26-99	76-100	71-100
HP kit Radim	81	90		
Roche MTP	94-99	83-86	88	90
HpG screen	83-93	68-91	66-84	84-100
Microstar	97	76	80	98
SIA sigma	85-90	80-98	76-96	88-100
HM cap EIA	83-98	80-96	76	86
Autozyme	89	52	58	87
Pyloragen	79	75	71	83
Enzygnost	80	74	70	83
Quidel EIA	89	66	68	89
Enzywell	90	71	71	91
Color Vue	88	66	63	87

Table 7 Sensitivity, specificity, positive predictive value (PPV), and negative predictive value (NPV) for selected point-of-care immunoassays.

Kit name	Sensitivity	Specificity	PPV	NPV
AccuStat	89	93	89	93
Helisal RBT	82-92	55-91	56-92	86-89
FlexSure HP	76-96	77-100	72-96	83-95
Quick Vue	78-89	70-93	70-82	86-88
Pyloriset LA	68-92	56-76	68-85	62-84
Pyloriset Dry	64-97	75-95	72-95	75-93
Pylori Screen	95	94	91	97
HpCheck	88	85	83	90
Quadratech	83	57	60	81
CLOser	95	72	80	93

recombinant immunoblot assay [RIBA]) and these may give additional information on clinical significance of colonization through the identification of Type I strains which are mostly associated with severe pathology. There is some doubt, however, as to the accuracy of these tests for this purpose (106).

2. Salivary antibody assays

Due to the ease of collection, particularly in children, salivary antibody assays may be particularly useful. In general, the salivary antibody assays are not as accurate as those for serum antibody although comparable sensitivity and specificity to serum assays has been achieved using the OraSure salivary device (Epitope Inc.) which facilitates collection (107).

3. Point-of-care testing

There is an increasing requirement for point-of-care testing as more patients are managed by general practitioners on a test-and-treat basis. There are several novel tests of this type that are available (108-116), but they tend to lack diagnostic accuracy when compared to laboratory ELISA. Most of the tests are one-step assays that use whole blood, but others require serum separation; the latter may therefore diminish their usefulness as near-patient kits. Also, there may be variations in sensitivity and specificity depending on whether capillary or venous blood is used. Currently available point-of-care tests are not recommended for use in screening (117).

4. Antigen detection

One of the most promising developments for the detection of H. pylori is fecal antigen detection because of its speed, technical simplicity, and ease of collection. The Premier Platinum HpSA EIA (Meridian Diagnostics, U.S.) uses an affinity-purified polyclonal antibody capture in microwell plate format. Fecal suspensions are added, and detection is completed by a peroxidase-conjugated antibody sandwich and substrate. This kit has been assessed in several studies, and it has a sensitivity and specificity of 80-94% and 75-100% respectively with a positive and negative predictive value of 93% and 92% (118-120).

5. Effect of population on serological results

It is recognized from seroepidemiological studies that different ethnic populations have widely differing prevalence of infection and that the assay cut-off value may require modification in order to account for this variability. Similarly, the positive and negative predictive values of the various serological tests may vary according to age, drug administration (such as non-steroidal anti-inflammatory drug usage), or co-existent disease in the population or individual under investigation (e.g., HIV or cystic fibrosis). Serological studies in a childhood population and in the elderly have shown a decreased specificity of the serological tests when compared to culture and histology. In the elderly, this can often be due to atrophic gastritis and reduction in colonization by H. pylori.

6. Diagnostic and management strategies

General considerations

Colonization by H. pylori is determined in the clinical context of dyspepsia investigations. There is currently no indication for H. pylori to be sought in asymptomatic patients except in the rare circumstance of individual patients who are concerned about the risk of developing gastric malignancy. In the future, however, studies of populations with high gastric cancer prevalence rates may provide indications for population screening and eradication. The patient populations for whom H. pylori eradication is advised are set out in the Maastrich criteria (121), and it is within these groups of patients that the diagnosis of H. pylori colonization should be made.

There are several key determinant factors for management of dyspepsia. Dyspepsia is a very common complaint and may be due to a number of conditions, only some of which are unambiguously linked to colonization by *H. pylori*. The role of *H. pylori* as a cause of NUD is not certain, and existing evidence is contradictory. PUD can be cured by eradication of *H. pylori*. PUD can only be diagnosed by endoscopy, and endoscopy is expensive. Given these issues, there are four principle strategies in dealing with a patient who suffers from dyspepsia:

I)   empiric treatment with *H. pylori* eradication therapy (T),
II)   endoscopy and then treatment if colonization is confirmed (ET),
III) testing for colonization with *H. pylori* through a non-invasive screening test and treatment if positive (TT), and
IV)   testing for colonization with a non-invasive screening test, and thereafter following with endoscopy and subsequently treatment if indicated (TET).

These strategies will be conditional on the age of the patient, where the consultation is taking place, and the clinical group to which the patient belongs, i.e., whether they are presenting for the first time or whether they are presenting with recurrent symptoms.

For a patient who is over 45 years or who exhibits emergent symptoms (e.g., anemia, weight loss, bleeding) endoscopy is mandatory. Among those less than 45 years and without such alarm symptoms, given that endoscopy is expensive and time-consuming and given the need to decrease the endoscopy workload, screening strategies have been introduced (TT, TET) either to select for those patients who do not require endoscopy or those who should proceed directly to treatment. Screening prior to endoscopy has been shown to be cost-effective without significant loss of diagnostic accuracy in the majority of populations. In deciding between options TT and TET, the cost-benefit is conditional on the prevalence of PUD, the percentage of patients with NUD that improve on eradication of *H. pylori*, and the ulcer relapse rate that occurs as a consequence of treatment failure or re-infection. The TET approach avoids more endoscopies if seropositive patients are not endoscoped than if seronegatives are not endoscoped, but the difference is marginal, and the advantage of endoscopy for seropositive patients is that the definitive diagnosis of PUD, as distinct from NUD, can be made. Unnecessary antibiotics can thereby be avoided.

Screening tests

Screening can be performed either by serology (laboratory-based or point-of-care), antigen detection, or the urea breath test. A critical consideration in the screening strategy will be the negative predictive value of the test. Point-of-care serological tests that are currently available have lower sensitivities and specificities than laboratory-based ELISA tests. Overall, they are not as accurate and thus are currently not generally recommended. In populations where the seroprevalence of *H. pylori* is low, however, the negative predictive value of the point-of-care testing may be adequate to reassure the patient that they do not have PUD. The role of antigen detection as a screening test or for follow up is as yet undecided in part due to the lack of sufficient prospective study. The UBT has higher sensitivity and specificity than most serological tests particularly those of point-of-care, and it also has a high NPV. UBT also provides evidence for current infection where serology does not. A decision-analysis mathematical model of the non-invasive screening methods (122) found that, for a prevalence of 30%, the fecal antigen test had comparable cost-effectiveness to point-of-care serological (not whole blood) tests.

If the patient is a child or pregnant female, screening with radioactive UBT should not be performed. One test that appears to have a particular advantage for use in children is the HpSA fecal antigen test, but again, prospective studies are required to confirm. Similar comments apply to the detection of *H. pylori* in feces by PCR.

Management strategies (Figure 5)

In patients who are presenting for the first time in a primary health care (PHC) setting, a TT strategy is usually adopted, although the patient may also be referred to an open-access endoscopy clinic (TET strategy) where an eradication regimen is given if PUD is confirmed. This latter approach has the advantage in that PUD can be distinguished from NUD. An accurate diagnosis will allow for a reduction in the antibiotic burden. If endoscopy is performed, there is a strong argument that biopsies should be taken as a routine both for histology and culture (susceptibility tests if culture-positive). As this is likely to be done in the context of recurrent symptoms, the antibiotic sensitivity of the isolate may be invaluable for guiding treatment. Recurrent dyspeptic symptoms are common, and over 50% of patients return to their physician with complaints following a course of eradication therapy. In such circumstances, the patient may proceed directly to endoscopy (ET) or a TET strategy may be adopted using either the UBT or HpSA as evidence of current infection rather than serology, particularly if the patient is known to have previously had PUD. Rather than being used as a screening test under these circumstances, however, the test would be diagnostic, and perhaps would complement endoscopy-based assessments, RUT, and culture, as the latter may suffer from sampling errors and may provide false negative results if only small numbers of organisms are present following treatment. Endoscopy is important in this group of patients not only to offer reassurance to the patient but also to establish the diagnosis of reflux disease, to determine whether any pre-malignant histopathological condition such as intestinal metaplasia exists, and importantly in those who are colonized, to obtain specimens for culture and sensitivity testing of the organism.

7.   Future prospects in diagnosis

An unmet clinical need is quite clearly the accurate determination of the presence of ulceration or gastric atrophy without the aid of an endoscopy because of its cost and potential side effects for the patient. An additional unmet clinical need is to have available an accurate, economical, real-time, and noninvasive diagnostic test that provides information on the active status of colonization, i.e., a better alter-

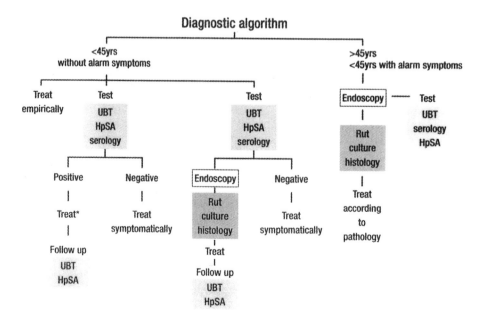

Figure 5   An algorithm of management strategies for *H. pylori*-associated diseases.

native than the urea breath test. One such prospect may already exist in the format of the fecal antigen test, but there are alternatives that potentially have greater diagnostic scope.

Quartz crystal microbalances (QCM) - the 'urea-less' breath test

Quartz crystal microbalances are essentially sensors which weigh gas partitioning of a volatile compound on a coating sensor. A wide range of coatings, often gas chromatographic stationary phases, are available whose sorbent properties are well-characterized and which can maximize more than one type of interaction. The design of specific sensors that maximize all of the common types of chemical interaction will result in a general purpose chemical profiling array (Figure 6). The array instrument incorporates on-line data processing including principal component analysis, discriminant function analysis, and Kohonen and Back-propagation networks. Preliminary work using such an instrument for the analysis of volatile products in breath can distinguish between patients who are colonized by *H. pylori* from those who are not colonized. The latter can be accomplished without the need for any urea test meal (123).

Serological markers of inflammation

H. pylori infection is associated with a set of well-recognized disturbances to normal gastric physiology. Plasma gastrin and pepsinogen levels are both elevated in the course of infection. Pepsinogen I (PG I) levels are even further elevated in PUD compared to those without PUD, and the elevation is correlated with the degree of inflammation. Variation in the levels and the ratio of PG I to pepsinogen II (PG II) can be used to predict the presence of more serious gastric pathology. When used as a screening test in an asymptomatic population, a low PG I combined with seropositivity to the bacterium can predict gastric atrophy with a sensitivity and specificity of 88% and 92% respectively (124). A high serum anti-*H. pylori* IgA antibody level, when associated with a decreased PGI (<50 ng./ml.), correlates with an increased risk of gastric cancer: Odds Ratio - 5.96; 95% Confidence Interval 2.02-17.57 (125).

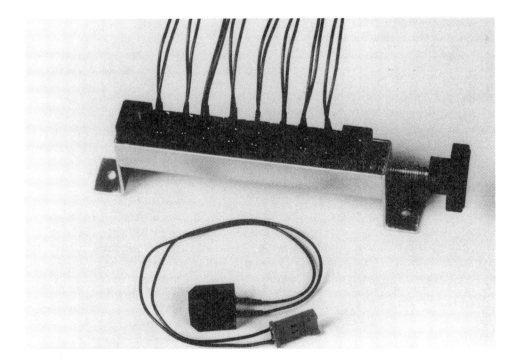

Figure 6   An array of quartz crystal microbalances.

VII. SUSCEPTIBILITY TESTING

A. Eradication of *H. pylori*

Many combinations of antibiotics and anti-ulcer agents have been used in order to eradicate *Helicobacter*, beginning with single agents, and then moving on to two agents and finally triple or even quadruple therapy. With the increased number of therapeutic agents, there has been a decrease in the length of treatment from 4-6 weeks to 7-10 days or even shorter periods. Currently, the regimens that are commonly used include an anti-ulcer agent such as ranitidine, bismuth citrate, or a proton pump inhibitor (e.g., omeprazole, pantoprazole), and a combination of two antibiotics from either metronidazole, clarithromycin, or amoxycillin (126).

A significant problem, however, in current treatment strategies is the increasing resistance to antibiotics, particularly metronidazole. Resistance to metronidazole in a large multi-centre study ranged from 16-42% with resistance to clarithromycin ranging from 1-5% (127). The eradication success rate is influenced by primary resistance to these antibiotics, and thus, it is arguable that antibiotic susceptibility should be determined prior to treatment, particularly in areas where resistance is known to be considerable.

B. Traditional methods

Antibiotic susceptibility testing of *H. pylori* thus far has not been standardized, and there is no consensus at a national or international level for methodology, testing media, the time of incubation or the standards which determine susceptibility and resistance phenotypes, i.e., break-points. A variety of methods (time-kill curves, E-test, agar dilution, broth dilution, and disc diffusion), a variety of media (Muller-Hinton, Brucella, Isosensitest, egg yolk agar with triphenyltetrazolium chloride), a variety of inocula (10^4-10^8 CFU/ml.), a variety of incubation times (36-120 hrs.), and several different interpretative methods have all been assessed. The slow growth of *H. pylori* makes the determination of susceptibility by disc diffusion questionable, and although tempting to use it as a routine, it does have poor correlation with the agar dilution method. The standard broth or agar dilution method for determining minimum inhibitory and bactericidal concentrations, though more accurate, are labour-intensive and not applicable for routine sensitivity testing although they are considered by many to be the reference method. Comparison of different methods for testing susceptibility has shown an excellent correlation between the E-test and agar dilution for clarithromycin and amoxycillin but a poor correlation for metronidazole. Culture of primary isolates from a biopsy specimen on multi-sector plates of antibiotic-containing media can provide a more rapid estimation of the antibiotic susceptibility profile compared to the traditional routine of subculturing (128); the latter is a subject for further evaluation.

C. Molecular methods

Further developments of molecular techniques may be useful for the detection of antibiotic resistance *H. pylori*. Clarithromycin-resistant bacteria have A-G, A-C point mutations in the 23S rRNA gene (129), and these can be detected by PCR or In Line Probe Assays (LiPA). In LiPA, biotinylated primers are used to amplify target sequences. The biotinylated amplicon is then hybridized with specific oligonucleotide targets which are immobilized on membranes. After hybridization, the immobilized amplicons are visualized by the addition of enzyme-labeled streptavidin (130). The A-G point mutations in the 23S rRNA gene may also be detected by PCR and RFLP as these mutations introduce new restriction sites into the genome (131). In addition, the A-C mutation may be detected using 3'-mismatched PCR (132). Finally, as these point mutations will decrease the speed of heteroduplex formation in the wild-type, the mutations can be detected by a preferential homoduplex formation assay (PHFA) where unlabelled strain amplicons compete with a labelled heteroduplex, and thus the presence of the mutation is detected by slow annealing (133). LightCycler technology has also been used to detect clarithromycin resistance.

REFERENCES

1. Warren JR, Marshall B. Unidentified curved bacilli on gastric epithelium in active chronic gastritis. Lancet 1983; i:1273-1275.
2. Goodwin CS, Armstrong JA, Chilvers T, Peters M, Collins MD, Sly T, McConnell W, Harper WES. Transfer of *Campylobacter pylori* and *Campylobacter mustelae* to *Helicobacter* gen. nov. as *Helicobacter pylori* comb nov. and *Helicobacter mustelae* comb nov. Int J Syst Bacteriol 1989; 16:397-405.
3. Tomb JF, White O, Kerlavage AR, Clayton RA, Sutton GG, Fleischmann RD, Ketchum KA, Klenk HP, Gill S, Dougherty BA, Nelson K, Quackenbush J, Zhou L, Kirkness EF, Peterson S, Loftus B, Richardson D, Dodson R, Khalak HG, Glodek A, McKenney K, Fitzegerald LM, Lee N, Adams MD, Hickey EK, Berg DE, Gocayne JD, Utterback TR, Peterson JD, Kelley JM, Cotton MD, Weidman JM, Fujii C, Bowman C, Watthey L, Wallin E, Hayes WS, Borodovsky M, Karp PD, Smith HO, Fraser CM, Venter C. The complete genome sequence of the gastric pathogen *Helicobacter pylori*. Nature 1997; 388:539-547.
4. Vandamme P, Falsen E, Rossau R, Hoste B, Segers P, Tytgat R, De Ley J. Revision of *Campylobacter, Helicobacter* and *Wolinella* taxonomy: amendation of generic descriptions and proposals of *Arcobacter* gen. nov. Int J Syst Bacteriol 1991; 41:88-103.
5. Paster BJ, Lee A, Fox LG, Dewhirst FE, Tordoff LA, Fraser GJ, O'Rouke J, Taylor NS, Ferrero R. Phylogeny of *Helicobacter felis* sp. nov., *Helicobacter mustelae*, and related bacteria. Int J Syst Bacteriol 1991; 41:31-38.
6. Bronsdon MA, Goodwin CS, Sly LI, Chilvers T, Schoenknecht FD. *Helicobacter nemestrinea* sp. nov. a spiral bacterium found in the stomach of a pigtailed macaque (Macaca nemestrina). Int J Syst Bacteriol 1991; 41:148-153.
7. Lee A, Phillips MW, O'Rouke JL, Paster BJ, Dewhirst FE, Fraser GJ, Fox JG, Sly LI, Romaniuk PJ, Trust TJ, Kouprach S. *Helicobacter muridarum* sp. nov. a microaerophilic helical bacterium with a novel ultrastructure isolated from the intestinal mucosa of rodents. Int J Syst Bacteriol 1992; 42:27-36.
8. Eaton KA, Dewhirst FE, Radin MJ, Fox JG, Paster BJ, Krakowka S, Morgan DR. *Helicobacter acinonyx* sp. nov. isolated from cheetahs with gastritis. Int J Syst Bacteriol 1993; 43:99-106.
9. Stanley J, Linton D, Burness AP, Dewhirst FE, Owen RJ, Porter A, On SLW, Costas M. *Helicobacter canis* sp. nov. a new species from dogs: an integrated study of phenotype and genotype. J Gen Microbiol 1993; 139:2495-2504.
10. Fox JG, Dewhirst FE, Tully JG, Paster BJ, Yan L, Taylor NS, Collins MJ, Gorelick PL, Ward JM. *Helicobacter hepaticus* sp. nov. a microaerophilic bacterium isolated from livers and intestinal mucosal scrapings from mice. J Gen Microbiol 1994; 32:1238-1245.
11. Dewhirst FE, Seymour C, Fraser GJ, Paster BJ, Fox JG. Phylogeny of *Helicobacter* isolates from bird and swine feces and description of *Helicobacter pametensis* sp. nov. Int J Syst Bacteriol 1994; 44:553-560.
12. Stanley J, Linton D, Burnens AP, Dewhirst FE, On SLW, Porter A, Owen RJ, Costas M. *Helicobacter pullorum* sp. nov. genotype and phenotype of a new species isolated from poultry and from human patients with gastroenteritis. Microbiology 1994; 140: 3441-3449.
13. Fox JG, Yan LL, Dewhirst FE, Paster BJ, Shames B, Murphy JC, Hayward A, Belcher JC, Mendes EN. *Helicobacter bilis* sp. nov. a novel *Helicobacter* species isolated from bile, livers and intestines of aged, inbred mice. J Clin Microbiol 1995; 33:445-454.
14. Hanninen ML, Happonen I, Saari S, Jalava K. Culture and characteristics of *Helicobacter bizzozeroni*, a new canine gastric *Helicobacter* sp. Int J Syst Bacteriol 1996; 46:160-166.
15. Mendes EN, Queiroz DMM, Dewhirst FE, Paster BJ, Moura SB, Fox JG. *Helicobacter trogontum* sp. nov., isolated from the rat intestine. Int J Syst Bacteriol 1996; 46:916-921.
16. Franklin CL, Beckwith CS, Livingstone RS, Riley LK, Gibson SV, Besch-Williford CL, Hook RR. Isolation of a novel *Helicobacter* species, *Helicobacter cholecystus* sp. nov. from the gallbladder of Syrian hamsters with cholangiofibrosis and centrilobular pancreatitis. J Clin Microbiol 1996; 34:2952-2958.
17. Trivett-Moore NL, Rawlinson WD, Yuen M, Gilbert GL. *Helicobacter westmeadii* sp. nov., a new species isolated from blood cultures of two AIDS patients. J Clin Microbiol 1997; 35:1144-1150.

18. McNulty CAM, Dent JC, Curry A, Uff JS, Ford GA, Gear MWL, Wilkinson SP. New spiral bacterium in gastric mucosa. J Clin Pathol 1989; 42:585-591.

19. Andersen LP, Boye K, Blom J, Holck S, Norgaard A, Elsborg L. Characterization of a culturable *"Gastrospirillum hominis"* (*Helicobacter heilmannii*) strain isolated from human gastric mucosa. J Clin Microbiol 1999; 37:1069-1076.

20. Queiroz DMM, Rocha GA, Mendes EN, Moura SB, Oliveira AMR, Miranda D. Association between *Helicobacter* and gastric ulcer disease of the pars esophagea in swine. Gastroenterology 1996; 111:19-27.

21. Stolte M, Kroher G, Meining A, Morgner A, Bayerdorffer E, Bethke B. A comparison of *Helicobacter pylori* and *Helicobacter heilmannii* gastritis: a matched control study involving 404 patients. Scand J Gastroenterol 1997; 32:28-33.

22. Dixon MF, Genta RM, Yardley JH, Correa P. Classification and grading of gastritis: the updated Sydney system. International Workshop on the Histopathology of Gastritis. Am J Surg Pathol 1996; 20:1161-1181.

23. McColl K, Murray L, El-Omar E, Dickson A, El-Nujumi A, Wirz A, Kelman A, Penny C, Knill-Jones R, Hilditch T. Symptomatic benefit from eradicating *Helicobacter pylori* infection in patients with nonulcer dyspepsia. N Engl J Med 1998; 339:1869-1874.

24. Blum AL, Talley NJ, O'Morain C, van-Zanten SV, Labenz J, Stolte M, Louw JA, Stubberod A, Theodors A, Sundin M, Bolling-Sternevald E, Junghard O. Lack of effect of treating *Helicobacter pylori* infection in patients with nonulcer dyspepsia: omeprazole plus clarithromycin and amoxicillin effect one year after treatment (OCAY) study group. N Engl J Med 1998; 339:1875-1881.

25. NIH Consensus Conference. *Helicobacter pylori* in peptic ulcer disease: NIH consensus development panel on *Helicobacter pylori* in peptic ulcer disease. JAMA 1994; 272:65-69.

26. IARC Working Group on the Evaluation of Carcinogenic Risks to Humans. Schistosomes, liver flukes and *Helicobacter pylori*. IARC Monogr Eval Carcinog Risks Hum 1994; 61:1-241.

27. Forman D. Helicobacter pylori and gastric cancer. Scand J Gastroenterol 1996; 220:S23-S26.

28. Parsonet J, Hansen S, Rodriguez L, Gelb AB, Warnke RA, Jellem E, Orentreich N, Vogelman JH, Friedman GD. *Helicobacter pylori* infection and gastric lymphoma. New Engl J Med 1994; 330:1267-1271.

29. Gasbarrini A, Franceschi F, Armuzzi A, Ojetti V, Candelli M, Sanz Torre E, De Lorenzo A, Anti M, Pretolani S, Gasbarrini G. Extra-digestive manifestations of *Helicobacter pylori* gastric infection. Gut 1999; 45:S9-S13.

30. Webb PM, Knight T, Greaves S, Wilson A, Newell DG, Elder J, Forman D. Relation between infection with *Helicobacter pylori* and living conditions in childhood: evidence for person to person transmission in early life. Br Med J 1994; 308:750-753.

31. Lambert JR, Lin SK, Sievert W, Nicholson L, Schembri M, Guest C. High prevalence of *Helicobacter pylori* antibodies in an institutionalized population: evidence for person-to-person transmission. Am J Gastroenterol 1995; 90:2167-2171.

32. Kosunen TU, Hook J, Rautelin HI, Myllyla G. Age-dependent increase of *Campylobacter pylori* antibodies in blood donors. Scand J Gastroenterol 1989; 24:110-114.

33. Thomas JE, Gibson GR, Darboe MK, Dale A, Gibson GR. Isolation of *Helicobacter pylori* from human feces. Lancet 1992; 340:1194-1195.

34. Hulten K, Han SW, Enroth H, Klein PD, Opekun AR, Gilman RH, Evans DG, Engstrand L, Graham DY, El-Zaatari FA. *Helicobacter pylori* in the drinking water in Peru. Gastroenterology 1996; 110:1031-1035.

35. Aspinall GO, Monteiro MA, Pang H, Walsh EJ, Moran AP. Lipopolysaccharide of the *Helicobacter pylori* type strain NCTC 11637 (ATCC 43504): structure of the O antigen chain and core oligosaccharide regions. Biochemistry 1996; 35:2489-2497.

36. Kuwahara H, Miyamoto Y, Akaike T, Kubota T, Sawa T, Okamoto S, Maeda H. *Helicobacter pylori* urease suppresses bactericidal activity of peroxynitrite via carbon dioxide production. Infect Immun 2000; 68:4378-4383.

37. Piotrowski J, Skrodzka D, Slomiany A, Slomiany BL. *Helicobacter pylori* lipopolysaccharide induces gastric epithelial cells apoptosis. Biochem Mol Biol Int 1996; 40:597-602.

38. Peek RM, Wirth HP, Moss SF, Yang M, Abdalla AM, Tham KT, Zhang T, Tang LH, Modlin IM, Blaser MJ. *Helicobacter pylori* alters gastric epithelial cell cycle events and gstrin secretion in Mongolian gerbils. Gastroenterology 2000; 118:48-59.

39. Shirin H, Sordillo EM, Kovelska TK, Hibshoosh H, Kawabata Y, Oh SH, Kuebler JF, Delohery T, Weghorst CM, Weinstein IB, Moss SF. Chronic *Helicobacter pylori* infection induces an apotosis-resistant phenotype associated with decreased expression of p27^{kip1}. Infect Immun 2000; 68:5321-5328.

40. Cover TL The vacuolating cytotoxin of *Helicobacter pylori*. Mol Microbiol 1996; 20:241-246.

41. Moss SF, Legon S, Bishop AE, Polak JM, Calam J. Effect of *Helicobacter pylori* on gastrin and somatostatin in duodenal ulcer disease. Lancet 1992; 340: 930-932.

42. Segal ED, Lange C, Covacci A, Tompkins LS, Falkow S. Induction of host signal transduction pathways by *Helicobacter pylori*. Proc Natl Acad Sci USA 1997; 94:7595-7599.

43. Covacci A, Falkow S, Berg DE, Rappuoli R. Did the inheritance of a pathogenicity island modify the virulence of *Helicobacter*. Trends Microbiol 1997; 5:205-208.

44. Appelmelk BJ, Negrini R, Moran AP, Kuipers EJ. Molecular mimicry between *Helicobacter pylori* and the host. Trends Microbiol 1997; 5:70-73.

45. Kamiya K, Arisawa T, Goto H, Shibayama K, Horii T, Hayakawa T, Ohta M. Are autoantibodies against Lewis antigens involved in the pathogenesis of *Helicobacter pylori* induced peptic ulcers? Microbiol Immunol 1999; 43:403-408.

46. Faller G, Steininger H, Appelmik B, Kirchner T. Evidence of novel pathogenic pathways for the formation of antigastric autoantibodies in *Helicobacter pylori* gastritis. J Clin Pathol 1998; 51:244-245.

47. El Omar EM, Carrington M, Chow WH, McColl KEL, Bream JH, Young HA, Herrera J, Lissowska J, Yuan CC, Rothman N, Lanyon G, Martin M, Fraumenl JF, Rabkin CS. Interleukin-1 polymorphisms associated with increased risk of gastric cancer. Nature 2000; 404:398-402.

48. Alkpout AM, Blackwell CC, Weir DM. Increased inflammatory response of persons of blood group O to *H. pylori*. J Infect Dis 2000; 181:1364-1369.

49. Sutton P. Kolesnikow T, Danon S, Wilson J, Lee A. Dominant nonresponsiveness to *Helicobacter pylori* infection is associated with production of interleukin 10 and not gamma interferon. Infect Immun 2000; 68:4802-4804.

50. Mitchell HM, Hazell SL, Kolesnikow T, Mitchell J, Frommer D. Antigen recognition during progression from acute to chronic infection with a *cagA* positive strain of *Helicobacter pylori*. Infect Immun 1996; 64:1166-1172.

51. Aucher P, Petit ML, Mannant PR, Pezennec L, Babin P, Fauchere JL. Use of immunoblot assay to define serum antibody patterns associated with *Helicobacter pylori* infection and with *Helicobacter pylori*-related ulcers. J Clin Microbiol 1998; 36:931-936.

52. Sorberg M, Engstrand L, Strom M, Jonsson KA, Jorbeck H, Granstrom M. The diagnostic value of enzyme immunoassay and immunoblot in monitoring eradication of *Helicobacter pylori*. Scand J Infect Dis 1997; 29:147-151.

53. Hala MT, El-Zimaity K, Wu J, Graham DY. Modified Genta triple stain for identifying *Helicobacter pylori*. J Clin Pathol 1999; 52 693-694.

54. Christensen AO, Gjorup T, Hilden J, Fenger C, Henriksen B, Vyberg M, Osteraard K, Hansen BF. Observer homogeneity in the histological diagnosis of *Helicobacter pylori*. Scand J Gastroenterol 1992; 27:933-939.

55. Misawa K, Kumagai T, Ahimizu T, Furihata K, Ota H, Akamatsu T, Katsuyama T. A new histological procedure for re-evaluation of the serological test of *Helicobacter pylori*. Eur J Clin Microbiol Infect Dis 1998; 17:14-19.

56. Salmenkyla S, Hyvarinen H, Halonen K, Sipponen P. Frozen-section biopsy in per-endoscopic diagnosis of *Helicobacter pylori*. Helicobacter 1997; 2:123-126.

57. Queiroz DMM., Mendes EN, Rocha GA. Indicator medium for *Campylobacter pylori* J Clin Microbiol 1987; 25:2378-2379.

58. Dent JC, McNulty CAM. Evaluation of a new selective medium for *Campylobacter pylori*. Eur J Clin Microbiol Infect Dis 1988; 7:555-568.

59. Glupczynski Y, Labbe M, Thiabaumont F. Comparative evaluation of a new selective culture medium for improved isolation of *Campylobacter pylori* from gastric biopsy secimens. In: Megraud F, Lamouliatte H, eds. Gastroduodenal Pathology and *Campylobacter pylori*. Amsterdam:Elsevier Science, 1989:3-6.

60. Westblom TU, Madan E, Midkiff BR. Egg yolk emulsion agar, a new medium for the cultivation of *Helicobacter pylori*. J Clin Microbiol 1991; 29:819-821.

61. Cellini L, Allocati N, Piccolomini R, DiCampli E, Dainelli B. New plate medium for growth and detection of urease activity of *Helicobacter pylori*. J Clin Microbiol 1992; 30:1351-1353.

62. Olivieri R, Bugnoli M, Armellini D, Bianciardi S, Rappuoli R, Bayeli PF, Abate L, Esposito E, DeGregorio L, Aziz J, Basagni C, Figura N. Growth of *Helicobacter pylori* in media containing cyclodextrins. J Clin Microbiol 1993; 31:160-162.

63. Veenendaal RA, Lichtendahl-Bernards AT, Pena AS, Endtz HP, van Boven CPA, Lamers CBHW. Effect of transport medium and transportation time on culture of *Helicobacter pylori* from gastric biopsy material. J Clin Pathol 1993; 46:561-563.

64. Laine L, Lewin D, Naritoku W, Estrada R, Cohen H. Prospective comparison of commercially available rapid urease tests for the diagnosis of *Helicobacter pylori*. Gastrointest Endosc 1996; 44:523-526.

65. Roda A, Piazza F, Pasini P, Baraldini M, Zambonin L, Fossi S, Bazzoli F, Rose E. Development of a chemiluminescent urease activity assay for *Helicobacter pylori* in gastric mucosa biposies. Anal Biochem 1998; 264:47-52.

66. Sato T, Fujino MA, Kojima Y, Ohtsuka H, Ohtaka M, Kubo K, Nakamura T, Morozumi A, Nakamura M, Hosaka H. Endoscopic urease sensor system for detecting *Helicobacter pylori* on gastric mucosa. Gastrointest Endosc 1999; 49:32-38.

67. Morotomi M, Hoshina S, Green P, Neu HC, LoGerfo P, Watanabe I, Mutai M, Weinstein IB. Oligonucleotide probe for detection and identification of *Campylobacter pylori*. J Clin Microbiol 1989; 27:2652-2655.

68. Lage AP, Fauconnier A, Burette A, Glupczynski Y, Bollen A, Godfroid E. Rapid colorimetric hybridization assay for detecting amplified *Helicobacter pylori* DNA in gastric biopsy specimens. J Clin Microbiol 1996; 34:530-533.

69. Owen RJ, Slater ER, Xerry J, Peters TM, Teare EL, Grant A. Development of a scheme for genotyping *Helicobacter pylori* based on allelic variation in urease subunit genes. J Clin Microbiol 1998; 36:3710-3712.

70. Li C, Ha T, Chi DS, Ferguson DA Jr, Jiang C, Laffan JJ, Thomas E. Differentiation of *Helicobacter pylori* strains directly from gastric biopsy specimens by PCR-based restriction fragment length polymorphism analysis without culture. J Clin Microbiol 1997; 35:3021-5302.

71. Gibson JR, Slater E, Xerry J, Tompkins DS, Owen RJ. Use of an amplified-fragment length polymorphism technique to fingerprint and differentiate isolates of *Helicobacter pylori*. J Clin Microbiol 1998; 36:2580-2585.

72. Weiss J, Mecca J, da Silva E, Gassner D. Comparison of PCR and other diagnostic techniques for detection of *Helicobacter pylori* infection in dyspeptic patients. J Clin Microbiol 1994; 32:1663-1668.

73. Valentine JL, Arthur RR, Mobley HL, Dick JD. Detection of *Helicobacter pylori* by using the polymerase chain reaction. J Clin Microbiol 1991; 29:689-695.

74. Hammar M, Tyszkiewicz T, Wadstrom T, O'Toole PW. Rapid detection of *Helicobacter pylori* in gastric biopsy material by polymerase chain reaction. J Clin Microbiol 1992; 30:54-58.

75. Clayton CL, Kleanthous H, Coates PJ, Morgan DD, Tabaqchali S. Sensitive detection of *Helicobacter pylori* by using polymerase chain reaction. J Clin Microbiol 1992; 30:192-200.

76. Lage AP, Godfroid E, Fauconnier A, Burette A, Butzler JP, Bollen A, Glupczynski Y. Diagnosis of *Helicobacter pylori* infection by PCR: comparison with other invasive techniques and detection of *cagA* gene in gastric biopsy specimens. J Clin Microbiol 1995; 33:2752-2756.

77. Bamford KB, Lutton DA, O'Loughlin B, Coulter WA, Collins JS. Nested primers improve sensitivity in the detection of *Helicobacter pylori* by the polymerase chain reaction. J Infect 1998; 36:105-110.

78. Husson MO, Gottrand F, Vachee A, Dhaenens L, dela Salle EM, Turck D, Houcke M, Leclerc H. Importance in diagnosis of gastritis of detection by PCR of the *cagA* gene in *Helicobacter pylori* strains isolated from children. J Clin Microbiol 1995; 33:3300-3303.

79. Atherton JC, Cao P, Peek RM Jr.,Tummuru MK, Blaser MJ, Cover TL. Mosaicism in vacuolating cytotoxin alleles of *Helicobacter pylori*: association of specific *vacA* types with cytotoxin production and peptic ulceration. J Biol Chem 1995; 270 :17771-17777.

80. Rudi J, Kolb C, Maiwald M, Kuck D, Sieg A, Galle PR, Stremmel W. Diversity of *Helicobacter pylori vacA* and *cagA* genes and relationship to *vacA* and *cagA* protein expression, cytotoxin production, and associated diseases. J Clin Microbiol 1998; 36:944-948.

81. van Doorn LJ, Figueiredo C, Rossau R, Jannes G, van Asbroek M, Sousa JC, Carneiro F, Quint WG. Typing of *Helicobacter pylori vacA* gene and detection of *cagA* gene by PCR and reverse hybridization. J Clin Microbiol 1998; 36:1271-1276.

82. van Doorn LJ, Figueiredo C, Sanna R, Pena S, Midolo P, Ng EK, Atherton JC, Blaser MJ, Quint WG. Expanding allelic diversity of *Helicobacter pylori vacA*. J Clin Microbiol 1998; 36:2597-2603.

83. Atherton JC, Cover TL, Twells RJ, Morales MR, Hawkey CJ, Blaser MJ. Simple and accurate PCR-based system for typing vacuolating cytotoxin alleles of *Helicobacter pylori* J Clin Microbiol 1999; 37:2979-2982.

84. Monteiro L, Cabrita J, Megraud F. Evaluation of performances of three DNA enzyme immunoassays for detection of *Helicobacter pylori* PCR products from biopsy specimens. J Clin Microbiol 1997; 35:2931-2936.

85. Allardyce RA, Chapman BA, Tie AB, Burt MJ, Yeo KJ, Keenan JI, Bagshaw PF. 37 kBq 14C-urea breath test and gastric biopsy analyses of *H. pylori* infection. Aust N Z J Surg 1997; 67:31-34.

86. Logan RP, Dill S, Bauer FE. The European 13C-urea breath test for the detection of *Helicobacter pylori*. Gut 1991; 3:915-921.

87. Hildebrand P, Beglinger C. Nondispersive infrared spectrometry: a new method for the detection of *Helicobacter pylori* infection with the 13C-urea breath test. Clin Infect Dis 1997; 25:1003-1005.

88. Minoli G, Prada A, Schuman R, Murnick D, Rigas B. A simplified urea breath test for the diagnosis of *Helicobacter pylori* infection using the LARA system. J Clin Gastroenterol 1998; 26:264-6.

89. Graham DY, Runke D, Anderson SY, Malaty HM, Klein PD. Citric acid as a test meal for the 13C urea breath test. Am J Gastroenterol 1999; 94:1214-1217.

90. Mock T, Yatscoff R, Foster R, Hyun JH, Chung IS, Shim CS, Yacyshyn B. Clinical validation of the Helikit: a 13C urea breath test used for the diagnosis of *Helicobacter pylori* infection. Clin Biochem 1999; 32:59-63.

91. Moayyedi P, Braunholtz D, Heminbrough E, Clough M, Tompkins DS, Mapstone NP, Mason S, Dowell AC, Richards ID, Chalmers DM, Axon AT. Do patients need to fast for a 13C-urea breath test? Eur J Gastroenterol Hepatol 1997; 9:275-7.

92. Cadranel S, Corvaglia L, Bontems P, Deprez C, Glupczynski Y, Van Riet A, Keppens E. Detection of *Helicobacter pylori* infection in children with a standardized and simplified 13C-urea breath test. J Pediatr Gastroenterol Nutr 1998; 27:275-280.

93. van den Oever HL, Loffeld RJ, Stobberingh EE. Usefulness of a new serological test (Bio-Rad) to diagnose *Helicobacter pylori*-associated gastritis. J Clin Microbiol 1991; 29:283-286.

94. Goossens H, Glupczynski Y, Burette A, Van den Borre C, DePrez C, Bodenmann J, Keller A, Butzler JP. Evaluation of a commercially available complement fixation test for diagnosis of *Helicobacter pylori* infection and for follow-up after antimicrobial therapy. J Clin Microbiol 1992; 30:3230-3233.

95. Aguirre PM, Pascual CY, Merino FJ, Velasco AC. Evaluation of two commercial enzyme immunoassays for the diagnosis of *Helicobacter pylori* infection. Eur J Clin Microbiol Infect Dis 1992; 11:634-639.

96. Trautmann M, Moldrzyk M, Vogt K, Korber J, Held T, Marre R. Use of a receiver operating characteristic in the evaluation of two commercial enzyme immunoassays for detection of *Helicobacter pylori* infection. Eur J Clin Microbiol Infect Dis 1994; 13:812-819.

97. Granberg C, Mansikka A, Lehtonen OP, Kujari H, Gronfors R, Nurmi H, Raiha I, Stahlberg MR, Leino R. Diagnosis of *Helicobacter pylori* infection by using Pyloriset EIA-G and EIA-A for detection of serum immunoglobulin G (IgG) and IgA antibodies. J Clin Microbiol 1995; 31:1450-1453.

98. Marchildon PA, Ciota LM, Zamaniyan FZ, Peacock JS, Graham DY. Evaluation of three commercial enzyme immunoassays compared with the 13C urea breath test for detection of *Helicobacter pylori* infection. J Clin Microbiol 1996; 34:1147-1152.

99. Talley NJ, Kost L, Haddad A, Zinsmeister AR. Comparison of commercial serological tests for detection of *Helicobacter pylori* antibodies. J Clin Microbiol 1992; 30:3146-3150.

100. van de Wouw BA, de Boer WA, Jansz AR, Roymans RT, Staals AP. Comparison of three commercially available enzyme linked immunosorbent assays and biopsy dependent diagnosis for detecting *Helicobacter pylori* infection. J Clin Microbiol 1996; 34:94-97.

101. Wilcox MH, Dent TH, Hunter JO, Gray JJ, Brown DF, Wight DG, Wraight EP. Accuracy of serology for the diagnosis of *Helicobacter pylori* infection: a comparison of eight kits. J Clin Pathol 1996; 49:373-376.

102. Feldman RA, Deeks JJ, Evans SJW, and the *Helicobacter pylori* Serology Study Group. Multi-laboratory comparison of eight commercially available *Helicobacter pylori* serology kits. Eur J Clin Microbiol Infect Dis 1995; 14:428-433.

103. Hoek FJ, Noach LA, Rauws AJ, Tytgat GNJ. Evaluation of the performance of commercial test kits for detection of *Helicobacter pylori* antibodies in serum. J Clin Microbiol 1992; 30:1525-1528.

104. Jensen AKV, Andersen LP, Wachmann CH. Evaluation of eight commercial kits for *Helicobacter pylori* IgG antibody detection. APMIS 1993; 101:795-801.

105. Schembri MA, Lin SK, Lambert JR. Comparison of commercial diagnostic tests for *Helicobacter pylori* antibodies. J Clin Microbiol 1993; 31:2621-2624.

106. Yamaoka Y, Kodama T, Graham DY, Kashima K. Comparison of four serological tests to determine the *cagA* or *vacA* status of *Helicobacter pylori* strains. J Clin Microbiol 1998; 36:3433-3434.

107. Malaty HM, Peacock JS, Marchildon P, Passaretti N. OraSure salivary test for the screening of *Helicobacter pylori* infection in asymptomatic children. Gut 1998; 43 (Suppl. 2): A53.

108. Midolo PD, Lambert JR, Russell EG, Lin SK. A practical single sample dry latex agglutination test for *Helicobacter pylori* antibody detection. J Clin Pathol 1995; 48:969-971.

109. Moayyedi P, Carter AM, Catto A, Heppell RM, Grant PJ, Axon ATR. Validation of a rapid whole blood test for diagnosing *Helicobacter pylori* infection. Br Med J 1997; 314:119.

110. Borody TJ, Andrews P, Shortis NP. Evaluation of whole blood antibody kit to detect active *Helicobacter pylori* infection. Am J Gastroenterol 1996; 91:2509-2512.

111. Stevens M, Livsey SA. MDA Evaluation Reports No. 41, 43, 44, 48, 58, 60, 62, 63, 64, 65, 74, 82, 83, 85, 89. HMSO Norwich, UK. 1996.

112. Stevens M, Livsey SA. MDA Evaluation Reports No. 15, 16, 17, 37, 43. HMSO Norwich, UK. 1997.

113. Mowat C, Murray L, Hilditch TE, Kelman A, Oien K, McColl KE. Comparison of Helisal rapid blood test and 14C-urea breath test in determining *Helicobacter pylori* status and predicting ulcer disease in dyspeptic patients. Am J Gastroenterol 1998; 93:20-25.

114. Oksanen A, Veijola L, Sipponen P, Schauman KO, Rautelin H. Evaluation of Pyloriset Screen, a rapid whole-blood diagnostic test for *Helicobacter pylori* infection. J Clin Microbiol 1998; 36:955-957.

115. Duggan AE, Hardy E, Hawkey CJ. Evaluation of a new near patient test for the detection of *Helicobacter pylori*. Eur J Gastroenterol Hepatol 1998; 10:133-136.

116. Anderson JC, Cheng E, Roeske M, Marchildon P, Peacock J, Shaw RD. Detection of serum antibodies to *Helicobacter pylori* by an immunochromatographic method. Am J Gastroenterol 1997; 92:1135-1139.

117. Anon. *Helicobacter pylori* testing kits. Drug Ther Bull 1997; 35:23-24.

118. McNamara D, Whelan H, Hamilton H, Beattie S, O'Morain C. HpSA: assessment of a new non-invasive diagnostic assay for *Helicobacter pylori* infection in an Irish population. Ir J Med Sci 1999; 168:111-113.

119. Vaira D, Malfertheiner P, Megraud F, Axon AT, Deltenre M, Hirschl AM, Gasbarrini G, O'Morain C, Garcia JM, Quina M, Tytgat GN. Diagnosis of *Helicobacter pylori* infection with a new non-invasive antigen-based assay. Lancet 1999; 354:30-33.

120. Chang MC, Wu MS, Wang HH, Wang HP, Lin JT. *Helicobacter pylori* stool antigen (HpSA) test: a simple, accurate and non-invasive test for detection of *Helicobacter pylori* infection. Hepatogastroenterology 1999; 46:299-302.

121. European Helicobacter Pylori Study Group. Current European concepts in the management of *Helicobacter pylori* infection. The Maastricht Consensus Report. Gut 1997; 41:8-13.

122. Vakil N. Cost effectiveness of new non-invasive testing methods for *Helicobacter pylori* in dyspeptic patients in Europe and the USA. Gut (Suppl. 3) 1999; 45:A125.

123. May IP, Slater JM, Holton J, Bloom SL. Detection of *Helicobacter pylori* volatile breath components using quartz crystal microbalances: the urea-less breath test. Gut (Suppl. 1) 1999; 44:A114.

124. Knight T, Wyatt J, Wilson A, Greaves S, Newell D, Hengels K, Corlett M, Webb P, Forman D, Elder J. *H. pylori* gastritis and serum pepsinogen levels in a healthy population: development of a biomarker strategy for gastric atrophy in high risk groups. Br J Cancer 1996; 73:819-824.

125. Aromaa A, Kosunen TU, Knekt P, Maatela J, Teppo L, Heinonen OP, Harkonen M, Hakama MK. Circulating anti-*Helicobacter pylori* immunoglobulin A antibodies and low serum pepsinogen I levels are associated with increased risk of gastric cancer. Am J Epidemiol 1996; 144:142-149.

126. de Boer WA, Tytgat GN. Treatment of *H. pylori* infection. BMJ 2000; 320:31-34.

127. Megraud F, Lehn N, Lind T, Bayerdorffer E, O'Morain C, Spiller R, Unge P, Veldhuyzen van Zanten S, Wrangstadh M, Burman CF. Antimicrobial susceptibility testing of *H. pylori* in a large multicenter trial: the MACH 2 study. Antimicrob Agents Chemother 1999; 43:2747-2752.

128. Oderda G, Para A, Ronchi B, Zavallone A, Marinello D, Vaira D, Bona G. A fast and easy to perform test for antibiotic susceptibility of *Helicobacter pylori*. Gut (Suppl. 3) 1999; 45:A97.

129. Versalovic J, Osato MS, Spakovsky K, Dore MP, Reddy R, Stone GG, Shortridge D, Flamm RK, Tanaka SK, Graham DY. Point mutations in the 23S rRNA gene of *Helicobacter pylori* associated with different levels of clarithromycin resistance. J Antimicrob Chemother 1997; 40:283-286.

130. van Doorn LJ, Debets-Ossenkopp YJ, Marais A, Sanna R, Megraud F, Kusters JG, Quint WGV. Rapid detection by PCR and reverse hybridization of mutations in the *Helicobacter pylori* 23S rRNA gene associated with macrolide resistance. Antimicrob Agents Chemother 1999; 43:1779-1782.

131. Szczebara F, Dhaenens L, Vincent P, Husson MO. Evaluation of rapid molecular methods for detection of clarithromycin resistance in *Helicobacter pylori*. Eur J Clin Microbiol Infect Dis 1997; 16:162-164.

132. Alarcon T, Domingo D, Prieto N, Lopez-Brea M. Polymerase chain reaction using 3' mismatched primers to detect mutation to clarithromycin in *Helicobacter pylori* clinical isolates. Gut (Suppl. 2)1998; 43:A9.

133. Maeda S, Yoshida H, Ogura K, Matsunaga H, Kawamata O, Shiratori Y, Omata M. Detection of *Helicobacter pylori* 23S rRNA gene mutation associated with clarithromycin resistance using preferential homoduplex formation assay. Gut (Suppl. 2) 1998; 43:A7.

21

Legionellosis

Janet E. Stout
Infectious Disease Division, Pittsburgh VA Healthcare System, University of Pittsburgh, Pittsburgh, Pennsylvania

John D. Rihs
Special Pathogens Laboratory, Department of Laboratory Medicine and Pathology, VA Medical Center, Pittsburgh, Pennsylvania

I. HISTORICAL BACKGROUND

Legionnaires' disease was first recognized as a clinical entity following an outbreak of pneumonia that occurred among delegates to the American Legion convention in Philadelphia in 1976 (1). A total of 182 persons contracted pneumonia and 34 died. More than six months would pass before investigators from the Centers for Disease Control and Prevention (CDC) would isolate a previously unidentified bacterium from autopsy lung specimens. The bacterium was ultimately named *Legionella pneumophila*. Sera stored in CDC freezers from unsolved outbreaks of pneumonia revealed antibody seroconversion to *L. pneumophila*, suggesting that this was not a new disease. Retrospectively identified epidemics of Legionnaires' disease included outbreaks that occurred at the same Philadelphia hotel during a convention in 1974, an outbreak at a psychiatric hospital in Washington, D.C., U.S.A. in 1965 (2), and another at a meat-packing plant in Minnesota in 1957 (3). One *Legionella* species was isolated from specimens that dated back to 1947 (4).

II. CLINICAL ASPECTS

Pontiac Fever and Legionnaires' disease (pneumonia) are two different forms of infections attributed to *Legionella* species. It is not known why there are two different forms, but the infectious dose of the organism, differing modes of transmission, and host factors may lead to the occurrence of these two disease entities.

Pontiac fever is an acute, self-limiting, flu-like illness without pneumonia which derived its name from an outbreak of the disease in Pontiac, Michigan in 1968 (5,6). The incubation period is 24-48 hours, and the attack rate of those exposed is generally 90% or higher. The predominant symptoms are malaise, myalgias, fever, chills, and headache. The chest x-ray remains clear. Complete recovery occurs within one week without antibiotic therapy. Pontiac fever has been attributed to exposure to several *Legionella* species; *L. pneumophila* serogroups 1, 6, and 7, *L. micdadei*, *L. feelei*, and *L. anisa*

(6-9). Diagnosis has been made by establishing seroconversion to the implicated strain. Pontiac Fever has been linked to aerosol exposure from evaporative condensers, cooling towers, air conditioners, and whirlpools. Simultaneous occurrence of both Pontiac Fever and Legionnaires' disease has been reported after exposure to a common source (7,9,10).

Unlike Pontiac Fever, the incubation period for Legionnaires' disease typically ranges from 2-10 days. Legionnaires' disease is essentially a pneumonia that is caused by *Legionella* spp. Legionnaires' disease should be suspected in a patient with pneumonia if: a) the Gram stain of respiratory secretions shows abundant neutrophils, and no typical organisms are seen, b) serum sodium is less than 130 mEq/ml., and c) the patient has failed to respond to beta-lactam and aminoglycoside antibiotics.

The disease usually begins with non-specific symptoms including fever, malaise, myalgia, anorexia, and headache. Symptoms range from a mild, slightly productive cough and mild fever to stupor with widespread pulmonary infiltrates and multisystem organ failure. Fever is almost always present and often exceeds 40°C. In one series, 19% of patients had temperatures in excess of 40.5°C (6). Sputum may be streaked with blood, but gross hemoptysis is uncommon. Chest pain, occasionally pleuritic, can be prominent, and when coupled with hemoptysis can be mistaken for a pulmonary embolus.

Gastrointestinal symptoms, especially diarrhea, occur in 25-50% of infections (11). It has been suggested that the combination of abdominal pain and loose stools and/or diarrhea is indicative of Legionnaires' disease in a patient with community-acquired pneumonia (12). Change in mental status is the most common neurological abnormality. Bradycardia relative to temperature elevation is seen most often among elderly patients with advanced pneumonia, and is probably overemphasized as a diagnostic finding for Legionnaires' disease (13).

Most importantly, clinical manifestations and laboratory abnormalities during pneumonia caused by *L. pneumophila* are non-specific compared to those that are seen with pneumonia caused by other organisms (14,15). Abnormalities in liver function tests, hypophosphatemia, hematuria, and hematological abnormalities do not occur significantly more frequently in Legionnaires' disease than in pneumonias of other etiology. Hyponatremia (serum sodium less than 130 mmol/L.) occurs significantly more often in Legionnaires' disease than in other types of pneumonia (14,16).

Extrapulmonary legionellosis is rare, but cases have been documented in immunosuppressed patients. These infections include cellulitis, sinusitis, perirectal abscess, pericarditis, pyelonephritis, peritonitis, pancreatitis, and endocarditis (17). Wound infections following cardiothoracic surgery have resulted from contamination of the wound by water that has been colonized with *Legionella*. *Legionella* prosthetic valve endocarditis has also been described in one hospital (18).

The majority of patients with Legionnaires' disease have abnormal chest radiographic findings on presentation. Respiratory symptoms and fever, however, may predate the visualization of the pulmonary infiltrate (19). The initial involvement is usually unilateral and often has lower lobe predominance, but can progress to more widespread consolidation over the next several days despite appropriate antibiotic therapy. Pleural effusions can be seen in one-third of patients and may occasionally precede the radiographic appearance of the infiltrate (11). Nodular infiltrates, cavitation, and abscess are not uncommon in the immunosuppressed host who is receiving corticosteroids (20,21). This radiological presentation has been confused with fungal pneumonia in immunocompromised patients (22). Cavitation may occur up to fourteen days after presentation and even after appropriate antibiotic therapy and apparent clinical response. Radiographic improvement usually lags behind clinical improvement, and complete clearing of the infiltrate can take as long as 1-4 months.

Unfortunately, the mortality rates for *Legionella* pneumonia are high: 20-30% for community-acquired cases and 30-50% for nosocomial cases (23,24). Inappropriate specific treatment or delay in appropriate antimicrobial therapy is related to poor outcome (25).

Patients with community-acquired Legionnaires' disease are significantly more likely to be admitted to an intensive care unit after presentation than patients with other types of pneumonia. Guidelines from the Infectious Disease Society of America recommend the use of antimicrobial agents that are active against *Legionella* for the empiric therapy of patients who require admission to the ICU. The specific recommendation includes erythromycin, azithromycin, or a fluoroquinolone plus cefotaxime, ceftriaxone, or a beta-lactam/beta-lactamase inhibitor combination (26).

III. EPIDEMIOLOGY OF INFECTION

Legionnaires' disease does not occur from direct person-to-person transmission. Water that contains the bacterium gains access to the respiratory tract either by inhalation of aerosols or aspiration after direct contact between contaminated water and the upper airway.

Legionella species are found in nearly undetectable numbers in natural bodies of water including surface water, rivers, lakes, and groundwater. L. pneumophila has been demonstrated in water from a wide-range of environmental conditions: temperature, 0-63°C; pH, 5.0-8.5; dissolved oxygen, 0.2-15.0 mg./L. (27).

Legionella are relatively chlorine-tolerant (28,29). This enables the organism to survive the water treatment process and to pass into water distribution systems, but again only in small numbers. Studies have shown that legionellae are present in all segments of community water supplies including water treatment facilities (30-33).

Man-made water systems provide Legionella with favorable growth conditions such as warm temperatures, symbiotic microorganisms, and nutrient rich biofilms. Aerosol-generating systems that have been linked to disease transmission include cooling towers, respiratory therapy equipment (humidifiers), and whirlpool spas (11). Water distribution systems that are colonized with Legionella are now recognized as the primary source for nosocomial infections and are a significant source for sporadic community-acquired cases (27,34,35). Acquisition of Legionnaires' disease has been linked to contamination of water supplies in residencies, rehabilitation centers, nursing homes, and industrial water reservoirs (34). In fact, there is growing evidence that Legionnaires' disease is a significant nosocomial pathogen in rehabilitation centres (J.E. Stout, unpublished data; 36).

Water distribution systems harbour symbiotic microorganisms including amoebae and commensal water bacteria that provide Legionella with the nutrients that are necessary for growth (37,38). L. pneumophila can infect and multiply within amoebae and ciliated protozoa (39). When the protozoan host ruptures, large numbers of motile Legionella are freed. It has been suggested that Legionella could be transmitted to humans via inhalation of these amoebic vesicles (40). Amoebic cysts may also contribute to its survival in unfavourable environmental conditions, e.g., in the presence of elevated chlorine levels.

Colonization of water distribution systems by L. pneumophila is dependent on a combination of several factors including water temperature, sediment accumulation, and commensal microflora (27). Temperature appears to be a particularly critical parameter. Hot water tanks with temperatures below 140°F were significantly more likely to be culture-positive for L. pneumophila (41,42). L. pneumophila is found in the biofilm that coats the inner surfaces of fixtures and pipes in water systems. Studies have shown that Legionella can form biofilms on a variety of materials including metallic piping surfaces (43,44). Biofilm-associated bacteria, including L. pneumophila, are presumably less sensitive to biocides than free-floating (planktonic) bacteria (43). This may explain the persistence of the organism even after disinfection attempts.

After multiplication in man-made water systems, Legionella can be transmitted to humans either by aerosolization, aspiration, or direct instillation into the lungs. The earliest evidence for transmission of Legionella via aerosolization came from the 1968 outbreak of Pontiac Fever in an office building (5). L. pneumophila was isolated from the lungs of guinea pigs that were exposed to the air at the facility.

Another study by CDC investigators convincingly demonstrated aerosol transmission in an outbreak at a Louisiana grocery store. The outbreak of Legionnaires' disease was linked to exposure with aerosols that were generated by an ultrasonic mist machine in the grocery store (45).

Although showers have often been cited as sources for aerosol dissemination of Legionella, simulation studies have shown that only small numbers of Legionella are aerosolized and then only for short distances (inches) (46,47). Epidemiological investigations have reported both positive and negative associations between showering and the acquisition of Legionnaire's disease (14,48-50).

Aspiration as a mode of transmission of Legionnaires' is now accepted as an alternate mode of transmission particularly in hospitalized patients. Surgical patients undergoing general anesthesia are a well-established risk group and have a high propensity for aspiration (51,52). Nasogastric tubes have been linked to nosocomial legionellosis in several studies; the presumed mode of entry was micro-aspiration of contaminated water (48,53-55).

The incidence of Legionnaires' disease not only depends on the degree of contamination of the aquatic reservoir, but also the susceptibility of the persons exposed to that water. The risk of developing Legionnaires' disease following exposure to a contaminated water source increases dramatically in persons of advanced age with chronic lung disease, hematologic malignancy, end-stage renal disease, and immunosuppression. Cigarette smoking is consistently identified as an important risk factor for this disease. Excess alcohol intake and renal failure have been noted in some studies. Surgery is a major predisposing factor in nosocomial infection with transplant recipients at highest risk (56,57).

This disease has also been diagnosed in children (58,59). The most common presentation is hospital-acquired pneumonia in neonates, immunosuppressed children, and children with underlying pulmonary disease. A few sporadic cases of community-acquired pneumonia in immunocompetent infants have been documented (60). Epidemiological investigations have consistently shown a link to the hospital water supply (61).

Legionella infection does occur in AIDS patients (62,63), but infections are rare. When they occur, they are often progressive with extrapulmonary manifestations including bacteremia and lung abscess (64).

Legionnaires' disease can be prevented with the eradication of the bacterium from its reservoir. Currently there are two approaches for the prevention of hospital-acquired legionellosis. Pittsburgh investigators recommend a proactive approach which begins with performing routine environmental cultures of the hospital water system (65). The results of environmental cultures are used to guide both clinical decision-making and the focus for laboratory testing. This approach was first advocated by the Allegheny County Health Department in Pittsburgh, Pennsylvania, who published the guide "Approaches to Prevention and Control of *Legionella* Infection in Allegheny County Health Care Facilities" in 1993 (66).

Alternatively, the CDC guidelines for "Prevention of Nosocomial Pneumonia" emphasize patient surveillance with a recommendation that environmental surveillance be performed only after cases are diagnosed. The main weakness of this strategy is that it relies on physicians to make the diagnosis of Legionnaires' disease among their patients. Unfortunately, numerous studies have documented that that Legionnaires' disease is often unrecognized and undiagnosed (67,68).

An extensive review of the various approaches for controlling *Legionella* in water systems has been published elsewhere (27). We have found copper-silver ionization to be the most effective method to date, and superior to thermal eradication and hyperchlorination (69,70).

IV. NATURE OF THE BACTERIUM, PATHOGENESIS, AND CLINICAL MANIFESTATIONS

Members of the *Legionellaceae* family are thin and faintly-staining Gram negative rods that require L-cysteine for growth on primary isolation. Fry et al. used 16S ribosomal RNA analysis to demonstrate that the family *Legionellaceae* is a single monophylogenetic subgroup within the gamma subdivision of the *Proteobacteria* (71). These organisms are aerobic non-spore-forming unencapsulated bacilli that measure 0.3 to 0.9 um. in width and 2-20 um. in length. The organisms are small coccobacilli that measure 1-2 um. when seen in tissue and clinical specimens. Elongated filamentous forms may be seen after growth on some culture media.

Legionella spp. are motile (except for *L. oakridgensis*), oxidase-negative or weakly positive, weakly catalase-positive, nitrite-negative, and urease-negative, and they liquefy gelatin. Carbohydrates are not fermented or oxidized. *L. pneumophila* and a few other *Legionella* species hydrolyze hippurate. Some members of the genus fluoresce blue-white, yellow-green, or red when exposed to long wave ultraviolet light. Reference laboratories can best identify these organisms to the species level using serological methods.

Currently, there are more than 42 species in the family *Legionellaceae*. Seven species can be further divided into serogroups with *L. pneumophila* alone accounting for 15 different serogroups (72). *L. pneumophila* is responsible for about 90% of the infections that are caused by members of *Legionellaceae*. Eighteen of the 42 species have been linked to human disease (73). *L. pneumophila* serogroups 1, 4, and 6, however, account for the overwhelming majority of strains that are implicated in human infection (24).

Techniques that are used to classify *Legionella* species include biochemical methods, fatty acid and ubiquinone analysis, molecular methods, and serological methods (72). Molecular methods can be used to identify *Legionella* to the species level based on hybridization studies or amplification of DNA or RNA (71,74). Subtyping of *L. pneumophila* with molecular fingerprinting methods have been useful for epidemiological investigations. Numerous molecular typing methods have been applied, but restriction enzyme analysis by PFGE has been the most widely used (75-77). For epidemiological investigations, a combination of phenotypic and genotypic methods may be necessary for maximal discrimination because some studies have suggested that the variability of the *L. pneumophila* genome is limited (78,79).

Most clinical laboratories presumptively identify *Legionella* species on the basis of colony morphology, staining characteristics, and the organism's dependence for L-cysteine. Colonies of *Legionella pneumophila* have an iridescent edge with a ground-glass internal morphology when grown on buffered charcoal-yeast extract agar (BCYE). It is for this reason that culture plates should be reviewed with the use of a dissecting microscope that has oblique lighting (Figure 1).

The organism can be visualized by Gram stain with some difficulty in clinical specimens; basic fuchsin serves as a better counterstain than safranin. The organism is more effectively visualized using the Gimenez stain which is as rapid as the Gram stain. Silver stains, including the Dieterle and Warthin-Starry stains, allow visualization of *Legionella* in paraffin-fixed tissues.

The organism is nutritionally fastidious and does not grow on standard bacteriological media. Charcoal-yeast extract agar that is buffered to pH 6.9 is the base medium that is used for isolation of these organisms. L-cysteine is a critical ingredient in culture, while keto-acids and ferric ions together stimulate growth. The activated charcoal can absorb and detoxify fatty acids and oxygen radicals as well as prevent the oxidation of cysteine (80). Addition of alpha-ketoglutaric acid promotes the growth of *Legionella* possibly by stimulating production of oxygen-scavenging enzymes (81).

Legionella produce a diffusable melanin-like brown pigment on media that contain tyrosine and a fluorescent yellow-green pigment on agar media when exposed to long-wave ultraviolet light (82). Ultrastructural features which are typical of Gram negative bacilli include: an inner trilaminar cytoplasmic membrane, a peptidoglycan layer, and an outer trilaminar membrane (83). A single polar flagellum and multiple fimbriae (pili) are present among most strains on primary isolation (84).

L. pneumophila contains a major outer membrane protein with a molecular weight of 24-29 kD. This protein forms ion-permeable channels in contact with lipid membranes as is characteristic for porins (85). The lipopolysaccharide of *L. pneumophila* serogroup 1 is tightly bound to this protein. Antibodies, as detected by indirect immunofluorescence, are directed primarily at the lipopolysaccharide (86).

Legionella enters the lung via inhalation of aerosols or via aspiration. After *Legionella* enters the upper respiratory tract, clearance is normally accomplished by intact pulmonary immunity and by cilia on respiratory epithelial cells. The consistent epidemiological association of increased risk of Legion-

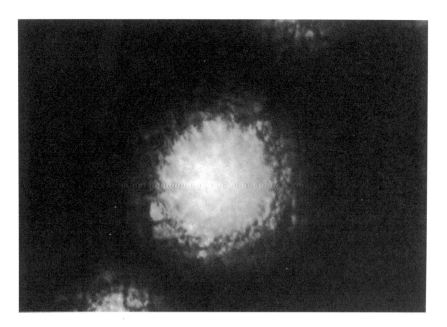

Figure 1   Colony of *Legionella pneumophila* as observed using a dissecting microscope. *Legionella* colonies have a distinctive ground glass morphology.

naires' disease among cigarette smokers, patients with chronic pulmonary diseases, and alcoholics suggests that aspiration and impaired mucociliary clearance increases the risk of infection. Virulent *Legionella* have been shown to be flagellated and to adhere to human respiratory epithelial cells via pili (84). A *Legionella* gene has homology to the type IV pilin genes that are found in other pathogenic bacteria, and mutation of this gene reduces adherence to respiratory tract epithelial cells in vitro (87). *Legionella* then enters and replicates within respiratory epithelial cells. Although it is well established that *Legionella* replicates within alveolar macrophages, alveolar epithelial cells may provide an alternate site for replication which contributes to the development of adult respiratory distress syndrome that is seen in many patients with Legionnaires' disease (87).

Alveolar macrophages readily phagocytose *Legionella*, although the process is more avid in the presence of specific opsonizing antibody (88). After entry, virulent *L. pneumophila* inhibits phagosome-lysosome fusion and acidification (89). The ribosome-studded phagosome allows *Legionella* to escape the normal degradative mechanisms of these organelles, and intracellular replication proceeds until the macrophage ruptures (89,90). The liberated bacteria are taken up by newly recruited cells, and the cycle of ingestion, multiplication, and liberation with cell lysis begins again.

Phagocytosis by human monocytes is mediated by complement receptors. The major outer membrane protein of *Legionella* fixes C3, and the alternate pathway of complement is activated (88). Polymorphonuclear (PMN) leukocytes ingest *Legionella* efficiently only in the presence of specific antibody or complement. Given that neutropenic patients do not have an undue predilection for Legionnaires disease, the role of the PMNs in host defense against *Legionella* is unclear. Although *L. pneumophila* is susceptible to oxygen-dependent microbicidal systems in vitro, *L. pneumophila* resists killing by polymorphonuclear leukocytes. Unlike monocytes, however, intracellular replication of the organism fails to occur within polymorphonuclear leukocytes. One possible role for neutrophils is the lysis of infected macrophages. *Legionella*-infected macrophages can become targets for lymphokine-activated killer cells and natural killer cells (88,91-93).

In both infected patients and animals, mononuclear cells respond to *L. pneumophila* antigens with proliferation and with the generation of monocyte-activating cytokines including gamma interferon, interleukin 1 and 2, and tumor necrosis factor (88,94,95). Natural killer-like cells triggered by interleukin 2 have been shown to kill mononuclear cells that are infected by *L. pneumophila*. Tumor necrosis factor-alpha (TNF) stimulates resistance of alveolar macrophages and neutrophils to *L. pneumophila* and mediates endogenous interleukin-12 and gamma interferon release (96). Depletion of TNF has been shown to decrease pulmonary host defense against *Legionella* (95). Gamma-interferon decreases the multiplication rate of *Legionella* by limiting the availability of iron to the organism. Interleukin-10 (IL-10) reverses the protective effects of gamma-interferon, thus enhancing growth of *Legionella* within human monocytes (97). As a result, *Legionella* may have a greater ability to replicate within newly recruited monocytes due to increased concentrations of IL-10 in the infected lung.

L. pneumophila strains clearly differ in virulence. For example, among the cases of Legionnaires' disease that are reported to the U.S. Centers for Disease Control and Prevention, the vast majority are caused by *L. pneumophila* (24). Although multiple strains of *L. pneumophila* may colonize water distribution systems, only a few strains are likely to cause disease in patients exposed to this water (103-105). A surface epitope of *L. pneumophila* serogroup 1 that is recognized by one particular antibody (Mab-2) may be associated with virulence. *L. pneumophila* serogroup 6 is more common in nosocomial strains and more likely to be associated with poor outcome. Agar-passaged strains which lose their virulence are more serum-sensitive, unable to multiply in monocytes or inhibit phagosome-lysosome fusion, and less able to kill guinea pigs (106). Virulence may be enhanced by replication within amoebae (107).

Several research groups have identified *Legionella* virulence factors by producing genetically-engineered mutants. Two types of mutants have been identified that have altered ability to replicate intracellularly or that affect trafficking of the phagosome. These genes are *mip* (for macrophage infectivity potentiator protein), *icm* (for intracellular multiplication), and *dot* (for defective organelle trafficking) (108).

Other putative virulence factors include exoproteases (zinc metallo-protease), hemolytic enzymes, and monoclonal antibody reactive epitopes (37,106,109-111). The organism produces a number of enzymes and potential toxins that can be detected in culture supernates or in lysates of intact bacteria including hemolysins, proteases, esterases, phosphatases, aminopeptidases, and endonucleases (110). The role of these products in pathogenesis and tissue damage is questionable since many of these products are produced by strains that are avirulent for experimental animals.

V. IMMUNOLOGY OF INFECTION

Humoral immunity appears to play a secondary role in host defense against *Legionella* (98). In vitro studies have shown that anti-*L. pneumophila* antibody in the presence of complement enhances uptake, but does not promote killing of *L. pneumophila* either by complement or by phagocytes (polymorphonuclear leukocytes, monocytes, or alveolar macrophages). Patients with Legionnaires' disease do produce type-specific anti-*Legionella* antibody usually with immunoglobulin M initially and then followed by immunogobulin G. Antibody titres are usually measurable within the first several weeks of infection. Moreover, immunized animals develop a specific antibody response with subsequent resistance to *Legionella* challenge (99,100). Serum antibodies appear to activate antibody-dependent cellular cytotoxicity in host cells (88). Diminished growth of *L. pneumophila* was observed in mice that were inoculated with opsonized bacteria. Decreased recovery may be due to complement-independent factors such as enhanced secretion of inflammatory mediators (96).

Legionnaires' disease is more common and more severe for patients with depressed cell-mediated immunity including transplant recipients, patients receiving corticosteroids, diabetics, and AIDS patients (24). Legionnaires' disease has frequently been noted among patients with hairy cell leukemia which is a malignancy that is associated with monocyte deficiency and dysfunction (101,102).

VI. LABORATORY DIAGNOSIS

Legionnaires' disease has been aptly described as underdiagnosed but over-treated (112). Although the CDC estimates that 18,000-25,000 cases of Legionnaires' disease occur annually in the United States, these figures well underestimate the true incidence of Legionnaires' disease. Cases of Legionnaires' disease go unrecognized because it is not clinically possible to distinguish between Legionnaires' disease and other causes of pneumonia, and because diagnostic tests for *Legionella* are not routinely ordered.

The tests that are currently available for establishing the diagnosis of Legionnaires' disease include culture of respiratory secretions, direct fluorescent antibody (DFA) staining, serum antibody testing, and *Legionella* urinary antigen testing. The reported sensitivity of these tests varies widely depending on the study. The sensitivities of culture, DFA, serology and the urinary antigen test have been reported to be 40-80%, 25-75%, 40-75%, and 70-90% respectively (11,113,114). These tests should be performed by experienced microbiologists in order to achieve optimal sensitivity and specificity. Many laboratories have inadequate experience with these tests, and thus often refer specimens to a reference laboratory. In fact, laboratories that do perform in-house *Legionella* diagnostic testing may not do it well. A College of American Pathologists survey of laboratories showed that only 32% of laboratories successfully identified a pure culture of *Legionella pneumophila* (113). Culture is the most sensitive diagnostic method. Optimal recovery of *Legionella* from culture is accomplished by using multiple selective media and acid-buffer pretreatment of sputum specimens, but for many smaller laboratories, this is often impractical.

A. Urinary antigen test

The urinary antigen test is a practical alternative to culture for the diagnosis of Legionnaires' disease due to *L. pneumophila* serogroup 1. In fact, reports from the CDC and others indicate that the introduction of the urinary antigen test into some hospital laboratories has resulted in the detection of unrecognized endemic nosocomial outbreaks of Legionnaires' disease (67,68). The urinary antigen test has several advantages over culture. For many patients with Legionnaires' disease, obtaining an adequate sputum specimen is difficult if not impossible. Urine, on the other hand, is easily obtained. The test format is an enzyme immunoassay (EIA) and is available commercially from two U.S. suppliers (Wampole Laboratories and Bartels). The results of the urinary antigen test can be available within hours, whereas culture results require 3-5 days (115). The disadvantage of the urinary antigen test is that it is specific for *L. pneumophila* serogroup 1 only. Since the majority of cases of Legionnaires' disease are caused by this species and serogroup, this limitation has not been considered a major disadvantage of the test.

The antigen of *L. pneumophila* serogroup 1 in urine is believed to be the lipopolysaccharide portion of the cell wall. Although the antibody used in the test has specificity for *L. pneumophila* serogroup 1, there have been reports of cross-reactivity to other serogroups of *L. pneumophila* (116). The antigen can be detected in a patient's urine even after antibiotic treatment has been initiated. In our experience, most patients will remain positive for *Legionella* urinary antigen for weeks, and on rare occasions even months. In our laboratory, among 66 culture-confirmed cases of Legionnaires' disease caused by *L. pneumophila* serogroup 1 the sensitivity of the urine antigen test was approximately 85% with a specificity of 100% (117).

A new rapid urinary antigen test has been made available that yields results in less than 15 minutes. This test is the Binax NOW *Legionella* Urinary Antigen Test (Binax). The test is an immunochromatographic membrane assay that is performed with a swab that has been dipped in urine and which is inserted into the card-type test device. The reaction is read as a presence or absence of a visually detectable pink to purple-colored line that results from the antigen-antibody reaction. A thorough review of the *Legionella* urinary antigen test can be found elsewhere (119).

B. Culture

Gram stain of normally sterile sites (transtracheal aspirate, lung biopsy, and pleural fluid) can occasionally raise suspicion for diagnosis, but the definitive method for diagnosis of *Legionella* infection is the isolation of organism from respiratory secretions.

Unlike most other respiratory pathogens, *Legionella* does not colonize the respiratory tract. Thus, even a single colony isolate will confirm the diagnosis of Legionnaires' disease. Appropriate specimens for culture include: expectorated sputum, tracheal suction, bronchial washings and biopsies, bronchoaveolar lavage fluid, pleural fluid, and lung tissue. We have found that with the routine use of selective media for sputum specimens, expectorated sputum, and bronchoscopy specimens can give a similar yield. The fact that bronchoscopy specimens may sometimes give the first clue to an outbreak of legionellosis is probably because culture is more likely to be performed for bronchoscopy specimens in most hospitals (57,119). Experience has shown that even poor quality sputum samples may reveal the organism (120). For that reason, laboratories should not reject samples for *Legionella* that do not pass classical sputum Gram stain criteria.

Specimens that are submitted for culture should be collected by usual methods and delivered to the laboratory as promptly as possible. If a delay in culturing is expected, samples should be refrigerated. As per standard laboratory practice, samples should be processed in a biological safety cabinet. Sputum and suctioned material can be plated directly onto the media using a sterile swab and then streaked for isolation. If the sample contains areas of purulence or blood, they should be selected and cultured. Clear body fluids and diluted bronchial specimens can be concentrated by centrifugation. After concentration, the sediment is resuspended before plating. Tissue samples are homogenized with the use of a small amount of sterile nutrient broth.

Heavily contaminated specimens may be overgrown with organisms like *Pseudomonas*, yeast, or antibiotic-resistant *Enterobacteriaceae*. When this occurs, it is unlikely that the isolation of *Legionella* will be successful. Recovery can be enhanced by acid-buffer pre-treatment of the specimen with a KCl-HCl buffer (pH 2.2) (121). This procedure may be completed at the time of initial culture, or the sample may be processed directly without decontamination, and the remaining sample can be refrigerated and saved. If the direct culture reveals bacterial overgrowth, the sample can be retrieved, decontaminated, and re-cultured. Decontamination includes the dilution of sample (1:5) with the acid buffer and subsequent vortexing. The sample should then be allowed to incubate at room temperature for four minutes. After the incubation period, the sample should be immediately cultured on selective and non-selective BCYE media.

The standard medium for *Legionella* isolation is buffered charcoal-yeast extract agar (BCYE) that is supplemented with polymyxin, anisomycin, vancomycin, and dyes; the antimicrobial agents prevent the overgrowth of *Legionella* by competing organisms, while the dyes impart a distinctive color to the *Legionella* organisms (119). For maximal sensitivity, we recommend the simultaneous use of three media: 1) BCYE, 2) BCYE with polymyxin, anisomycin, and cefamandole, and 3) BCYE with polymyxin, anisomycin, vancomycin, and dyes. All of these three media are commercially available.

If there is a pleural effusion, thoracentesis should be performed, and the fluid should be evaluated by DFA, culture, and the *Legionella* antigen assay that is used for urine (122). *Legionella* has also been isolated from pericardial fluid, peritoneal fluid, rectal abscess, and wounds.

Blood cultures may also be obtained, but they should not be used in place of respiratory cultures. When bacteremia occurs, it tends to be the final insult in the severely-ill patient (123). Patients often have succumbed to their disease by the time blood cultures have been determined as positive. Blood cultures for *Legionella* should be processed using blood lysis-centrifugation, and they should be plated directly to BCYE. Conventional blood culture bottles will not usually support the growth of *Legionella*. The bacteria will remain viable in both the aerobic and anaerobic bottles, but they will go undetected unless blind subcultures are made onto BCYE. To increase recovery, 0.5 ml. of the blood-broth mixture should be transferred and spread over entire plates (123).

The inoculated plates are incubated at 35-37°C in humidified room air, and they should be held for seven days. The plates should be examined using a stereoscopic microscope and then illuminated with a light source which is directed at a slight angle. Typical colonies are usually apparent in 3-4 days. Mature colonies are about 3-4 mm. in diameter, convex, circular, and have a frosted-glass internal appearance (Figure 1). Very young colonies have a speckled green, blue, or pinkish-purple iridescence. Older colonies will develop grayish-white centers with iridescence around the outer periphery. Suspicious colonies that reveal thin Gram negative rods on Gram stain should be tested to determine if L-cysteine is required for growth. This can be done easily by subculturing the isolates in parallel to 5% sheep blood agar and BCYE. Bacteria that grow on both media can be ruled out as *Legionella* spp. Isolates that grow on BCYE, but fail to grow on 5% sheep blood agar, and that have typical colony morphology and staining characteristics can presumptively be identified as *Legionella.*

C. Gram stain

Gram stains can be useful. Fluid or pus from a normally-sterile sites such as pleural fluid, blood, transtracheal aspirate, or lung can yield small, pleomorphic faintly-staining, Gram negative bacilli (64). In sputum, the organisms are poorly visualized and, if visible, cannot be differentiated from *Haemophilus influenzae* or oropharyngeal flora. A useful clinical clue is the presence of numerous leukocytes with few, if any, organisms seen. This type of Gram stain is similar to those that are seen with other types of "atypical" pneumonia including mycoplasma, chlamydia, and viral pneumonias.

D. Direct fluorescent antibody stain (DFA)

A major drawback to this rapid diagnostic test is the fact that the sensitivity is less than that of culture since positive results depend on the presence of large numbers of organisms in the specimen. The DFA is more likely to be positive when multilobar infiltrates are present on the chest roentgenogram (124). Cross-reactions to non-*Legionella* organisms occur rarely; false-positive DFA tests are usually due to laboratory technique or contaminated reagents rather than cross-reacting bacteria. Monoclonal antibody reagents are superior to polyclonal reagents in that background staining is improved, and the test is technically easier to perform. In addition, the monoclonal reagent will detect all serogroups of *L. pneumophila* (Genetic Systems). DFA reagents for the newer species and serogroups are not available commercially.

E. Antibody detection by serology

Indirect fluorescent antibody and enzyme-linked immunosorbent assays have been the most commonly-used methodologies. The CDC recommends that only IFA results for *L. pneumophila* serogroup 1 be used for diagnostic purposes due to insufficient information on the sensitivity and specificity of tests for other serogroups and species (113,125). Diagnosis is made on a four-fold rise in antibody titre to 1:128; thus, both acute and convalescent sera are needed because 4-12 weeks is often required to detect an antibody response (117). Some patients' sera never demonstrate a four-fold increase in titre. Taken together, these facts show that the utility of serology as a diagnostic tool is quite poor. Serology is useful in epidemiological studies, but it is less helpful to the clinician in making an immediate diagnosis of Legionnaires' disease for an individual patient. On the other hand, if the seroprevalence of *L. pneumophila* antibody titres within the community is known to be low, a single elevated titre (1:256) may indicate the presence of acute disease. Some 25-40% of patients may have elevated titres in the first week of disease (126). False-positive results can rarely occur as a result of cross-reacting antibody to other Gram negative organisms. The use of IgM and IgG assays gives maximal sensitivity, although IgM antibodies are significantly more likely to be elevated during the disease phase. Finally, a single elevated titre does not confirm a case of Legionnaires' disease because IFA titres of $\geq$1:256 have been found in 1-16% of healthy adults (125).

F. Polymerase chain reaction (PCR)

DNA amplification of *Legionella* by PCR has been reported from patients with pneumonia using throat swab specimens, bronchoalveolar lavage (BAL), urine, and serum (127-129). Primer sequences of the macrophage infectivity potentiator (*mip*) gene of *L. pneumophila* and the 5S rRNA have been utilized in PCR assays. Clinical experience has not shown that PCR is more sensitive than culture, and therefore, the CDC does not recommend the routine use of genetic probes or PCR for detection of *Legionella* in clinical samples (125). A PCR kit has been used successfully to detect *Legionella* in both clinical and environmental samples, but it is not commercially available (130,131).

VII. SUSCEPTIBILITY TESTING

Legionella is an intracellular pathogen, and antibiotics which achieve high intracellular/tissue concentrations are more efficacious in humans than those agents that have poor intracellular penetration (132,133). Therefore, intracellular systems using cell culture models or animal models are the most valid systems for the in vitro evaluation of antimicrobial efficacy. These models confirm that the macrolides, quinolones, rifampin, trimethoprim-sulfamethoxazole, and tetracyclines are effective agents in vivo against *Legionella*. Penetration of the aforementioned antibiotics into phagocytic cells is the presumed basis for their clinical superiority over beta-lactam and aminoglycoside agents.

Broth dilution susceptibility testing with buffered yeast extract broth is the most frequently-used method for *Legionella* susceptibility testing (Table 1) (134,135). Agar dilution with BCYE agar is also used to evaluate comparative susceptibility, but it should be noted that quinolone agents are significantly inhibited by the presence of charcoal in the agar media.

Clinical studies of antibiotic efficacy in the treatment of Legionnaires' disease are rare and have largely been case studies and retrospective analyses. When the diagnosis was made by isolation of *Legionella* from culture rather than by serological methods, the data which supports efficacy has been more convincing. Antibiotics that have fulfilled this criterion include azithromycin, ciprofloxacin, levofloxacin, rifampin, trimethoprim-sulfamethoxazole, and tetracycline (136,137). In a study of 625 episodes of community-acquired pneumonia, 500 mg. daily of levofloxacin resulted in clinical improvement or cure in 92% of the 26 patients with a diagnosis of Legionnaires' disease (138).

Erythromycin has been the standard therapy for Legionnaires' disease, but it has a higher frequency of adverse effects when compared to the newer macrolides. These include ototoxicity, gastrointestinal symptoms, and thrombophlebitis at the intravenous site. In elderly patients with heart and lung disease, the large fluid volume that is required for erythromycin administration is especially problematic.

As a result, the newer macrolides (especially azithromycin) and the quinolones (especially ciprofloxacin and levofloxacin) are now the antibiotics of choice for Legionnaires' disease (132,133). Antimicrobial agents that are currently licensed by the FDA for the treatment of Legionnaires' disease include azithromycin (intravenous), levofloxacin, trovafloxacin, erythromycin, and dirithromycin.

Table 1   Susceptibility of *Legionella pneumophila* to antimicrobial agents by a broth dilution method. Some MIC values represent the means of the MICs for several strains.

Antimicrobial	MIC_{50} (mg./L.)	MIC_{90} (mg./L.)	MIC range (mg./L.)
Azithromycin	0.06-1.39	1.65-2.77	0.12-7.80
Clarithromycin	0.007	0.008-0.013	<0.001-0.125
Dirithromycin	-	-	0.50-8.0
Roxithromycin	0.0625	-	0.06-0.25
Ciprofloxacin	0.016	0.032	0.008-0.032
Levofloxacin	-	-	0.015-0.06
Ofloxacin	0.0157	-	0.015-0.06
Sparfloxacin	≤0.003	-	-
Piperacillin	0.25	-	-
Imipenem	0.0157	-	-
Rifampicin	<0.001	<0.001	≤0.001-0.062
Doxycycline	1.76-2.48	3.65-4.95	0.24-31.25
Minocycline	0.03	-	-

(Source: references 134,135,137)

REFERENCES

1. Fraser DW, Tsai T, Orenstein W, Parkin WE, Beecham HJ, Sharrar RG, Harris J, Mallison GF, Martin SM, McDade JE, Shepard CC, Brachman PS. Legionnaires' disease: description of an epidemic of pneumonia. N Engl J Med 1977; 297:1189-1197.
2. Thacker SB, Bennet JV, Tsai T. An outbreak in 1975 of severe respiratory illness caused by Legionnaires' disease bacteriium. J Infect Dis 1978; 238:512-519.
3. Osterholm MT, Chin TD, Osborne DO, Dull HB, Dean AG, Fraser DW, Hayes PS, Hall WN. A 1957 outbreak of Legionnaires' disease associated with a meat packing plant. Amer J Epidemiol 1983; 117:60-67.
4. McDade JE, Brenner DJ, Bozeman FM. Legionnaires' disease bacterium isolated in 1947. Ann Intern Med 1979; 90:659-661.
5. Glick TH, Gregg MB, Berman B, Mallison G, Rhodes WW, Kassanoff I. Pontiac fever. An epidemic of unknown etiology in a health department. I. Clinical and epidemiologic aspects. Amer J Epidemiol 1978; 107:149-160.
6. Vergis EN, Yu VL. Legionellosis. In: Fishman AP, ed. Fishman's Pulmonary Diseases and Disorders. New York:McGraw-Hill, 1998:2235-2296.
7. Luttichau HR, Vinther C, Uldum SA, Moller J, Faber M, Jensen JS. An outbreak of Pontiac fever among children following use of a whirlpool. Clin Infect Dis 1998; 26:1374-1378.
8. Fallon RJ, Rowbotham TJ. Microbiological investigations into an outbreak of Pontiac fever due to *Legionella micdadei* associated with use of a whirlpool spa. J Clin Pathol 1990; 43:479-483.

9. Thomas DL, Mundy LM, Tucker PC. Hot tub legionellosis: Legionnaires' disease and Pontiac fever after a point-source exposure to *Legionella pneumophila*. Arch Intern Med 1993; 153:2597-2599.

10. Ackelsberg J, LoHff C, Kondracki S, Hennessey, MD, Wong S, Schoonmaker-Bopp D, Zaki S, Fields BS, Torok T, Wallace B. Large simultaneous outbreaks of Legionnaires' disease and Pontiac Fever: need for improved hospital cooling tower standards. 37th Annual Meeting of the Infectious Disease Society of America, 1999: Abstract 559.

11. Stout JE, Yu VL. Current concepts: Legionellosis. N Engl J Med 1997; 337:682-687.

12. Cunha BA. Clinical features of Legionnaires' disease. Semin Resp Infect 1998; 13:116-127.

13. Fang GD, Fine M, Orloff J, Arisumi D, Yu VL, Kapoor W, Grayston JT, Wang SP, Kohler R, Muder RR, Yee YC, Rihs JD, Vickers RM. New and emerging etiologies for community-acquired pneumonia with implications for therapy: a prospective multicenter study of 359 cases. Medicine 1990; 69:307-316.

14. Yu VL, Kroboth FJ, Shonnard J, Brown A, McDearman S, Magnussen MH. Legionnaires' disease: New clinical perspective from a prospective pneumonia study. Amer J Med 1982; 73:357-361.

15. Sopena N, Sabria-Leal M, Pedro-Botet ML, Padilla E, Dominguez J, Morera J, Tudela P. Comparative study of the clinical presentation of *Legionella* pneumonia and other community-acquired pneumonias. Chest 1998; 113:1195-1200.

16. Miller AC. Hyponatremia in Legionnaires' disease. BMJ 1982; 284:558-559.

17. Lowry PW, Tompkins LS. Nosocomial legionellosis: a review of pulmonary and extrapulmonary syndromes. Am J Infect Cont 1993; 21:21-27.

18. Tompkins LS, Roessler BJ, Redd SC, Markowitz LE, Coehn ML. *Legionella* prosthetic-valve endocarditis. N Engl J Med 1988; 318:530-535.

19. Muder RR, Reddy S, Yu VL, Kroboth FJ. Pneumonia caused by Pittsburgh pneumonia agent: radiologic manifestations. Radiology 1984; 150:633-637.

20. Ebright JR, Tarakji E, Brown WJ, Sunstrum J. Multiple bilateral lung cavities caused by *Legionella pneumophila*: case report and review. Infect Dis Clin Pract 1993; 2:195-199.

21. Muder RR, Yu VL, Parry M. Radiology of *Legionella* pneumonia. Semin Resp Infect 1987; 2:242-254.

22. Harrington RD, Woolfrey AE, Bowden R, McDowell MG, Hackman RC. Legionellosis in a bone marrow transplant center. Clin Infect Dis 1996; 18:361-368.

23. Carratala J, Gudiol F, Pallares R, Verdaguer R, Ariza J, Manresa F. Risk factors for nosocomial *Legionella pneumophila* pneumonia. Am J Respir Crit Care Med 1994; 149:625-629.

24. Marston BJ, Lipman HB, Breiman RF. Surveillance for Legionnaires' disease. Risk factors for morbidity and mortality. Arch Intern Med 1994; 154:2417-2422.

25. el-Ebiary M, Sarmiento X, Torres A, Nogue S, Mesalles E, Bodi M, Almirall J. Prognostic factors of severe *Legionella* pneumonia requiring admission to ICU. Am J Crit Care Med 1997; 156:1467-1472.

26. Bartlett JG, Breiman RF, Mandell LA, File TM, Jr. Community-acquired pneumonia in adults: guidelines for management. Clin Infect Dis 1998; 26:811-838.

27. Lin YE, Vidic RD, Stout JE, Yu VL. *Legionella* in water distribution systems. J Amer Water Works Assoc 1998; 90:112-121.

28. Kuchta JM, States SJ, McNamara AM. Susceptibility of *Legionella pneumophila* to chlorine in tap water. Appl Environ Microbiol 1983; 46:1134-1139.

29. Kuchta JM, States SJ, McGlaughlin, Overmeyer JH, Wadowsky RM, McNamara AM, Wolford RS, Yee RB. Enhanced chlorine resistance of tap water-adapted *Legionella pneumophila* as compared with agar medium-passaged strains. J Appl Microbiol 1985; 50:21-26.

30. Colbourne JS, Dennis PJ, Trew R, Berry C, Vesey G. *Legionella* and public water supplies. Water Sci Tech 1988; 20:5-10.

31. Colbourne JS, Dennis PJ. The ecology and survival of *Legionella pneumophila*. Thames Water Authority Journal of the Institution of Water and Environmental Management 1989; 3:345-350.

32. Voss L, Button K, Lorenz RC, Tuovinen O. *Legionella* contamination of a pre-operational treatment plant. J Amer Water Works Assoc 1986; 78:70-75.

33. States SJ, Conley L, Kuchta JM, Oleck BM, Lipovich MJ, Wolford RS, Wadowsky RM, McNamara AM, Sykora JL, Keleti G, Yee RB. Survival and multiplication of *Legionella pneumophila* in municipal drinking water systems. Appl Environ Microbiol 1987; 53:979-986.

34. Stout JE, Yu VL, Muraca P, Joly J, Troup N, Tompkins LS. Potable water as the cause of sporadic cases of community-acquired Legionnaires' disease. N Engl J Med 1992; 326:151-154.

35. Straus WL, Plouffe JF, File TM, Lipman HB, Hackman BH, Salstrom SJ, Benson RF, Breiman RF. Risk factors for domestic acquisition of Legionnaires' disease. Arch Intern Med 1996; 156:1685-1692.

36. Nechwatal R, Ehret W, Klatte OJ, Zeissler HJ, Prull A, Lutz H. Nosocomial outbreak of legionellosis in a rehabilitation center. Demonstration of potable water as a source. Infection 1993; 21:235-240.

37. Shuman HA, Purcell M, Segal G, Hales L, Wiater LA. Intracellular multiplication of *Legionella pneumophila*: human pathogen or accidental tourist? Curr Top Microbiol Immunol 1998; 225:99-112.

38. Barker J, Brown MRW. Trojan horses of the microbial world: protozoa and the survival of bacterial pathogens in the environment. Microbiol 1994; 140:1253-1259.

39. Fields BS. *Legionella* and protozoa: interaction of a pathogen and its natural host. In: Barbaree JM, Breiman RF, Dufour AP, eds. *Legionella*: Current Status and Emerging Perspectives. Washington, DC:American Society for Microbiology, 1993:129-136.

40. Rowbotham TJ. Current views on the relationships between amoebae, legionellae, and man. Isr J Med Sci 1986; 22:678-689.

41. Vickers RM, Yu VL, Hanna SS, Muraca P, Diven W, Carmen N, Taylor FB. Determinants of *Legionella pneumophila* contamination of water distribution systems: 15 hospital prospective study. Infect Cont 1987; 8:357-363.

42. Plouffe JF, Webster LR, Hackman B. Relationship between colonization of hospital buildings with *Legionella pneumophila* and hot water temperatures. Appl Environ Microbiol 1983; 46:769-770.

43. Wright JB, Ruseska I, Athar M, Corbett S, Costerton JW. *Legionella pneumophila* grows adherent to surfaces in vitro and in situ. Infect Control Hosp Epidemiol 1989; 10:408-415.

44. Rogers J, Doowsett AB, Dennis PJ, Lee JV, Keevil CW. Influence of plumbing materials on biofilm formation and growth of *Legionella pneumophila* in potable water systems. Appl Environ Microbiol 1994; 60:1842-1851.

45. Mahoney FJ, Hoge CW, Farley TA, Barbaree JM, Breiman RF, Benson RF, McFarland LM. Community-wide outbreak of Legionnaires' disease associated with a grocery store mist machine. J Infect Dis 1992; 165:736-739.

46. Bollin GE, Plouffe JF, Para MF, Hackman B. *Legionella pneumophila* generated by shower heads and hot water faucets. Appl Environ Microbiol 1986; 50:1128-1131.

47. Woo AH, Yu VL, Goetz A. Potential in-hospital mode of transmission for *Legionella pneumophila*: demonstration experiments for dissemination by showers, humidifiers, and rinsing of ventilation bag apparatus. Amer J Med 1986; 80:567-573.

48. Blatt SP, Parkinson MD, Pace E, Hoffman P, Dolan D, Lauderdale P, Zajac RA, Melcher GP. Nosocomial Legionnaires' disease: aspiration as a primary mode of transmission. Am J Med 1993; 95:16-22.

49. Breiman R, Fields B, Sanden G, Volmer L, Meier A, Spika JS. Association of shower use with Legionnaires' disease: possible role of amoebae. JAMA 1990; 263:2924-2926.

50. Hanrahan JP, Morse D, Scharf V, Debbie JG, Schmidt GP, McKinney RM, Shayegani M. Community hospital legionellosis outbreak linked to hot water showers. In: Thornsberry C, Balows A, Feeley JC, Jakubowski W, eds. *Legionella* - Proceedings of the 2nd International Symposium. Washington, DC:American Society for Microbiology, 1984:224-225.

51. Johnson JT, Yu VL, Best M, Vickers RM, Goetz A, Wagner R, Wicker H, Woo A. Nosocomial legionellosis uncovered in surgical patients with head and neck cancer: implications for epidemiologic reservoir and mode of transmission. Lancet 1985; 2:298-300.

52. Korvick J, Yu VL. Legionnaires' disease: an emerging surgical problem. Ann Thor Surg 1987; 43:341-347.

53. Loeb M, Simor AE, Mandell L, Krueger P, McArthur M, James M, Walter S, Richardson E, Lingley M, Stout J, Stronach D, McGeer A. Two nursing home outbreaks of respiratory infections with *Legionella sainthelensi*. J Am Geriatric Soc 1999; 47:547-552.

54. Marrie TJ, Haldane D, Macdonald S. Control of endemic nosocomial Legionnaires' disease by using sterile potable water for high risk patients. Epidemiol Infect 1991; 107:591-605.

55. Venezia RA, Agresta MD, Hanley EM, Urquhart K, Schoonmaker D. Nosocomial legionellosis associated with aspiration of nasogastric feedings diluted in tap water. Infect Control Hosp Epidemiol 1994; 15:529-533.

56. Chow J, Yu VL. *Legionella*: a major opportunistic pathogen in transplant recipients. Sem Resp Infect 1998; 13:132-139.

57. Knirsch CA, Jakob K, Schoonmaker D, Kiehlbauch JA, Wong SJ, Della-latta P, Whittier S, Layton M, Scully B. An outbreak of *Legionella micdadei* pneumonia in transplant patients: education, molecular epidemiology, and control. Am J Med 2000; 108:290-295.

58. Green M, Wald ER, Dashefsky B, Barbadora K, Wadowsky RM. Field inversion gel electrophoretic analysis of *Legionella pneumophila* strains associated with nosocomial legionellosis in children. J Clin Microbiol 1996; 34:175-176.

59. Carlson NC, Kuskie MR, Dobyns EL, Wheeler MD, Roe MIT, Abzug MJ. Legionellosis in children: an expanding spectrum. Infect Dis J 1990; 9:133-137.
60. Famiglietti RF, Bakerman PR, Saubolle MD, Rudinsky M. Cavitary legionellosis in two immunocompetent infants. Peds 1997; 99:899-903.
61. Luck PC, Dinger D, Helbig JH, Thurm V, Keuchel H, Presch C, Ott M. Analysis of *Legionella pneumophila* strains associated with nosocomial pneumonia in a neonatal intensive care unit. Eur J Clin Microbiol Infect Dis 1994; 13:565-571.
62. Morley JN, Crocker Smith L, Baltch AL, Smith RP. Recurrent infection due to *Legionella pneumophila* in a patient with AIDS. Clin Infect Dis 1994; 19:1130-1132.
63. Bangsborg JM, Jensen BN, Friis-Moller A, Bruun B. Legionellosis in patients with HIV infection. Infection 1990; 18:342-346.
64. Babe KS, Reinhardt JF. Diagnosis of *Legionella* sepsis by examination of a peripheral blood smear. Clin Infect Dis 1994; 19:1164-1165.
65. Yu VL. Resolving the controversy on environmental cultures for *Legionella*. Infect Cont Hosp Epid 1998; 19:893-897.
66. Allegheny County Health Department. Approaches to Prevention and Control of Legionella Infection in Allegheny County Health Care Facilities (Second Edition). Allegheny County Health Department 1997; Pittsburgh, PA:1-15.
67. Lepine LA, Jernigan DB, Butler JC, Pruckler JM, Benson RF, Kim G, Hadler JL, Cartter ML, Fields BS. A recurrent outbreak of nosocomial Legionnaire's disease detected by urinary antigen testing: evidence for long-term colonization of a hospital plumbing system. Infect Control Hosp Epidemiol 1998; 19:905-910.
68. Kool JL, Fiore AE, Kioski CM, Brown EW, Benson RF, Pruckler JM, Glasby C, Butler JC, Cage GD, Carpenter JC, Mandel RM, England B, Breiman RF. More than ten years of unrecognized nosocomial transmission of Legionnaires' disease among transplant patients. Infect Control Hosp Epidemiol 1998; 19:898-904.
69. Stout JE, Lin YSE, Goetz AM, Muder RR. Controlling *Legionella* in hospital water systems: experience with the superheat-and-flush method and copper-silver ionization. Infect Control Hosp Epidemiol 1998; 19:911-914.
70. Mietzner S, Schwille RC, Farley A, Wald ER, Ge JH, States SJ, Libert T, Wadowsky RM. Efficacy of thermal treatment and copper-silver ionization for controlling *Legionella pneumophila* in high-volume hot water. Am J Infect Cont 1997; 25:452-457.
71. Fry N K, Warwick S, Saunders NA, Embley TM. The use of 16S ribosomal RNA analysis to investigate the phylogeny of the family *Legionellaceae*. J Gen Microbiol 1991; 137:1215-1222.
72. Benson RF, Fields BS. Classification of the genus *Legionella*. Semin Resp Infect 1998; 13:90-99.
73. Lo Presti F, Riffard S, Vandenesch F, Reyrolle M, Ronco E, Ishai P, Etienne J. The first clinical isolate of *Legionella parisiensis*. J Clin Microbiol 1997; 35:1706-1709.
74. Bangsborg JM, Gerner-Smidt P, Colding H, Fiehn NE, Brunn B, Hoiby N. Restriction fragment length polymorphism of rRNA genes for molecular typing of members of the family *Legionellaceae*. J Clin Micro 1995; 33:402-406.
75. Saunders NA, Harrison TG, Haththotuwa A, Kachwalla N, Taylor AG. A method for typing strains of *Legionella pneumophila* serogroup 1 by analysis of restriction fragment length polymorphisms. J Med Microbiol 1990; 31:45-55.
76. Pruckler JM, Mermel LA, Benson RF. Comparison of *Legionella pneumophila* isolates by arbitrarily primed PCR and pulsed-field gel electrophoresis: Analysis from seven epidemic investigations. J Clin Microbiol 1995; 33:2872-2875.
77. Lawrence C, Ronco E, Dubrou S, Leclero R, Nauciel C, Matsiota-Bernard P. Molecular typing of *L. pneumophila* serogroup 1 isolates from patients and the nosocomial environment by arbitrarily primed PCR and pulsed-field gel electrophoresis. J Med Microbiol 1999; 48:327-333.
78. Struelens MJ, Maes N, Rost F, Deplano A, Jacobs F, Liesnard C, Bornstein N, Grimont F, Lauwers S, McIntyre MP, Serruys E. Genotypic and phenotypic methods for the investigation of a hospital-acquired *Legionella pneumophila* outbreak and efficacy of control measures. J Infect Dis 1992; 166:22-30.
79. Drenning S, Stout JE. Analysis of pulsed-field gel electrophoresis (PFGE) patterns of clinical isolates of *Legionella pneumophila* serogroup 1: similarity breeds contempt. Interscience Conference on Antimicrobial Agents and Chemotherapy 1997; Abstract #K-10.
80. Hoffman PS, Pine L, Bell S. Production of superoxide and hydrogen peroxide in medium used to culture *L. pneumophila*: catalytic composition by charcoal. Appl Environ Microbiol 1983; 45:784-791.

81. Pine L, Hoffman PS, Malcolm GB, Benson RF, Franzus MJ. Role of keto acids and reduced oxygen-scavenging enzymes in the growth of *Legionella* species. J Clin Microbiol 1986; 23:33-42.
82. Vickers RM, Yu VL. Clinical laboratory differentiation of *Legionellaceae* family members with pigment production and fluorescence on media supplemented with aromatic substrates. J Clin Microbiol 1984; 19:583-587.
83. Hebert GA, Callaway C, Ewing EP. Comparison of *Legionella pneumophila*, *L. micdadei*, *L. bozemanii*, and *L.. dumoffi* by transmission electron microscopy. J Clin Microbiol 1984; 19:116-121.
84. Bosshardt SC, Benson RF, Fields BS. Flagella are a positive predictor for virulence in *Legionella*. Microbiol Pathogenesis 1997; 23:107-112.
85. Gabay J, Blake M, Niles WD, Horwitz MA. Purification of *Legionella pneumophila* major outer membrane protein and demonstration that it is a porin. J Bacteriol 1985; 162:85-91.
86. Ciesielski CA, Blaser MJ, Wang WLL. Serogroup specificity of *Legionella pneumophila* is related to lipopolysaccharide characteristics. Infect Immun 1986; 51:397-404.
87. Stone BJ, Kwaik YA. Expression of multiple pili by *Legionella pneumophila*: identification and characterization of a type IV pilin gene and its role in adherence to mammalian and protozoan cells. Infect Immun 1998; 66:1768-1775.
88. Friedman H, Yamamoto Y, Newton C, Klein T. Immunologic response and pathophysiology of *Legionella* infection. Semin Resp Infect 1998; 13:100-108.
89. Horwitz MA. Toward an understanding of host and bacterial molecules mediating *L. pneumophila* pathogenesis. In: Barbaree JM, Breiman RF, Dufour AP, eds. *Legionella*: Current Status and Emerging Perspectives. Washington, DC:American Society for Microbiology, 1993:55-62.
90. Vogel JP, Andrews HL, Wong SK, Isberg RR. Conjugative transfer by the virulence system of *Legionella pneumophila*. Science 1998; 279:873.
91. Blanchard DI, Friedman H, Klein TW, Djeu JY. Induction of interferon-gamma and tumor necrosis factor by *Legionella pneumophila* - augmentation of human neutrophil bactericidal activity. J Leukocyte Biol 1989; 45:538-545.
92. Blanchard DK, Stewart WE, Klein TW. Cytolytic activity of human peripheral blood leukocytes against *Legionella pneumophila* - infected monocytes: characaterization of effector. J Immunol 1987; 139:551-556.
93. Blanchard DK, Friedman H, Stewart WE, Klein TW, Djeu JY. Role of gamma interferon in induction of natural killer activity by *Legionella pneumophila* in vitro an in an experiment murine infection model. Infect Immun 1988; 56:1187-1193.
94. Skerrett SJ, Martin TR. Tumor necrosis factor and lipopolysaccharide potentiate gamma interferon-induced resistance of alveolar macrophages to *Legionella pneumophila*. In: Barbaree JM, Brieman RF, Dufour AP, eds. *Legionella*: Current Status and Emerging Perspectives. Washington, DC:American Society for Microbiology, 1993:105-106.
95. Skerrett SJ, Bagby GJ, Schmidt RA, Nelson S. Antibody-mediated depletion of tumor necrosis factor-alpha impairs pulmonary host defenses to *Legionella pneumophila*. J Infect Dis 1997; 176:1019-1028.
96. Brieland JK, Remick DG, LeGendre ML, Engleberg NC, Fantone JC. In vivo regulation of replicative *Legionella pneumophila* lung infection by endogenous interleukin-12. Infect Immun 1998; 66:65-69.
97. Park DR, Skerrett SJ. IL-10 enhances the growth of *Legionella pneumophila* in human mononuclear phagocytes and reverses to protective effect of IFN-γ. J Immunol 1996; 157:2528-2538.
98. Brieland JK, Heath LA, Huffnagle GB, Remick DG, McClain MS, Hurley MC, Kunkel RK, Fantone JC, Engleberg C. Humoral immunity and regulation of intrapulmonary growth of *Legionella pneumophila* in the immunocompetent host. J Immunol 1996; 157:5002-5008.
99. Breiman RF, Horwitz MA. Guinea pigs sublethally infected with aerosolized *Legionella pneumophila* develop humoral and all-mediated immune responses. J Exp Med 1987; 164:799-811.
100. Yoshido S, Groto Y, Mizuguchi Y, Skamene E. Genetic control of natural resistance in mouse macrophages regulating replication in vitro. Infect Immun 1991; 59:428-423.
101. Cordonnier C, Farcet JP, Desforges L. Legionnaires' disease and hairy-cell leukemia. Arch Int Med 1984; 144:2373-2375.
102. Korvick J, Yu VL. Simultaneous infection with *Cryptococcus neoformans* and *Legionella pneumophila*: in vivo expression of common defects in immunity. Respiration 1988; 53:132-136.
103. Dournon E, Bibb WF, Rajagopalan P, Desplaces N, McKinney RM. Monoclonal antibody reactivity as a virulence marker for *Legionella pneumophila* serogroup 1 strains. J Infect Dis 1988; 157:496-501.
104. Stout JE, Joly J, Para M, Plouffe J, Ciesielski C, Blaser MJ, Yu VL. Comparison of molecular methods for subtyping patients and epidemiologically-linked environmental isolates of *L. pneumophila*. J Infect Dis 1988; 157:486-495.

105. Bollin GE, Plouffe JE, Para MF. Difference in virulence of environmental isolates of *Legionella pneumophila*. J Clin Microbiol 1985; 21:674-677.

106. Dowling JN, Saha AK, Glew RH. Virulence factors of the family *Legionellaceae*. Microbiol Rev 1992; 56:32-60.

107. Cirillo JD, Falkow S, Tompkins LS. *Legionella pneumophila* in *Acanthamoeba castellani* enhances invasion. Infect Immun 1994; 62:3254-3261.

108. Roy CR. Trafficking of the *Legionella pneumophila* phagosome. ASM News 1999; 65:416-421.

109. Shuman HA, Horwitz MA. *Legionella pneumophila* invasion of mononuclear phagocyte. Curr Top Microbiol Immunol 1996; 209:99-112.

110. Hacker J, Ott M, Wintermeyer E, Ludwig B, Fischer G. Analysis of virulence factors of *Legionella pneumophila*. Zbl Bakteriol 1993; 278:348-358.

111. Quinn FD, Keen MG, Tompkins LS. Genetic, immunological, and cytotoxic comparisons of *Legionella* proteolytic activities. Infect Immun 1989; 57:2719-2725.

112. Bartlett JG. Legionnaires' disease: overtreated, underdiagnosed. J Crit Illness 1993; 8:755-768.

113. Edelstein PH. Legionnaires' disease. Clin Infect Dis 1993; 16:741-749.

114. Kashuba ADM, Ballow CH. *Legionella* urinary antigen testing: potential impact on diagnosis and antibiotic therapy. Diagn Microbiol Infect Dis 1996; 24:129-139.

115. Kazandjian D, Chiew R, Gilbert GL. Rapid diagnosis of *Legionella pneumophila* serogroup 1 infection with the Binax enzyme immunoassay urinary antigen test. J Clin Microbiol 1997; 35:954-956.

116. Chang FY, Jacobs SL, Colodny SM, Stout JE, Yu VL. Nosocomial Legionnaires' disease caused by *Legionella pneumophila* serogroup 5: laboratory and epidemiological infection. J Infect Dis 1996; 174:1116-1119.

117. Vickers RM, Yee YC, Rihs JD, Wagener MM, Yu VL. Prospective assessment of sensitivity, quantitation, and timing of urinary antigen, serology, and direct fluorescent antibody for diagnosis of Legionnaires' disease. 93rd Meeting of the American Society for Microbiology 1994; Abstract C17

118. Stout JE. Laboratory diagnosis of Legionnaires' disease: the expanding role of the *Legionella* urinary antigen test. Clin Microbiol Newsletter 2000; 22:62-64.

119. Muder RR, Stout JE, Yu VL. Nosocomial *Legionella micdadei* infection in transplant patients: fortune favors the prepared mind. Am J Med 2000; 108:346-348.

120. Ingram JG, Plouffe J. Danger of sputum purulence screens in culture of *Legionella* species. J Clin Microbiol 1994; 32:209-210.

121. Buesching WJ, Brust RA, Ayers LW. Enhanced primary isolation of *Legionella pneumophila* from clinical specimens by low-pH treatment. J Clin Microbiol 1983; 17:1153-1155.

122. Oliverio MJ, Fisher MA, Vickers RM, Yu VL, Menon A. Diagnosis of Legionnaires' disease by radioimmunoassay of *Legionella* antigen in pleural fluid. J Clin Microbiol 1991; 29:2893-2894.

123. Rihs JD, Yu VL, Zuravleff JJ, Goetz A, Muder RR. Isolation of *Legionella pneumophila* from blood using the BACTEC: a prospective study yielding positive results. J Clin Microbiol 1985; 22:422-424.

124. Zuravleff JJ, Yu VL, Shonnard J, Davis B, Rihs JD. Diagnosis of Legionnaires' disease: an update of laboratory methods with new emphasis on isolation by culture. JAMA 1983; 250:1981-1985.

125. Centers for Disease Control. Guidelines for prevention of nosocomial pneumonia. MMWR 1997; 46:1-79.

126. Yu VL. *Legionella pneumophila* (Legionnaires' disease). In: Mandell GL, Bennett JE, Dolin R, eds. Principles and Practice of Infectious Diseases. New York:Churchill Livingstone, 1995:2087-2097.

127. Ramirez JA, Ahkee S, Tolentino A, Miller RD, Summersgill JT. Diagnosis of *Legionella pneumophila*, *Mycoplasma pneumoniae*, or *Chlamydia pneumoniae* lower respiratory infection using the polymerase chain reaction on a single throat swab specimen. Diagn Microbiol Infect Dis 1996; 24:7-14.

128. Jonas D, Rosenbaum A, Weyrish S, Bhakdi S. Enzyme-linked immunoassay for detection of PCR-amplied DNA of legionellae in bronchoalveolar fluid. J Clin Microbiol 1995; 33:1247-1252.

129. Murdoch DR, Walford EJ, Jennings LC, Light GJ, Schousboe MI, Chereshsky AY, Chambers ST, Town GI. Use of polymerase chain reaction to detect *Legionella* DNA in urine and serum samples from patients with pneumonia. Clin Infect Dis 1996; 23:475-480.

130. Matsiota-Bernard P, Pitsouni E, Legakis N, Nauciel C. Evaluation of commercial amplification kit for detection of *Legionella pneumophila* in clinical samples. J Clin Microbiol 1994; 32:1503-1505.

131. Martin WT, Fields BS, Hutwagoner LC. Comparison of culture and polymerase chain reaction to detect legionellae in environmental samples. In: Barbaree JM, Breiman RF, Dufour AP, eds. *Legionella*: Current Status and Emerging Perspectives. Washington, DC:American Society for Microbiology, 1993:175.

132. Edelstein PH. Antimicrobial chemotherapy for Legionnaires' disease: time for a change. Ann Intern Med 1998; 129:328-330.

133. Dedicoat M, Venkatesan P. The treatment of Legionnaires' disease. J Antimicrob Chemother 1999; 43:747-752.

134. Stout JE, Arnold B, Yu VL. Comparative activity of ciprofloxacin, ofloxacin, levofloxacin, and erythromycin against *Legionella* species by broth microdilution and intracellular susceptibility testing in HL-60 cells. Diagn Microbiol Infect Dis 1998; 30:37-43.

135. Stout JE, Arnold B, Yu VL. Activity of azithromycin, clarithromycin, roxithromycin, dirithromycin, quinupristin/dalfopristin and erythromycin against *Legionella* species by intracellular susceptibility testing in HL-60 cells. J Antimicrob Chemother 1998; 41:289-291.

136. Woodhead MD, MacFarlane JT, Rodgers FG, Lavenick A, Pilkington R, Macrae AD. Aetiology and outcome of severe community-acquired pneumonia. J Infect 1985; 10:204-210.

137. Vergis EN, Yu VL. *Legionella* species. In: Yu VL, Merigan TC, Barriere SL, eds. Antimicrobial Therapy and Vaccines. Baltimore, MD:Lippincott Williams and Wilkins, 1999:257-272.

138. Williams RR, Stout JE, Yu VL, Greenberg RN, Kojak C. Levofloxacin is safe and effective in the management of community-acquired pneumonia due to *Legionella*. 36th Annual Meeting of the Infectious Disease Society of America, Denver, CO 1998; Abstract 167Sa .

22

Bartonellosis

Anna Sander
Department of Medical Microbiology and Hygiene, University of Freiburg, Freiburg, Germany

I. HISTORICAL BACKGROUND

For several decades, the genus *Bartonella* consisted of a single species, *Bartonella bacilliformis*, which is the agent of Carrión's disease, a unique biphasic infection that is endemic to the valleys of the South American Andes in Peru, Columbia, and Ecuador. In endemic regions, members of indigenous populations usually show symptoms of verruga peruana, the secondary eruptive phase of Carrión's disease, whereas visitors to these regions develop a primary febrile hemolytic illness termed Oroya fever. Probably the most dramatic outbreak of Oroya fever occurred during the construction of the railroad from Lima to La Oroya between 1869 and 1873. La Oroya is a rich mining center 5000 metres above sea level. At the time, more than 10,000 labourers were hired mainly from Chile and the coastal cities of Peru which were areas where *B. bacilliformis* infections were not endemic. It was estimated that at least 8,000 workers contracted an illness that was characterized by fever and anemia and that most of them died. The "Puente de Verrugas", a viaduct of the trans-Andean railroad in this area, bears witness to this epidemic. The biphasic nature of the disease confused many investigators. Even railroad company physicians and Peruvians believed that the two stages were caused by two different etiological agents (1,2). A 26-year-old Peruvian medical student, Daniel Alcides Carrión, set out to demonstrate that both phases were caused by the same pathogen. In August 1885, he heroically inoculated himself with secretions from a skin lesion of a patient with verruga peruana. Three weeks after inoculation, he developed fever and anemia; his red blood cell count decreased precipitously. Daniel Carrión died a few weeks later, and the illness now bears his name (2,3).

Carrión's disease has been present in Peru since ancient times, and typical morphological characteristics of verruga peruana have been found in a rehydrated Inca mummy (4). Epidemics were reported in 1540 and 1630 during the colonial period (1,2), and outbreaks of Carrión's disease still occur today having been reported in Peru as recently as 1998 (5).

In 1916, during World War I, a *Bartonella* infection completely different from Oroya fever was first reported. Werner and Hiss, two German military physicians, described a newly recognized disease which began to spread throughout the German army in Wolhynia on the eastern front in a region which is today part of the Ukraine (6). After an incubation period of two to three weeks, various symptoms including relapsing fever with temperatures up to 40°C (usually 6 to 10 attacks of fever), weakness, weight loss, headache, myalgia, bone pain (especially in the tibia), back- and joint- pain, hepatospleno-megaly, and moderate anemia occurred. More than 400,000 soldiers suffered from this "trench fever" during World War I, and new epidemics occurred during World War II. Due to the five-day (four to eight day range) periodic nature of the fever, the disease was known as febris quintana or five-day fever, as well as Werner-Hiss' disease, Wolhynia fever, or trench fever (7,8). Werner and Benzler inoculated themselves with blood from an febrile patient and demonstrated the infectious nature of the disease (9). Despite the chronic course of the infection, no deaths from trench fever have been reported. The agent of trench fever, *Rickettsia quintana,* was first described in 1917 by Schmincke et al. (10). A few months later, Jungmann and Kuczynski described the agent as *Rickettsia wolhynica* (11). Henry da Ro-cha Lima first demonstrated that, in contrast to *Rickettsia prowazekii,* the agent of trench fever only multiplies extracellularly in the bowels of the louse (8). Da Rocha Lima introduced the name *Rickettsia pediculi.* In 1961, Vinson and Fuller (12) successfully isolated this bacterium on solid media, and the agent of trench fever was renamed *Rochalimaea quintana* in honor of da Rocha Lima.

In 1990, Relman et al. (13) first found evidence of another *Rochalimaea* species which they ob-tained by means of polymerase chain reaction amplification of *R. quintana*-like DNA from bacillary angiomatosis lesions of AIDS patients. Soon afterwards, independent of each other, Slater et al. (14,15) and Regnery et al. (16) isolated this bacterium from the blood cultures of immunosuppressed patients. In 1992, the organism was named *R. henselae* after Diane Hensel who was highly involved in the identi-fication of this organism (15).

One year later, in 1993, a new *Rochalimaea* species was isolated from the blood of a patient with endocarditis. The isolate was named *R. elizabethae* (17) after Saint Elizabeth's Hospital (Brighton, Massachusetts) where the organism was isolated. This new species was most closely related to *R. vin-sonii* which was first isolated from the spleen of the Canadian vole in 1946 (18).

Until 1993, the genera *Bartonella* (including the only species *B. bacilliformis*) and *Rochalimaea* (including the species *R. quintana, R. vinsonii, R. henselae,* and *R. elizabethae*) had been classified as belonging to the two different families, *Bartonellaceae* and *Rickettsiaceae,* of the order *Rickettsiales.* On the basis of DNA relatedness data, 16S rRNA sequencing, guanine-plus-cytosine contents, and phe-notypic characteristics, the genus *Rochalimaea* was united with the genus *Bartonella* in the family *Bartonellaceae* and removed from the order *Rickettsiales.* All *Rochalimaea* species were transferred to the genus *Bartonella* (19). In 1995, on the basis of molecular relatedness and phenotypical characteris-tics, the genera *Grahamella* (containing the species *G. talpae, G. peromysci,* and three unnamed spe-cies) and *Bartonella* were unified, and the name *Bartonella* was retained (20).

In the last few years, the number of identified *Bartonella* species has increased rapidly, and the *Bartonellaceae* family currently contains 14 species and 3 subspecies (Table 1). Recent investigations demonstrated the widespread occurrence of further, yet uncharacterized, *Bartonella* species in the bloodstream of most investigated mammals (30,31). Furthermore, *Bartonella*-DNA was also detected in 60% of *Ixodes ricinus* ticks in the Netherlands (32). We can expect that additional new *Bartonella* spe-cies will be described in the near future.

II. CLINICAL ASPECTS

A. Carrión's disease: Oroya Fever and verruga peruana

Carrión's disease, once referred to as bartonellosis, is caused by *B. bacilliformis* and manifests as a di-phasic illness. Ihler (33) has recently proposed that the name bartonellosis is inappropriate today be-cause many *Bartonella* species cause human disease.

After an incubation period of approximately 21 days (one to four weeks), the acute septicemic stage of the infection, termed Oroya fever, typically commences with a high fever and severe acute hemolytic anemia. Patients may suffer from general malaise, anorexia, headache, and an enlargement of lymph nodes, liver, and spleen. *B. bacilliformis* penetrates red blood cells, and the rapid progression of disease is usually caused by severe hypochromic macrocytic anemia; red cell counts drop in some patients to below 10^{12}/L. (34,35). This stage is additionally characterized by variably-induced immunosuppression, and opportunistic infections such as generalized toxoplasmosis, tuberculosis, salmonellosis, and shigellosis may follow (36-38).

The acute phase of the disease is followed by a latency period of several weeks to several years. Subsequently, the second, cutaneous phase of the disease (termed verruga peruana) may occur. Superficial and/or subcutaneous nodules, representing tumor-like proliferations of vascular endothelial cells,

Table 1   Currently recognized *Bartonella* spp. reservoirs and associated human diseases.

Bartonella species and date isolated (reference)	Natural host	Naturally occurring human diseases
B. bacilliformis, 1905 (21)	human	Carrión's disease
B. talpae, 1911 (22)	mole	none reported
*B. quintana,*1917 (10)	human	Trench Fever, endocarditis, bacillary angiomatosis-peliosis
B. peromysci, 1942 (23)	deer, mouse	none reported
B. vinsonii subsp. *vinsonii,* 1946 (18)	vole	none reported
B. henselae, 1992 (15, 16)	cat	cat scratch disease, endocarditis, bacillary angiomatosis-peliosis
B. elizabethae, 1993 (17)	rat	endocarditis, neuroretinitis
B. grahamii, 1995 (20)	mouse, vole	none reported
B. taylorii, 1995 (20)	mouse, vole	none reported
B. doshiae, 1995 (20)	vole	none reported
B. vinsonii subsp. *berkhoffii,* 1996 (24)	dog	none reported
B. clarridgeiae, 1996 (25)	cat	cat scratch disease
B. tribocorum, 1998 (26)	rat	none reported
*B. alsatica,*1999 (27)	rabbit	none reported
*B. koehlerae,*1999 (28)	cat	none reported
B. vinsonii subsp. *arupensis,* 1999 (29)	mouse	bacteremia, fever

occur in numerous forms, in variable numbers and sizes, and are unrelated to previous treatment with antibiotics. Skin lesions may occur as multiple small papules (miliary form), as larger pedunculated and erosive eruptions (mular form), or as deeper nodular forms. These lesions are in general painless but may bleed easily. They are primarily localized on the face and extremities, but may also be generalized (1). The verrugas are self-limiting and gradually disappear after several months.

B. Cat scratch disease

The typical clinical presentation of cat scratch disease (CSD) was first recognized more than 50 years ago by Debré, a French physician, who described several patients with suppurative adenitis which occurred from cat scratches (39). It was soon recognized that cats play a major role in the transmission of this disease. Most patients with CSD have a history of cat scratches, bites, or mere contact with a cat, often a newly acquired kitten. Transmission of the infectious agent by cat fleas is also suspected.

Until 1992, many organisms had been suspected of causing CSD: chlamydiae, acid-fast bacteria, *Pasteurella*, *Rothia dentocariosa*, Herpes simplex-like virus, and many other feline bacterial and viral agents. In 1988, *Afipia felis* was isolated from the lymph nodes of a few patients with symptoms similar to CSD (40). At present, however, there is no laboratory evidence which indicates that cats are a reservoir for *A. felis*.

The isolation of *B. henselae* in 1992 from the blood of an asymptomatic cat was soon followed by serological investigations of patients with CSD by Regnery et al., and these studies first demonstrated the link between *B. henselae* and CSD (41,42). One year later, Dolan cultured the first strain of *B. henselae* from the lymph nodes of patients with CSD (43). In the meantime, a great number of serological and molecular-based studies have demonstrated that the main agent of CSD is indeed *B. henselae*. The most frequent clinical manifestation of CSD, presenting as a primary skin lesion at the site of inoculation along with typical regional lymphadenopathy, is known as typical CSD, whereas other rather rare organ manifestations have been designated as atypical CSD.

Typical cat-scratch disease is usually found in immunocompetent patients and follows a characteristic clinical course. The first clinical manifestation is a primary lesion at the site of inoculation which appears three to ten days after contact with a cat. It may be a vesicular, erythematous, or often red-brown papular skin lesion of one to several millimeters in diameter, and it may persist from only a few days to several weeks. About two weeks after inoculation, one or more of the regional lymph nodes which drain this area enlarge as much as several centimeters in two to three weeks. Fever, especially a high fever of up to 40°C, is rather rare and occurs only in about one-third of all patients. Usually, the lymph node enlargement remains unchanged for another two to three weeks and then resolves thereafter. The usual duration of the disease is approximately two to four months, but in some circumstances, it may last longer. Late in the course of the illness, lymph nodes may redden and fluctuate; suppuration occurs in approximately 10 to 15% of CSD patients. Decompression and hence the prevention of the rupture of such lymph nodes may be facilitated by needle aspiration (44).

The location of the lymphadenopathy in CSD depends on the site of inoculation. In an overview which was based on the study of 1,200 patients, Carithers (45) reported that, in approximately 45% of patients, adenopathy develops in the axilla. The cervical or submandibular regions are involved in about 26%, and the inguinal lymph nodes in about 17%. Less commonly, the adenopathy may develop at epitrochlear, femoral, or supraclavicular sites. Eighty-seven percent of the patients in this study were 18 yrs. old or younger. In other studies, adults were observed to contract the disease just as often as children. In an assessment of 246 patients by Hamilton et al. (46), the site most commonly infected was the neck (43%), followed by the axilla (38%) and groin (20%). Thirty-seven percent of the patients reported lymphadenopathy at more than one site. These authors found a broader age distribution of CSD; approximately one-half of their patients were adults.

Atypical CSD occurs in 5-25% of all infections, and it presents as Parinaud's oculoglandular syndrome or as systemic CSD with involvement of various organs such as the liver, spleen, central nervous system, skin, bones, among others. The recognition of atypical CSD has apparently increased in the last few years. This fact may be explained by the availability of specific diagnostic tools which have been developed since the initial identification of the etiological agent of CSD in 1992.

Parinauds's oculoglandular syndrome (POGS), first described in 1889 by Henri Parinaud (47), is the most common atypical presentation of CSD and occurs in 2-17% of all patients (48,49). POGS is manifested as unilateral, nonsuppurative conjunctivitis with focal granulomatous reactions, and it is usually associated with ipsilateral preauricular or submandibular lymphadenopathy. Granulomatous lesions may be observed on the conjunctivae of the eyelids as small red to yellow nodules of 2-3 mm. in diameter and possibly up to 1-2 cm. (48). POGS is thought to occur after direct inoculation of the eye or when the organism has been transmitted to the eye by the hand of a patient after contact with an infected cat. Diagnosis of POGS may be performed by using Warthin-Starry staining methods as reported by Wear et al (50), but false-negative results have also been recognized (51,52). Grando et al. (51) were recently able to culture the first isolate of *B. henselae* from a patient with POGS some twenty-one days after incubation. Since isolation of *B. henselae* from clinical material is difficult to achieve, detection of *B. henselae*-specific DNA in tissues with conjunctival lesions (52, 53) and then serological testing for antibodies against this agent (51, 54, 55) are the most successful procedures for diagnosis. Recently, other ocular features of bartonellosis have been reported; mainly unilateral neuroretinitis and pan-uveitis (55,56). Patients may suffer from a decrease of visual acuity. Ophthalmoscopic findings include vitritis, disc edema, retinal edema, intraretinal infiltrates, dilated retinal vessels, and macular star exudates. Fluorescein angiography may demonstrate leakage from the optic disc and retinal vessels. The prognosis for normal vision following ocular manifestations of *Bartonella* infections is very good, and the disease runs a prolonged but self-limiting generally benign course. Corticosteroids alleviate the associated inflammatory reaction. The role of antibiotics in ocular bartonellosis also has to be clarified (55). Some authors postulate that early antibiotic therapy may shorten the course of infection and hasten visual recovery (57).

Recently, Leber's neuroretinitis, caused by *B. elizabethae*, was reported for the first time (58). The diagnosis was based on a low serological titre (1:128) against *B. elizabethae* and negative serology for other *Bartonella* species.

Systemic *B. henselae* infection (disseminated CSD) generally shows initial symptoms of prolonged fever or fever of unknown origin (FUO); the latter may often be associated with malaise, fatigue, myalgia, weight loss, headache, chills, and vomiting with or without peripheral lymphadenopathy. Fever and abdominal pain seem to be important symptoms in visceral, especially hepatosplenic, involvement. Ultrasonic observations of the abdomen reveal single or multiple hypoechogenic lesions in the liver and/or spleen which suggest that abscesses may be due to *B. henselae* infection. Hepatosplenic involvement may be found even in children suffering from typical CSD who lack apparent systemic clinical symptoms (59-62).

Neurological complications which are associated with CSD occur in 2-3% of patients; the most frequently reported manifestations being encephalopathy, encephalitis, myelitis, radiculitis, cerebral arteritis, and compressive neuropathy (63). Encephalitis is the most common neurological manifestation, and symptoms usually occur abruptly, approximately 1-6 weeks after the initial manifestations of CSD (64). Patients may develop headaches and convulsions, become confused and disorientated, and progress to a comatose state. Cerebrospinal fluid examination demonstrates mononuclear pleocytoses in only 20-30% of circumstances (63). Status epilepticus as the initial clinical presentation of CSD (with normal cerebrospinal fluid data), however, has been reported (65,66).

Bone involvement in systemic CSD, such as paravertebral abscesses or osteomyelitis, has been occasionally reported (67,68). A large number of other atypical clinical symptoms are rarely observed in CSD patients: pneumonia, pleural effusions, panaritia, erythema nodosum, and musculoskeletal manifestations (44,69-71).

Chronic lymphadenopathy of cervical or mediastinal lymph nodes caused by *B. quintana* has been reported (72,73), but at present, it is unclear if these illnesses represent chronic CSD or a different clinical entity of *Bartonella* infections.

Recently, two case reports implicated *B. clarridgeiae* as another possible agent of CSD. The first case of typical CSD due to *B. clarridgeiae* was reported of a veterinarian (74). The patient was bitten on the left index finger by his young kitten and developed headaches, fever, and left axillary lymphade- nopathy within 3 weeks. The patient's blood cultures remained sterile, but blood cultures from his cat yielded *B. clarridgeiae*. Sera from the patient showed high antibody titres to the feline isolate and were not reactive against other human pathogenic species of *Bartonella* (74). The second case report de- scribes a patient who presented with an upper chest wall abscess that extended into the axilla (75). The diagnosis was based on a low antibody titre against *B. clarridgeiae*, although *Streptococcus pneumoniae* was cultured from the pus of a spontaneously ruptured abscess. Unfortunately, no molecular diagnostics were applied to confirm the etiological agent. *B. clarridgeiae* was isolated from the blood culture of the patient's cat.

C. Bacillary angiomatosis – peliosis (BAP)

In 1983, Stoler et al. (76) first described bacillary angiomatosis as atypical subcutaneous lesions in an HIV-infected patient. The disease occurs mainly in immunocompromised patients. Most of these pa- tients suffer from AIDS, but some have cancer or have undergone organ transplantation. Bacillary an- giomatosis has rarely, however, been reported among immunocompetent individuals. The lesions are vasculo-proliferative and usually manifest as cutaneous tumors, although they may be observed in other organs such as lymph nodes, spleen, bones, brain, and bronchi (77,78). Skin lesions may be solitary or multiple (up to 1,000) and are usually red to purple. They may develop from small papules to form nod- ules or tumors which resemble pyogenic granulomas, hemangiomas, or Kaposi's sarcoma (79). In- volvement of the liver is known as bacillary peliosis hepatis. The term bacillary angiomatosis-peliosis (BAP) was coined because bacillary angiomatosis and bacillary peliosis hepatis are different organ manifestations of the same pathology (80,81). Fever, chills, night sweats, poor appetite, vomiting, and weight loss are the clinical symptoms most often reported along with extracutaneous manifestations (79). Findings of a study performed by Mohle-Boetani et al. (80) demonstrated that HIV-infected pa- tients with BAP were more severely immunocompromised than controls, with median CD4 lymphocyte counts of 2.1×10^7/L. The disease occurs late in the course of HIV infection, and it is therefore consid- ered an AIDS-defining opportunistic infection.

Two human pathogenic *Bartonella* species, *B. henselae* and *B. quintana*, have been shown to be involved in BAP. Since culture and species identification of the etiological agent may be difficult, most BAP cases have been diagnosed histologically, and in most studies, the infecting *Bartonella* species has not been identified. Investigations by Koehler et al. (81) showed that both species, *B. henselae* and *B. quintana*, were equally likely to be involved in BAP (53% and 47% respectively) and in skin lesions. Subcutaneous and lytic bone lesions, however, have been strongly associated with *B. quintana*, whereas lymph node, liver, and spleen infections have mainly been caused by *B. henselae*. Interestingly, organs that are diseased in *B. henselae* infections among patients with BAP correspond to those that are mainly involved in CSD which suggests some species-specific affinity for certain tissues.

D. Bacteremia and endocarditis

In recent years, an increasing number of diseases caused by *Bartonella* spp. have been identified. Bacte- remia due to *B. henselae* was first reported in 1990 (14). Immunocompromised, mostly HIV-infected patients, were affected (16). An outbreak of ten patients with *B. quintana* bacteremia was reported among homeless, alcoholic individuals in Seattle (82).

In 1993, Spach et al. (83) reported the first episode of endocarditis caused by *B. quintana* in an HIV-infected patient. In the same year, Hadfield et al. (84) described the first patient with endocarditis caused by *B. henselae* and Daly et al. (17) published the only case observed to date of an endocarditis caused by *B. elizabethae* in an immunocompetent patient. Since then, more than forty illnesses of *Bar- tonella* endocarditis have been reported in the literature. Homeless and chronically alcoholic individuals are particularly susceptible to the disease. It is estimated that *Bartonella* species account for 3-4% of all cases of endocarditis. Homeless, chronically alcoholic individuals with no history of valvulopathy appear more likely to become infected with *B. quintana*, whereas patients with a history of valvulopathy are more likely to have *B. henselae* (85). Despite antibiotic therapy, surgical removement of the infected valves was necessary in most cases.

III. EPIDEMIOLOGY OF INFECTION

Only six of the fourteen *Bartonella* species are known to be pathogenic to humans (Table 2).

   B. bacilliformis is endemic to the Andes of South America and is transmitted to humans by the bite of hematophagous female sandflies of the genus *Lutzomyia*, especially the species *Lutzomyia verrucarum*. These sandflies have their natural habitats in regions that are 500 to 3000 m. above the sea level, from 5°5″ latitude north to 13° latitude south (1). In recent outbreaks of Oroya fever in Peru, most patients were children (5, 86). Most of the native population acquires a degree of immunity during childhood. Those who are not native to the area are most likely to suffer from severe infections (2). Historically, the most dramatic outbreaks were seen among immigrants. Outside of South America, Carrión's disease has only been observed in patients who have recently been traveling in South America (87). Long-term bacteremia (5-15 months), however, has been reported to follow Oroya fever (33,86,88). To date, humans in endemic regions are the only known reservoir for this agent. In recent studies, asymptomatic bacteremia with *B. bacilliformis* has been described in up to 8-15% of those patients who have recovered from Oroya fever and in 22% of those patients who suffer from verruga peruana (86,89). Seroepidemiological studies in an endemic area of Peru have revealed a seroprevalence of 38% (90). Similar data were reported in another study with 41% of the native people in an endemic region of Peru having a history of Carrión's disease (86). Thus, asymptomatic bacteremic patients represent the main reservoir for *B. bacilliformis* and play an important role in the transmission of Carrión's

Table 2   Epidemiology of human pathogenic *Bartonella* species.

Bartonella species	Geographic distribution	Mode of Transmission
B. bacilliformis	Peru, Ecuador, Columbia	sandfly
B. quintana	worldwide	body louse
B. henselae	worldwide	cat scratches or bites, cat flea
B. clarridgeiae	worldwide	cat scratches or bites, cat flea
B. elizabethae	unknown (probably worldwide)	unknown
B. vinsonii subsp. *arupensis*	unknown	unknown

disease. Although several different strains of *Bartonella* have been identified in blood cultures of wild and domestic animals in endemic regions of Peru, these animals do not seem to be infected by the human pathogen *B. bacilliformis* (91,92). Since *B. bacilliformis* has been experimentally transmitted to *Macaca mulatta* via sandflies (93), an as yet unidentified animal reservoir cannot be definitively excluded.

Regarding *B. quintana* infections, it was quickly recognized by H. da Rocha Lima that body lice (*Pediculus humanus*) played an important role in the transmission of trench fever. During World War I, da Rocha Lima was able to find *B. quintana* in 73% of the body lice that were obtained from patients who suffered from trench fever, but only in 18% of healthy controls (8). Nevertheless, body lice were present both before and after World Wars I and II. Trench fever apparently disappeared in the decades following these wars, but in recent years, an increase of *B. quintana* infections has been observed among individuals who are living under poor social conditions especially the homeless population, among individuals with chronic alcohol abuse, and among HIV-infected people (94,95). It was shown that homeless people in Marseille and Moscow were infested with body lice in 4 and 12% respectively (96). Additionally, recent investigations of body lice, which have been collected from infested individuals in Africa and Europe, have demonstrated the presence of *B. quintana* in up to 14% of these vectors. As with *B. bacilliformis*, humans are presently the only known reservoir for *B. quintana*.

Bartonella henselae is found worldwide, and CSD is the most common *Bartonella* infection in humans. Little data is available concerning the incidence rate of CSD. In the United States, it is estimated that 24,000 cases occur yearly with an incidence rate of 9.3/100,000 ambulatory patients per year (97). Seasonal differences are reported, and most cases of CSD occur in late fall or winter. Cats form a large reservoir for *B. henselae*. Impounded or stray cats, as well as young pet cats (less than one year of age), were more likely to be bacteremic than adult pet cats (98-100). Chomel et al. (99) showed that antibodies to *B. henselae* were higher in bacteremic than in nonbacteremic cats. These animals seem to be infected worldwide. Results from different studies regarding the prevalence of *B. henselae* bacteremia in cats are reviewed in Table 3. In summary, domestic cats have a frequency of bacteremia varying from 4-48%, and the frequency for impounded or stray cats is higher at 16-89%. Interestingly, *B. henselae* is able to remain in the bloodstream of healthy cats for several months (98,100,112). *B. henselae* could not be found, however, in gingival swabs of animals. Although *B. henselae* might be transmitted by cat bites, it seems to be unlikely that it is a component of the normal buccal flora (100).

A large number of serological studies have been performed to examine the antibody prevalence to *B. henselae* in cats (Table 4). There is an overall seropositivity rate of 4-100% among the animals so investigated. Serological screening for *Bartonella* antibodies may not be useful for the identification of bacteremic cats, but the lack of antibodies to *B. henselae* seems to be highly predictive of the absence of bacteremia (99). The seroprevalence in cats correlates with the geographic region and climatic conditions; higher infection rates being observed in warm and humid areas (117). Infections with *Toxoplasma gondii*, feline leukemia virus (FeLV), feline immunodeficiency virus (FIV), feline coronavirus (FCoV), or feline spumavirus (FeSFV) were not associated with bacteremia or seropositivity for *B. henselae* in cats (99,121,122).

Epidemiological studies of the risk factors that are associated with CSD have demonstrated a role for cat fleas, *Ctenocephalides felis*, in the transmission of the disease. *B. henselae* has been detected in cat fleas with the use of PCR techniques (98), and bacteremic cats were more likely to be infested with fleas than nonbacteremic animals (99). It was experimentally shown that cat fleas which were removed from bacteremic cats may transmit *B. henselae* to uninfected animals (102). Infection of domestic cats with *B. henselae* could also be achieved by intradermal injection of infected flea feces (124), by intradermal and subcutaneous inoculation of whole bacteria (125), and by transmission of blood from infected animals (126). In contrast, bacteremia or seroconversion could not be induced by intramuscular application of urine sediment from infected cats (126), and cats that were inoculated with *B. quintana* remained abacteremic as well (127). It has been demonstrated that *B. henselae* is not transmitted transplacentally or in colostrum or milk, since fetuses and kittens of infected cats were not bacteremic and

Table 3   World-wide prevalence of *B. henselae* bacteremia in cats.

Country	Cats investigated	Bacteremia %	(n)	Reference
USA, California	impounded	41	(25/61)	(98)
USA	cats from patients with CSD	89	(17/19)	(101)
	domestic	28	(7/25)	
USA, Davis	domestic	4.4	(3/68)	(99)
San Francisco	domestic	47.7	(21/44)	
Davis	impounded	53	(26/49)	
Sacramento	impounded	70.4	(31/44)	
USA	impounded	89	(42/47)	(102)
Japan	domestic	9.1	(3/33)	(103)
Australia	domestic	16	(3/18)	(104)
	stray	40	(24/59)	
Germany	domestic	13	(13/100)	(100)
France	stray	16	(15/94)	(105)
The Netherlands	impounded	8	(9/113)	(106)
USA	domestic	12	(1/8)	(107)
Zimbabwe	domestic	8	(2/25)	(108)
Indonesia	stray	21	(3/14)	(109)
Philippine	domestic	19	(6/31)	(110)
Japan	domestic	8.2	(37/450)	(111)

did not produce anti-*B. henselae* antibodies (128).

Recent studies have demonstrated that cats serve as a reservoir for an additional *Bartonella* species, namely *B. clarridgeiae*. This new species was first described in 1996 by Lawson and Collins (25) and was isolated from the cat of a patient with *B. henselae* septicemia. In the meantime, *B. clarridgeiae* has been isolated worldwide from various apparently healthy cats. An overview of the prevalence of *B. clarridgeiae* in blood cultures from cats is given in Table 5. Coinfections with both species, as well as with two different 16S rRNA- genotypes of *B. henselae,* are reported (129). Furthermore, *B. clarridgeiae* DNA was detected in cat fleas using PCR-methods (106), and it therefore seems quite probable that these ectoparasites transmit both *Bartonella* species in the same way.

IV. NATURE OF THE BACTERIUM AND PATHOGENESIS

The members of the family *Bartonellaceae* belong to the α-2 subdivision of the *Proteobacteria*. Phylogenetic analyses have demonstrated a close evolutionary relationship between *Bartonella* species and members of the genus *Brucella*. The 16S rRNA similarity values between *B. abortus* and *Bartonella* species are between 94.74 and 95.58%. Two other bacteria that are closely related to *Bartonella* species are the plant pathogens *Rhizobium melitoti* and *Agrobacterium tumefaciens* (130). *Bartonella* species are genetically and phenotypically closely related. It was shown, however, that *B. henselae* and *B.*

Table 4   World-wide seroprevalence of *B. henselae* antibody in cats.

Country	Cats investigated	Seroprevalence % (n)	Reference
U.S.	cats of patients with CSD	81 (39/48)	(113)
	domestic	38 (11/29)	
U.S., Baltimore	impounded	14.7 (87/592)	(114)
U.S.	impounded	41 (25/61)	(98)
U.S., Texas	impounded	37.9 (199/567)	(115)
Maryland	impounded and pet	13.2 (81/612)	
Georgia	domestic	47.9 (35/73)	
Maine	domestic	65.4 (34/52)	
Kansas	domestic	50 (5/10)	
Egypt	domestic	11.9 (5/42)	
Portugal	domestic	6.7 (1/14)	
Austria	NA	33 (32/96)	(116)
U.S., Davis	domestic	61.8 (42/68)	(99)
San Francisco	domestic	86.4 (38/44)	
Davis	impounded	85.7 (42/49)	
Sacramento	impounded	100 (44/44)	
U.S., Southeast	domestic	54.6 (53/97)	(117)
Hawaii	domestic	47 (9/19)	
California	domestic	40 (32/80)	
South central	domestic	37 (22/60)	
Northwest	domestic	34 (24/70)	
Northeast	domestic	27 (20/74)	
Southwest	domestic	15 (6/40)	
Midwest	domestic	7 (4/60)	
Alaska	domestic	5 (1/20)	
Rocky Mountains	domestic	4 (4/108)	
Japan	domestic	15.1 (30/199)	(118)
South Africa	domestic	24 (28/119)	(119)
Zimbabwe	domestic	21 (11/52)	
U.S., N. Carolina	NA	40 (46/114)	(120)
Israel	NA	40 (45/114)	
The Netherlands	impounded	50 (57/113)	(106)
	domestic	56 (28/50)	
Switzerland	healthy	7.2 (22/304)	(121)
	sick	9.2 (39/424)	

Table 4 cont'd.

Country	Cats investigated	Seroprevalence % (n)	Reference
Japan	impounded and pet	9.1 (43/471)	(122)
Indonesia	stray	54 (40/74)	(109)
Philippines	domestic	68 (73/107)	(110)
Singapore	stray	47.5 (38/80)	(123)

NA = not available

Table 5   Prevalence of *B. clarridgeiae* in cats.

Country	Cats investigated	Bacteremia % (n)	Reference
France	stray	16 (15/94)	(105)
The Netherlands	impounded	8 (9/113)	(106)
USA	domestic	12 (1/8)	(107)
Indonesia	stray	21 (3/14)	(109)
Philippines	domestic	19 (6/31)	(110)
Japan	domestic	1.3 (6/450)	(111)

quintana may have pili, whereas *B. clarridgeiae* and *B. bacilliformis* possess multiple unipolar flagellae. The *Fla*A-gene of *B. clarridgeiae* has a 77.8% DNA sequence homology to the *Fla*A-gene of *B. bacilliformis* (131). A dendrogram analysis of several flagellin sequences demonstrated that the *B. bacilliformis* flagellin, together with the *Azospirillum, R. meliloti, A. tumefaciens,* and *Caulobacter crescentus* flagellins, form a cluster that is different from all other flagellins, including that of *E. coli* (132).

The genomes of various *Bartonella* species were estimated to be approximately 2.005, 1.700, 2.174, 1.600, and 2.082 Mb for *B. henselae, B. quintana, B. elizabethae, B. bacilliformis,* and *B. vinsonii,* respectively (33,133). The guanine-plus-cytosine content of the genomes ranges from 39-41% (70). A linear extrachromosomal double-stranded DNA fragment of 14 kb, a bacteriophage-like particle, has been found in *B. henselae* and *B. bacilliformis* (134,135).

A.   DNA fingerprinting of *Bartonella* isolates

Studies which are based on different target genes and on the whole genomes of *B. henselae* and *B. quintana* have shown evidence of intraspecies differences within a number of isolates.

1. The 16S ribosomal RNA (16S rRNA) gene as target molecule

On the basis of the 16S rRNA gene, *Bartonella* species are closely related and have interspecies similarities of 98.10-99.62% (28). Recent investigations, using partial 16S rRNA sequence analysis, indicated the presence of two *B. henselae* genotypes (I and II) which differ by five nucleotides as located at positions 172 to 176 in the 16S rRNA gene (136). Using specific primers, *B. henselae* genotype I was detected in 78, 15, and 59% and *B. henselae* genotype II in 17, 85, and 23% of the CSD-patient lymph nodes that were examined in the Netherlands, Switzerland, and Germany respectively (136,137,138). In contrast, most cats in Europe have been infected with *B. henselae* genotype II (56% in the Netherlands, 51% and 71% in France, and 94% in Germany). 100% of cat isolates from the Phillipines were genotype II (110). No obvious clinical differences have been found among patients who suffer from CSD that is caused by one genotype or the other (139). No differences in the 16S rRNA gene in other *Bartonella* species have yet been described.

2. The 16S-23S rRNA intergenic spacer region as target molecule.

The size of the 16S-23S rRNA intergenic spacer region that is described in most bacteria is between 250 and 500 bp. The corresponding regions in *Bartonella* species have been shown to be longer than those in other bacteria: 1.382, 1.331, 1.378, 1.648, and 0.906 kb for *B. henselae, B. quintana, B. vinsonii, B. elizabethae,* and *B. bacilliformis* respectively. The intergenic spacer region of the *Bartonella* species contains the genes encoding tRNA^{Ile} and tRNA^{Ala}, but most are currently considered to be nonfunctional (133,140,141). Sequence analysis of the 16S-23S spacer region revealed a low mutation rate of 0.5-4% for *B. henselae* and 0.6% for *B. quintana* (133).

Using a PCR-based restriction fragment length polymorphism (RFLP) analysis of the 16S-23S rRNA intergenic spacer region and digestion of the amplicons with the restriction endonucleases *Alu*I and *Hae*II, Matar et al. (142) were able to differentiate between various *Bartonella* species, and they obtained six different restriction patterns among eleven *B. henselae* isolates, mostly from patients suffering from BA. *Alu*I RFLP analysis of the spacer PCR products revealed only two *B. henselae* RFLP variants among Dutch patients with CSD (136) and as well among Dutch and German cat isolates (106, 143). The correlation between the *Alu*I RFLP patterns and the 16S rRNA genotype was 100% in both studies although each typing method is based on polymorphisms in different parts of the bacterial genome. These results suggest that different *B. henselae* subtypes might be involved in CSD and in BA. Analysis of *B. quintana* isolates by this method revealed two different variants (133). It was shown in some studies that 16S-23S spacer RFLP typing may be useful for rapid species identification of *Bartonella* isolates (133,142), but it does not seem to be reliable enough for isolate identification and epidemiological studies (133,143).

3. The citrate synthase gene (glt*A*) as target molecule

RFLP-analysis of PCR products of the citrate synthase gene in different *Bartonella* isolates was shown to be a useful method for species identification. Multiple restriction endonuclease digests of PCR products from various *B. henselae* isolates, however, failed to differentiate bacteria within the same species (16,144). Comparison of the glt*A* sequences of different *Bartonella* species revealed that the levels of similarity between the sequences were 83.8-93.5% whereas the similarity between isolates of the same species were more than 99.8% (145).

4. The riboflavin gene as target molecule

Sequence analysis of the riboflavin synthesis genes indicated that these could provide an excellent tool for differentiation between *Bartonella* species. Comparing the sequences of the riboflavin C gene from 17 different *B. henselae* strains, two different genotypes could be detected (146).

5.   The whole Bartonella genome as target molecule

Typing methods that are based on the whole genome should be used in epidemiological studies. The application of these methods for *Bartonella* species, however, is limited by the difficulties that are encountered when attempting to isolate bacteria from clinical specimens.

Rep-PCR (ERIC- and REP-PCR)

Repetitive element sequence-based PCR (rep-PCR), such as ERIC (enterobacterial repetitive intergenic consensus)-PCR and REP (repetitive extragenic palindromic)-PCR, has been successfully used for the identification of *Bartonella* strains on the species level; showing different band patterns for *B. henselae, B. quintana, B. elizabethae, B. vinsonii, B. bacilliformis*, and *B. clarridgeiae* (147, 148,149). Through the combination of both PCR methods, discrimination among 17 isolates of *B. henselae* and 5 strains of *B. quintana* yielded five different *B. henselae* fingerprint profiles, whereas only a unique profile could be demonstrated for *B. quintana* (148). Similar results were obtained in another study where 18 strains of *B. henselae* clustered in 4 different patterns (143). Both studies showed that ERIC-PCR was more discriminatory than REP-PCR.

Arbitrarily primed (AP)-PCR

The core sequence of phage M13 was used for AP-PCR as single primer to differentiate between 18 *B. henselae* strains. The patterns so obtained by this method showed a clear differentiation between the four clusters as seen with ERIC- and REP- PCR (143).

Major advantages of PCR-based fingerprint methods (ERIC-, REP-, and AP- PCR) are technical simplicity, wide availability of equipment and reagents, and rapid feasibility.

Pulsed-field gel electrophoresis (PFGE)

PFGE has been shown to be a suitable method for the differentiation of *Bartonella* strains at the species level. Digestion of genomic *Bartonella* DNA with different restriction endonucleases has revealed specific band patterns for each of the analyzed species. The subtyping of seven *B. quintana* and four *B. henselae* strains revealed a specific profile for each of the isolates (133,150) depending on the restriction endonucleases that are used. Furthermore, among 18 strains of *B. henselae*, 10 different patterns were obtained with PFGE by *Sma*I digestion of the DNA (143).

In comparing several different typing methods, PFGE was shown to provide the highest discriminatory potential for subtyping of 18 *B. henselae* strains (143; Table 6). Therefore, PFGE seems to be the most reliable typing method for epidemiological and clinical follow-up studies. The latter is more expensive and time-consuming, however, than PCR-based fingerprinting methods.

B.   Pathogenesis

The hemotropic potential may be a distinguishing feature of *Bartonella* species. Intracellular growth of *B. bacilliformis* in erythrocytes was first described by Barton in 1905 (21). Almost all of the symptoms of Oroya fever (fever, anemia, hepatosplenomegaly, and circulatory collapse) arise as a consequence of infection of red cells; in severe cases, essentially 100% of the red cells can be parasitized (151). *B. bacilliformis* is highly motile having multiple unipolar flagella. Isolation and characterization of the flagella revealed a 42 kD Fla A protein as a major component. Antiflagellin antibodies tended to inhibit the invasion of human erythrocytes (152). A second (67 kD) protein, called deformin, was found to be secreted by *B. bacilliformis*, and it is responsible for producing deep invaginations within the erythrocyte membrane (153). Hemolytic activity of *B. bacilliformis* was detected by incubation with red cells, and it has been suggested that deformin might be the hemolysin (33). Other *Bartonella* spp. have not yet been found in human erythrocytes. Electron microscopic examination of feline erythrocytes, however, has revealed intracellular *B. henselae* in 2.9-6.2% (112).

Table 6 Comparison of different typing methods for *Bartonella henselae* isolates (modified after 143,146). Abbreviations are detailed in the above text.

Isolate	PFGE	ERIC	REP	M13	AluI RFLP	16S rRNA genotype	Riboflavin genotype	Proposed variant
FR96/BK3	P1	E1.1	R1	M1	A2	16S-2	Ribo-1	I
FR96/BK8	P2	E1	R1	M1	A2	16S-2	Ribo-1	I
FR96/BK75II	P1	E1	R1	M1	A2	16S-2	Ribo-1	I
FR96/BK77	P3	E1	R1	M1	A2	16S-2	Ribo-1	I
FR96/BK78	P1	E1	R1	M1	A2	16S-2	Ribo-1	I
FR96/BK79	P4	E1	R1	M1	A2	16S-2	Ribo-1	I
FR96/BK26II	P5	E2	R2	M2	A2	16S-2	Ribo-2	II
FR96/BK36	P5	E2	R2	M2	A2	16S-2	Ribo-2	II
FR96/BK36II	P6	E2	R2	M2	A2	16S-2	Ribo-2	II
FR96/BK38	P7	E2	R2	M2	A2	16S-2	Ribo-2	II
FR96/BK74	P5	E2	R2	M2	A2	16S-2	Ribo-2	II
FR96/BK75	P6	E2	R2	M2	A2	16S-2	Ribo-2	II
FR96/K2	P5	E2	R2	M2	A2	16S-2	Ribo-2	II
FR96/K4	P6	E2	R2	M2	A2	16S-2	Ribo-2	II
FR96/K5	P5	E2	R2	M2	A2	16S-2	Ribo-2	II
FR96/K6	P8	E2	R2	M2	A2	16S-2	Ribo-2	II
FR97/K7	P9	E3	R3	M3	A1	16S-1	Ribo-1	III
Houston-1 (ATCC 49882)	P10	E4	R4	M4	A1	16S-1	Ribo-1	IV

Another flagellated human pathogen *Bartonella* species is *B. clarridgeiae*, and a 41 kD protein could be identified as the flagellin filament protein (FlaA). Western blot analysis showed that 3.9% of patients with lymphadenopathy had antibodies against this protein (131) thus suggesting that *B. clarridgeiae* might indeed be involved in CSD.

The most striking pathological feature of *Bartonella* infections is the ability of these bacteria to produce angioproliferative lesions. Histological investigation of verruga peruana and BAP shows typical proliferations of capillaries with large cuboidal endothelial cells as a result of *B. bacilliformis*, *B. henselae*, or *B. quintana* infections (154-156). Extracts of these three species have been reported to induce vasoproliferative growth and to stimulate human umbilical vein endothelial cell proliferation in vitro (157). *B. henselae* and *B. quintana* possess pili which appear to play an important role in the adhesion to human epithelial cells (158). Interestingly, *Bartonella* spp. are the only known bacteria that have the ability to cause neovascularization in humans. The immune status of patients, as well as the variation of virulence among strains, may determine the different clinical manifestations of *Bartonella* infections.

V. IMMUNOLOGY OF INFECTION

In vitro, *B. henselae* is very sensitive to serum- or complement-mediated cytolysis. The organisms are able to activate complement and to stimulate phagocytosis and an oxidative burst in polymorphonuclear leukocytes (159). *B. henselae* activates both classical and alternative complement pathways. Western blot analysis of *B. henselae* antigen preparations with sonicated whole cell organisms indicated that nonimmune sera contain antibodies that react with several of the components of *B. henselae* (159). Screening of sera from CSD patients for immunoglobulin isotype-specific, as well as for the IgG subclass-specific reactivity against *B. henselae*, has revealed that predominant antigen recognition was limited to IgG_1 (160).

Present knowledge indicates that *Bartonella*-specific IgM antibodies are produced early in the initial infection and persist only for a short time. In many cases, diagnosis of CSD is performed late in the course of the illness thus resulting in negative values for IgM antibodies. In general, IgG antibodies are detectable when clinical symptoms are present, they persist for several months, and they gradually decrease. Life-long immunity against *Bartonella*-infection is unlikely; relapses or reinfections may occur.

VI. LABORATORY DIAGNOSIS

Until recently, CSD was diagnosed by exclusion and required the presence of at least three of the following four criteria: a history of cat contact and the presence of a scratch or a primary lesion, a regional lymphadenopathy with negative results for other causes of lymphadenopathy, characteristic histopathological features in lymph node biopsy specimens, and a positive cat scratch disease skin test reaction. The skin test was never standardized, however, and it is not commercially available. Skin test antigen was historically prepared from the lymph nodes of patients with CSD. Compared to serology and PCR, the skin test lacks specificity and sensitivity (161). It also carries the risk that other infections may be transmitted to the patient. In the last few years, reliable serological tests and molecular-based methods for diagnosis of CSD have been established worldwide. The skin test is therefore no longer recommended for the diagnosis of CSD. The presence of a *Bartonella*-infection should be considered among patients with lymphadenopathy and culture-negative endocarditis. Immunocompromised patients with lesions that are consistent with BAP or fever of unknown origin (FUO) are also likely candidates.

A. Serological diagnosis

Serological testing should be the first step in the diagnosis of typical and atypical CSD and *Bartonella*-endocarditis. In contrast, many immunocompromised patients who suffer from BAP may fail to produce antibodies against *Bartonella* species. In episodes of clinically suspect CSD, a negative serological test result does not necessarily rule out current or recent infection, and a second serum sample should be tested later in the course of illness. In some patients, seroconversion was reported as late as the third week after onset of illness (162). Antibody titres to *B. henselae* were highest, however, in the early weeks after the onset of lymphadenopathy, and they declined over time often resulting in borderline titres after 25-28 weeks post-illness (113). There have been reports of patients with initial negative serum titres and positive lymph node cultures for *B. henselae,* as well as initially negative serum titres followed by a four-fold titre increase in convalescent sera (163).

Serological differentiation between *B. henselae* and *B. quintana* is definitely not possible, and cross-reactivity between both *Bartonella* species was shown to be very high in many studies, specifically 95-100% (160,162,164).

1. B. henselae and B. quintana

Indirect immunofluorescent antibody assay (IFA)

Remarkably, antigen preparation from plate-grown *Bartonella* species may lead to false-negative results and excessively low antibody titres when compared with antigens prepared from organisms co-cultivated with cell cultures (165). It was shown that co-cultivation improves the detection of IgG against *B. henselae* (166,167). Since genetic heterogeneity among *B. henselae* strains is high (143), strain related variation of antibody titres may occur (168,169).

Two commercial IFAs are presently available: one that is based on human larynx carcinoma cells that are co-infected with *B. henselae* Houston 1 (ATCC 49882) (BION Enterprises, Park Ridge, Illinois), and one that is based on Vero cells that are co-infected with *B. henselae* or *B. quintana* (MRL Diagnostics, Cypress, California). A large number of diagnostic laboratories, however, use their own IFA or antigen which they have obtained from the CDC, Atlanta, Georgia, where this test was initially developed (42). Very high sensitivities of nearly 100% are observed in groups of patients with histologically proven CSD, patients with a positive skin test, and in studies with a strict clinical case definition of CSD (regional lymphadenopathy and cat scratch or bite with a primary skin lesion distal to the lymph node, or at least a history of intimate contact with a cat that frequently bites, licks, or scratches) (162,163). In patients with a broad clinical definition of CSD, where the illness is only suspected on the basis of regional lymphadenopathy (with or even without contact to cats), sensitivities dropped to 80% or less, suggesting that some patients with clinically suspected CSD have probably not been diagnosed correctly (162). Serological titres in patients with CSD were usually high (>1:256). Titres >1:256 were generally found 1-26 weeks after onset of illness and decline slowly thereafter (113,162). In healthy controls, however, there is a reported *B. henselae* seroprevalence of 20-30 % (164,170) and even as high as 60% (166,171,172). Antibody titres in healthy controls are usually low (between 1:64 and 1:256), and exceed a titre of 1:256 in only about 1-3 % of all cases (42,164,166,170-172). Interpretation of such low titres may be difficult in patients suffering from lymphadenopathy. These titres could indicate the onset or the final stage of CSD or even prior contact with *B. henselae*. It was shown in a group of eleven children with regional lymphadenopathy other than CSD (staphylococci, group A beta-hemolytic streptococci, or *Mycobacterium avium-intracellulare*) that nearly half of the patients had low (1:64 to 1:256) antibody titres to *B. henselae* (171). There are patients with histologically-diagnosed lymphomas and low antibody titres to *B. henselae* (A. Sander, unpublished data). Therefore, if CSD is clinically suspected, a titre increase in a second serum sample obtained 2-4 weeks later should confirm the diagnosis. In circumstances where an increase of antibody titre does not appear, fine needle aspiration or surgical removal of the lymph node for histopathological and molecular-based diagnostic procedures is strongly recommended.

IgM antibodies were detected in 66% (53/80) of patients with clinically suspected CSD and in 73% (41/56) of patients with positive skin tests (173). In another study, IgM antibodies have been less frequently detected in patients with histologically-diagnosed CSD than in patients with primary and clinically suspected CSD (164). Since lymph node extirpation is usually performed in a later stage of the illness, it seems possible that IgM antibodies were no longer present.

Low serological titres alone (1:64 to 1:256) are not indicative of *Bartonella* infection. The seroprevalence in healthy people is high and one has to be careful not to overdiagnose *Bartonella* infections in such patients. Owning a cat in itself is a risk factor for CSD, but not every low antibody titer in cat owners is indicative of CSD. In atypical clinical illnesses, a large number of infectious (toxoplasmosis, borreliosis, cytomegalovirus, tuberculosis, atypical mycobacteria, and actinomycosis) and non-infectious agents (malignant and benign lymphadenopathies) should be considered in the differential diagnosis.

Enzyme-linked immunoassay (EIA)

Less experience has been reported with the use of an EIA for serological diagnosis of CSD. The results that have been obtained by different investigators are conflicting. Whereas Barka et al. (174) described a highly specific (99%) and sensitive (95%) EIA for the detection of IgG antibodies, serological investigations by Szelc-Kelly et al. (173) clearly demonstrated that IgG EIA was less sensitive (sensitivities of 32-35 %) than IFA (sensitivities of 83-93%). Similar results were also obtained by Bergmans et al. (175) with very low sensitivities in both IFA and EIA assays. Using outer membrane proteins as antigen, an EIA developed by Litwin et al. (176) showed 98.6% and 91.4% agreement with an indirect fluorescence test for IgG and IgM antibodies respectively.

Western blot analysis (WB)

In a recent study, an 83 kD *B. henselae* protein (Bh83) was found to react with all CSD sera and with the sera of patients with *B. quintana* infections. CSD sera failed, however, to recognize this protein when tested against the *B. quintana* antigen (160). A recombinant expressed 17 kD protein was shown to be reactive on immunoblot with individual serum samples from patients with CSD (177). Furthermore, reactivity to an 8 kD band showed a correlation with the positive results that were obtained using IgM IFA and EIA (176).

In unselected serum samples of patients with CSD, however, immunodominant proteins are not present in every sample. Using *B. henselae* whole cell antigen for WB, multiple proteins cross-reacted with antisera from patients who suffered from other bacterial infections (*Ehrlichia chaffeensis, Mycoplasma pneumoniae, Escherichia. coli, Francisella tularensis, Treponema pallidum, Chlamydia spp., Coxiella burnetii* and *Rickettsia rickettsii)* (160,178,179).

In conclusion, further studies are needed to evaluate the reliability of EIA and Western blot analysis for the diagnosis of CSD. In the meantime, IFA is the most frequently-used serological method for diagnosing CSD. Non-specific cross-reactions can be minimized by detecting antibodies to *Bartonella* that are co-cultivated with infected cells.

2. *B. bacilliformis*

Currently, there are no commercially available or generally accepted assays for the serological diagnosis of *B. bacilliformis* infections. ELISA and IFA which detect antibodies to *B. bacilliformis* were first described by Knobloch et al. (180). It was shown that crude antigen cross-reacted with anti-*Chlamydia psittaci* antibodies as well as with antibodies against other agents (181). Using a cut-off point of 1:256 or higher, a recently developed IFA was shown to be 74% sensitive and 92% specific when compared with a gold standard of culture-confirmed infection (182).

B. Histopathological examination

1. *Carrión's disease*

Diagnosis of acute Oroya fever is usually performed by detection of intraerythrocytic *B. bacilliformis* in Giemsa-stained blood films or by isolation of the organisms from blood cultures. In patients suffering from verruga peruana, *B. bacilliformis* usually appears as coccobacilli within the erythrocytes. Verruga peruana is histopathologically characterized by a lobular vascular proliferation in the dermis or subcutis (154).

2. Cat scratch disease and BAP

Whereas during Carrión's disease a large number of erythrocytes are infected, the level of bacteremia due to *B. henselae* or *B. quintana* seems to be too low for direct microscopic detection of these bacilli in blood smears.

Histopathological examination of the lymph nodes from patients with CSD shows three evolutionary stages. The first stage is characterized by an enlargement that is caused by the expansion of the cortex and hyperplasia of the germinal centers with epithelioid granulomas and Langhans' giant cells. Later in the course of the disease, granulomas enlarge, fuse with each other, and become infiltrated with polymorphonuclear leukocytes thereafter developing central necrosis with progressive suppuration and sinus formation. In the third stage, many pus-filled sinuses are present, and rupture of the capsule may occur. Although these findings are typical, however, they are not specific for CSD. Similar lesions may also occur in sarcoidosis, infectious mononucleosis, mycobacterial infections, lymphogranuloma venereum, brucellosis, and tularemia (183).

Histological findings of BAP are similar to those of verruga peruana; they appear as tumor-like capillary proliferations in a fibromyxoid stroma with plump endothelial cells that protrude into the vascular lumina. The surrounding stroma contains mixed inflammatory cells, neutrophils, histiocytes, nuclear debris, and amphophilic material. The most important diseases which should be considered in the differential diagnosis of BAP include Kaposi's sarcoma, pyogenic granuloma, epithelioid hemangioma, and angiosarcoma.

Warthin-Starry silver staining of fixed tissue sections was performed successfully for some patients with CSD and BAP and demonstrated the presence of the organisms. In patients with CSD, bacilli may be detected by Warthin-Starry staining during the early stages of lymphadenopathy, but not in the later granulomatous stage of the illness (184). Warthin-Starry staining is not specific for *Bartonella* spp., however, and lacks sensitivity. In a study performed by Demers et al. (163), positive results were obtained by this method in only 4 (12.5%) of 32 patients with CSD and in 4 of 7 patients with BAP (185).

Immunohistochemical staining of *Bartonella* spp. is used in some cases for detection of the organisms in tissue sections, but this method is only available in specialized laboratories.

C. Polymerase chain reaction (PCR)-based diagnostic methods

PCR-amplification of a *Bartonella* DNA fragment from human specimens is widely used to diagnose *Bartonella* infections. Several different PCR-based assays have been described using primer pairs with different target genes. In 1990, Relman et al. (13) developed the first primer pair (p24E-p12B) for the detection of *Bartonella* DNA. This permits amplification of a 241 bp fragment of the 16S rRNA. *Bartonella* species identification must be performed by sequencing or hybridization (161,186). In 1994, Anderson et al. (187) developed the primers CAT1 and CAT2 which are based on the sequence of the *htr*A gene (60 kD heat-shock protein gene). Using these primers, they were able to amplify a 414 bp fragment from the two major human pathogens *B. henselae* and *B. quintana* but not from *B. elizabethae*, *B. vinsonii*, or *B. bacilliformis*. Dot-blot hybridization with species-specific, digoxigenin-labeled oligonucleotide probes (RH1 and RQ1) permits differentiation between the two species. Other primer pairs that are described for the detection of *Bartonella* DNA utilize the citrate synthase gene (*glt*A) as a target (144) or the gene coding for the cell division protein FtsZ (*fts*Z) (188). In order to distinguish between the human pathogenic species, *B. henselae*, *B. quintana*, *B. clarridgeiae*, and *B. bacilliformis*, primer sets that are based on the riboflavin synthesis genes have been developed (146). Genus and species-specific primer sets for the detection of *B. henselae*, *B. quintana*, *B. bacilliformis*, and *B. elizabethae* have also been developed on the basis of the 16S-23S intergenic spacer (IST) region (189). Detection of *B. bacilliformis* DNA in human specimens by PCR was already described in 1992 (190). A large number of other *Bartonella* species were described after 1992, however, and it remains to be seen whether the primers described in that report also amplify other *Bartonella* spp. Another sensitive method is the amplification of a part of the 16S rRNA gene with universal primers (broad-range PCR) that is followed by direct sequencing of the PCR product; this allows detection of all *Bartonella* and other bacterial species in normally sterile clinical specimens (191).

Large differences were found in the sensitivities of these assays depending on the primers used and on whether fresh (sensitivities ranging from 60-100%) or formalin-fixed, paraffin-embedded (sensitivities ranging from 43-78%) tissues were investigated (138).

Using a semi-quantitative, species-specific PCR-enzyme immunoassay, the approximate numbers of CFU (colony forming units) in clinical specimens from patients with CSD or BAP were calculated to range between 10^3-10^6 CFU/ml. (186).

D. Isolation and culture of *Bartonella* spp.

The number of positive diagnoses for *Bartonella* infections has increased dramatically in the recent years. Most diagnoses are obtained with the use of serological or PCR-based methods. *Bartonella* species are difficult to cultivate. Only a few *B. henselae* isolates have been obtained worldwide from the lymph nodes of patients who suffer from CSD (43,163,192). Blood cultures of these patients are usually sterile. Recently, the first isolate of *B. henselae* was cultured from a patient with Parinaud's oculoglandular syndrome (51). Two *B. quintana* isolates were obtained from two patients with chronic lymphadenopathy: one isolate from a blood culture and one isolate from an osteomedullar biopsy sample (192). Most human *Bartonella* isolates were isolated from blood cultures or biopsies of patients with BAP (81,147,192) and some isolates are obtained from untreated patients with *Bartonella* endocarditis (83,84,192). Successful isolation of organisms from human specimens requires the collection of specimens very early in the course of illness and before antibiotic treatment. Attempts to isolate *Bartonella* from blood cultures (especially in immunocompromised patients, patients with FUO, or systemic CSD) or homogenized tissues (biopsies or aspirates from lymph nodes, liver, spleen, skin, and bone marrow) should be encouraged, however, in order to provide isolates for further clinical, drug resistance, and epidemiological studies.

1. Culture on solid media

Growth of *Bartonella* species is hemin-dependent, and growth occurs best on blood-enriched media in a humid atmosphere containing 5-10% CO_2. The plates are incubated at 35-37°C except in the case of *B. bacilliformis* which prefers a growth temperature of 25-30°C and a hemin- and cysteine-containing blood agar. A large number of different agar formulations have been reported which facilitate the isolation of *B. henselae* and *B. quintana*: standard chocolate agar plates, commercial brain heart infusion agar (BHIA) containing 5% sheep blood, tryptic soy agar (TSA) supplemented with 5% sheep blood, heart infusion agar (HIA) containing 5% rabbit blood, and Columbia blood agar (15,16,192,193). The quality and the origin (sheep or rabbit) of the blood that is used may influence the growth of *Bartonella* spp., but it is more important to use agar plates which are as fresh as possible (preferably less than four days old) and to preserve the moisture content of the medium by sealing the plates with parafilm or shrink seal after the first 24 hrs. of incubation. This procedure additionally prevents the plates from becoming environmentally contaminated with molds or other rapidly-growing bacteria which could destroy the cultures during the long incubation period.

Isolation of *Bartonella* species from human specimens is quite difficult, time-consuming, and unreliable, and it requires special laboratory procedures. *Bartonella* species are very fastidious, slow-growing bacteria, and successful primary isolation requires a prolonged incubation time of at least 4-6 weeks. Routine bacterial culture protocols usually do not result in the isolation of *Bartonella* strains. Primary isolates are not detectable before 6-12 days of incubation (81,100), and isolation after prolonged incubation periods of up to 21-45 days have been reported (150). Repeated subcultures reduce the time that is necessary for visible growth from two weeks to 3-4 days. Primary cultures of *Bartonella* spp. on solid media yield colonies that are very small (0.2-3.0 mm in diameter), grow very heterogen-

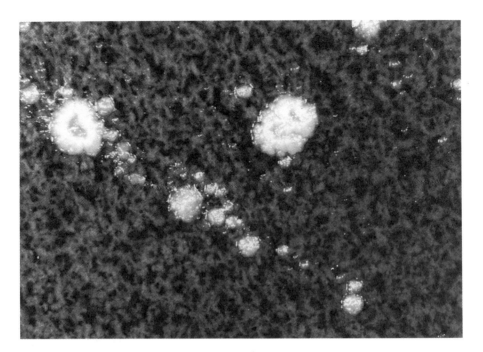

Figure 1   Rough and smooth colonies of *B. clarridgeiae* as cultured on Columbia blood agar plates for ten days at 37°C.

eously, and form irregular rough (cauliflower-like) and/or circular smooth colonies (Figure 1). They are whitish-cream colored, often highly adherent, and deeply imbedded in the agar. Therefore, the first sub-cultivation may be very difficult. Even experienced laboratories have lost isolates due to the inability to obtain further subcultures (100,129,192). After several (4-5) successful passages, however, the isolates adapt to the agar medium and can be easily subcultured; the colonies become smooth, shiny, and less adherent.

2.   Blood culture systems

Most isolates of *B. henselae* and *B. quintana* from blood have been obtained by collecting blood in EDTA or, preferably, in lysis-centrifugation systems (Isolator™ blood-lysis tubes, Wampole, Cranbury, New Jersey). Isolator™ tubes contain saponin which lyses erythrocytes and leukocytes; this is a procedure which seems to be effective since *B. henselae* and *B. bacilliformis* are known to reside within erythrocytes (112,151). The lysis-centrifugation system has been reported to be more sensitive than the direct plating of EDTA-blood onto agar plates. Lysing the erythrocytes by freezing the EDTA-blood samples was even more effective than using the Isolator™ tubes (194). Automated blood culture systems (BacT/Alert™, Bactec™) for isolation of *Bartonella* species have also been used successfully (195,196), but bacterial growth usually is not indicated in the system because of the low amount of CO_2 produced. Bacterial presence can be demonstrated by the detection of twitching, motile, pleomorphic bacilli on wet preparations or by routine acridine orange staining (195,196). Subculturing onto solid media is recommended after one week of incubation in these automated systems. The use of Isolator™ tubes seems to be the optimal procedure for the isolation of *Bartonella* species from blood cultures. Within a few hours, the centrifuged sediment should be plated onto freshly prepared agar plates, preferably both chocolate agar plates and rabbit heart infusion agar plates.

3. Cell culture systems

Isolation of *Bartonella* species by co-cultivation in different cell cultures has been described. These include bovine endothelial cells (78) and immortalized human endothelial cells (165). Subculturing of the isolates onto agar plates for further identification, however, was reported to be difficult; routine microbiological laboratories may lack the systems that are required. Co-cultivation on cell culture systems may be used as an additional method to enhance recovery of *Bartonella* species.

There is to date no gold standard for the diagnosis of *Bartonella* infections. Therefore, it may be necessary to combine serological, PCR-based, culture, and histopathological investigations in order to confirm the diagnosis of a *Bartonella* infection.

E. Identification of *Bartonella* isolates.

1. Microscopic examination

Bartonella spp. are Gram negative, pleomorphic, small, slightly curved rods measuring 0.6 to 1.0 μm. (Figure 2). They tend to auto-adhere and form clumps on microscopic slides. *B. henselae* and *B. quintana* may have pili and appear to have a twitching motility on wet preparations. *B. clarridgeiae* and *B. bacilliformis* possess multiple, unipolar flagellae.

2. Biochemical characteristics

Bartonella spp. are fastidious bacilli and, in general, biochemically inert. They are catalase, oxidase, indole, and urea negative, and do not produce acid from carbohydrates such as glucose, fructose, lactose, inositol, maltose, mannose, mannitol, melibiose, raffinose, rhamnose, and sucrose in conventional biochemical test systems. Gelatin hydrolysis, esculin hydrolysis, citrate, and indole production, as well as the Voges-Proskauer reactions, are negative. Enzyme activities are detectable using test kits which are primarily designed for anaerobic organisms (Table 7). None of the various commercially available identification systems contain *Bartonella* spp. in their databases, but identification to the genus level seems to be possible in some systems. Gram staining of the isolate is absolutely necessary because some strains of *Corynebacterium* species may have identical reaction profiles (100). A reliable differentiation

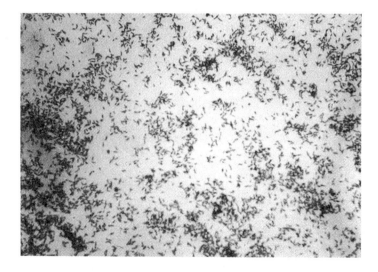

Figure 2   Gram-stained *B. henselae* showing pleomorphic, slightly curved, small rods.

Table 7 Biotype codes of different commercial systems for identification of human pathogenic *Bartonella* spp.

System	Biotype codes				
	B. henselae	*B. quintana*	*B. clarridgeiae*	*B. elizabethae*	*B. bacilliformis*
RapID ANA II System	000671	00067/41	004671	00067/61	00067/41
Rapid ID 32 A	0000073705	0000073705	0001073705	0000073705	0000073705
MicroScan Rapid Anaerobe Panel	10077640	10077/3640	ND	ND	10077240
An-IDENT System	0004032	0004032	ND	ND	0004032
Rapid-STREP	0040000	0040000	0040000	0040000	0040000

ND = not done

on the species level is not possible in any of these systems. Concerning the RapID ANA II System, enzymatic hydrolysis of proline-ß-naphthylamide (PRO) and phenylalanine-ß-naphthylamide (PAL) is usually less pronounced, and the intensity of the reaction depends on the density of the inoculum. The reactions are clearly positive, however, when they are compared with those in the IDS RapID ANA II System color chart. A strong enzymatic hydrolysis of leucyl-glycine-ß-naphthylamide (LGY), glycine-ß-naphthylamide (GLY), arginine-ß-naphthylamide (ARG), and serine-ß-naphthylamide (SER) is detectable (193). Biochemical testing, especially detection of enzyme activities, should be performed only on young (not older than four to maximum five days) well-grown colonies, because false negative results have been observed with older cultures.

3. Protein profiles (SDS-PAGE analysis)

Each of the *Bartonella* species has been shown to have its own protein profile. *B. bacilliformis* and *B. clarridgeiae* are flagellated, and the FlaA proteins of these species have been characterized as 42 kD and 41 kD proteins respectively. Distinct protein profiles were demonstrated for *B. henselae, B. quintana, B. clarridgeiae, B. bacilliformis*, and *B. elizabethae*, whereas very similar protein profiles were found in different isolates of the same species (193).

4. Cellular fatty acid analysis

Whole-cell fatty acid analysis provides a useful tool for the identification of *Bartonella* at the genus level. Organisms are cultivated on blood-containing agar plates. Well-grown colonies should be harvested after four to five days of incubation. Gas-liquid chromatography profiles are relatively typical for *Bartonella* species, and the major fatty acids include *cis*-11-octadecanoic acid (C18:1ω7c), octadecanoic acid (C18:0), and hexadecanoic acid (C16:0) (15-17,43,100,147, 149). Fatty acid profiles of *B. henselae, B. quintana*, and *B. clarridgeiae* are very similar, and CFA analysis cannot be used to distinguish between the three species(149). The three species mentioned each contain a large amount of C18:0, whereas *B. elizabethae* has a higher proportion of C17:0. The fatty acid composition of *B. bacilliformis* differs completely from that of the other species, and maintains more C16:1ω7c and very few C18:0 acids (149,193). The major fatty acids found in *Bartonella* species are shown in Table 8.

5. PCR-based methods

Identification of *Bartonella* isolates by PCR-based methods are already described in IV. A. and VI. C. sections. All of the fingerprint methods presented, as well as the PCR-based diagnostic methods, are useful for species identification. Since biochemical methods, determination of protein profiles, and CFA-analysis of *Bartonella* isolates cannot be considered suitable for the differentiation of species, molecular-based methods remain so far the only effective way to identify *Bartonella* spp.

VII. SUSCEPTIBILITY TESTING

A. In vitro susceptibility

Bartonella species are fastidious slow-growing bacteria, and standardized susceptibility testing guidelines are not as yet recommended (e.g., by committees such as or corresponding to the National Committee for Clinical Laboratory Standards, U.S.). Due to the limited number of strains that have been isolated worldwide, very little susceptibility testing data has been obtained for *Bartonella* spp.

Determination of the minimum inhibitory concentrations (MICs) of four *B. bacilliformis* isolates with the use of an agar dilution technique showed high susceptibility to most beta-lactams (except oxacillin, cephalothin, and cefotetan), macrolides (erythromycin, azithromycin, clarithromycin, and roxithromycin), rifampin, doxycycline, fluoroquinolones (ciprofloxacin and sparfloxacin), and aminoglycosides. Fosfomycin, colistin, clindamycin, and vancomycin have been rather ineffective in inhibiting bacterial growth (197).

Using an antibiotic agar dilution method which is based on a Columbia agar base that is supplemented with 5% horse blood (198), or a Mueller-Hinton agar supplemented with 5% sheep blood (199), comparable antibiotic susceptibilities have been shown for isolates of *B. henselae*, *B. quintana*, *B. vinsonii*, and *B. elizabethae*. In vitro, the different *Bartonella* spp. were highly susceptible to penicillin G, aminopenicillins, third-generation cephalosporins, macrolides, ciprofloxacin, tetracyclines, trimethoprim-sulfamethoxazole, and rifampicin. Penicillinase-resistant penicillins, first-generation cephalospo-

Table 8 Whole-cell fatty acid analysis of human pathogenic *Bartonella* spp. (149,193).

	16:1ω7c	16:0	17:0	18:1ω7c/ω9t/ω12t	18:0
		% CFA methyl ester			
B. henselae	0-1	16-23	0-3	48-59	19-36
B. quintana	0-1	15-23	0-5	48-56	16-32
B. clarridgeiae	0-1	12-19	2-3	39-57	23-26
B. elizabethae	1	24-25	14-19	38-41	11-12
B. bacilliformis	17-21	22-28	0	40-52	2

rins, and clindamycin have been less effective. Ciprofloxacin and sparfloxacin were the most potent of the fluoroquinolones, and of the aminoglycosides, gentamicin was shown to be more active than amikacin.

Similar results were obtained by using the Etest™ method (AB Biodisk, Solna, Sweden) for susceptibility testing of feline *B. henselae* isolates. Due to the fastidious nature of the bacteria, a longer incubation time is required (mean 4 to 5 days) before bacterial growth becomes visible. Of the 10 and 16 *B. henselae* isolates that were tested on chocolate agar plates in two different studies (200 and 100, respectively), the MICs were < 0.016 mg./L. for azithromycin, <0.016-0.023 mg./L. for both erythromycin and doxycycline, 0.016-1.00 mg./L. for tetracycline, 0.25-5.0 mg./L. for ciprofloxacin, 0.003-0.012 mg./L. for rifampicin, and 1-6 mg./L. for vancomycin. Surprisingly, vancomycin, which is only known to be effective against Gram positive bacteria, showed MICs close to the break point of 4 mg./L. for most of the isolates tested.

These data should be considered critically, however, because of the limited number of strains tested. In vitro results may not necessarily correlate with clinical responses, and therefore should not be used exclusively as a guide for therapy. The facultative intracellular life-style of *Bartonella* spp., and the actual immune status of infected patients may influence the outcome of antibiotic therapy. Development of resistance, particularly in the case of relapsing infection, has not yet been investigated.

B. Treatment of *Bartonella* infections

Untreated Oroya fever has one of the highest fatality rates of all infectious diseases and will result in death in 40-88% of patients. This high death rate is due to the rapidly progressing acute hemolysis, a variably induced immune deficiency, and in some cases, late diagnosis of the illness (1,33,201). Although *B. bacilliformis* is highly susceptible to many antibiotics in vitro, chloramphenicol was selected for successful treatment of Oroya fever in 1955, and since then, it has been the most commonly-used drug. It is the drug of choice, given in a daily dosage of 2 gm. or more for a minimum of 7 days (202). Chloramphenicol, a highly effective broad-spectrum antimicrobial agent, is very active against many Gram positive and Gram negative bacteria, including *Salmonella* and other agents of secondary infections which may accompany the acute stage of Carrion's disease. In an outbreak of Oroya fever in Peru in 1990, 14 of 16 patients (88%) who received no antibiotic treatment died, whereas no deaths occurred in the ten patients treated with chloramphenicol (201). Penicillin G, tetracyclines, and, more recently, macrolides (erythromycin and roxithromycin) as well as ciprofloxacin have been used successfully in the treatment of Oroya fever (197,203). Fever usually disappears within 24 hrs., although bacteremia may persist for a longer time (202). Chloramphenicol does not prevent the appearance of verruga peruana, however, and it seems to be ineffective in the treatment of verrugas (203). Streptomycin (2 mg./kg. of body weight/day for 10 days) is considered the drug of choice in this second stage of Carrión's disease, and rifampin has been proposed as an alternative (197,203). The benefit of chemotherapy, however, has not been clearly proven since verrugas usually disappear spontaneously within several months.

Trench fever was successfully treated in the past with tetracyclines and chloramphenicol, but relapses have been observed in some patients. Chloramphenicol is no longer recommended for the treatment of *B. quintana* infections, however, because it causes side effects like bone marrow toxicity, and because newer antimicrobial agents are available.

B. quintana and *B. henselae* are both etiological agents of BAP. Antimicrobial therapy of BAP, which occurs mostly in immunocompromised patients, is absolutely indicated. Erythromycin in a dose of 250 to 500 mg; four times/day is considered the drug of choice. Alternatively, newer macrolides (azithromycin) and tetracyclines (doxycycline and minocycline) have been successfully used. In severely ill patients, erythromycin or doxycycline may be used in combination with rifampin. A few case reports have described the successful treatment of BAP with third-generation cephalosporins, trimethoprim-sulfamethoxazole, or quinolones, but there has been no widespread use of these antibiotics for this purpose. Penicillins and first-generation cephalosporins are not effective. Of crucial significance is the duration of treatment. Relapses of *Bartonella* infections often occur when the period of treatment has been too short. In patients who suffer only from cutaneous BA, an antimicrobial treatment lasting at least two months is indicated. Patients with peliosis hepatis or other organ involvement (e.g., osteomyelitis) should receive antibiotics for at least four months. A Jarisch-Herxheimer reaction after initiation of therapy is described (204). If relapse occurs in HIV-infected patients, however, extended treatment with erythromycin or doxycycline is recommended (204).

Treatment of cat scratch disease depends on the severity of the illness. Antibiotic therapy in immunocompetent patients who suffer from typical CSD is usually not indicated. In general, lymph nodes resolve spontaneously within two to four months with or without antibiotic treatment. Conservative, symptomatic treatment is recommended for the majority of patients with mild or moderate CSD (205). Due to the self-limiting nature of CSD, it is very difficult to judge the effectiveness of an antimicrobial therapy in these patients. In suppurative lymph nodes, needle aspiration may be of value for decompression. Antibiotic treatment is indicated in patients with prolonged high fever and severe systemic symptoms, malaise, headache, or blindness (atypical CSD). In a retrospective study of 268 patients, for which eighteen different antimicrobials had been prescribed, only four were shown to be seemingly effective: rifampin (oral, 87%), ciprofloxacin (oral, 84%), trimethoprim-sulfamethoxazole (oral, 58%), and gentamicin (intramuscular, 73%) (205). Collipp (206) summarized the treatment of 101 patients with CSD and reported good therapeutic results in patients who were treated with trimethoprim-sulfamethoxazole. Based on the in vitro bactericidal activity of aminoglycosides, gentamicin is recommended by some authors for antibiotic therapy of CSD (207). Due to the ototoxicity, nephrotoxicity, and low intracellular penetration of aminoglycosides, however, they should not be considered as the drugs of choice for treatment of typical CSD. Additionally, ciprofloxacin should probably not be prescribed for children or adolescents under the age of eighteen years because of possible arthropathy.

Recently, the first prospective randomized, double-blind, placebo-controlled study on the treatment of typical CSD with azithromycin was reported (208). Oral azithromycin taken for 5 days (500 mg. on day one and 250 mg. on days 2-5 as single daily doses) was shown to provide some clinical benefit by decreasing lymph node size to 20% of the initial volume within the first 4 weeks of treatment (in 7 of 14 azithromycin-treated patients and in only 1 of 15 placebo-treated patients, respectively). In some patients in the azithromycin-treated group, however, new enlarged lymph nodes appeared and some increased in size during therapy. In the placebo-treated group, all lymph nodes resolved within 140 days, whereas in the azithromycin-treated group, twelve had lymph node hypertrophy that resolved within 130 days. In the last two patients, resolution took 190 and 210 days respectively. All together these results should encourage the use of this antibiotic for the treatment of symptomatic cases of CSD even if the lymph node enlargements do not disappear within a few days.

Few patients with *Bartonella*-induced endocarditis are reported in the literature, and the diagnosis was obtained in many cases retrospectively by the detection of *Bartonella*-DNA in the native valves. Although most of these illnesses have been treated as recommended for culture-negative endocarditis, with an aminoglycoside and ß-lactam compound, valve replacement could not be prevented. In some cases, surgical treatment was followed by long-term therapy with erythromycin.

REFERENCES

1. Cáceres-Ríos H, Rodríguez-Tafur J, Bravo-Puccio F, Mauina-Vargas C, Sanguineti Díaz C, Ramos DC, Patarca R. Verruga Peruana: an infectious endemic angiomatosis. Crit Rev Oncog 1995; 6:47-56.
2. Garcia-Caceres U, Garcia FU. Bartonellosis. An immunodepressive disease and the life of Daniel Alcides Carrión. Am J Clin Pathol 1991; 95 (Suppl 1):S58-S66.
3. Schultz MG. Daniel Carrion's experiment. N Engl J Med 1968; 278:1323-1326.
4. Allison MJ, Pezzia A, Gerszten E, Mendoza D. A case of Carrión's disease associated with human sacrifice from the Huari culture of southern Peru. Am J Phys Anthropol 1985; 41:295-300.

5. Ellis BA, Rotz LD, Leake JA, Samalvides F, Bernable J, Ventura G, Padilla C, Villaseca P, Beati L, Regnery R, Childs JE, Olson JG, Carillo CP. An outbreak of acute bartonellosis (Oroya fever) in the Urubamba region in Peru, 1998. Am J Trop Med Hyg 1999; 61:344-349.
6. Werner H, Haenssler E. Über Fünftagefieber, febris quintana. Münch med Wochenschrift 1916; 63:1020-1023.
7. Munk F, da Rocha-Lima H. Klinik und Aetiologie des sogen. „Wolhynischen Fiebers". (Werner-Hissche Krankheit) I. Klinischer Teil. Münch Med Wochenschr 1917; 64:1357-1361.
8. Munk F, da Rocha-Lima H. Klinik und Aetiologie des sogen. „Wolhynischen Fiebers". (Werner-Hissche Krankheit). II. Ergebnis der ätiologischen Untersuchung und deren Beziehung zur Fleckfieberforschung. Münch Med Wochenschr. 1917; 64:1422-1426.
9. Werner H, Benzler F, Wiese O. Zur Aetiologie des Fünftagefiebers. Münch Med Wochenschrift 1916; 63:1359-1370.
10. Schmincke RA. Histopathologischer Befund in Roseolen der Haut bei Wolhynischem Fieber. Münch Med Wochenschr 1917; 64:961.
11. Jungmann P, Kuczynski MH. Zur Klinik und Aetiologie der Febris wolhynica (His-Wernersche Krankheit). Dtsch med Wochenschr 1917; 12:358-62.
12. Vinson JW, Fuller HS. Studies on trench fever. 1. Propagation of rickettsia-like organisms form a patients blood. Pathol Microbiol 1961; 24:S152-S166.
13. Relman DA, Loutit JS, Schmidt TM, Falkow S, Tompkins LS. The agent of bacillary angiomatosis. An approach to the identification of uncultured pathogens. N Engl J Med 1990; 323:1573-1580.
14. Slater LN, Welch DF, Hensel D, Coody DW. A newly recognized fastidious gram-negative pathogen as a cause of fever and bacteremia. N Engl J Med 1990; 323:1587-1593.
15. Welch DF, Pickett DA, Slater LN, Steigerwalt AG, Brenner DJ. *Rochalimaea henselae* sp. nov., a cause of septicemia, bacillary angiomatosis, and parenchymal bacillary peliosis. J Clin Microbiol 1992; 30:275-280.
16. Regnery RL, Anderson BE, Clarridge JE, Rodriguez-Barradas MC, Jones DC, Carr JH. Characterization of a novel *Rochalimaea* species, *R. henselae* sp. nov., isolated from blood of a febrile, human immunodeficienty virus-positive patient. J Clin Microbiol 1992; 30:265-274.
17. Daly JS, Worthington MG, Brenner DJ, Moss CW, Hollis DG, Weyant RS, Steigerwalt AG, Weaver RE, Daneshvar MI, O'Connor SP. *Rochalimaea elizabethae* sp. nov. isolated from a patient with endocarditis. J Clin Microbiol 1993; 31:872-881.
18. Baker JA. A rickettsial infection in Canadian voles. J Exp Med 1946; 84:37-50.
19. Brenner DJ, O'Connor SP, Winkler HH, Steigerwalt AG. Proposals to unify the genera *Bartonella* and *Rochalimaea*, with descriptions of *Bartonella quintana* comb. nov., *Bartonella vinsonii* comb. nov., *Bartonella henselae* comb. nov., and *Bartonella elizabethae* comb. nov., and to remove the family *Bartonellaceae* from the order *Rickettsiales*. Int J Syst Bacteriol 1993; 43:777-786.
20. Birtles RJ, Harrison TG, Saunders NA, Molyneux DH. Proposals to unify the genera *Grahamella* and *Bartonella*, with descriptions of *Bartonella talpae* comb. nov., *Bartonella peromysci* comb. nov., and three new species, *Bartonella grahammii* sp. nov., *Bartonella taylorii* sp. nov., and *Bartonella doshiae* sp. nov. Int J Syst Bacteriol 1995; 45:1-8.
21. Barton AL. Cuerpos endoglobulares en la sangre verrucosa. Gaceta de los Hospitales 1905; 18:35-39.
22. Brumpt E. Note sur le parasite des hematies de la taupe: *Grahamella talpae* n.g. n.sp. Bull Soc Pathol Exot 1911; 4:514-517.
23. Tyzzer EE. A comparison study of *Grahamellae*, *Haemobartonellae* and *Eperythrozoa* in small mammals. Proc Am Phil Soc 1942; 85:359-398.
24. Kordick DL, Swaminathan B, Greene CE, Wilson KH, Whitney AM, O'Connor S, Hollis DG, Matar GM, Steigerwalt AG, Malcolm GB, Hayes PS, Hadfield TL, Breitschwerdt EB, Brenner DJ. *Bartonella vinsonii* subsp. *berkhoffii* subsp. nov., isolated from dogs; *Bartonella vinsonii* subsp. *vinsonii*; and emended description of *Bartonella vinsonii*. Int J Syst Bacteriol 1996; 46:704-709.
25. Lawson PA, Collins MD. Description of *Bartonella clarridgeiae* sp. nov. isolated from the cat of a patient with *Bartonella henselae* septicemia. Med Microbiol Lett 1996; 5:64-73.
26. Heller R, Riegel Ph, Hausmann Y, Delacour G, Bermond D, Dehio C, Lamarque F, Monteil H, Chomel B, Piemont Y. *Bartonella tribocorum* sp. nov., a new *Bartonella* species isolated from the blood of wild rats. Inter J Syst Bacteriol 1998; 48:1333-1339.
27. Heller R, Kubina M, Mariet P, Riegel P, Delacour G, Dehio C, Lamarque F, Kasten R, Boulouis H-J, Monteil H, Chomel B, Piemont Y. *Bartonella alsatica* sp. nov., a new *Bartonella* species isolated from the blood of wild rabbits. Int J Syst Bacteriol 1999; 49:283-288.

28. Droz S, Chi B, Horn E, Steigerwalt AG, Whitney AM, Brenner DJ. *Bartonella koehlerae* sp. nov., isolated from cats. J Clin Microbiol 1999; 37:1117-1122.

29. Welch DF, Carroll KC, Hofmeister EK, Persing DH, Robinson DA, Steigerwalt AG, Brenner DJ. Isolation of a new subspecies, *Bartonella vinsonii* subsp. *arupensis*, from a cattle rancher: identity with isolates found in conjunction with *Borrelia burgdorferi* and *Babesia microti* among naturally infected mice. J Clin Microbiol 1999; 37:2598-2601.

30. Heller R, Bermond D, Delacour G, Boulouis HJ, Chomel B, Piemont Y. Distribution of *Bartonella* in European wild mammals. 1st International Conference on *Bartonella* as Emerging Pathogens. Tübingen, Germany, March 5-7, 1999. J Microbiol Meth 1999; 37:279-280.

31. Chomel BB, Kasten RW, Yamamoto K, Chang C, Honadel TE, Kikuchi Y. Epidemiology of *Bartonella* infections in domestic and wild carnivores and ruminants. 1st International Conference on *Bartonella* as Emerging Pathogens. Tübingen, Germany, March 5-7, 1999. J Microbiol Meth 1999; 37:280-281.

32. Schouls LM, van de Pol I, Rijpkema SGT, Schot CS. Detection and identification of *Ehrlichia*, *Borrelia burgdorferi* sensu lato, and *Bartonella* species in Dutch *Ixodes ricinus* ticks. J Clin Microbiol 1999; 37:2215-2222.

33. Ihler GM. *Bartonella bacilliformis*: dangerous pathogen slowly emerging from deep background. FEMS Microbiol Lett 1996; 144:1-11.

34. Hurtado A, Musso J, Merino C. La maladie de la enfermedad de Carrión (verruga peruana). Anales de la Facultad de Medicina de Lima 1938; 28:154-168.

35. Ricketts WE. Clinical manifestations of Carrión's disease. Arch Intern Med 1949; 84:751-781.

36. Irrivaren J, Carcelen A, Gotuzzo E. Toxoplasmosis en Bartonellosis. XIV Congreso: de TBC y Torax Arequipa Peru 1981; 189.

37. Pinkerton H, Weinman D. *Toxoplasma* infection in man. Arch Pathol 1940; 30:374-392.

38. Weiss P. Hacia una concepción de la verruga peruana. Annals of the Faculty of Medicine of Lima 1926; 9:279-300.

39. Debré R, Lamy M, Jammet ML, Costil L, Mozziconacci P. La maladie des griffes de chat. Bull Mem Soc Med Hop Paris 1950; 66:76-79.

40. English CJ, Wear DJ, Margileth AM, Lissner CR, Walsh GP. Cat-scratch disease: isolation and culture of the bacterial agent. JAMA 1988; 259:1347-1352.

41. Regnery R, Martin M, Olson J. Naturally occuring "Rochalimaea henselae" infection in domestic cats. Lancet 1992; 340:557-558.

42. Regnery RL, Olson JG, Perkins BA, Bibb W. Serological response to "Rochalimaea henselae" antigen in suspected cat-scratch disease. Lancet 1992; 339:1443-1445.

43. Dolan MJ, Wong MT, Regnery RL, Jorgensen JH, Garcia M, Peters J, Drehner D. Syndrome of *Rochalimaea henselae* adenitis suggesting cat scratch disease. Ann Intern Med 1993; 118:331-336.

44. Bass JW, Vincent JM, Person DA. The expanding spectrum of *Bartonella* infections: II Cat-scratch disease. Pediatr Infect Dis J 1997; 16:163-179.

45. Carithers HA. Cat scratch disease: an overview based on a study of 1200 patients. Am J Dis Child 1985; 139:1124-1133.

46. Hamilton DH, Zangwill KM, Hadler HL, Cartter ML. Cat-scratch disease–Connecticut, 1992-1993. J Infect Dis 1995; 172:570-573.

47. Parinaud H. Conjonctivite infectieuse transmise par les animaux. Annales d'Oculistique 1889; 101:252-253.

48. Carithers HA. Oculoglandular disease of Parinaud. A manifestation of cat scratch disease. Am J Dis Child 1978; 132:1195-1200.

49. Margileth AM. Cat scratch disease as a cause of the oculoglandular syndrome of Parinaud. Pediatrics 1957; 20:1000-1005.

50. Wear DJ, Malaty RH, Zimmermann LE, Hadfield TE, Margileth AM. Cat scratch disease bacilli in the conjunctiva of patients with Parinaud's oculoglandular syndrome. Ophthalmolology 1985; 92:1282-1287.

51. Grando D, Sullivan LJ, Flexman JP, Watson MW, Andrew JH. *Bartonella henselae* associated with Parinaud's oculoglandular syndrome. Clin Infect Dis 1999; 28:1156-1158.

52. Dondey JC, Sullivan TJ, Robson JMB, Gatto J. Application of polymerase chain reaction assay in the diagnosis of orbital granuloma complicating atypical oculoglandular cat scratch disease. Ophthalmology 1997; 104:1174-1178.

53. Le HH, Paslay DA, Anderson B, Steinberg JP. Conjunctival swab to diagnose ocular cat scratch disease. Am J Ophthalmol 1994; 118:249-250.

54. Kessler DF, Cruz OA. Serologic confirmation of *Rochalimaea* in cat scratch disease. Ann Ophthalmol 1995; 27:33-35.

55. Kerkhoff FT, Ossewaarde JM, de Loos WS, Rothova A. Presumed ocular bartonellosis. Br J Ophthalmol 1999; 83:270-275.

56. Ness T, Pünder M, Sander A. Ocular Manifestations of *Bartonella* Infection. 1st International Conference on Bartonella as Emerging Pathogens. Tübingen, Germany. March 5-7, 1999. J Microbiol Meth 1999; 37:270.

57. Reed BJ, Scales DK, Wong MT, Lattuada CP, Dolan MJ, Schwab IR. *Bartonella henselae* neuroretinitis in cat scratch disease. Diagnosis, management and sequelae. Ophthalmology 1998; 105:459-466.

58. O'Halloran HS, Draud K, Minix M, Rivard AK, Pearson PA. Leber's neuroretinitis in a patient with serological evidence of *Bartonella elizabethae*. Retina 1998; 18:276-278.

59. Arisoy ES, Correa AG, Wagner ML, Kaplan SL. Hepatosplenic cat scratch disease in children: Selected clinical features and treatment. Clin Infect Dis 1999; 28:778-784.

60. Ventura A, Massei F, Not T, Massimetti M, Bussani R, Maggiore G. Systemic *Bartonella henselae* infection with hepatosplenic involvement. J Pediatr Gastroenterol Nutr 1999; 29:52-56.

61. Dunn MW, Berkowitz FE, Miller JJ, Snitzer JA. Hepatosplenic cat-scratch disease and abdominal pain. Pediatr Infect Dis J 1997; 16:269-272.

62. Jacobs RF, Schutze GE. *Bartonella henselae* as a cause of prolonged fever and fever of unknown origin in children. Clin Infect Dis 1998; 26:80-84.

63. Marra CM. Neurologic complications of *Bartonella henselae* infection. Curr Opin Neurol 1995; 8:164-169.

64. Carithers HA, Margileth AM. Cat-scratch disease: acute encephalopathy and other neurological manifestations. Am J Dis Child 1991; 145:98-101.

65. Easley RB, Cooperstock MS, Tobias JD. Cat-scratch disease causing status epilepticus in children. South Med J 1999; 92:73-76.

66. Noah DL, Bresee JS, Gorensek MJ, Rooney JA, Cresanta JL, Regnery RL, Wong J, del Toro J, Olson JG, Childs JE. Cluster of five children with acute encephalopathy associated with cat scratch disease in south Florida. Pediatr Infect Dis J 1995; 14:866-869.

67. Waldvogel K, Regnery RL, Anderson BE, Caduff R, Caduff J, Nadal D. Disseminated cat-scratch disease: detection of *Rochalimaea henselae* in affected tissue. Eur J Pediatr 1994; 153:23-27.

68. Robson JMB, Herte GH, Osborne DRS, McCormack JG. Cat-scratch disease with paravertebral mass and osteomyelitis. Clin Infect Dis 1999; 28:274-278.

69. Sander A, Frank B. Paronychia caused by *Bartonella henselae*. Lancet 1997; 350:1078.

70. Anderson BE, Neuman MA. *Bartonella* spp. as emerging human pathogens. Clin Microbiol Rev 1997; 10:203-219.

71. Spach DH, Koehler JE. *Bartonella*-associated infections. Emerg Infect Dis 1998; 12:137-155.

72. Drancourt M, Moal V, Brunet P, Dussol B, Berland Y, Raoult D. *Bartonella* (*Rochalimaea*) *quintana* infection in a seronegative hemodialyzed patient. J Clin Microbiol 1996; 34:1158-1160.

73. Raoult D, Drancourt M, Carta A, Gastaut JA. *Bartonella* (*Rochalimaea*) *quintana* isolation in a patient with chronic adenopathy, lymphopenia and a cat. Lancet 1994; 343:977.

74. Kordick DL, Hilyard EJ, Hadfield TL, Wilson KH, Steigerwald AG, Brenner DJ, Breitschwerdt EB. *Bartonella clarridgeiae*, a newly recognized zoonotic pathogen causing inoculation papules, fever, and lymphadenopathy (cat scratch disease). J Clin Microbiol 1997; 35:1813-1818.

75. Margileth AM, Baehren DF. Chest-wall abscess due to cat-scratch disease (CSD) in an adult with antibodies to *Bartonella clarridgeiae*: case report and review of the thoracopulmonary manifestations of CSD. Clin Infect Dis 1998; 27:353-357.

76. Stoler MH, Bonfiglio TA, Steigbigel MT, Pereira M. An atypical subcutaneous infection associated with acquired immune deficiency syndrome. Am J Clin Pathol 1983; 80:714-718.

77. Koehler JE, Tappero JW. Bacillary angiomatosis and bacillary peliosis in patients with human immunodeficiency virus. Clin Infect Dis 1993; 17:612-624.

78. Koehler JE, Quinn FD, Berger TG, LeBoit PE, Tappero JW. Isolation of *Rochalimaea* species from cutaneous and osseous lesions of bacillary angiomatosis. N Engl J Med 1992; 327:1625-1631.

79. Cockerell CJ. Bacillary angiomatosis and related diseases caused by *Rochalimaea*. J Am Acad Dermatol 1995; 32:783-790.

80. Mohle-Boetani JC, Koehler JE, Berger TG, LeBoit PE, Kemper CA, Reingold AL, Plikaytis BD, Wenger JD, Tappero JW. Bacillary angiomatosis and bacillary peliosis in patients infected with human immunodeficiency virus: clinical characteristics in a case control study. Clin Infect Dis 1996; 22:794-800.

81. Koehler JE, Sanchez MA, Garrido CS, Whitfeld MJ, Chen FM, Berger TG, Rodriguez-Barradas MC, LeBoit PE, Tappero JW. Molecular epidemiology of *Bartonella* infections in patients with bacillary angiomatosis-peliosis. N Engl J Med 1997; 337:1876-1883.

82. Jackson LA, Spach DH, Kippen DA, Sugg NK, Rergnery RL, Sayers MH, Stamm WE. Seroprevalence to *Bartonella quintana* among patients at a community clinic in downtown Seattle. J Infect Dis 1996; 173:1023-1026.

83. Spach DH, Callis KP, Paauw DS, Houze YB, Schoenknecht FD, Welch DF, Rosen H, Brenner DJ. Endocarditis caused by *Rochalimaea quintana* in a patient infected with human immunodeficiency virus. J Clin Microbiol 1993; 31:692-694.

84. Hadfield TL, Warren R, Kass M, Brun E, Levy C. Endocarditis caused by *Rochalimaea henselae*. Hum Pathol 1993; 24:1140-1141.

85. Fournier PE, Raoult D. Cat-scratch disease and an overview of other *Bartonella henselae*-related infections. In: Schmidt A, ed. *Bartonella* and *Afipia* Species Emphasizing *Bartonella henselae*. Basel:Karger, 1998:32-62.

86. Laughlin L, Chamberlin J, Ponce C, Gonzales H, Romero S, Gonzalo A, Watts D, Carillo C. Epidemiology of bartonellosis in Peru: prospective population-based study. 1st International Conference on *Bartonella* as Emerging Pathogens. Tübingen, Germany. March 5-7. 1999. J Microbiol Meth 1999; 37:270-271.

87. Matteelli A, Castelli F, Spinetti A, Bonetti F, Graifenberghi S, Carosi G. Verruga peruana in an Italian traveller from Peru. Am J Trop Med Hyg 1994; 50:143-144.

88. Herrer A. Carrión's disease. II. Presence of *Bartonella bacilliformis* in the peripheral blood of patients with the benign form. Am J Trop Med Hyg. 1953; 2:645-649.

89. Herrer A. Epidemiologia de la verruga peruana. Lima, Pribaceb 1990.

90. Chamberlin J, Gordon S, Laughlin L, Regnery R, Olson J, Romero S, Gonzalo A. Diagnosis of human bartonellosis by indirect fluorescence antibody test. 1st International Conference on *Bartonella* as Emerging Pathogens. Tübingen, Germany, March 5-7, 1999. J Microbiol Meth 1999; 37:275-276.

91. Birtles RJ, Canales J, Alvarez E, Guerra H, Llanos-Cuentas A, Raoult D, Doshi N, Harrison TG. Survey of Bartonella species infecting intradomicillary animals in the Huayllacallan valley Ancash, Peru, a region of endemic for human bartonellosis. Am J Trop Med Hyg 1999; 60:799-805.

92. Carney WP, Gordon SW, Hohenhaus GS, Gozalo A, Watts D, Gonzales A, Regnery RL, Olson JC, Rooney J, Marston EL. Epidemiology of bartonellosis in Peru: Animal reservoirs studies. 1st International Conference on Bartonella as Emerging Pathogens. Tübingen, Germany, March 5-7, 1999. J Microbiol Meth 1999; 37:283-284.

93. Herrer A, Christensen HA. Implication of *Phlebotomus* sand flies as vectors of bartonellosis and leishmaniasis as early as 1764. Science 1975; 190:154-155.

94. Jackson LA, Spach DH. Emergence of *Bartonella quintana* infection among homeless persons. Emerg Infect Dis 1996; 2:141-142.

95. Spach DH, Kanter AS, Dougherty MJ, Larson AM, Coyle MB, Brenner DJ, Swaminathan B, Matar GM, Welch DF, Root RK, Stamm WE. *Bartonella* (*Rochalimaea*) *quintana* bacteremia in inner-city patients with chonic alcoholism. N Engl J Med 1995; 332:424-428.

96. Roux V, Raoult D. Body lice as tools for diagnosis and surveillance of re-emerging diseases. J Clin Microbiol 1999; 37:596-599.

97. Jackson LA, Perkins BA, Wenger JD. Cat scratch disease in the United States: An analysis of three national databases. Am J Public Health 1993; 83:1707-1711.

98. Koehler JE, Glaser CA, Tappero JW. *Rochalimaea henselae* infection. A new zoonosis with the domestic cat as a reservoir. JAMA 1994; 271:531-535.

99. Chomel BB, Abbott RC, Kasten RW, Floyd-Hawkins KA, Kass PH, Glaser CA, Pedersen NC, Koehler JE. *Bartonella henselae* prevalence in domestic cats in California: risk factors and association between bacteremia and antibody titers. J Clin Microbiol 1995; 33:2445-2450.

100. Sander A, Bühler C, Pelz K, von Cramm E, Bredt W. Detection and identification of two *Bartonella henselae* variants in domestic cats in Germany. J Clin Microbiol 1997; 35:584-587.

101. Kordick DL, Wilson KH, Sexton DJ, Hadfield TL, Berkhoff HA, Breitschwerdt EB. Prolonged *Bartonella* bacteremia in cats associated with cat-scratch disease patients. J Clin Microbiol 1995; 33;3245-3251.

102. Chomel BB, Kasten RW, Floyed-Hawkins K, Chi-Yamamoto B, Roberts-Wilson J, Gurfield AN, Abbott RC, Pedersen NC, Koehler JE. Experimental transmission of *Bartonella henselae* by the cat flea. J Clin Microbiol 1996; 34:1952-1956.

103. Maruyama S, Nogami S, Inoue I, Naamba S, Asanome K, Katsube Y. Isolation of *Bartonella henselae* from domestic cats in Japan. J Vet Med Sci 1996; 58:81-83.

104. Branley J, Wolfson C, Waters P, Gottlieb T, Bradbury R. Prevalence of *Bartonella henselae* bacteremia, the causative agent of cat scratch disaese, in an Australian cat population. Pathology 1996; 28:262-265.

105. Heller R, Artois M, Xémar V, De Briel D, Géhin H, Jaulhac B, Monteil H, Piémont Y. Prevalence of *Bartonella henselae* and *Bartonella clarridgeiae* in stray cats. J Clin Microbiol 1997; 35:1327-1331.

106. Bergmans AMC, de Jong DMA, van Amerongen G, Schot CS, Schouls LM. Prevalence of *Bartonella* species in domestic cats in The Netherlands. J Clin Microbiol 1997; 35:2256-2261.

107. Kordick DL, Breitschwerdt EB. Persistent infection of pets within a household with three *Bartonella* species. Emerg Infect Dis 1998; 4:325-328.

108. Kelly PJ, Rooney JJA, Marston EL, Jones DC, Regnery RL. *Bartonella henselae* isolated from cats in Zimbabwe. Lancet 1998; 351:1706.

109. Marston EL, Finkel B, Regnery RL, Winoto IL, Ross Graham R, Wignal S, Simanjuntak G, Olson JO. Prevalence of *Bartonella henselae* and *Bartonella clarridgeiae* in an urban Indonesian cat population. Clin Diagn Lab Immunol 1999; 6:41-44.

110. Chomel BB, Carlos ET, Kasten RW, Yamamoto K, Chang C-C, Carlos RS, Abenes MV, Pajares CM. *Bartonella henselae* and *Bartonella clarridgeiae* infection in domestic cats from the Philippines. Am J Trop Med Hyg 1999; 60:593-597.

111. Maruyama S, Tanaka S, Sakai T, Katsube Y. Prevalence of *Bartonella* species among pet cats in Japan. 1st International Conference on *Bartonella* as Emerging Pathogens. Tübingen, Germany, March 5-7, 1999. J Microbiol Meth 37:284-285.

112. Kordick DL, Breitschwerdt EB. Intraerythrocytic presence of *Bartonella henselae*. J Clin Microbiol. 1995; 33:1655-1656.

113. Zangwill KM, Hamilton DH, Perkins BA, Regnery RL, Plikaytis BD, Hadler JL, Cartter ML, Wenger JD. Cat scratch disease in Connecticut. N Engl J Med 1993; 329:8-13.

114. Childs JE, Rooney JA, Cooper JL, Olson JG, Regnery RL. Epidemiologic observations on infection with *Rochalimaea* species among cats living in Baltimore, MD. J Am Vet Med Assoc 1994; 204:1775-1778.

115. Childs JE, Olson JG, Wolf A, Cohen N, Fakile Y, Rooney JA, Bacellar F, Regnery RL. Prevalence of antibodies to *Rochalimaea* species (cat-scratch disease agent) in cats. Vet Rec 1995; 136:519-520.

116. Allerberger F, Schönbauer M, Regnery RL, Dierich M. Prävalenz von Rochalimaea henselae-Antikörpern bei Katzen in Österreich. Wien Tierärztl Mschr 1995; 82:40-43.

117. Jameson P, Greene C, Regnery R, Dryden M, Marks A, Brown J, Cooper J, Glaus B, Greene R. Prevalence of *Bartonella henselae* antibodies in pet cats throughout regions of North America. J Infect Dis 1995; 172:1145-1149.

118. Ueno H, Muramatsu Y, Chomel BB, Hohdatsu T, Koyama H, Morita C. Seroepidemiological survey of *Bartonella* (*Rochalimaea*) *henselae* in domestic cats in Japan. Microbiol Immunol 1995; 39:339-341.

119. Kelly PJ, Matthewman LA, Hayter D, Downey S, Wray K, Bryson NR, Raoult D. *Bartonella* (*Rochalimaea*) *henselae* in southern Africa – evidence for infections in domestic cats and implications for veterinarians. J S Afr Vet Assoc 1996; 67:182-187.

120. Baneth G, Kordick DL, Hegarty BC, Breitschwerdt EB. Comparative seroreactivity to *Bartonella henselae* and *Bartonella quintana* among cats from Israel and North Carolina. Vet Microbiol 1996; 50:95-103.

121. Glaus T, Hofmann-Lehmann R, Greene C, Glaus B, Wolfensberger C, Lutz H. Seroprevalence of *Bartonella henselae* in cats in Switzerland. J Clin Microbiol 1997; 35:2883-2885.

122. Maruyama S, Hiraga S, Yokoyama E, Naoi M, Tsuruoka Y, Ogura Y, Tamura K, Namba S, Kameyama Y, Nakamura S, Katsube Y. Seroprevalence of *Bartonella henselae* and *Toxoplasma gondii* infections among pet cats in Kanagawa and Saitama Prefectures. J Vet Med Sci 1998; 60:997-1000.

123. Nasirudeen AMA, Thong ML. Prevalence of *Bartonella henselae* immunoglobulin G antibodies in Singaporean cats. Pediatr Infect Dis J 1999; 18:276-278.

124. Foil L, Andress E, Freeland RL, Roy AF, Rutledge R, Triche PC, O'Reilly KL. Experimental infection of domestic cats with *Bartonella henselae* by inoculation of *Ctenocephalides felis* (*Siphonaptera*: *Pulicidae*) feces. J Med Entomol 1998; 35:625-628.

125. Greene CE, McDermott M, Hameson PH, Atkins JCL, Marks AM. *Bartonella henselae* infection in cats: evaluation during primary infection, treatment, and rechallenge infection. J Clin Microbiol 1996; 34:1682-1685.

126. Kordick DL, Breitschwerdt EB. Relapsing bacteremia after blood transmission of *Bartonella henselae* to cats. Am J Vet Res 1997; 58:492-497.

127. Regnery RL, Rooney JA, Johnson AM, Nesby SL, Manzewitsch P, Beaver K, Olson JG. Experimentally induced *Bartonella henselae* infections followed by challenge exposure and antimicrobial therapy in cats. Am J Vet Res 1996; 57:1714-1719.

128. Guptil L, Slater L, Wu C-C, Lin T-L, Glickman LT, Welch DF, Tobolski J, HogenEsch H. Evidence of reproductive failure and lack of perinatal transmission of *Bartonella henselae* inexperimentally infected cats. Vet Immunol Immunopathol 1998; 65:177-189.

129. Gurfield N, Boulouis HJ, Chomel B, Heller R, Larsen RW, Yamamoto K, Piemont Y. Co-infection by *Bartonella clarridgeiae* and *Bartonella henselae* and different *Bartonella henselae* strains in domestic cats. J Clin Microbiol 1997; 35:2110-2113.

130. Marston EL, Sumner JW, Regnery RL. Evaluation of intraspecies genetic variation within the 60 kDa heat-shock protein gene (groEL) of *Bartonella* species. Int J Syst Bacteriol. 1999; 49:1015-1023.

131. Sander A, Zagrosek A, Bredt W, Bereswill S, Lanz C, Schilz E, Dehio C. Characterization of *Bartonella clarridgeiae* flagella and detection of antiflagellin antibodies in patients with lymphadenopathy. (Submitted for publication)

132. Moens S, Michiels K, Keijers V, Van Leuven F, Vanderleyden J. Cloning, sequencing, and phenotypic analysis of laf 1, encoding the flagellin of the lateral flagella of *Azospirillum brasilense* Sp 7. J Bacteriol 1995; 177:5419-5426.

133. Roux V, Raoult D: Inter- and intraspecies identification of *Bartonella* (*Rochalimaea*) species. J Clin Microbiol 1995; 33:1573-1579.

134. Anderson BE, Goldsmith CS, Johnson AJ, Padmalayam I, Baumstark BR. Bacteriophage-like particle of *Rochalimaea henselae*. Mol Microbiol 1994; 13:67-73.

135. Umemori E, Sasaki Y, Amano K, Amano Y. A phage in *Bartonella bacilliformis*. Microbiol Immunol 1992; 36:731-736.

136. Bergmans AMC, Schellekens JFP, van Embden JDA, Schouls LM. Predominance of two *Bartonella henselae* variants among cat-scratch disease patients in The Netherlands. J Clin Microbiol 1996; 34:254-260.

137. Box ATA, Sander A, Perschil I, Goldenberger D, Altwegg M. Cats are probably not the only reservoir for infections due to *Bartonella henselae*. J Microbiol Meth 1996; 27:101-102.

138. Sander A, Posselt M, Boehm N, Ruess M, Altwegg M. Detection of *Bartonella henselae* DNA by two different PCR assays and determination of the genotype in histologically defined cat scratch disease. J Clin Microbiol 1999; 37:993-997.

139. Sander A, Ruess M, Deichmann K, Böhm N, Bredt W. Two different genotypes of *Bartonella henselae* in children with cat-scratch disease and their pet cats. Scand J Infect Dis 1998; 30:387-391.

140. Minnick MF, Strange JC, Williams KF. Characterization of the 16S-23 rRNA intergenic spacer of *Bartonella bacilliformis*. Gene 1994; 143:149-150.

141. Roux V, Raoult D. The 16S-23S rRNA intergenic spacer region of *Bartonella* (*Rochalimaea*) species is longer than usually described in other bacteria. Gene 1995; 165:107-111.

142. Matar GM, Swaminathan B, Hunter SB, Slater LN, Welch D. Polymerase chain reaction-based restriction fragment length polymorphism analysis of a fragment of the ribosomal operon from *Rochalimaea* species for subtyping. J Clin Microbiol 1993; 31:1730-1734.

143. Sander A, Ruess M, Bereswill S, Schuppler M, Steinbrückner B. Comparison of different fingerprint techniques for molecular typing of *Bartonella henselae* isolates. J Clin Microbiol 1998; 36:2973-2981.

144. Norman AF, Regnery R, Jameson P, Greene C, Krause DC. Differentiation of *Bartonella*-like isolates at the species level by PCR-restriction fragment length polymorphism in the citrate synthase gene. J Clin Microbiol 1995; 33:1797-1803.

145. Birtles RJ, Raoult D. Comparison of partial citrate synthase gene (gltA) sequences for phylogenetic analysis of *Bartonella* species. Int J Syst Bacteriol 1996; 46:891-897.

146. Bereswill S, Hinkelmann S, Kist M, Sander A. Molecular analysis of riboflavin synthesis genes in the human pathogen *Bartonella henselae* and use of the ribC gene for differentiation of *Bartonella* species by PCR. J Clin Microbiol 1999; 37:3159-3166.

147. Schmidt HU, Kaliebe T, Poppinger J, Bühler C, Sander A. Isolation of *Bartonella quintana* from an HIV-positive patient with bacillary angiomatosis. Eur J Clin Microbiol Infect Dis 1996; 15:736-741.

148. Rodriguez-Barradas MC, Hamill RJ, Houston ED, Georghiou PR, Clarridge JE, Regnery RL, Koehler JE. Genomic fingerprinting of *Bartonella* species by repetitive element PCR for distinguishing species and isolates. J Clin Microbiol 1995; 33:1089-1093.

149. Clarridge JE, Raich TJ, Pirwani D, Simon B, Tsai L, Rodriguez-Barradas MC, Regnery RL, Zollo A, Jones DC, Rambo C. Strategy to detect and identify *Bartonella* species in routine clinical laboratory yields *Barton-*

ella henselae from human immunodeficiency virus-positive patient and a unique *Bartonella* strain form his cat. J Clin Microbiol 1995; 33:2107-2113.

150. Maurin M, Roux V, Stein A, Ferrier F, Viraben R, Raoult D. Isolation and characterization by immunofluorescence, sodium dodecyl sulfate-polycrylamide gel electrophoresis, western blot, restriction fragment length polymorphism-PCR, 16S rRNA gene sequencing, and pulsed field gel electrophoresis of *Rochalimaea quintana* from a patient with bacillary angiomatosis. J Clin Microbiol 1994; 32:1166-1171.

151. Reynafarje C, Ramos J. The hemolytic anemia of human human bartonellosis. Blood 1961; 17:562-678.

152. Scherer DC, DeBuron-Connors I, Minnick MF. Characterization of *Bartonella bacilliformis* flagella and effect of antiflagellin antibodies on invasion of human erythrocytes. Infect Immun 1993; 61:4962-4971.

153. Mernaugh G, Ihler GM. Deformation factor: an extracellular protein synthesized by *Bartonella bacilliformis* that deforms erythrocyte membranes. Infect Immun 1992; 60:937-943.

154. Arias-Stella J, Lieberman PH, Erlandson RA. Histology, immunochemistry, and ultrastructure of the verruga in Carrion's disease. Am J Surg Pathol 1986; 10:595-610.

155. Leboit PE, Berger TG, Egbert BM, Beckstead JH, Yen BTS, Stoler MH. Bacillary angiomatosis. The histopathology and differential diagnosis of a pseudoneoplastic infection in patients with human immunodeficiency virus disease. Am J Surg Pathol 1989; 13:909-920.

156. Perkocha LA, Geaghan SM, Yen TSB, Nishimura SL, Chan SP, Garcia-Kennedy R, Honda G, Stoloff AC, Klein HZ, Goldman RL, van Meter S, Ferrel LD, Leboit PE. Clinical and pathological features of bacillary peliosis hepatis in association with human immunodeficiency virus infection. N Engl J Med 1990; 323:1581-1586.

157. Dehio C. Pathogenensis of *Bartonella* (*Rochalimaea*) infections. Bull Inst Pasteur 1997; 95:197-207.

158. Batterman HJ, Peek JA, Loutit JS, Falkow S, Tompkins LS. *Bartonella henselae* and *Bartonella quintana* adherence to and entry into cultured human epithelial cells. Infect Immun 1995; 63:4553-4556.

159. Rodriguez-Barradas MC, Bandres JC, Hamill RJ, Trial J, Clarridge JE, Baughn RE, Rossen RD. In vitro evaluation of the role of humoral immunity against *Bartonella henselae*. Infect Immun 1995; 63:2367-2370.

160. McGill SL, Regnery RL, Karem KL. Characterization of human immunoglobulin (Ig) Isotype and IgG subclass response to *Bartonella henselae* infection. Infect Immun 1998; 66:5915-5920.

161. Bergmans AMC, Groothedde JW, Schellekens JFP, von Embden JDA, Ossewaarde JM, Schouls LM. Etiology of cat scratch disease: comparison of polymerase chain reaction detection of *Bartonella* (formerly *Rochalimaea*) and *Afipia felis* DNA with serology and skin test. J Infect Dis 1995; 171:916-923.

162. Dalton MJ, Robinson LE, Cooper J, Regnery RL, Olson JG, Childs JE. Use of *Bartonella* antigens for serologic diagnosis of cat-scratch disease at a national referral center. Arch Intern Med 1995; 155:1670-1676.

163. Demers DM, Bass JW, Vincent JM, Person DA, Noyes DK, Staege CM, Samlaska CP, Lockwood NH, Regnery RL, Anderson BE. Cat scratch disease in Hawaii: etiology and seroepidemiology. J Pediatr 1995; 126:23-26.

164. Sander A, Posselt M, Oberle K, Bredt W. Seroprevalence to *Bartonella henselae* in patients with CSD and in healthy controls. Evaluation and comparison of two commercial serological tests. Clin Diagn Lab Immunol 1998; 5:486-490.

165. Drancourt M, Mainardi J, Brouqui P, Vandenesch F, Carta A, Lehnert F, Etienne J, Goldstein F, Acar J, Raoult D. *Bartonella* (*Rochalimaea*) *quintana* endocarditis in three homeless men. N Engl J Med 1995; 332:419-423.

166. Zbinden R, Michael N, Sekulowski M, von Graevenitz A, Nadal D. Evaluation of commercial slides for detection of immunoglobulin G against *Bartonella henselae* by indirect immunofluorescence. Eur J Clin Microbiol Infect Dis 1997; 16:648-652.

167. Zbinden R, Höchli M, Nadal D. Intracellular location of *Bartonella henselae* cocultivated with Vero cells and used for an indirect fluorescent-antibody test. Clin Diagn Lab Immunol 1995; 2:693-695.

168. Drancourt M, Birtles R, Chaumentin G, Vandenesch F, Etienne J, Raoult D. New serotype of *Bartonella henselae* in endocarditis and cat-scratch disease. Lancet 1996; 347:441-443.

169. Cimolai N, Benoit L, Hill A, Lyons C. *Bartonella henselae* IFA serology: observer concordance and the effect of utilizing wild–type substrate. 1st International Conference on Bartonella as Emerging Pathogens. Tübingen, Germany, March 5-7, 1999. J Microbiol Methods 1999; 37:276.

170. Rath PM, von Recklinghausen G, Ansorg R. Seroprevalence of immunoglobulin G antibodies to *Bartonella henselae* in cat owners. Eur J Clin Microbiol Infect Dis 1997; 16:326-327.

171. Nadal D, Zbinden R. Serology to *Bartonella* (*Rochalimaea*) *henselae* may replace traditional diagnostic criteria for cat-scratch disease. Eur J Pediatr 1995; 154:906-908.

172. Cimolai N, Benoit L, Hill A, Lyons C. Will endemic seropositivity for *Bartonella henselae* lead to considerable overdiagnosis? 1st International Conference on *Bartonella* as Emerging Pathogens. Tübingen, Germany, March 5-7, 1999. J Microbiol Methods 1999; 37:276-277.

173. Szelc-Kelly CM, Goral S, Perez-Perez GI, Perkins BA, Regnery RL, Edwards KM. Serologic responses to *Bartonella* and *Afipia* antigens in patients with cat scratch disease. Pediatrics 1995; 96:1137-1142.

174. Barka NE, Hadfield T, Patnaik M, Schwarzmann WA, Peter JB. EIA for detection of *Rochalimaea henselae*-reactive IgG, IgM and IgA antibodies in patients with suspected cat-scratch disease. J Infect Dis 1993; 167:1503-1504.

175. Bergmans AMC, Peeters MF, Schellekens JFP, Vos MC, Sabbe LJM, Ossewaarde JM, Verbakel H, Hooft HJ, Schouls LM. Pitfalls and fallacies of cat scratch disease serology: Evaluation of *Bartonella henselae*-based indirect fluorescence assay and enzyme-linked immunoassay. J Clin Microbiol 1997; 35:1931-1937.

176. Litwin CM, Martines TB. Hill HR. Immunologic response to *Bartonella henselae* as determined by enzyme immunoassay and western blot analysis. Am J Clin Pathol 1997; 108:202-209.

177. Anderson B, Lu E, Jones D, Regnery R. Characterization of a 17-kilodalton antigen of *Bartonella henselae* reactive with sera from patients with cat scratch disease. J Clin Microbiol 1995; 33:2358-2365.

178. La Scola B, Raoult D. Serological cross-reaction between *Bartonella quintana, Bartonella henselae*, and *Coxiella burnetii*. J Clin Microbiol 1996; 34:2270-2274.

179. Maurin M, Eb F, Etienne J, and Raoult D. Serologic cross-reactions between *Bartonella* and *Chlamydia* species: implications for diagnosis. J Clin Microbiol 1997; 35:2283-2287.

180. Knobloch J, Solano L, Alvarez O, Delgado E. Antibodies to *Bartonella bacilliformis* as determined by fluorescence antibody test, indirect haemagglutination and ELISA. Trop Med Parasitol 1985; 36:183-185.

181. Knobloch J. Analysis and preparation of *Bartonella bacilliformis* antigens. Am J Trop Med Hyg 1988; 39:173-178.

182. Chamberlin J, Gordon S, Laughlin L, Regnery R, Olson J, Romero S, Gonzalo A. Diagnosis of human bartonellosis by indirect fluorescence antibody test. 1st International Conference on *Bartonella* as Emerging Pathogens. Tübingen, Germany, March 5-7, 1999. J Microbiol Methods 1999; 37:275-276.

183. Kaschula ROC. Infectious diseases. In: Berry C, ed. Paediatric Pathology. London:Springer, 1996:729-820.

184. Welch DF, Slater LN. *Bartonella* and *Afipia*. In: Murray PR, Baron EJ, Pfaller MA, Tenover FC, Yolken RH, eds. Manual of Clinical Microbiology. Washington, DC:American Society for Microbiology, 1999:638-646.

185. Gasquet S, Maurin M, Brouqui P, Lepidi H, Raoult D. Bacillary angiomatosis in immunocompromised patients. AIDS 1998; 12:1793-1803.

186. Sander A, Penno S. Semiquantitative Species-specific detection of *Bartonella henselae* and *Bartonella quintana* by PCR-enzyme immunoassay. J Clin Microbiol 1999; 37:3097-3101.

187. Anderson B, Sims K, Regnery R, Robinson L, Schmidt MJ, Goral S, Hager C, Edwards K. Detection of *Rochalimaea henselae* DNA in specimens from cat scratch disease patients by PCR. J Clin Microbiol 1994; 32:942-948.

188. Kelly TM, Padmalayam I, Baumstark BR. Use of the cell division protein FtsZ as a means of differentiating among *Bartonella* species. Clin Diagn Lab Immunol 1998; 5:766-772.

189. Minnick MF, Barbian KD. Identification of *Bartonella* using PCR; genus- and species-specific primer sets. J Microbiol Methods 1997; 31:51-57.

190. Maas M, Schreiber M, Knobloch J. Detection of *Bartonella bacilliformis* in cultures, blood and formalin-preserved skin biopsies by use of polymerase chain reaction. Trop Med Parasitol 1992; 43:191-194.

191. Goldenberger D, Schmidheini T, Altwegg M. Detection of *Bartonella henselae* and *Bartonella quintana* by a simple and rapid procedure using broad-range PCR amplification and direct single-strand sequencing of part of the 16S rRNA gene. Clin Microbiol Infect 1997; 3:240-245.

192. La Scola B, Roult D. Culture of *Bartonella quintana* and *Bartonella henselae* from human samples: a 5-year experience (1993 to 1998). J Clin Microbiol 1999; 37:1899-1905.

193. Sander A. Microbiological diagnosis of *Bartonella* species and *Afipia felis*. In: Schmidt A, ed. *Bartonella* and *Afipia* Species Emphasizing *Bartonella henselae*. Basel:Karger, 1998:98-112.

194. Brenner SA, Rooney JA, Manzewitsch P, Regnery RL. Isolation of *Bartonella* (*Rochalimaea*) *henselae*: Effects of methods of blood collecting and handling. J Clin Microbiol 1997; 35:544-547.

195. Tierno PM, Inglima K, Parisi MT. Detection of *Bartonella* (*Rochalimaea*) *henselae* bacteremia using BacT/Alert blood culture system. Am J Clin Pathol 1995; 104:530-536.

196. Larson AM, Dougherty MJ, Nowowiejski DJ, Welch DF, Matar GM, Swaminathan B, Coyle MB. Detection of *Bartonella* (*Rochalimaea*) *quintana* by routine acridine orange staining of broth blood cultures. J Clin Microbiol 1994; 32:1492-1496.

197. Sobraques M, Maurin M, Birtles R, Raoult D. In vitro susceptibilities of four *Bartonella bacilliformis* strains to 30 antibiotic compounds. Antimicrob Agents Chemother 1999; 43:2090-2092.
198. Maurin M, Gasquet S, Ducco C, D. Raoult. MICs of 28 antibiotic compounds for 14 *Bartonella* (formerly *Rochalimaea*) isolates. Antimicrob Agents Chemother 1995; 39:2387-2391.
199. Maurin M, D. Raoult. Antimicrobial susceptibility of *Rochalimaea quintana*, *Rochalimeae vinsonii*, and the newly recognized *Rochalimaea henselae*. J Antimicrob Chemother 1993; 32:587-594.
200. Wolfson C, Branley J, Gottlieb T. The E test for antimicrobial susceptibility testing of *Bartonella henselae*. J Antimicrob Chemother 1996; 38:963-968.
201. Gray GC, Johnson A, Thornton SA, Smith WA, Knobloch J, Kelley PW, Escudero LO, Huayda MA, Wignall FS. An epidemic of Oroya fever in the Peruvian Andes. Am J Trop Med 1990; 42:215-221.
202. Urteaga O, Payne EH. Treatment of the acute febrile phase of Carrion's disease with chloramphenicol. Am J Trop Med 1955; 4:507-511.
203. Maguina Vargas C. Bartonellosis o enfermedad de Carrion. Nuevos aspectos de una vieja enfermedad. Lima, Peru: A. F. A. Editores Importadores S.A., 1998.
204. Spach D, Koehler JE. *Bartonella*-associated infections. Emerg Infect Dis 1998; 12:137-155.
205. Margileth AM. Antibiotic therapy for cat-scratch disease: clinical study of therapeutic outcome in 268 patients and review of the literature. Pediatr Infect Dis J 1992; 11:474-478.
206. Collipp PJ. Cat-scratch disease: therapy with trimethoprim-sulfamethoxazole. Am J Dis Child 1992; 146:397-399.
207. Maurin M, Raoult D. Minimal inhibitory concentration determination in *Bartonella henselae*. In: Schmidt A, ed. *Bartonella* and *Afipia* Species Emphasizing *Bartonella henselae*. Basel:Karger, 1998:164-175.
208. Bass JW, Treitas BC, Treitas AD, Sisler CL, Chan DS, Vincent JM, Person DA, Claybaugh JR, Wittler RR, Weisse ME, Regnery RL, Slater LN. Prospective randomized double blind placebo-controlled evaluation of azithromycin for treatment of cat-scratch disease. Pediatr Infect Dis J 1998; 17:447-452.

23

Whooping Cough (Pertussis)

James C. Paton
Department of Molecular Biosciences, Adelaide University, Adelaide, South Australia, Australia.

I. HISTORICAL INTRODUCTION AND NATURE OF THE ETIOLOGICAL AGENT

Whooping cough (pertussis) derives its name from the characteristic sound which is caused by the rapid influx of air past the glottis at the end of paroxysmal coughing fits among patients with the disease. This clinical presentation is quite distinctive, and the disease was first recognized in the Middle Ages, with the first documented epidemic occurring in Paris in 1578 as cited in (1). The principal causative organism, now known as *Bordetella pertussis*, was first isolated by Bordet and Gengou in 1906 (2). It is a small, aerobic Gram-negative coccobacillus, and because of its preference for culture media with high concentrations of blood, it was placed in the genus *Haemophilus* for many years. The organism, however, does not require X and V factors for growth, a characteristic of other members of this genus, and so in the 1960s, it was given its current name in honour of Bordet.

In addition to *B. pertussis*, the genus *Bordetella* includes *B. parapertussis*, *B. bronchiseptica*, and *B. avium*, as well as three recently recognized species, *B. hinzii* (previously referred to as "*B. avium-like*"), *B. holmesii* (previously classified as "CDC non-oxidizer group 2"), and *B. trematum* (3). *B. parapertussis* is also capable of causing whooping cough in humans. *B. bronchiseptica* is a common cause of respiratory disease in rodents, dogs, and pigs; human infections are very uncommon, although there are a number of reports of respiratory infections, including pneumonia in HIV-infected and other immunocompromised individuals. Human infections with *B. holmesii* and *B. trematum* have also been reported. *B. avium* causes coryza in turkeys, but it is yet to be associated with human disease. *B. hinzii* also occurs in the respiratory tract of birds and has been isolated from humans, but does not appear to cause disease in either host (3).

In spite of the availability of a whole-cell vaccine since the late 1940s, and more recently a less reactogenic acellular formulation, whooping cough continues to be a major cause of morbidity and mortality worldwide. The World Health Organization has estimated that globally, there are in the order of 45 million illnesses and over 400,000 deaths each year (4). As might be expected, the impact of the disease is most severe in infants and young children, particularly those who have not received a full course of immunizations. There is a high incidence in developing countries, but even in developed countries with high vaccination rates, whooping cough is an important cause of morbidity.

II.   CLINICAL ASPECTS

Whooping cough is acquired by inhalation of aerosols or other direct contact with infected materials due to *B. pertussis*. There is an incubation period of approximately seven to ten days which is followed by a catarrhal stage that involves mild respiratory symptoms, occasionally with a slight fever, and may be virtually indistinguishable from the common cold.   This stage lasts for one to two weeks during which time the patient is highly infectious. He or she develops an irritating cough, which initially may be dry, but as the disease progresses, mucus production increases and the bouts of coughing become more severe. A spasmodic or paroxysmal stage follows and is characterized by fits of coughing during which the face becomes increasingly cyanotic as more and more air is forced from the lungs by the rapid succession of coughs. As the final cough in one of these episodes subsides, the glottis relaxes and air rushes back into the lungs making the characteristic whooping sound. This may be followed by emesis. There may be many such spasmodic coughing episodes each day, and the frequency usually increases at night. These classical clinical manifestations of whooping cough are distressing, exhausting, and virtually diagnostic of the disease. In neonates, very young infants, older children, and adults, however, whooping may be absent. In very young children, an important manifestation is apnea. The paroxysmal stage lasts at least one, usually two to three weeks, after which the frequency and severity of the coughing spasms gradually diminish. Coughing (without whooping or vomiting) may continue during convalescence for months (5).

The most severe cases of whooping cough occur in unvaccinated children less than one year old, and this group accounts for the bulk of mortality. Serious neurological sequelae, induced at least in part by anoxia during coughing paroxysms, also occur more frequently in this age group. Respiratory complications include bronchopneumonia (usually secondary), which was presumably responsible for the majority of whooping cough deaths during the pre-antibiotic era, and lung collapse (5). In older children and adults, the disease is usually less severe; the classical symptoms are less obvious or absent, and a diagnosis of whooping cough is largely dependent on laboratory analysis. Nevertheless, establishing this diagnosis is very important from the infection control and public health perspectives.

Although generally less prevalent than *B. pertussis*, *B. parapertussis* is now recognized as a significant cause of respiratory disease in humans. The clinical spectrum ranges from asymptomatic carriage to severe infections which are characterized by coughing paroxysms that are indistinguishable from those that are associated with classical pertussis. Fatal infections have also been reported, although it is possible that at least some of these may have been among patients who were also co-infected with *B. pertussis* (6). Notwithstanding the capacity to cause life-threatening disease, *B. parapertussis* infections are usually less severe and are associated with lesser frequency of paraoxysmal coughing and with a shorter mean duration of illness (7). In the majority of patients, infections include a bronchitis which includes a dry, non-paroxysmal cough. Such symptoms are likely to be attributed to viral infection and not further investigated, thereby contributing to an under-recognition of the true incidence of *B. parapertussis* infections (6).

III.   EPIDEMIOLOGY OF INFECTION

Whooping cough is an endemic disease throughout the world, although the overall incidence is higher in temperate and cooler climates. Epidemic cycles are superimposed on this with a periodicity of roughly two to five years, corresponding to the time taken for herd immunity to diminish after the previous epidemic. It is a highly contagious disease; 90-100% of susceptible household contacts that are exposed to an infected person will develop frank disease, and many immunized contacts will develop mild or subclinical infections (8). Humans are the only known host for *B. pertussis*, and so it is theoretically possible to eliminate the disease if a vaccine that is capable of providing long-term protection against acquisition of infection, as opposed to limitation of the severity of illness, can be developed and administered to a high proportion of the population. In the years before the widespread availability of pertussis vaccines, the peak incidence was in children aged from two to six years, and a similar age distribution is seen today in countries that do not include pertussis in childhood vaccination programs. In countries with high rates of vaccine uptake, incidence, as well as clinical severity, is greatest in children less than six months of age who are yet to receive a full course of vaccine, and in undervaccinated preschool children (8). Notwithstanding this, significant rates of infection occur in older children and adults in whom the disease is usually (but not always) less severe, may present atypically, or may be subclinical. Frequently, the diagnosis goes unrecognized in such individuals and they probably act as an important reservoir for infection (9).

Introduction of pertussis vaccines into childhood immunization programs has undoubtedly resulted in a significant reduction in morbidity and mortality, and differences in incidence between geographically and socioeconomically similar countries can largely be attributed to differences in vaccination policies and vaccine uptake. In several countries with consistently high rates of vaccination, however, the incidence of pertussis has increased steadily since the early 1980s. The most likely explanation for this is an increase in the size of the susceptible adult population, who were vaccinated as children, but who are no longer protected. Unlike earlier (pre-vaccine) cohorts, this group had been protected against childhood pertussis which may have induced stronger and longer lasting (albeit not lifelong) protection. In addition to contributing to reported cases in their own right, this group undoubtedly is responsible for transmitting infection to many younger incompletely vaccinated contacts, further adding to the overall incidence of disease (8).

IV. PATHOGENESIS

The pathogenesis of whooping cough is a complex multi-step process requiring the expression of a range of virulence factors, many of which are coordinately regulated in response to environmental signals by a two-component signal transduction system [reviewed in (10)]. *B. pertussis* is known to undergo phase variation from a virulent phase, during which all the major virulence factors required for establishment of an infection are expressed, to an avirulent phase which is believed to favour survival of the organism during nutrient depletion in vitro, and which may contribute to intracellular survival in vivo (10). The first stage in pathogenesis, after inhalation of droplets containing *B. pertussis*, is adherence of the organism to the ciliae of respiratory epithelial cells. A number of virulence factors are involved in this process, the most important of which are filamentous hemagglutinin (FHA) and pertussis toxin (PT) (functioning as cooperative adhesins) (11). Other factors which are believed to contribute include fimbriae, pertactin, tracheal colonization factor, and serum resistance factor (1,10).

Proliferation of *B. pertussis* in the respiratory tract is facilitated by evasion of host defences. Key virulence factors that are involved in this include the adenylate cyclase and PT, which inhibit host immune-effector cell function and bacterial clearance (1). PT also induces expression of integrin, which acts as a receptor for FHA and mediates phagocytosis via the macrophage CR3 receptor; *B. pertussis* organisms taken up in this manner do not trigger an oxidative burst and are able to survive and multiply intracellularly (12). Serum resistance factor (the *BrkA* and *BrkB* proteins) also confers resistance to the bactericidal effects of serum (13).

Local tissue damage at the site of infection is presumed to cause the symptoms of pertussis. The tracheal cytotoxin, a muramyl peptide derived from the cell wall peptidoglycan, is largely responsible for this and thus generating marked respiratory ciliated epithelial cytopathology including ciliostasis and extrusion of ciliated cells. The precise mode of action, however, is not understood (10). Dermonecrotic toxin, lipopolysaccharide (LPS), and PT may also contribute to local damage, albeit to a much lesser extent. Studies in mice have shown that PT, which acts by ADP-ribosylation of G proteins, also generates a variety of systemic effects including lymphocytosis, hyperinsulinemia, hypoglycemia, and sensitization to histamine. Both lymphocytosis and hyperinsulinemia are seen in humans with pertussis, and it has been postulated that convulsions and encephalopathy, which are associated with the illness, could be due to PT-induced hypoglycemia. There is insufficient direct evidence to support this, and it seems most probable that these complications are caused by anoxia due to the paroxysms and respiratory damage (1). The involvement of PT as a *sine qua non* of virulence is also disproven by the fact that *B. parapertussis*, which does not produce PT, is also capable of causing whooping cough (6).

V. IMMUNOLOGY OF INFECTION AND VACCINATION

Neither natural infection with *B. pertussis* nor vaccination confer life-long protection against whooping cough, although both clearly limit the clinical severity of subsequent infections. Primary infection of non-vaccinees elicits immune responses to a range of *B. pertussis* antigens, with serum antibodies usually becoming detectable 1-2 weeks after onset of symptoms (14). More than 90% of infected individuals respond to PT and FHA, whereas only 30-60% respond to other antigens such as pertactin, LPS, and fimbriae (15). Infection elicits antibodies of all isotypes, although IgG antibodies (principally of the IgG1 subclass) are found in the highest frequency; roughly 90% of infected persons have IgG responses to PT or FHA, and 30-60% have IgG responses to pertactin and fimbriae. IgA responses are somewhat less frequent; the proportions of infected patients that respond to the various antigens are 20-40% for PT, 30-50% for FHA, and 20-40% for pertactin and fimbriae (14). Nevertheless, IgA responses are valuable serological markers of current or recent infection (discussed later), as they are not usually elicited by vaccination (16). After an infection, the levels of antibody to the various *B. pertussis* antigens gradually diminish over 1-3 years. Detectable levels of antibody however may persist for many years, perhaps as a consequence of subclinical reinfections (14).

Vaccines which consist of killed and partially detoxified *B. pertussis* cells became widely available in the late 1940s, and typically have been administered to infants as a primary course of three injections (usually commencing at about 3 months of age) in combination with tetanus and diphtheria toxoids. Booster doses are required at approximately 15-18 months of age and again at 4-5 years if immunity is to be maintained into school age (1). Antibodies that are elicited by a full course of the whole cell vaccine are mostly of the IgG isotype, and although these are directed against a range of antigens, antibodies to outer membrane proteins and fimbriae predominate (14). Whole cell pertussis vaccines are estimated to be at least 80-90% efficacious in preventing symptomatic disease, and those vaccinees who do become infected usually have a milder illness. The protective efficacy is highlighted by the massive reduction in the mortality rate from pertussis which has followed the introduction of vaccination programs, and the close inverse relationship between the overall incidence of pertussis and infant vaccination rates. This is illustrated by the experience of countries such as the United Kingdom, Japan, and Sweden which had high vaccination rates in the mid-1970s, and concomitant low rates of disease. Subsequent reduction in immunization rates (and in Sweden, complete withdrawal of the whole cell vaccine in 1979) was closely followed by a massive increase in the severity of epidemics of pertussis. The epidemics were controlled in the United Kingdom and Japan by renewed promotion of vaccination, but not in Sweden where it was not reintroduced (1). It should be noted, however, that although the amplitude of epidemics can be minimized by high rates of vaccination with the whole cell vaccine, the underlying 2-5 year periodicity of epidemics remains largely unchanged, indicating that the vaccine is controlling severity of illness rather than the prevalence of *B. pertussis* in the community (1). Clearly, a vaccine capable of blocking transmission of the organism will be required if the disease is to be eliminated, as has been achieved for smallpox.

Notwithstanding their efficacy, the whole cell vaccines are quite reactogenic, due largely to the presence of LPS (endotoxin) and incompletely inactivated toxins. The reactions which can be unequivocally attributed to the vaccine include redness, pain, and swelling at the injection site, as well as systemic reactions such as fever, drowsiness, irritability, anorexia, and vomiting (1,10). In the 1970s and early 1980s much controversy surrounded the possibility that whole cell pertussis vaccines were also responsible for rare neurological events which occurred during the immediate post-vaccination period. Exhaustive epidemiological studies however have shown that, although fever which results from the residual traces of endotoxin, might trigger febrile convulsions in susceptible infants, the so-called 'pertussis vaccine encephalopathy' is a myth (1,17). Nevertheless, adverse publicity concerning the safety and reactogenicity of the vaccine, combined with a perception among parents that whooping cough was a disease of the past, caused a marked decline in vaccination rates in many countries, the consequences of which have been discussed above.

The ongoing problems (both real and imagined) that have been associated with the whole cell vaccines have provided powerful selective pressure for development of safer and less reactogenic vaccines which include purified *B. pertussis* virulence factors. A variety of these so-called 'acellular vaccines' that contain various combinations of toxoided PT, FHA, pertactin, and fimbriae have been developed. The common finding from numerous clinical trials is that acellular vaccines are indeed less reactogenic than whole cell vaccines although the problem has not been eliminated altogether (18). Assessment of the comparative immunogenicity and protective efficacy of acellular and whole cell vaccines is complicated by the wide variety of different acellular formulations (in terms of preparation method, composition, and actual dose of individual components). Moreover, the performance of different whole cell vaccine formulations is by no means uniform. Early efficacy trials in Sweden of monovalent (PT) and bivalent (PT + FHA) acellular vaccines were somewhat disappointing with levels of protection being less than that which were historically observed with whole cell vaccines although they clearly were effective in ameliorating the severity of illness (19). Analysis of immunogenicity data from a number of more recent trials indicates that for each of the components, antibody levels elicited by acellular formulations exceeded those elicited by whole cell vaccines (18). Moreover, large efficacy trials in Italy and Sweden demonstrated that three-component and five-component acellular vaccines were more efficacious than either a whole cell vaccine or a two-component acellular formulation (20, 21), although in a separate study, a different whole cell vaccine was as protective as the five-component acellular vaccine (22). Multivariate analysis has shown that clinical protection against pertussis correlates best with high levels of antibody that is directed against pertactin, fimbriae (both Fim2 and Fim3), and PT, in that order (23,24). Acellular vaccines are now licensed for primary immunization of infants and for boosting of older children in many countries. Moreover, the lower reactogenicity of these vaccines may in due course enable their incorporation into diphtheria-tetanus booster formulations for use in adults. This may reduce the incidence of mild or atypical disease as well as asymptomatic carriage in this age group which is now recognized as an important reservoir of *B. pertussis* in the community.

VI. LABORATORY DIAGNOSIS

Timely and accurate laboratory diagnosis of whooping cough is increasingly being recognized as a vital component of effective stategies to combat the disease in the community. During the paroxysmal phase of the disease in young unvaccinated children, symptoms are sufficiently distinctive for a diagnosis to be made on clinical grounds with a degree of confidence. It should be remembered however that other pathogens such as *Mycoplasma pneumoniae*, *Chlamydia pneumoniae*, and adenovirus among other respiratory viruses can also cause pertussis-like episodes (25). Furthermore, the mild or atypical disease as seen in vaccinees, older children, and adults with pertussis frequently goes unrecognized. Infections in these latter groups are far more common than was once thought, and failure to diagnose such infections undoubtedly contributes towards the spread of *B. pertussis* to susceptible contacts. Laboratory diagnosis requires either isolation of *B. pertussis* (or *B. parapertussis*) from respiratory secretions, demonstration of specific antigens or nucleic acids in said secretions, or detection of a serological response to infection. Each of these approaches has its strengths and weaknesses, as outlined below.

A. Culture

Culture of *B. pertussis* has long been considered the "gold standard" diagnostic method. This title may be appropriate given the fact that specificity is essentially 100%. The sensitivity of culture, however, is suboptimal and is influenced by a range of factors, including stage of illness, quality of the specimen, prior antimicrobial therapy, among other things. Certain of the other diagnostic procedures described in this chapter are superior to culture in particular circumstances, and as a consequence frequently yield true positive results when culture is negative.

1. Specimen collection and processing

The importance of specimen collection and processing to the success of subsequent microbiological analyses cannot be overestimated. *B. pertussis* is a very delicate organism and may lose viability rapidly after a specimen is obtained from the patient. In circumstances of whooping cough, *B. pertussis* is present in the respiratory tract from the nose to the bronchi, but the nasopharynx usually has high numbers of bacteria that are brought up from the lower respiratory tract by coughing. Secretions from this site are easily collected either by aspiration or by swabbing. Conventional throat swab cultures and cough plates which are held in front of the patient's mouth are unsuitable samples for pertussis culture because they will be heavily contaminated with commensals. There is general agreement that aspiration is the optimal method for collection of nasopharyngeal secretions (3,14,25,26). This is achieved by the introduction of a flexible plastic tube, connected via a mucus trap to a suction source, into one nostril and then insertion along the nasopharyngeal floor as far as the posterior pharynx. After aspiration, the catheter is withdrawn and the tubing is flushed with 1 mL of sterile saline. Alternatively, the tubing can be flushed with a liquid transport medium such as 1% casamino acids in phosphate-buffered saline (PBS). Washes may also be acquired by instillation of saline and subsequent aspiration. Nasopharyngeal (pernasal) swabs are also commonly used, but the yield of *B. pertussis* is usually lower as inevitably some bacteria remain adherent to the fibre tip. It is much more difficult to divide the latter specimens if additional diagnostic tests (see below) are to be employed. Pernasal swabs which are used for this purpose have a long flexible shaft and are tipped with either dacron, calcium alginate, or cotton. Cotton tips are the least suitable for culture as the fibres, or contaminants therein, can possibly inhibit growth of the organism. Alginate tips appear to be optimal for culture as the fibres are partially soluble thereby more easily releasing the bacteria, and they are relatively free of growth inhibitors (3). Dacron-tipped swabs should be used if the sample is also to be tested by PCR because alginate fibres are known to inhibit such assays (27).

    B. pertussis loses viability if exposed to low temperatures, and although not always practicable, the best isolation rates are obtained when nasopharyngeal specimens are plated directly on to an appropriate agar medium within minutes of collection. If a delay between collection and plating is unavoidable, use of a transport medium is essential. As mentioned above, 1% casamino acids in PBS is a convenient medium in which to collect nasopharyngeal aspirates (NPAs). If the delay is more than a few hours, however, the specimen should be placed in a tube containing Regan-Lowe transport medium (28). This is particularly important for swabs which should never be transported dry. The tips of catheters that are used for collection of NPAs can also be placed in a transport tube. Regan-Lowe medium consists of half-strength charcoal agar which is supplemented with 10% horse blood and 40 mg./L. cephalexin; the latter enables multiplication of *B. pertussis* while inhibiting commensal nasopharyngeal flora. Pre-incubation for 1-2 days at 36°C is recommended if a specimen has to be transported any great distance (e.g., by post or courier). The increased survival of *B. pertussis* that is afforded by this step, however, is counterbalanced by the risk of overgrowth by cephalexin-resistant commensals which might preclude subsequent isolation of the pathogen. This can be limited by refrigerated transport, but low temperatures may lead to a significant reduction in viability of *B. pertussis* (14).

2. Media and culture conditions

The medium of choice for isolation of *B. pertussis* is unquestionably charcoal agar supplemented with 10% horse blood and 40 mg./L. cephalexin (CHB-ceph). Some laboratories also inoculate specimens on to non-selective CHB plates because of concerns that the cephalexin is slightly inhibitory to growth of *B. pertussis*, although this extra step is probably not warranted (14). Use of an enrichment step, however, has been shown to improve the yield of *B. pertussis* by up to 14% (25). After inoculation of primary culture plates, the remainder of the specimen (including the swab or aspiration catheter tip where present) can be inoculated into Regan-Lowe medium (or returned to the original transport tube), incubated for 48 hours, and then replated.

Agar media should be incubated at 35-36°C in air, and need to be kept moist during the long incubation period. For this reason, they should not be poured too thin, and they should be incubated in a closed container (e.g., a candle jar minus the candle). Plates should be examined daily and *B. pertussis* colonies should become apparent after 3-4 days; *B. parapertussis* colonies grow faster and are usually visible after 1-2 days. Plates should be incubated for at least 7 days, however, before a specimen is pronounced culture-negative; indeed, one study has demonstrated improved isolation rates for both *B. pertussis* and *B. parapertussis* by extending incubation to 12 days (29).

3.   Identification

B. pertussis has a typical morphology on CHB agar; colonies are small, round and convex, greyish-white in colour, and have a shiny surface. *B. parapertussis* colonies are slightly larger, more grey in colour, and older cultures develop a brown pigmentation. Suspicious colonies should be Gram stained (both species are small Gram negative coccobacilli) and tested for oxidase and urease (*B. pertussis* is oxidase-positive and urease-negative, while *B. parapertussis* is oxidase-negative and urease-positive). The capacity of *B. parapertussis* to grow on routine blood agar is an additional distinction between the two species. Presumptive identification should then be confirmed by slide agglutination with commercially available specific antisera. Sometimes agglutination reactions are complicated by difficulty in emulsifying the bacteria, but this can usually be overcome by testing fresher subcultures. Cross-reactions between *B. pertussis* and *B. parapertussis* can occur with commercial antisera, and so to avoid confusion, only oxidase-positive colonies should be tested for agglutination with anti-*B. pertussis*, and only oxidase-negative colonies should be tested with anti-*B. parapertussis*. Alternatively, confirmation of identification for both species can be achieved by PCR if this technology is available.

4.   Serotyping

B. pertussis can be divided into serotypes on the basis of reactions with antisera specific for three so-called agglutinogens. The precise nature of these surface antigens is uncertain, but agglutinogen 2 is believed to be fimbrial, and the same may possibly be true for agglutinogen 3. Pertactin may also act as an agglutinogen (10). Clinical isolates of *B. pertussis* usually belong to serotypes 1,2 and 1,3. Serotyping has little value clinically. Agglutinogens 2 and 3, however, appear to be important protective components of whole cell pertussis vaccines; formulations lacking agglutinogen 2 have poor clinical efficacy against serotype 1,2 strains, and those lacking agglutinogen 3 have poor efficacy against type 1,3 strains (10). Thus, serotype surveillance may provide useful epidemiological information including an indication of type-specific vaccine performance, and investigation of clinical isolates to reference laboratories for this purpose should be encouraged.

B.   Direct antigen detection

The inevitable delay of 3 to 7 days between collection of a sample and the availability of a result is a serious deficiency of culture-based methods for diagnosis of whooping cough. Detection of *B. pertussis* or *B. parapertussis* by direct fluorescent antibody (DFA) staining, however, has the capacity to provide a same-day result. Moreover, it has the capacity to detect non-viable bacteria. The test involves application of nasopharyngeal secretions (aspirates or swabs) on a slide, fixation, and then direct staining with commercially available FITC-conjugated polyclonal or (more recently) monoclonal antibodies. The slides are then examined under a fluorescence microscope for the presence of small coccobacilli with brightly fluorescing outer surfaces. Several studies have reported major problems with false-positives when the polyclonal reagents are used as these can cross-react with other pharyngeal flora which may closely resemble *Bordetella* spp. microscopically (14,30). Thus, the accuracy of DFA is highly dependent on the skill and experience of laboratory personnel who are examining the slides. In recent years, a monoclonal DFA reagent that is specific for the LPS of *B. pertussis* has become commercially available, and this has largely overcome the problem with false positives (31). This has also been combined in a dual fluorochrome DFA assay with another monoclonal antibody conjugate that is specific for *B. parapertussis* (3).

Notwithstanding the improved specificity of monoclonal DFA reagents, the sensitivity of the test is significantly lower than culture. Less than 40% of culture-positive samples were DFA-positive in a recent large and well-controlled Swedish study (25), and similar poor sensitivities with respect to culture have also been reported in a number of earlier studies using polyclonal DFA reagents [cited in (14)]. Specimens with low numbers of *B. pertussis* are particularly problematic. Scanty *B. pertussis* colonies growing on a CHB-ceph plate may be readily recognizable, but similar numbers on a DFA slide are extremely hard to find, even after systematic (and very time-consuming) examination of a large number of high-power fields. In addition, many laboratories will impose a threshold of about four fluorescent bacteria with the correct morphology for a result to be classified as positive; no such threshold applies to culture. Consequently, DFA is reliable only for specimens which ultimately yield a moderate to heavy growth of *B. pertussis*. Thus, DFA is becoming a diagnostic dinosaur and is increasingly being replaced by PCR even in routine clinical laboratories.

C.   PCR

The advent of PCR technology has revolutionized diagnosis of many infectious diseases (see Chapter 5), and the technique is ideally suited to organisms such as *B. pertussis*, which are slow-growing and which readily lose viability after specimen collection if not handled appropriately. This, and the continued occurrence of epidemics of whooping cough, prompted the early application of PCR technology to pertussis diagnosis (32,33). Indeed, our own laboratory introduced a pertussis PCR assay into routine diagnostic service in 1989 (in lieu of DFA), and this test has been performed in parallel with culture throughout the last decade. Large clinical trials of various acellular pertussis vaccines as conducted in recent years have also provided an opportunity for further evaluation of pertussis PCR assays. Several other studies in which various PCR assays have been compared with culture and/or DFA and/or serology for diagnosis of pertussis have also been described [reviewed in (14)]. They vary considerably in terms of study population and the precise methodologies employed, and so there is little to be gained from a detailed comparison of the findings of each. A universal feature, however, is that PCR is highly sensitive, yielding unequivocal positive results in the vast majority of culture-positive cases as well as detecting a significant number of additional cases which were culture-negative; in some studies, this increased the number of positive diagnoses several-fold. In most studies, a high proportion of these culture-negative, PCR-positive samples were collected from patients who had a persistent cough and who had either been in close contact with a confirmed case or had serological evidence of infection such that they satisfied the case definition of pertussis as recommended by the WHO (34). Importantly, PCR can provide a same-day, or at the latest, a next-day result, with a very high positive and negative predictive value, thus enabling early implementation of appropriate antimicrobial therapy and other interventions to minimize spread of the disease to contacts. It is not yet possible to recommend any one of the published pertussis PCR assays for adoption as a standard protocol, as there have been few if any direct comparisons. The relative theoretical merits, however, of alternative methodologies for each stage of the process are considered below.

1.   Specimen preparation

As was the case with culture, NPAs are the preferred specimen for pertussis PCR. These can be easily divided for separate culture analysis and the aspirates can be stored at 4°C for short periods (< 1 day) or frozen at -15°C or -70°C prior to batch processing without loss of sensitivity. Of course, it is preferable to process samples immediately, or at least on a daily basis, given the importance of a rapid result. Nasopharyngeal swabs can also be used for PCR; dacron-tipped swabs are preferable, as those tipped with alginate have been shown to inhibit PCR reactions (27). Swabs should be vortexed in a small volume (about 0.5 ml) of buffer (e.g., Tris-EDTA, or PBS-EDTA) and then applied against the wall of the tube to extract as much potential PCR template as possible. Methods for subsequent template preparation vary markedly amongst published studies. PCR assays are most efficient, and hence most sensitive, when purified DNA templates are tested because complex biological specimens such as nasopharyngeal secretions may contain potential inhibitors of the polymerase reaction itself, or nucleases which could degrade template DNA. Extensive purification protocols, however, are incompatible with staff workloads in all but the most fortunate clinical laboratories, and so a balance has to be struck between speed, simplicity, material cost, and ultimate sensitivity.

In several studies, NPAs have simply been boiled before PCR (35,36,37,38). In our laboratory, we continue to digest NPAs with proteinase K at 65°C for 1 hour, followed by boiling for 20 min, as described in our original study (32), and this method has been used by others (39). Sensitivity, however, can be improved by including an ethanol precipitation step, which apart from further removal of potential inhibitors, permits concentration of the sample prior to assay. Several studies have gone further and have extracted crude nasopharyngeal lysates with phenol/chloroform (40,41) or guanidine thiocyanate (42) prior to isopropanol and/or ethanol precipitation. It is not clear, however, just how many additional positive samples are detected as a consequence of the use of these additional purification steps which would add significantly to labour costs in the routine clinical laboratory setting. A simpler alternative is addition of Chelex beads (a weak anion exchange resin) to proteinase K-digested NPAs to remove potentially inhibitory cations (43,44). Use of Chelex has been shown to increase the proportion of PCR-positives when NPAs were tested, but intriguingly, it actually reduced the end-point sensitivity when pure culture extracts or control DNA were analysed (44). Clearly, this reduced efficiency of amplification caused by the Chelex was more than offset by its capacity to remove potent inhibitors from the more complex clinical samples. An alternative method for preparation of PCR template from NPAs involves treatment with a mucolytic agent (N-acetyl cysteine and NaOH) which is followed by centrifugation, resuspension of the pellet in a small volume of buffer, and boiling (45). This has the theoretical advantage of concentrating B. pertussis cells that are released from mucus and of removing soluble inhibitors (14), but any DNA released from non-viable cells will be lost in the supernatant fraction thereby reducing sensitivity.

If NPAs are being tested, use of the proteinase K digestion/boiling protocol (32) probably represents an appropriate balance between simplicity and sensitivity for a routine clinical laboratory. If the specimen, however, has been collected using an alginate-tipped swab, or has been sent to the laboratory in transport medium (regardless of swab type), more extensive DNA extraction should be employed.

2. Selection of target sequence and amplification conditions

The majority of PCR assays for B. pertussis described to date are targeted at either the repetitive DNA element known as IS481 (32,33,35,40) or the promoter region of the gene encoding PT (33,39,41) although sequences upstream of the porin gene (45) and the adenylate cyclase gene (46) have also been used. IS481 is an attractive target for a diagnostic PCR because it is present in about 80 copies per cell thereby potentially enhancing sensitivity over that which is achieved by using single copy targets. On the basis of DNA hybridization studies, IS481 appears to be absolutely specific for B. pertussis, with the exception of B. bronchiseptica, which contains a single copy of a closely related element (32). Of course, PCR assays targeted at this sequence will not detect cases caused by B. parapertussis which is responsible for a small proportion of cases of whooping cough. B. parapertussis, however, also contains a specific repetitive element designated IS1001 which can be used as a PCR target (47), and sensitive IS481/IS1001 multiplex PCR assays that are capable of simultaneous detection and discrimination between the two species have been developed (37,38,48). The PT promoter region, although a single copy target, has the advantage that flanking sequences are conserved between B. pertussis, B. parapertussis, and *B. bronchiseptica* thus enabling detection of all three species with a single primer pair; sequence differences within the amplicons enables species discrimination by restriction analysis (44). A shared primer PCR which is specific for sequences upstream of the porin gene can also simultaneously detect and discriminate between *B. pertussis* and *B. parapertussis* (45). These species-discriminating PCR assays can also be used to confirm identification of presumptive isolates of *Bordetella* spp., particularly in cases where biochemical or serological reactions have yielded equivocal results (49). Indeed, during the initial characterization of our IS*481*-specific PCR assay (32) using extracts from about 100 preserved *B. pertussis* clinical isolates, we detected two isolates which were PCR-negative; these cultures were retested by slide agglutination and were found to be *B. parapertussis*.

Most of the PCR assays that are described for pertussis use 30-35 amplification cycles; if fewer than this are used, suboptimal sensitivity is likely to result, particularly if single copy sequences are the target. Even with the higher number of cycles, however, improved sensitivity may be achieved by using the IS element targets if specimens contain inhibitors which reduce the efficiency of amplification. Apart from the primers themselves, a host of factors influence performance of PCR assays. These include the precise denaturation, annealing, and elongation temperatures and incubation times, the type and quality of thermostable polymerase used (most use *Taq* polymerase), and the quality/purity of the template prepared from the nasopharyngeal specimen among others. Composition of the PCR assay buffer can also influence sensitivity. Basic PCR buffers typically comprise 10 mM Tris-HCl (pH 8.3), 50 mM KCl, and roughly 2 mM MgCl$_2$. In addition, we routinely include 0.1% gelatin, 0.1% Tween 20, and 0.1% Nonidet P-40 in our assay buffer; the detergents appear to improve performance with "dirty" templates, and the gelatin helps to protect the *Taq* polymerase from any residual proteinase K activity in the boiled NPA extract. In theory, use of nested PCR systems can also improve both sensitivity and specificity (35,44,48). This involves two rounds of PCR, the second of which is performed using primers specific for sequences within the amplicon that are obtained during the initial round. A small aliquot of the first PCR reaction mix is used as the template for the second step, thus effectively diluting any inhibitors which might have been present in the original assay.

3. PCR product detection

By far the most common method of PCR product detection is agarose gel electrophoresis and subsequent staining with ethidium bromide. This is a relatively quick and cheap procedure, and confirmation of the size of the PCR product is a check on specificity. Additional confirmation can be obtained by dot-blot or Southern hybridization analysis using labelled DNA or oligonucleotide probes which are specific for sequences within the amplified DNA fragment (14,39,46). Alternatively, digoxigenin-11-dUTP can be included in the original PCR amplification mix; after amplification, aliquots are spotted onto a filter and digoxigenin label that is incorporated into the PCR product can be detected by dot-immunoblot (45). These procedures undoubtedly increase sensitivity, although the additional steps increase the overall cost and will delay the result. As more and more PCR assays are introduced into routine clinical laboratory service, however, alternative product detection systems are becoming available which increase sensitivity and more readily lend themselves to automation. Two such examples involve immobilization of capture oligonucleotide probes that are specific for a portion of the amplified pertussis DNA in wells of a microtitre plate; after PCR has been performed, the product is denatured and then allowed to hybridize to the immobilized capture probe. In one case, PCR product is detected by fluid phase hybridization with an alkaline phosphatase-conjugated detector oligonucleotide (45); in the other example, the original PCR was carried out using a 5'-biotinylated primer for the strand which is complementary to the capture oligonucleotide, and then bound product is detected using a streptavidin-enzyme conjugate (36). In both cases, the microtitre plates were developed using chromogenic enzyme substrates and absorbance was measured spectrophotometrically, thereby enabling implementation of an objective positive cut-off value.

4. Quality control of PCR reactions

There are two principal areas for concern relating to the use of PCR assays for diagnosis of pertussis which warrant specific mention. First, specimen preparation methods may be such that inhibitors remain in some samples, resulting in false-negative results. If simple boiling is used to prepare extracts, roughly 5-10% will inhibit the PCR reaction. One way to control for the presence of such inhibitors is to include primers that are specific for a portion of a human gene such as that encoding β-actin in the PCR assay which direct amplification of a different size PCR product as compared to that directed by the pertussis primers (50). Nasopharyngeal specimens are almost certain to contain small amounts of human DNA, and so failure to amplify the β-actin fragment in a given sample is a potentially reliable indicator of the presence of inhibitors. Overlap extension PCR can also be used to construct synthetic internal control DNAs for use in pertussis PCR assay, which utilize the same primers as the target DNA (51). In many cases, inhibition can be overcome simply by diluting the original nasopharyngeal extract 5- to 10-fold and thereafter retesting it (50), although further purification (e.g., by phenol-chloroform extraction) may be necessary for recalcitrant samples.

The other major concern is the possibility of false-positive reactions caused by contamination of PCR reactions. In the overwhelming majority of cases, this contamination emanates from previous PCR reactions. Contamination of a batch of reagents is easily detected by the presence of a PCR product in negative control reactions that are included in each PCR run, but spot-contamination of individual tubes is harder to identify. Nevertheless, careful adherence to appropriate work practices and physical separation of the areas, where pre- and post- amplification steps are performed, can minimize these problems. Ideally, specimens and reagents should be prepared and reactions can be set up in a dedicated room, distantly located as far away as possible from the place where the thermal cycler is housed and the PCR products are detected. This 'PCR clean' room should be fitted with an ultraviolet light to facilitate decontamination, and work surfaces and equipment should be regularly cleaned with hypochlorite or dilute HCl. Staff should wash their hands and remove potentially contaminated gowns or lab coats worn elsewhere in the laboratory before entering; they should apply clean gowns and gloves once inside. Items of equipment and consumables that are taken into the clean room should be decontaminated beforehand (by exposure to UV, or swabbing with hypochlorite) wherever practicable. Equipment items such as micropipettes and microfuges should be dedicated to the facility. We have adopted these procedures in our own clinical laboratory, and in a decade of routine pertussis PCR testing that includes analysis of over 20,000 specimens, we have experienced contamination problems only once. On this occasion, the problem was traced to contamination of the inside of a micropipette (which presumably had been used previously for handling PCR product), and was solved by dismantling and cleaning the bore and piston of the pipette with hypochlorite. Of course, the risk of carryover from aerosols in micropipettes can be virtually eliminated by the use of plugged pipette tips, although these are more expensive than conventional ones. A further means of preventing false-positives involves inclusion of uracil-N-glycosylase and substitution of dUTP for dTTP in the PCR reaction mix. Thus, all PCR products will contain uracil, and predigestion of PCR reactions with the glycosidase will destroy any contaminating PCR product prior to amplification; the enzyme is then heat-inactivated during the first denaturation step of the PCR cycle. Native DNA, of course, will not be affected, as it is not a substrate for the glycosylase. Many of the pertussis PCR studies described in the literature have employed this system. For nested PCR assays, however, it can only be used during the secondary amplification step, and the assay will remain vulnerable to contamination with the larger primary PCR product.

D. Serology

Serological responses to *B. pertussis* are an important means of confirming a diagnosis of whooping cough. The immune response to primary infection in unvaccinated subjects (particularly infants) is slow and antibodies may not be detectable until well into the paroxysmal phase. Thus, serodiagnosis in this group involves the demonstration of rising antibody levels between paired "acute" and "convalescent" sera (usually collected at first presentation and 2-4 weeks later). In vaccinees and older children or adults with prior exposure to the organism, however, anemnestic responses may by sufficiently strong and rapid for antibody levels to have already peaked by the time pertussis is suspected and the first serum specimen has been collected. In such cases, a serological diagnosis can be made if the antibody levels in the acute specimen exceed a preset threshold. Antibodies to *B. pertussis* persist for many weeks after onset of symptoms, and so serological analysis will yield positive results long after the organism has been eliminated from the nasopharynx and hence is no longer detectable by culture or PCR. Such retrospective diagnosis is of little clinical value to the patient in question, but it may facilitate earlier recognition of pertussis in close contacts with respiratory symptoms. Serological diagnosis has also played a very important role in the analysis of the protective efficacy of acellular pertussis vaccines in several recent clinical trials (25).

In the past, whole cell agglutination assays, which measured mainly antibodies to fimbrial antigens, pertactin, and LPS have been used for serodiagnosis, but these have now been superseded by more sensitive enzyme-linked immunosorbent assays (ELISAs) (14). These assays also have the capacity to measure isotype-specific responses, which is important because immunization elicits few if any IgA antibodies, and so their presence is highly indicative of current or recent infection. A typical ELISA is performed by reacting one or more dilutions of sera with *B. pertussis* antigen which is immobilized on a solid phase support (usually wells of microtitre trays). Bound human immunoglobulins are then quantitated by reaction with isotype-specific second antibody-enzyme conjugates, and an appropriate (usually chromogenic) substrate. Absorbance values for each well are measured spectrophotometrically, and after correcting for serum dilution, are converted to arbitrary units as calculated with reference to readings that are obtained for the various standard sera which are included in each assay. Use of common standard sera, against which additional in-house control sera can be calibrated, enables comparison of results between laboratories, and such reference materials are available from the Laboratory of Pertussis, U.S. Food and Drug Administration (25).

The choice of *B. pertussis* antigen has a significant impact on the sensitivity and the specificity of ELISA assays. Some assays use sonicated whole cell lysates, and commercial kits that make use of crude sonicated antigen are available. Interpretation of such assays, however, is complicated by the potential for cross-reactions with other organisms. The development of acellular pertussis vaccines has resulted in the more widespread commercial availability of purified *B. pertussis* antigens, including PT, FHA, pertactin, and fimbriae. ELISA assays that use purified antigens are more specific and more sensitive than those which use sonicated cell lysates (52). PT is probably the most useful diagnostic antigen, because it is absolutely specific for *B. pertussis*, and roughly 90% of infected persons respond to it. There is a similarly high prevalence of responses to FHA, although it is somewhat less specific; FHA is also produced by *B. parapertussis* and it has epitopes in common with non-typable *H. influenzae* (14). Responses to other antigens such as pertactin and fimbriae occur with slightly lesser frequency (30-60%) (15,25). Antibodies elicited by infection are principally IgG, and the more diagnostically significant IgA responses are somewhat less frequent, occurring in only about 40% of patients (14). In view of this, most of the published serological studies have involved measurement of IgG and IgA responses to either PT alone, PT and FHA, or in some cases PT, FHA, and pertactin (25,40,53,54,55,56).

Interpretation of the diagnostic significance of serological data can be problematic, particularly in highly immunized populations. For a diagnosis to be made on the basis of the antibody titre in the acute serum, ELISA values for a given antigen and isotype need to exceed a cut-off which is calculated with reference to antibody levels in healthy persons that do not have the history of recent exposure to pertussis. Due to marked age-related differences in pertussis antibody levels, separate background serological data sets must be obtained for a series of age-groups which are selected on the basis of routine immunization schedules in a given country, and such that the effect of recent vaccination on baseline antibody levels can be accounted for. Background antibody levels will also be affected by changes in vaccines as is occurring in many parts of the world at present with the introduction of acellular pertussis formulations. A further complication is that antibody levels in a population may drift with time in accordance with herd immunity that results from the natural epidemic cycle of pertussis. Thus, ideally, the serological status of the 'healthy' population needs to be sampled regularly. For each of the healthy control groups, the mean serum ELISA titre for each isotype and antigen is then calculated. In most studies, the cut-off has been set at a level which is three standard deviations above the mean of the age-matched healthy controls, and a result is positive if this is exceeded for at least one (sometimes two) of the isotype/antigen combinations tested. In some studies, a result was also considered positive if the ELISA titre exceeded a cut-off that is set at two standard deviations above the mean for two or more isotype/antigen combinations. If ELISA titres in the acute specimen do not reach the diagnostic threshold, then a second sample can be collected and tested (in parallel with the first sample) to determine whether the patient has seroconverted. The second specimen should be collected a minimum of two weeks after the first, and in young children, this should be at least 6 weeks from the date of onset of symptoms, to allow sufficient time for seroconversion (37). There is marked variation in the literature regarding what is considered a significant rise in antibody levels. In some studies, rises of at least 4- or even 8-fold were required (37), whereas others determined the cut-off on the basis of an assessment of the intra-assay coefficients of variation for the ELISA assays employed. On these bases, increases of 1.5-fold to 2-fold (depending on the isotype being assayed) were defined as positive (53).

E.   Synopsis

Of the three principal methodologies for laboratory diagnosis of whooping cough, culture has always been considered the 'gold standard' against which the performance of the others was measured. Although the superior performance of PCR for pertussis diagnosis was first demonstrated a decade ago (32), there has been a reluctance to adopt this technology in routine laboratories. One reason for this has been concern about the possibility of false-positive reactions due to PCR product contamination as discussed above. Another contributing factor has been an inability to advocate adoption of a standard methodology because direct comparisons of the various published pertussis PCR assays have not been performed (57). This reluctance, however, ignores the fact that in virtually every study published to date, PCR has out-performed culture, regardless of the precise methodologies employed for either technique. Indeed, in one study, PCR increased the number of positive pertussis diagnoses nearly 4-fold (58). PCR has the capacity to detect non-viable organisms; this is consistent with several studies which have demonstrated that PCR-positive, culture-negative results are more likely to occur in samples from vaccinees, patients with mild or atypical disease, or those who had received prior erythromycin therapy (58,59). Indeed, analysis of follow-up specimens from antibiotic-treated patients have demonstrated that PCR remained positive for up to a week longer than culture (59). Thus, PCR provides a significant number of additional diagnoses, particularly in samples from patient groups in whom diagnosis on clinical grounds alone is most difficult. PCR detects a higher proportion of positive samples than culture, regardless of duration or severity of symptoms, age of patient, vaccination status, or antibiotic treatment (37). In addition, a positive or negative pertussis PCR result should be available in less than 24 hours, whereas a positive culture result is unlikely to be available earlier than 3 days from the date of collection, and may take up to 7 days; a specimen cannot be confirmed as culture-negative in under 10 days. A properly controlled and competently executed pertussis PCR assay is as specific as culture, and is much faster and more sensitive, but it involves a higher labour cost. This should, however, be balanced against the improvements in the quality of patient care that result from the use of PCR technology (e.g., earlier therapeutic intervention in atypical cases, better infection control, etc.) which in the hospital setting will have associated cost benefits. PCR has already replaced DFA testing in many clinical laboratories, and it is likely to become even more widespread in use once commercial kits become available. On the basis of its performance in a large number of studies, it deserves to replace culture as the 'gold standard' for pertussis diagnosis. Indeed, were it not for the occasional and epidemiological desirability of obtaining isolates of *B. pertussis* for antimicrobial susceptibility and serotype/biotype surveillance, persistence with routine pertussis culture in laboratories that are equipped for PCR would appear to serve little purpose.

Serology also has an important role to play as a complement to culture and PCR in the diagnosis of pertussis, although as discussed above, interpretation of ELISA results is complicated. Culture and PCR are likely to be positive from the early catarrhal stage (or even during incubation) until the end of the paroxysmal stage for culture and early convalescence for PCR (3). Serological diagnosis, on the other hand, is usually only possible from the mid-paroxysmal stage, but may continue to yield positive results well into the convalescent stage and weeks after all traces of the organism and residual nucleic acid sequences have been eliminated (3). In cases where serological results are equivocal, information regarding the vaccination status of the patient, clinical presentation, duration of illness relative to the dates that sera were collected, antibiotic exposure, etc., can aid interpretation, but unfortunately, these clinical details are not always available. Thus, optimal diagnosis of pertussis requires deployment of at least two complementary methodologies to detect early and advanced cases. For laboratories with appropriate facilities, maximal speed and sensitivity will be achieved by using a combination of PCR and serology; use of culture as a back-up for PCR is desirable, but not essential. Laboratories without access to PCR technology should continue to perform both culture and serological analyses.

VII. SUSCEPTIBILITY TESTING

Antibiotic therapy plays an important role in the management of cases of whooping cough and has two goals; firstly to ameliorate the symptoms and limit the duration of the disease, and secondly to prevent subsequent transmission of the infection by eliminating the organism from the respiratory tract. In both cases, therapy is most effective when commenced early in the course of disease, i.e., before it reaches the paroxysmal phase, and prophylaxis of close contacts of cases during the incubation period has been shown to be protective (60). Some clinical benefit as well as reduction in transmission, however, may still result when therapy is commenced during the paroxysmal phase (61). Erythromycin, particularly as the estolate form, is the antibiotic of choice for therapy for whooping cough, the recommended pediatric doses being 40 mg./kg./day as administered for two weeks (9,61). This drug has been the mainstay of therapy for many years, and erythromycin-resistant isolates of B. pertussis are extremely rare. New macrolides such as azithromycin and clarithromycin are equally active against B. pertussis in vitro, and although clinical data are limited, they should be highly effective in vivo as they are pharmacokinetically superior to erythromycin and can reach higher concentrations at the respiratory mucosa (9,61). Cotrimoxazole is also capable of eradicating B. pertussis from the nasopharynx, and has been used to successfully treat a patient that is infected with an erythromycin-resistant strain (62). It may also be more effective than erythromycin for the treatment of B. parapertussis infections (61).

Antimicrobial susceptibility testing for B. pertussis is not standardized, and given the extreme rarity of isolates that are resistant to erythromycin (the drug of choice), it cannot routinely be justified on clinical grounds. For erythromycin, agar dilution using Mueller-Hinton agar that is supplemented with 5% horse blood was found to be the most reliable method. Limited studies for cotrimoxazole also have suggested that the agar dilution method yields results which are more consistent with the associated in vivo efficacy than does the broth dilution method (3,61). Poor growth of B. pertussis also complicates the reading of E test plates, and standardized methods for disc diffusion are not available. Although growth of the bacterium is better on charcoal agar, this medium is unsuitable for susceptibility testing as it over estimates MIC values, presumably due to inactivation or adsorption of antibiotic (61).

REFERENCES

1. Cherry JD. Historical review of pertussis and the classical vaccine. J Infect Dis 1996; 174(Suppl 3):259-263.
2. Bordet J, Gengou O. Le microbe de la coqueluche. Annales de l'Institut Pasteur 1906; 20:731-741.

3. Hoppe JE. Bordetella. In: Murray PR, Baron EJ, Pfaller MA, Tenover FC, Yolken RH, eds. Manual of Clinical Microbiology, 7th edition. Washington, D.C.:ASM Press, 1999:614-624.

4. World Health Organization. In: V & B Annual report, 1998; Department of Vaccines and Other Biologicals. WHO/V&B/99.01, p. 34. WHO, Geneva, Switzerland; 1999.

5. Christie AB. Infectious Diseases: Epidemiology and Clinical Practice. 2nd ed. Edinburgh: Churchill Livingstone, 1974.

6. Hoppe JE. Update on respiratory infection caused by *Bordetella parapertussis*. Pediatr Infect Dis J 1999; 18:375-381.

7. Heininger U, Stehr K, Schmitt-Grohé S, Lorenz C, Rost R, Christenson PD, Überall M, Cherry JD. Clinical characteristics of illness caused by *Bordetella parapertussis* compared with illness caused by *Bordetella pertussis*. Pediatr Infect Dis J 1994; 13:306-309.

8. Black S. Epidemiology of pertussis. Pediatr Infect Dis J 1997; 16:S85-S89.

9. Hoppe JE. Update on epidemiology, diagnosis, and treatment of pertussis. Eur J Clin Microbiol Infect Dis 1996; 15:189-193.

10. Kerr JR, Matthews RC. *Bordetella pertussis*: pathogenesis, diagnosis, management, and the role of protective immunity. Eur J Clin Microbiol Infect Dis 2000; 19:77-88.

11. Tuomanen EI, Hendley JO. Adherence of *Bordetella pertussis* to human respiratory epithelial cells. J Infect Dis 1983; 148:125-130.

12. Sandros J, Tuomanen EI. Attachment factors of *Bordetella pertussis*: mimicry of cell recognition molecules. Trends Microbiol 1993; 1:192-196.

13. Fernandez RC, Weiss AA. Cloning and sequencing of a *Bordetella pertussis* serum resistance locus. Infect Immun 1994; 62:4727-4738.

14. Müller F-MC, Hoppe JE, von König C-HW. Laboratory diagnosis of pertussis: state of the art in 1997. J Clin Microbiol 1997; 35:2435-2443.

15. Meade BD, Mink CM, Manclark CR. Serodiagnosis of pertussis. In: Manclark CR, ed. Proceedings of the Sixth International Symposium on Pertussis. DHHS publication no. (FDA) 90-1164. Bethesda, MD:Food and Drug Administration, 1990:322-329.

16. Nagel J, Poot-Scholtens EJ. Serum IgA antibody to *Bordetella pertussis* as an indicator of infection. J Med Microbiol 1983; 16:417-426.

17. Cherry JD. "Pertussis vaccine encephalopathy": it is time to recognize it as the myth that it is. JAMA 1990; 263:1679-1680.

18. Pasternack MS. Pertussis in the 1990s: diagnosis, treatment and prevention. Curr Clin Top Infect Dis 1997;17:24-36.

19. Ad Hoc Group for the Study of Pertussis Vaccines. Placebo-controlled trial of two acellular pertussis vaccines in Sweden - protective efficacy and adverse reactions. Lancet 1988; i:955-960.

20. Greco D, Salmaso S, Mastrantonio P, Giuliano M, Tozzi AE, Anemona A, Ciofi degli Atti ML, Giammanco A, Panei P, Blackwelder WC, Klein DL, Wassilak SG. A controlled trial of two acellular vaccines and one whole cell vaccine against pertussis. N Engl J Med 1996; 334:341-348.

21. Gustafsson L, Hallander HO, Olin P, Reizenstein E, Storsaeter J. A controlled trial of a two-component acellular, a five-component acellular, and a whole cell pertussis vaccine. N Engl J Med 1996; 334:349-355.

22. Olin P, Rasmussen F, Gustafsson L, Hallander HO, Heijbel H. Randomized controlled trial of two-component, three-component, and five-component acellular pertussis vaccines compared with whole-cell pertussis vaccine. Ad Hoc Group for the Study of Pertussis Vaccines. Lancet 1997; 350:1569-1577.

23. Cherry JD, Gombein J, Heininger U, Stehr K. A search for serological correlates of immunity to *Bordetella pertussis* cough illnesses. Vaccine 1998; 16:1901-1906.

24. Storsaeter J, Hallander HO, Gustafsson L, Olin P. Levels of anti-pertussis antibodies related to protection after household exposure to *Bordetella pertussis*. Vaccine 1998; 16:1907-1916.

25. Hallander HO. Microbiological and serological diagnosis of pertussis. Clin Infect Dis 1999; 28(Suppl 2):99-106.

26. Hallander HO, Reizenstein E, Renemar B, Rasmuson G, Mardin L, Olin P. Comparison of nasopharyngeal aspirates with swabs for culture of *Bordetella pertussis*. J Clin Microbiol. 1993; 31:50-52.

27. Wadowsky RM, Laus S, Libert T, States SJ, Ehrlich GD. Inhibition of PCR-based assay for *Bordetella pertussis* by using calcium alginate fiber and aluminium shaft components of a nasopharyngeal swab. J Clin Microbiol 1994; 32:1054-1057.

28. Regan J, Lowe F. Enrichment medium for the isolation of *Bordetella*. J Clin Microbiol 1977; 6:303-309.

29. Katzko G, Hofmeister M, Church D. Extended incubation of culture plates improves recovery of *Bordetella* spp. J Clin Microbiol 1996; 34:1563-1564.

30. Ewanowich CA, Chui LWL, Paranchych MG, Peppler MS, Marusyk RG, Albritton WL. Major outbreak of pertussis in northern Alberta, Canada: analysis of discrepant direct fluorescent-antibody and culture results by using polymerase chain reaction technology. J Clin Microbiol 1993; 31:1715-1725.

31. McNicol P, Giercke SM, Gray M, Martin D, Brodeur B, Peppler MS, Williams T, Hammond G. Evaluation and validation of a monoclonal immunofluorescent reagent for direct detection of *Bordetella pertussis*. J Clin Microbiol 1995; 33:2868-2871.

32. Glare EM, Paton JC, Premier RR, Lawrence AJ, Nisbet IT. Analysis of a repetitive DNA sequence from *Bordetella pertussis* and its application to the diagnosis of pertussis using the polymerase chain reaction. J Clin Microbiol 1990; 28:1982-1987.

33. Houard S, Hackel C, Herzog A, Bollen A. Specific identification of *Bordetella pertussis* by the polymerase chain reaction. Res Microbiol 1989; 140:477-487.

34. World Health Organization. WHO meeting on case definition of pertussis. Geneva, 10-11 January, 1991. MIN/EPI/PERT/91.1, pp. 4-5.

35. Bäckman A, Johansson B, Olcén P. Nested PCR optimized for detection of *Bordetella pertussis* in clinical nasopharyngeal samples. J Clin Microbiol 1994; 32:2544-2548.

36. Buck GE. Detection of *Bordetella pertussis* by rapid-cycle PCR and colorimetric microwell hybridization. J Clin Microbiol 1996; 34:1355-1358.

37. Van der Zee A, Agterberg C, Peeters M, Mooi F, Schellekens J. A clinical validation of *Bordetella pertussis* and *Bordetella parapertussis* polymerase chain reaction: comparison with culture and serology using samples from patients with suspected whooping cough from a highly immunized population. J Infect Dis 1996; 174:89-96.

38. Lind-Brandberg L, Welinder-Olsson C, Lagergård T, Taranger J, Trollfors B, Zackrisson G. Evaluation of PCR for diagnosis of *Bordetella pertussis* and *Bordetella parapertussis* infections. J Clin Microbiol 1998; 36:679-683.

39. Grimpel E, Bégué P, Anjak I, Betsou F, Guiso N. Comparison of polymerase chain reaction, culture, and western immunoblot serology for diagnosis of *Bordetella pertussis* infection. J Clin Microbiol 1993; 31:2745-2750.

40. He Q, Mertsola J, Soini H, Skurnik M, Ruuskanen O, Viljanen MK. Comparison of polymerase chain reaction with culture and enzyme immunoassay for diagnosis of pertussis. J Clin Microbiol 1993; 31:642-645.

41. He Q, Schmidt-Schläpfer G, Just M, Matter HC, Nikkari S, Viljanen MK, Mertsola J. Impact of polymerase chain reaction on clinical pertussis research: Finnish and Swiss experiences. J Infect Dis 1996; 174:1288-1295.

42. Nelson S, Matlow A, McDowell C, Roscoe M, Karmali M, Penn L, Dyster L. Detection of *Bordetella pertussis* in clinical specimens by PCR and a microtiter plate-based DNA hybridization assay. J Clin Microbiol 1997; 35:117-120.

43. Mastrantonio P, Stefanelli P, Giuliano M. Polymerase chain reaction for the detection of *Bordetella pertussis* in clinical nasopharyngeal aspirates. J Med Microbiol 1996; 44:261-266.

44. Reizenstein E, Lindberg L, Möllby R, Hallander HO. Validation of nested *Bordetella* PCR in pertussis vaccine trial. J Clin Microbiol 1996; 34:810-815.

45. Li Z, Jansen DL, Finn TM, Halperin SA, Kasin A, O'Connor SP, Aoyama T, Manclark CR, Brennan MJ. Identification of *Bordetella pertussis* infection by shared-primer PCR. J Clin Microbiol 1994; 32:783-789.

46. Douglas E, Groote JG, Parton R, McPheat W. Identification *of Bordetella pertussis* in nasopharyngeal swabs by PCR of a region of the adenylate cyclase gene. J Med Microbiol 1993; 38:140-144.

47. Van der Zee A, Agterberg C, van Agterveld M, Peeters M, Mooi FR. Characterization of IS1001, an insertion element of *Bordetella parapertussis*. J Bacteriol 1993; 175:141-147.

48. Farrell DJ, Daggard G, Mukkur TKS. Nested duplex PCR to detect *Bordetella pertussis* and *Bordetella parapertussis* and its application in diagnosis of pertussis in nonmetropolitan southeast Queensland, Australia. J Clin Microbiol 1999; 37:606-610.

49. Stefanelli P, Giuliano M, Bottone M, Spigaglia P, Mastrantonio P. Polymerase chain reaction for the identification of *Bordetella pertussis* and *Bordetella parapertussis*. Diagn Microbiol Infect Dis 1996; 24:197-200.

50. Wadowsky RM, Michaels RH, Libert T, Kingsley LA, Ehrlich GD. Multiplex PCR-based assay for detection of *Bordetella pertussis* in nasopharyngeal swab specimens. J Clin Microbiol 1996; 34:2645-2649.

51. Müller FM, Schnitzler N, Cloot O, Kockelkorn P, Haase G, Li Z. The rationale and method for constructing internal control DNA used in pertussis polymerase chain reaction. Diagn Microbiol Infect Dis 1998; 31:517-523.

52. He Q, Mertsola J, Himanen JP, Ruuskanen O, Viljanen MK. Evaluation of pooled and individual components of *Bordetella pertussis* as antigens in an enzyme immunoassay for diagnosis of pertussis. Eur J Clin Microbiol Infect Dis 1993; 12:690-695.

53. Hallander HO, Storsaeter J, Möllby R. Evaluation of serology and nasopharyngeal cultures for diagnosis of pertussis in a vaccine efficacy trial. J Infect Dis 1991; 163:1046-1054.

54. Marchant CD, Loughlin AM, Lett SM, Todd CW, Wetterlow LH, Bicchieri R, Higham S, Etkind P, Silva E, Siber GR. Pertussis in Massachusetts, 1981-1991: incidence, serologic diagnosis, and vaccine effectiveness. J Infect Dis 1994; 169:1297-1305.

55. Giammanco A, Taormina S, Genovese M, Mangiaracina G, Giammanco G, Chiarini A. Serological responses to infection with *B. pertussis*. Dev Biol Stand 1997; 89:213-220.

56. Wirsing von König CH, Schmitt HJ. Epidemiological aspects and diagnostic criteria for a protective efficacy field trial of a pertussis vaccine. J Infect Dis 1996; 174(Suppl 3):281-286.

57. Meade BD, Bollen A. Recommendations for use of the polymerase chain reaction in the diagnosis of *Bordetella pertussis* infections. J Med Microbiol. 1994; 41:51-55.

58. Schläpfer G, Cherry JD, Heininger U, Überall M, Schmitt-Grohé S, Laussucq S, Just M, Stehr K. Polymerase chain reaction identification of *Bordetella pertussis* infections in vaccinees and family members in a pertussis vaccine efficacy trial in Germany. Pediatr Infect Dis J 1995; 14:209-214.

59. Edelman K, Nikkari S, Ruuskanen O, He Q, Viljanen M, Mertsola J. Detection of *Bordetella pertussis* by polymerase chain reaction and culture in the nasopharynx of erythromycin-treated infants with pertussis. Pediatr Infect Dis J 1996; 15:54-57.

60. Sprauer MA, Cochi SL, Zell ER, Sutter RW, Mullen JR, Englender SJ, Partriarca PA. Prevention of secondary transmission of pertussis in households with early use of erythromycin. Am J Dis Child 1992; 146:177-181.

61. Hoppe JE. State of art in antibacterial susceptibility of *Bordetella pertussis* antibiotic treatment of pertussis. Infection 1998; 26:242-246.

62. Lewis K, Saubolle MA, Tenover FC, Rudinsky MF, Barbour SD, Cherry JD. Pertussis caused by an erythromycin-resistant strain of *Bordetella pertussis*. Pediatr Infect Dis J 1995; 14:388-391.

24

Anaerobic Infections

Nevio Cimolai

Children's and Women's Health Centre of British Columbia, Vancouver, British Columbia, Canada

I. HISTORICAL BACKGROUND

Some knowledge of the existence of anaerobic life forms was already apparent as early as the late 1800s. The culture of these bacteria was promoted by the use of the anaerobic jar by the early 1900s (1). Yet much of the very important knowledge in this area of diagnostic bacteriology and its practical application was realized mainly within the last 25 years or so. An exponential growth of interest and science occurred during the 1970s and 1980s, and although of great relevance to contemporary medicine, the theme of anaerobic bacteriology seemingly has achieved a plateau in the last few years apart from numerous changes in the applied systematics. It is certain that the number of bacteria that are currently recognized and which are currently cultured with existing methods may represent only a fraction of the bacteria that are present in humans even in the normal state. Genetic methods have continued to emphasize that there are genomes in existence among normal flora samplings that are unaccounted for and thus likely represent previously unrecognized bacteria (2); see also Chapter 6. Anaerobes are good prospects among the latter. This area of diagnostic bacteriology has not been spared from the numerous name changes that have arisen from the advancements in applied systematics (Table 1) (3), and it is conceivable that the study of anaerobic bacteriology will receive considerable attention once more.

What is an 'anaerobe'? The definition must be accepted for the arbitrary explanation that one can propose. There are evidently bacteria that span a spectrum of aerotolerance and growth atmosphere requirements that vary from the extreme of strict exclusion of oxygen to growth in routine atmospheric air. Anaerobes will grow much better in existing anaerobic environments than aerobes or facultative bacteria. The 'much better' aspect is variable however as some will grow exclusively in the anaerobic milieu, e.g., fastidious fusobacteria or *A. israelii*, whereas others will grow much better anaerobically but will nevertheless become adaptable to microaerophilic atmosphere after subculture, e.g., some *Actinomyces* spp. or propionibacteria. Included in the definition of an anaerobe may also be the criteria of requirement for reduced oxygen tension and the inability to grow in an atmosphere of air that is supplemented by 10% CO_2. The criterion of atmospheric requirement is distinct from the issue of actual aerotolerance since many anaerobes tolerate exposure to atmospheric air for hours (4,5). Otherwise, it has been very difficult to define anaerobes on the basis of some other unique structural, physiological, or biochemical attribute(s). It must be reconciled therefore that the term is a crude yet useful categorization that favourably impacts on the diagnostic bacteriology laboratory as well as clinical medicine.

Table 1   Changes in the applied systematics of anaerobes that are relevant to the review of existing literature.

Former designation	Current designation
CDC group 1	*Actinomyces neuii*
(some) *Bacteroides* spp.	*Prevotella* spp. (*P. disiens, P. bivia, P. melaninogenica,* etc.)
(some) *Bacteroides* spp.	*Porphyromonas* spp. (e.g., *P. gingivalis, P. asaccharolyticus*)
Bacteroides ochraceus	*Capnocytophaga ochracea*
Bacteroides pneumosintes	*Dialister pneumosintes*
Wolinella recta	*Campylobacter rectus*
Wolinella curva	*Campylobacter curvus*
Bacteroides gracilis	*Campylobacter gracilis*
Arachnia propionica	*Propionibacterium propionicus*
(some) *Fusobacterium necrophorum*	*Fusobacterium varium*
(some) *Campylobacter gracilis*	*Sutterella wadsworthensis*
Hallella seregans (*Mitsuokella*)	*Prevotella dentalis*

Whereas a critical role in many diseases is undisputed, anaerobes also play a very important part in the establishment and maintenance of the healthy normal flora at most body sites where such bacteria usually exist (6). In the bowel, some *Bacteroides* spp. participate in the bioavailability of vitamin K, and others serve to create the resident normal flora that are somewhat detrimental to the establishment of enteric pathogens. The total quantitation of anaerobes markedly outnumbers the facultative and aerobic bacteria in the large bowel. The positive contributions that are gained from anaerobes in the bowel are largely under-recognized, but their benefit becomes apparent when they are suppressed by antibiotics and thereby allow for unusual patterns of microbial colonization that may lead to disease. In the vagina and mouth, anaerobes are part of the normal flora but in controlled numbers; in the vagina, high quantitations and the loss of normal lactobacilli (that may also in part exist as anaerobes) are associated with bacterial vaginosis, and imbalances of anaerobes in the mouth may be associated with (although not necessarily causative of) abnormalities of the gums and dentition.

Antimicrobial resistance among anaerobes has been a topic of interest to some, but not nearly to the extent that it has been for many facultative and aerobic bacteria. Trends in resistance have been followed over the last three decades especially, but although some interesting forms of resistance have emerged, anaerobic bacteria have generally appeared to be somewhat stable in this regard. A good example is the continuing susceptibility of Gram negative anaerobes to metronidazole.

Anaerobes continue to be major components of some infections, especially those relating to the intestines and mucous membranes, but great strides have occurred in the control of several. For example, tetanus is a rarity in developed countries where vaccine is routinely used and where other preventative measures can be implemented. The proper processing of foods has markedly reduced the occurrence of botulism, and the liberal use of antibiotics and the calibre of their activity has lessened the occurrence of clostridial gas gangrene. Several aspects of anaerobic bacteriology continue to be subjects for scientific inquiry. The tetanus toxin in its inactive form (toxoid) is an excellent immunogen, and it can be linked with modern technology to less immunogenic (especially carbohydrate) antigens in order to raise the immunological response to the latter. *Clostridium difficile* became recognized as a cause of antibiotic-associated diarrhea in the age of availability of potent broad spectrum antibiotics; it still is a problem, especially in hospitals, and it is capable of spreading in outbreak form in this milieu. Bacterial vaginosis is seemingly an infection, but it is associated with an imbalance in normal flora of the vagina; a role for anaerobes or a single anaerobe has been postulated and not entirely ruled out, and a single etiological agent, if it exists, has escaped discovery. Perhaps most important among this progress in the understanding of anaerobic bacteria is the contribution they have made to the evolution of various pathophysiological processes in general. From the laboratory's perspective, the great era of discovery in anaerobic bacteriology is being followed by a reconciliation with what truly needs to be performed for cost-effective services.

Table 2 outlines anaerobes that have been found in clinical specimens. Among clinical specimens from human infections, the most common isolates belong to the *Bacteroides fragilis* group, *Prevotella* spp., *Porphyromonas* spp., *Fusobacterium* spp., *Peptostreptococcus* spp., and *Clostridium* spp. There are many more anaerobes that have been found among animals and the environment; these are not the subject of this chapter.

II. CLINICAL ASPECTS

A. General concepts

1. Anaerobic infections are often mixed

Although there are many anecdotes of anaerobic infections in which a single bacterium has been isolated, most anaerobic infections are inclusive of a mixed bacteriology. The components of and predominance within this mixture will depend on the site of infection, the source of the infection, and the influence of prior antibiotic therapy. Infections that are contiguous to mucosal surfaces such as mouth or bowel commonly include aerobic or facultative organisms; the most common of these are members of the *Enterobacteriaceae*, microaerophilic streptococci, haemophili, and *S. aureus*. Multiple anaerobes in an infection arise also most likely from a pathological process that is near a mucosal surface. Polymicrobial bacteremia, which includes anaerobes, not uncommonly arises from the gastrointestinal tract and trauma thereof.

The presence of an anaerobe should raise the suspicion that other anaerobes may also be involved in the disease process, especially when multiple bacteria are present which indicate that a mucosal site, that is inclusive of mixed aerobic and anaerobic flora, has been the source.

2. Contributor or by-stander?

For infections that are seemingly caused by a single agent, it is evident that the disease is principally caused by that bacterium. In other circumstances where multiple bacteria have been isolated, it may be more difficult to ascribe causation. For example, in an abdominal abscess, anaerobes such as clostridia, *Bacteroides* spp., fusobacteria, and anaerobic Gram positive cocci are common often and in combination. Although the latter bacteria may have arisen from a common origin, it is conceivable that some, perhaps much less pathogenic on their own, are merely present as a consequence of the suitable environment that they have achieved rather than as the principal instigators of the disease process. Other bacteria, such as enterococci, may also participate more as by-standers than disease-causing agents when some anaerobes or even facultative enteric Gram negative rods are present.

The potential for bacteria to synergize and hence to accentuate a localized process must also be considered. Certainly there is at least a role for facultative bacteria to help initiate a cascade of pathological events which culminate in the creation of a suitable environment, with low red-ox potential, that favours the growth ofanaerobes. The treatment of most, rather than all, bacteria that are present may therefore have great impact.

Table 2   A simplified schema of anaerobes that are acquired from clinical samples.

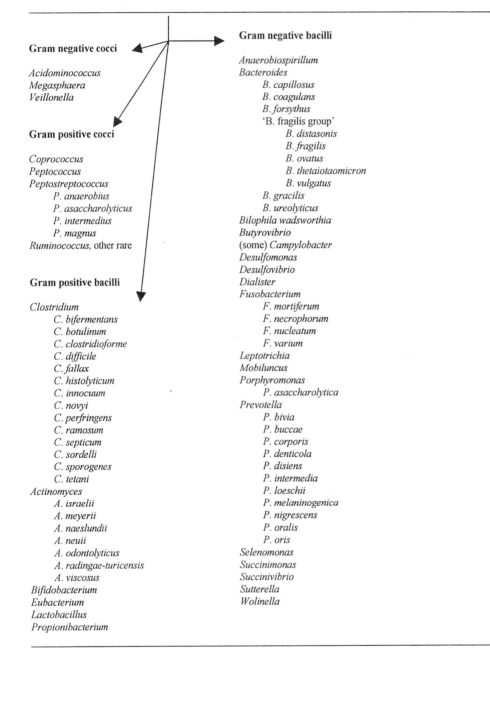

Gram negative cocci

Acidominococcus
Megasphaera
Veillonella

Gram positive cocci

Coprococcus
Peptococcus
Peptostreptococcus
  P. anaerobius
  P. asaccharolyticus
  P. intermedius
  P. magnus
Ruminococcus, other rare

Gram positive bacilli

Clostridium
  C. bifermentans
  C. botulinum
  C. clostridioforme
  C. difficile
  C. fallax
  C. histolyticum
  C. innocuum
  C. novyi
  C. perfringens
  C. ramosum
  C. septicum
  C. sordelli
  C. sporogenes
  C. tetani
Actinomyces
  A. israelii
  A. meyerii
  A. naeslundii
  A. neuii
  A. odontolyticus
  A. radingae-turicensis
  A. viscosus
Bifidobacterium
Eubacterium
Lactobacillus
Propionibacterium

Gram negative bacilli

Anaerobiospirillum
Bacteroides
  B. capillosus
  B. coagulans
  B. forsythus
  'B. fragilis group'
    B. distasonis
    B. fragilis
    B. ovatus
    B. thetaiotaomicron
    B. vulgatus
  B. gracilis
  B. ureolyticus
Bilophila wadsworthia
Butyrovibrio
(some) *Campylobacter*
Desulfomonas
Desulfovibrio
Dialister
Fusobacterium
  F. mortiferum
  F. necrophorum
  F. nucleatum
  F. varium
Leptotrichia
Mobiluncus
Porphyromonas
  P. asaccharolytica
Prevotella
  P. bivia
  P. buccae
  P. corporis
  P. denticola
  P. disiens
  P. intermedia
  P. loeschii
  P. melaninogenica
  P. nigrescens
  P. oralis
  P. oris
Selenomonas
Succinimonas
Succinivibrio
Sutterella
Wolinella

Table 3 Common sites for anaerobic infections.

Head and Neck	Obstetrical/Gynecological
gum disease	vulvovaginal infections
necrotizing mucositis	endometritis
periodontal infections	tubo-ovarian infections
deep tissue infections	chorioamnionitis
peritonsillar abscess	pelvic thrombophlebitis
chronic sinusitis	? bacterial vaginosis
chronic otitis media	
actinomycosis (also abdominal and thoracic)	**Miscellaneous**
subdural infections	skin/soft tissue abscesses
brain abscess	diabetic foot ulcers
	decubitus ulcers
Pulmonary	burn wound infections
aspiration pneumonia	bite wounds (animal/human sources)
lung abscess	cellulitis
empyema	fasciitis
	myonecrosis
Abdominal	osteomyelitis
generalized peritonitis	
intra-abdominal abscess (e.g., peritoneal, liver)	
ascending biliary infections	
perirectal abscess	
antibiotic-associated diarrhea	

3. Variable sites for infection

Table 3 outlines common sites and types of anaerobic infections. The site of infection is often related to the distribution of nearby human flora, and anaerobic infections can arise directly as a consequence of such proximity. Thus, infections that arise from gut flora will often include the *B. fragilis* group, clostridia, and anaerobic Gram positive cocci, whereas anaerobic infections of the head and neck will especially include other *Bacteroides* spp., *Prevotella*, *Porphyromonas*, and fusobacteria. Anaerobic infections that arise from human or animal bites include both bacteria from human skin as well as those (both aerobic and anaerobic) that are present in the perpetrator's oral flora. The bloodstream potentially acts as a conduit for spread to distal sites as is seen for other infections, e.g., to the brain and resulting in a brain abscess. Spread through fascial planes occurs in some limb infections.

4. Anaerobic infections may signal other pathological processes

Systemic or deep anaerobic infections may be a marker of pathology or specific underlying illnesses. For example, anaerobic brain infections may occur as a consequence of direct spread from nearby structures such as the middle ear and sinuses. Dental pathology may lead to anaerobic infection of nearby bone, deep tissue in the mouth or neck, or the nearby venous sinuses. Anaerobic bacteremias may develop from diseased tissue that is part of or nearby malignancies. Aspiration pneumonia (which often includes anaerobes as one component of the mixed bacteriology) may signal problems related to deglutition or abnormal gastric reflux. Pelvic inflammatory disease may indicate risk for sexually transmitted diseases. Decubiti or inflammatory bowel disease may be the underlying risk factors for an anaerobic pelvic osteomyelitis. Essentially, latent complicating features should be considered when the source of the anaerobic infection is not evident; the actual anaerobe may also be more suggestive of an underlying problem, e.g., clostridia and bowel cancer.

5. Devitalized tissue and medical procedures carry risk for infection

The presence of compromised tissue is of major benefit to the establishment of an anaerobic infection since this environment may be relatively deplete of oxygen. Tissue, blood, serous fluid, and other body substances are a wealth of growth substrates for most anaerobes. These substances are also substrates for non-anaerobes which may initiate the process of infection and which thereafter may create a context that is suitable for anaerobes. Devitalized tissue is likely to be present after significant trauma (with or without skin puncture), surgery, vaginal delivery of a newborn, and other elective or emergency medical procedures. Direct surgery which involves a mucosal site that is normally and heavily laden with bacteria, including anaerobes, provides an obvious opportunity for bacteria to enter deep tissue regardless of whether antibiotics have been administered.

The normal delivery of an infant provides a good example of the opportunity for anaerobes in the context of weakened tissue. During pregnancy, the structure of the uterus is markedly altered. The membranes which are near the cervix are essentially in direct contact with a pool of vaginal microbes that are considerably diverse; the membranes too must endure a growth process, and they become weakened closer to the time for delivery. The delivery itself is accompanied by great forces within the uterus which attempt to expulse a newborn, membranes, and a placenta. The interactive site between the uterus and the placenta is severed, and the membranes too are torn from the uterine wall. Thereafter, blood and serous fluid drain from the uterus into the vagina for several days. Retained bits of membrane and placenta may remain for a variable period or indeed until purposely removed through a medical procedure if necessary. The lining of the uterus has been markedly altered. The cervix will have been stretched considerably if not torn, and its status will allow for greater reflux of bacteria from the vaginal pool. Both aerobes and anaerobes from the vagina, which are high in numbers and which comprise a very diverse spectrum, may then act together. It is not surprising, therefore, that some patients will develop an ascending mixed microbial infection which includes anaerobes, e.g., post-partum endometritis, and it is perhaps even more surprising that such infections are not more common than actually occur.

6. Abscess formation is not acute

Many anaerobic infections present as abscesses, especially those that are of mixed bacterial cause and those that are related to mucosal sites. Abscesses represent collections of inflammatory cells which are largely polymorphonuclear cells. Whereas many pathogenic bacteria may elicit an inflammatory response within hours, the formation of an abscess per se usually requires several days. For example, after abdominal bowel surgery, intrapelvic abscesses become recognized usually within 5-7 days. Abscess formation in this context is therefore a manifestation of a more chronic infection. Although some clostridial infections may be manifest with acute symptomatology, anaerobes are not uncommonly associated with subacute or chronic infections.

7. Antibiotics may select for anaerobes

When infection is suspected and empiric antibiotics are first administered, the spectrum of antimicrobial activity may be insufficiently broad to cover anaerobic agents. The latter may especially be the case when an aminoglycoside (that will essentially lack any anti-anaerobe activity at usual doses and blood levels) is combined with a beta-lactam agent. Such treatment of intra-abdominal, gynecological, and oral mixed infections may selectively encourage the growth of anaerobes. In the current era, the use of antibiotics with an increasingly greater spectrum of activity has in part diminished such opportunity.

Although metronidazole is an excellent anti-anaerobic agent, it may have little activity against several non-spore forming anaerobic Gram positive bacilli, and it may select for them when they are present in a minority among other bowel source bacteria. Clindamycin also has excellent anti-anaerobic activity, yet it can be responsible for selectively inhibiting some anaerobes and allowing others, e.g., *C. difficile* in the bowel, to emerge. Others antibiotics may have a general role of suppressing both aerobic and anaerobic bowel flora so that the overgrowth of *C. difficile* will become manifest as antibiotic-associated enterocolitis. Along with this suppression of normal anaerobic flora, there may be a loss of the salutatory contributions of anaerobes in the healthy state.

B. Actinomycosis

Actinomycosis is a chronic infection that progresses slowly over many weeks to months (7). Although it is traditionally discussed in the context of *Actinomyces* spp., the infections are commonly mixed with bacteria that arise from the same source as the *Actinomyces* spp. (i.e., mouth, gastrointestinal tract, and genital tract). The infection can occur among previously healthy individuals although immunosuppression is an important risk factor.

The major sites for actinomycosis are the cervicofacial region, the thorax, and the abdomen (including the uterus) (7). Infection of the cervicofacial area is the most common form. It begins as a mixed infection with bacteria from the mouth due to dental problems or after trauma or surgery (8). Initially, there may be a pain-free mass which may be remittent, and there is often a lack of fever. There may be a paucity of reaction in the surrounding tissue, but the mass may drain to the skin surface; this drainage is often serous and a sinus tract may result. The infection may also spread to nearby mandibular bone or other structures, superficial and deep, of the head and neck. Antibiotic treatment, if given, may temporarily suppress the infection, but relapses and the tendency to chronicity are common. Thoracic actinomycosis usually arises as a consequence of aspirated oral microbes, although rarely it may extend from the cervicofacial region. The infection initially involves the lung tissue itself, but spread can occur to other thoracic structures and to the chest wall (even as a chest wall fistula). Patients may have fever, cough, and hemoptysis. The lung will appear to have a mass lesion with or without disease in the pleural space. Again, the illness is chronic and will have evolved over many weeks to months. It will often be confused with tuberculosis, nocardiosis, and malignancy. Abdominal actinomycosis arises from the presence of *Actinomyces* spp. in the gastrointestinal tract and its spread from a bowel perforation or other pathology which traumatized the integrity of the intestinal mucosa (9). The disease will progress over months to years. It will be indolent with variable fever, abdominal pain, and some constitutional symptoms. From the local infection, the bacterium may create sinus tracts to any contiguous site within the abdomen and even to the skin, e.g., perianal fistulae. It may also disseminate via blood to the kidney or other distant foci. A variation of abdominal actinomycosis (pelvic actinomycosis) is that which involves the uterus as a consequence of the long-term presence of an intrauterine contraceptive device (10). Patients with the latter may have some localized lower abdominal pain, bleeding via the cervix, and seemingly genital discharge. A secondary endometritis can follow, and occasionally, extension to bladder and bowel can occur.

Rarely, *Actinomyces* spp. may cause infection of the skin (localized) (11), bone (secondary to trauma), or central nervous system, and may disseminate via blood.

C. Bacterial vaginosis

Although it is difficult to ascribe this illness purely to an anaerobic infection, there is sufficient evidence at this time to believe that anaerobes have a large if not causative role. If defined solely by a major derangement of normal vaginal bacterial flora, the process can exist in both asymptomatic and symptomatic forms. In the symptomatic form, the patient will often have vaginal irritation and a thin homogenous non-purulent discharge which has a bad odor. The vaginal pH is elevated (usually >4.5-4.7). For either symptomatic or asymptomatic forms, an amine odor may be released after the vaginal fluid secretion is admixed with a drop of 10% KOH on a microscope slide (12). Clue cells (epithelial cells which are studded with adherent Gram negative or Gram variable forms) are apparent, and the Gram stain of the vaginal discharge or of a vaginal swab will show that the usual lactobacilli forms are relatively missing and that they have been replaced by a greater quantitation of Gram negative or Gram variable, especially curved, morphotypes (13). The vaginal fluid contains an excess of putrefactive amines and shows a change in the predominance of organic acids (i.e., much less lactic acid and proportionately more succinic acid).

The anaerobic bacteriology of bacterial vaginosis has been well-studied. Lactobacilli are usually present in high proportions in the normal vagina (~10^7-10^9/ml. of vaginal fluid). As a consequence of bacterial vaginosis, these numbers are reduced by several logarithms. There are large quantities of anaerobes such as *Mobiluncus* spp., *Bacteroides* spp., anaerobic Gram positive cocci, *Prevotella* spp., and fusobacteria. Both the quantity and variety of anaerobes are increased, although there tends to be a paucity of anaerobic spore-forming Gram positive bacilli and 'B. fragilis group' organisms. As an illustration of the latter change, it has been documented that *Mobiluncus* spp. are usually present in less than 5% of the female population, but this frequency increases to 30-90% among those with bacterial vaginosis.

The role of *G. vaginalis* is disputed as is the sole role for *Mobiluncus* spp. (see Chapter 13)(14) The inoculation of either alone into the vaginae of volunteers leads to variable disease, but the application of both simultaneously leads to a compatible illness quite often. The beneficial effect of metronidazole also in part lends credibility to the role of anaerobes in this disease process.

D. Clostridial infections

1. Tetanus

Tetanus is an acute neurotoxic illness due to *C. tetani* that especially affects the inhibitory cells of the central nervous system and hence is associated with muscular spasms. There is a high frequency of death, but it is almost totally preventable with the widespread use of tetanus toxoid vaccine (15).

Tetanus can be localized or generalized. In the localized form, only the musculature at the site of infection (i.e., the site of initial inoculation) may be affected. For example, in the cephalic variant, the cranial nerves may be involved. The localized form may then give rise to the generalized illness. In the generalized form, the uptake of toxin from the site of infection leads to a disorder of muscle groups throughout the body. Initially, the latter may seemingly include only the muscles of the face with contraction of the jaw muscles or those about the face. Abdominal rigidity then ensues, and posturing of the arms and limbs occurs as well. These muscle groups are involved in intense spasms with or without pain, and the spasmodic episodes tend to have several stimuli. The patient generally remains conscious apart from some anoxic episodes that may occur when the diaphragmatic musculature is also affected. The illness may last for weeks. Neonatal tetanus is a generalized tetanus that arises from infection at the umbilical stump when there is poor hygiene and when the mother is not immune and therefore has not transferred protective antibody to the newborn via the placenta (16). Initially the child is weak or floppy and does not appear to feed, but this is soon followed by intense muscular spasms, rigidity, and apnea. Again, the death rate is very high (>90%) (17).

2. Botulism

Botulism is an acute neurotoxic illness due to *C. botulinum* which predominantly affects the peripheral neuromuscular and autonomic nerve junctions and leads to a paralysis (18). The toxic illness is most often acquired from foods where pre-formed toxin has developed. The toxin is absorbed through the gastrointestinal tract, is disseminated via blood, and then causes systemic paralysis. Infant botulism essentially evolves in similar mechanism to the latter except that spores develop into vegetative bacteria in the gastrointestinal tract; toxin is thus produced in vivo rather than having been previously produced in food. In wound botulism, the toxin is absorbed from the site of infection. Occasionally the source may not be apparent.

In food-borne botulism, there is usually a period of 12-24 hrs. between ingestion and overt physiological effects. Patients may experience dry mouth and cranial nerve dysfunction. Diarrhea or constipation are variable. The patient then develops generalized and progressive symmetrical weakness in the absence of sensory changes. Cranial nerve palsies especially involved the periocular sites, e.g., ptosis, e.g., facial paresis, and dysphagia and dysarthria may also become apparent. Weakness spreads to the upper limbs, the trunk, and then the lower limbs. Diaphragmatic involvement may compromise respiration. Recovery may require 1-2 months depending on the initial quantity of toxin that was absorbed. There is some evidence that supports a variation of symptomatology depending on the type of botulin toxin that is present. For infant botulism, the illness has a slower onset (19,20). The infant may not want to feed, may be constipated, and becomes hypotonic. The illness will self-resolve over 1-2 weeks in most circumstances, but it may also relapse. In wound botulism, the absorption of toxin occurs from a lesion at a time when it appears that the initial wound is healing (21).

3. Antibiotic-associated diarrhea

Diarrhea is not an uncommon consequence of antibiotic administration, and it is reported in 5-25% of antibiotic usages (22). The frequency is a function of the length of therapy as well as the type of antibiotic. C. difficile is the major cause of severe forms of antibiotic-associated diarrhea, but it is not necessarily the only cause. For patients with mild diarrheal episodes, up to 30% will have an illness that is associated with C. difficile, whereas the bacterium may be found in up to ¾ of those who develop a colitis. More than 90% of pseudomembranous colitides, however, can be attributed to C. difficile. Other microbial causes of antibiotic-associated diarrhea have included S. aureus, C. perfringens, and yeast. The association of C. difficile with disease is complicated also by the occurrence of asymptomatic carriage of bacterium and the potential presence of measurable fecal toxin among well patients, especially young children.

The diarrheal illness usually begins within 3-10 days of antibiotic use, whether oral or parenteral (22-24). The illness may be mild and brief; it may cease on the same day that the antibiotic use is terminated. It may become progressive for others and may be associated with considerable water and electrolyte loss. A severe watery diarrhea may progress further to a colitis with blood loss, and in its most severe form, present as a pseudomembranous colitis. Fever, abdominal pain, and leucocytosis are variably present. When the bowel is severely affected, it may result in a toxic megacolon and pose a risk for bowel perforation. In rare circumstances, a reactive arthritis may follow (25). Overall, most illnesses would be difficult to differentiate from other infectious and non-infectious colitides were it not for the history of antibiotic use. The illness may also occur after the use of some antineoplastic chemotherapeutic agents rather than antibiotics (26). Although many such illnesses will resolve after discontinuation of the antibiotic, others will require purposeful anti-C. difficile therapy. Relapses among high risk patients are not uncommon. There is also the potential for C. difficile to produce disease mainly in the cecal area and right colon; such a focal illness may not be accompanied by diarrhea.

4. C. perfringens food poisoning

Strains of this bacterium may be capable of producing a pre-formed toxin in foods (27,28). The onset of the illness is usually within 6-12 hrs. of ingestion but as long as 24 hrs. later. Patients often have a watery diarrhea with or without pain and cramps. Nausea is common but unlike some food poisonings that are caused by S. aureus or B. cereus, there is generally a much lesser emetic effect. The illness resolves without specific treatment in 12-24 hrs. after onset.

5. Clostridial gas gangrene (myonecrosis)

This rapidly progressive and serious disease is often associated with C. perfringens, but indeed it may be caused by a number of other clostridia or by a mixture of other aerobic and anaerobic bacteria (even in the absence of clostridia).

The illness will often begin at a site of traumatic injury or recent surgery. In general, the site of infection will have tissue that has been compromised and that has been seeded with C. perfringens and/or other bacteria. The uterus may also be at risk for such an infection after a septic miscarriage or after delivery.

The site of infection will often be painful. The site may become quickly edematous and tender. Gas may be evident in the soft tissue. The overlying skin may be discoloured, and superficial bullae may appear. A light watery discharge with or without blood-tinging may be apparent, but there is distinctly a lack of purulence. Systemically, the patient will appear toxic as the disease progresses; sweating, fever, rapid heart rate, disseminated intravascular coagulation, hypotension, and shock may all follow within a few hours. The infection will break through fascial planes, and the underlying muscle may undergo necrosis. In the initial phases of the illness, it may be difficult to distinguish from streptococcal necrotizing fasciitis. Progression of the area involved may continue after appropriate antibiotics are given.

6.   Other clostridial infections

The sites of clostridial infections encompass a broad spectrum, and the etiological agents can include many of the *Clostridium* spp. Common sites for clostridial infections include abdominal abscesses, biliary tract, superficial soft tissue, and lung. Bacteremias especially occur among oncology patients, but occasionally the bacterium may be present in blood cultures as a contaminant. Neutropenic cecitis in oncology patients is likely caused by a mixture of bacteria, but clostridia are believed to play a role in many circumstances. Although not recognized in developed countries, it has been accepted that some *C. perfringens* strains may be causative of a necrotizing small bowel enteritis.

E.   Disease associations for common anaerobes

The combination of anaerobic species and sites of infection are numerous. The following highlights define more common associations:

Head and Neck: *Bacteroides* spp., *Prevotella* spp., *Porphyromonas* spp., *Fusobacterium* spp., *Peptostreptococcus* spp.
Central Nervous System: *Bacteroides* spp., *Prevotella* spp., *Fusobacterium* spp., *Peptostreptococcus* spp., *Actinomyces* spp.
Abdominal: *B. fragilis* group, *Peptostreptococcus* spp., other *Bacteroides* spp., *Fusobacterium* spp., *Clostridium* spp., non-spore forming Gram positive anaerobic bacilli
Female Genital Tract: *Bacteroides* spp., *Prevotella* spp., *Porphyromonas* spp., *Peptostreptococcus* spp., *Actinomyces* spp., *Clostridium* spp.
Soft Tissue: *Clostridium* spp., *B. fragilis* group, other *Bacteroides* spp., *Fusobacterium* spp., *Prevotella* spp., *Peptostreptococcus* spp., *Peptococcus*, non-spore forming Gram positive anaerobic bacilli
Lung: *Prevotella* spp., *Peptostreptococcus* spp., *Fusobacterium* spp.
Blood-borne: *B. fragilis* group, *Peptostreptococcus* spp., various less common anaerobes
Bone: Peptostreptococcus spp., Fusobacterium spp., Bacteroides spp.

III. EPIDEMIOLOGY OF INFECTION

The vast majority of anaerobic infections are acquired from the endogenous microbial flora, although the environment and other living species may also harbour some pathogenic anaerobic bacteria.

A.   Exogenous sources

Clostridia are abundant in the environment and are especially found in soil and decaying vegetation. They are also commonly found in the intestinal lumena of vertebrates and invertebrates. Minor fecal contamination of meat during the packing process is capable of ensuring that the organisms are present prior to cooking, e.g., for *C. perfringens*. There are several clostridia that are found in the environment and which are pathogenic, but most notable among these is *C. perfringens*, hence its prominent role in the anaerobic infection of puncture wounds. Both *C. botulinum* and *C. tetani* are also common in soil.

The epidemiology of *C. difficile* has been studied considerably, and a role for acquisition from the hospital environment may be important in some settings.

All mammals carry an abundance of anaerobes in their normal bacterial flora analogous to the pattern of humans, albeit with variations in the actual constitution and quantity. Therefore, animal bites often serve to initiate mixed infections which include anaerobes, and the saliva and other excreta of animals also have the potential to contaminate foods or inanimate objects.

Although a single definitive cause of bacterial vaginosis is yet to be defined, the bacteria that are associated with this disease can be transmitted to sexual contacts, whether anaerobes or *G. vaginalis*, and the urethrae of male partners often harbour these bacteria.

B. Endogenous sources – normal microbial flora

The skin maintains an abundant microbial flora although the spectrum of bacteria is relatively narrow compared to other sites. Propionibacteria and to a lesser extent peptostreptococci can be found on the skin; their numbers vary according to site. The perianal area and groin are not usually permanent sources of anaerobes, but soilage from urethral, vaginal, and especially fecal pools is not uncommon. The magnitude of such contamination depends on the state of the host, but there are many examples where the compromised patient, e.g., bed-ridden, e.g., neurologically impaired, may have near permanent soilage. It is evident that very young children will often have fecal anaerobes on their skin due to diapering. Those who suffer from chronic skin ulcers, such as diabetics on their lower limbs or immobile patients with decubiti, may have a continuous presence of anaerobes at the site rather than actual infection.

The vaginal pool may contain up to 10^5-10^7 bacteria per ml. of secretion (29); among these are a diversity of anaerobes which, although in smaller number individually, include *Bacteroides* spp., fusobacteria, peptostreptococci, clostridia, *Eubacterium* spp., *Porphyromonas* spp., *Actinomyces* spp., *Bifidobacterium* spp., and propionibacteria.

The mouth and nares have a very complex bacteriology. There may be up to 10^8 bacteria/ml. of saliva, and there may be a diverse spectrum of aerobes and anaerobes. The quantitation and complexity of anaerobes may be greater in the periodontal sulci. Common anaerobes of the mouth include peptostreptococci, fusobacteria, *Bacteroides* spp., *Prevotella* spp., and *Porphyromonas* spp., but other anaerobes such as *Leptotrichia*, *Actinomyces* spp., *Selenomonas*, former *Wollinella* (now *Campylobacter*), *Bifidobacterium* spp., *Eubacterium* spp., and *Veillonella* among others may also be present. The nares have lesser quantities and a lesser spectrum of diversity; propionibacteria will also be more common at the latter site.

Despite the influence from swallowed saliva, the upper gastrointestinal tract is relatively deplete of bacteria in large part due to the influence of gastric pH which inhibits most species. Thereafter, the bacterial population increases gradually in numbers and diversity as one descends from the upper small bowel to the colon. In the distal duodenal and upper jejunal regions, bacterial counts vary from 10^2 to 10^4/ml. Anaerobes initially are represented in a minor proportion of this total. The number of total bacteria/ml. gradually increases to 10^4-10^6 in the ileum where anaerobes now equal other total bacterial counts. In the large intestine, anaerobes usually predominate, and the total count may exceed 10^{10}/ml. *Enterobacteriaceae* and enterococci are prominent in the large bowel, and yet anaerobes may exceed the total number of facultative bacteria in ratios of 100:1 – 1000:1. The anaerobic flora of the large bowel are tremendously diverse, but more common representation includes *B. fragilis* group, clostridia, non-spore forming Gram positive bacilli, peptostreptococci, and fusobacteria. There are likely many more anaerobic bacteria within the gastrointestinal tract than can be appreciated by routine culture techniques (2). Genetic studies have suggested that *B. thetaiotaomicron*, *C. clostridioforme*, *E. limosum*, *E.*

rectale, *F. prausnitzii*, and *P. productus* are among the most common individual species in the large bowel (2,30,31).

Given the above complement of anaerobes at such accessible sites, the selection of adequate samples for anaerobic culture can be complicated.

C. Special clostridial infections

Due largely to vaccination and post-puncture prophylaxis, tetanus is a rarity in developed countries. Neonatal tetanus in underdeveloped countries and tetanus among injection drug users, however, continue to be of concern.

C. botulinum isolates produce one of six toxins, labelled A-F, and the different toxigenic isolates are associated with different sources (32). Type E-producing isolates are not uncommonly acquired from fish. Wound botulism is often associated with types A and B, and infant botulism with types A, B, and F. The majority of food acquisitions are from canned or fermented foods. There are linkages between the consumption of honey and infant botulism, and although *C. botulinum* spores can occasionally be isolated from honey, such a linkage does not explain the majority of incidences.

The intestinal carriage of *C. difficile*, as assessed by culture, increases considerably after antibiotic use (33), and it is inversely related to the presence of fecal lactobacilli (34). Antibiotic-associated diarrhea has been recorded with almost all antibiotics, but among the most common associations are clindamycin, broad-spectrum penicillins, and broad-spectrum cephalosporins. Antibiotics least likely to be associated are sulphas (including cotrimoxazole), chloramphenicol, and tetracycline. The rate of culture-proven carriage is usually less than 10% in healthy adults, but this may rise to 10-25% simply after a hospital admission (22). Risks otherwise for carriage and disease include a chronic illness, uremia, old age, malignancy, gastrointestinal surgery, and the use of antimotility pharmacological agents. As the frequency of carriage increases, so too does the frequency of stool specimens that have detectable free toxin, although the two are not synonymous. Asymptomatic presence of toxin, even in high titres, does occur. Although humans are likely to be the source of the bacterium for other patients, there is an apparent role for the patients' environment; bacterium has been cultured from the hands of caregivers and inanimate objects and floors. In outbreak settings, such presence may give rise to commonality among isolates, but in many putative outbreaks, isolates are heterogeneous. *C. difficile* can also be found among the enteric flora of various animals and in the non-hospital environment.

IV. NATURE OF THE BACTERIUM, PATHOGENESIS, AND CLINICAL MANIFESTATIONS

For many years, traditional methods of classification have served anaerobic bacteriology well, and this classification along with knowledge of pathogenesis and generalizations regarding susceptibility testing have been generally sufficient for clinicians. There have been many reclassifications and, furthermore, many new species that have been named. Much of this change can be attributed to the application of molecular techniques for the purposes of applied systematics, e.g., 16S rRNA sequencing (35) and cellular fatty acid analysis.

One area in particular that has contributed considerably to a broader appreciation of anaerobic bacteriology is the study of dental sciences (36). For example, interests in the area of periodontitis and its pathogenesis have stimulated the research of anaerobic bacteriology and gingival crevices (37). A progression of Gram positive flora to mainly Gram negative flora is associated with the induction of inflammation in periodontitis (38). Anaerobic bacteria may also promote the presence of other non-anaerobic periodontal pathogens by facilitating interspecies adherence (39).

Anaerobic infections generally elicit a pyogenic response which is heavily weighted with polymorphonuclear cells. Exceptions to this generalization include toxin-mediated diseases (i.e., of clostridia) and actinomycosis.

A. Anaerobic Gram positive cocci

These bacteria often appear in pairs and chains on Gram stains, although some may be nearly cocco-bacillary. There is limited variation in the predominant organic acid by-products as assessed by GLC. The latter do however contrast to the predominance of lactic acid from truly anaerobic streptococci; the latter are also resistant to metronidazole.

Anaerobic Gram positive cocci are closely related to clostridia from a phylogenetic perspective. Within the genera, a number of important events have taken place over the last few decades. Initially, there were several *Peptococcus* spp., but most of these have been transferred to the *Peptostreptococcus* genus; only *Peptococcus niger* remains in the former genus. There have been several new species added to the *Peptostreptococcus* genus over the last decade. Among the more important of these species are: *P. anaerobius*, *P. asaccharolyticus*, *P. indolicus*, *P. magnus*, *P. micros*, *P. prevotii*, and *P. productus* (3,40).

A role for capsule in the pathogenesis of infection has been examined for some of these bacteria (41,42).

B. Non-spore forming anaerobic Gram positive bacilli

Some of these bacteria may stain variably in the Gram process. As well, they may appear irregular or in branching forms. With few exceptions (e.g., some *Actinomyces* spp. and propionibacteria), these bacteria are catalase-negative. Although many *Actinomyces* isolates are very strict anaerobes (e.g., especially *A. israelii*), some may be microaerophilic as may be many lactobacilli and propionibacteria (hence the discussion of the latter in part in Chapter 13). Genetic links to clostridia are evident for many of these genera (43).

Colonies of pathogenic *Actinomyces* spp. may maintain the classic 'molar tooth' appearance. *A. viscosus* and *A. neuii* are catalase-positive. The disease in actinomycosis often requires co-pathogens to initiate the process, and these are often facultative commensals of the mouth. The pathology includes chronic inflammation with accompanying fibrosis that surrounds the disease centres, and the disease may spread through tissue strata despite normal tissue boundaries. Individual lesions, mimicking hard abscesses, may be multiple but interconnected. The lesions may have a purulent core reaction with many polymorphonuclear cells, but they also often contain a mixture of other cells including macrophages, plasma cells, eosinophils, and multinucleated giant cells. 'Sulphur granules' are small circular concretions that may be found in the inflammatory core or along the sinus tracts that subsequently form; they are composed of amorphous crystalline material and some bacteria. The presence of the latter from the infected sites should specifically raise the concern for actinomycosis.

There are several *Lactobacillus* spp., but few are obtained from clinical infections. The predominance of lactic acid as a by-product of metabolism is a key feature.

Pseudoramibacter alactolyticus has been named from one of the former *Eubacterium* spp. (3).

Mobiluncus spp. are motile Gram variable or Gram negative curved rods. They share cell wall attributes with both Gram positive and Gram negative bacteria, and they are phylogenetically somewhat related to the *Actinomyces* spp. The two species that are currently recognized include *M. curtisii* and *M. mulieris* (44). Virulence factors per se are not currently evident, and the exact contribution to bacterial vaginosis awaits clarification.

C. Clostridia

Clostridia are sometimes easily decolorized in the Gram stain when cultures are used, but this may be more common among Gram stains of clinical specimens that contain these bacteria. The bacilli are usually long and relatively square-ended, and thus they may be mistaken initially for *Bacillus* spp. when the Gram stain is over-decolorized. Spores are not apparent among bacilli that are seen in direct stains from clinical specimens. Spores are variably placed in the bacillus, and their placement may be used for the purposes of speciation. Spores are an important attribute since they allow for persistence despite exposure to extremes of heat and decontaminating agents, e.g., alcohol. Most clostridia are motile, and they are catalase-negative and oxidase-negative. There is a spectrum to the degree of aerotolerance among species and isolates of a species. For example, *C. tertium* may grow in an atmosphere with enhanced CO_2, although growth is truly better anaerobically.

Overall, the clostridia are a very diverse group in the phylogenetic sense, and indeed they are ubiquitous in the environment and among animals. It is apparent, however, that most clinically-relevant species belong to a more narrow cluster. Furthermore, there are some very interesting genetic relationships to anaerobic Gram negative (and non-spore-forming) rods, e.g., *Tissierella*. Figure 1 illustrates some relationships among these and other bacteria (45,46). There are several non-clostridial Gram positive and Gram negative bacteria that appear to be taxonomically related to clostridia. Clostridial species have consistent production of some short chained fatty acids when they are cultivated in a standard broth medium. They also have unique cell wall fatty acids; the pattern may be exploited for classification.

Common species in this genus include *C. bifermentans*, *C. clostridioforme*, *C. difficile*, *C. histolyticum*, *C. innocuum*, *C. novyi*, *C. perfringens*, *C. ramosum*, *C. septicum*, *C. tertium*, *C. sordelli*, and *C.*

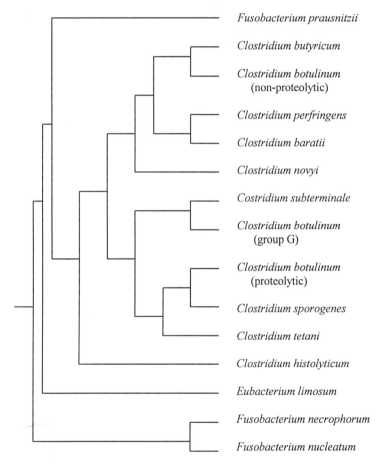

Figure 1 Inter-relationships among select clostridia and related bacteria as shown by dendrogram clusters. Adapted from Collins et al. (45) and from Wang et al. (46).

sporogenes. Although important as major toxin producers, *C. botulinum* and *C. tetani* are uncommon as clinical pathogens in developed countries. The latter bacteria as well as *C. difficile* and *C. perfringens* are often thought of as toxigenic clostridia, but this is somewhat of a misnomer since many other clostridia are indeed toxigenic. The complexity of toxigenicity among clostridia is comprehensively captured in the review by Hatheway (47).

1. C. botulinum

The production of toxin is critical to the pathogenesis of botulism (48). Some toxin-mediating genes can be phage-borne. Toxin can be serologically differentiated into seven types (named A-G), but only a portion of these (types A, B, E, and F) are seen among isolates from humans. Toxin is released from the bacterial cell during lysis, and it initially takes the form of a ~150 kD protein that is cross-linked by sulfhydryl bonds. The singular peptide is cleaved into ~50 kd and ~100 kD fragments which continue to be linked by the same bonds. The toxin is pre-formed in most cases (except infant botulism), and it is absorbed systemically. It crosses the presynaptic membrane of the nerve cell and is internalized. Among peripheral nerves, the toxin interacts with proteins that are responsible in part for the migration of neurotransmitter vesicles as they approach the terminal membrane. Effectively, then, there is a blockade in the release of the neurotransmitter acetylcholine.

Although uncommonly cited, there are reports of other clostridia that have been found to produce botulinum toxins: *C. baratii* (type F) and *C. butyricum* (type E) (49,50).

From the perspective of toxin structure, there is considerable similarity to the tetanus toxin, but each have very unique neurological functions; it is conceivable that a common ancestry is relevant in these regards with subsequent evolutionary modification.

2. C. difficile

Although *C. difficile* is present normally in the gastrointestinal tract, its numbers are suppressed in the milieu of the other normal flora by unknown factors. It flourishes during the alterations that are invoked with antibiotic use. During such growth, *C. difficile* releases toxins. Most human isolates release two toxins named toxin A and toxin B (51). Some isolates will not produce either toxin, and a lesser number may produce one or the other alone (52,53). Both toxins have a high molecular weight ~400-500 kD. Toxin A is recognized as an enterotoxin which causes fluid accumulation, is lethal to mice, and increases vascular permeability. It is also a cytotoxin, but these effects are comparatively minor and much less potent than the cytotoxic activity of toxin B (54). Toxin B is a potent cytotoxin which has the ability to affect a broad spectrum of cell lines; it is also lethal to mice and increases vascular permeability. Toxins A and B are partially homologous in composition. Similar toxins have been described for *C. sordellii*.

Colonic cells have a receptor for toxin A. *C. difficile* toxins are internalized into the cytoplasm, and they subsequently inactivate Rho proteins and interrupt the cytoskeleton (55,56). Signal transduction is affected, and cells round after the induction of apoptotic events (57,58). Through these events, the intestinal epithelial cell layer becomes disrupted, and the initial inflammatory events cause edema and an infiltration of polymorphonuclear cells. As more inflammatory mediators are activated (59), the mucosa becomes visually inflamed and swollen. Small discrete lesions form on the intestinal membrane and eventually coalesce to form pseudomembranes which are essentially composed of leukocytic infiltrate, mucin, fibrin, and other debris from cell degradation. Disruption of the mucosa may also lead to the leakage of capillaries with the subsequent entry of blood into the intestinal lumen.

3. C. perfringens

On blood agar, a hallmark of this species is the evidence of a double zone of beta-hemolysis. The inner zone is caused by the theta-toxin, whereas the outer zone is attributed to the alpha-toxin. These toxins are only a few of the many major and minor toxins that are produced by this bacterium.

Five toxin types A-E are distinguished on the basis of the production of one or more of four specific toxins that may be lethal to laboratory animals; these are labelled as alpha-, iota-, epsilon-, and beta-toxins (47). The alpha-toxin is also known as phospholipase C, and it is probably the most important single toxin. The other minor toxins have a very broad range of tissue active toxicity including lipases, DNAases, other hemolysins, hyaluronidases, collagenases, neuraminidases, and proteases (60).

The active agent in *C. perfringens* food poisoning is a 35 kD polypeptide enterotoxin that is produced throughout the growth cycle (although it was classically considered a toxin that was especially generated during sporulation) (61,62). Receptors on mucosal cells have been defined predominantly in the small intestine. It has the capacity to alter intestinal epithelium, and it has been studied as a possible superantigen.

4. *C. tetani*

This species is strictly anaerobic. By way of motility, it has the capability of swarming on blood agar, and the spreading growth may appear as a film.

The major toxin is classically referred to as tetanospasmin. Its production is due to a gene that is harboured on a single large plasmid. Like the botulinum toxins, it is ~150 kD and is released after cell lysis. Proteolytic cleavage renders two peptides of 50 kD and 100 kD which are joined by sulfhydryl bonds. Its effect may be seen locally at the site of initial toxin absorption, i.e., affecting lower motor neurons, or it may enter the neuronal axon and ascend to the central nervous system through the neuronal fibres and body. In either case, tetanospasmin blocks the release of the gamma-aminobutyric acid neurotransmitter. When affecting the inhibitory cell terminals, there is a resulting disinhibition of motor nerve transmissions which leads to repetitive spasms of the musculature. The autonomic nervous system is also potentially affected.

Tetanolysin is an oxygen-sensitive hemolysin; its absence will not change the course of tetanus.

D. Pigmented anaerobic Gram negative bacilli

These include the genera of *Prevotella* and *Porphyromonas* which fluoresce red after younger cultures are exposed to ultraviolet excitation. As colonies become mature, they may develop a black pigmentation that is apparent in light. A few species have been entered into this group on the basis of genetic studies and they may not necessarily have such pigment; these are more likely to occur among the oral *Porphyromonas* spp.

Common *Prevotella* spp. and *Porphyromonas* spp. are listed in Table 2 (3). There is usually a greater presence of some species in different body sites. For example, *P. buccae* is common among the respiratory tract flora, whereas *P. bivia* and *P. disiens* have been more commonly isolated among flora of the female genital tract. New species continue to be identified especially from the gingival crevices (64).

A number of these bacteria produce tissue active enzymes. *P. melaninogenica* has been studied for its capsule. Although possessing the classic double membrane structure of Gram negative organisms that is detailed for *Enterobacteriaceae* in Chapter 15, the potency of endotoxin from these bacteria is much less.

E. *Bacteroides*

Historically, there were many *Bacteroides* spp., but the genus was split into several groups in the 1980s particularly. For example, the genera of *Prevotella* and *Porphyromonas* were derived. The common species in the *Bacteroides* genus are listed in Table 2. The most prominent of these from a clinical perspective is the 'B. fragilis group' (includes the species *B. distasonis, B. fragilis, B. ovatus, B. thetaiotaomicron,* and *B. vulgatus*) which are resistant to bile; indeed such resistance has been used as a time-honoured preliminary mechanism to define members of this genus. It is believed that several more re-

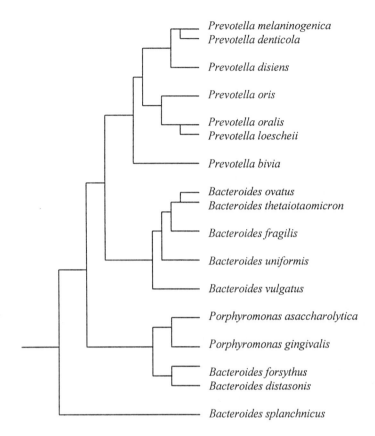

Figure 2 Phylogenetic tree which illustrates the clustering of select anaerobic Gram negative bacilli and crudely shows their interrelationships. Adapted from Paster et al. (63).

classifications of *Bacteroides* species to other or new genera will occur given the diversity that remains despite what has already taken place to refine the applied systematics in this area (Figure 2)(63).

With the Gram stain, these bacteria appear as short rods or often coccobacillary. Again, the Gram negative endotoxin is not potent, but a role for it in the pathogenesis of mixed anaerobic infections and their sequelae cannot be entirely dismissed. Adherence to eukaryotic cells is facilitated by fimbriae, and adherence is thought to be more common among pathogenic isolates (65). The capsule of *B. fragilis* has been studied considerably, and it appears to be important in adherence, abscess formation, and the inhibition of phagocytosis (42).

Several enzymes have been deemed tissue-active, but the most intriguing at this time is the toxin that has been associated with *B. fragilis*. Termed *B. fragilis* toxin or fragilysin, this toxin is a 20 kD metalloprotease toxin which acts like an enterotoxin: it stimulates the secretion of fluid in ligated animal intestinal loops and it alters the morphology of intestinal epithelial cell lines (67). It may effect damage by altering the cellular cytoskeleton (68). The gene for the toxin exists on a putative pathogenicity island (69). The responses of human colonic cells to the toxin are variable (70). Nevertheless, it appears that the toxin is produced only by isolates that are associated with diarrheal illnesses (71). A full understanding of a role for these toxigenic bacteria in human disease is yet to be had, but fragilysin has proteolytic activity (72).

F. Fusobacteria

Fusobacteria are often seen as thin and elongated Gram negative rods when visualized from the direct stains of specimens. *F. nucleatum* often has tapering ends like some *Capnocytophaga* spp. From a blood culture, usually from an oncology patient, such a Gram stain morphology will highly suggest either of these latter two genera, but the morphology is not clearly suggestive of either alone. More variable Gram stain morphology is seen among the other *Fusobacterium* spp. which may be swollen and stain irregularly.

These bacteria are fermentative and have unique organic acid product profiles. The common clinical species are listed in Table 2 (73).

Both *F. necrophorum* and *F. nucleatum* have been studied with respect to virulence factors (74,75). *F. nucleatum* forms aggregates with other suspected pathogens in periodontal disease. *F. necrophorum* has several potential virulence factors, although the endotoxin and leukotoxin seem more important. Nevertheless the endotoxin from species of this genus is not very potent as it may be for some non-anaerobic Gram negative bacilli. Overall, fusobacteria usually act synergistically with other bacteria in producing infection.

G. Other non-spore forming Gram negative bacilli

There are a number of genera represented here including *Anaerobiospirillum, Anaerorhabdus, Bilophila, Butyrovibrio, Centipeda, Desulfomonas, Desulfovibrio, Dialister, Selenomonas, Sutterella,* and *Tissierella* (76). Former *Wolinella* spp. have been transferred to the *Campylobacter* genus even though they are normal bowel inhabitants rather than actual causes of diarrhea, although a recent study has raised some interest in determining whether *Campylobacter concisus* and *Sutterella wadsworthensis* are enteric pathogens (77). Recent work has shown how these new *Campylobacter* spp. are related to similar bacteria (Figure 3). *Sutterella wadsworthensis* has been named from the study of unusual *Campylobacter gracilis* isolates (78). There are several unique attributes for these species. For example, *Bilophila* is bile-resistant and catalase-positive. *Desulfovibrio* reduces sulphur compounds to hydrogen sulphide. *Butyrivibrio, Succinivibrio, Anaerovibrio, Desulfovibrio,* and *Anaerobiospirillum* all have unique morphology as their names suggest. *Selenomonas* spp. are also curved rods. Some are quite rare clinical isolates, and some are more likely to be isolated from particular body sites, e.g., *Selenomonas* from the mouth, e.g. *Butyrivibrio* from the gastrointestinal tract. When obtained from clinical samples, they are most often mixed with multiple other bacteria and anaerobes in particular. Isolation in pure form from a clinical infection is very unusual.

H. Anaerobic Gram negative cocci

Three genera of anaerobic Gram negative cocci include *Veillonella, Acidaminococcus,* and *Megasphaera.* They are not commonly isolated from clinical specimens, and when present, they are usually in the company of other anaerobes. *Veillonella* has small cocci, and colonies will fluoresce red with ultraviolet excitation. When colonies of *Veillonella* are small, they may be mistaken for large colony mycoplasmas (e.g., *M. hominis*) and vice-versa. Both *Acidominococcus* and *Megasphaera* do not fluoresce, and *Megasphaera* cocci may be somewhat large cells. The profile of organic acid products is helpful in identification if necessary.

V. IMMUNOLOGY OF INFECTION

Since abscess formation requires many days to occur, it is possible to develop an immune response to anaerobes during this time, but antibody responses to anaerobes are nevertheless slow to develop. Both antibody and cell-mediated immuneresponses may be important in anaerobic infections. The complexity of the immune response may be increased since non-anaerobic bacteria not uncommonly accompany

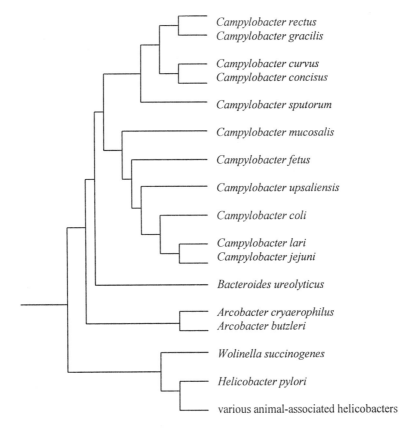

Figure 3   Phylogenetic tree which illustrates the relationships among campylobacters and campylobacter-like organisms. Adapted from Vandamme et al. (79).

anaerobes in infections. Antibody and the subsequent fixation of complement are bactericidal for many anaerobes, but the ability of both of these factors to penetrate the sites of anaerobic infections is compromised. Anaerobes are generally susceptible to phagocytosis by polymorphonuclear cells and macrophages, and polymorphonuclear cell function does occur under anaerobic conditions.

A.   Clostridia

The humoral response to *C. tetani* toxoid vaccine is excellent, but some immunity may be lost after many years. Thus, booster vaccinations are recommended in adulthood. Immunity also is diminished after treatment regimens for malignancies or bone marrow transplantation. Human immune sera may reduce the severity of tetanus although cell-bound toxin will be spared from antibody binding. After significant exposure in a non-immune subject, the use of both booster immunization and human immune globulin are advocated.

Protective humoral immunity does not develop after clinical botulism. Illnesses may benefit from the administration of trivalent horse anti-toxin.

The use of horse-derived anti-toxin for *C. perfringens*-associated gas gangrene was contemplated many decades ago, but its use was abandoned. During gas gangrene, there is a noticeable absence of polymorphonuclear cells in the tissue. This absence is likely to be a function of polymorphonuclear cell lysis from bacterial toxin, impedance of phagocytic cell migration by toxin, and a general lack of potent factors to attract the same immune cells.

The existence of antibody to *C. difficile* toxins is common in the general population (80,81). The latter antibody can be neutralizing but is mainly IgA rather than IgG (82). Humoral responses also occur to non-toxin proteins of *C. difficile* (83). Anecdotally, oral IgA has been used to treat recurrent infection. Recurrent disease is possible, and thus, it appears that mucosal protection may be difficult to achieve. Nevertheless, it is has been proposed that neutralizing antibody and particularly antibody to toxin B are somewhat protective. In animal models of infection, systemic vaccination provides protection (84). Toxin differentially affects white blood cell subsets (85).

B. Other anaerobes

Antibodies develop to the capsule of *Bacteroides* spp. and they may act with complement to achieve lysis. Much experimental work, however, has indicated that T cell activation is critical in the development of abscesses (86,87). The capsule of *B. fragilis* cross-reacts with *H. influenzae* type b.

Antibody to various periodontal pathogens has been examined, and quantities are elevated among diseased patients when compared to well children and adults (88,89). It has been suspected that the humoral response may have some role in the pathogenesis of periodontal disease (90).

There is a differential immune response to *Actinomyces* spp. (91) which may explain why *A. israelii* may be more likely associated with actinomycosis in contrast to some of the *Actinomyces* spp. that are mainly found in the gingival spaces.

Systemic antibody does develop to *Mobiluncus* spp. during bacterial vaginosis (92), but it does not appear that such a response is accompanied by mucosal protection.

VI. LABORATORY DIAGNOSIS

A. Specimen collection

Recommendations for the proper collection of specimens that are intended for anaerobic culture are provided in Chapter 3. Essentially, it is desirable to acquire samples in a fashion that limits contamination from the normal anaerobic flora of the body. The use of an anaerobic transport container is often beneficial but must be tempered by the context of the medical site.

B. Specimen transport

Recommendations relating to the transport of specimens that are intended for anaerobic culture are also discussed in Chapter 3. Overall, it is desirable to use a transport container that is free of oxygen so that bacteria are spared from oxygen-induced toxicity.

An anaerobically pre-gassed and rubber stoppered tube (Hungate tube) which does not have media was historically proposed as the preferred transport mechanism. This vehicle required the inoculation of the tube with a needle and syringe since the opening of the stoppered cap might allow for dispersion of the internal anaerobic gases. There are also many specimens that are not amenable to such inoculation including swabs which are perhaps the most common form of sample that is sent to the bacteriology laboratory. Aspiration of an abscess with needle and syringe has been recommended, although some have recently argued against this method given the potential for biohazard when health care workers process specimens with needles. Aspiration may not be possible for some samples despite a worthy concern for anaerobic culture. Also, oxygen may diffuse into a syringe if it is being held for many hours prior to processing.

Pre-reduced anaerobically sterilized (PRAS) media have also been touted for anaerobic transport and continue to be commonly used (93-95). These consist of tubes with agar media that have been sterilized and have maintained a reduced anaerobic environment under seal. Components of the medium sufficiently support the anaerobic state even when the tube cap is removed as a swab is inserted. As the deep part of the tube especially continues to be anaerobic even when the top is exposed to atmospheric air, the swab that is plunged through the agar medium to the deep is sufficiently protected.

The Vacutainer™ transporter has now been used for several decades and continues to be favoured by some. It consists of an agar free tube within a tube. A sterile swab and holder are removed from the first tube initially. When the specimen has been collected, this swab is pushed along with the inner tube through to the larger tube which has an anaerobic gas environment; the latter contains a mixture of hydrogen, carbon dioxide, and nitrogen. A catalyst within the larger tube also facilitates the conversion of oxygen and hydrogen to water.

There is good agreement that anaerobic transport mechanisms should be used for specimens that are submitted over distances and over lengthy periods of time. The transport issue may be a subject for healthy debate, however, when specimens are delivered over short courses and when they are to be processed with little delay. As previously suggested, many common anaerobes are relatively tolerant to room air, and such tolerance may be accentuated when the bacteria are in the milieu of the clinical sample. Furthermore, while it is desirable to have the best transport method and to ensure the utmost which will maximize the culture of anaerobes, there are some samples which probably do not justify such a rigid view, e.g., intra-abdominal abscesses after previous bowel surgery or catastrophe. The latter specimens will invariably yield anaerobes, and anaerobes are usually present in a mixture such that anaerobe-targeted therapy is likely to be given regardless of the total number that are actually isolated. A routine swab is not preferable, but yet it should not be automatically discarded when it arrives in the laboratory only a short time after collection from the operating room even though anaerobic culture is indicated. The refusal to process specimens for anaerobic culture must take several factors into consideration, especially the fact that a privileged specimen may not be easily recollected. There are circumstances, however, where prior knowledge of the clinical disease may prompt strict attention to collection and transport, e.g., actinomycosis, e.g., previous known *Fusobacterium* spp. infection.

Tissue, when acquired, will usually be forwarded to a laboratory that, in addition to performing histopathological examination, will be able to process the specimen for anaerobic culture. Tissue may be transported in anaerobic bags, but such an approach is not generally warranted. It is best to handle the tissue expeditiously.

C. Initial processing and culture

1. Working conditions

Specimens should be handled promptly during set-up, again in order to reduce exposure to oxygen. This initial processing can take place on the bench top, although anaerobic chambers (discussed below) have been devised for initial and final processing (96,97). Pre-reduced media which are maintained anaerobically are optimal for initial set-up (93,98-100), and inoculated media from the bench top made be held in an anaerobic holding chamber (box) (101) until formally incubated since it may be useful to pool the media so that anaerobic jars (for example) can be optimally used. Anaerobic plastic bags which have reducing agents can also serve to maintain anaerobic solid media especially when the specimen number is small. Anaerobic jars are probably the most feasible culture chamber.

The mincing of tissue, when submitted, is not known to adversely affect the ability to recover anaerobes. It is essential, however, that the tissue sample be representative of the infection core. For example, peripheral tissue from an actinomycotic focus may not always yield the bacterium.

2. Growth atmosphere

The intent of the anaerobic culture vessel is to provide an atmosphere that is deprived of oxygen; these variably contain 5-10% CO_2, 5-10% H_2, and 80-90% N_2. The production of an anaerobic atmosphere has been considerably simplified by the use of commercial gas generating pouches ('gas packs') which generate H_2 and CO_2 after the admixture of water, sodium borohydrate, citric acid, and sodium bicarbonate. Alternatively, the atmosphere may be created with repetitive evacuation of an anaerobic jar and replenishment of the atmosphere with an equivalent gas mix that is obtained from commercial cylinders. The latter alternative may prove to be more economical when compared to other options. Alumina pellets are conventionally used as catalysts in order to remove residual O_2, but these tend to be inactivated over time by the water by-product. Accordingly, the catalysts need periodic rejuvenation with dry oven heat. Anaerobic vessels may be controlled with the use of methylene blue or reazurin indicators which are colourless in the anerobic state; when the indicators are newly opened and initially exposed to air, they may remain coloured for several hours even though the anaerobic environment has been adequately achieved. Anaerobic plastic pouches for solid medium culture have been commercialized (102); they have gas generating ampoules and an impermeable plastic. The latter are restricted by the limitation in space such that only a few solid media may be held at any one time.

The anaerobic chamber, usually in the configuration of a large box-like structure, was initially designed to provide a large working area in an anaerobic environment so that there would be a minimum of specimen and culture medium handling; most if not all work could essentially be performed in the chamber (103,104). Material within the chamber can be handled with long gloves that are sealed to a see-through plastic cover. The chamber provides proper incubation temperature, atmosphere, and humidity. It provides for continuous culture and is continuously monitored with anaerobic indicators. A small step-down box allows for the transport of specimens in and out of the larger chamber without the peril of introducing atmospheric oxygen. Although the chamber may have its advantages for several purposes, it is relatively costly and may consume more time overall given the maintenance that is required. It also will require a dedicated space. Problems with gas leakage/seals or system break-downs are not uncommon, and there should be a provision for alternate culture apparati if this system fails and cannot be repaired for several days.

3. Growth media

The pattern of practice relating to the selection of growth media for the purposes of anaerobic culture should be dictated by the given needs that are generally experienced in a particular context. This may include considerations for additional anaerobic media when specific concerns arise. In addition, it must be acknowledged that anaerobic culture is in most circumstances an adjunct to the overall culture process which in many circumstances is just as likely, if not more likely, to yield other bacteria.

With respect to anaerobic culture, both solid and liquid media should be used in order to maximize the yield. The media may include non-selective, selective, and/or differential ones. Routine non-selective anaerobic media are generally supplemented with 5% blood; heme (5 mg./L.) and vitamin K (10 mg./L.) are also common supplements. Non-selective solid media include Brucella blood agar, Schaedler blood agar, Columbia blood agar, and Anaerobic blood agar; these may be enriched with yeast extract. Non-selective broth media include supplemented thioglycollate medium, chopped-meat glucose broth, and supplemented anaerobic brain-heart infusion broth.

The addition of selective media may be standard for some specimens that commonly yield anaerobes, but may be added selectively depending on the nature of the specimen and perhaps the Gram stain in some circumstances. Bile tends to select for some Gram negative anaerobes, especially those of the 'Bacteroides fragilis group'. Gram negative anaerobes are also selected by the addition of aminoglycosides and vancomycin to the solid media (e.g., kanamycin-vancomycin laked-blood agar). The use of PEA medium inhibits facultative Gram negative rods and thus allows for better recognition of anaerobic Gram positive cocci. Clostridia may be purposely screened on neomycin-egg yolk agar which provides differential phenotypes for those which have enzymes that affect the lipids. Overall, the anaerobic environment suppresses growth of yeast and other fungi, and their plentiful growth on anaerobic solid media in part may define problems with the anaerobic atmosphere. Bacteroides-Bile Esculin agar (105) has been used to especially select and differentiate for members of the 'B. fragilis group'. Cycloserine-cefoxitin fructose agar (106) is among many that have been used for the selection of *C. difficile*. Spore selection has also been used for *C. difficile* culture. Various studies of complex anaerobic flora have defined a number of other selective and differential media that are not commonly used for the purposes of routine clinical specimens; these have included media that are tailored for *Bifidobacterium* spp., lactobacilli, oral *Actinomyces* spp., fusobacteria, and *Veillonella*.

4. Incubation time and temperature

Since the generation time may be slow for some anaerobes, it is generally recommended that anaerobic cultures be incubated for a minimum of two days prior to assessment. Thus, anaerobic jars, if used, would be opened and the media inspected after 48 hrs., but re-incubated for another 48-72 hrs. thereafter as some fastidious anaerobes such as some fusobacteria and *Actinomyces* spp. may require 4-7 days of culture. Nevertheless, members of the 'B. fragilis group' and several clostridia grow so well that they may be reasonably sized after 18-24 hrs., and it may be useful to inspect some anaerobic cultures this early if the need to know about gas gangene pathogens is real. Cultures which are purposely sent for *Actinomyces* spp. detection can be dealt with in two stages: one solid medium may be viewed at 5-7 days, and the other duplicate can be viewed at 10-14 days.

Enrichment media should be assessed over a 7-day period if cultures are apparently negative otherwise. Both anaerobic pouches and the anaerobic chambers allow for visualization of the solid media while work is in progress; accordingly, interventions such as subculture can be decided on proactively.

Cultures are maintained at 35-37°C, and the use of lower or higher temperatures is not applicable to anaerobic bacteriology.

D. Specimen staining

Anaerobic bacteria should be considered when there is a discrepancy between the Gram stain which shows numerous bacteria and when routine culture does not yield facultative bacteria within the first 18-24 hrs. in the absence of antibiotic treatment. In anaerobic pneumonia, commonly due to aspiration of bacteria that are refluxed from the upper gastrointestinal tract or due to salivary secretions that cannot properly drain, the Gram stain of endobronchial aspirates may show plenty of bacteria and polymorphonuclear cells in the relative absence of epithelial cells which would indicate salivary contamination.

With respect to individual bacterial morphotypes, several generalizations can be made. *Actinomyces* may appear as branched and filamentous Gram variable or Gram positive elements. *Veillonella* appears as tiny Gram negative cocci but are often overshadowed by other bacterial forms. Some fusobacteria are defined by their spindle-shaped, elongated, and tapered Gram negative rod morphology. *Bacteroides* spp. may appear as coccobacillary forms or as coliform-like Gram negative rods. Clostridia may appear Gram negative or Gram positive (107), and the bacilli are usually quite regular and square-ended. Propionibacteria are often diphtheroidal. *Leptotrichia* commonly appears as very long and plump Gram negative bacilli and at times almost fusiform; they are more likely to be seen in the Gram stains of clinical samples that have been contaminated with mouth flora.

The sulphur granules of actinomycosis, when present, are usually evident to the eye unless passed over casually as tissue debris. These may be crushed and then Gram stained to demonstrate mats of actinobacilli amidst amorphous material.

E. Determinate processing

1. General

Initially, the main requisite is to prove that the isolate is indeed an anaerobe as defined (see I. Historical Background). It may be evident that a colony, which is found on the anaerobic media but not on the other routine bacteriological media, may indeed be an anaerobe. Experience with the recognition of common anaerobe colonies will allow in some circumstances a short-cut to the next level of identification. Otherwise, anaerobic dependency is demonstrated by confirming that the isolate does not grow on chocolate medium in an atmosphere with 5-10% CO_2.

The morphology of anaerobic bacterial colonies has been described in detail in some reference anaerobic bacteriology manuals, but outside of a few more typical colonies, the relatively inexperienced technologist will not make much use of these descriptions. Observation of colonies with the aid of an inverted microscope may be of value, however, in the early detection of pigment.

The degree of identification must be influenced by the given needs and by the actual pattern of growth that is evident (108). For most circumstances, knowledge that anaerobes exist and a description to the genus level are often satisfactory. Unique contexts may arise, however, when speciation is desirable, e.g., blood cultures where contamination is dubious, e.g., monomicrobial anaerobic infections of deep tissue such as CSF, abscesses in unique sites such as brain, or bone infections. Furthermore, speciation may be of some value when the sampled site is one that has not responded to conventional antimicrobial therapy including anti-anaerobic agents. For some infections where there are several anaerobes from a likely mucosal source, it may be best to simply indicate that such a mixture exists, since even the identification of the several isolates may not give justice to the actual complexity of anaerobic bacteriology that may have existed, e.g., report 'mixed fecal flora present' when a mixture of aerobic and anaerobic bacteria of bowel origin are cultured. When the perceived work is likely to be considerable for a given specimen, it may be prudent to ensure that the patient's status warrants that such laboratory resource be consumed. The identification of anaerobes is best handled on a multi-tiered basis which will allocate priority to those specimens and organisms that so deserve it.

Most bacteriology laboratories should have the capacity to identify common anaerobes with the use of some relatively simple assays. These will include the Gram reaction, colony morphology (for some), hemolysis on blood agar, observations of swarming growth or pitting of the agar media, spore formation, catalase determination (10%, not the conventional 3%), motility, indole, and susceptibility to three antibiotic discs (kanamycin 1000; colistin 10; vancomycin 5). In addition, simple tests for nitrate, growth on 20% bile, urease, SPS disc susceptibility, fluorescence of colonies on laked blood agar under uv excitation, lecithinase, and lipase are usually within the reach of most modest-sized diagnostic laboratories. The combination of these tools along with some commercial anaerobic identification kits will suffice to identify up to 80-90% of common isolates. A crude scheme for such identification steps is illustrated in Figure 4.

More definitive identification can be undertaken with the assistance of several methods. Pre-reduced anaerobically sterilized (or equivalent) biochemicals can be used for assessing fermentation patterns and a few other determinations; they may be purchased or prepared in-house. Commercial biochemical systems come in two forms – some require 24-48 hr. of incubation and are largely dependent on microbial growth and subsequent reactions over this time. Although labeled at times as rapid kits, these methods often require heavy inocula which mandates the use of a reasonable growth from subculture plates. Other kits utilize enzyme substrates which give rapid results over several hours on the basis of pre-formed enzymes. In general, these test kits include substrates for proteolytic enzymes, saccharolytic enzymes, carbohydrate fermentation, indole, nitrate, arginine dehydrolase, among others. On a cautionary note, some of the latter commercial systems do not perform well for particular genera and species, and their limitations should be understood in advance. The databases often lag behind the published changes in applied systematics. As for other such kits that are used for bacterial identification, some reactions can subjective and thus prone to variability ininterpretation. Experience in kit interpretation must be had. There are several commercial kits for anaerobic identification, and examples of these include AN-IDENT, Rapid ID 32 A, RapID ANA II, and Vitek ANI card (113-118).

The determination by gas-liquid chromatography (GLC) of volatile and non-volatile acid products from growth in modestly well-defined media is a time-honoured tertiary method which has served anaerobic bacteriology well (119). Patterns of expected products are published (110), and the method is among the last resorts once other more simple methods for characterization are practically exhausted.

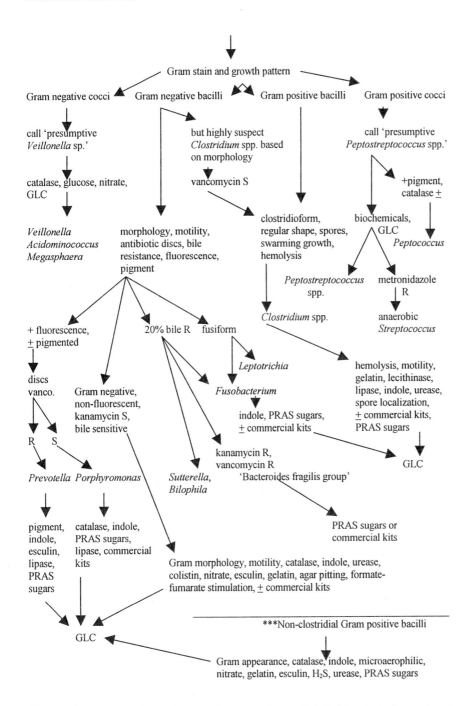

Figure 4 An overview scheme of presumptive and definitive techniques for characterization of anaerobic isolates. Adapted from several sources (109-112).

The method is time-consuming and should be reserved for those isolates that are truly deserving of extensive characterization. The determination of long chain fatty acids through a commercial instrument has also be used for several years but not to the extent of GLC. Early uses were hindered by the limitation of the profile database, but the database has been enlarged considerably. Some reports also detailed the application of GLC to direct assessment of clinical material (120). It is inevitable that 16S rRNA sequencing will become available in a practical form for the speciation of anaerobes, since much of the recent renovation in applied systematics in this area has depended on such technology.

2. Anaerobic Gram positive cocci

On a practical basis, the absolute speciation for this group of bacteria is not commonly required in the clinical diagnostic realm. Mere definition to the level of the generic identification of anaerobic Gram positive cocci will suffice because the speciation in itself does not have any prognostic or diagnostic impact and because the susceptibility of this group of bacteria is fairly predictable.

There are several *Peptostreptococcus* spp., but only one *Peptococcus* species; the latter may be suspected on the basis of a weak catalase reaction (10-15% peroxide) and the finding of pigment when colonies are view under a dissecting microscope and when the isolate is fresh. Anaerobic streptococci mimic other anaerobic Gram positive cocci in many ways, but they are commonly fermentative and produce a strong lactic acid peak when GLC is applied. At least four other genera of anaerobic cocci exist, and these are rarely found in clinical samples: *Coprococcus, Ruminococcus, Atopobium*, and *Sarcina*. The most common *Peptostreptococcus* species include *P. anaerobius, P. magnus*, and *P. asaccharolyticus*. Anaerobic Gram positive cocci are found in up to 1/3 of all clinical specimens that yield anaerobes.

These anaerobes are relatively aerotolerant. Their morphology may be variable at times. In addition, care must be taken to ensure that variation in the Gram stain does not allow for Gram positive anaerobic cocci to be confused with Gram negatives and vice-versa. The papers of Murdoch give comprehensive descriptions of species and as well detail the biochemical schemata that may be used to define these (40,121). It is accepted that changes in the nomenclature of existing peptostreptococci are forthcoming. Biochemical identification is most useful especially with the inclusion of peptidase assays since many of the sugar reactions are non-reactive for this subset of anaerobes. There are particular problems with the speciation of butyrate-producing isolates. Commercial kits have variable performance outcomes for species of this group, but the success rate is ~70-90%. Again, the actual need for the latter is dubious in the majority of isolates. GLC has some limited benefit, but it is mainly adjunctive in a minor role to biochemical identification otherwise.

3. Non-spore forming anaerobic Gram positive bacilli

The definition of this group of bacteria to the species level is not commonly warranted, but there are particular short-cuts that may be taken, and there may be circumstances where the more definitive identification may be desirable. For example, an anaerobic non-spore forming Gram positive rod may deserve more attention if it is a relatively pure isolate from a site where actinomycosis is possible and perhaps even clinically suspect. On a practical basis, *P. acnes* is one of the most common clinical isolates from this group. Although true infection is possible, most isolations reflect contamination from skin. Thus, the quick differentiation of *P. acnes* on the basis of diphtheroidal appearance, positive indole, and positive catalase is indicative of skin contamination especially when this is applied to blood cultures; *P. acnes* is grown from the anaerobic bottle after 4-7 days, and it is the second most common blood culture contaminant (after coagulase-negative staphylococci) in several recent series. Differentiation in samples from intra-abdominal abscesses is a circumstance where excessive work should not be done.

Among the broad anaerobic groups, this one generally is most problematic to apply commercial kits for speciation. Depending on the species, ~20-90% accuracy is obtained, and the least accuracy is achieved usually for those isolates that are most desirable to seek speciation. GLC is, however, very useful for this group. Lactobacilli have a strong lactic acid peak. Propionic acid is largely produced on a proportionate basis for *Propionibacterium* spp. *Bifidobacterium* spp. produce a balance of acetic acid and lactic acid.

Lactobacilli generally have regularly shaped rods. *Bifidobacterium* spp. may show bifurcated ends in Gram stains, although such an appearance is not entirely specific. *Mobiluncus* spp. are motile but may stain Gram variable. Species within the genera of *Eubacterium*, *Bifidobacterium*, and *Mobiluncus* can be identified mainly with biochemicals, and GLC may be a useful adjunct in some cases. The definition of *Mobiluncus* spp. in vaginal fluids is not of practical value for defining bacterial vaginosis. Rather, in addition to clinical symptoms and a few simple tests, the Gram stain of vaginal smears is most important (122); two schemata which detail the anticipated profiles have been devised and are widely used (123,124).

Actinomyces spp. are often mixed, and the separation from other bacteria may be tedious. If the histopathology and clinical circumstances are sufficiently consistent with actinomycosis, it may be wise to accept a role for *Actinomyces* spp. and not proceed with the lengthy culture protocol and isolation that may be needed. When *Actinomyces* spp. are particularly sought, media should be set with the anticipation that they may be viewed once or twice over 5-14 days. Blood agar and PEA are usually adequate, and the addition of metronidazole may provide for some selection. Although it is commonly written that *Actinomyces* spp. often have 'molar tooth' colonies, some colonies are smooth. Biochemicals are used to differentiate the species in this genus; two species may be particularly aerotolerant and catalase-positive.

The lactobacilli and propionibacteria are particularly microaerophilic (see Chapter 13), and they may become even more so after repetitive culture and some adaptation.

4. Clostridia

The location of spores has been used to assist in identification since some species have very predictable central or subterminal patterns (110). In addition, however, there may at times be some difficulty in confirming spore presence, and the use of heat or alcohol spore selection may be used to confirm that one is dealing with a spore-forming anaerobe (125).

C. perfringens can be reliably identified on the basis of its double-zoned hemolysis and little else may be required. Otherwise, speciation of clostridia may include lipase and lecithinase reactions on egg yolk agar, gelatin hydrolysis, indole reaction, fermentation patterns, and GLC profiles. Commerical kits perform very well for identifying *C. perfringens* and a few other common species, but their performance may be quite variable for some others. If such speciation is required, it may be prudent to ensure that kit identifications are supported by reactions from some more time-honoured assessments.

The laboratory diagnosis of botulism is dependent on the form of the illness that is being investigated. In infant botulism, there is usually very little circulating toxin, and thus, it is very difficult to detect by using serum toxin analyses. It is preferable to have a sufficient stool sample in order to detect either bacterium by culture or toxin. In food-borne botulism, toxin and bacterium are possibly detected in the food item of origin. Furthermore, toxin may be detected in serum, stool, or vomitus. Toxin assays are biological ones that use mice; extracts with and without co-administration of antitoxin are administered intraperitoneally. By necessity, such an assay may require 24 hrs. or more. Suspect bacterial isolates from stool should also be tested for toxigenicity, although PCR detection for toxin genes is also described (126,127).

For *C. perfringens* food poisoning, assays of bacterial toxin have also been detailed, but these are not commonly used. Rather, it is practical for most laboratories to simply examine bacterial counts of suspect food or patient's stool. Counts >10^5/gm. are generally regarded as significant. Since *C. perfringens* can normally be found in stool, its mere presence cannot be taken to indicate a cause-and-effect relationship.

C. difficile-associated diarrhea

Among all of the diagnostic issues which pertain to anaerobes, it may very well be that *C. difficile*-associated diarrhea as a sole entity has received the most attention in recent times (128). Progress in this area as well as a fundamental appreciation of current methods depend on having understood the sequence of events over the last twenty or more years. In the 1970s, it became apparent that some antibiotic use was associated with the development of symptomatic enteritis; clindamycin was particularly implicated by some. A varying degree of clinical illness was recognized, and the search for a specific enteric pathogen led to the discovery that *C. difficile* overgrowth in the large bowel and its liberation of a potent toxin were largely responsible. By the late 1970s, it was accepted that a major marker for advanced disease was the detection of free cytotoxic activity in stool with the use of various susceptible eukaryotic cell lines. Specificity of the toxin detection was maintained by the simultaneous assessment that such activity could be neutralized by an animal anti-toxin antibody. For those patients with advanced enteric illness such as pseudomembranous colitis, the presence of cytotoxin was found in more than 95% of stool specimens (129). For those patients with an illness of lesser intensity, the frequency of cytotoxin presence was not as common. Detection of cytotoxin by this approach then became established as the single standard. Despite this gain, there were several issues which posed concern. Since not all patients who had an apparent antibiotic-associated diarrhea would yield stool specimens which had such toxin activity, it was proposed that perhaps other markers of *C. difficile*-induced disease should be sought. Furthermore, it was noted that the presence of neutralization-confirmed toxin was not confined to patients with disease. For example, young infants in the absence of antibiotic use or asymptomatic individuals who received antibiotics might have measurable free toxin in the absence of illness. In a population of such individuals, free toxin activity could be measured in a range of ~2-15% (130,131). The mere presence of stool cytotoxin was by no means an absolute indicator of disease activity or of prognostic importance. Commercial tissue culture cytotoxin assays became available, and they continue to be used.

The other single marker that became of use was the simple presence of *C. difficile* in stool through the assessment of culture. The culture of *C. difficile* was thoroughly studied, and there is the potential to use several selective media (134), although CCFA (cycloserine-cefoxitin fructose agar) has emerged as one of the more popular (132). In addition, *C. difficile* culture could also be facilitated with the use of spore selection (either heat or alcohol) with and without subsequent selective media. It was realized soon, however, that the presence of *C. difficile* as a spore or vegetative bacterium in stool was considerably non-specific for diagnostic purposes since normal carriage must be present given the role of this bacterium at times in the normal enteric flora. Nevertheless, it is a sensitive marker. In order to enhance the sensitivity overall, some chose to combine toxin detection with culture for all assessments. Yet others chose to use the culture as the sole diagnostic measure given its high sensitivity, while yet another strategy was to use culture as a screening method which could be followed by cytotoxin testing of stool for confirmation (since the latter was seen as a cumbersome technique to have in diagnostic bacteriology laboratories which most often did not maintain cell culture capability). The use of culture alone was also complicated by the recognition that not all *C. difficile* isolates were toxigenic. Thus, it was proposed that bacterial isolates should be toxin tested, and that toxin-positive status only would merit concern. The speciation of *C. difficile* is not overly difficult and requires the combination of colony characteristics, association with a particular pungent odour, various biochemicals, and fluorescence on solid media. Commercial kits vary in their ability to speciate this bacterium, but there are some examples which perform very well in this regard (133). Very rarely do other maneuvers need to be used, and again, it is possible to use the cytotoxin assay of broth culture supernatants in order to confirm the presence of a toxigenic strain. Indeed in current times, PCR-based or other genetic detection methods can be used to demonstrate toxigenicity potential (135). Overall, the detection of toxin and the culture of toxigenic bacterium were available, but there was some controversy over which approach in particular was the most sensitive while balancing the issue of specificity. As well, laboratories also required some consideration for which method or pattern they would choose given time and cost concerns.

As rapid agglutination and enzyme immunoassay techniques became increasingly used in diagnostic bacteriology, it seemed sensible that their application to the detection of bacterial toxin would be of value. Initially, latex agglutination was commercially available for this purpose (136,137). There were many supportive trials which touted latex agglutination as an equal (but much less costly and less time consuming) to stool cytotoxicity determination. Others found the latex agglutination and similar assays to be insufficiently sensitive (~50-80%), and this led some to advocate the conjoined use of latex agglutination and culture. As the use of latex agglutination for this purpose became somewhat well-popularized, it was discovered that the antibody predominantly recognized non-toxin antigen(s), especially glutamate dehydrogenase (138). It was apparent, however, that although toxin itself was not being detected, there was nevertheless a good correlation with the presence of high numbers of bacteria although differentiation of toxigenic and non-toxigenic bacterium was now not possible with this method alone. Non-specific agglutination with some stool specimens was a problem, and the inability to be definitive about some agglutinations (i.e., equivocal agglutination; in up to 5-10%) posed as an additional complicating factor. The polyclonal antibody that was used in latex agglutination was also used in an EIA format; the promises and pitfalls were essentially like those of the latex agglutination.

As the above events were proceeding, knowledge of the nature of the cytotoxic activity was advancing too, and such insight was translated into new methods of toxin detection since it was desirable to have an efficient, accurate, portable, and less costly approach to diagnosis (139). In particular, the recognition of two major toxins as previously detailed was then used to design EIA systems that could detect toxin A, toxin B, or both. The recognition of toxin A as an enterotoxin suggested that its detection might in itself serve to define the presence of the actual principally-responsible virulence factor and thus be more accurate as a diagnostic marker. To the contrary, since the time-honoured standard in part was to assess cytotoxicity, yet others believed that EIA detection of toxin B was an effective surrogate. Both of the latter approaches had their pitfalls, and the production of toxin A/B EIAs also emerged. Overall, EIA detection of *C. difficile* toxins is not as sensitive as cell culture cytotoxicity, but the good correlation as well as the technical advantages have been sufficient for many laboratories to choose EIA. Given the EIA configuration, however, it must be acknowledged that some colourimetric readings will fall in an equivocal zone; this may include up to 10% of assays. Rapid membrane immunoassays have also been commercially developed (140). The sensitivity and specificity of EIAs range ~50-90% and 70-95% respectively (141-149). Overall, EIA is less sensitive than the cell culture cytotoxicity assay.

Although an uncommon event, there continue to be episodes whereby a putative *C. difficile*-associated illness, even very severe, occurs in the context of negative assays for stool toxin regardless of what method is used. Some of these illnesses have been supported by the endoscopic finding of pseudomembranous colitis. In relevance to the latter, right-sided colonic illness in the absence of left-sided colonic illness has been detailed (150). Due to such concerns, some have advocated that methods should be chosen so to maximize sensitivity (i.e., combination of culture and toxin assay whether conventional or EIA-based). The outstanding concern with such an approach is that the frequency of false-positives will out-number the few circumstances where laboratory diagnostic testing will miss true disease. Of more fundamental importance is the definition of disease association. It is apparent that any one method alone will be subject to some interpretive error or limitation. It is imperative therefore that diagnostic testing be assessed in the clinical context and with knowledge of such limitations. Thus, knowledge of antibiotic use, clinical course, response to antibiotic cessation if it occurs, previous such illness, status of the patient regarding other medical conditions and risk factors, other laboratory data, endoscopic findings if pursued, among other things should be considered. In most circumstances, diagnostic information relating to *C. difficile* is being acquired because the patient is symptomatic. Investigation should not be an automatism if only an enteric illness occurs in the presence of antibiotic use. Many antibiotic-associated diarrheas will resolve even when the antibiotic is continued. Most others will resolve when the antibiotic course is complete or interrupted. Investigation is most likely to be needed when it is desirable to assist in a complex investigation or when therapeutic intervention is likely to be warranted. For most such illnesses, the use of the cell culture cytotoxin assay alone will be sufficient as a single test. When the disease continues and is severe, it may be warranted that culture for toxigenic *C. difficile* be attempted, but it is quite likely that endoscopy will have already been performed. A positive or for that matter negative assay will only be considered in the context of the clinical illness. When diagnostic assays are being compared, it is critical to see how the standard for diagnosis is defined; a combination of laboratory and clinical criteria are most apt. As well, even if the single assay being assessed is not perfect, the study should determine what frequency of clinically-important disease would be missed if the assay is falsely negative; the latter assessment necessitates the follow-up of many patients. Otherwise, most comparisons of assays basically reflect a simplified method-to-method analysis. There is also the possibility that non-*C. difficile* causes may be important in antibiotic-associated diarrhea and that a significant change in bowel flora alone may be the initial trigger of the illness. There is also endoscopic pathology which can mimic pseudomembranous colitis, and pseudomembranous colitis may be a response to more than just *C. difficile*-induced disease.

Typing of *C. difficile*

Relapsing illnesses in some patients, but especially the commonality of illness in some hospitals or other health care centres, has historically prompted interest in examining the epidemiology of infection with a typing method of sorts. Several approaches have been taken, and these have included both phenotypic (e.g., serotyping, immunoblot typing, S^{35}-methionine labelling/SDS-PAGE typing, pyrolysis mass spectrometry) and genotypic (e.g., PCR ribotyping, RAPD-PCR, REA, RFLP) methods (151-156). The correlation among these methods is generally quite good (157).

Comparisons and applications of these fingerprinting methods have indicated that there is reason to believe that cross-infection can occur among patients who are in a common area and especially among those that have risk factors (158). Nevertheless, there is considerable heterogeneity among community-acquired isolates, and several studies of hospital isolates, including those from initially putative outbreaks, have shown heterogeneity as well (159).

Apart from maintaining good infection control techniques, there is usually little need for routine typing of isolates even in small outbreaks since a particular pattern of clinical response is required regardless.

5. Pigmented anaerobic Gram negative bacilli

These bacteria are characterized by the production of visibly black-pigmented colonies and/or the evidence of pink to red fluorescence under uv light (160). The ability to produce pigment is variable among *Prevotella* spp., and they may require several weeks for this to be evident; some *Prevotella* may not be pigmented. *Prevotella* spp. are usually resistant to both vancomycin and kanamycin but sensitive to colistin. *Porphyromonas* are susceptible to vancomycin discs but resistant to colistin.

KVLB medium will select for *Prevotella* but may be inhibitory to *Porphyromonas* unless the concentration of vancomycin is reduced. The growth of some isolates in this group may be delayed up to 5-7 days. Commercial kits are variable in their application to this group, and the databases may not have several newer species.

6. Bacteroides

Members of the 'B. fragilis group' grow very well and hardy colonies are noted within 24 hrs. Commercial kits perform well for identifying this cluster of bacteria, but such support is often not required since several other simple assessments may be used. KVLB medium is selective for members of the 'B. fragilis group', and they are resistant to all three antibiotic discs and 20% bile. Most species produce black colonies on Bacteroides-Bile Esculin agar.

Other *Bacteroides* spp. are usually resistant to kanamycin and vancomycin discs and bile, but susceptibility to colistin is variable. There remains some debate about the most appropriate placement for the *B. ureolyticus* group. Some *Bacteroides* spp. are supported in growth by fumarate-formate substrates.

The presence of *B. fragilis* toxin can be determined with biological or genetic detection techniques (161,162).

7. Fusobacteria

Fusobacteria are resistant to vancomycin but susceptible to kanamycin and colistin. *F. nucleatum* may have the typical fusiform morphology, but this may be less apparent for other species. Some fusobacteria may grow on Bacteroides-Bile Esculin medium. Commercial identification kits are not often required (163).

8. Other non-spore forming Gram negative bacilli

Commercial kits are not often useful for identifying this broad group. Some species are motile.

The long and wide cells with pointed tips are consistent among *Leptotrichia*, and a strong lactic acid peak is identified with GLC.

Sutterella is bile-resistant but catalase- and urease-negative. *Bilophila* is also bile-resistant but catalase- and often urease-positive. Both genera are resistant to vancomycin but susceptible to kanamycin and colistin.

Desulfomonas and *Desulfovibrio* are colistin-resistant and kanamycin-susceptible.

Anaerobiospirillum is a spiral organism and motile.

Selenomonas is motile and crescent-shaped.

9. Anaerobic Gram negative cocci

On a practical basis, anaerobic Gram negative cocci may be referred to as *Veillonella* spp. without any consequence regarding clinical outcome of therapy. Differentiation can be achieved with catalase, glucose, nitrate, and GLC as well as some colony and Gram stain characteristics as mentioned in section IV.H. There is no need here for the use of commercial identification kits.

VII. SUSCEPTIBILITY TESTING

A. General issues

Susceptibility testing has been studied considerably, and indeed many refinements have been made in order to create more applicable and standardized testing methods. The use of susceptibility testing for anaerobes, however, is not relevant for many anaerobic infections (164). Firstly, anaerobes are often one component of mixed infections. Although antibiotic therapy may be targeted towards anaerobes in the latter context, therapy towards other facultative bacteria may be more important relatively speaking, and not all of the anaerobes necessarily need to be targeted. Furthermore, many anaerobic infections may have surgical therapy which may be more important than or at least equally to the administration of antibiotics. Secondly, there are many clinical trials which have examined the use of single broad spectrum or combinations of antibiotics, and the currently available regimens may not depend on knowledge of susceptibility testing with few exceptions. In addition, experience and pre-existing science have provided insight regarding which antibiotics may penetrate the sites of anaerobic infections and which antibiotics may generally be regarded as anti-anaerobic agents. Anti-anaerobic agents generally include metronidazole, clindamycin, and chloramphenicol, but a number of beta-lactams may have broad activity as well such as cefoxitin, cefotetan, imipenem, meropenem, and combinations of beta-lactams and beta-lactamase inhibitors (165). Sulphas and aminoglycosides should be avoided. Although the new quinolones of the 1980s and early 1990s generally have not had good anti-anaerobic activity, e.g., ciprofloxacin, more recent and novel variants have improved in this regard and are actively being studied for this purpose.

The need for susceptibility testing continues to be controversial (166), and most laboratories will need to assess individual priorities which indeed may be infection-site specific. Indications for susceptibility testing of select isolates may include at least the following, although not necessarily on a routine basis: a) context of serious infections and limited pathogen numbers where the testing is more to provide a measure of confidence rather than being an absolute prognostic indicator in itself, b) presence of an unusual pathogen especially when alone, c) circumstances of ongoing infection despite seemingly appropriate therapy and relevant surgical intervention, d) need to assess the potential role for second-line agents in critical cases, and e) confirm the likelihood of a high-level resistance in a circumstance where the clinical team may want to use a particular antimicrobial for other reasons. In addition to these select circumstances, it is of value for a few sentinel laboratories to keep some form of invigilation over resistance patterns for routinely-isolated anaerobes (167). Some trends have emerged when the latter approach has been taken, and it is prudent to continue to do so given the overall trend in antimicrobial resistance that has emerged on a global basis.

B. Methods

Susceptibility testing has been hindered by the variation in anaerobe requirements for growth whether media, time for growth, or culture conditions. Examples such as the 'B. fragilis group' grow quickly and yield relatively consistent patterns of apparent susceptibility. Standard criteria for susceptibility testing methods have evolved over the last three decades (168), and standards for testing are now published, e.g., NCCLS recommendations. Break-points for susceptibility, inoculum standards, prescribed media (Wilkins-Chalgren agar), recommended control bacteria, and interpretation of results are all detailed (169). Nevertheless, sufficiently detailed studies which examine the correlation of in vitro data with in vivo correlation, i.e., validation data, are not generally available. Perhaps the latter is largely due to the fact that anaerobic infections are usually polymicrobial. Such methods, however, are not necessarily applicable to all anaerobes, and thus it must be acknowledged that the results of any given method must be seen as a guide at best, perhaps even to a lesser extent than would be gleaned from the susceptibility testing of facultative bacteria (170).

A variety of testing methods have been assessed, and the ones that have been recommended or are currently widely-used include agar dilution, microbroth dilution, and Etest (171-173). Given the infrequency of anaerobic susceptibility testing that may be required, the agar dilution method is cumbersome to use on an ad hoc basis even though the test conditions are perhaps the best standardized of all methods, especially for rapid-growing anaerobes. This method is perhaps best dedicated to periodic cumulative susceptibility testing reviews or research studies since it has the potential to handle multiple isolates at one time. Broth microdilution requires the availability of pre-made antibiotic panels which will support the growth of anaerobes. This method correlates very well with agar dilution and can be used for individual isolates. Disc diffusion (analogous to modified Kirby-Bauer testing) has been used by some (174), but the problems which are inherent to its use for facultative bacteria are increased due to the slow growth of many anaerobes. This method is not generally recommended.

The broth disc elution was described many years ago (175,176), and it facilitates the testing of single isolates on an ad hoc basis to a limited group of antibiotics (177). It is essentially a form of macrobroth dilution. Antibiotic discs are used to provide a fixed (i.e., critical) concentration of antibiotic to a broth (e.g., thioglycollate or equivalent), and a standardized inoculum is added. Growth is compared to a control tube without antibiotic. The practicality of this approach lent itself to use by small laboratories which likely carried both the antibiotic discs and the liquid medium. Despite its popularity, however, and despite initial recommendations for its use, some authorities recommended removal from routine use. The latter was largely due to the unreliable results which were most often seen with the testing of beta-lactamase producers (e.g., 'B. fragilis group') with beta-lactamase antibiotics (178,179). This dilemma was perhaps more so a function of the fact that susceptibility often fell close to the break-point for this combination of antimicrobial and bacterium (180). The methodological details for this method are relatively simple, and thus the reproducibility is fairly good. Some have argued that this method may still yet have its role in routine practice given the crude information that is generally sought in anaerobic susceptibility testing, and indeed argue that other methods are not much better in having the science of their application verified. This debate, however, may be one of the past now that the Etest has been shown to be correlating well with currently recommended methods (181,182). Etest may be problematic to use with fastidious growers. Perhaps it is possible to examine the results of both Etest and a single broth disc elution for further support when a unique opportunity arises to test a given drug-bacterium combination. Again, the actual need must be placed in context.

The medical and scientific literature contains many reports of anecdotal information relating to the treatment of anaerobic infections, and the accumulation of such data will provide a valuable source for consideration and may even obviate the need for susceptibility testing.

Beta-lactamase testing by itself also has some value, and may represent the only method invoked in some circumstances. For example, although commonly susceptible to penicillin, both fusobacteria and *Prevotella* do occasionally produce a beta-lactamase. In this setting, it would be of some interest to know whether an important isolate is beta-lactamase positive. The chromogenic cephalosporin assay for beta-lactamase testing performs well for anaerobes.

Some anaerobic bacteria are capable of inactivating chloramphenicol due to the presence of a nitroreductase, but determination of such capability by an enzymatic method is not practically available. As well, chloramphenicol is not widely used in developed countries for the treatment of anaerobic infections given the alternatives.

Commercial methods for anaerobic susceptibility testing continue to be explored (183).

C. Specific bacterial groups

1. *Anaerobic Gram positive cocci*

Species of this group are commonly susceptible to penicillin, and many other beta-lactams including newer generation cephalosporins and meropenem (40). Beta-lactamases are essentially not found in this group (184), and there is no specific need for beta-lactam:beta-lactamase inhibitor combinations.

Anaerobic Gram positive cocci are also usually susceptible to vancomycin, metronidazole, clindamycin, and chloramphenicol. Rare isolates have been found to be penicillin-, metronidazole-, and clindamycin-resistant. When tested and when unusual patterns of resistance are determined, it is critical to ensure that the isolate is not a microaerophilic or anaerobic streptococcus.

2. *Anaerobic non-spore forming Gram positive bacilli*

These bacteria are usually susceptible to penicillin, chloramphenicol, and clindamycin. Lactobacilli may be vancomycin-resistant and may therefore confuse the laboratory when grown as a vancomycin-resistant microaerophile. *Propionibacterium* spp. are very penicillin-susceptible.

Several species, including *Propionibacterium* spp., *Lactobacillus* spp., and *Actinomyces* spp., are metronidazole-resistant and indeed may be selected for in a mixed infection if this antimicrobial is used.

Actinomycosis is a chronic infection, and it requires prolonged therapy. In addition to the *Actinomyces* isolates, acintomycosis is not uncommonly a polymicrobial infection (especially when odontogenic), and thus, it may be warranted to include a broader spectrum of antimicrobial coverage in addition to that which is specifically targeted to the *Actinomyces*. Treatment of monomicrobial actinomycosis usually involves intravenous penicillin for several weeks as well as prolonged treatment with oral penicillin for months. Options have included clindamycin, erythromycin, and tetracycline. Metronidazole should be avoided as a sole agent.

3. *Clostridia*

Most clostridia are penicillin- and vancomycin-susceptible. Occasional isolates of *C. ramosum* and *C. clostridioforme* have been beta-lactamase positive and penicillin-resistant (184). Some *C. perfringens* isolates have shown intermediate susceptibility to penicillin but it is not clear that the latter has clinical relevance (185). In addition, the latter may show increasing resistance to cefoxitin. Clostridia are still very susceptible to metronidazole and chloramphenicol. Most are also susceptible to clindamycin, but resistance has been noted among isolates of *C. difficile*, *C. sporogenes*, *C. tertium*, *C. subterminale*, some *C. perfringens*, and *C. innocuum*; this resistance is the basis at least for *C. difficile* selection and associated disease when clindamycin is used clinically. Several species may be resistant to cephalosporins.

Both oral metronidazole and oral vancomycin have been quite effective in the treatment of *C. difficile*-associated enteritis. Oral metronidazole is a cheap alternative, whereas vancomycin is much more expensive, and its use has been linked to the development of vancomycin-resistant enteric flora which are becoming an increasingly problematic nosocomial issue. Despite seemingly adequate therapy, relapses of *C. difficile*-associated diarrhea are not uncommon, and re-treatments are sometimes required; this is more likely to be seen among patients who have chronic underlying diseases and who are at risk for the infection initially. Alternative treatments include oral bacitracin, fusidic acid, and teichoplanin.

4.   Anaerobic Gram negative bacilli

Increasing resistance has been documented especially over the last two decades, but these bacteria have uniformly remained susceptible to metronidazole. Most attention has been directed to the 'B. fragilis group'.

Beta-lactamase positivity is common among the 'B. fragilis group' (186). Resistance to advanced cephalosporins and clindamycin has been seen but more so to the former. These bacteria remain susceptible to chloramphenicol, beta-lactam:beta-lactamase inhibitor combinations, and meropenem and imipenem. Some species within the group may show resistance more often than others – for example, *B. distasonis* more commonly shows high level resistance to beta-lactams and even in the absence of beta-lactamase production. Mechanisms of resistance have been best studied among members of this group (66). There are some potent beta-lactamases, and among some isolates, reduced affinity to beta-lactams also has been documented.

Up to 30-50% of *Prevotella* spp. are beta-lactamase positive (184), but susceptibility remains to metronidazole, clindamycin, chloramphenicol, beta-lactam:beta-lactamase inhibitor combinations, and new generation cephalosporins. *Porphyromonas* spp. are also susceptible to these antibiotics and are much less likely to produce beta-lactamase.

Fusobacteria are also generally susceptible to most antibiotics as above, but beta-lactamase positivity has been observed among some species (184), and these may have an accompanying resistance to new generation cephalosporins. Several other anaerobic Gram negative bacilli may be beta-lactamase positive and hence should be tested for the same, e.g., *Bilophila*. *Sutterella* may be resistant to metronidazole (~25%). The motile anaerobic Gram negative bacilli are usually metronidazole, clindamycin, and chloramphenicol susceptible, but may have some variability in penicillin susceptibility, e.g., *Campylobacter gracilis* is often penicillin-resistant.

Although not strictly an anaerobic Gram negative bacillary infection, bacterial vaginosis responds to oral or topical (vaginal) metronidazole or clindamycin, but no form of susceptibility is indicated, e.g., for *Mobiluncus* or other anaerobes. There is a variable outcome for beta-lactam agents such as ampicillin and cephalosporins. Given the imbalance in vaginal anaerobes, some have attempted recolonization using lactobacilli with variable success.

5.   Anaerobic Gram negative cocci

These bacteria are very susceptible to penicillin, metronidazole, and clindamycin.

REFERENCES

1. McIntosh J, Fildes P. A new apparatus for the isolation and cultivation of anaerobic micro-organisms. Lancet 1916; I:768-770.

2. Suau A, Bonnet R, Sutren M, Godon JJ, Gibson GR, Collins MD, Dore J. Direct analysis of genes encoding 16S rRNA from complex communities reveals many novel molecular species within the human gut. Appl Environ Microbiol 1999; 65:4799-4807.

3. Jousimies-Somer H. Recently described clinically important anaerobic bacteria: taxonomic aspects and update. Clin Infect Dis 1997; 25:S78-S87.

4. Tally FP, Stewart PR, Sutter VL, Rosenblatt JE. Oxygen tolerance of fresh clinical anaerobic bacteria. J Clin Microbiol 1975; 1:161-164.

5. Loesche WJ. Oxygen sensitivity of various anaerobic bacteria. Appl Microbiol 1969; 18:723-727.

6. Hentges DJ. The anaerobic microflora of the human body. Clin Infect Dis 1993; 16 (Suppl 4):S175-S180.

7. Smego RA, Foglia G. Actinomycosis. Clin Infect Dis 1998; 26:1255-1261.

8. Zitsch RP, Bothwell M. Actinomycosis: a potential complication of head and neck surgery. Am J Otolaryngol 1999; 20:260-262.

9. Cintron JR, Del Pino A, Duarte B, Wood D. Abdominal actinomycosis. Dis Colon Rectum 1996; 39:105-108.

10. Lippes J. Pelvic actinomycosis: a review and preliminary look at prevalence. Am J Obstet Gynecol 1999; 180:265-269.

11. Warren NG. Actinomycosis, nocardiosis, and actinomycetoma. Dermatol Clin 1996; 14:85-95.

12. Chen KCS, Amsel R, Eschenbach DA, Holmes KK. Biochemical diagnosis of vaginitis: determination of diamines in vaginal fluid. J Infect Dis 1982; 145:337-345.

13. Amsel R, Totten PA, Spiegel CA, Chen KCS, Eschenbach D, Holmes KK. Nonspecific vaginitis: diagnostic criteria and microbial and epidemiologic associations. Am J Med 1983; 74:85-90.

14. Catlin BW. Garnerella vaginalis: characteristics, clinical considerations, and controversies. Clin Microbiol Rev 1992; 5:213-237.

15. Bleck TP. Tetanus: pathophysiology, management, and prophylaxis. Dis Mon 1991; 37:545-603.

16. Stoll BJ. Tetanus. Pediatr Clin North Am 1979; 26:415-431.

17. Ernst ME, Klepser ME, Fouts M, Marangos MN. Tetanus: pathophysiology and management. Ann Pharmacother 1997; 31:1507-1513.

18. Cherington M. Clinical spectrum of botulism. Muscle Nerve 1998; 21:701-710.

19. Pickett J, Berg B, Chaplin E, Brunstetter MA. Syndrome of botulism in infancy: clinical and electrophysiologic study. N Engl J Med 1976; 295:770-772.

20. Midura TF. Update: infant botulism. Clin Microbiol Rev 1996; 9:119-125.

21. Swedberg J, Wendel TH, Deiss F. Wound botulism. West J Med 1987; 147:335-338.

22. Bartlett JG. *Clostridium difficile*: history of its role as an enteric pathogen and the current state of knowledge about the organism. Clin Infect Dis 1994; 18 (Suppl 4):S265-S272.

23. Cleary RK. *Clostridium difficile*-associated diarrhea and colitis: clinical manifestations, diagnosis, and treatment. Dis Colon Rectum 1998; 41:1435-1449.

24. Knoop FC, Owens M, Crocker IC. *Clostridium difficile*: clinical disease and diagnosis. Clin Microbiol Rev 1993; 6:251-265.

25. Putterman C, Rubinow A. Reactive arthritis associated with *Clostridium difficile* pseudomembranous colitis. Semin Arthritis Rheum 1993; 22:420-426.

26. Anand A, Glatt AE. *Clostridium difficile* infections associated with antineoplastic chemotherapy: a review. Clin Infect Dis 1993; 17:109-113.

27. Meer RR, Songer JG, Park DL. Human disease associated with *Clostridium perfringens* enterotoxin. Rev Environ Contam Toxicol 1997; 150:75-94.

28. Nakamura M, Schulze JA. *Clostridium perfringens* food poisoning. Ann Rev Microbiol 1970; 24:359-372.

29. Masfari AN, Duerden BI, Kinghorn GR. Quantitative studies of vaginal bacteria. Genitourin Med 1986; 62:256-263.

30. Wang RF, Cao WW, Cerniglia CE. PCR detection and quantitation of predominant anaerobic bacteria in human and animal fecal samples. Appl Environ Microbiol 1996; 62:1242-1247.

31. Wang RF, Cao WW, Cerniglia CE. Phylogenetic analysis of *Fusobacterium prausnitzii* based upon the 16S rRNA gene sequence and PCR confirmation. Int J Syst Bacteriol 1996; 46:341-343.

32. Hatheway CL. Botulism: the present status of the disease. Curr Top Microbiol Immunol 1995; 195:55-75.

33. Mitty RD, LaMont JT. *Clostridium difficile* diarrhea: pathogenesis, epidemiology, and treatment. Gastroenterologist 1994; 2:61-69.

34. Naaber P, Klaus K, Sepp E, Bjorksten B, Mikelsaar M. Colonization of infants and hospitalized patients with *Clostridium difficile* and lactobacilli. Clin Infect Dis 1997; 25 (Suppl 2):S189-S190.

35. Tanner A, Maiden MF, Paster BJ, Dewhirst FE. The impact of 16S ribosomal RNA-based phylogeny on the taxonomy of oral bacteria. Periodontol 2000 1994; 5:26-51.
36. Thaller MC, Passariello C. Taxonomy and identification of periodontopathogenic bacteria and related species. New Microbiol 1997; 20:161-176.
37. Trowbridge HO, Stevens BH. Microbiologic and pathologic aspects of pulpal and periapical disease. Curr Opin Dent 1992; 2:85-92.
38. Holt SC, Bramanti TE. Factors in virulence expression and their role in periodontal disease pathogenesis. Crit Rev Oral Biol Med 1991; 2:177-281.
39. Yao ES, Lamont RJ, Leu SP, Weinberg A. Interbacterial binding among strains of pathogenic and commensal oral bacterial species. Oral Microbiol Immunol 1996; 11:35-41.
40. Murdoch, DA. Gram-positive anaerobic cocci. Clin Microbiol Rev 1998; 11:81-120.
41. Brook I, Walker PI. The role of encapsulation in the pathogenesis of anaerobic Gram-positive cocci. Can J Microbiol 1985; 31:176-180.
42. Brook I. The role of encapsulated anaerobic bacteria in synergistic infections. FEMS Microbiol Rev 1994; 13:65-74.
43. Willems A, Collins MD. Phylogenetic relationships of the genera *Acetobacterium* and *Eubacterium* sensu stricto and reclassification of *Eubacterium alactolyticum* as *Pseudoramibacter alactolyticus* gen. nov., comb. nov. Int J Syst Bacteriol 1996; 46:1083-1087.
44. Tiveljung A, Forsum U, Monstein HJ. Classification of the genus *Mobiluncus* based on comparative partial 16S rRNA gene analysis. Int J Syst Bacteriol 1996; 46:332-336.
45. Collins MD, Lawson PA, Willems A, Cordoba JJ, Fernandez-Garayzabal J, Barcia P, Cai J, Hippe H, Farrow JAE. The phylogeny of the genus *Clostridium*: proposal of five new genera and eleven new species combinations. Int J Syst Bacteriol 1994; 44:812-826.
46. Wang RF, Cao WW, Cerniglia CE. Phylogenetic analysis of *Fusobacterium prausnitzii* based upon the 16S rRNA gene sequence and PCR confirmation. Int J Syst Bacteriol 1996; 46:341-343.
47. Hatheway CL. Toxigenic clostridia. Clin Microbiol Rev 1990; 3:66-98.
48. Maselli RA. Pathogenesis of human botulism. Ann NY Acad Sci 1998; 841:122-139.
49. Hall JD, McCroskey LM, Pincomb BJ, Hatheway CL. Isolation of an organism resembling *Clostridium barati* which produces type F botulinal toxin from an infant with botulism. J Clin Microbiol 1985; 21:654-655.
50. McCroskey LM, Hatheway CL, Fenicia L, Pasolini B, Aureli P. Characterization of an organism that produces type E botulinal toxin but which resembles *Clostridium butyricum* from the feces of an infant with type E botulism. J Clin Microbiol 1986; 23:201-202.
51. Bongaerts GP, Lyerly DM. Role of toxins A and B in the pathogenesis of *Clostridium difficile* disease. Microb Pathog 1994; 17:1-12.
52. Kato H, Kato N, Watanbe K, Iwai N, Nakamura H, Yamamoto T, Suzuki K, Kim SM, Chong Y, Wasito EB. Identification of toxin A-negative, toxin B-positive *Clostridium difficile* by PCR. J Clin Microbiol 1998; 36:2178-2182.
53. Cohen SH, Tang YJ, Hansen B, Silva J. Isolation of a toxin B-deficient mutant strain of *Clostridium difficile* in a case of recurrent *C. difficile*-associated diarrhea. Clin Infect Dis 1998; 26:410-412.
54. Riegler M, Sedivy R, Pothoulakis C, Hamilton G, Zacherl J, Bischof G, Cosentini E, Feil W, Schiessel R, Lamont JT, et al. *Clostridium difficile* toxin B is more potent than toxin A in damaging human colonic epithelium in vitro. J Clin Invest 1995; 95:2004-2011.
55. Pothoulakis C. Pathogenesis of *Clostridium difficile*-associated diarrhoea. Eur J Gastroenterol Hepatol 1996; 8:1041-1047.
56. Borriello SP. Pathogenesis of *Clostridium difficile* infection. J Antimicrob Chemother 1998; 41(Suppl C):S13-S19.
57. Jefferson KK, Smith MF, Bobak DA. Roles of intracellular calcium and NF-kappa B in the *Clostridium difficile* toxin A-induced up-regulation and secretion of IL-8 from human monocytes. J Immunol 1999; 163:5183-5191.
58. Fiorentini C, Fabbri A, Falzano L, Fattorossi A, Matarrese P, Rivabene R, Donelli G. *Clostridium difficile* toxin B induces apoptosis in intestinal cultured cells. Infect Immun 1998; 66:2660-2665.
59. Linevsky JK, Pothoulakis C, Keates S, Warny M, Keates AC, Lamont JT, Kelly CP. IL-8 release and neutrophil activation by *Clostridium difficile* toxin-exposed human monocytes. Am J Physiol 1997; 273:1333-1340.
60. Rood JI, Cole CT. Molecular genetics and pathogenesis of *Clostridium perfringens*. Microbiol Rev 1991; 55:621-648.

61. Kokai-Kun JF, McClane BA. The *Clostridium perfringens* enterotoxin. In: Rood JI, McClane BA, Songer JG, Titball RW, eds. The Clostridia: Molecular Biology and Pathogenesis. New York, NY:Academic Press, Inc., 1997:325-357.

62. McClane BA. New insights into the genetics and regulation of expression of *Clostridium perfringens* enterotoxin. Curr Top Microbiol Immunol 1998; 225:37-55.

63. Paster BJ, Dewhirst FE, Olsen I, Fraser GJ. Phylogeny of *Bacteroides, Prevotella, Porphyromonas* spp. and related bacteria. J Bacteriol 1994; 176:725-732.

64. Moore LV, Johnson JL, Moore WE. Descriptions of *Prevotella tannerae* sp. nov. and *Prevotella enoeca* sp. nov. from the human gingival crevice and emendation of the description of *Prevotella zoogleoformans*. Int J Syst Bacteriol 1994; 44:599-602.

65. Guzman CA, Biavasco F, Pruzzo C. Adhesiveness of *Bacteroides fragilis* strains isolated from feces of healthy donors, abscesses, and blood. Curr Microbiol 1997; 34:332-334.

66. Finegold SM. Mechanisms of resistance in anaerobes and new developments in testing. Diagn Microbiol Infect Dis 1989; 12 (Suppl 4):S117-S120.

67. Sears CL, Myers LL, Lazenby A, Van Tassell RL. Enterotoxigenic *Bacteroides fragilis*. Clin Infect Dis 1995; 20:S142-S148.

68. Koshy SS, Montrose MH, Sears CL. Human intestinal epithelial cells swell and demonstrate actin rearrangement in response to the metalloprotease toxin of *Bacteroides fragilis*. Infect Immun 1996; 64:5022-5028.

69. Moncrief JS, Duncan AJ, Wright RL, Barroso LA, Wilkins TD. Molecular characterization of the fragilysin pathogenicity islet of enterotoxigenic *Bacteroides fragilis*. Infect Immun 1998; 66:1735-1739.

70. Sanfilippo L, Baldwin TJ, Menozzi MG, Borriello SP, Mahida YR. Heterogeneity in responses by primary adult human colonic epithelial cells to purified enterotoxin of *Bacteroides fragilis*. Gut 1998; 43:651-655.

71. Ferreira R, Alexandre MC, Antunes EN, Pinhao AT, Moraes SR, Ferreira MC, Domingues RM. Expression of *Bacteroides fragilis* virulence markers in vitro. J Med Microbiol 1999; 48:999-1004.

72. Obiso RJ, Bevan DR, Wilkins TD. Molecular modeling and analysis of fragilysin, the *Bacteroides fragilis* toxin. Clin Infect Dis 1997; 25 (Suppl 2):S153-S155.

73. Bennett KW, Eley A. Fusobacteria: new taxonomy and related diseases. J Med Microbiol 1993; 39:246-254.

74. Bolstad AI, Jensen HB, Bakken V. Taxonomy, biology, and periodontal aspects of *Fusobacterium nucleatum*. Clin Microbiol Rev 1996; 9:55-71.

75. Tan ZL, Nagaraja TG, Chengappa MM. *Fusobacterium necrophorum* infections: virulence factors, pathogenic mechanism and control measures. Vet Res Commun 1996; 20:113-140.

76. Johnson CC, Finegold SM. Uncommonly encountered, motile, anaerobic Gram-negative bacilli associated with infection. Rev Infect Dis 1987; 9:1150-1162.

77. Engberg J, On SL, Harrington CS, Gerner-Smidt P. Prevalence of *Campylobacter, Arcobacter, Helicobacter*, and *Sutterella* spp. in human fecal samples as estimated by a re-evaluation of isolation methods for campylobacters. J Clin Microbiol 2000; 38:286-291.

78. Wexler HM, Reeves D, Summanen PH, Molitoris E, McTeague M, Duncan J, Wilson KH, Finegold SM. *Sutterella wadsworthensis* gen. nov., sp. nov., bile-resistant microaerophilic *Campylobacter gracilis*-like clinical isolates. Int J Syst Bacteriol 1996; 46:252-258.

79. Vandamme P, Daneshvar MI, Dewhirst FE, Paster BJ, Kersters K, Goosens H, Moss CW. Chemotaxonomic analyses of *Bacteroides gracilis* and *Bacteroides ureolyticus* and reclassification of *B. gracilis* as *Campylobacter gracilis* comb. nov. Int J Syst Bacteriol 1995; 45:145-152.

80. Aronsson B, Granstrom M, Mollby R, Nord CE. Serum antibody response to *Clostridium difficile* toxins in patients with *Clostridium difficile* diarrhoea. Infection 1985; 13:97-101.

81. Kelly CP. Immune response to *Clostridium difficile* infection. Eur J Gastroenterol Hepatol 1996; 8:1048-1053.

82. Johnson S. Antibody responses to clostridial infection in humans. Clin Infect Dis 1997; 25:S173-S177.

83. Pantosti A, Cerquetti M, Viti F, Ortisi G, Mastrantonio P. Immunoblot analysis of serum immunoglobulin G response to surface proteins of *Clostridium difficile* in patients with antibiotic-associated diarrhea. J Clin Microbiol 1989; 27:2594-2597.

84. Giannasca PJ, Zhang ZX, Lei WD, Boden JA, Giel MA, Monath TP, Thomas WD. Serum antitoxin antibodies mediate systemic and mucosal protection from *Clostridium difficile* disease in hamsters. Infect Immun 1999; 67:527-538.

85. Daubener W, Leiser E, von Eichel-Streiber C, Hadding U. *Clostridium difficile* toxins A and B inhibit human immune response in vitro. Infect Immun 1988; 56:1107-1112.

86. Shapiro ME, Kasper DL, Zaleznik DF, Spriggs S, Onderdonk AB, Finberg RW. Cellular control of abscess formation: role of T cells in the regulation of abscesses formed in response to *Bacteroides fragilis*. J Immunol 1986; 137:341-346.

87. Crabb JH, Finberg R, Onderdonk AB, Kasper DL. T cell regulation of *Bacteroides fragilis*-induced intraabdominal abscesses. Rev Infect Dis 1990; 12:S178-S184.

88. Hall ER, Martin SA, Suzuki JB, Falkler WA. The gingival immune response to periodontal pathogens in juvenile periodontitis. Oral Microbiol Immunol 1994; 9:327-334.

89. Mouton C, Hammond PG, Slots J, Genco RJ. Serum antibodies to oral *Bacteroides asaccharolyticus* (*Bacteroides gingivalis*): relationship to age and periodontal disease. Infect Immun 1981; 31:182-192.

90. Ishikawa I, Nakashima K, Koseki T, Nagasawa T, Watanabe H, Arakawa S, Nitta H, Nishihara T. Induction of the immune response to periodontopathic bacteria and its role in the pathogenesis of periodontitis. Periodontol 2000 1997; 14:79-111.

91. Behbehani MJ, Heeley JD, Jordan HV. Comparative histopathology of lesions produced by *Actinomyces israelii*, *Actinomyces naeslundii*, and *Actinomyces viscosus* in mice. Am J Pathol 1983; 110:267-274.

92. Schwebke JR, Morgan SC, Hillier SL. Humoral antibody to *Mobiluncus curtisii*, a potential serological marker for bacterial vaginosis. Clin Diagn Lab Immunol 1996; 3:567-569.

93. Peterson LR. Effect of media on transport and recovery of anaerobic bacteria. Clin Infect Dis 1997; 25 (Suppl 2):S134-S136.

94. Brook I. Comparison of two transport systems for recovery of aerobic and anaerobic bacteria from abscesses. J Clin Microbiol 1987; 25:2020-2022.

95. Hudspeth MK, Citron DM, Goldstein EJC. Evaluation of a novel specimen transport system (Venturi Transystem) for anaerobic bacteria. Clin Infect Dis 1997; 25 (Suppl 2):S132-S133.

96. Cox ME, Kohr RJ, Samia CK. Comparison of quality control results with use of anaerobic chambers versus anaerobic jars. Clin Infect Dis 1997; 25 (Suppl 2):S137-S138.

97. Downes J, Mangels JI, Holden J, Ferraro MJ, Baron EJ. Evaluation of two single-plate incubation systems and the anaerobic chamber for the cultivation of anaerobic bacteria. J Clin Microbiol 1990; 28:246-248.

98. Mangels JI, Douglas BP. Comparison of four commercial brucella agar media for growth of anaerobic organisms. J Clin Microbiol 1989; 27:2268-2271.

99. Sondag JE, Ali M, Murray PR. Relative recovery of anaerobes on differential isolation media. J Clin Microbiol 1979; 10:756-757.

100. Murray PR. Growth of clinical isolates of anaerobic bacteria on agar media: effects of media composition, storage conditions, and reduction under anaerobic conditions. J Clin Microbiol 1978; 8:708-714.

101. Martin WJ. Practical method for isolation of anaerobic bacteria in the clinical laboratory. Appl Microbiol 1971; 22:1168-1171.

102. Downes J, Mangels JI, Holden J, Ferraro MJ, Baron EJ. Evaluation of two single-plate incubation systems and the anaerobic chamber for the cultivation of anaerobic bacteria. J Clin Microbiol 1990; 28:246-248.

103. Wren MW. The culture of clinical specimens for anaerobic bacteria: a comparison of three regimens. J Med Microbiol 1977; 10:195-201.

104. Doan N, Contreras A, Flynn J, Morrison J, Slots J. Proficiencies of three anaerobic culture systems for recovering periodontal pathogenic bacteria. J Clin Microbiol 1999; 37:171-174.

105. Livingston SJ, Kominos SD, Yee RB. New medium for selection and presumptive identification of the *Bacteroides fragilis* group. J Clin Microbiol 1978; 7:448-453.

106. George WL, Sutter VL, Citron D, Finegold SM. Selective and differential medium for isolation of *Clostridium difficile*. J Clin Microbiol 1979; 9:214-219.

107. Johnson MJ, Thatcher E, Cox ME. Techniques for controlling variability in Gram staining of obligate anaerobes. J Clin Microbiol 1995; 33:755-758.

108. Rosenblatt JE. Can we afford to do anaerobic cultures and identification? A positive point of view. Clin Infect Dis 1997; 25 (Suppl 2):S127-S131.

109. Baron EJ, Citron DM. Anaerobic identification flowchart using mimimal laboratory resources. Clin Infect Dis 1997; 25 (Suppl 2):S143-S146.

110. Holdeman LV, Cato EP, Moore WEC – eds. Anaerobe Laboratory Manual, 4th Edn. Blacksburg, VA:Virginia Polytechnic Institute and State University, 1977.

111. Summanen P, Baron EJ, Citron DM, Strong C, Wexler HM, Finegold SM. Wadsworth Anaerobic Bacteriology Manual, 5th Edition. Belmont, CA:Star Publishing, 1993.

112. Rodloff AC, Appelbaum PC, Zabransky RJ. Practical Anaerobic Bacteriology, Cumitech 5A. Washington, DC:American Society for Microbiology, 1991.

113. Burlage RS, Ellner PD. Comparison of the PRAS II, AN-Ident, and RapID-ANA systems for identification of anaerobic bacteria. J Clin Microbiol 1985; 22:32-35.

114. Head CB, Ratnam S. Comparison of API ZYM system with API AN-Ident, API 20A, Minitek Anaerobe II, and RapID-ANA systems for identification of *Clostridium difficile*. J Clin Microbiol 1988; 26:144-146.

115. Quentin C, Desailly-Chanson MA, Bebear C. Evaluation of AN-Ident. J Clin Microbiol 1991; 29:231-235.

116. Moll WM, Ungerechts J, Marklein G, Schaal KP. Comparison of BBL Crystal ANR ID Kit and API RapidID 32 A for identification of anaerobic bacteria. Zentralbl Bakteriol 1996; 284:329-347.

117. Schreckenberger PC, Celig DM, Janda WM. Clinical evaluation of the Vitek ANI card for identification of anaerobic bacteria. J Clin Microbiol 1988; 26:225-230.

118. Gulletta E, Amato G, Nani E, Covelli I. Comparison of two systems for identification of anaerobic bacteria. Eur J Clin Microbiol 1985; 4:282-285.

119. Hauser KJ, Zabransky RJ. Modification of the gas-liquid chromatography procedure and evaluation of a new column packing material for the identification of anaerobic bacteria. J Clin Microbiol 1975; 2:1-7.

120. Phillips KD, Tearle PV, Willis AT. Rapid diagnosis of anaerobic infections by gas-liquid chromatography of clinical material. J Clin Pathol 1976; 29:428-432.

121. Murdoch DA, Mitchelmore IJ. The laboratory identification of gram-positive anaerobic cocci. J Med Microbiol 1991; 34:295-308.

122. Eschenbach DA, Hillier S, Critchlow C, Stevens C, DeRouen T, Holmes KK. Diagnosis and clinical manifestations of bacterial vaginosis. Am J Obstet Gynecol 1988; 158:819-828.

123. Spiegel CA. Diagnosis of bacterial vaginosis by direct Gram stain of vaginal fluid. J Clin Microbiol 1983; 18:170-177.

124. Nugent RP, Krohn MA, Hillier SL. Reliability of diagnosing bacterial vaginosis is improved by a standardized method of Gram stain interpretation. J Clin Microbiol 1991; 29:297-301.

125. Koransky JR, Allen SD, Dowell VR. Use of ethanol for selective isolation of sporeforming micro-organisms. Appl Environ Microbiol 1978; 35:762-765.

126. Takeshi K, Fujinaga Y, Inoue K, Nakajima H, Oguma K, Ueno T, Sunagawa H, Ohyama T. Simple method for detection of *Clostridium botulinum* type A to F neurotoxin genes by polymerase chain reaction. Microbiol Immunol 1996; 40:5-11.

127. Aranda E, Rodriquez MM, Asensio MA, Cordoba JJ. Detection of *Clostridium botulinum* types A, B, E and F in foods by PCR and DNA probe. Lett Appl Microbiol 1997; 25:186-190.

128. Bartlett JG. *Clostridium difficile*: history of its role as an enteric pathogen and the current state of knowledge about the organism. Clin Infect Dis 1994; 18 (Suppl 4):S265-S272.

129. George WL, Rolfe WL, Finegold SM. *Clostridium difficile* and its cytotoxin in feces of patients with antimicrobial agent-associated diarrhea and miscellaneous conditions. J Clin Microbiol 1982; 15:1049-1053.

130. Bartlett JG. Antibiotic-associated diarrhea. Clin Infect Dis 1992; 15:573-581.

131. Bartlett JG. *Clostridium difficile*: clinical considerations. Rev Infect Dis 1990; 12:S243-S251.

132. Mundy LC, Shanholtzer CJ, Willard KE, Gerding DN, Peterson LR. Laboratory dectection of *Clostridium difficile*: a comparison of media and incubation systems. Am J Clin Pathol 1995; 103:52-56.

133. Bate G. Comparison of Minitek Anaerobe II, API An –Ident, and RapID ANA systems for identification of *Clostridium difficile*. Am J Clin Pathol 1986; 85:716-718.

134. Marler LM, Siders JA, Wolters LC, Pettigrew Y, Skitt BL, Allen SD. Comparison of five cultural procedures for isolation of *Clostridium difficile* from stools. J Clin Microbiol 1992; 30:514-516.

135. Arzese A, Trani G, Riul L, Botta GA. Rapid polymerase chain reaction method for specific detection of toxigenic *Clostridium difficile*. Eur J Clin Microbiol Infect Dis 1995; 14:716-719.

136. Mattia AR, Doern GV, Clark J, Holden J, Wu L, Ferraro MJ. Comparison of four methods in the diagnosis of *Clostridium difficile* disease. Eur J Clin Microbiol Infect Dis 1993; 12:882-886.

137. Kelly WF, Wait KJ, Gilligan PH. Evaluation of the latex agglutination test for detection of *Clostridium difficile*. Arch Pathol Lab Med 1992; 116:517-520.

138. Lyerly DM, Barroso LA, Wilkins TD. Identification of the latex test-reactive protein of *Clostridium difficile* as glutamate dehydrogenase. J Clin Microbiol 1991; 29:2639-2642.

139. Lyerly DM, Krivan HC, Wilkins TD. *Clostridium difficile*: its disease and toxins. Clin Microbiol Rev 1988; 1:1-18.

140. Staneck JL, Weckbach LS, Allen SD, Siders JA, Gilligan PH, Coppitt G, Kraft JA, Willis DH. Multicenter evaluation of four methods for *Clostridium difficile* detection: Immunocard C. *difficile*, cytotoxin assay, culture, and latex agglutination. J Clin Microbiol 1996; 34:2718-2721.

141. Lyerly DM, Neville LM, Evans DT, Fill J, Allen S, Greene W, Sautter R, Hnatuck P, Torpey DJ, Schwalbe R. Multicenter evaluation of the *Clostridium difficile* TOX A/B TEST. J Clin Microbiol 1998; 36:184-190.

142. Siarakas S, Tambosis E, Robertson GJ, Funnell GR, Bradbury R, Gottlieb T. Comparison of two commercial enzyme immunoassays with cytotoxicity assay and culture for the diagnosis of *Clostridium difficile* related diarrhea. Pathology 1996; 28:178-181.

143. Riederer KM, Lawson P, Held MS, Petrylka K, Briski LE, Khatib R. Diagnosis of *Clostridium difficile* associated diarrhea: comparison of three rapid methods employing different markers for detection. Can J Microbiol 1995; 41:88-91.

144. Merz CS, Kramer C, Forman M, Gluck L, Mills K, Senft K, Steiman I, Wallace N, Charache P. Comparison of four commercially available rapid enzyme immunoassays with cytotoxin assay for detection of *Clostridium difficile* toxin(s) from stool specimens. J Clin Microbiol 1994; 32:1142-1147.

145. Altaie SS, Meyer P, Dryja D. Comparison of two commercially available enzyme immunoassays for detection of *Clostridium difficile* in stool specimens. J Clin Microbiol 1994; 32:51-53.

146. Whittier S, Shapiro DS, Kelly WF, Walden TP, Wait KJ, McMillon LT, Gilligan PH. Evaluation of four commercially available enzyme immunoassays for laboratory diagnosis of *Clostridium difficile*-associated diseases. J Clin Microbiol 1993; 31:2861-2865.

147. Barbut F, Kajzer C, Planas N, Petit JC. Comparison of three enzyme immunoassays, a cytotoxicity assay, and toxigenic culture for diagnosis of *Clostridium difficile*-associated diarrhea. J Clin Microbiol 1993; 31:963-967.

148. Doern GV, Coughlin RT, Wu L. Laboratory diagnosis of *Clostridium difficile*-associated gastrointetinal disease: comparison of a monoclonal antibody enzyme immunoassay for toxins A and B with a monoclonal antibody enzyme immunoassay for toxin A only and two cytotoxicity assays. J Clin Microbiol 1992; 30:2042-2046.

149. Fedorko DP, Engler HD, O'Shaughnessy EM, Williams EC, Reichelderfer CJ, Smith WI. Evaluation of two rapid assays for detection of *Clostridium difficile* toxin A in stool specimens. J Clin Microbiol 1999; 37:3044-3047.

150. Gould PC, Khawaja FI, Rosenthal WS. Antibiotic-associated hemorrhagic colitis. Am J Gastroenterol 1982; 77:491-493.

151. Tabaqchali S. Epidemiological markers of Clostridium difficile. Rev Infect Dis 1990; 12:S192-S199.

152. Mulligan ME, Peterson LR, Kwok RYY, Clabots CR, Gerding DN. Immunoblots and plasmid fingerprints compared with serotyping and polyacrylamide gel electrophoresis for typing *Clostridium difficile*. J Clin Microbiol 1988; 26:41-46.

153. Clabots CR, Johnson S, Bettin KM, Mathie PA, Mulligan ME, Schaberg DR, Peterson LR, Gerding DH. Development of a rapid and efficient restriction endonuclease analysis typing system for *Clostridium difficile* and correlation with other typing schemes. J Clin Microbiol 1993; 31:1870-1875.

154. O'Neill GL, Ogunsola FT, Brazier JS, Duerden BI. Modification of a PCR ribotyping method for application as a routine typing scheme for *Clostridium difficile*. Anaerobe 1996; 2:205-209.

155. Brazier JS, Delmee M, Tabaqchali S, Hill LR, Mulligan ME, Riley TV. Proposed unified nomenclature for *Clostridium difficile* typing. Lancet 1994; 343:157.

156. Magee JT, Brazier JS, Hosein IK, Ribeiro CD, Hill DW, Griffiths A, Da Costa C, Sinclair AJ, Duerden BI. An investigation of nosocomial outbreak of *Clostridium difficile* by pyrolysis mass spectrometry. J Med Microbiol 1993; 39:345-351.

157. Brazier JS, Mulligan ME, Delmee M, Tabaqchali S, and the International *Clostridium difficile* Study Group. Preliminary findings of the international typing study on *Clostridium difficile*. Clin Infect Dis 1997; 25 (Suppl 2):S199-S201.

158. Djuretic T, Wall PG, Brazier JS. *Clostridium difficile*: an update on its epidemiology and role in hospital outbreaks in England and Wales. J Hosp Infect 1999; 41:213-218.

159. Wullt M, Laurell MH. Low prevalence of nosocomial *Clostridium difficile* transmissioin, as determined by comparison of arbitrarily primed PCR and epidemiological data. J Hosp Infect 1999; 43:265-273.

160. Jousimies-Somer HR. Update on the taxonomy and the clinical and laboratory characteristics of pigmented anaerobic Gram-negative rods. Clin Infect Dis 1995; 20 (Suppl 2):S187-S191.

161. Weikel C, Grieco F, Reuben J, Myers LL, Sack RB. Human colonic epithelial cells HT29/C1 treated with crude *Bacteroides fragilis* enterotoxin dramatically alter their morphology. Infect Immun 1992; 60:321-327.

162. Shetab R, Cohen SH, Prindiville T, Tang YJ, Cantrell M, Rahmani D, Silva J. Detection of *Bacteroides fragilis* enterotoxin gene by PCR. J Clin Microbiol 1998; 36:1729-1732.

163. Bennett KW, Duerden BI. Identification of fusobacteria in a routine diagnostic laboratory. J Appl Bacteriol 1985; 59:171-181.

164. Rosenblatt JE, Brook I. Clinical relevance of susceptibility testing of anaerobic bacteria. Clin Infect Dis 1993; 16 (Suppl 4):S446-S448.

165. Wexler HM, Molitoris E, Molitoris D. Susceptibility testing of anaerobes: old problems, new options? Clin Infect Dis 1997; 25 (Suppl 2):S275-S278.

166. Wexler HM. Susceptibility testing of anaerobic bacteria: myth, magic, or method? Clin Microbiol Rev 1991; 4:470-484.

167. Baquero F, Reig M. Resistance of anaerobic bacteria to antimicrobial agents in Spain. Eur J Clin Microbiol Infect Dis 1992; 11:1016-1020.

168. Wexler HM. Susceptibility testing of anaerobic bacteria – the state of the art. Clin Infect Dis 1993; 16 (Suppl):S328-S333.

169. Wilkins TD, Chalgren S. Medium for use in antibiotic susceptibility testing of anaerobic bacteria. Antimicrob Agents Chemother 1976; 10:926-928.

170. Brook I. In vitro susceptibility vs. in vitro efficacy of various antimicrobial agents against the *Bacteroides fragilis* group. Rev Infect Dis 1991; 13:1170-1180.

171. Heizmann W, Werner H, Herb B. Comparison of four commercial microdilution systems for susceptibility testing of anaerobic bacteria. Eur J Clin Microbiol Infect Dis 1988; 7:758-763.

172. Jones RN, Barry AL, Cotton JL, Sutter VL, Swenson JM. Collaborative evaluation of the micro-media systems anaerobe susceptibility panel: comparisons with reference methods and test reproducibility. J Clin Microbiol 1982; 16:245-249.

173. Duerden BI. Role of the reference laboratory in susceptibility testing of anaerobes and a survey of isolates referred from laboratories in England and Wales during 1993-1994. Clin Infect Dis 1995; 20 (Suppl 2):S180-S186.

174. Horn R, Bourgault AM, Lamothe F. Disk diffusion susceptibility testing of the *Bacteroides fragilis* group. Antimicrob Agents Chemother 1987; 31:1596-1599.

175. Kurzynski TA, Yrios JW, Helstad AG, Field CR. Aerobically incubated thioglycollate broth disk method for antibiotic susceptibility testing of anaerobes. Antimicrob Agents Chemother 1976; 10:727-732.

176. Wilkins TD, Thiel T. Modified broth-disk method for testing the antibiotic susceptibility of anaerobic bacteria. Antimicrob Agents Chemother 1973; 3:350-356.

177. Finegold SM, Rolfe RD. Susceptibility testing of anaerobic bacteria. Diagn Microbiol Infect Dis 1983; 1:33-40.

178. Wexler HM, Finegold SM. Media- and method-dependent variation in MIC values for ceftizoxime for clinical isolates of the *Bacteroides fragilis* group. Clin Ther 1990; 12 (Suppl C):13-24.

179. Aldridge KE, Henderberg A, Schiro DD, Sanders CV. Discordant results between the broth disk elution and broth microdilution susceptibility tests with Bacteroides fragilis group isolates. J Clin Microbiol 1990; 28:375-378.

180. Jorgensen JH, Redding JS, Howell AW. Evaluation of broth disk elution methods for susceptibility testing of anaerobic bacteria with the newer beta-lactam antibiotics. J Clin Microbiol 1986; 23:545-550.

181. Rosenblatt JE, Gustafson DR. Evaluation of the Etest for susceptibility testing of anaerobic bacteria. Diagn Microbiol Infect Dis 1995; 22:279-284.

182. Bolmstrom A. Susceptibility testing of anaerobes with Etest. Clin Infect Dis 1993; 16 (Suppl 4):S367-S370.

183. Dubreuil L, Houcke I, Singer E. Susceptibility testing of anaerobic bacteria: evaluation of the redesigned (Version 96) bioMerieux ATB ANA device. J Clin Microbiol 1999; 37:1824-1828.

184. Nord CE, Hedberg M. Resistance to beta-lactam antibiotics in anaerobic bacteria. Rev Infect Dis 1990; 12 (Suppl 2):S231-S234.

185. Williamson R. Resistance of *Clostridium perfringens* to beta-lactam antibiotics mediated by a decreased affinity of a single essential penicillin-binding protein. J Gen Microbiol 1983; 129:2339-2342.

186. Hill GB, Ayers OM, Everett BQ. Susceptibilities of anaerobic Gram-negative bacilli to thirteen antimicrobials and beta-lactamase inhibitor combinations. J Antimicrob Chemother 1991; 28:855-867.

25

Borrelioses

Nevio Cimolai
Children's and Women's Health Centre of British Columbia,Vancouver, British Columbia, Canada

Jarmo Oksi
Department of Medicine, Turku University Central Hospital, and Department of Medical Microbiology, Turku University, Turku, Finland

Matti K. Viljanen
Department in Turku, National Public Health Institute, Finland

I. HISTORICAL BACKGROUND

Borrelioses are arthropod-borne illnesses that are caused by spirochetes of the *Borrelia* genus and that may be acquired world-wide. Two major forms of borreliosis are clinically manifest: 1) relapsing fever - a febrile illness with a recurrent fever pattern but generally few other systemic manifestations for most patients, and 2) Lyme disease - a potentially multi-system illness that may have several clinical presentations depending on which organ system is sufficiently diseased. Both of these illnesses are modestly well-studied, especially Lyme disease which is endemic in most well-developed countries. Although borrelioses may be considered by some to be emerging diseases, they are by no means new infections. Indeed there are several early descriptions of each that have been published many decades or even a century before the discovery of the causative spirochete and the interest that has grown exponentially over the last two decades. Relapsing fever has been recognized on most continents, but citations of infection have been generally few on a yearly basis in westernized countries. Large outbreaks in underdeveloped Africa continue, but many outbreaks were recorded in the past, mostly associated with the military or the impoverished during times of war (1). Lyme spirochetes have been detected by genetic amplification techniques in archived European ticks which date back to 1884 (2). Lyme disease was essentially recognized in its complexity by the 1980s when the etiological agent, *Borrelia burgdorferi*, was discovered and then exploited for diagnostic purposes. Lyme disease is now both a fascinating disease and a relatively common illness in several regions of the world. Although there have been many interesting findings and publications that explored relapsing fever spirochetes much before the recent interest in Lyme disease, it was the emergence of the latter which placed research and endeavour in the area of borrelioses to the forefront. Whereas much of the exploratory science is contemporary, the spirochetes and their vectors are likely to have existed in nature for as long as animals have inhabited the earth. One can clearly attribute activity in this field to the new discoveries from the last two decades, but one must one must acknowledge that growing and spreading human populations have also forced the contact of people with elements in nature to an unprecedented level.

Relapsing fever may be either louse- or tick-borne, but its historical impact probably lays on the louse-borne epidemics that plagued individuals in the context of poverty or during times of war (1). Louse-borne spread is dependent on the body louse, *Pediculus humanus*, which is spread from person-to-person and which is more likely to persist among people and populations when hygiene is severely compromised (1). In current times, louse-borne relapsing fever is much less common than tick-borne, and contemporary epidemics seem to be mainly reported from the continent of Africa (3). Tick-borne relapsing fever has been cited in small epidemics and often only affecting a few individuals who have been exposed to infected ticks in the wild. Since ticks do not infest large populations nor do they persist on the human body, this sporadic and relatively infrequent occurrence of the disease will likely continue into the future. Apart from the history of disease among humans, it should be recognized that the study of relapsing fever borreliae has had a significant, albeit under-recognized, role in the study of pathogenesis of spirochetal infections. The relapsing nature of the illness and the results of subsequent brief studies with animal models led to the proposal that the changing of surface "coats", and hence changing antigenicity, could serve as a virulence factor. This theme of spontaneous antigenic variation in vivo has subsequently been pursued and confirmed in a number of other infections, whether bacterial, viral, fungal, or parasitic.

Lyme disease seemingly has a very contemporary history. An association of arthritis with the history of tick bite among a group of children in Connecticut led to a co-ordinated search for an infectious etiological agent which subsequently proved to be *B. burgdorferi* (4,5). Initially, the illness appeared to be endemic mainly to the northeast United States, but the availability of diagnostic techniques soon thereafter led to the recognition of disease throughout the North American continent and beyond to most other continents. With the more complete realization of the disease spectrum, it was also apparent, however, that various manifestations of Lyme disease had been recognized as particularly unique entities in Europe for decades. Erythema chronicum migrans (EM), first demonstrated by a Swedish physician Afzelius in 1909, was coined historically as an enlarging rash which often originated from an apparent tick bite; its faster resolution after the use of antibiotics, rather than without them, led to the hypothesis of an infectious origin much before the etiological agent was defined in the early 1980s (6). Already a century before the discovery of *B. burgdorferi*, a chronic skin manifestation, termed acrodermatitis chronica atrophicans (ACA), was described (7,8), and in the early 1920s, a painful meningoradiculitis, later termed Bannwarth's syndrome (9), was reported by French scientists Garin and Bujadoux. Both of these manifestations constitute examples of the varied cutaneous and neurological complications of what is now recognized as Lyme disease. In the United States alone, mainly in the northeast, there have been well over 100,000 infections reported to date. Whereas the initial excitement of a newly recognized infection led to the diagnosis of thousands of illnesses in a few years, it is now accepted that the recent discovery was followed by a period of marked over-diagnosis among both children and adults (10,11). The issue of over-diagnosis and chronic disease is one with considerable impact on health care resources (12-14). Simultaneously with the recognition of pitfalls in the diagnostics and hence over-diagnosis, concerns about the chronic sequelae of Lyme disease and possible unsuccessful eradication of the spirochete from some of the patients have been realized. The frequency of chronicity and relapses of infection with *B. burgdorferi* is currently a very controversial issue. The present needs for clinical purposes and more accurate diagnosis underline the importance of focusing research on development of reliable diagnostic tests.

The availability of molecular tools has quickly led to a new era in the study of borrelioses. This has made the development of new diagnostic methods, differentiation of isolates, and the discovery of new species possible, and has contributed to the epidemiology of disease both among humans and in nature. Although relapsing fever and Lyme disease still continue to constitute the major forms of borreliosis, the discoveries in recent decades probably are only an introduction to the complex presentations of borreliosis in the ecosystem.

II. CLINICAL ASPECTS

A. Relapsing fever

The awareness of the complex biology of the relapsing fever spirochetes is improving, and as a consequence of this new knowledge, there will emerge some deeper understanding of differences among the illnesses that are caused by relapsing fever borreliae. As of yet, however, clinical cases with different causative agents in the developed world are not frequent enough in order to gather considerable comparative data. It is apparent, however, that the louse-borne relapsing fever is somewhat different from tick-borne relapsing fevers (1).

After the initial infestation is carried out by an arthropod, the spirochete will typically penetrate the skin of the host; for louse-borne disease, this is likely to occur after the body louse is inadvertently crushed on the skin and spirochetes afterward penetrate, whereas with tick-borne illnesses, the spirochetes are directly released into the dermis via the tick bite. Shortly thereafter, there is systemic dissemination of the bacterium most likely through the bloodstream. An initial incubation period of 5-14 days is needed before clinical manifestations are apparent; primarily an illness of high fever that may or may not be associated with rigors, photophobia, headache, myalgias, and/or cough. The onset of illness is correlated with bacterial sepsis which can often be seen microscopically as high grade spirochetemia. Following dissemination of the bacterium, the patient will experience a variable number of afebrile and febrile episodes; hence the terminology of "relapsing fever". The initial episode of fever may last for 3-5 days, and resolution can be accompanied by hypotension or shock which are presumably related to bacterial lysis which resembles artificially-induced lysis that is caused by appropriate antibiotic therapy. The patient is then otherwise well until the next febrile episode which typically occurs after approximately one week. The next febrile relapse will also last several days but tends to be shorter in duration. Each of the subsequent relapses, if they occur, will also last several days but tend to be of shorter duration and intensity than the previous episodes. The total number of relapses is variable; typically there will be 1-3 of these, but the number can be as many as a dozen or more in rare instances. The change in quality of relapses and their eventual resolution are probably caused by effective humoral immunity that arises during each episode. During the resolution of the febrile episodes, the bacterium maintains itself in a protected state in tissue where it can hide beyond the most powerful attack of antibodies due to the poor penetration of antibody to certain tissue sites. Each relapse is associated with further recruitment of the humoral response and then ultimately protection. Tick-borne relapsing fever is associated with more relapses than the louse-borne form. Since fever is seemingly the only manifestation of the majority of illnesses, it is quite likely that these febrile episodes will be under-recognized as borrelia infections.

Other complications of relapsing fever are either uncommon or under-appreciated (1,15). Their occurrence is a direct consequence of bacterial spread outside of the bloodstream. Hepatitis (mostly subclinical) occurs in up to one-third of patients. The main causative agent for hepatitis in relapsing fevers is the agent of louse-borne disease, *B. recurrentis*, which may, in fact, cause a more advanced disease in the liver than other borreliae and lead to jaundice (1). The enlargement of the liver and spleen are more common than clinical hepatitis. The frequency of all types of neurological manifestations varies by *Borrelia* species, from none to >50%. *Borrelia turicatae* and *Borrelia duttonii*, the agents of tick-borne relapsing fever in southwestern North America and sub-Saharan Africa respectively, cause neurological disease as often as *B. burgdorferi* in Lyme disease. The louse-borne agent, *B. recurrentis*, appears to invade the brain or meninges less commonly. The most commonly reported neurological complications of relapsing fever are meningitis and facial nerve involvement. Less common are encephalitis, myelitis, radiculitis, and neuropsychiatric disturbances (15). A truncal rash is seen in some patients towards the termination of the initial febrile episode. Less commonly, patients may have central nervous system illness, a respiratory illness, or hemorrhagic diatheses; transplacental infection has been reported. The possibility to present with complications such as a severe Jarisch-Herxheimer reaction increases with louse-borne borreliosis (1), and mortality may reach 15-30%. It is unclear whether death is directly attributable only to the consequences of infection or whether the underlying diseases or factors affecting the general health of a patient have a major role in susceptibility. The louse-borne agent, *B. recurrentis*, currently is encountered in areas of Africa where individuals are already compromised by disparate social circumstances, malnutrition, other intercurrent infections, among other things (1). In contrast, death is uncommon in tick-borne relapsing fever (<2-3%). A recent study of louse-borne relapsing fever from northern Somalia illustrated that borreliosis is a common cause of pyrexia of unknown origin (3). In this community-based study, however, there were no fatal cases.

Heterogeneity in clinical illness is certainly dependent on host variability, and this has been documented through experiments in animal models. The potential for the bacteria to change antigens of the outer membrane in vivo probably has a role in the spectrum of clinical manifestations as is also seen during the sequence of relapsing fever episodes. The nature of relapsing fever borreliae is such that one might anticipate the potential for chronic illness analogous to Lyme disease or syphilis. A chronic course of illness, however, has not been described in relapsing fevers. In Lyme disease, the chronic manifestations do not develop until several months have elapsed since the acquisition of the infection. Relapsing fevers are more quickly evolving infections with a high burden of spirochetes in the bloodstream and also a more rapid rise of antibodies against the causative spirochete than is seen with Lyme disease. The potential for chronic manifestations from relapsing fever, however, remains a possibility and deserves further study.

B. Lyme disease

Despite plenty of similarities in the biology of the different borreliae, it is of considerable curiosity that the clinical illness which is termed Lyme disease is very distinct from relapsing fever, although both may affect several organs or organ systems of the body.

In general terms, Lyme disease is notable for its involvement mainly of skin, joint, neurological system, and the heart (16,17). The specific manifestations, however, are quite variable (see Table 1). The progression of Lyme disease takes place in stages from superficial to disseminated to chronic infection. Although some may dislike the comparison of Lyme disease to clinical syphilis due to the sexual transmission of the latter and hence varied negative connotations, the sequential progression and the spectrum of illness among target organs are phenomenally similar with each other. The first stage is an acute localized infection (chancre in syphilis versus EM in Lyme disease), the second stage is a disseminated infection, and the third stage includes late cardiac and central nervous system (CNS) lesions in syphilis, and rheumatological, neurological, cardiac, or skin complications in Lyme disease. The three stages of Lyme disease, however, greatly overlap. The first and second stages are considered early stages and the third stage a late or chronic stage. EM may still be present while manifestations of the second stage are developing a few weeks, usually not more than three months, after the onset of infection. On the other hand, the occasional spirochetemia and frequent systemic symptoms in patients with the first stage indicate very early spread of spirochetes from the skin to other organs. There is no consensus about the exact interval between stages, but the third stage often begins in one year after the onset of infection.

Meningitis, however, which is generally considered a manifestation of the second stage, may develop after arthritis which is a manifestation of the third stage. Thus, the staging may be difficult, and it may be practical and pathophysiologically valid to divide the manifestations of Lyme disease into EM (early localized infection) and disseminated manifestations (18). Furthermore, patients with Lyme disease evidently may undergo a latent phase of the disease as is the case in syphilis.

Most patients will never have the initial site of tick bite recognized. This site may be the focus for the sentinel clinical manifestation which initiates as EM in the first stage of disease. EM, an expanding skin lesion, arises at the site of the inoculation of *B. burgdorferi* in 60-80% of infected patients (19). The incubation period (time interval between tick bite and onset of EM) varies between 1-3 days and 4 months but is commonly 1-2 weeks (20,21). About 70% of patients with EM do not recall a preceding

Table 1 The disease spectrum of Lyme disease.

Dermatological	Ocular
erythema migrans (single or multiple)	conjunctivitis
borrelia lymphocytoma	iritis
urticaria	interstitial keratitis
panniculitis	chorioretinitis
morphea and sclerotic changes of the skin	retinal vasculitis
acrodermatitis chronica atrophicans	
	Neurological
Cardiac	meningitis
myocarditis	radiculitis
pericarditis	encephalitis
A-V conduction disturbances	cranial nerve involvement
dilated cardiomyopathy	epilepsy
	peripheral neuropathy
Musculoskeletal	chronic encephalopathy
myalgia	psychiatric disease
arthralgia and arthritis	stroke
tendinitis	vasculitis
myositis	
osteomyelitis	Other
fibromyalgia	hepatitis
	splenomegaly
	orchitis
	adult respiratory distress syndrome
	congenital infection

tick bite (5,20). In a few instances, patients may recall a sting of a flying insect (21,22). The low number of recalled preceding tick bites is probably due to the fact that tiny and easily unnoticed nymphal ticks transmit the majority of clinical infecitons. EM generally begins as a red macula or papula that enlarges centrifugally to form an erythematous patch with or without central clearing. Most EM lesions reported from both Europe and America, however, are homogeneous and lack the central clearing; a finding also in a recent large American prospective cohort study (23,24). EM is presumabley related to the spread of the organism, since spirochetes can be isolated from its leading margin (21,25). EM lesions may be asymptomatic or pruritic, and they are often warmer than the surrounding normal skin. Some of them may have a purpuric appearance or vesicular center. EM margins are usually regular and generally not elevated from the surrounding skin. Scaling is uncommon. If untreated, the EM usually expands and reaches a diameter of 15 cm. or more. Exceptionally, EM lesions may measure less than 4 cm. in diameter and hardly expand (20). EM usually resolves spontaneously in a few weeks or months, although it may re-emerge when untreated. Furthermore, it has become clear that the disappearance of EM should not be interpreted as proof of the eradication of the spirochete or cure of the disease. *B. burgdorferi* can be cultured from skin biopsy specimens 1-6 months after the disappearance of EM or at the site of a previous tick bite (26). Secondary similar lesions, although usually smaller smaller than the initial EM, may occur elsewhere as a consequence of blood and lymphatic spread. Early reported frequencies of multiple EM were as high as 48% of patients with EM (5). Recently, rates below 25% have been reported from the U.S. Since most multiple EM lesions develop after hematogenous spread of the spirochete (comparable to secondary lesions of syphilis), these lesions are now regarded as components of stage II disease. In Europe, about 4-8% of patients have multiple concurrent EM-like lesions. Along with the EM, some patients may experience an acute febrile illness with or without general symptoms such as fatigue, malaise, myalgia, arthralgia, headache, and stiff neck; these symptoms will be variable and intermittent. In Europe, one or more of these symptoms are associated with EM in 20-70% of patients. Objective physical findings other than regional lymphadenopathy or fever, however, are infrequent in patients with EM (21). The onset of EM must necessarily coincide with the period when tick transmission can occur; in most areas of endemicity, this time will vary from late spring to early fall.

Early in the course of infection, *B. burgdorferi* may disseminate to several organs via blood circulation. The low frequency at which *B. burgdorferi* can be cultured from the blood suggests that the spirochetes are rapidly cleared from the circulation. From the perspective of clinical manifestations, the preferred sites of infection will include other regions of skin, the nervous system, the heart, and joints. Neurological disease is quite variable in its presentation: Lyme disease may affect peripheral nerves, cranial nerves, the meningeal lining of the CNS, and the CNS parenchyma itself (27,28). The CNS tends to be infected early in Lyme disease (29). Meningeal irritation may progress to meningitis, but *B. burgdorferi* can be cultured from the CSF in only approximately 10% of patients (18). Lyme meningitis resembles aseptic meningitis and is usually acute, but it may also take a long-term or relapsing course (30). Vasculitis and deeper cortical involvement may also occur and lead to encephalopathies, psychoses, and neurovascular disease (31-33). The three most typical manifestations of Lyme neuroborreliosis are lymphocytic meningitis, cranial neuritis (particularly involving the facial nerve), and radiculoneuritis. This triad was the first extracutaneous complex of symptoms to be associated with *B. burgdorferi* infection (34,35). Virtually any of the cranial nerves may be affected, but most frequently the seventh nerve is involved and results in a facial palsy which may be unilateral or bilateral (36,37). Lymphocytic meningoradiculitis usually starts as a painful limb disorder, with subsequent remissions and exacerbations that often last for 5-6 mo. (38). Dysesthesia and distressing migrating pain are the main symptoms, frequently mimicing those caused by a herniated intervertebral disc. The sensory symptoms can be accompanied by motor symptoms and peripheral nerve paresis. Peripheral motor or sensory neuropathies may result as a consequence of direct nerve infiltration or vasculitis of the epineural vessels (18,28,39,40). Less frequently, acute myelitis, encephalitis with or without seizures, or ataxia may be the most prominent features even in the early disseminated stage of Lyme disease (41). Months to years after disease onset, chronic encephalomyelitis may appear. Spinal or cerebral symptoms and signs may predominate or co-exist. Magnetic resonance imaging may show focal abnormalities that usually involve the white matter and may be difficult to distinguish from lesions that are found in multiple sclerosis (31,32,42). Case reports of Lyme neuroborreliosis with stroke-like manifestations or focal or general vasculitis in the CNS have been published (32). Encephalopathy associated with Lyme disease may be common, but prevalence estimates vary depending on how this entity is defined. It may occur even without CNS infection, perhaps being mediated by inflammatory host reactions, e.g., production of cytokines and their systemic influence. Patients with chronic Lyme encephalopathy, however, have been shown to have multifocal reductions in cerebral blood flow and to objectively benefit from antibiotic therapy (43). The neuro-ophthalmical and ocular manifestations of Lyme disease show characteristics that resemble those of syphilis, and include cranial neuropathies, optic nerve disease, meningitis and papilledema, neuroretinitis, retinal vasculitis, vitreitis, uveitis, keratitis, and conjunctivitis (44,45). Joint disease is also variable from person to person (46). Arthralgia and myalgia are early musculoskeletal symptoms of Lyme disease. In the U.S., about 60% of untreated patients with EM experience brief attacks of monoarticular or oligoarticular arthritis which usually develop several months after the onset of the infection, tend to be intermittent, and mostly affect the large joints (19). The arthritic attacks may continue to last for several months but most often subside eventually. Chronic and erosive forms of arthritis may develop in about 10% of patients with untreated EM (19). The reportedly higher frequency of arthritis in the U.S. may be due to the occurrence of one genospecies of *B. burgdorferi* sensu lato (in contrast to three in Europe) and due to a possible tropism of this to joints or neurological manifestations (47). Acute arrhythmias may occur, especially atrioventricular block, which are usually transient but may often require a temporary pacemaker. Myopericarditis is a relatively common form of cardiac manifestation. Dilated cardiomyopathy caused by, and an association of coronary artery disease with, *B. burgdorferi* infection have been reported (48,49). Besides EM, other dermatological manifestations of Lyme disease, especially in European patients, include borrelial lymphocytoma (a bluish-red tumor-like skin infiltrate) and acrodermatitis chronica atrophicans (chronic skin involvement which becomes atrophic gradually and often many years, or even decades, after onset of infection) (50). Again, the remitting and relapsing nature of illnesses as well as the diverse distribution has many parallels to secondary syphilis. *B. burgdorferi* infection may sometimes lead to sclerotic changes of the skin, e.g. morphea, and has occasionally been linked to urticaria (51). The third stage of illness essentially constitutes the persistence of bacterium in skin, joint, and central nervous system. It will be manifest in months to years after the initial infection.

Overall, there is considerable variation in Lyme disease; this diversity is evident in children as it is in adults (52). Many infections will be asymptomatic and may thus present as interpretive dilemmae when positive serology is present in the absence of active disease. Single foci of involvement may be prominent for some whereas multisystem disease may be apparent for others. It is not clear what variables interact to either contain or facilitate the dissemination of the spirochete, but specific host genetic factors have been proposed as being linked with the occurrence of arthropathy in some. Differences in the presentations of Lyme disease between the continents of Europe and North America had been observed. These had initially been attributed to population differences, but subsequent molecular work has determined that "*B. burgdorferi*" (*B. burgdorferi* sensu lato) isolates are heterogeneous (53); at least four genomospecies are now recognized as Lyme spirochetes in Europe: *B. burgdorferi* sensu strictu, *B. garinii*, *B. afzelii*, and *B. valaisiana*.

Considering the tremendous diversity among clinical illnesses, it is not surprising therefore that Lyme disease might be contemplated when individuals have a chronic systemic illness or an isolated but cryptic illness especially when of joint or when neurological. Lyme disease will necessarily be considered in the differential diagnosis of many illnesses, and individuals will necessarily be keen to have a diagnosis made when the prospect of treatment with an antibiotic is possible. These considerations have led to considerable overdiagnosis from a clinical perspective (10-14). Such excess anxiety prompts more laboratory testing which, if fallible, may be associated with many false diagnoses when predictive values are low.

III. EPIDEMIOLOGY OF INFECTION

A. Relapsing fever

Tick-borne relapsing fever spirochetes cause infection among humans worldwide, and spirochetemia has also been documented among avians. There are many species that are geographically restricted by the specificity for particular ticks which are also geographically limited. It is not apparent that significant differences between strains exist among the louse-borne spirochetes, but this area is not as well studied as vector-spirochete connections in tick-borne diseases.

Human-to-human transmission, with the body louse as the intermediate, is important for the acquisition of *B. recurrentis*. The louse feeds on an infected human and acquires the spirochetes from the blood meal. The bacteria then multiply in the arthropod midgut and thereafter invade the systemic body fluids. It is believed that bacteria re-enter the next human after the infected louse gains parasite status and is inadvertently crushed, hence releasing live motile spirochetes which are able to invade skin (1). Thus, unlike tick-borne infection, the spirochete is not actually transferred during the arthropod feed. Given the locale for most recognized disease and the human reservoir, it is not surprising to see a lack of seasonality in the occurrence of infection. Conditions of poor hygiene and over-crowding have much to contribute to the continuation of louse-borne disease in endemic areas. Given the differences in spirochete-vector association and in clinical features of louse-borne and tick-borne diseases, it is of considerable interest, however, that *B. recurrentis* (louse-borne) and *B. duttonii* (tick-borne) are closely related genetically.

Tick-borne borreliae are carried in nature by soft ticks, mainly of the *Ornithodoros* spp., which parasitize mammals in the wild (30). For example, in the Pacific northwest of the North American continent, *B. hermsii* and *B. parkeri* are transmitted by *O. hermsii* and *O. parkeri* respectively; *B. duttonii* is transmitted by *O. duttonii* in several African locales whereas *B. venezuelensis* is carried by *O. venezuelensis* in South and Central America. There are over twenty *Borrelia* spp. that are currently recognized to be tick-borne. It is not well understood how borreliae maintain tick specificity. Small mammals, e.g., rodents, particularly serve as the natural reservoirs, e.g., rodents, and these animals serve to carry the ticks (and thus spirochetes) when they are mobile. When the spirochete enters the tick gut after a blood feed, it quickly infects all arthropod tissues, and therefore may infect the next mammal or indeed human during the subsequent feeding process. It is possible, although not very common, that the spirochetes are vertically transmitted to tick progeny. In many areas of the world where tick-borne illness is endemic, the extreme of climatic conditions during the year force both tick and human to be more active during warm periods; hence, there is a much greater likelihood for the transmission to occur from late spring to early fall (and the disease to be manifest after the appropriate incubation period). In North America in particular, infection is associated with camping in infested areas or habitation of cabins (55) that are infiltrated by infected rodents. As the soft ticks are often night-feeders, the feed on a human host will often pass unnoticed.

Overall, the containment of these illnesses will mainly depend on either good hygiene (louseborne) or vector control (tick-borne). In the case of louse-borne disease, however, it is also possible that accurate and timely diagnosis may have some contribution to the spread of the infection that is due to the human-to-human transmission.

B. Lyme disease

Hard ticks, at this time mainly recognized as *Ixodes* spp., are the important arthropods for the transmission of spirochetes causing Lyme disease (54). Again, the specific ixodid tick may vary geographically: e.g., *I. ricinus* – Europe, *I. persulcatus* – Asia, *I. pacificus* – Pacific North America. Other hard ticks including *Argas* spp., *Amblyomma* spp., and *Rhipicephalus* spp. have also been implicated as vectors although not as frequently as is the case with the ixodids. Very early in the understanding of Lyme disease, most of the work focused on what was believed to be the major if not only spirochete causing Lyme disease – *B. burgdorferi* sensu stricto. Further work has now made it clear that differences between genospecies causing Lyme disease can be demonstrated with molecular techniques, and the cluster of these spirochetes have been termed *B. burgdorferi* sensu lato which covers *B. burgdorferi* sensu stricto, *B. garinii*, and *B. afzelii* among other candidates (56). These other candidates initially were termed VS116 (and M19) and a Japanese variant *B. burgdorferi*. They have now been designated *B. valaisiana* (57) and *B. japonica* (58) respectively. It may be that other genomospecies from this group are yet to be identified. In Europe, there is considerable heterogeneity among *B. burgdorferi* sensu lato, i.e., several of the genomospecies have been identified from human infections (59), but *B. burgdorferi* in North America is much more homogeneous. The potential for simultaneous infection by several genomospecies in Europe has been published (37,60). Clinically manifest disease can be seen among humans and domestic animals, but illness among mammals in nature is much less evident even though the wild animals may be highly infected. The spirochetal infestation rate of ticks in any given area is quite variable (61,62) as is also the frequency of ticks. Therefore, the frequency of infected mammals also greatly varies. Kirstein et al. demonstrate such variability in an interesting study from Ireland where both geographic and species heterogeneity were observed (63). These facts along with the issue of frequent or infrequent human contact with ticks affect the prevalence of Lyme disease. Whereas it may be anticipated that contact with ticks should occur most often in regions where vegetation is conducive, there is the real possibility that land development and urbanization among other things may be affecting arthropod dynamics (64). Transmission of *B. burgdorferi* can occur when ticks are questing, and this occurs typically during the peak summer months.

Essentially all stages of the hard tick may be capable of transmitting the disease. The nymphal stage, which already is frequently carrying the spirochete but small enough to go unnoticed by the victim, is probably the major origin of human disease. In general, though, adult ticks are more likely to parasitize large mammals. The likelihood to transfer the bacterium from arthropod to human is greatly influenced by the length of time of tick attachment. Borreliae are activated during feeding and migrate from the intestine to other organs of the tick such as the salivary glands thus facilitating the possibility of rapid transmission of *B. burgdorferi* to the host during feeding (65). Both mammals and birds may serve to carry ticks widely through nature; the potential for birds to mobilize ticks intercontinentally exists (66).

IV. NATURE OF THE BACTERIUM, PATHOGENESIS, AND CLINICAL MANIFESTA-TIONS

Borreliae are quite unique among the bacterial kingdom, and it is unlikely that they will be confused with other bacteria that infect humans. The study of spirochetes in this area has opened a new field for microbiology in general; whereas the human pathogens are quickly studied for medical and others purposes, it is becoming apparent that there are likely numerous other spirochetes in nature which have not been recognized and which will require study.

Borreliae are not stained well with the Gram stain, but numerous other stains may be used to identify these bacteria in tissue, including silver stains. These stains are not capable of facilitating the differentiation of *Borrelia* species or different genospecies of *B. burgdorferi* sensu lato. Borreliae have a G+C content of approximately 30% (67) and are quite well segregated as a distinct group on the basis of rRNA gene sequencing. Bacterial length varies from 10-30 um. and the length includes 4-10 spirals. The endoflagellae, which are located in the periplasmic space, are essential for the spirochete motility. Structural features facilitate differentiation from leptospires (Figure 1).

Borreliae are limited in their ability to grow in current artificial media; this limitation is consistent with the predicted biochemical limitations that were realized soon after the full sequencing of *B*.

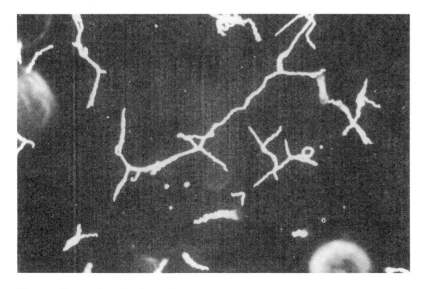

Figure 1 *B. burgdorferi* spirochetes from culture media as visualized by darkfield microscopy (photo: M. Viljanen).

burgdorferi was accomplished. Kelly's medium (68) is time-consuming to prepare, and some variations of it have been taken to experimental and diagnostic use (e.g., BSK, BSKII); serum and some form of long chain fatty acids appear to be prequisites for optimum growth conditions. Generation times in vitro approach twenty-four hours. The growth time in vitro must certainly be longer than in vivo since very high grade spirochetemia evolves over a short period of time during episodes of relapsing fever. Borreliae are capable of fermenting carbohydrates and appear to thrive best in microaerophilic conditions.

These bacteria have a typical limiting plasma membrane and a cell wall. An interesting structure is the outer membrane of the borreliae that exists external to the flagella. The outer membrane is capable of considerable variability and, through the use of the antigenic repertoire, allows for changing expression of antigens on its surface. The genes which code for outer membrane proteins reside on multiple linear plasmids which are also unique among bacteria (69). The unsheathed flagella are multiple and attach subterminally to each pole (70). Contractility leads to movement but is also responsible for the spirochetal shape in the resting state. Motility is of a cork-screw nature and will assist the bacterium in invading and then penetrating tissue.

Pulse field gel electrophoresis, and now sequencing studies, have placed the size of the long linear chromosome at approximately 900-950 kbp (71). Both linear and circular plasmids exist; these may vary in absolute number (e.g., 5-20) for any given bacterial isolate, and they may also vary in size (72). The plasmids may contribute another 500 kbp of DNA (71). It is unclear what ongoing exchange exists between the main chromosome and the plasmid DNA, but it is evident that interactions must occur in order to account for the antigenic variability at the level of the outer membrane.

A. Relapsing fever

The exact mechanisms which account for antigenic variation during relapsing illnesses are largely unknown, but research in this area has considerably explored the genetics of protein expression (69,73,74). Whereas it is evident that variability occurs among the outer membrane surface proteins and that these are regulated by events within the linear plasmids, it is not clear how immune selection facilitates the ongoing changes. Given the considerable variability for number of and quality of relapses, the actual relapse and the subsequent clinical manifestation quite likely occur as a result of a complex interaction between bacterium and host. Antigenic expression will vary as a consequence of temperature change and whether the bacterium is in the mammalian or arthropod host (75).

The most important feature of pathogenesis certainly is the ability of the bacterium to penetrate tissue and remain sequestered. This privileged time must then allow for recombination or regulation pathways to activate a new armour of surface proteins which allow the bacterium to evade the existing immune response. It is accepted that bactericidal antibody is protective; this antibody recruits complement and achieves bacterial killing ability in the periphery. The antibody response will be variably directed against the antigens that are present in the outer membrane structure at the time – hence a variable number of relapses to follow.

Tissue pathology, for the time being, has been poorly investigated for tick-borne borreliosis. This is true partly by the rarity of documented cases of patients with fatal outcomes of the disease, and partly by the sparse number of spirochetes that exist in infected tissue. More information in this regard is available from louse-borne disease (1); the number of patients are greater, and there is a higher mortality rate during the initial bacteremia. Although more widely thought of as bacteremic illnesses with only limited distribution to different organs, relapsing fevers do indeed affect several body tissues. Liver involvement with histopathological necrosis, hemorrhage within the central nervous system, myocarditis, and gastrointestinal lesions are some of the peripheral manifestations. On a clinical basis, however, most of these other organ involvements are not recognized. The molecular pathogenesis of these events warrants further study, but it appears that the pattern of clinical manifestations may vary as a consequence of the particular bacterial strain (73). Although borreliae have extractable components which in many ways mimic gram negative bacterial endotoxin, it is not certain that such structures are as important as the mere ability of the bacterium to penetrate tissue. The occurrence of a Jarisch-Herxheimer reaction after therapy of relapsing fever is frequent (76); the pathophysiology of this occurrence is not well understood, but it is postulated that massive release of tumor necrosis factor is contributory in large part (77). Some researchers propose a more complex interaction of cytokines and infection (78). In addition to tissue penetration, borreliae are able to enter cells. Whereas actual resistance to phagocytosis is not demonstrated for relapsing fever borreliae (79), it is conceivable that some form of immune evasion in addition to frank sequestration is likely to exist. Antibiotic treatment may increase the ability of polymorphonuclear cells to engulf these bacteria (79).

B. Lyme disease

Growth of Lyme disease-causing spirochetes is generally as restricted as the relapsing fever bacteria. Cultivation is accomplished with Barbour-Stoenner-Kelly liquid medium at 33°C which is essentially a variation of Kelly's original medium.

The full sequencing of *B. burgdorferi* certainly provides a new era of understanding in regards to the molecular biology of the organism and the disease mechanisms (71). Essentially all of the North American isolates can be referred to as *B. burgdorferi* sensu stricto, but many European isolates which were formerly called *B. burgdorferi* are now inclusive of *B. afzelii*, *B. garinii*, *B. burgdorferi* sensu stricto, and *B. valaisiana*. These genetic variations seem to correlate with clinical differences. The applied systematics are far from being concluded in regards to these borreliae. For instance, variability within *B. burgdorferi* sensu stricto and *B. garinii* have been reported (80,81). These differences may simply reflect intragenic heterogeneity, but possibly also new genomospecies will be named (82). *B. burgdorferi* can lose plasmids during laboratory passage, but otherwise its genome has been found to be reasonably stable despite extensive in vitro culture (83).

Antigenic variation at the outer membrane occurs analogous to the shift that is seen with relapsing fever spirochetes (84-86). This potential must also be crucial to varying antigenic coats that appear during active disease, sequestration, and relapse; indeed, variations in outer membrane proteins have been determined for isolates which have been obtained from different sites of infection (87). Unlike relapsing fever, however, a periodic fever pattern is not commonly seen in Lyme disease although it has been described. Different outer membrane proteins of *B. burgdorferi*, labeled as OspA to OspF, have been identified and used in immunodiagnostics. OspA has been studied as a vaccine candidate and furthermore implemented as an effective immunogen for clinical use; it has gained U.S. FDA approval as a vaccine. Osp proteins range in size from 19-36 kD, are encoded by the plasmids, and are among the first antigens to be recognized in the immune response. The flagellar (41 kD) and heat-shock proteins of *B. burgdorferi* have also been characterized.

Although Lyme disease-related deaths are very uncommon, and thus post-mortem tissue is generally lacking, the histopathology of Lyme disease has been now reasonably well-defined due to the availability of tissue especially from skin and joint. EM has been particularly well-characterized because of the availability of biopsy material. Animal models have also improved the understanding of the infection and mechanisms of disease. Spirochetes can be recovered from infected tissue decades after the transmission. The yield of culture, however, is very low in disseminated stages of the infection and only moderate from biopsies of EM lesions. Also, histopathological methods for visualization of the bacterium in diseased tissue are at best difficult. In contrast to relapsing fever spirochetes, Lyme disease-causing spirochetes seem to evade phagocytosis to some extent. The bacteria are capable of tissue and cellular penetration, although it is unclear as to what extent the latter occurs in vivo. There appears to be a relative tropism of the spirochete for tissue of skin, joints, and central nervous system (88); tissue receptors for the bacterium have been studied. Tissue infiltration with bacterium is accompanied by a lymphocytic response that may be focally manifest by a congregation of cells such as the development of lymphocytomata (89). Diseased tissue is associated with a mild vasculitis. There may be different patterns of injury in the peripheral and central nervous systems (28,32), but the complex interaction of bacterium and host is not well understood (90). As a consequence of central nervous system infection, the cerebrospinal fluid may reveal lymphocytic pleocytosis. The ability of *B. burgdorferi* to sequester within tissue for prolonged periods with the potential for subsequent relapse is consistent with the variable course of clinical illness for different patients. Evasion of the immune response due to the intracellular location, for both immune and non-immune system cells, is postulated to promote bacterial persistence (91-93). One possibility for the cascade of events during infection is that *B. burgdorferi* promotes a shift in the immune response of the host, and possibly is able to turn off the activation of Th2 cells and shift the balance towards Th1 cell type activation with subsequent production of increased quantities of IFN-gamma which is a potent activator of a proinflammatory cascade (94). On a theoretical basis, considerable down-regulation of major histocompatibility markers that participate in bacterial antigen presentation could play a role in part (95).

V. IMMUNOLOGY OF INFECTION

The immune responses after both relapsing fever and Lyme disease are reasonably well-studied, but there are several issues which complicate these observations in general. It is accepted that antigenic diversity among species occurs, and this is highlighted by the antigenic variation among outer membrane proteins. The initial humoral response will thus vary depending on which antigens have been recognized first. Antibody does not develop as rapidly as is seen with other micro-organisms. For example, many primary immune responses will be apparent after common viral infections by approximately 10-14 days. In borrelioses, this phase of response may require several more weeks. There is cross-reactivity to some extent between borrelia species whether tick- or louse-borne (70). Furthermore, there is some cross-reactivity between borrelia and other pathogenic and non-pathogenic spirochetes (96). The flagellar proteins, for example, have some common epitopes. Although lymphocytic responses are prominent in diseased tissue, the study of cell-mediated immunity in these illnesses is incomplete.

A. Relapsing fever

After initiation of the infection, the antibody response can be measured by a variety of conventional techniques such as complement fixation, immunofluorescence, and agglutination (97). Due to the antigenic variability of relapsing fever borreliae, the patterns of humoral immune response can be variable especially when considering that which is directed to outer membrane proteins; responses to flagellar and heat-shock proteins are not uncommon however. Bactericidal antibody is likely to be critical for host protection, but it is not necessarily measured by any of the previously mentioned techniques. In louse-borne relapsing fever, passive immunization with immune sera has been found to induce a crisis among infected patients (1). In the presence of complement, antibody is lytic when bacteria are exposed to it (1). Both complement and antibody may facilitate opsonization of spirochetes (98).

Heterophilic antibodies do occur during infection in some patients. For example, antibodies to Proteus OXK agglutinogens are recognized. False-positive assays for syphilis antibody occur in 5-10% of patients with relapsing fever.

B. Lyme disease

The level of antibodies can be measured by several conventional techniques during and after infection. The most common methods are immunofluorescence and enzyme immunoassay. Antibody quantitation will usually decline after antibiotic treatment although not disappear altogether. Since antibodies can persist indefinitely, a diagnostic dilemma is created in endemic areas where patients may be repeatedly tested over a lifetime. Bactericidal antibody (complement-activating) is a component of this humoral response, but it does not seem to have the same role in protection that is seen in relapsing fever. Nevertheless, Callister et al. have found that borreliacidal antibody may serve as a more sensitive indicator in early Lyme disease than other methods (99). For both experimental and diagnostic purposes, the sequence of anti-*B. burgdorferi* antibody development has been extensively followed by immunoblotting studies (see Serology). Although there can be considerable variability overall in the humoral response, there are some antigens that are consistently recognized. OspC, a flagellar protein (41 kD) (100), and a heat-shock protein (58 kD) are commonly targets of antibodies, and the peak of antibody response (i.e., IgG maximum) commonly includes a recognition of OspA and OspB. The anti-OspA antibody especially is prominent as the disease enters the third stage, e.g., as arthritic symptoms become chronic. It is interesting to note that some patients with large amounts of anti-OspA and anti-OspB antibody and with particular HLA types do not seem to respond to antibiotic therapy as well as others; it is unclear whether there is some cause-and-effect relationship here or whether the association is simply a marker for chronicity. Intrathecal production of antibodies can be measured by a capture-assay in patients with a central nervous system disease. Not all patients with neuroborreliosis, however, have detectable amounts of intrathecally-produced antibodies. In turn, intrathecal antibodies may be detectable for years after treatment and do not always reflect disease activity.

The entity of seronegative Lyme disease is controversial with the exception of the EM phase of the disease where one-half of all patients are seronegative. This entity, however, remains feasible as it is apparent that early infection can be associated with a relatively weak humoral immune response or even suppression of it, and that early insufficient treatment may also cause seronegativity later in the disease. In some circumstances, delayed antibody production may be responsible for this apparent seronegativity (101), but it is conceivable that antigenic variation might also have a role. As well, it is self-evident that methodologies which have a high cut-off level for antibody positivity may cause false-negative results (102). The differences between antigens of the infecting genospecies and those that are used in the test that measures the antibody level may cause marked insensitivity. Low or negative antibody levels may also result from the formation of immune complexes (104). Dattwyler and others have suggested that patients with seronegative Lyme disease have vigorous T cell proliferative responses in the absence of detectable antibody (103). Huppertz and colleagues have assessed lymphoproliferative responses among children and suggest that a contribution of this assessment to the diagnosis for a seronegative pediatric patient is possible (105). Seronegative Lyme disease is relatively uncommon, however, if patients are indeed assessed over a long period of time, and therefore, this diagnostic entity must be viewed cautiously (106). Infection may also be associated with a non-specific polyclonal humoral response, and a small percentage of patients may have false-positive tests for syphilis.

T cell proliferative responses are detected several weeks after initiation of infection, and some of these responses may be quite prominent. Borreliae may induce cytokine responses by activating mononuclear cells and hence cascade a number of important physiological events (88). Of concern, some of these T cell responses may be or become directed to autoantigens, but a cause-and-effect relationship for systemic disease, e.g., of joint, e.g., of central nervous system (90), is far from acknowledged. Lymphoid reactions are prominent in most diseased tissue, especially heart, skin, and central nervous system, but the joint commonly has a predominance of polymorphonuclear cells.

The frequency of disease in some areas of the world along with the potential for serious multisystem illnesses has necessarily led to the development of vaccines. A vaccine which includes purified OspA has been assessed in laboratory models, and is now implemented for use among humans (107,108). Protective efficacy is apparently substantial, but the vaccine's use will have some role in confusing the assessment of antibody responses for diagnostic purposes (109). It has been postulated, however, that heterogeneity even within the same genospecies of *B. burgdorferi* sensu lato, especially in Europe, may warrant a vaccine that is multivalent in contrast to the current OspA vaccine (110). The experimental data from Barthold are intriguing and address a key issue in natural infection and vaccine production (111). Animals that were challenged with varied isolates of *B. burgdorferi*, *B. afzelii*, and *B. garinii* were protected against subsequent homologous challenge, but cross-protection from heterologous species or strains was not achieved (111).

VI. LABORATORY DIAGNOSIS

A. Relapsing fever

1. Microscopy

Given the paucity of relapsing fever illnesses, the diagnosis is not uncommonly made by the accidental finding of spirochetes in blood count films. Whereas the bacteria do not stain well by the Gram method, they may be stained by a number of vital stains which are otherwise used for the purposes of complete blood counts – these include the stains of Wright, Romanowsky, and Giemsa among others. None of the latter are particularly superior to one or another. Alternatively, a wet film may also be of help in visualizing spirochetes. Spirochetemia is high (>1000/ml.) when the bacteria are seen via the aforementioned methods, and this usually correlates with an initial febrile episode or with a relapse. There does not appear to be a definitive correlation between quantitative spirochetemia and quality of disease, but it is unclear if the lack of such correlation is artifactual and methodology dependent (1). During the afebrile intervals, neither live nor inactivated bacteria may be detected, although there have been a few reports of circulating spirochetes during the afebrile phase (1). In addition to vital stains or direct mounts, acridine orange has been used to stain these bacteria in blood films; this technique is identical to that which is generally applied to the finding of bacteria in positive blood cultures. The diagnosis of relapsing fever is not often considered when patients are suffering from the initial episode. As relapses occur, the bacterial burden in blood progressively diminishes. For many, the consideration of relapsing fever will be a retrospective one, and direct bacterial detection by microscopy may be of little value. It is possible to use fluorescent-labeled antisera for direct detection, but the infrequency of illnesses and therefore the lack of sufficient experience (and likelihood therefore to maintain reagents) preclude the widespread availability of these.

Blood smears are the preferred specimens for direct examination. It is unlikely that invasive specimens are otherwise acquired, and spirochetes are not commonly seen in other more easily acquired body secretions.

It is possible for the disease to be accompanied by a meningitis that resembles aseptic meningitides of other causation; a lymphocytic predominance of leucocytes is detected in the cerebrospinal fluid.

2. Culture

Culture of relapsing fever borreliae requires special media, and due to the prolonged time which is required, liquid media are preferred. The original medium of Kelly contains buffers, peptones, albumin, gelatin, and 6% rabbit serum (68). The subsequent modification to Barbour-Stoenner-Kelly medium (BSK) was made (112), and a new variation, BSKII, is now commonly used. The latter utilizes tissue culture medium (CMRL-1066 with glutamine) as well as yeast hydrolysate in addition to gelatin, albumin, and rabbit serum (5). Bacteria are cultured at 33°C for 4-6 weeks, and the broth is inspected with a wet mount periodically; growth is variable, and may be apparent at any time after the first week. Subcultures can be maintained by subsequent passage to another BSKII or by freezing at –70°C. On a practical basis, however, it is uncommon to have BSKII readily available for bacterial culture when the diagnosis of relapsing fever is being considered, and therefore, a culture is uncommonly used for diagnostic purposes. Rather, culture is more likely to be used to obtain a strain for academic purposes. Liquid media are also used for the purposes of culturing spirochetes from the innards of ticks, again mainly during academic or experimental endeavours; both antibacterial and antifungal agents are usually needed in the medium. It is possible to maintain relapsing fever spirochetes in their tick hosts for a lengthy period of time, but this potential is of academic interest rather than of major diagnostic value.

Blood is the specimen of choice when culture is desirable; again, the favourable period is when fever and maximal spirochetemia are present. Apart from culturing the bacteria from ticks, they may also be found in animal blood. Laboratory animals may also be used as a primary culture mechanism. After inoculation of the animal with the suspect blood sample, the animal's peripheral blood can then be monitored for spirochetemia on an intermittent basis.

Repetitive subculture may be associated with changes in bacterial antigenic structure whether in vitro or in vivo, and such changes may be cumulative. The outer membrane proteins are most susceptible to such change.

Identification of the spirochete after successful culture will remain a challenge for most laboratories, but on practical grounds, the speciation may be extrapolated on the basis of the epidemiology, e.g., the likelihood for a given tick vector in a particular geographic region will give a high probability for the tick-specific *Borrelia* spp. to exist. Some regions may have overlapping domains for varied ticks, however, and a more precise speciation may be desirable; again, this is largely academic when the treatment courses of relapsing fevers caused by different *Borrelia* spp. are fairly similar to each other. In the current era, definitive speciation is best accomplished by partial sequencing of DNA that encodes the 16S rRNA gene. Species-specific monoclonal antibodies are not available for the entire diversity of borreliae, and they may be limited in determining new species or variants; nevertheless, some such reagents have been described (113).

3. Serology

Serology is of limited value in the diagnosis of relapsing fever and is mainly of some interest in circumstances where multiple relapses of illness continue or in retrospect when a cryptic illness is yet to be diagnosed. Serology is also somewhat hampered by the large number of different relapsing fever borreliae species. Cross-reactive epitopes may allow for the detection of illnesses using a single *Borrelia* species as an antigen in serology, but the ability to do so is inconsistent and not overly reliable.

The availability of serology is limited to a few reference centres, and serology generally makes use of the IFA format. Paired sera may be required for serological diagnosis. Cross-reactivity with Lyme disease borreliae must be considered in endemic areas for Lyme disease (96). The use of IFA on a historical basis for other bacterial serologies has been met with several problems, the most common of which is the interpretive standard for assessing positive fluorescence. Persistence of antibody after a previous infection must also be acknowledged in areas where relapsing fever is endemic.

Given the low frequency of relapsing fever and hence its diagnostic consideration, EIA or Western blots have not been used for diagnostic purposes. Furthermore, the variability in relapsing fever borreliae is likely to significantly complicate the interpretation of Western blot patterns. Schwan and others have defined an antigen which appears to be capable of differentiating responses to *B. burgdorferi* and relapsing fever spirochetes (114); conceivably such differentiation may have value in areas where both forms of borreliosis are of concern.

4. Genetic detection

Direct detection with first generation probes is more useful for speciation of bacterium in isolation. Detection by polymerase chain reaction has been detailed and is conceivably applicable to clinical samples with spirochetemia. On a practical basis, such determination, which will undoubtedly be limited in availability, may have little impact on the course of an illness. The treatment of relapsing fever is standard and is likely to be given at the time that a direct detection by microscopy is made.

B. Lyme disease

1. Microscopy

Microscopy is generally unrewarding when samples are acquired from acute illnesses. Although the bacterium may occasionally be recovered from blood by culture, high grade spirochetemia is not apparent, neither during the first or second stage of illness. When vital stains or silver stains are used, it is generally very difficult to visualize spirochetes in tissue. Silver stains (115) and direct fluorescence antibody stains have been used to detect borreliae in tissue with modest success. Despite active disease, the quantity of spirochetes is low, and only those who are most experienced with these techniques are likely to find the bacteria. Given the general problems with background artifact during silver staining, there is always the potential of making false-positive diagnoses.

2. Culture

Although blood samples are considerably less likely to yield viable spirochetes in Lyme disease than in relapsing fever illnesses (116), cultivation from blood and several other tissues may occasionally yield the bacterium. The most success is achieved with samples that are obtained during the first stage of Lyme disease and to a lesser extent the second stage. Yield is highest with biopsy samples of EM lesions, but even so, the frequency may barely reach 50% (117); these are best acquired from within the margins of spreading lesions. Samples such as cerebrospinal fluid, synovial fluid, splenic tissue, urine, and biopsies from endomyocardium, bone, tendon, and iris have also yielded Lyme disease borreliae (118). The cultivation of Lyme disease-causing spriochetes utilizes the same general conditions as those detailed for relapsing fever spirochetes, and BSKII medium or similar variations (119) has been favoured. Blood culture for spirochetes is approximately 3-4 times less sensitive than PCR detection of the same specimen (116).

Animal inoculation can be used for culture of the bacterium, but it is not generally required to the same extent as may be needed in relapsing fever.

Identification of *B. burgdorferi* can be accomplished with direct fluorescence antibody reagents, and such identification is likely to be highly specific in endemic areas where it is unlikely that other spirochetes exist. Otherwise, currently available 16S rRNA sequencing techniques are the most reliable methods for the identification of *B. burgdorferi*. Overall, reference laboratories are likely to be called on to assume such tasks.

3. Serology

Of all the diagnostic maneuvers, serology is by far the most practical and therefore the most widely available. Its use is, however, problematic due to the potential for false-positive and false-negative results. Antibody development after onset of disease is quite variable and is in general delayed in comparison to the response in other infections. The detection of antibody does not necessarily establish current active versus past infection. The use of antibiotics may delay or prevent antibody development altogether; many patients for whom there is a suspicion of disseminated infection will already have received some form of antibiotic therapy especially prior to having been referred to specialty clinics. Cross-reactivity with other spirochetes yields sufficient measurable antibody in some to cause false-positive assays (96). Nevertheless, it may be possible to use immunoblotting to enhance differentiation of cross-reactive serology between syphilis and Lyme disease; immune responses against low molecular antigens appear to be sufficiently distinct from each other in these two spirochetal diseases (120). In highly endemic areas, there may be a significant background positivity among a population perhaps with seroprevalences as high as 20-30% which then complicate the diagnostic decision-making when using serological results. In general, such problems lead to variability and hence inconsistency in standardization between laboratories (121). Concern about accuracy in this regard and its potential impact on appropriate health care has led some to organize proficiency testing programs for Lyme disease serology (122).

Antigenic variation is a real concern, and this is best exemplified by the divergence among what was initially believed to be *B. burgdorferi* in both Europe and North America. Clinical differences among patients with Lyme disease was inferred on the basis of the prominence of particular clinical manifestations of disease. The recognition of differences was then followed by the findings of antigenic variation among *B. burgdorferi* sensu lato from both continents. Ultimately, it was determined that there was sufficient difference in genotypes such that several genospecies were defined (as previously detailed), although mainly outside of North America (especially Europe). Among North American *B. burgdorferi* isolates, however, antigenic variation is also known to occur. Whereas much of the prominent antibody response may be directed to particular dominant outer surface proteins, variation in the expression of these or the absolute absence of some of them may lead to variable antibody responses.

Three main assays have been used for serodiagnosis: indirect immunofluorescence (IFA), enzyme immunoassay (EIA), and Western blotting (immunoblotting); hemagglutination has also been used to a lesser degree. IFA was already being used for relapsing fever serology at the time that *B. burgdorferi* was first cultivated, and therefore, there was a natural tendency to apply this method to another borrelia. Furthermore, the IFA technology had already been used and relatively standardized. EIA had the potential to be more standardized given the lack of need for a subjective observer, and it also is amenable to high volume testing and can be automated. As problems with specificity for both IFA and EIA became apparent during the 1980s, a "confirmatory" form of assay was desirable and immunoblotting emerged to potentially fill this role. The latter arose at a time when intensive research efforts were being employed to establish confirmatory assays for EIA and for other methods that were being used as the state-of-the-art in HIV diagnostics.

For IFA, there was some debate over what titre should be used as the break-point; 1:256 was initially proposed, but individual preference also often extended this interpretive breakpoint to the range of 1:128-1:512. It was clear that a titre acquired in one laboratory was not necessarily reproduced in another (123,124). This and other inconsistencies with IFA had been learned many times over in other bacterial diagnostics. Nevertheless, some believe that IgM-IFA is better than either EIA or immunoblotting for the diagnosis in early disease (125). The sensitivities for IFA and EIAs have been found to vary markedly (126): in early stages of Lyme disease as much as 8-62% and in late-staged disease as much as 62-86% (127).

For EIA (most assays initially indirect EIAs), different antigens may be used: whole cell lysates, partially purified antigens, or recombinant antigens (128). Given the number of different EIA approaches, let alone the varied sources and quality of reagents, it is not surprising that the results with these assays were not always comparable. Furthermore, the type of antigen used on different continents also poses potential problems. Some have determined that the use of any one of three genospecies (i.e., *B. burgdorferi* sensu stricto, *B. garinii*, or *B. afzelii*) yields generally equivalent EIA results (129,130), although there did exist some variation which could affect performance for some patients. It has been suggested that the use of *B. afzelii* as an antigen for EIA substrate in Europe may enhance the differentiation between those infected and uninfected controls (131).

Both IgM- and IgG- EIA have been designed to be used individually or in a complementary fashion. Cut-off values and grey-zone (indeterminate) intervals are difficult to establish. Early in the illness, the level of antibodies frequently is low or undetectable, yet low grade positivity may also be present in populations as a consequence of endemic seropositivity, cross-reactive antigens, or other less well understood reasons. As the threshold for positivity is lowered in order to gain sensitivity, there is an increase in non-specific and thus false-positive results; as the threshold is increased in order to eliminate false positives, sensitivity is compromised (132). Predictive values are then also affected by the frequency of the infection among the patient population so sampled. The problems in dealing with the latter issues in themselves might lead to considerable overdiagnosis. For example, in some populations, the majority of positive EIA may be associated with negative immunoblots (133). Whereas the initial need was for the development of a sensitive serological assay which could be used to diagnose a new disease, this was soon followed by a period where many false diagnoses were made purely by the misuse of IFA or EIA or even serology in general. A partial solution to this problem has been the use of immunoblotting as a confirmatory test. Immunoblots provide evidence that the perceived seroreactivity, as assessed by IFA or EIA, truly reflects antibody recognition of bacterial specific antigens.

Both IgM and IgG immunoblotting were designed by several groups and eventually commercialized (134). The immunoblot responses are considerably variable, but there are several antigens that are likely to be recognized by the majority of sera. IgG immunoblotting has then, at least in the U.S., been included within the proposed recognition patterns that are acceptable for confirmatory diagnosis. IgM should be assessed in early disease rather than late second or third stages when antibody may have declined; negative assays very early on may simply be a reflection of the delayed antibody response, and so negative assays in contexts of high suspicion should be followed by repeat specimens 3-6 weeks later. It is critical to recall that conventional immunoblotting is based on the resolution of bacterial antigens (hydrophilic mainly; especially polypeptides) by SDS-PAGE; the spectrum of what one perceives as an immune response is thus limited, and indeed varied hydrophobic antigens may also be recognized (135).

There is considerable controversy about the bands of identity as well as the number of them that should be required to indicate a specific response to *B. burgdorferi*. Steere and colleagues have recommended that a minimum of 2 of 8 common bands (to include among 18, 21, 28, 37, 41, 45, 58, and 93 kD) for IgM and 5 of 10 common bands (to include among 18, 21, 28, 30, 39, 41, 45, 58, 66, and 93 kD) for IgG be considered diagnostic. In Europe, the presence of three or more genomospecies has complicted recommendations for Western blot criteria. For example (136), when examining for IgM responses, it has been proposed that recognition bands should include at least one of 39 kD, OspC, 17 kD, or a strong 41 kD band for *B. afzelii* infection, and at least one band among 39 kD and OspC, or a strong 41 kD band for *B. garinii* infection. For IgG banding, at least two bands out of 14, 17, 21, OspC, 30, 39, 43, 58, and 83/100 kD are recommended for *B. afzelii* and at least one from 17b, 21, OspC, 30, 39, and 83/100 kD for *B. garinii*. It was concluded from this study that *B. afzelii* is probably the best substrate for immunoblotting in Europe (136). Others have suggested that all three genomospecies be used as antigens in immunoblotting (137). Among these antigens, whether for North America or European isolates, it has been determined that the 39 kD antigen is a relatively specific marker and is indeed distinct from the 41 kD (flagellar) antigen (138). The 18, 21, and 83 kD bands are also apparently highly specific for Lyme disease (139).

The acceptance of any two positive IgM bands for diagnosis in early Lyme disease has been proposed (140), but any such implementation must be carefully considered in its context. Among controls for either endemic or non-endemic areas, there may be a pre-existing and modest frequency of positive IgM immunoblot (or IgG) assessments (141). These responses are often directed to the 41 kD (flagellar) or heat-shock proteins (141). In fact, the specificity of a Western blot test alone may be lower than that of EIA (142,143). Therefore, the Western blot should not be used as a screening assay. Perhaps it is crucial to realize that criteria for positive Western blots may vary depending on whether one is dealing with early versus late stages of disease (144). In Europe, for the time being, it may be premature to be definitive about criteria for Western blots due to the reasons discussed previously.

Overall, then, a prudent strategy, at least in America, would be to use either IFA or EIA as a screening or first-step method; positive or borderline positive assays would then be followed by an immunoblot. This approach is analogous to the use of screening and confirmatory serology which is currently advocated for the diagnosis of syphilis, HIV infection, and hepatitis C infection. There is a good argument, however, against the labelling of the immunoblot as a "confirmatory" assay because of the aforementioned issues. Rather, it has been recommended that it be termed a "supplementary" assay in a two-staged process (134). Soon after a large number of commercial serological assays were being marketed, Magnarelli proposed that serological diagnosis in general should be emphasized as a secondary and supportive tool, but that clinical diagnosis should remain paramount (145). A full decade later, and despite much progress in the field, others continue to stress that serology is but an adjunct to clinical diagnosis (146). It is conceivable that the application of serology will continue to be problematic. The diagnosis of EM does not usually require serology, but most of the problems in the establishment of diagnoses are those among patients with non-classical manifestations.

Central nervous system infection may be confirmed by the comparison of CSF to serum antibody quantitation, i.e., "Antibody Index" (147). This is perhaps better achieved with an EIA method for which quantitative readings can be obtained. There are also commercial kits using capture assay by which the result of intrathecal production of antibodies can be readily seen from a positive index. Care must be taken to ensure that the CSF which is submitted for testing is not significantly tainted with blood during the acquisition since the measure may therefore largely reflect serum antibody. Both IgG and IgM are produced intrathecally; the IgG may be detected, despite clinical cure, for a considerable period of time after the treatment (148). Antibody may become detectable as late as 6-8 weeks after the onset of neurological symptoms (149). Serum IgG and IgM titres tend to be relatively high in patients with neuroborreliosis and may take many months and years respectively to return to a non-detectable level (150). A positive assay therefore does not imply active disease. Intrathecal antibody production is commonly observed even for those who suffer from facial nerve palsy (36) although this may be less common among children (151). Although a positive assay for intrathecal antibody is helpful in assessing neuroborreliosis, it must be accepted that a negative assessment does not absolutely rule out such an illness. Oligoclonal banding of CSF protein is also a predictive marker for neuroborreliosis (147).

Despite the aforementioned difficulties with serology, it is estimated that up to 30-40% of patients will have positive serology when the disease is early and manifest simply as EM. When followed for another 2-4 weeks, this frequency may increase to 50-75%. Given the variation among methodologies, even when of the same format, it is prudent to have follow-up serology performed by the same laboratory which is assessing the sample with the same methodology (152). The persistence of a positive level of antibodies after treatment is common but highly variable (153).

The advent of OspA vaccination for individuals of high risk for disease acquisition poses some problems for serodiagnosis (109). In highly endemic areas, there are vaccinated individuals who have a high probability of being assessed sometime later for infection whether for primary or re-infection. The whole cell lysates or partially purified antigens (e.g., outer membrane proteins) generally contain OspA, and thus seroreactivity will not be able to differentiate vaccination from infection. Immunoblotting will be of value here in further differentiation, but it may pose some problems when OspA itself is one of the few antigens that are being recognized. Antigens from OspA-negative mutants may serve to eliminate this concern (154). Given that the vaccine is not fully protective, however, it is quite likely that other more complex vaccines will be used (110), and again, this diagnostic dilemma will be confronted.

Seronegative Lyme disease is a subject of considerable controversy (106) as previously indicated.

4.   Genetic detection

Varied PCR methods have been detailed for the direct detection of Lyme disease borreliae from clinical specimens. Readers are directed to the recent and extensive review as published by Schmidt (155). Genetic amplification has been applied to the detection of Lyme spirochetes from humans, animals, and even tick reservoirs (in lieu of culture).

The targets for amplification have been variable and have included sequences within the OspA gene, OspB gene, other genes on the linear plasmids, "clone 2H1", Lyl gene, flagellin gene, 16S/23S rRNA gene, and the *hbb* (histone) gene. For some of these, numerous target variants on the same gene have been assessed. Both standard and nested PCR procedures have been examined (156), and although the latter may seem more sensitive on the basis of in vitro data, in fact both approaches have given comparable yields from various clinical samples. There have been many variations on the theme of sample processing, e.g., extraction of DNA. Fresh samples of fluid and tissue are preferred, although positive results can be obtained, however with a low frequency, from formalin-fixed paraffin-embedded material. The PCR product has been detected directly through visualization on ethidium bromide-stained agarose gels or through hybridization techniques with ^{32}P-label, digoxigenin label, or chemiluminescent label. As for other bacterial amplifications and with similar specimens, inhibitors can be anticipated. Such a cause for false-negative assays should be controlled for with eukaryotic gene amplifications (of host cell within the specimen) or with bacterium controls. Controls for inhibition are somewhat more difficult to achieve for solid tissue such as skin biopsies. It is surprising that fluids as apparently simple as CSF may contain a high frequency of inhibitors. Non-specific amplification products are not uncommon due to the high eukaryotic DNA load in several of the clinical samples.

With the use of nucleic acid detection methods, there are fundamental problems which must be considered. Firstly, in clinical samples, the number of bacteria (and hence DNA copies) is often low. The spirochetes are expected to be in higher amounts in skin biopsy specimens or even blood samples during EM or during early dissemination, however, in contrast to later phases of the infection. Discordance is common between pioneering development in the laboratory and the clinical application of the technique. The definition of a gold standard for comparison is problematic because culture is of low yield. The use of a second (or more) alternate and independent genetic amplification may serve to overcome the latter. Nevertheless, direct comparisons of independent PCR assays are limited. Given the differences among isolates of *B. burgdorferi* sensu lato in Europe, concern has been expressed about the applicability of some targets to all genomospecies (156); this concern seems founded for OspA-PCR.

Bacterium has been detected particularly in skin, blood, joint fluid, and cerebrospinal fluid; urine has also been used as an indirect indicator with some success. For biopsy specimens take from EM lesions, PCR may be more sensitive than either culture or serology (157-159), although for culture, some researchers have proposed equivalency when superior culture media are used (119). Patients with EM have also been found to have positive results with PCR in urine (159), breast milk (160), and plasma specimens. Analysis of skin biopsy specimens with PCR may also be rewarding when assessing patients with acrodermatitis chronica atrophicans. In neuroborreliosis, PCR may be positive in patients with meningitis, cranial nerve palsies, polyneuritis, meningoencephalitis, and encephalopathy. Among the neurological illnesses, PCR is more often positive in the second stage than in the third stage (161). PCR diagnostics, however, are much less likely to be positive among children with neuroborreliosis, especially those with facial palsy (162,163). The differences may reflect technical difficulties, however, rather than true differences in the pathophysiology of the infection. Although it is uncommon to have culture-positive joint fluids in Lyme arthritis, a reasonable number have been PCR-positive (164). In general, the frequencies of PCR-positives either equal to or exceed those of culture for various specimens. Blood samples have served as a surrogate for other more difficult samples although consistency of results is a problem. The frequencies for detection of borreliae with PCR, however, have been somewhat inconsistent in different studies, and it is evident that it cannot be expected that genetic detection will replace all other methods. The major limitation with the use of PCR in the diagnostics of Lyme borreliosis is the minimal and transient occurrence of borrelial DNA in clinical specimens. The capture of sufficient DNA in the small aliquot of sample that is used for PCR may be difficult (165).

There may be an inverse correlation of serology and PCR positivity (166). Whether this is a reflection of the acquisition of more intense infection by hosts that cannot respond sufficiently due to their humoral immune system, or of the binding of antibodies to immune complexes in patients with high spirochetal burden, or some other factors, is largely unknown. PCR has been considered as the sole method for test of cure after appropriate antibiotics. In particular, long term positive detection by PCR may correlate with treatment failure and associated relapse (167).

Problems that are faced with serology include the delay in seroconversion, frequent slow evolution of the humoral immune response thus resulting in low levels of seropositivity or even seronegativity, immunoblot patterns that are inconclusive, and background seropositivity in the population. The major problem with culture is low yield. Genetic amplification methods, e.g., PCR, may be an adjunct to these, but will not replace them. Nevertheless, there are circumstances when tissue samples are not available, when the amount of bacterium is insufficient even for genetic amplification, and when the disease has already been partially or fully treated. The application of PCR must be considered carefully in a given context and with the detailed knowledge of clinical stage and serodiagnostic results. A negative result with PCR never can exclude Lyme borreliosis. Apart from the availability of PCR in several centres within endemic areas, the techniques are likely to be left to reference centres in large part due to the high standards that are required for laboratory hygiene and due to the other expertise that is required with the technique.

VII. SUSCEPTIBILITY TESTING

Borrelioses are in large part highly responsive to antibiotic therapy. Although both relapsing fever and Lyme disease may resolve without any form of antimicrobial intervention, antibiotics, given at the earliest opportunity, may interrupt the course of an illness.

In relapsing fever, early antibiotic therapy will terminate the cyclic febrile pattern. As for borrelioses and other spirochetoses in general, however, caution with even appropriate therapy is warranted since an immediate reaction to antibiotics with hypotension, chills, and potentially shock may follow the lysis of circulating spirochetes (Jarisch-Herxheimer reaction) (1). An appropriate use of antibiotics is rarely followed by relapse, and chronic illnesses are unlikely. Acute mortality with relapsing fever is uncommon but nevertheless possible; this has been recorded much more often with louse-borne relapsing fever than with the tick-borne illnesses. It had been recognized well before antimicrobial susceptibility testing was available for these bacteria that tetracyclines, penicillins, chloramphenicol, and erythromycin were active in clinical illnesses. This experience correlates with relatively exquisite susceptibility in vitro (168). At this time, the development of resistance is highly unlikely given the infrequency of human disease and hence its treatment, and the lack of antibiotic use for animal vectors in the wild. Perhaps the potential for such resistance to emerge might be greatest for *B. recurrentis* since humans appear to be the reservoir; this has not been documented. It must be emphasized that many relapsing fevers are not specifically diagnosed and thus are often untreated intentionally with antibiotics.

In contrast to the above, Lyme disease may be relatively over-diagnosed and over-treated (10-14) depending on geographical location given the variations in endemicity or non-endemicity, and also depending on public awareness of the disease and its manifestations. It is probable that marked differences between continents and different countries in both public awareness and treatment policies occur. Lyme borreliosis is also much more likely to leave a residual subacute or chronic illness if not treated or if only partially treated. Given the vast numbers of infections that have been treated or are likely to be treated in the future, and the need for relatively long courses of antibiotics, one might conjecture that the potential for antimicrobial resistance is significantly greater for Lyme disease than for relapsing fever borreliae. While the resistance to antibiotics is seemingly possible, it is somewhat unlikely since the source for most Lyme borreliosis in the wild is the continuing cycle in nature rather than the human who has been exposed to an antibiotic. In vitro, *B. burgdorferi* is susceptible to penicillins, tetracyclines, erythromycin, and extended spectrum cephalosporins, but resistant to sulphonamides, aminoglycosides, rifampin, and quinolones. The antibiotic resistance phenotypes have not been well-studied for molecular mechanisms of resistance, but knowledge of resistance is of value in creating selective media especially for the isolation of spirochetes from sources in nature, e.g., ticks. Despite this rudimentary in vitro data, however, the therapy of Lyme disease is complicated in large part due to the variety of clinical manifestations and due to the diverse body sites where the spirochetes may reside and indeed sequester (169). Lyme disease in its early stages is susceptible to various antibiotics that have now had evident success through clinical experience. For example, both first and second stage disease will often respond to amoxicillin, doxycycline, erythromycin, and extended spectrum oral cephalosporins. Although treatment for 10 days may generally be successful for early disease, most authorities recommend treatment for 14 days and some for even 21 days. Treatment regimens will be prolonged when more invasive disease is apparent or when a chronic illness occurs. As well, chronic and invasive illnesses may warrant the use of intravenous rather than oral antibiotics. For example, neurological manifestations and arthritis with an advanced or chronic course may be treated with intravenous penicillin, ceftriaxone, or cefotaxime. For disseminated disease, most authorities recommend a therapy for 2-4 weeks either with intravenous or oral regimens depending on the clinical manifestations. Some prefer to use intravenous therapy for all disseminated manifestations and thereafter occasionally follow this with oral therapy for a few of months. It should be stated that, at least thus far, there is no convincing evidence showing that long-term treatment necessarily prevents treatment failures. In many ways, again, the treatment requisites mirror those for syphilis in that standard forms of therapy may be sufficient with primary disease, but the more deep-seated and invasive forms of infection often require prolonged and intensive therapy. In Lyme disease, the Jarisch-Herxheimer reactions, when present, are usually milder than are seen among relapsing fever patients; they may also develop later, be prolonged for several days, and be difficult to distinguish from allergic reactions (179).

Since culture of different types of specimens has poor sensitivity and since antibodies may remain detectable or even high for a long period of time, a possible laboratory test of cure rests with PCR. The use of PCR for monitoring treatment efficacy continues to be studied, but it must be recognized that PCR-positivity may continue for a variable time after appropriate therapy since the assay does not distinguish between viable and dead spirochete.

In vitro susceptibility testing methods are obviously complicated by the unusual growth requirements of borreliae. One may generalize for all borreliae that agar-based susceptibility testing methods are not feasible. Slow growth of these bacteria along with their particular nutritional requirements complicates such assessment. Broth dilution techniques are favoured (170-172), but the interpretation is complicated by the prolonged culture times (173). The assessment of broth dilution end-points may be accomplished by subculturing the broth dilutions. A microtitre format has been studied (174). Alternate proposals for assessment have been made (175), but it is acknowledged at this time that there is a need for a uniform approach in order to ensure that data from different studies are comparable (176). It must also be acknowledged that in vivo susceptibility, or for that matter resistance, may have very little to do with the modification of treatment regimens. For example, penicillin activity in vitro is relatively unimpressive when compared to other antibiotics, but yet penicillin is quite active in vivo (176). The minimum inhibitory concentrations are generally the same as the minimum bactericidal concentrations even for antibiotics (e.g., azithromycin and doxycycline) which are considered bacteriostatic for other bacteria (174).

Two major problems remain: a) penetration of an antibiotic that should be effective, and to which the bacterium is susceptible, to the site of infection that may be relatively secluded (177) and may thus require a high dosage and/or a long course of the antibiotic, and b) the treatment of an illness that is wrongly diagnosed as Lyme disease and draws considerable concern and/or anxiety due to its chronic nature and gives the patient an irrelevant hope of permanent cure (10-14). Accurate diagnosis therefore is at this time much more impactful than the need for susceptibility testing. As well, for any given patient, it is uncommon for the diagnosis to be established by bacterial isolation, and hence to have the isolate available for susceptibility testing.

Several treatment dilemmae continue to provide concern for physicians: the possible use of prophylaxis after tick exposure, definition of the best agents, length of therapy, and route of antibiotic administration (178).

REFERENCES

1. Bryceson ADM, Parry EHO, Perine PL, Warrell DA, Vukotich D, Leithead CS. Louse-borne relapsing fever: a clinical and laboratory study of 62 cases in Ethiopia and a reconsideration of the literature. Q J Med 1970; 39:129-170.
2. Matuschka FR, Ohlenbusch A, Eiffert H, Richter D, Spielman A. Characteristics of Lyme disease spirochetes in archived European ticks. J Infect Dis 1996; 174:424-426.
3. Brown V, Larouze B, Desve G, Rousset JJ, Thibon M, Fourrier A, Schwoebel V. Clinical presentation of louse-borne relapsing fever among Ethiopian refugees in northern Somalia. Ann Trop Med Parasitol 1988; 82:499-502.
4. Burgdorfer W, Barbour AG, Hayes SF, Benach JL, Grunwaldt E, Davis JP. Lyme disease – a tick borne spirochetosis? Science 1982; 216:1317-1319.
5. Steere AC, Grodzicki RL, Kornblatt AN, Craft JE, Barbour AG, Burgdorfer W, Schmid GP, Johnson E, Malawista SE. The spirochetal etiology of Lyme disease. N Engl J Med 1983; 308:733-740.

6. Berger BW, Clemmensen OJ, Gottlieb GJ. Spirochetes in lesions of erythema chronicum migrans. Am J Dermatopathol 1982; 4:4:556.

7. Thyresson N. The penicillin treatment of acrodermatitis atrophicans chronica (Herxheimer). Acta Derm Venereol 1949; 29:572-621.

8. Asbrink E, Brehmer-Andersson E, Hovmark A. Acrodermatitis chronica atrophicans – a spirochetosis. Am J Dermatopathol 1986; 8:209-219.

9. Bannwarth A. Zur klinik und pathogenese der "chronischen lymphocytaren meningitis". Arch Psychiatr Nervenkr 1944; 117:161-185.

10. Steere AC, Taylor E, McHugh GL, Logigian EL. The overdiagnosis of Lyme disease. JAMA 1993; 269:1812-1816.

11. Rose CD, Fawcett PT, Gibney KM, Doughty RA. The overdiagnosis of Lyme disease in children residing in an endemic area. Clin Pediatr 1994; 33:663-668.

12. Sigal LH. The Lyme disease controversy. Social and financial costs of misdiagnosis and mismanagement. Arch Intern Med 1996; 156:1493-1500.

13. Svenungsson B, Lindh G. Lyme borreliosis – an overdiagnosed disease? Infection 1997; 25:140-143.

14. Reid MC, Schoen RT, Evans J, Rosenberg JC, Horwitz RI. The consequences of overdiagnosis and overtreatment of Lyme disease: an observational study. Ann Intern Med 1998; 128:354-362.

15. Cadavid D, Barbour AG. Neuroborreliosis during relapsing fever: review of the clinical manifestations, pathology, and treatment of infections of humans and experimental animals. Clin Infect Dis 1998; 26:151-164.

16. Nadelman RB, Wormser GP. Lyme borreliosis. Lancet 1998; 352:557-565.

17. Cooke WD, Dattwyler RJ. Complications of Lyme borreliosis. Ann Rev Med 1992; 43:93-103.

18. Halperin JJ. Neuroborreliosis. Am J Med 1995; 98:S52-S56.

19. Steere AC. Lyme disease. N Engl J Med 1989; 321:586-596.

20. Weber K, Burgdorfer W. Therapy of tick bite. In: Weber K, Burgdorfer W, eds. Aspects of Lyme Borreliosis. Berlin:Springer-Verlag, 1993:350-351.

21. Nadelman RB, Wormser GP. Erythema migrans and early Lyme disease. Am J Med 1995; 98:S15-S23.

22. Oksi J, Helander I, Ahho H, Marjamaki M, Viljanen MK. *Borrelia burgdorferi* shown by PCR from skin biopsy specimen after a fly bite. In: Axford JS, Rees DHE, eds. Lyme Borreliosis. New York:Plenum Press, 1994:45-48.

23. Nadelman RB, Novakowski J, Forester G, Goldberg NS, Bittker S, Cooper D, Aguero-Rosenfeld M. The clinical spectrum of early Lyme borreliosis in patients with culture-confirmed erythema migrans. Am J Med 1996; 100:502-508.

24. Smith RP, Schoen RT, Parenti DL, Rahn DW, Holman MS, Steere AC. Clinical characteristics of 120 microbiologically confirmed cases of early Lyme disease. VIII International Conference of Lyme Borreliosis and Other Emerging Tick-Borne Diseases. Munich, Germany, 1999:18.

25. Asbrink E, Hovmark A. Lyme borreliosis: aspects of tick-borne *Borrelia burgdorferi* infection from a dermatologic viewpoint. Semin Dermatol 1990; 9:277-291.

26. Kuiper H, van Dam AP, Spanjaard L, Dejogh BM, Widjojokusumo A, Ramselaar TCP, Cairo I, Vos K, Dankert J. Isoaltion of *Borrelia burgdorferi* from biopsy specimens taken from healthy-looking skin of patients with Lyme borrelioisis. J Clin Microbiol 1994; 32:715-720.

27. Garcia-Monco JC, Benach JL. Lyme neuroborreliosis. Ann Neurol 1995; 37:691-702.

28. Haass A. Lyme neuroborreliosis. Curr Opin Neurol 1998; 11:253-258.

29. Garcia-Monco JC, Fernendez-Villar B, Alen JC, Benach JL. Borrelia burgdorferi in the central nervous system: experimental and clinical evidence for early invasion. J Infect Dis 1990; 161:1187-1193.

30. Pachner AR. Early disseminated Lyme Disease: Lyme meningitis. Am J Med 1995; 98:S30-S37.

31. Halperin JJ. Neuroborreliosis: central nervous system involvement. Semin Neurol 1997; 17:19-24.

32. Oksi J, Kalimo H, Marttila RJ, Marjamaki M, Sonninen P, Nikoskelainen J, Viljanen MK. Inflammatory brain changes in Lyme borreliosis. A report on three patients an dreview of literature. Brain 1996; 119:2143-2154.

33. Oksi J, Kalimo H, Marttila RJ, marjamaki M, Sonninen P, Nikoskelainen J, Viljanen MK. Intracranial aneuryms in three patients with disseminated Lyme borreliosis: cause or chance association? J Neurol Neurosurg Psych 1998; 64:636-642.

34. Garin C, Bujadoux C. Paralysie par les tiques. J Med Lyon 1922; 71:765-767.

35. Bannwarth A. chronische lymphocytare meningitis, entzundliche polyneuritis und "rheumatismus". Beitrag zum problem "Allergi und nervensystem". Arch Psychiatr Nervenkr 1941; 113:284-376.

36. Smouha EE, Coyle PK, Shukri S. Facial nerve palsy in Lyme disease: evaluation of clinical diagnostic criteria. Am J Otol 1997; 18:257-261.

37. Oksi J, Marjamaki M, Koski K, Nikosalainen J, Viljanen MK. Bilateral facial palsy and meningitis caused by borrelia double infection. Lancet 1995; 345:1583-1584.
38. Ackermann R, Hortrup P, Schmidt R. Tick-borne meningopolyneuritis (Grain-Bujadoux, Bannwarth). Yale J Biol Med 1984; 57:485-490.
39. Logigian EL. Peripheral nervous system Lyme borreliosis. Semin Neurol 1997; 17:25-30.
40. Camponovo F, Meier C. Neuropathy of vasculitic origin in a case of Garin-Bujadoux-Bannwarth syndrome with positive borrelia antibody response. J Neurol 1986; 233:69-72.
41. Garcia-Monco JC, Benach JL. Lyme neuroborreliosis. Ann Neurol 1995; 37:691-702.
42. Halperin JJ, Luft BJ, Anand AK, Roque CT, Alvarez O, Volkman DJ, Dattwyler RJ. Lyme neuroborreliosis: central nervous sytem manifestations. Neurology 1989; 39:753-759.
43. Logigian EL, Kaplan RF, Steere AC. Successful treatment of Lyme encephalopathy with intravenous ceftriaxone. J Infect Dis 1999; 180:377-383.
44. Balcer LJ, Winterkorn JM, Galetta SL. Neuro-ophthalmic manifestations of Lyme disease. J Neuroophthalmol 1997; 17:108-121.
45. Karma A, Seppala I, Mikkila H, Kaakkola S, Viljanen M, Tarkkanen A. Diagnosis and clinical characteristics of ocular Lyme borreliosis. Am J Ophthalmol 1995; 119:127-135.
46. Sigal LH. Musculoskeletal manifestations of Lyme arthritis. Rheum Dis Clin North Am 1998; 24:323-351.
47. Nagi KS, Joshi R, Thakur RK. Cardiac manifestations of Lyme disease: a review. Can J Cardiol 1996; 12:503-506.
48. Stanek G, Klein J, Bittner R, Glogar D. Isolation of *Borrelia burgdorferi* from the myocardium of a patient with longstanding cardiomyopathy. N Engl J med 1990; 322:249-252.
49. Oksi J, Voipio-Pulkki LM, Uksila J, Pulkki K, Laippala P, Viljainen MK. *Borrelia burgdorferi* infection in patients with suspected acute myocardial infarction. Lancet 1997; 350:1447-1448.
50. Asbrink E. Cutaneous manfestations of Lyme borreliosis. Clinical definitions and differential diagnoses. Scand J Infect Dis 1991; 77:S44-S50.
51. Berger BW. Dermatologic manifestations of Lyme disease. Rev Infect Dis 1989; 11(Suppl. 6):S1475-S1481.
52. Prose NS, Abson KG, Berg D. Lyme disease in children: diagnosis, treatment , and prevention. Semin Dermatol 1992; 11:31-36.
53. Filipuzzi-Jenny E, Blot M, Schmid-Berger N, Meister-Turner J, Meyer J. Genetic diversity among *Borrelia burgdorferi* isolates: more than three genospecies? Res Microbiol 1993; 144:295-304.
54. Schwan TG. Ticks and *Borrelia*: model systems for investigating pathogen-arthropod interactions. Infect Agents Dis 1996; 5:167-181.
55. Trejevo RT, Schriefer ME, Gage KL, Safranek TJ, Orloski KA, Pape WJ, Montenieri JA, Campbell GL. An interstate outbreak of tick-borne relapsing fever among vacationers at a Rocky Mountain cabin. Am J Trop Med Hyg 1998; 58:743-747.
56. Marti Ras N, Postic D, Foretz M, Baranton G. *Borrelia burgdorferi* sensu stricto, a bacterial species "made in the USA"? Int J Syst Bacteriol 1997; 47:1112-1117.
57. Wang G, van Dam AP, Le Fleche A, Postic D, Peter O, Baranton G, de Boer R, Spanjaard L, Dankert J. Genetic and phenotypic analysis of *Borrelia valaisiana* sp. nov. (*Borrelia* genomic groups VS116 and M19). Int J Syst Bacteriol 1997; 47:926-932.
58. Wang G, van Dam AP, Spanjaard L, Dankert J. Molecular typing of *Borrelia burgdorferi* sensu lato by randomly amplified polymorphic DNA fingerprinting analysis. J Clin Microbiol 1998; 36:768-776.
59. Hulinska D, Votypka J, Valesova M. Persistence of *Borrelia garinii* and *Borrelia afzelii* in patients with Lyme arthritis. Zentralbl Bakteriol 1999; 289:301-318.
60. Demaerschalck I, Ben Massaoud A, De Kesel M, Hoyois B, Lobet Y, Hoet P, Bigaignon G, Bollen A, Godfroid E. Simultaneous presence of different *Borrelia burgdorferi* genospecies in biological fluids of Lyme disease patients. J Clin Microbiol 1995; 33:602-608.
61. Gustafson R. Epidemiological studies of Lyme borrelioses and tick-borne encephalitis. Scand J Infect Dis 1994; 92:S1-S63.
62. Junttila J, Peltomaa M, Soini H, Marjamaki M, Viljanen MK. Prevalence of *Borrelia burgdorferi* in *Ixodes ricinus* ticks in urban recreational areas of Helsinki. J Clin Microbiol 1999; 37:1361-1365.
63. Kirstein F, Rijpkema S, Molkenboer M, Gray JS. Local variations in the distribution and prevalence of *Borrelia burgdorferi* sensu lato genomospecies in *Ixodes ricinus* ticks. Appl Environ Micro 1997; 63:1102-1106.
64. Steere AC. Lyme disease: a growing threat to urban populations. Proc Natl Acad Sci USA 1994; 91:2378-2383.
65. Piesman J. Dispersal of the Lyme disease spirochete *Borrelia burgdorferi* to salivary glands of feeding nymphal *Ixodes scapularis* (*Acari*: *Ixodidae*) J Med Entomol 1995; 32:519-521.

66. Olsen B, Jaenson TG, Bergstrom S. Prevalence of *Borrelia burgdorferi* sensu lato-infected ticks on migrating birds. Appl Environ Microbiol 1995; 61:3082-3087.

67. Cutler SJ, Moss J, Fukanaga M, Wright DJ, Fekade D, Warrell D. *Borrelia recurrentis* characterization and comparison with relapsing fever, Lyme-associated, and other *Borrelia* spp. Int J Syst Bacteriol 1997; 47:958-968.

68. Kelly R. Cultivation of *Borrelia hermsii*. Science 1971; 173:443-444.

69. Restrepo BI, Barbour AG. Antigen diversity in the bacterium *B. hermsii* through "somatic" mutations in rearranged vmp genes. Cell 1994; 78:867-876.

70. Charon NW, Greenberg EP, Koopman MB, Limberger RJ. Spirochete chemotaxis, motility, and the structure of the spirochetal periplasmic flagella. Res Microbiol 1992; 143:597-603.

71. Fraser CM, Casjens S, Huang WM, Sutton GG, Clayton R, Lathigra R, White O, Ketchum KA, Dodson R, Hickey EK, Gwinn M, Dougherty B, Tomb TF, Fleischmann RD, Richardson D, Peterson J, Kerlavage AR, Quackenbush J, Salzberg S, Hanson M, van Vugt, Palmer N, Adams MD, Gocayne J, Weidman J, Utterback T, Watthey L, McDonald L, Artiach P, Bowman C, Garland S, Fujii C, Cotton MD, Horst K, Roberts K, Hatch B, Smith HO, Venter JC. Genomic sequence of a Lyme disease spirochaete, *Borrelia burgdorferi*. Nature 1997; 390:580-586.

72. Samuels DS, Marconi RT, Garon CF. Variation in the size of the OspA-containing linear plasmid, but not the linear chromosome, among the three *Borrelia* species associated with Lyme disease. J Gen Microbiol 1993; 139:2445-2449.

73. Pennington PM, Cadavid D, Barbour AG. Characterization of VspB of *Borrelia turicatae*, a major outer membrane protein expressed in blood and tissues of mice. Infect Immun 1999; 67:4637-4645.

74. Hinnebusch BJ, Barbour AG, Restrepo BI, Schwan TG. Population structure of the relapsing fever spirochete *Borrelia hermsii* as indicated by polymorphism of two multigene families that encode immunogenic outer surface lipoproteins. Infect Immun 1998; 66:432-440.

75. Schwan TG, Hinnebusch BJ. Bloodstream- versus tick-associated variants of a relapsing fever bacterium. Science 1998; 280:1938-1940.

76. Warrell DA, Perine PL, Krause DW, Bing DH, MacDougal SJ. Pathophysiology and immunology of the Jarisch-Herxheimer-like reaction in louse-borne relapsing fever: comparison of tetracycline and slow-release penicillin. J Infect Dis 1983; 147:898-909.

77. Vidal V, Scragg IG, Cutler SJ, Rockett KA, Fekade D, Warrell DA, Wright DJ, Kwiatkowski D. Variable major lipoprotein is a principal TNF-inducing factor of louse-borne relapsing fever. Nature Med 1998; 4:1416-1420.

78. Cuevas LE, Borgnolo G, Hailu B, Smith G, Almaviva M, Hart CA. Tumour necrosis factor, interleukin-6 and C-reactive protein in patients with louse-borne relapsing fever in Ethiopia. Ann Trop Med Parasitol 1995; 89:49-54.

79. Butler T, Aikawa M, Habte-Michael A, Wallace C. Phagocytosis of *Borrelia recurrentis* by blood polymorphonuclear leukocytes is enhanced by antibiotic treatment. Infect Immun 1980; 28:1009-1013.

80. Belfaiza J, Postic D, Bellenger E, Baranton G, Girons IS. Genomic fingerprinting of *Borrelia burgdorferi* sensu lato by pulsed-field gel electrophoresis. J Clin Microbiol 1993; 31:2873-2877.

81. Will G, Jauris-Heipke S, Schwab E, Busch U, Rossler D, Soutschek E, Wilske B, Preac-Mursic V. Sequence analysis of OspA genes shows homogeneity within *Borrelia burgdorferi* sensu stricto and *Borrelia afzelii* strains but reveals major subgroups within *Borrelia garinii* species. Med Microbiol Immunol 1995; 184:73-80.

82. Wang G, van Dam AP, Dankert J. Phenotypic and genetic characterization of a novel *Borrelia burgdorferi* sensu lato isolate from a patient with Lyme borreliosis. J Clin Microbiol 1999; 37:3025-3028.

83. Busch U, Will G, Hizo-Teufel C, Wilske B, Preac-Mursic V. Long-term in vitro cultivation of *Borrelia burgdorferi* sensu lato strains: influence on plasmid patterns, genome stability and expression of proteins. Res Microbiol 1997; 148:109-118.

84. Wilske B, Barbour AG, Bergstrom S, Burman N, Restrepo BI, Rosa PA, Schwan T, Soutschek E, Wallich R. Antigenic variation and strain heterogeneity in *Borrelia* spp. Res Microbiol 1992; 143:583-596.

85. Zhang JR, Hardham JM, Barbour AG, Norris SJ. Antigenic variation of Lyme disease borreliae by promiscuous recombination of VMP-like sequence cassettes. Cell 1997; 89:275-285.

86. Stevenson B, Casjens S, Rosa P. Evidence of past recombination events among the genes encoding the *Erp* antigens of *Borrelia burgdorferi*. Microbiology 1998; 144:1869-1879.

87. Seinost G, Dykhuizen DE, Dattwyler RJ, Golde WT, Dunn JJ, Wang IN, Wormser GP, Schriefer ME, Luft BJ. Four clones of *Borrelia burgdorferi* sensu stricto cause invasive infection in humans. Infect Immun 1999; 67:3518-3524.

88. Garcia-Monco JC, Benach JL. Mechanisms of injury in Lyme neuroborreliosis. Semin Neurol 1997; 17:57-62.

89. Pohl-Koppe A, Wilske B, Weiss M, Schmidt H. *Borrelia* lymphocytoma in childhood. Pediatr Infect Dis 1998; 17:423-426.
90. Sigal LH. Immunologic mechanisms in Lyme neuroborreliosis: the potential role of autoimmunity and molecular mimicry. Semin Neurol 1997; 17:63-68.
91. Ma Y, Sturrock A, Weis JJ. Intracellular localization of *Borrelia burgdorferi* within human endothelial cells. Infect Immun 1991; 59:671-678.
92. Montgomery RR, Nathanson MH, Malawista SE. The fate of *Borrelia burgdorferi*, the agent for Lyme disease, in mouse macrophages: destruction, survival, recovery. J Immunol 1993; 150:909-915.
93. Girschick HJ, Huppertz HI, Russmann H, Krenn V, Karch H. Intracellular persistence of *Borrelia burgdorferi* in human synovial cells. Rheumatol Int 1996; 125-132.
94. Oksi J, savolainen J, Pene J, Bousquet J, Laippala P, Viljanen MK. Decreased interleukin-4 and increased gamma inerferon production by peripheral blood mononuclear cells of patients with Lyme borreliosis. Infect Immun 1996; 64:3620-3623.
95. Aberer E, Koszik F, Silberer M. Why is chronic Lyme borreliosis chronic? Clin Infect Dis 1997; 25:S64-S70.
96. Magnarelli LA, Anderson JF, Johnson RC. Cross-reactivity in serological tests for Lyme disease and other spirochetal infections. J Infect Dis 1987; 156:183-187.
97. Dodge RW. Human serological response to louse-borne relapsing fever. Infect Immun 1973; 8:891-895.
98. Spagnuolo PJ, Butler T, Bloch EH, Santoro C, Tracy JW, Johnson RC. Opsonic requirements for phagocytosis of *Borrelia hermsii* by human polymorphonuclear leukocytes. J Infect Dis 1982; 145:358-364.
99. Callister SM, Jobe DA, Schell RF, Pavia CS, Lovrich SD. Sensitivity and specificity of the borreliacidal-antibody test during early Lyme disease: a "gold standard"? Clin Diagn Lab Immunol 1996; 3:399-402.
100. Gilmore RD, Murphee RL, James AM, Sullivan SA, Johnson BJ. The *Borrelia burgdorferi* 37-kilodalton immunoblot band (P37) used in serodiagnosis of early Lyme disease is the *flaA* gene product. J Clin Microbiol 1999; 37:548-552.
101. Cinco M, Trevisan G, Agolzer A. Isolation of *Borrelia burgdorferi* from a Lyme seronegative patient in northern Italy: expression of OspB immunodominant proteins on the isolated strain. Microbiologica 1992; 15:95-98.
102. Liegner KB, Shapiro JR, Ramsay D, Halperin AJ, Hogrefe W, Kong L. Recurrent erythema migrans despite extended antibiotic treatment with minocycline in a patient with persisting *Borrelia burgdorferi* infection. J Am Acad Dermatol 1993; 28:312-314.
103. Dattwyler RJ, Volkman DJ, Luft BJ, Halperin JJ, Thomas J, Golightly MG. Seronegative Lyme disease: dissociation of specific T- and B- lymphocyte responses to *Borrelia burgdorferi*. N Engl J Med 1988; 319:1441-1446.
104. Schutzer SE, Coyle PK, Belman AL, Golightly MG, Drulle J. Sequestration of antibody to *Borrelia burgdorferi* in immune complexes in seronegative Lyme disease. Lancet 1990; 335:312-315.
105. Huppertz HI, Mosbauer S, Busch DH, Karch H. Lymphoproliferative responses to *Borrelia burgdorferi* in the diagnosis of Lyme arthritis in children and adolescents. Eur J Pediatr 1996; 155:297-302.
106. Steere AC. Seronegative Lyme disease. JAMA 1993; 270:1369.
107. Sigal LH, Zahradnik JM, Lavin P, Patella SJ, Bryant G, Haselby R, Hilton E, Kunkel M, Adler-Klein D, Doherty T, Evans J, Molloy PJ, Seidner AL, Sabetta JR, Simon HJ, Klempner MS, Mays J, Marks D, Malawista SE. A vaccine consisting of recombinant *Borrelia burgdorferi* OspA to prevent Lyme disease: recombinant OspA Lyme disease vaccine study consortium. N Engl J Med 1998; 339:216-222.
108. Wormser GP, Nowakowski J, Nadelman RB, Schwartz I, McKenna D, Holmgren D, Aguero-Rosenfeld M. Efficacy of an OspA vaccine preparation for prevention of Lyme disease in New York State. Infection 1998; 26:208-212.
109. Schutzer SE, Luan J, Coyle PK. Detection of Lyme disease after OspA vaccine. N Engl J Med 1997; 337:794-795.
110. Wormser GP. Prospects for a vaccine to prevent Lyme disease in humans. Clin Infect Dis 1995; 21:1267-1274.
111. Barthold SW. Specificity of infection-induced immunity among *Borrelia burgdorferi* sensu lato species. Infect Immun 1999; 67:36-42.
112. Barbour AG. Isolation and cultivation of Lyme disease spirochetes. Yale J Biol Med 1984; 57:521-525.
113. Schwan TG, Gage KL, Karstens RH, Schrumpf ME, Hayes SF, Barbour AG. Identification of the tick-borne relapsing fever spirochete *Borrelia hermsii* by using a species-specific monoclonal antibody. J Clin Microbiol 1992; 30:790-795.
114. Schwan TG, Schrumpf ME, Hinnebusch BJ, Anderson DE, Konkel ME. GlpQ: an antigen for serological discrimination between relapsing fever and Lyme borreliosis. J Clin Microbiol 1996; 34:2483-2492.

115. De Koning J, Bosma RB, Hoogkamp-Korstanje JA. Demonstration of spirochetes in patients with Lyme disease with a modified silver stain. J Med Microbiol 1987; 23:261-267.
116. Goodman JL, Bradley JF, Ross AE, Goellner P, Lagus A, Vitale B, Berger BW, Luger S. Bloodstream invasion in early Lyme disease: results from a prospective, controlled, blinded study using the polymerase chain reaction. Am J Med 1995; 99:6-12.
117. Berg D, Abson K, Prose NS. The laboratory diagnosis of Lyme disease. Arch Dermatol 1991; 127:866-870.
118. Oksi J, Mertsola J, Reunanen M, Marjamaki M, Viljanen MK. Subacute multiple-site osteomyelitis caused by *Borrelia burgdorferi*. Clin Infect Dis 1994; 19:891-896.
119. Picken MM, Picken RN, Han D, Cheng Y, Ruzic-Sabljic E, Cimperman J, Maraspin V, Lotric-Furlan S, Strle F. A two year prospective study to compare culture and polymerase chain reaction amplification for the detection and diagnosis of Lyme borreliosis. Mol Pathol 1997; 50:186-193.
120. Rath PM, Marsch WC, Brade V, Fehrenbach F. Serological distinction between syphilis and Lyme borreliosis. Zentralbl Bakteriol 1994; 280:319-324.
121. Schwartz BS, Goldstein MD, Ribeiro JMC, Schulze TL, Shahied SI. Antibody testing in Lyme disease: a comparison of results in four laboratories. JAMA 1989; 262:3431-3434.
122. Bakken LL, Callister SM, Wand PJ, Schell RF. Interlaboratory comparison of test results for detection of Lyme disease by 516 participants in the Wisconsin State Laboratory of Hygiene/College of American Pathologists proficiency testing program. J Clin Microbiol 1997; 35:537-543.
123. Hedberg CW, Osterholm MT, MacDonald KL, White KE. An interlaboratory study of antibody to *Borrelia burgdorferi*. J Infect Dis 1987; 155:1325-1327.
124. Luger SW, Krauss E. Serologic tests for Lyme disease: interlaboratory variability. Arch Intern Med 1990; 150:761-763.
125. Mitchell PD, Reed KD, Aspeslet TL, Vandermause MF, Melski JW. Comparison of four immunoserologic assays for detection of antibodies to *Borrelia burgdorferi* in patients with culture-positive erythema migrans. J Clin Microbiol 1994; 32:1958-1962.
126. Corpouz M, Hilton E, Lardis MP, Singer C, Zolan J. Problems in the use of serologic tests for the diagnosis of Lyme disease. Arch Intern Med 1991; 151:1837-1840.
127. Nohlmans MK, Blaauw AA, van den Bogaard AE, van Boven CP. Evaluation of nine serological tests for diagnosis of Lyme borreliosis. Eur J Clin Microbiol Infect Dis 1994; 13:394-400.
128. Magnarelli LA, Fikrig E, Padula SJ, Anderson JF, Flavell RA. Use of recombinant antigens of *Borrelia burgdorferi* in serologic tests for diagnosis of Lyme borreliosis. J Clin Microbiol 1996; 34:237-240.
129. Dressler F, Ackermann R, Steere AC. Antibody responses to the three genomic groups of *Borrelia burgdorferi* in European Lyme borreliosis. J Infect Dis 1994; 169:313-318.
130. Magnarelli L, Anderson JF, Johnson RC, Nadelman RB, Wormser GP. Comparison of different strains of *Borrelia burgdorferi* sensu lato used as antigens in enzyme-linked immunosorbent assays. J Clin Microbiol 1994; 32:1154-1158.
131. Hauser U, Krahl H, Peters H, Fingerle V, Wilske B. Impact of strain heterogeneity on Lyme disease serology in Europe: comparison of enzyme-linked immunosorbent assays using different species of *Borrelia burgdorferi* sensu lato. J Clin Microbiol 1998; 36:427-436.
132. Oksi J, Uksila J, Marjamaki M, Nikoskelainen J, Viljanen MK. Antibodies against whole sonicated *Borrelia burgdorferi* spirochetes, 41-kilodalton flagellin, and P39 protein in patients with PCR- or culture-proven late Lyme borreliosis. J Clin Microbiol 1995; 33:2260-2264.
133. Pachner AR, Ricalton NS. Western blotting in evaluating Lyme seropositivity and the utility of a gel densitometric approach. Neurology 1992; 42:2185-2192.
134. Wormser GP, Aguero-Rosenfeld ME, Nadelman RB. Lyme disease serology: problems and opportunities. JAMA 1999; 79-80.
135. Wheeler CM, Garcia Monco JC, Benach JL, Golightly MG, Habicht GS, Steere AC. Nonprotein antigens of *Borrelia burgdorferi*. J Infect Dis 1993; 167:665-674.
136. Hauser U, Lehnert G, Wilske B. Validity of interpretation criteria for standardized Western blots (immunoblots) for serodiagnosis of Lyme borreliosis based on sera collected throughout Europe. J Clin Microbiol 1999; 37:2241-2247.
137. Cinco M, Murgia R, Ruscio M, Andriolo B. IgM and IgG significant reactivity to *Borrelia burgdorferi* sensu stricto, *Borrelia garinii* and *Borrelia afzelii* among Italian patients affected by Lyme arthritis and neuroborreliosis. FEMS Immunol Med Microbiol 1996; 14:159-166.
138. Ma B, Christen B, Leung D, Vigo-Pelfrey C. Serodiagnosis of Lyme borreliosis by Western immunoblot: reactivity of various significant antibodies against *Borrelia burgdorferi*. J Clin Microbiol 1992; 30:370-376.

139. Kowal K, Weinstein A. Western blot band intensity analysis: application to the diagnosis of Lyme arthritis. Arthritis Rheum 1994; 37:1206-1211.

140. Sivak SL, Aguero-Rosenfeld ME, Nowakowski J, Nadelman RB, Wormser GP. Accuracy of IgM immunoblotting to confirm the clinical diagnosis of early Lyme disease. Arch Intern Med 1996; 156:2105-2109.

141. Cooke WD, Bartenhagen NH. Seroreactivity to Borrelia burgdorferi antigens in the absence of Lyme disease. J Rheumatol 1994; 21:126-131.

142. Karlsson M, Mollegard I, Stiernstedt G, Wretlind B. Comparison of Western blot and enzyme-linked immunosorbent assay for diagnosis of Lyme borreliosis. Eur J Clin Microbiol Infect Dis 1989; 8:871-877.

143. Karlsson M. Aspects of diagnosis of Lyme borreliosis. Scand J Infect Dis 1990; 67:1-59.

144. Zoller L, Cremer J, Faulde M. Western blot as a tool in the diagnosis of Lyme borreliosis. Electrophoresis 1993; 14:937-944.

145. Magnarelli LA. Laboratory diagnosis of Lyme disease. Rheum Dis Clin North Am 1989; 15:735-745.

146. Brown SL, Hansen SL, Langone JJ. Role of serology in the diagnosis of Lyme disease. JAMA 1999; 282:62-66.

147. Kaiser R, Lucking CH. Intrathecal synthesis of specific antibodies in neuroborreliosis: comparison of different ELISA techniques and calculation methods. J Neurol Sci 1993; 118:64-72.

148. Hammers-Berggren S, Hansen K, Lebech AM, Karlsson M. Borrelia burgdorferi-specific intrathecal antibody production in neuroborreliosis: a follow-up study. Neurology 1993; 43:169-175.

149. Hansen K. Lyme neuroborreliosis: improvements of the laboratory diagnosis and a survey of epidemiological and clinical features in Denmark 1985-1990. Acta Neurol Scand 1994; 151:S1-S44.

150. Hammers-Berggren S, Lebech AM, Karlsson M, Svenungsson B, Hansen K, Stiernstedt G. Serological follow-up after treatment of patients with erythema migrans and neuroborreliosis. J Clin Microbiol 1994; 32:1519-1525..

151. Zbinden R, Goldenberger D, Lucchini GM, Altwegg M. Comparison of two methods for detecting intrathecal synthesis of Borrelia burgdorferi-specific antibodies and PCR for diagnosis of Lyme neuroborreliosis. J Clin Microbiol 1994; 32:1795-1798.

152. Hofmann H. Lyme borreliosis – problems of serological diagnosis. Infection 1996; 24:470-472.

153. Hammers-Berggren S, Lebech AM, Karlsson M, Andersson U, Hansen K, Stiernstedt G. Serological follow-up after treatment of Borrelia arthritis and acrodermatitis chronica atrophicans. Scand J Infect Dis 1994; 26:339-347.

154. Zhang YQ, Mathiesen D, Kolbert CP, Anderson J, Schoen RT, Fikrig E, Persing DH. Borrelia burgdorferi enzyme-linked immunosorbent assay for discrimination of OspA vaccination from spirochete infection. J Clin Microbiol 1997; 35:233-238.

155. Schmidt BL. PCR in laboratory diagnosis of human Borrelia burgdorferi infections. Clin Microbiol Rev 1997; 10:185-201.

156. Valsangiacomo C, Balmelli T, Pifferetti JC. A nest polymerase chain reaction for the detection of Borrelia burgdorferi sensu lato based on a multiple sequence analysis of the hbb gene. FEMS Microbiol Lett 1996; 136:25-29.

157. Moter SE, Hofmann H, Wallich R, Simon MM, Kramer MD. Detection of Borrelia burgdorferi sensu lato in lesional skin of patients with erythema migrans and acrodermatitis chonica atrophicans by ospA-specific PCR. J Clin Microbiol 1994; 32:2980-2988.

158. Schwartz I, Wormser GP, Schwartz JJ, Cooper DA, Weissensee P, Gazumyan A, Zimmerman E, Goldberg NS, Bittker S, Campbell GL, Pavia CS. Diagnosis of early Lyme disease by polymerase chain reaction amplification and culture of skin biopsies from erythema migrans lesions. J Clin Microbiol 1992; 30:3082-3088.

159. Brettschneider S, Bruckbauer H, Klugbauer N, Hofmann H. Diagnostic value of PCR for detection of Borrelia burgdorferi in skin biopsy and urine samples from patients with skin borreliosis. J Clin Microbiol 1998; 36:2658-2665.

160. Schmidt BL, Aberer E, Stockenhuber C, Kladed H, Breier F, Luger A. Detection of Borrelia burgdorferi DNA by polymerase chain reaction in the urine and breast milk of patients with Lyme borreliosis. Diagn Microbiol Infect Dis 1995; 21:121-128.

161. Nocton JJ, bloom BJ, Rutledge BJ, Persing DH, Logogian EL, Schmid CH, Steere AC. Detection of Borrleia burgdorferi DNA by polymerase chain reaction in cerebrospinal fluid in Lyme neuroborreliosis. J Infect Dis 1996; 174:623-627.

162. Christen HJ, Eiffert H, Ohlenbusch A, Hanefeld F. Evaluation of the polymerase chain reaction for the detection of Borrelia burgdorferi in cerebrospinal fluid of children with acute peripheral facial palsy. Eur J Pediatr 1995; 154:374-377.

163. Issakainen J, Gnehm HE, Lucchini GM, Zbinden R. Value of clinical symptoms, intrathecal specific antibody production and PCR in CSF in the diagnosis of childhood Lyme neuroborreliosis. Klin Padiatr 1996; 208:106-109.

164. Nocton JJ, Dressler F, Rutledge BJ, Rys PN, Persing DH, Steere AC. Detection of *Borrelia burgdorferi* DNA by polymerase chain reaction in synovial fluid from patients with Lyme arthritis. N Engl J med 1994; 330:229-234.

165. Pachner AR. Pathogenesis of neuroborreliosis – lessons from a monkey model. Wien Klin Wochenschr 1998; 110:870-873.

166. Mouritsen CL, Wittwer CT, Litwin CM, Yang L, Weis JJ, Martins TB, Jaskowski TD, Hill HR. Polymerase chain reaction detection of Lyme disease. Am J Clin Pathol 1996; 105:647-654.

167. Oksi J, Marjamaki M, Nikoskelainen J, Viljanen MK. *Borrelia burgdorferi* detected by culture and PCR in clinical relapse of disseminated Lyme borreliosis. Ann Med 1999; 31:225-232.

168. Johnson RC, Kodner C, Russell M. In vitro and in vivo susceptibility of Lyme disease spirochete, *Borrelia burgdorferi*, to four antimicrobial agents. Antimicrob Agents Chemother 1987; 31:164-167.

169. Anonymous. Treatment of Lyme disease. Med Lett Drugs Ther 1997; 39:47-48.

170. Dever LL, Jorgensen JH, Barbour AG. In vitro antimicrobial susceptibility testing of *Borrelia burgdorferi*: a microdilution MIC method and time-kill studies. J Clin Microbiol 1992; 30:2692-2697.

171. Agger WA, Callister SM, Jobe DA. In vitro susceptibilities of *Borrelia burgdorferi* to five oral cephalosporins and ceftriaxone. Antimicrob Agents Chemother 1992; 36:1788-1789.

172. Preac-Mursic V, Wilske B, Schierz G, Sub E, Grob B. Comparative antimicrobial activity of the new macrolides against *Borrelia burgdorferi*. Eur J Clin Microbiol Infect Dis 1989; 8:651-653.

173. Dever LL, Jorgensen JH, Barbour AG. In vitro susceptibility testing of *Borrelia burgdorferi* by a dialysis culture method. Antimicrob Agents Chemother 1997; 41:1208.

174. Baradaran-Dilmaghani R, Stanek G. In vitro susceptibility of thirty *Borrelia* strains from various sources against eight antimicrobial chemotherapeutics. Infection 1996; 24:60-63.

175. Hammers-Stiernstedt S, Wretlind B. Dialysis culture enables more accurate determination of MIC of benzylpenicillin for *Borrelia burgdorferi* than does conventional procedure. Antimicrob Agents Chemother 1996; 40:2882-2883.

176. Hammers-Stiernstedt S, Wretlind B. In vitro susceptibility testing of *Borrelia burgdorferi* by a dialysis culture method. Antimicrob Agents Chemother 1997; 41:1208-1209.

177. Brouqui P, Badiaga S, Raoult D. Eucaryotic cells protect *Borrelia burgdorferi* from the action of penicillin and ceftriaxone but not from the action of doxycycline and erythromycin. Antimicrob Ag Chemother 1996; 40:1552-1554.

178. Wormser GP. Controversies in the use of antimicrobials for the prevention and treatment of Lyme disease. Infection 1996; 24:178-181.

179. Oksi J, Nikoskelainen J, Viljanen MK. Comparison of oral cefixime and intravenous ceftriaxone followed by oral amoxicillin in disseminated Lyme borreliosis. Eur J Clin Microbiol Infect Dis 1998; 17:715-719.

26

Treponemal and Other Spirochetoses

Bruno L. Schmidt

Ludwig Boltzmann Institute of Dermato–Venerological Serodiagnostics, Hospital of the City of Vienna-Lainz, Vienna, Austria

I. HISTORICAL BACKGROUND

A. Syphilis

Syphilis was first recognized as a disease entity when it rapidly spread through Europe in the late fifteenth century, coinciding with the return of Columbus from the New World. It became one of the most prevalent and devastating infectious diseases of the world and was termed the Great Pox in the beginning of the sixteenth century. The disease received its present name from the poem by Girolamo Fracastoro in 1530 about the conflicted shepherd, Syphilus. One (environmental) theory postulates that venereal syphilis is merely a variant of another treponemal disease, yaws, which is known to be epidemic in Central and South America. Due to environmental changes in Europe, the pathogen may have evolved into a new and more virulent species. Many experts have long assumed that syphilis was spread from the New World to the Old (Columbian theory), but more arguments accumulate against this hypothesis (1).

B. Leptospirosis

Leptospirosis has been recognized fore more than 100 years, although the family *Leptospiraceae* have been described first in 1979. It is now being considered as one of the emerging infectious diseases (2).

II. CLINICAL MANIFESTATIONS

A. Syphilis

Syphilis, like other spirochetal diseases, is characterized by episodes of active clinical disease which are punctuated by periods of asymptomatic or latent infection.

Early syphilis includes primary and secondary disease as well as early latent stages (defined as less than 1 year duration in the United States and less than 2 years duration in Europe). A primary chancre, the first clinical manifestation, appears at the site of infection after approximately 2-6 weeks and is characteristically indurated and painless. It may persists for 2-6 weeks and then heal spontaneously. Within several weeks after, or concurrent with the healing of the chancre, patients will develop manifestations of the secondary stage of syphilis, which may include disseminated infectious rash, generalized lymphadenopathy, condyloma lata, and mucous patches. Again, these manifestations persist for several weeks or months and then heal spontaneously. The patient enters the latent stage, which can be interrupted by recurrent secondary manifestations. In most patients, however, the latent stage will persist for a lifetime if left untreated. The tertiary stage appears often decades after initial infection and may involve virtually any organ. In the pre-antibiotic era, approximately one-third of patients with untreated syphilis developed tertiary manifestations: symptomatic neurosyphilis (6.5%), cardiovascular syphilis (10%), or gummatous syphilis (16%). The last two forms of the disease, however, have now become exceedingly rare. Neurological manifestations, including syphilitic meningitis, may occur as early as three months post-infection, especially in patients with HIV-infections Thus, neurosyphilis should not be considered solely a late manifestation of the disease.

Congenital syphilis results from the transmission of *T. pallidum* across the placenta during pregnancy, and the illness may be evident as either early prenatal syphilis, where clinical signs develop within the first two years of life, or late-staged.

Yaws, pinta, and endemic syphilis are predominantly diseases of childhood and poverty, and about 70% of infections occur before the age of ten. Transmission is by direct contact of abraded skin with an infected lesion. In endemic syphilis, primary chancres are rarely noted because the inoculum is usually small. The presentation of endemic syphilis is similar to secondary syphilis. In pinta, clinical manifestations are confined to the skin; systemic symptoms, and cardiovascular and neurological involvement are absent. Yaws does not commonly involve the cardiovascular and nervous systems. Clinical manifestations of secondary and tertiary endemic syphilis are similar to that of venereal syphilis.

B. Leptospirosis

Leptospiroses occurs in two clinically recognizable syndromes: anicteric and icteric leptospirosis. The more common syndrome is the anicteric form which is a self-limited systemic illness that occurs in about 85% of the cases. There are two clearly defined stages in anicteric leptospirosis; the septicemic (first) stage and the immune (second) stage with aseptic meningitis as the most prevalent clinical finding. Icteric leptospiroses, or Weil's syndrome, are characterized by hepatic, renal, and vascular dysfunction.

The onset of the anicteric leptospirosis is abrupt and is characterized by fever, headache, severe myalgia, and chills with rigors. The septicemic stage lasts for 3-7 days, and the most common physical finding is conjunctival suffusion in the absence of purulent discharge. The duration of the immune stage ranges from 4-30 days with a preceding 1-3 day asymptomatic period. Fever, headache, and vomiting are less severe than during the first stage. The hemorrhagic diatheses are attributed to severe vasculitis which have endothelial damage and which result in injury of the capillaries. Renal insufficiency and failure are the result of tubular damage which may occur in the absence of interstitial inflammation. Pulmonary lesions are primarily hemorrhagic rather than inflammatory.

III. EPIDEMIOLOGY OF INFECTION

A. Syphilis

European syphilitic epidemics have been recorded since the late fifteenth century, and the disease was an extremely common one only a few decades past. During World War I, 13% of American military draftees were found to be infected with syphilis or gonorrhea. The widespread use of penicillin reduced the number of cases from 72 cases per 100,000 in 1943 to about 4 per 100,000 in 1956. After an epidemic rise in the 1960s, associated with relaxed sexual restraints, the rate of syphilis cases at any stage rose from 28.5 to 53.8 per 100,000 persons in 1990. The outbreak was occurring primarily among African-American heterosexual men and women in cities. The high number of infected young women has resulted in an alarming increase in new cases of congenital syphilis. Prenatal syphilis had declined from 4085 reported cases in 1962 to 287 in 1981, but peaked in 1991 with 4352 cases. In 1999, syphilis is not a very common disease in the United States and is estimated to infect about 10,000 people a year. Of importance, the genital sores lead to infected people being more vulnerable to a still more fatal infection with the human immunodeficiency virus.

In western European countries, the incidence of early syphilis dropped to 1.5 per 100,000 with the availability of penicillin. Due to the social, socio-economic, and behavioral changes in the Russian Federation, however, a huge increase of new syphilis cases had been reported reaching 263 cases per 100,000 persons in 1996 (3). As a result of this new epidemic, the incidence of syphilis has begun to increase also in the western European countries during the last years, and cases of congenital syphilis, which were absent in the past decades, have been reported from several countries.

The World Health Organization estimated that in 1995 there were approximately 12 million new cases of syphilis in adults worldwide with 5.8 million cases in South and Southeast Asia and 3.5 million in sub-Saharan Africa. The prevalence of syphilis in pregnant women attending antenatal clinics in major African cities ranges from 4 to 15 % (4).

Non-venereal treponematoses, which include yaws, endemic syphilis, and pinta constitute a group of potentially disabling infections which primarily afflict children in tropical and subtropical areas (Table 1). Foci where these diseases are endemic usually have a patchy distribution and are typically confined to communities with poor socio-economic conditions with limited access to health services. Pinta was widespread in South and Central America. Yaws is present in parts of Equatorial and West Africa, Latin America, South-East Asia, and some South Pacific Islands, while endemic syphilis (bejel) is present in Eastern Mediterranean, Asian, and African countries, particularly in arid regions. From 1948 to 1969, mass penicillin campaigns were undertaken by health administrations in 46 countries in the context of the WHO Treponematoses Programme. These activities almost eradicated the endemic treponematoses. No vaccines for human treponematoses are yet available.

B. Leptospirosis

Leptospirosis is an ubiquitous zoonotic disease (more common in wet climates) that affects most mammals. The organism is secreted in the urine of infected animals and may survive for days or months in freshwater, soil, or mud. Humans are dead-end hosts in the chain of transmission. There are important differences in the epidemiology of the disease in temperate and tropical regions. In Europe, North America, and other developed regions, the group at risk are those whose leisure activities expose them to immersion in water ('adventure tourism'), and people that come often in contact with animals (e.g., farmers, veterinarians). Only a sporadic pattern occurs in Europe and the United States, where the annual incidence is 0.05 cases per 100,000 population (Hawaii: 1.08 cases per 100,000).

Human vaccines are not widely used in Western countries, but in China, Korea, and Japan, polyvalent vaccines have been used extensively. A vaccine containing only the serovar *L. icterohaemorrhagiae* is licensed for human use in France.

Table 1   Characteristics of human treponematoses and leptospiroses.

	venereal syphilis	yaws	endemic syphilis	pinta	leptospiroses
synonyms	---	frambesia, pian	bejel,dichuwa	carate, cute	
infectious agent	T. pallidum subsp. pallidum	T. pallidum subsp. pertenue	T. pallidum subsp. endemicum	T. carataneum	Leptospira interrogans
distribution	worldwide	tropical areas, Africa, South America, Caribbean, Indonesia	arid areas, North Africa, Middle East	semiarid areas, Central or South America	worldwide
predominant age of onset	adolescents, adults	children	children, adults	children, adolescents	children, adults
transmission	sexual contact	skin contact	mucous membrane	skin contact	direct or indirect exposure to animal urine, or contaminated water or soil
transmissibility	high	high	high	low	high
congenital infection	yes	no	rarely	no	no

IV.   NATURE OF THE BACTERIA

A.   Syphilis

The causative agent of syphilis, *Treponema pallidum* subsp. pallidum, is a corkscrew-shaped prokaryotic microorganism, that belongs to the Order *Spirochaetales*, Family *Spirochaetaceae* and Genus *Treponema*. It measures between 8 and 20 μm. in length and has an amplitude of 0.15 μm. Darkfield microscopic examination of a wet preparation reveals a rotary motion with flexion, and back-and-forth motion. The organism is only pathogenic to humans.

Other treponemes include the animal pathogens *T. cuniculi* (rabbit syphilis), *T. fribourg-blanc* (monkey syphilis), and *T. hyodysenteriae* (swine dysentery), now reclassified as *Serpulina hyodysente-*

riae. Some human or animal nonpathogenic saprophytic treponemes, such as *T. microdentium, T. denticola,* or *T. vincentii,* are particularly abundant in the oral or anal cavities.

Despite numerous attempts, *T. pallidum* has not yet been cultured continuously in vitro. Consequently, the current knowledge of virulence mechanisms of the organism is limited. Most of our knowledge of the physiology, metabolism, and antigenic structure of *T. pallidum* are derived from study of the Nichols strain which has been maintained in rabbits since 1912. *T. pallidum* does not produce lipopolysaccharide or potent exotoxins. One characteristic feature is the paucity of immunogenic transmembrane proteins. By freeze-fracture electron microscopy, it could be shown that the density of intramembranous particles is extraordinarily low, approximately three orders of magnitude less than in *E. coli* (5) thus making research even more difficult.

A major breakthrough in syphilis research was the successful sequencing of the genome as recently completed (6). It comprises 1,138,006 base pairs containing 1041 predicted protein coding sequences, 28% thereof have yet no database match and hence may be novel genes. *T. pallidum* is unable to synthesize enzyme co-factors, fatty acids, and nucleotides de novo. Like *B. burgdorferi,* it lacks a respiratory electron transport chain, but in contrast to *B. burgdorferi,* it lacks genes which encode superoxide dismutase, catalase, or peroxidase, activities that protect against oxygen toxicity. Motility-associated genes are highly conserved in highly invasive spirochetes. *T. pallidum* has three core proteins (*FlaB1, FlaB2,* and *FlaB3*), a sheath protein (*FlaA*) and two yet uncharacterized proteins, whereas most other bacteria have only a core protein (7). Of special interest is a large family of duplicated genes (paralogs) (*tprA-L*) (8), that may function as porins and adhesins. The latter hypothesis is based on pairwise and multiple sequence alignments of the *T. pallidum* gene family to a major outer sheath protein (Msp) from *T. denticola* and is reminiscent of a 32-member paralog gene family encoding outer membrane proteins (omp) in *Helicobacter pylori.*

Treponema pallidum subsp. endemicum, *Treponema pallidum* subsp. pertenue and *Treponema carateum,* the causative organisms of endemic syphilis, yaws, and pinta cannot be distinguished from one another morphologically or by laboratory tests. Even with modern sequencing techniques, only minimal differences have been discovered (9).

B.   Leptospirosis

For leptospiroses, the pathogenic species in humans is *Leptospira interrogans.* More than 200 serovars that belong to 23 serogroups have been identified. Free-living nonpathogenic serovars comprise the species *L. biflexa,* of which at least 60 serovars are recognized. Members of the family *Leptospiraceae* are flexible helical rods of 0.1 μm. in diameter and 6 to 12 μm. in length. The helical conformation is right-handed with more than 18 coils per cell. Leptospires are aerobic bacteria and unique among spirochetes because they have terminal hooks. A helically-shaped cell cylinder and two periplasmic flagellae enable the organism to burrow into tissue.

V.   PATHOGENESIS AND IMMUNOLOGY OF SPIROCHAETAL INFECTIONS

A.   Syphilis

T. pallidum is transmitted by direct contact with an infectious lesion, and both primary and secondary syphilitic lesions contain numerous treponemes to facilitate this activity. The mechanism by which *T. pallidum* invades tissues is not well understood, and the organism has been shown to attach to eukaryotic cells. *T. pallidum* begins to multiply locally with one generation of approximately 30-33 hrs., but also may gain access to the blood and lymphatic systems and disseminates widely within the first several hours.

The knowledge of the immune response to syphilitic infection mostly results from studies of experimental syphilis in rabbits which is similar to that of humans at least in the beginning stages of the disease.

Upon intradermal inoculation, typical chancres develop in rabbits and intratesticular infection results in syphilitic orchitis. Both early and late lesions of syphilis are characterized by a pronounced mononuclear infiltration. In primary syphilitic orchitis, T lymphocytes can be detected at 6 days after infection and reach maximal numbers on day 10 to 13. At that time, also, the numbers of spirochetes reach a maximum. Macrophages first become apparent on day 10 and reach maximal numbers by day 13, just before a dramatic clearance of organisms from tissue occurs (10).

Communication between the cells of the immune system is effected by means of soluble factors called cytokines. During the primary stage, syphilitic patients are able to produce IL-2, IFN, TNF, and weakly IL-6 even before antibodies can be detected. The highest level of IL-6 is reached in secondary syphilis, where cells start to produce IL-10 which reaches a maximum in early latent syphilis (11). Increasing presence of IL-6 and IL-10 is then associated with diminished production of IL-2, IFN, and TNF. The suppression of Th1 cytokines was distinctly seen in early latent syphilis, when the level of IL-10 was highest. In the rabbit model, it has been demonstrated that on day 6-14 of infection, IL-2 production by T cells is diminished from its high level on day 4. This suppression is mediated by macrophages which produce prostaglandin (PGE-2). It has been proposed that the down-regulation of Th1 cytokines might favor the survival of treponemes (12).

Antibody is produced early in the course of syphilis infection and provides the basis for serological diagnosis. Both immunoglobulin M (IgM) and immunoglobulin G (IgG) appear during primary infection, and here the intensity of reactivity is generally proportional to the duration of clinical symptoms. With the exception of early primary syphilis, IgG reaches far higher titres than does IgM, although both classes of immunoglobulins are produced throughout infection. In secondary and early latent syphilis, a full range of treponemal antigens is recognized and with high titers. Therapeutic intervention at any stage causes a generalized loss of antibody against individual antigens, and the rate and degree of loss depends on the duration of infection prior to therapy. The major antigens which display strong reactivity with specific antibody include: TpN47 (a penicillin-binding lipoprotein which was earlier claimed to be surface-exposed), TpN37, TpN35, TpN33 and TpN30 (which belong to the flagellin complex), and TpN15 and TpN17 (with yet no known functions). Reactivity to the 37 and 47 kD antigens develops very soon after experimental infection, and is followed by reactivity to the core endoflagellar molecules, and lastly, to the two low molecular weight lipoproteins (13).

One of the central paradoxes of syphilis is the fact that the immune system has the capacity to eliminate millions of treponemes from the primary site of infection (14), yet some organisms evade the immune response and survive to cause a persistent infection which can last for decades. Several hypotheses have been raised to explain this ability to survive:

i) the theory of an 'immunoprotective niche': *T. pallidum* has the capacity to disseminate to many different anatomical locations, including the nervous system, the eye, and the fetus via the placenta. Each of these sites is considered to be immunologically privileged and may serve as reservoirs in which treponemes might escape the immune system. In addition, *T. pallidum* can maintain sequestration in non-phagocytic cells in vivo which might then protect the organism from exposure to antibodies and antibiotics(15).

ii) the theory of the critical antigenic mass necessary to trigger the local response: The presence of low numbers of organisms with no resultant pathology can be an explanation for the persistence during latency. In addition, the surface of *T. pallidum* contains only a paucity of proteins, making the organism immunologically inert. It has been demonstrated that organisms carefully extracted from infected tissue are only poorly reactive with antibody (16).

iii) the theory of specific suppression of the immune response: Cellular immune response studies using peripheral blood lymphocytes from humans have shown depressed responses to treponemal antigens, T-cell mitogens, and both (17), although studies of spleen and lymph-node lymphocytes from infected rabbits have demonstrated an impressive specific anti-*T. pallidum* proliferative response (13). It has been postulated that premature down-regulation of the local immune response by macrophages, perhaps from early PEG-2 production, permit some organisms to escape clearance mechanisms. In chronic infections, this shift of the balance from Th1 (protective, delayed-type hypersensitivity-based response) to Th2 (non-protective antibody-based mechanism) cytokines determines the maintenance of latency (12). In humans, pharmacological immunosuppression (post-transplant) and concurrent HIV infection are examples of impaired cellular immune response which result in more severe clinical manifestations of early syphilis and more frequent symptomatic neurological involvement (18).

iv) the theory of antigenic variation: By determining the nucleotide sequence of the complete genome of *T. pallidum*, a family of 12 related genes, called *tpr* genes (*tprA-L*), that encode predicted products with similarity to the major sheath protein (Msp) of *Treponema denticola* was found (19). Msp is highly immunogenic and has been found to bind to fibronectin and laminin and has porin-like activity. Although a similar surface array has not yet been found on T. pallidum, it can be speculated that the predicted tpr proteins of *T. pallidum* are surface located. The fact that there are multiple versions of the genes may reflect an antigenic variation system, common to pathogenic borreliae, *Neisseria gonorrhoeae*, and *Mycoplasma genitalium*.

B. Leptospirosis

Leptospires infect the human host by entering through cut or abraded skin, mucous membranes, or conjunctivae. Pathogenic leptospires rapidly invade the bloodstream after penetrating the mucous membranes. The organisms spread through all sites of the body and can penetrate tissues, including CNS and aqueous humor. The incubation period for leptospiroses is usually 7-12 days, and leptospires may enter the aqueous humor during the septicemic phase and may thereafter persist for months.

VI. LABORATORY DIAGNOSIS

A. Syphilis

The first test for the diagnosis of syphilis was introduced in 1906 by Wassermann and his colleagues, using the treponeme-gorged livers of stillborn infants who suffered from congenital syphilis. Decades ago, the *Treponema pallidum* immobilization (TPI) test was the yardstick of syphilis serology, but this test is no longer in use, due to lacking sensitivity and high costs. The most sensitive test is the rabbit infectivity test (RIT), being able to detect one or two treponemes in lesions, but requires 3 to 6 months to complete and accordingly is only used in research laboratories.

Routine tests for syphilis can be divided into direct tests for demonstrating the spirochete, which are used when lesions are present, and serological tests.

1.   Direct detection methods

Darkfield microscopy
Treponemes cannot be observed with the ordinary light microscope because of their narrow width. The use of darkfield illumination for examination of *T. pallidum* was first described in 1909. Viability of the treponeme is necessary to distinguish *T. pallidum* from morphologically similar saprophytic spirochetes within the genitalia (*T. phagedenis*, *T. refringens*) . Therefore, darkfield examination must be undertaken immediately after the specimen is obtained. Care should be taken when examining specimens of the oral cavity (*T. denticola*), sebaceous secretions, colon, and rectum, since a number of anaerobic treponemes and other spirochetes are parasites in humans.

Direct fluorescent antibody test for *T. pallidum* (DFA-TP)

The test detects and differentiates pathogenic from nonpathogenic treponemes by using a specific monoclonal antibody that is conjugated with a fluorochrome. The organism is not required to be motile, and samples collected from oral, rectal, or intestinal lesions can be examined. Samples are air-dried and fixed immediately before staining. A positive test is highly probable of infection but a negative result, like the in dark-field microscopy, does not exclude the diagnosis of syphilis. A modification of this test was developed to examine tissue sections (DFAT-TP).

Polymerase chain reaction (PCR)

Genes which are targeted for diagnostic PCR have included the genes coding for the proteins TpN47, TpN44,5 (*TmpA*), TpN39, and TpN19 (20). As well, RNA for the 16S rRNA may be targeted in a RT-PCR assay (21). Although the analytical sensitivity, demonstrated on buffer dilutions of specific RNA, was high (due to the high copy number, the RNA-equivalent of 0.001 treponemes could be detected in the RT-PCR assay), the clinical sensitivity is still insufficient. A PCR assay with primers for the gene encoding the 47 kD lipoprotein have been used to assess clinical specimens (amniotic fluid, neonatal sera, and neonatal CSF) and resulted in an overall sensitivity of 78% compared with results obtained by the RIT (22). The lack of sensitivity has generally be found to be associated with nonspecific inhibitors in clinical samples and furthermore due to losses of DNA or RNA during the extraction process. It can be anticipated, however, that these difficulties may be overcome, and thus, PCR should be become extremely valuable in diagnosing particularly problem illnesses of primary, congenital, and neuro-syphilis. A multiplex PCR for the detection of *T. pallidum*, Herpes simplex virus types 1 and 2, and *Haemophilus ducreyi* has been evaluated (23), and the simultaneous detection of sexually transmitted disease pathogens has the potential to reduce costs.

2. Serological assays

About two-thirds of the syphilis cases reported in the United States and Western countries are diagnosed at the latent (asymptomatic) stage, which underlines the importance of serology. Serological tests fall into one of two categories: nontreponemal (reagin or lipoidal tests) or treponemal. Nontreponemal tests are used for screening in the United States, are inexpensive, convenient to perform, and are useful for determining the efficacy of treatment by follow-up of declining titres. Treponemal tests have *T. pallidum* subsp. pallidum as antigen and are primarily used to verify reactivity in the nontreponemal tests or to confirm clinical impression in late syphilis when nontreponemal tests are negative. In Europe, treponemal tests are used also for screening.

Nontreponemal tests

Based on an antigen composed of an alcoholic solution containing cardiolipin, cholesterol, and lecithin, the nontreponemal tests measure IgM and IgG antibodies to lipoidal material which is released from damaged host cell as well as antibodies to lipoprotein-like material from treponemes. These antibodies can also be produced in about 1-2% of persons in response to autoimmune diseases, viral infections, pregnancy, and a variety of nontreponemal diseases of an acute or chronic nature during which tissue damage occurs (24).

The standard nontreponemal test is the Venereal Disease Research Laboratory (VDRL) test, in which flocculation of lipoidal particles (antigen, see before) with the patient's serum is visualized by microscopic examination. The unheated serum reagin (USR) test differs only slightly from the VDRL test in that unheated serum can be used and antigen does not need to be produced daily. The rapid plasma reagin (RPR) test and the toluidine red unheated serum test (TRUST) differ from the VDRL test in that these tests can be read visually due to the addition of coloured particles. Both tests can be used with plasma. Each of the nontreponemal tests can be performed as a quantitative assay by preparing serial dilutions of the patient's serum to reach an endpoint titre. The VISUWELL Reagin test and the Spirotec Reagin II test are indirect enzyme-linked immunosorbent assays (ELISA) in which VDRL antigen is coated to the solid phase of a microtitre plate. After incubation with patient's serum, antigen-

Table 2 Sensitivity (%) and specificity (%) of serological tests for *T. pallidum*.

	Sensitivity (%)				Specificity (%)
	primary syphilis	secondary syphilis	early latent syphilis	late syphilis	
Nontreponemal					
VDRL	78 (74-87)	100	95	71 (37-94)	98
RPR	76 (68-89)	100	98	73	98
USR	76 (69-86)	100	95		98
TRUST	74 (66-85)	100	98		98
ELISA	78 (69-87)	100	98		98
Treponemal					
MHA-TP	80 (69-87)	100	97	94 (97-100)	99
FTA-ABS	85 (70-95)	100	100	98 (97-100)	97
ELISA	84 (69-92)	100	100	99	98
Treponemal IgM					
Captia-M Syphilis	87 (80-91)	90	92	<25	91
19S IgM FTA-ABS	91 (89-93)	94	96	<25	97

(Source: adapted from (20) and own studies; abbreviations – see text)

antibody complexes are incubated with an labelled anti-human immunoglobulin conjugate. Results are read spectophotometrically. Limitations of the nontreponemal tests are their lack of sensitivity in the beginning of the disease and in late syphilis (Table 2). Prozone (false negative) reactions occur in 1-2% of patients with secondary syphilis and can be overcome by diluting the sera before testing. The causes of false-positive or better nonspecific reactive results are multiple (see above), and therefore every reactive reagin test has to be confirmed by a treponemal test. Data of sensitivity and specificity of nontreponemal tests are summarized in Table 2, and a detailed description of procedures and licenced status (standard or provisorial) in the United States has been published by the American Public Health Association (25).

Treponemal tests

Tests using *T. pallidum* subsp. pallidum as antigen can be subdivided according to the methodology employed. In the Fluorescent Treponemal Antibody-Absorption (FTA-ABS) test, the serum of the patient is first diluted 1:5 in sorbent (an extract from cultures of the nonpathogenic Reiter treponeme) to remove nonspecific group-antibodies. This mixture is layered on a microscope slide to which *T. pallidum* has been fixed. If specific antibodies are present in the serum, the formed antigen-antibody complexes are incubated with a FITC-labelled anti-human immunoglobulin, resulting in FITC-stained spirochetes which can be examined by fluorescence microscopy. A modification of the FTA-ABS test is the FTA-ABS double staining (FTA-ABS DS) test in which a second fluorochrome (tetramethylrhodamine isothiocyanate), which is attached to an anti-human IgG globulin, helps locate the treponemes by dark-field microscopy when the patient's serum does not contain specific antibodies. The FTA-ABS test is used as a confirmatory test although nonspecific results may occur due to cross-reaction with other spirochetes. A definite association has been made between a false-positive FTA-ABS test and the diagnosis of systemic, discoid, and drug-induced varieties of lupus erythematosus (20), resulting in an "atypical beading" fluorescence pattern.

Passive hemagglutination of erythrocytes which are sensitized with an antigen is an extremely simple method for the detection of antibody. Tanned sheep erythrocytes that are sensitized with ultra-sonicated material from *T. pallidum* are used in the microhemagglutination assay for antibodies to *T. pallidum* (MHA-TP). Modifications include the use of gelatin particles instead of erythrocytes, named the Treponema pallidum particle agglutination assay (TP-PA), and sensitized chicken erythrocytes in a test developed specifically for automation which is used in blood banking (Olympus TP-PK test). The patient's serum is first mixed with absorbing diluent that is made from non-pathogenic Reiter trepo-nemes and other absorbents and stabilizers. The serum is then placed in a microtitre plate and incubated with coated erythrocytes and gelatin particles respectively. Agglutination can be examined visually if specific antibodies are present in serum. The results are reported as reactive if agglutination occurs at a dilution of 1:80 or more. Quantitative evaluation is performed by serial dilution of the serum with ab-sorbing diluent. The sensitivity of the MHA-TP is superior to the VDRL and the FTA-ABS test except in primary syphilis, and specificity is extremely high (Table 2).

Several tests using the ELISA format have been developed. Sandwich assays have antigen coated to the solid phase, and after incubation with patient serum, bound complexes can be detected specto-photometrically with the addition of an enzyme-labelled anti-human globulin and substrate. Competi-tive assays have antigen bound to solid phase and, in addition, antitreponemal antibodies in the conju-gate. Lack of specific antibodies in patients serum results in a high absorbance by photometric reading. If specific antibodies are present, these antibodies in serum compete with antibodies in conjugate and thereby reduce measured absorbance.

With the availability of individual *T. pallidum* antigens as a consequence of the use of recombi-nant DNA techniques, new tests with cloned antigens have been developed. The use of recombinant *T. pallidum* antigens in place of poorly defined mixtures of antigens from Nichols strain of *T. pallidum*, which may be contaminated with rabbit testicular components, has the potential for improving the specificity of serological assays. Tests which are based on antigens that have been produced from single genes (*TmpA*) and tests using a combination of cloned antigens have become available (26,27). A spe-cial capture ELISA, ICE Syphilis, is able to detect specific antibodies in addition to the antigen. Both recombinant *T. pallidum* proteins (TpN15, TpN17, and TpN47) as well as capture antibodies for human immunoglobulins are fixed to the solid phase. The antitreponemal component of the captured antibodies is detected by a peroxidase-conjugated antigen (28). ELISAs can easily be automated thus allowing for the screen of large numbers of samples. Sensitivities and specificities are different in the various formats used (29), but are similar to other treponemal tests. A disadvantage is the higher cost compared to non-treponemal tests.

A test which allows for measure of reactivity to individual antigens is the Western Blot. Perform-ance is similar to the well-known confirmation of antibodies to HIV. Antibodies to the 15, 17, 44.5, and 47 kD antigens appear to be diagnostic for acquired syphilis. Unfortunately, this test is not available commercially and can only be performed in research laboratories.

Treponemal tests that are developed for the detection of specific IgM antibodies are the 19S FTA-ABS test and the Captia Syphilis M test. Anti-human IgM antibodies are bound to microtitre plates in the latter and therefore capture the human IgM fraction. Specificity is achieved by the addition of a conjugate which consists of *T. pallidum* components and a monoclonal antibody that is labelled with an enzyme. Sensitivity is comparable to the 19S IgM FTA-ABS test but the specificity is less (30). The procedure of the 19S IgM FTA-ABS assay is the same as in the FTA-ABS test except that an IgM frac-tion of the patient's serum is detected, and the conjugate is IgM-specific.

3. Diagnostic criteria for venereal syphilis

During primary syphilis, direct tests for the demonstration of the spirochete are most useful. Serous fluid from the lesion contains numerous treponemes. Darkfield microscopy can be positive days to weeks before serological tests become reactive. A negative test, however, does not exclude syphilis as the number of treponemes can be too low to be detected, or the lesion may be in the healing stage. Antibodies do not appear until the first week after the chancre has formed, and the humoral response can most easily be detected by specific IgM tests then followed by specific IgG tests days later. By about the sixth week of infection, generally all nontreponemal and treponemal tests are reactive regardless of whether clinical symptoms are present or not. Serology is highly sensitive in diagnosing early latent syphilis. By the secondary stage of syphilis, the organism has invaded every organ of the body. All serological tests are reactive, very often with high titers, and treponemes may be found in lesions. Symptoms of late or tertiary syphilis may occur 10 to 20 years after the initial infection. Treponemal tests are reactive, however, in one-third of infected patients lipoidal tests are nonreactive in this stage of the disease (Table 3). Patients with reactive treponemal tests in the absence of clinical and historical findings are defined as having late latent syphilis. At present, however, there is no test available which allows differentiation between solely long-lasting reactivity of treponemal tests after therapy and the actual remnant activity of the disease.

Diagnosis of cardiovascular syphilis is made on the basis of symptoms that indicate aortic insufficiency or aneurysm, reactive treponemal tests, and in the context of no known history of treatment.

The indication to perform a lumbar puncture in patients with reactive treponemal tests in serum include neurological or ophthalmological symptoms or signs, tertiary syphilis (e.g., aortitis, gumma, etc.), treatment failure, HIV-infection and neurological symptoms, and congenital infection. The diagnosis of neurosyphilis requires a reactive treponemal test result with a serum sample, a CSF cell count of more than five mononuclear cells per cubic millimeter, and a CSF total protein in excess of 40 mg./dl. A reactive VDRL in CSF indicates disease, but nonreactive VDRL results have been seen in up to 73% of patients with neurosyphilis, particularly in asymptomatic forms and in tabes dorsalis (31). A negative CSF FTA-ABS or negative MHA-TP test are useful to rule out neurosyphilis. The intrathecal synthesis of *T. pallidum*-specific antibodies can indicate active neurosyphilis. In order to discriminate

Table 3   Interpretation of serological tests for syphilis.

Serological tests			
Nontreponemal	Treponemal	Treponemal IgM	Interpretation
--	--	--	no syphilis (until 3-4 wks. before examination)
--	--	+	early primary syphilis
+	--	--	biological nonspecific reactive
--	+	+	early syphilis
+	--	+	early syphilis
+	+	+	early syphilis
--	+	--	late infection, treated syphilis
+	+	--	late infection, treated syphilis

antibodies that are transudated from serum as compared to intrathecally-produced ones, formulae which compare CSF results to blood-brain barrier are used.

$$\text{TPHA index} = \frac{\text{CSF MHA-TP titre}}{\text{albumin quotient} * 1000}$$

$$\text{albumin quotient} = \frac{\text{CSF albumin (mg./dL.)}}{\text{serum albumin (mg./dL.)}}$$

The TPHA-Index is defined as the quotient of the CSF MHA-TP titre and the albumin quotient (32). Values greater than 70 are diagnostic for neurosyphilis. A hyperbolic function for determining the relation of specific to nonspecific IgM, IgG, and IgA in CSF and serum was developed in Germany (33). Concentrations of immunoglobulins are determined by ELISA, and values greater than 2 are diagnostic for neurosyphilis.

To monitor the efficacy of treatment, nontreponemal tests are most useful. The rate of decline in titres depends on the stage of infection, the initial titre, and a history of previous syphilis. Patients with disease of longer duration or with previous episodes of syphilis infection show slower declines in titre and are less likely to become negative. A four-fold decline after 3 months can be expected after treatment of primary or secondary syphilis. Patients who are treated in the late stages show a more gradual decline in titre and low titres may persist longer than two years. The same is true for the TPHA–index which can persist above the diagnostic cut-off for up to two years after treatment. Reactivity in treponemal tests generally lasts for decades except in patients who received treatment in the very beginning of the disease. A graph of typical rise and decline of different serological tests over time is given in Figure 1 before and after adequate treatment of a patient with early syphilis.

4. Diagnostic criteria in HIV-infected patients

Syphilis can facilitate HIV-1 transmission by increasing either the infectiousness (*T. pallidum* lipoproteins have been shown to increase HIV-1 replication), the susceptibiliy of the partner, or both. This relation between syphilis or commonsexually transmitted diseases and HIV-1 has been called "epidemiological synergy" (34). The majority of patients who are co-incidently infected with HIV present with typical manifestations of syphilis and respond normally in serological tests for syphilis. Problems in the diagnosis of syphilis in HIV-infected patients have been related to: i) lack of serologic response after infection with *T. pallidum*, ii) failure in the decline of nontreponemal tests after treatment, iii) unusually high titres of nontreponemal tests according to B-cell activation, iv) the rapid progression to late stages of syphilis, and v) confusing clinical signs and symptoms (18). In the HIV-seropositive patient with early syphilis, a lumbar puncture should be seriously considered.

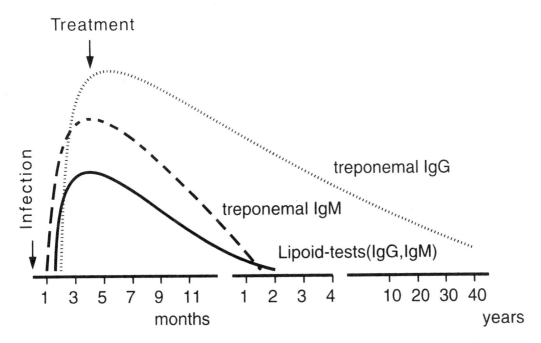

Figure 1   Reactivity (measured in relative units) of nontreponemal and treponemal tests before and after adequate treatment of a patient with early syphilis.

5.   Diagnostic criteria for congenital syphilis

The standard serological tests for syphilis, based on the measurement of IgG, reflect antibodies that are passively transferred from the mother to the infant. Reactivity of specific IgM tests of the serum of newborns is proof of prenatal syphilis in addition to clinical signs. At birth, however, up to 50% of infected infants can be asymptomatic, and reactivity in specific IgM tests can be delayed for several weeks especially in infants who are infected in late pregnancy. Sensitivity of PCR is equal to RIT when amniotic fluid is used as specimen (22). The diagnosis of congenital syphilis depends on a combination of physical, radiographic, serological, and direct microscopic or PCR-based criteria.

6.   Diagnostic criteria for other treponematoses

The standard serological tests for syphilis are uniformly reactive with yaws, pinta, and endemic syphilis, and to date, no routine test allows differentiation of the causative organisms. These diseases are most prevalent during childhood (Table 1), and diagnosis is based on clinical signs and routine syphilis tests.

B. Leptospirosis

Leptospires are present in blood and CSF during the first week of illness, and they appear in the urine after the first week. A presumptive identification of leptospires can be made by direct microscopic methods. Blood, CSF, and tissues may be screened by either darkfield microscopy or direct fluorescent-antibody assays. For urine and CSF, the sample is centrifuged at 1500 x g for 30 min, the supernatant is discarded, and a wet mount is prepared from the sediment. On a freshly-prepared slide, the characteristic hooked ends of the leptospires establish a presumptive diagnosis. A definite diagnosis is made by isolating leptospires from any clinical material by culture. Semi-solid media (Fletcher's, Ellinghausen's) should be incubated for 6 weeks at 28 to 30°C in the dark and under aerobic conditions. The inoculum volume for blood should be kept to a minimum (< 100 µl), due to the possible presence of inhibitors. For CSF, up to 0.5 ml. can be used per 5 ml. of medium. Cultures should be inspected weekly by dark-field microscopy.

Identification of leptospiral isolates can be approached by serological procedures with the use of the microscopic agglutination test (MAT) or molecular methods. The MAT is performed with isolates that have been passaged at least three times in liquid medium in order to dilute out agar granules that might produce agglutination artifacts. Paired serum samples, however, are often required for more definitive diagnosis. Large numbers of live antigen serovars must be maintained as well as hyperimmune rabbit antiserum, and reproducibility between laboratories is inconsistent. Inverse titers of 200-800 are commonly used to indicate infection, but even a threshold of 800 may persist for several months. MAT remains the definite serological assay, however, and it requires the use of techniques and reagents that are usually limited to reference laboratories.

PCR assays for the detection of leptospiral DNA in blood, serum, CSF, and urine have been developed. Sensitivity of PCR on urine samples is twice as high as with culture, and PCR can detect infection in the early stage of an illness when serology is negative (35).

In the U.S., a commercially-produced indirect hemagglutination assay has been the only diagnostic assay approved by the Food and Drug Administration for many years. In acute leptospirosis, this test was found to be 100% sensitive and 94% specific as compared to the MAT (36). Alternatives to the MAT, which use either ELISA or dipstick format, have been developed. By ELISA, IgM and IgG antibodies can be detected from the 2nd and 7th day of symptoms respectively (37). Results of an international multicentre evaluation of a dipstick assay for measuring specific IgM antibodies were concordant in 93.2% with results from ELISAs (38).

1.   Diagnostic criteria for leptospirosis

Evaluation of serological results in addition to clinical and epidemiological findings are the first step in the diagnosis of leptospirosis. A four-fold rise in the MAT titre to one or more serovars between acute- and convalescent- phase serum specimens, which have been run in parallel, confirm leptospirosis. Limitations of serological tests are due to the fact that delayed seroconversions are not uncommon, and cross-reactions with pathogens that are associated with syphilis, relapsing fever, Lyme borrelioses, or legionellosis can occur. Negative findings by direct examinations of specimens do not necessarily rule out acute disease. Molecular and ELISA-based methods offer rapid and sensitive new approaches, but further evaluations are needed before these methods can be widely adopted. Up to then, diagnosis will be mainly restricted to a few reference laboratories, the WHO/FAO Collaborating Center for Reference and Research on Leptospirosis at CDC (U.S.), Amsterdam, The Netherlands, and Brisbane, Australia.

VII.   OTHER HOST-ASSOCIATED SPIROCHETES

A number of spirochetes inhabit supragingival and subgingival plaques in humans. *T. denticola, T. socranskii, T. pectinovorum, T. vincentii,* and *T. medium* are parasites of the oral cavity. They are spiral-shaped with lengths between 5 and 16 µm, and diameters of 0.15 to 0.30 µm. These treponemes are considered commensal organisms and are difficult to isolate from healthy gums. They can be detected, however, in the subgingival plaque of approximately 90% of patients with periodontal disease. In vitro culture is possible. In contrast, pathogen-related oral spirochetes (PROS), found in necrotizing ulcerative gingivitis or periodontitis can only be detected by reactivity with monoclonal antibodies that are specific for *T. pallidum* antigens. Due to the difficulty for culture of PROS, little is known about structure, antigens, and virulence factors. Due to the successful sequencing of the complete genome of *T. pallidum* and the completion of sequencing the *T. denticola* genome in the near future, however, new insights in the differences between pathogenic and nonpathogenic treponemes will become available, and progress in diagnosis can be expected.

Treponemal species that inhabit the sebaceous secretions which are found beneath the prepuce and in other epithelial folds of the genital region include *T. phagedenis*, *T. refringens*, and *T. minutum*; these can be cultured in vitro and are nonpathogenic. Although homology of their DNA with *T. pallidum* is low, comparison of the 16S rRNA sequences indicates a relationship with pathogenic treponemes.

Human intestinal spirochetes are relatively short (3-6 μm.) and are 0.2 to 0.4 μm. in diameter. Two species can be separated: *Serpulina pilosicoli* and *Brachyspira aalborgii*. *S. pilosicoli* represents the vast majority of intestinal spirochetes and is related to *S. hyodysenteriae*. Association between intestinal spirochetes and disease has not yet been clarified; signs of tissue damage or inflammation are usually absent. Rectal swabs or fresh stool specimens should be examined by darkfield microscopy for the presence of spirochetes, and positive samples can be cultured under anaerobic conditions.

A spiral-formed bacterium, which has not yet been ordered into a taxonomic family is *Spirillum minus*, it is one cause of rat bite fever in China and Japan. Fever develops after an incubation period of 1-2 weeks, generally after the bite-lesion has healed. The disease has a lethality of about 10%. Diagnosis is usually made by dark-field microscopy of blood.

VIII. SUSCEPTIBILITY TESTING

Penicillins and tetracyclines are effective in treatment of *T. pallidum* and *L. interrogans* infections. Standardized procedures have not been developed for antimicrobial susceptibility testing of leptospires. No antibiotic resistance has yet been detected for *T. pallidum* to penicillins.

REFERENCES

1. Luger A. The origin of syphilis: Clinical and epidemiologic considerations on the Columbian theory. Sex Transm Dis 1993; 20:110-117.
2. Levett PN. Leptospirosis: re-emerging or re-discovered disease? J Med Microbiol 1999; 48:417-418.
3. Tichonova L, Borisenko K, Ward H, Meheus A, Gromyko A, Renton A. Epidemics of syphilis in the Russian Federation: Trends, origins, and priorities for control. Lancet 1997; 350:210-213.
4. Singh AE, Romanowski B. Syphilis: review with emphasis on clinical, epidemiologic, and some biologic features. Clin Microbiol Rev 1999; 12: 187-209.
5. Radolf JD, Robinson EJ, Bourell KW, Akins DR, Porcella SF, Weigel LM, Jones JD, Norgard MV. Characterization of outer membranes isolated from *Treponema pallidum*, the syphilis spirochete. Infect Immun 1995; 63:4244-4252.
6. Fraser CM, Norris SJ, Weinstock CM, White O, Sutton GG, Dodson R, Gwinn M, Hickey EK, Clayton R, Ketchum KA, Sodergren E, Hardham JM, McLeod MP, Salzberg S, Peterson J, Khalak H, Richardson D, Howell JK, Chidambaram M, Utterback T, McDonald L, Artiach P, Bowman C, Cotton MD. Complete genome sequence of *Treponema pallidum*, the syphilis spirochete. Science 1998; 281:375-388.
7. Norris SJ, Treponema Pallidum Polypeptide Research Group. Polypeptides of *Treponema pallidum*: Progress toward understanding their structural, functional, and immunologic roles. Microbiol Rev 1993; 57:750-779.
8. Weinstock GM, Hardham JM, McLeod MP, Sodergren EJ, Norris SJ. The genome of *Treponema pallidum*: new light on the agent of syphilis. FEMS Microbiol Rev 1998; 22:323-332.
9. Centurion-Lara A, Castro C, Van Voorhis WC, Lukehart SA. Two 16S-23S ribosomal DNA intergenic regions in different *Treponema pallidum* subspecies contain tRNA genes. FEMS Microbiol Lett 1996; 143:235-240.
10. Lukehart SA, Baker-Zander SA, Lloyd RMC, Sell S. Characterization of lymphocyte responsiveness in early experimental syphilis. II. Nature of cellular infiltration and *Treponema pallidum* distribution in testicular lesions. J Immunol 1980; 124:461-467.
11. Podwinska J, Lusiak M, Zaba R, Bowszyc. The pattern and level of cytokines secreted by Th1 and Th2 lymphocytes of syphilitic patients correlate to the progression of the disease. FEMS Immunol Med Microbiol 2000; 28:1-14.

12. Sell S, Hsu P-L. Delayed hypersensitivity, immune deviation, antigen processing and T-cell subset selection in syphilis pathogenesis and vaccine design. Immunol Today 1993; 14:576-582.

13. Baker-Zander SA, Hook EW, Bonin W, Handfield HH, Lukehart SA. Antigens of *Treponema pallidum* recognized by IgG and IgM antibodies during syphilis in humans. J Infect Dis 1985; 151:264-272.

14. Lukehart SA, Shaffer JM, Baker-Zander SA. A subpopulation of *Treponema pallidum* is resistant to phagocytosis: possible mechanism of persistence. J Infect Dis 1992; 166:1449-1453.

15. Sykes JA, Miller JN, Kalan AJ. *Treponema pallidum* within cells of a primary chancre from a human female. Br J Vener Dis 1974; 50:40-44.

16. Van der Sluis JJ, Kant M, Onvlee PC, Stolz E. The inaccessibility of the outer membrane of adherent *Treponema pallidum* (Nichols strain) to anti-treponemal antibodies, a possible role of proteins. Genitourin Med 1999; 66:165-170.

17. Schell RF, Musher DM, Jacobson K, Schwethelm P. Induction of acquired cellular resistance following transfer of thymus-dependent lymphocytes from syphilitic rabbits. J Immunol 1975; 114:550-553.

18. Musher DM, Baughn RE. Neurosyphilis in HIV-infected persons. N Engl J Med 1994; 331:1516-1517.

19. Haapasalo M, Muller KH, Uitto VJ, Leung WK, McBride BC. Characterization, cloning, and binding properties of the major 53-kilodalton *Treponema denticola* surface antigen. Infect Immun 1992; 60:2058-2065.

20. Larsen SA, Steiner BM, Rudolph AH. Laboratory diagnosis and interpretation of tests for syphilis. Clin Microbiol Rev 1995; 8:1-21.

21. Centurion-Lara A, Castro C, Shaffer JM, Van Voorhis WC, Marra CM, Lukehart SA. Detection of *Treponema pallidum* by a sensitive reverse transcriptase PCR. J Clin Microbiol 1997; 35:1348-1352.

22. Sanchez PJ, Wendel GD, Grimprel E, Goldberg MS, Hall M, Arencibia-Mireles O, Radolf JD, Norgard MV. Evaluation of molecular methodologies and rabbit infectivity testing for the diagnosis of congenital syphilis and neonatal central nervous system invasion by *Treponema pallidum*. J Infect Dis 1993; 167:148-157.

23. Orle KA, Gates CA, Martin DH, Body BA, Weiss JB. Simultaneous PCR detection of *Haemophilus ducreyi*, *Treponema pallidum*, and herpes simplex virus types 1 and 2 from genital ulcers. J Clin Microbiol 1996; 34:49-54.

24. Catterall RD. Systemic disease and the biological false positive reaction. Br J Vener Dis 1972; 48:1-12.

25. Larsen SA, Pope V, Johnson RE, Kennedy EJ. A Manual of Tests for Syphilis. 9th Ed. Washington, D.C.:American Public Health Association, 1998.

26. Ebel A, Bachelart L, Alonso JM. Evaluation of a new competitive immunoassay (BioElisa Syphilis) for screening for *Treponema pallidum* antibodies at various stages of syphilis. J Clin Microbiol 1998; 36:358-361.

27. Zrein M, Maure I, Boursier F, Soufflet L. Recombinant antigen-based enzyme immunoassay for screening of *Treponema pallidum* antibodies in blood bank routine. J Clin Microbiol 1995; 33:525-527.

28. Young H, Moyes A, Seagar L, McMillan A. Novel recombinant-antigen enzyme immunoassay for serological diagnosis of syphilis. J Clin Microbiol 1998; 36:913-917.

29. Schmidt BL, Edjlalipour M, Luger A. Comparative evaluation of nine different enzyme-linked immunosorbent assays for the determination of antibodies against *Treponema pallidum* in patients with early syphilis. J Clin Microbiol 2000; 38:1279-1282.

30. Schmidt BL, Luger A, Duschet P, Seifert W, Gschnait F. Spezifische IgM-teste in der syphilis-diagnose. Hautarzt 1994; 45:685-689.

31. Davis LE, Schmitt JW. Clinical significance of cerebrospinal fluid tests for neurosyphilis. Ann Neurol 1989; 25:50-55.

32. Luger A, Schmidt BL, Steyrer K, Schoenwald E. Diagnosis of neurosyphilis by examination of the cerebrospinal fluid. Br J Vener Dis 1981; 57:232-237.

33. Reiber H. External quality assessment in clinical neurochemistry: survey of analysis for cerebrospinal fluid (CSF) proteins based on CSF/Serum quotients. Clin Chem 1995; 41:256-263.

34. Wasserheit JN. Epidemiological synergy: interrelationships between human immunodeficiency virus infection and other sexually transmitted diseases. Sex Transm Dis 1992; 19:61-77.

35. Brown PD, Gravekamp C, Carrington DG. Evaluation of the polymerase chain reaction for early diagnosis of leptospirosis. J Med Microbiol 1995; 43:207-213.

36. Levett PN, Whittington CU. Evaluation of the indirect hemagglutination assay for the diagnosis of acute leptospirosis. J Clin Microbiol 1998; 36:11-14.

37. Silva MV, Camargo ED, Batista L, Vaz AJ, Brandao AP, Nakamura PM, Negrao JM. Behaviour of specific IgM, IgG and IgA class antibodies in human leptospirosis during the acute phase of the disease and during convalescence. J Trop Med Hyg 1995; 98:268-272.

38. Smits HL, Ananyina YV, Chereshsky A, Dancel L, Lai-A-Fat RF. International multicenter evaluation of the clinical utility of a dipstick assay for detection of *Leptospira*-specific immunoglobulin M antibodies in human serum specimens. J Clin Microbiol 1999; 37:2904-2909.

27

Chlamydiae

Lee Ann Campbell
Department of Pathobiology, University of Washington, Seattle, Washington

Jeanne M. Marrazzo
Division of Allergy and Infectious Diseases, Department of Medicine, University of Washington, Seattle, Washington

Walter E. Stamm
Division of Allergy and Infectious Diseases, Department of Medicine, University of Washington, Seattle, Washington

Cho-chou Kuo
Department of Pathobiology, University of Washington, Seattle, Washington

I. HISTORICAL BACKGROUND

There are four species of *Chlamydia*: *Chlamydia trachomatis*, *Chlamydia pneumoniae*, *Chlamydia psittaci*, and *Chlamydia pecorum*. Several significant disease processes in humans are caused by chlamydial infection with *C. trachomatis*, *C. pneumoniae*, and *C. psittaci*. Recognized as a cause of cervicitis, urethritis, and other anogenital infections only in the last three decades, *C. trachomatis* is a leading cause of sexually transmitted disease in the United States and the leading cause of preventable blindness in developing nations. Several recent advances in the understanding of the biology, natural history, and laboratory diagnosis of chlamydial infections deserve emphasis. These include: a) an increasing awareness of the magnitude of asymptomatic chlamydial infection in both men and women; b) evidence of the organism's role in pelvic inflammatory disease (PID), ectopic pregnancy, tubal infertility, and chronic pelvic pain; c) demonstration of the effectiveness of screening for chlamydial cervical infection in preventing subsequent symptomatic PID; d) the development of more sensitive diagnostic tests using nucleic acid amplification techniques; e) the successful use of these tests on new types of specimens including first void urine and self-collected vaginal swabs; and f) the relative insensitivity and laboratory-to-laboratory variability of chlamydial culture and other non-amplified diagnostic assays.

    C. pneumoniae is a human respiratory pathogen. It was isolated serendipitously in 1965 from the conjunctiva of a Taiwanese child who was participating in a trachoma vaccine trial (1). The isolation was in the yolk sac of an embryonated chicken egg which was the only method then available for growth of chlamydiae. The isolate, TW-183, was untypable as a trachoma strain of *C. trachomatis* by micro-immunofluorescence (micro-IF) antibody typing. In 1971, when cell culture methods became available, the organism was observed to form round, dense inclusions in HeLa cells which were more similar in morphology to those of *C. psittaci* than to those of *C. trachomatis* (C-C Kuo, unpublished data). Since the initial isolation, *C. pneumoniae* has not been isolated from the eye nor associated with eye infections.

TW-183 was first suspected to cause respiratory infection during an outbreak of pneumonia in military conscripts in Finland. Since these patients had complement-fixation (CF) antibodies against chlamydiae (2), human sera were tested by the micro-IF test against TW-183 and were found to be positive. The organism's role as a human pathogen was defined in 1983 when the first respiratory isolate (AR-39) was obtained in Seattle, Washington from a university student with pharyngitis (3). The isolates were designated TWAR which combines the code names of the first two isolates TW-183 and AR-39. A new species, *Chlamydia pneumoniae*, was established for these isolates in 1989 (4). The name TWAR has since been used synonymously with *Chlamydia pneumoniae*.

C. psittaci is an animal pathogen and includes strains that infect avian and mammalian species. *C. psittaci* is found in wild and domesticated animals. In general, infection in animals is a systemic disease with various clinical manifestations among animal hosts. *C. psittaci* infection in animals is often latent. Humans may be accidentally infected by sick animals. Avian strains are innately more virulent to humans than mammalian strains.

Psittacosis in humans is a generalized infection that is usually manifested as pneumonia and that is due to *C. psittaci* as contracted from infected psittacine birds (parrots or parakeets). Ornithosis is an equivalent term that was proposed by Meyer (5) to describe a similar infection which is contracted from animals other than psittacine birds. The ornithosis strains are thought to be less virulent to humans.

II. CLINICAL ASPECTS

A. Clinical manifestations of *C. trachomatis* infection

The common clinical syndromes caused by *C. trachomatis* are a consequence of its tropism for columnar or squamocolumnar epithelial cells of the adult cervix, urethra, rectum, and/or conjunctiva, and the infant respiratory tract. The clinical manifestations include urethritis and conjunctivitis in males and females, cervicitis, and neonatal pneumonia. The rectal epithelium may also be infected and thus give rise to proctitis (6). The sequestered intracellular and intravacuolar life cycle of chlamydiae, as well as the relative inertness of the extracellular elementary body (EB), contribute to the paucity of an inflammatory response and hence an asymptomatic nature of most chlamydial infections.

Among women infected with *C. trachomatis*, the organism generally gains entry through the endocervix. In the great majority (70-90%) of cervical infections, symptoms are either minimal or do not occur, and the cervix appears normal on examination. In fact, these infections may persist for months to years (7). When present, symptoms generally include abnormal vaginal discharge, or intermenstrual or post-coital bleeding. When signs are present, the most common cervical abnormalities include easily-induced endocervical bleeding, mucopurulent endocervical discharge, or edematous ectopy (6). Asymptomatic secondary infection of the urethra and/or rectum occurs in more than 50% of women who have cervical infections. In some instances, chlamydial infection of the female urethra may become symptomatic and may mimic the symptoms of acute bacterial cystitis which include dysuria, frequency, and hesitancy: the "acute urethral syndrome" (8). Absence of bacteriuria or a negative urine culture in a woman with this presentation and pyuria should prompt testing for *C. trachomatis*. Most women infected at the urethra, however, do not have urethral symptoms; equally important, 60-80% of women infected at the urethra are also infected at the cervix thus making endocervical testing a sufficient means of diagnosis in most cases. Between 20-40% of untreated endocervical infections ascend to the upper genital tract, and of these, approximately 10-40% subsequently develop symptoms which are consistent with PID (9,10). Infants born to women with endocervical infection at the time of delivery experience neonatal conjunctivitis in 15-35% and infantile pneumonia in 10-15% (11). Neonatal pulmonary infection may predispose to the eventual development of reactive airways disease in early childhood (12).

Numerous studies have shown a strong association between the occurrence of adverse pelvic sequelae and prior chlamydial infection. These sequelae include tubal infertility, ectopic pregnancy, and chronic pelvic pain. These are most likely a consequence of tubal damage which results from the immunopathology that is provoked by persistent or recurrent tubal infection. While many studies document an important role for *C. trachomatis* in symptomatic PID and its sequelae, asymptomatic upper genital tract inflammation which results from chlamydial infection probably occurs three times as often as does symptomatic chlamydial PID. In fact, asymptomatic PID is estimated to account for 50-75% of all PID (13). *C. trachomatis* has been implicated in the etiology of adverse pelvic sequelae in the absence of prior symptomatic pelvic disease in several studies (14-18). The role of recurrent chlamydial infection in potentiating upper genital tract disease in women has been supported by evidence from both animal models and epidemiological studies in humans (19-21). The predominantly cell-mediated immune response to infection, and the homology between chlamydial heat shock protein (CHSP-60) and human heat shock proteins, may underlie the subsequent immunopathology that damages Fallopian tubes. Sequential infection with different chlamydial serovars may confer an increased risk of tubal scarring (22), and specific major outer membrane protein (MOMP) genotypes may be associated with more invasive disease (23).

In men, *C. trachomatis* is the etiology in 10-40% of patients with non-gonococcal urethritis (NGU) (6,24). Many males with urethral chlamydial infection are thus symptomatic generally with dysuria or burning on urination; urethral discharge may be present. While this discharge is characteristically less frankly purulent than that caused by urethral infection with *Neisseria gonorrhoeae*, this feature is not sufficently consistent to reliably distinguish the two. Recent studies have revealed the substantial prevalence of asymptomatic or minimally symptomatic chlamydial urethral infections especially in adolescent men (25,26). Whether these infections were mildly symptomatic initially, or were never symptomatic, is not clear. In about 1% of infected males, the infection ascends to cause acute epididymitis.

Lymphogranuloma venereum (LGV), a sexually transmitted infection (STI) caused by *C. trachomatis* serovars L_{1-3}, is uncommon in the United States, but it occurs throughout Africa, Asia, and Central and South America. LGV begins as a single non-descript genital papule which is followed by the development of inguinal or femoral lymphadenopathy. An urethral, rectal, or cervical portal of entry may occur in some patients. Thus, the clinical presentation may be similar to that of chancroid or rectal herpes simplex virus infection in some cases. Diagnosis of LGV is made using a combination of clinical findings and a positive chlamydial serology as well as the elimination of other etiologies including herpes, syphilis, and chancroid (6).

C. trachomatis may also induce Reiter's syndrome which is a constellation of conjunctivitis, urethritis, oligoarthritis, and skin lesions that occur 3-6 weeks after genital infection. It predominantly affects males and particularly those of HLA-B27 genotype. Chlamydial antigens and DNA have been detected within both synovial tissue and joint fluid in affected individuals. Specific intra-articular T-cell responses to chlamydial antigens may underlie its pathogenesis (27-29).

B. Clinical manifestations of *C. pneumoniae* infection

The primary site of *C. pneumoniae* infection is the respiratory tract. Therefore, *C. pneumoniae* infection is first recognized by the development of acute symptoms of the upper and lower respiratory tract, i.e., symptoms of pharyngitis (sore throat), bronchitis (cough), and pneumonia (shortness of breath) as with infections that are caused by other bacterial and viral pathogens. The overt clinical manifestations that result from infections of other organ systems have not been described although the systemic dissemination of the organism from the lungs does occur (33). Systemic dissemination has been demonstrated by the presence of bacteremia in humans (34) and experimental animals (35) and by detection of the organism in human atherosclerotic arteries (36). In humans, the organism has been detected in peripheral blood mononuclear cells by PCR in as many as 50% of adults. Following intranasal inoculation in mouse models, *C. pneumoniae* was both cultured from PBMC and detected by PCR, thus indicating that bacteremia occurs during acute infection (37). Frequent detection of *C. pneumoniae* in the atheromata, but not in normal arteries, has suggested that *C. pneumoniae* may have a tropism for atherosclerotic lesions in the artery and may contribute to the pathogenesis of atherosclerosis.

Pneumonia and bronchitis are the most frequently-recognized illnesses that result from *C. pneumoniae* infection. Approximately 10% of patients with pneumonia and approximately 5% of adults with bronchitis and sinusitis will have their infection attributed to this organism (38). Asymptomatic infection or unrecognized, mildly symptomatic illnesses, however, are the most common result of infection. Although no set of symptoms uniquely define pulmonary infections with *C. pneumoniae*, there are several characteristics of the clinical presentation which may help to distinguish it from infection with other respiratory pathogens (38,39). A subacute onset often occurs. Pharyngitis, sometimes with hoarseness, is common early in the course of the illness. The illness may have a biphasic pattern: first demonstrating upper respiratory symptoms which are followed by lower respiratory tract involvement. Specifically, pharyngitis often resolves prior to the subsequent development of a more typical bronchitis or pneumonia syndrome. Symptoms of sinus infection often occur. A persistent cough is common. Although fever is often not present at examination, there may be a history of fever. Since symptoms are often mild but persistent, the period from onset to clinic visit is longer for *C. pneumoniae* infections than other acute respiratory infections. Most episodes of pneumonia are relatively mild and do not require hospital admission. Even in mild infections, however, complete recovery is slow despite appropriate antibiotic therapy, and cough and malaise may persist for many weeks after the acute illness. Older adults appear to have, on average, a more severe clinical course than do young adults. The outcome of *C. pneumoniae* infection can be aggravated by underlying illness and concurrent infection with other bacteria (40).

While the patient's leukocyte count is usually normal, the erythrocyte sedimentation rate is often elevated. A chest roentgenogram usually demonstrates a single subsegmental pneumonitis in milder, non-hospitalized patients while more extensive or bilateral pneumonitis may be seen in those who are admitted to hospital. In those with more severe disease, pleural effusions have also been demonstrated. The role of *C. pneumoniae* as an opportunistic pathogen among immunocompromised persons has not been well-defined, although *C. pneumoniae* has been isolated or detected by PCR from bronchoalveolar lavage specimens of human immunodeficiency virus (HIV)-infected and other immunocompromised patients (41,42). Moreover, *C. pneumoniae* has been implicated in severe respiratory infection in HIV patients by serology, by detection of antigen in respiratory specimens, and by response to treatment with anti-chlamydial therapy. It has also been found in acute respiratory infections among asymptomatic HIV-infected children by seroconversion (43,44).

C. pneumoniae has also been associated with other acute and chronic diseases. Among the acute illnesses are included purulent sinusitis (45), otitis media with effusion (46), endocarditis (47), and lumbosacral meningoradiculitis (48). Several chronic diseases that have been presumptively associated with *C. pneumoniae* are asthmatic bronchitis and asthma exacerbation (49), chronic obstructive pulmonary disease (50), erythema nodosum (51,52), Guillain-Barre syndrome (53), reactive arthritis or Reiter's syndrome (54), Alzheimer's disease (55), and multiple sclerosis (56).

Considerable attention has focused on the association of *C. pneumoniae* with coronary artery disease and other atherosclerotic syndromes including carotid stenosis, stroke, aortic aneurysm, and occlusion of the artery of the lower extremity (claudication) (57-60). The evidence of association has come from seroepidemiological studies which show an increased risk of cardiovascular disease and antibodies against *C. pneumoniae*, from detection of the organism in atherosclerotic lesions by immunocytochemistry (ICC) and PCR in approximately 50% of patients, and by isolation of the organism from atheromatous tissue. Whether the organism plays a causal role or contributes to the immunopathology of atherosclerosis has not been definitively determined. Rabbit and mouse model experiments which have shown that intranasal inoculation of hyperlipidemic animals with *C. pneumoniae* accelerates the progression of atherosclerosis, and pilot therapeutic trials in humans which show favorable outcomes from antibiotic therapy against *C. pneumoniae*, have provided some support for a putative role (59).

C. Clinical manifestations of *C. psittaci* infection

1. Avian psittacosis

The incubation time is usually 7 to 14 days, but it can range from 4 to 28 days. The primary manifestation in humans is pneumonia, although in severe infections disease is generalized. The clinical picture varies from inapparent infection to a febrile illness without localization to fulminant pneumonia.

Respiratory symptoms include cough, dyspnea, pleuritic chest pain, epistaxis, sore throat, and hemoptysis. Systemic symptoms may include fever, malaise, anorexia, shaking chills, sweats, nausea and vomiting, myalgia and arthralgia, headache, and abdominal pain.

Physical signs include rales, pulmonary consolidation, pleural friction rub, pulse-temperature deficit (relative bradycardia in spite of elevated temperature), pharyngeal erythema, hepatomegaly, splenomegaly, meningeal signs, and mental disturbance. Chest x-ray is characteristic of an atypical pneumonia pattern. The infiltration is usually unilateral and less commonly bilateral. Pleural reactions and hilar gland hyperplasia are common. Routine laboratory tests are of little help for diagnosis. Abnormal findings include increased blood sedimentation rate, leukocytosis or leukopenia, anemia, proteinuria, and abnormal liver enzyme tests.

Other rare primary manifestations are endocarditis (66-68) and myocarditis (69). Deaths due to psittacosis were not unusual in the pre-antibiotic era. The mortality rate was 20% or higher in some epidemics. Deaths had been reported in sporadic infections that were improperly treated. Causes of death have included pulmonary insufficiency, generalized toxemia, or cardiac failure.

In the differential diagnosis, other forms of pneumonia due to viruses, *Mycoplasma pneumoniae*, *C. pneumoniae*, and other bacteria should be sought by appropriate microbial and serological tests.

An effective vaccine for *C. psittaci* is not available. Therefore, quarantine of imported birds in combination with preventive antibiotic treatment remain the most important and practical preventive measures (70).

2. Mammalian psittacosis.

Mammalian psittacosis causes disease and latent infection in large and small mammals other than human (71). Both domestic (cattle, sheep, goats, horse, hogs, dogs, guinea pigs, hamsters, and mice) and wild (rodents, hares, koala, and seals) are affected. The common manifestations in animals are pneumonitis, enteritis, conjunctivitis, polyarthritis, encephalitis, and abortion (infection of placenta and fetus). These diseases may cause serious problems in animal husbandry including economic loss. Mammalian psittacosis is much less virulent than avian psittacosis; therefore, human infection (ornithosis) due to mammalian psittacosis is rare. It has been reported only in laboratory personnel or animal farmers. These case reports included pneumonia due to feline pneumonitis (72), sheep abortion (73), and bovine abortion (74) agents. An episode of keratoconjunctivitis in a laboratory worker due to the feline pneumonitis agent (75) and two illnesses of pregnancy which were complicated by the sheep abortion agent that was acquired from sheep (76) have been reported.

III. EPIDEMIOLOGY OF INFECTION

A. Epidemiology of *C. trachomatis* infection

C. trachomatis is now estimated to cause 3 million incident (new) cases of STI annually in the United States, and 89 million new cases worldwide (77-79). In 1995, infections with *C. trachomatis* were the most common of reportable bacterial diseases in the United States (79). Among females, the prevalence declines with increasing age, and it is thus highest in adolescents in whom it ranges from 7% to 25% depending on the population tested. Accurate estimates for chlamydial prevalence in males should soon become available with the advent of more extensive use of urine-based diagnostic testing particularly among asymptomatic men. While established screening programs have effected declines of *C. trachomatis* infection in some populations, overall detection and reporting of chlamydial infections remain suboptimal. This is a result not only of failure on the part of clinicians to test patients at risk, but also of laboratories to use appropriate diagnostic tests. A study of *C. trachomatis* testing in laboratories in Washington State, U.S., for example, unexpectedly revealed that insensitive rapid diagnostic tests, which are intended for point-of-care use, were actually the most commonly-used test in laboratories (80). Despite these concerns, diagnostic testing for *C. trachomatis* has gradually become more widespread, and the reporting has become more complete, thus resulting in increases of annually-reported cases of infection especially among women in whom most testing is currently done.

B. Epidemiology of *C. pneumoniae* infection

Seroepidemiological studies using the *C. pneumoniae*-specific micro-IF test have shown that antibody against *C. pneumoniae* is rare under the age of five in the United States and that it occurs more frequently in tropical countries (1). Antibody prevalence increases steeply from ages 5-14 yrs. at a 6% to 8% increment per year thus indicating that infections are acquired at school. By age 20, approximately 50% of persons have detectable levels of antibody to the organism. The seroprevalence continues to increase among older age groups, but at a slower rate, and it reaches approximately 75% in the elderly. This high seroprevalence indicates that most people are infected and reinfected throughout their life, and this is of interest considering that infection induces a time-limited antibody response (3-5 yrs.).

The frequency of *C. pneumoniae* antibody is the same in both sexes under fifteen years of age. The antibody prevalence in adult men, however, is higher than that among adult women. This pattern is different from that which is observed with other infectious respiratory diseases in which females are more frequently infected than males. No explanation for the increased frequency among males has been found.

C. pneumoniae infection is ubiquitous, although the prevalence of infection may vary by geographical locale (1). A higher prevalence has been noted in tropical, less developed countries than in more northern, developed countries.

Humans are the only known reservoir of *C. pneumoniae*, although genetically similar strains have been isolated from horse and koala (81,82). The incubation period of infection due to *C. pneumoniae* is about 3 weeks which is longer than that for many other respiratory pathogens. Transmission is believed to be from person to person via respiratory secretions. The periodicity of epidemics of *C. pneumoniae* infection is 6-8 years. Studies at the University of Washington and Finnish military outbreaks with documented *C. pneumoniae* infection indicate that the transmission is relatively inefficient, and the secondary transmission appears to be rare (1).

Laboratory studies have shown that *C. pneumoniae* can survive in aerosols at room temperature under conditions of high relative humidity. Although infectivity decreases within thirty seconds at room temperature, survival in these circumstances supports the possibility of direct person-to-person transmission under crowded conditions (83). Transfer from fomites may also occur as the organism can remain viable on inanimate objects for several hours (84).

C. Epidemiology of *C. psittaci* infection

The incidence of human psittacosis has been reduced drastically since the 1950s after quarantine procedures and preventive antimicrobial therapy of imported birds (with feeds that are impregnated with tetracycline) were implemented (70). Human psittacosis is still reported sporadically from households that own pet birds; these are spread most often from psittacine birds but also from other caged birds such as canaries and finches. The largest and most important reservoirs of infection in North America and Europe have been turkeys, ducks, and pigeons. Poultry infection incurs economic losses and involves risk for poultry breeders and processing workers. The poultry industry has become a source of outbreaks for human psittacosis in recent years.

Transmission of infection is by the airborne route, either by direct contact with birds or humans with psittacosis, or indirectly by inhalation of dust that is contaminated with the excreta of infected birds. The organisms resist drying and remain viable for a month at room temperature. The organism is destroyed within 3.5-5 min. at 56°C. Therefore, the risk of infection is eliminated by proper cooking of poultry. Spread of the disease from processed birds to consumers has not been reported.

IV. NATURE OF THE BACTERIUM AND PATHOGENESIS

A. Bacteriology

All chlamydiae possess DNA, RNA, and a cell wall that has characteristics of Gram negative bacteria, including the presence of lipopolysaccharide (LPS) (85). Unlike other Gram negative bacteria, however, peptidoglycan has not been found in the cell wall. The structural rigidity of the cell is maintained by the formation of disulfide-linked complexes among the cysteine-rich proteins in the outer membrane complex (86). None of the chlamydiae can be cultured on strictly artificial media, but all can be propagated in various cell lines (87,88). The organism takes two distinct forms. The elementary body (EB) is infectious, metabolically inert, and suited to survive in the extracellular environment. While the mechanisms by which chlamydiae attach to and enter columnar or squamocolumnar epithelial cells are still incompletely understood, electrostactic interactions and various other proposed adhesins which bind to moeities on the eukaryotic cell surface appear to be important. The EB then enters the eukaryotic cell in a phagolysosome which resists phagolysosomal fusion and allows for the subsequent formation of metabolically active, non-infectious reticulate bodies (RB). The RB divides by binary fission to form a large inclusion that occupies much of the host cell. The chlamydiae are in effect energy parasites; they do not possess the ability to make adenosine triphosphate or some amino acids, and thus must parasitize the host cell's metabolic machinery. Within 8-12 hours, the RB undergoes transformation to produce more EBs which are eventually released from the cell by rupture upon cell death to renew the infectious cycle. The intracellular life cycle lasts approximately 48-72 hours.

C. pneumoniae has some characteristics that are common to chlamydiae and others that distinguish it from the other chlamydial species. Common characteristics include the requirement for an intracellular environment, a developmental cycle, and sharing of a genus-reactive LPS antigen. This reactivity is detectable by the complement-fixation (CF) test or by reaction with a monoclonal antibody that recognizes the genus-specific epitope on LPS.

Characteristics that distinguish *C. pneumoniae* from other chlamydial species are DNA homology, ultrastructural morphology of the EB, and the presence of *C. pneumoniae* species-specific antigen which can be demonstrated by micro-IF serology and which is destroyed by methanol treatment (4,89). Different *C. pneumoniae* isolates have 94 to 100% DNA homology with each other but less than 5% DNA homology with *C. trachomatis* and less than 10% homology with *C. psittaci*. *C. pneumoniae* EBs have a characteristic pear-shaped ultrastructural morphology which is surrounded by a wide periplasmic space that is morphologically distinct from the round EBs of *C. trachomatis* and *C. psittaci* (Figure 1) (90). Although there have been a few reports of *C. pneumoniae* organisms with round-shaped EBs, the electron micrographs show the presence of a periplasmic space that is not observed with the other species, and these isolates are otherwise similar to other *C. pneumoniae* strains by molecular analysis (91).

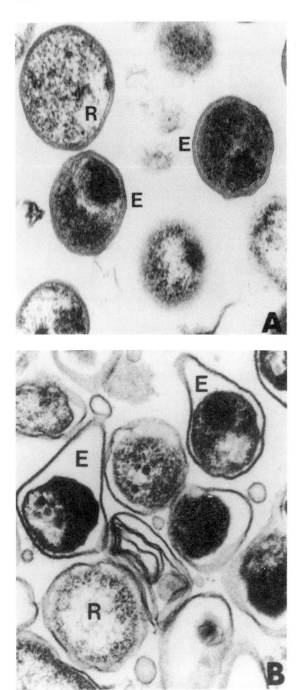

Figure 1 Ultrastructure of the elementary body of *C. trachomatis* and *C. pneumoniae*. The *C. trachomatis* EB (E) is round and dense with no visible periplasmic space (Panel A). The *C. pneumoniae* EB is pear-shaped with a large periplasmic space (Panel B). The RBs (R) of both are similar in ultrastructure. The RB is less electron dense and larger than the EB.

Structural analysis of *C. pneumoniae* cell wall demonstrated a 98 kD cysteine-rich protein in the outer membrane complex in addition to the three cysteine-rich outer membrane proteins of 60-, 40-, and 12-15 kD molecular masses found in chlamydiae (92). It has been postulated that the additional cysteine-rich outer membrane protein might provide a more rigid membrane structure to sustain a pear-shaped morphology. The initial discovery by electron microscopy of the presence of the organism within coronary atheromata was based on the identification of the unique pear-shaped structure, the latter which was later confirmed in the same specimens by direct detection methods (93).

B. Pathogenesis

Chlamydial infection is often asymptomatic and chronic or persistent. The acute symptoms result from active inflammatory reactions at the primary sites of infection. The acute inflammatory reactions usually subside even without antimicrobial therapy due to the host's immune response to contain, but not necessarily eradicate, the infection. If the infection persists or re-infection(s) occurs, perhaps because immunity is weak and short-lived, the infection may cause tissue damage at the site of infection and may result in structural damage and functional impairment of the affected organ. Two well-described human diseases due to *C. trachomatis* infection, blindness from trachoma (94) and infertility/ectopic pregnancy from salpingitis (95, 96), illustrate characteristics of chlamydial pathogenesis. The chronic and persistent nature of *C. pneumoniae* infection has been well-demonstrated by detection of *C. pneumoniae* by ICC and PCR at high frequency in human lung and atheromatous tissue which is removed at autopsy as well as from atherosclerotic artery tissues that are removed by surgery (33,36). Chronic diseases which are analogous to those which result from *C. trachomatis* infection, however, have not been described for *C. pneumoniae*. An association of *C. pneumoniae* chronic pulmonary diseases such as chronic obstructive pulmonary disease or adult-onset asthma might be predicted since the primary site of infection is the lung. Indeed, several studies have demonstrated an association with these pulmonary diseases. The clinical significance, however, has yet to be established (97).

An important attribute of *C. pneumoniae* in pathogenesis is its capability to disseminate from the lungs to the atherosclerotic artery via infected monocytes/macrophages by hematogenous and/or lymphatic routes and to establish persistent infection in atherosclerotic lesions of the artery (98, 99). Within the atherosclerotic lesion, the organism has been localized to macrophage-derived foam cells and smooth muscle cells. Thus, during the acute stage of infection, the bronchial ciliated epithelial cells of the lungs are the primary cells that are infected. The cells that play a central role in the pathogenesis of infection, however, are macrophages, and these can disseminate infection and may serve as a reservoir of chronic infection.

V. IMMUNOLOGY OF INFECTION

The immune response to chlamydial infection is critical not only in immune protection. It likely also plays a major role in immunopathology as well. For *C. trachomatis*, the major outer membrane protein (MOMP) appears to be an important determinant of immunity through elicitation of both specific neutralizing antibody and T cell-mediated immune responses (32). Four variable regions of the MOMP nucleotide sequence define at least eighteen serovars of *C. trachomatis*; each is defined by a distinct MOMP sequence and is recognizable by specific monoclonal antibodies that are used for typing. Serovars D-K are responsible for most oculogenital sexually transmitted infections. Immunity to *C. trachomatis* appears to be serovar-specific; consequently, sequential infection with different serovars can occur. Allelic variation in the MOMP gene occurs frequently either by point mutation or through recombinational events (100,101). This polymorphism may represent a form of immune evasion since even single amino acid changes in MOMP may abrogate the effectiveness of neutralizing antibodies (100). Recurrent infections with different serovars may be important in inducing the immunopathology that is involved in producing the sequelae of chlamydial infection in women. Also critical in this pathology is

CHSP-60 which is a 60 kD heat shock protein that elicits cell-mediated immune responses in humans (101) and, with repeated exposures, marked inflammatory response and immunopathology in animals. Underlying these complex phenomena may be the considerable (50%) homology between CHSP-60 and human heat shock proteins (102). A higher proportion of women with PID, tubal infertility, and ectopic pregnancy demonstrate antibody to CHSP-60 relative to controls (103,104). Furthermore, women with the greatest degree of tubal pathology that is associated with PID and/or the presence of perihepatitis have markedly elevated titres of antibody to CHSP-60. Whether elevation of antibody to CHSP-60 in these situations reflects a causative role for HSP-60 and/or persistent chlamydial infection by inciting immunopathology is not yet clear (105). The immune response to HSP-60 may be restricted by human leukocyte antigen (HLA) class I type and by the inability to generate a Th1 type immune response (32,106). Tumor necrosis factor (TNF) and gamma-interferon (INF-γ) may also mediate tubal inflammation possibly by stimulation of fibroblast proliferation (107).

C. pneumoniae infection also induces humoral and cellular immune responses. Infection with C. pneumoniae induces serum IgM, IgG, and IgA responses (1). These antibodies can be detected by standard serological tests using the fluorescence antibody and EIA techniques. Although the infection of cell culture with C. pneumoniae can be neutralized with C. pneumoniae-specific monoclonal antibodies, it is unknown how the neutralizing antibodies contribute to immunity against C. pneumoniae infection (108). In contrast to C. trachomatis, MOMP is not the immunodominant antigen that is recognized during human infection (109). A feature that distinguishes C. pneumoniae from C. trachomatis and C. psittaci is the genetic homogeneity of the MOMP gene (110-113) in contrast to the multiple serovars that have been reported for the other chlamydial species; only one serovar has been reported for C. pneumoniae which is consistent with the conserved MOMP gene sequences. Reactivities against several C. pneumoniae specific antigens (including 42, 54, and 98 kD) are observed by immunoblot analysis (109, 114, 115). No clearly consistent patterns, however, have been observed that would aid serological diagnosis.

As with C. trachomatis, CHSP60 has received attention for a potential participatory role in immunopathology. Interestingly, CHSP60 co-localizes with human HSP60 in atheromata (116).

A cell-mediated immune response to C. pneumoniae infection can also be demonstrated by the lymphocyte transformation assay with peripheral blood lymphocytes (117). Lymphocyte transformation activity is associated with the number of organisms shed from the cervix in C. trachomatis infection (118). The role of cellular immunity, however, in resistance against C. pneumoniae is unknown.

C. pneumoniae infection of macrophages results in the production of pro-inflammatory cytokines such as TNF-α, IL-1β, IL-6, and IL-8 as well as expression of CD14 molecules (119,120).

Some immunological diseases have been associated with C. pneumoniae such as sarcoidosis (121,122), erythema nodosum (51,52), and reactive arthritis or Reiter's syndrome (54). The evidence for an association of C. pneumoniae with these diseases is weak. Therefore, whether C. pneumoniae infection induces autoimmune disease is still questionable.

VI. LABORATORY DIAGNOSIS

A. Laboratory diagnosis of *C. trachomatis* infection

1. Cell culture isolation

While cell culture has long been considered the "gold standard" for detection of C. trachomatis, it requires stringent technical expertise and specimen transport conditions which often present a challenge for settings in which neither a cold chain nor a cell culture system can be maintained. The specimen collection method and technique also affect the integrity of the culture; an adequate sample of columnar epithelial cells from the cervix or urethra is necessary for successful isolation. Specimens that contain predominantly polymorphonuclear cells, or are abundant in mucopurulent discharge, do not suffice. Specimens may be collected with a cotton-tipped swab (those with wooden sticks should not be used). In some studies, use of a cytobrush for collection of endocervical specimens has been associated with an increase in culture sensitivity presumably by increasing the amount of endocervical columnar cells that are collected (123). Specimens for culture must be placed in specific transport media, SPG or 2SP (see below under *C. pneumoniae*), and refrigerated. They should be inoculated within 24 hrs. onto cell culture plates that contain any of several cell lines (McCoy cells are most frequently used). After incubation, a direct fluorescent monoclonal antibody (DFA) is generally used to visualize inclusions and elementary bodies that are present (124).

2. Antigen detection assays

While chlamydial culture has been an important research tool, its technical difficulties and high cost have made it impractical for use in public health screening programs. For this reason, non-culture diagnostic tests for *C. trachomatis* have been developed, and many are now commercially available (Table 1) (125). Methodologies which use antigen detection of either chlamydial LPS or MOMP emerged first as a means of detecting EBs in genital specimens. The DFA and enzyme immunoassay (EIA) tests are currently the most widely used of these tests largely because of their relatively low cost, ease of automation, and rapid results (usually within 1-2 days). MOMP-specific monoclonal antibody reagents are employed in the DFA test, while the EIA tests utilize detection of genus-specific LPS antigen. While the latter enhances sensitivity due to the generally high amounts of LPS in clinical specimens, cross-reactivity with other bacterial LPS requires that a confirmatory assay with a blocking antibody be used to rule out false positive EIA results. When applied to either endocervical specimens from women or urethral specimens from symptomatic men, both the DFA and EIA detect 60-85% of infections relative to culture. The performance of the various EIAs, in particular, vary somewhat by individual assay (125). Like most diagnostic tests for *C. trachomatis*, sensitivity of both DFA and EIA tests on urethral speci-

Table 1 Comparative performances of selected diagnostic tests in the detection of *Chlamydia trachomatis*.

Methods of detection	Sensitivity*	Specificity	Detectability level**
Enzyme immunoassay	40-60%	99.5%***	1000-10000
Non-amplified genetic probe	40-65%	99.0%	1000-10000
Direct fluorescent	50-80%	99.8%	50-1000
Cell culture	50-90%	99.9%	10-100
Ligase chain reaction	81-100% (cervix) 69-96% (female urine) 90-96% (male urine)	99.7%	1-10
Polymerase chain reaction	60-92% (cervix) 82-93% (female urine) 87-100% (male urine)	99.6%	1-10

* - relative to expanded gold standard
** - number of elementary bodies; defined using a combination of different test methodologies, including culture, DFA, and PCR or LCR that are directed against a target sequence that is distinct from that used in the routine PCR or LCR assays
*** - specificity using confirmatory assays

mens from asymptomatic men is lower than on specimens from symptomatic men, possibly because the antigenic load as reflected in the number of EBs is about one log lower than in symptomatic individuals (126). Performance of the DFA test is highly operator-dependent; it is optimal when performed by an experienced technician and with careful collection of an adequate specimen (127). In addition to being highly specific (99%), the DFA test also has the advantage of allowing for concurrent assessment of specimen adequacy by permitting observation of the number of columnar epithelial cells on the slide.

3.   DNA probes

The GenProbe assay, which detects but does not amplify chlamydial DNA, was the first commercially-available diagnostic test for *C. trachomatis* which utilizes nucleic acid hybridization. Its performance on endocervical and urethral specimens is similar to that of DFA and is superior to EIAs (125). DFA, EIA, and GenProbe all cost less than culture, and are relatively easy to use when transport or maintenance of specimens at colder temperatures is problematic. The sensitivities of all of these tests, however, remain lower than culture, and when applied to urine or vaginal swabs are unacceptably low (129).

4.   Nucleic acid amplification assays

A major advance in chlamydia diagnostics has been the development of newer automated methods to detect amplified *C. trachomatis* nucleic acids (DNA or RNA), thus termed nucleic acid amplified tests (NAATs). The most widely-used methods are ligase chain reaction (LCR) and polymerase chain reaction (PCR), both of which can be used for cervical, vaginal, urethral, and urine specimens from females, and urine and urethral specimens from men. These tests markedly increase the sensitivity of detection for *C. trachomatis* while maintaining excellent specificity (>99%) (125). LCR and PCR target nucleotide sequences on the *C. trachomatis* plasmid which is present in multiple copies within each elementary body. Transcription-mediated assay (TMA), another NAAT which targets and amplifies chlamydia ribosomal RNA, and a signal nucleic acid hybridization test, which uses signal amplification to increase sensitivity (hybrid-capture), have been developed more recently and appear to have performance characteristics similar to LCR and PCR (130-133). The lower limit of detection of all of these tests is in the range of 1-10 EBs as compared to 10,000 EBs for EIA. Specimens for NAATs are stable during transport, and results can be available within a day.

Since the NAATs were the first chlamydia diagnostic assays that were more sensitive than culture, their evaluation presented new analytic challenges. To define their performance, an alternative gold standard beyond that of cell culture was necessary. Initially, when only one NAAT (LCR) was available, an approach termed 'discrepant analysis' was used. This required confirmation of specimens that were negative by culture but positive by LCR (the test under evaluation). Confirmation was first sought using DFA (which is highly specific in experienced hands) and this was followed by LCR that is directed against a target sequence other than the plasmid DNA (a chromosomal MOMP gene sequence). While this approach has been criticized because only discrepancies are selectively retested, because the test under evaluation plays a role in defining "true positives," and because a variant of the test being evaluated (LCR-plasmid) is used for discrimination (LCR-MOMP), subsequent analyses have shown that the approach provided an accurate estimate of specificity, and that is only modestly increased estimates of sensitivity. Now that additional amplification assays are available, an alternative approach generally being used is to perform several assays on all specimens, thus defining 'true-positives' as those positive in two or more assays.

Using expanded gold standards in multicentre field studies, LCR applied to first-catch urine (FCU; the first 10-30 ml. of stream) has a sensitivity of approximately 90-96% for the detection of chlamydial urethritis in males (133,134) and 69-96% for chlamydial urethritis and/or cervicitis in females (135-137). Sensitivity of LCR which is performed on endocervical specimens has ranged from 81-100% (135,138,139). Compared to the performance of cell culture at all sites, LCR has detected 15-43% more infected patients. LCR performed on endocervical specimens is consistently more sensitive than culture, and its performance on FCU is sensitive enough to provide a means of non-invasive testing for the diagnosis of chlamydial infection of the urethra and the cervix. Most recently, NAATs have been applied to self-collected vaginal swab samples from women. This approach may be as accurate as NA-ATs which are performed on female urine specimens, and may offer the advantage of off-site collection given the more convenient specimen for transport (for example, mailing in swabs for laboratory testing) (140-141).

Among males, the sensitivity of PCR when performed on FCU has generally been good; achieving sensitivities in the range of 87-100% (142-147) and detecting up to ~40% more infections than urethral culture in some studies (144). In at least one study, however, PCR performed on male urine specimens was significantly less sensitive than LCR (133), possibly due to PCR-specific inhibitors present in fresh urine. Among females, PCR performed on FCU has demonstrated a sensitivity of 82-93% (128,144). Particularly in earlier studies, performance of PCR on endocervical specimens has been somewhat more variable with sensitivities ranging from 60-92% (128,144-146). The presence of PCR inhibitors in endocervical mucous is thought to be responsible for much of this variability in PCR sensitivity; in one study, this translated into a reduction of sensitivity by 15% (128). In an in vitro study of urine samples that were spiked with $C.$ $trachomatis$, the performances of PCR, TMA, and LCR were variably inhibited by the presence of hemoglobin, beta-human chorionic gonadotrophin (β-HCG), nitrites, and crystals (148). Inhibition was abrogated either by diluting or freezing the samples before the NAATs were run. The potential effect of these inhibitors in clinical settings has been studied in only a relatively small number of patients, and its importance is unknown. One study suggested that sensitivity of LCR varied with the menstrual cycle (149); another found that PCR sensitivity was significantly reduced in pregnant women (150). For now, no specific recommendations regarding NAATs in these populations exist. While the effect of inhibitors requires further study, it is likely that the overall increase in NAAT sensitivity, coupled with improvements in laboratories' ability to diminish or eliminate inhibitors, will make NAATs ones of choice in all patient populations. The only factors that prevent their more widespread use have been their relatively high cost compared with earlier tests and the low throughput of some assays.

5.   Rapid diagnostic tests for Chlamydia

Due to the failure to successfully inform infected patients about their positive test results or due to the failure to seek treatment even if informed, the ideal diagnostic test for $C.$ $trachomatis$ would be one that could be performed on-site and that could provide immediate results while the patient is in the clinic. While such rapid antigen detection tests are also available, their performance has been disappointing; most have yielded unacceptably low sensitivities relative to culture and their use is discouraged until performance can be improved (151). Newer versions of these tests may prove to be more useful and are under study (152).

6.   Serology

While serological tests for $C.$ $trachomatis$ are available, they are not generally recommended for routine diagnosis of acute genital infection (6). The complement fixation (CF) test recognizes antibodies to the LPS antigen that is common to the genus $Chlamydia$, and thus, it is not species-specific. The CF test is most appropriate when serial measurements are used to assist in the diagnosis of acute psittacosis or LGV, both of which elicit high titres of antibodies. The CF test is not applicable to trachoma biovar infection as it is insensitive. The micro-immunofluorescence (micro-IF) test recognizes antibodies to the $C.$ $trachomatis$ MOMP, is more sensitive than the CF test, and is species-specific. Specific methodologies for performing and interpreting the micro-IF test are given below. It is particularly useful for the diagnosis of neonatal disease due to $C.$ $trachomatis$. Seroconversion occurring in association with genital chlamydial infection other than LGV is variable, and it appears to be dependent on the number and serotype of prior chlamydial infections, degree of systemic infection, timing of specimen collection, and gender (higher titres are seen in women). In women with PID and/or perihepatitis, high antibody titers as measured by micro-IF are generally present and can be useful if an etiology for the clinical syndrome is in question (105).

7. Selection of a diagnostic test

Test performance, cost, considerations of specimen transport and storage, and ease of implementation all contribute to decisions about which diagnostic test to employ in a given clinical or public health setting. In general, the specificities of the available diagnostic tests are high (>99%) so that the likelihood of false-positive tests is low even in low prevalence populations. The NAATs certainly represent the most sensitive assays that are available, but their higher cost makes routine use unattainable in some settings. As noted, a major advantage of the NAATs is their excellent performance on urine specimens and self-collected vaginal swabs which expands the opportunities for innovative approaches to chlamydiae screening in asymptomatic populations. The non-amplified diagnostic test specimens (DFA, EIA, and genetic probe) are stable in transport over varying conditions and results can be obtained quickly, but their sensitivity is low especially for urine specimens. One approach to preserve the low cost of these tests and improve their sensitivity is the use of NAATs to confirm EIA assays that may fall just below the cutoff for positivity (the "negative grey zone" concept). Another approach for cost reduction is the pooling of samples; 4-10 individual urine specimens for NAAT testing. A positive result for the pool mandates that each sample then be tested individually, but a negative test for the pool is reasonably specific in predicting that all specimens that contributed to the pool also represent uninfected specimens (153-155). The optimal number of samples that are pooled depends on the prevalence of chlamydial infection in the population being tested, but generally is between 4-10. While further validation is undertaken, this approach may prove to be especially useful in populations with a low prevalence of chlamydial infection where the benefit of testing many persons to detect relatively fewer infected may not appear to outweigh the cost.

B. Diagnosis of *C. pneumoniae* infection

1. Cell culture isolation

The most sensitive cell lines for isolation are HL (human line) (156,157) and HEp-2 (158,159). Cell lines which are commonly-used for isolation of *C. trachomatis*, such as McCoy and HeLa 229 cells, are not sufficiently sensitive for *C. pneumoniae* culture (160,161). Centrifugation of the inoculum onto cell monolayers and incorporation of cycloheximide into the culture medium to inhibit host cell metabolism are critical to enhance the sensitivity of isolation. After the isolates have been adapted to grow in cell culture and the titres have been increased by serial passages, *C. pneumoniae* can be grown in large culture vessels without centrifugation. The most commonly-used medium for growing *C. pneumoniae* is the Eagles' minimum essential medium which has been supplemented with 10% fetal calf serum. Detection of inclusions in cell cultures is best performed by the use of fluorescein-conjugated *C. pneumoniae*-specific or *Chlamydia* genus-specific (against LPS) monoclonal antibodies. Giemsa staining is less sensitive than detection by immunofluorescence, and the finding of inclusions is difficult due to lack of contrast with stained cells.

Specimens for isolation are usually obtained from swabs of the oropharynx. Tissue samples are homogenized before inoculation. Swab specimens should be placed in chlamydial transport medium, SPG (sucrose, 75 gm.; KH_2PO_4, 0.52 gm.; $NaHPO_4$, 1.22 gm.; glutamic acid, 0.72 gm.; H_2O to 1 L.; pH 7.4-7.6), or 2SP (sucrose, 68.47 gm.; KH_2PO_4, 0.6 gm.; K_2HPO_4 2.83 gm.; H_2O to 1 L.; pH7.4-7.6). Addition of 10% fetal calf serum to the transport medium has been shown to further enhance the stability of chlamydial organisms (162). *C. pneumoniae* organisms are sensitive to temperature and freeze-thawing (160). Therefore, if isolation can be done within 24 hrs. after specimen collection, specimens should be stored in a refrigerator (4°C) without freezing. If isolation cannot be performed within 24 hours, the specimens should be stored for 1-4 hours at 4°C prior to slow freezing below -65°C. For thawing, organisms should be 'quick-thawed' by submerging in lukewarm water (no higher than 37°C).

2. Method of cell culture isolation

Either shell vials or multi-well plates have been used. For shell vial culture, 1-dram glass vial shell (outside diameter, 15 mm.; height, 45 mm.) containing a round cover slip (diameter, 12 mm.) and plugged with a No. 0 non-toxic silicone rubber stopper is seeded with 2 x 10^5 HL or HEp-2 cells. Usually, three vials per specimen are inoculated. The vial is incubated overnight to obtain a confluent cell monolayer. Prior to the inoculation of organism or the clinical specimen, the culture medium is removed and 0.1 ml. of specimen is added. The vials are centrifuged at 900X g for 60 min. at 20 to 25° C. After centrifugation, the inoculum is removed, and 1 ml. of culture medium containing cycloheximide (0.6 µg./ml. for HL cells) is added. The vials are incubated for three days at 35° C. One vial is used for staining with fluorescent antibody (either *C. pneumoniae* species-specific or *Chlamydia* genus-specific monoclonal antibody) and is scanned for chlamydial inclusions under a fluorescent microscope. The cell monolayers of the remaining vials are harvested in chlamydial transport medium SPG by scraping with a Pasteur pipette. The amount of SPG that is used varies, but smaller volumes are desired for successful passage, e.g., 0.5 ml. per 2 vials and 2.5 ml. per 150 cm.² flask. The harvested material is either inoculated into the new culture vials immediately or is frozen at -75° C. The number of vials that can be inoculated are dependent on the infectivity as estimated by inclusion count.

3. Serial passages in cell culture and growth in flask

A detailed description is provided due to the difficulty that laboratories have experienced in growing *C. pneumoniae*. Keys to success in serial passages, so to raise the titre from the first isolation in vial culture to growth in flask culture for large-scale production of organisms, are "slow expansion" and the use of minimum inoculum volume. Infection should be passed every three days using the same number of vials until more than 50% of cells are infected before increasing the number of vials. When high infection frequency is achieved, harvests from 20 to 30 vials should be used to infect a 1-day old cell monolayer in a small size (75 cm.²) flask with the use of a 0.5 ml. inoculum. Inoculation is accomplished by first removing culture medium and then rinsing the cells with Hanks' balanced salt solution (HBSS). Adsorption is carried out at room temperature or in a 35° C incubator for 2 to 2.5 hr. with intermittent rolling of the bottle. No centrifugation is necessary for flask cultures. After adsorption, 80 ml. of culture medium per 150 cm.² size flask is added, and the bottle is incubated for three days at 35° C. Harvest is achieved by discarding the medium and adding sterile 4-mm. diameter glass beads with 10 ml. of HBSS. This results in cell detachment and rupture. The cell suspension is transferred to a 30 ml. centrifuge tube. The bottle is rinsed with HBSS, and the fluid is added to the cell suspension. The cell suspension is sonicated briefly for 20 sec. and is then submitted to one cycle of differential centrifugation (500X g for 10 min. and 30,000X g for 20 min.). The cell pellet is resuspended in SPG and inoculated into fresh cell cultures or stored at –75° C. Passages should be continued in small flasks to raise the titre before going to large flasks (150 cm.²). After titres have increased significantly, the number of infected bottles can be increased as describe above for vial cultures. Titres should be periodically checked at harvest as a guide for expansion. To ensure good infection, cultures should be inoculated with greater than one multiplicity of infection. A culture flask of 150 cm.² surface area (~1 x 10^7 cells) with 100% infection should yield greater than 1 x 10^8 inclusion forming units/ml. per flask after purification.

4. Direct detection

Two methods for direct detection of *C. trachomatis* in clinical specimens, immunofluorescence and EIA, have not proven to be sufficiently sensitive and specific for *C. pneumoniae* (163). Our limited experience with direct fluorescence antibody detection of *C. pneumoniae* EBs in throat smears, using a *C. pneumoniae*-specific monoclonal antibody, showed a sensitivity of 50% (five smears positive from ten culture-positive samples). This is due to small number of EBs contained in swab specimens. Of 30 isolations, 25 (84%) contained fewer than 100 inclusion-forming units.

PCR is a sensitive and specific direct detection method for *C. pneumoniae* (164). It can be performed with swab specimens, bronchoalveolar lavage, sputum, peripheral blood mononuclear cells, and fresh or formalin-fixed and paraffin-embedded tissues. Several *C. pneumoniae*-specific primers have been used in PCR detection of organisms. Primers which have been used for *C. pneumoniae* amplification have been derived from several target genes including a *C. pneumoniae*-specific sequence of polymerized gene (164), 16S rRNA gene sequence (165), and the MOMP gene (166). Currently, there are no commercially-available DNA diagnostic kits for *C. pneumoniae* diagnosis, although such efforts are underway.

5. Sensitivity of detection methods

The sensitivity of cell culture for the diagnosis of acute *C. pneumoniae* respiratory infection is reasonable (approximately 60%). In our studies of serologically confirmed acute respiratory infections, including pneumonia, bronchitis, and pharyngitis, the isolation rates from throat swabs were 24/49 (59%) in students at the University of Washington, Seattle, Washington, and 25/43 (58%) in a military epidemic of *C. pneumoniae* in Kajaani, Finland (167,168). The sensitivity of PCR for the diagnosis of *C. pneumoniae* from throat swabs in the respiratory infection was 18/19 (95%) during the acute stage in patients who were both isolation- and serology- positive and 16/35 (46%) during the chronic stage in patients who were serology-positive but isolation-negative. None of 132 patients who were both isolation- and serology- negative were positive by PCR, thus indicating that PCR is specific.

Isolation of the organism from the chronic stage of infection is much more difficult. Culture is often negative, while PCR may be positive. This is evident from the fact that very few isolates have been obtained from atherosclerotic lesions in the artery, although *C. pneumoniae* is detected by ICC and/or PCR in 50% of samples. The likely reasons for difficulty in the isolation during chronic stages of infection are: 1) infection in the chronic stage involves deeper tissues, such as lung interstitial macrophages, arterial wall macrophages, and smooth muscle cells, 2) titres of the organism are low due to poor growth in these cells and due to immune suppression of multiplication and maturation of the organism, and 3) these sites are often not readily accessible by routine sample collection methods.

6. Serology

The micro-IF test, which was devised in 1970 for *C. trachomatis* (169), is the only sensitive and specific serological assay for any of the chlamydiae and remains the gold standard for the serological diagnosis of *C. pneumoniae* infection. The micro-IF test can distinguish between antibodies in the IgM, IgG, and IgA class. In this test, formalin-fixed purified whole *C. pneumoniae* EBs (or *C. trachomatis*) are used. Use of antigen that is prepared with *C. pneumoniae* which has been isolated from the geographic region where the patient resides has been suggested to be more sensitive for detection of *C. pneumoniae* antibody (170,171). No significant difference, however, in detection between assays that are performed with *C. pneumoniae* isolates from geographically diverse areas has been found (172).

The criteria for the serological diagnosis of *C. pneumoniae* by micro-IF are four-fold titre rises between acute and convalescent samples, IgM titres of ≥1:16, or IgG titres of ≥1:512 for acute antibody; and IgG titres from 1:8 to 1:256 for chronic antibody. The appearance of micro-IF antibody is slow and may take three to four weeks to appear. Therefore, it is recommended that convalescent sera be obtained at 3-4 week intervals in contrast to the conventional two week interval that is typically recommended for other infectious diseases (1). Failure to detect micro-IF antibodies in sera from patients from whom *C. pneumoniae* was isolated may occur (62), but this usually due to the slow antibody response (1). For this reason, a third serum sample that is obtained two months after onset may be useful. Since false-positive micro-IF IgM antibody tests may occur if patients have circulating rheumatoid factor, removal of IgG rheumatoid factor for micro-IF IgM-positive sera is recommended (173).

IgA antibody has been considered to represent chronic *C. pneumoniae* infection by some investigators. Such claims, however, have not been definitively proven. The kinetics of IgA antibody appearance usually mirrors IgG antibody and appears in lower titre and frequency than IgG antibody.

Method of micro-IF serology

The micro-IF test is an indirect fluorescent antibody technique in which serial 2-fold serum dilutions are tested against formalin-fixed (0.02%) purified chlamydial EBs which have been placed on a microscope slide (174). To facilitate the adherence of EBs onto the glass slide, EBs are mixed with 3-5% of formalinized chicken yolk sac membrane homogenates.

Using a guide template that is placed under the slide, 16 antigen dots arranged in 4 x 4 with 5 mm. distances from each other are applied on the slide using a dip pen point. A single slide allows for the testing of eight dilutions of two different sera starting at 1:8 to 1:1024. If more than one chlamydial species or serotype strain are to be tested, different antigens can be dotted next to each other in each of 16 spots in the exact order. The slides are air-dried and then fixed for 15 min. in pure acetone (methanol fixation inactivates reactivity to *C. pneumoniae* species-specific antigen, but not *C. trachomatis* serotype-specific antigen). The fixed slides should be used on the same day in order to obtain the best quality of reaction. Each serial dilution of serum is applied onto separate antigen dots using a bacterial loop from the highest dilution downward. The bacterial loop is then flamed, cooled, and used for applying the next dilution. The slides are incubated in a moist chamber for 30 min. at 37° C, and then subsequently rinsed gently by dipping and draining in four jars of phosphate-buffered saline, followed by three jars of distilled water. After the slides are air-dried, fluorescein-conjugated anti-human antiserum (anti-IgM, IgG, or IgA) which includes a counterstain (rhodamine-conjugated bovine albumin or Evans Blue) is applied with a bacterial loop. The slides are incubated in a moist chamber for 30 min. at 37° C. The washing step is repeated. Finally, the air-dried slides are covered with mounting fluid and a cover slip, and are viewed with epifluorescence microscopy. The antigen dots are first located by low power (10X) and then read at a high power objective (40X). The end-point is defined by the highest dilution giving definite fluorescence. A positive reaction is the sharp crispy fluorescence that is associated with EBs.

Complement fixation test

CF antibody is often positive in primary *C. pneumoniae* infection when a prompt chlamydial CF antibody response is seen (1). In the CF test, a four-fold titre rise or a titre equal to or greater than 1:64 is indicative of acute antibody. *C. pneumoniae* micro-IF IgM antibody appears later, about three weeks after the onset of illness. Antibody in the IgG fraction may not appear until six to eight weeks after onset. In reinfection, CF and IgM antibody may not appear or may appear only at low titres. The IgG antibody titre rises quickly, often in one to two weeks, and may reach a value of 1:512 or more.

EIA serology

EIA serology with whole EB, recombinant protein, or LPS antigens have been used for *C. pneumoniae* serology. The sensitivity and specificity of these EIA tests, however, have not been defined.

C. Diagnosis of *C. psittaci* infection

1. *Cell culture*

Diagnosis is established by isolation of the organism in cell culture. Specimens for isolation include sputum, throat swab, buffy coat of blood, or tissues of the viscera (lung, spleen, and intestine) which have been obtained from necropsy.

2.   Serology

The only available serological test is the CF test as described above. Both acute and convalescent (two or three weeks later) sera should be obtained. Criteria for positive CF tests are seroconversion, a four-fold rise or fall in titres, and high titres without an increase or fall. Serological differentiation of CF-positive sera due to *C. psittaci* rather than *C. pneumoniae* and *C. trachomatis* can be achieved by the micro-IF test. Although strain-specific micro-IF tests are possible for *C. psittaci* using formalin-fixed elementary bodies of common avian psittacosis strains including parrot, turkey, duck, and pigeon strains (S.-P. Wang, personal communication), antigens are not commercially available. EIA using LPS antigen may be used; however, this test cannot differentiate infection from that of *C. pneumoniae* and *C. tra-chomatis*.

Since cell culture and serology are often not available and since the test results are not known early enough to institute the specific therapy, the single most valuable diagnostic clue is a history of exposure to birds, especially parrots or parakeets. Inquiries about contact with pet, wild, and farm birds are especially helpful in making a presumptive diagnosis, because it is important that treatment be initiated as soon as psittacosis is suspected.

VII.   SUSCEPTIBILITY TESTING

A.   Antimicrobial chemotherapy for *C. trachomatis* infection

The unique biology of *C. trachomatis* imposes specific requirements on antibiotic therapy. Since extracellular elementary bodies are metabolically inert and resistant to killing, the intracellular locale of the actively dividing reticulate body requires that an antibiotic with good intracellular penetration be used. The relatively long life cycle of *C. trachomatis* must also be considered, and either a proportionately prolonged course of therapy or an antibiotic with a long half-life must be used. Doxycycline, generally given for seven days, accomplishes these goals, but new alternatives are now available (30). In particular, azithromycin, with a half-life of 5-7 days and excellent intracellular and tissue penetration, offers the advantage of single-dose therapy (31). Its efficacy in the treatment of chlamydial cervical infection and non-gonococcal urethritis is equal to that of doxycycline (31,32). Ofloxacin, a fluoroquinolone that is also active against gonococci and other bacteria, is currently recommended as an alternative therapy; it must, however, be given for a full week. It is contraindicated during pregnancy, lactation, and in individuals less than 16 years of age, and it is costly (30).

Since cure rates of lower genital tract infection are generally considered high in compliant non-pregnant patients who are treated with azithromycin, doxycycline, or ofloxacin, a test of cure is not indicated. In pregnancy, erythromycin given as a 2 gm. daily dose achieves cure in 84-94% of treated women (31-32), but up to one-half of women develop significant gastrointestinal side effects and cannot complete the course of therapy (30). Single-dose azithromycin, while not yet studied extensively, probably achieves a cure of cervical infection in most pregnant women. Although clinically meaningful antimicrobial resistance to tetracyclines, macrolides, and fluoroquinolones has been considered rare among *C. trachomatis* strains tested to date, at least four instances of clinical treatment failure that are associated with drug resistance have recently been reported. Thus, test of cure is indicated where symptoms persist or recur.

B.   Antimicrobial chemotherapy for *C. pneumoniae* infection

Like other chlamydial species, *C. pneumoniae* is susceptible to macrolide and tetracycline antibiotics (61). Since *C. pneumoniae* infection frequently recurs after short or conventional courses of appropriate antibiotics and since persistent infection has been documented by culture even after treatment, intensive long-term treatment is recommended (62). Treatment regimens may include the following: tetracycline

500 mg. four times daily for 14 days; doxycycline 100 mg. twice daily for 14 days; or erythromycin 500 mg. four times daily for 14 days or 250 mg. four times daily for 21 days if the higher dose is not tolerated (1). If symptoms such as cough or malaise persist after one treatment regimen, a second course may be useful. Unless the drug is contraindicated, tetracycline or doxycycline is recommended for the second course.

Clarithromycin and azithromycin are also effective against *C. pneumoniae* (63,64). Since these drugs are associated with fewer gastrointestinal side effects, they are better tolerated than erythromycin. Azithromycin achieves a very high intracellular concentration and has a longer duration of action than clarithromycin which may therefore allow for a shorter course of therapy. The recommended dosages for the treatment of acute respiratory infection are: clarithromycin 250 mg. twice daily for 2 weeks and a single dose of azithromycin 500 mg. on day 1 followed by 250 mg. daily for 2 to 5 days for a total of 5 days therapy (65).

C. Antimicrobial chemotherapy for *C. psittaci* infection

Tetracyclines are the drugs of choice. For successful treatment, it is essential that antibiotic treatment is started early in the disease and is given in high doses for a long period. A dose of 500 mg. every 6 hrs. by mouth or 20 to 40 mg./kg./day for children, for fourteen days, or at least seven days after clinical recovery, is recommended. In severe infections, a longer period of medication may be required. Inadequate treatment may lead to relapse and the establishment of a carrier state. Some patients have responded to erythromycin which may be the first choice in children. Since psittacine birds and some poultry have been fed with tetracyclines for many years, the emergence of tetracycline-resistant strains is a possibility; however, this aspect has not yet been investigated. Some of the newer tetracyclines and macrolides may be effective, but such antibiotics have not been extensively tested in vitro and in vivo against *C. psittaci*.

D. General considerations

Assessment of chlamydiae for resistance to antimicrobials is challenging given the organisms' stringent culture requirements and the fact that most treated persons do not have test of cure cultures obtained. Clinically-evident antimicrobial resistance appears to be rare perhaps because the actively replicating form of the organism is sequestered in an intracellular vacuole and has little genetic interaction with other organisms that have resistance genes. Selection of isolates that are resistant to tetracycline has been demonstrated with successive cell passage in the laboratory setting (175). More recently, three examples of relapsing or persistent chlamydial genital infections that were resistant to multiple antibiotics, including doxycycline, azithromycin, and ofloxacin have been reported (176). Whether such events represent isolated occurrences remains to be seen.

Antibiotic susceptibility testing for chlamydial species has been traditionally performed in cell culture because of the ease of such testing (61,177). After inoculation of cell culture with *C. trachomatis* or *C. pneumoniae*, inoculated cells are incubated with media that contain serial two-fold dilutions of antibiotics. After three days of incubation, inclusion staining is done to determine the infectivity titre (first passage). Unstained parallel cultures are harvested, passed to new cells, and cultured in the absence of the antibiotic (second passage). The minimum inhibitory titre is defined by the dilutions (concentration) of antibiotics at which inclusion formation is completely inhibited. The first passage end-point is traditionally defined as the minimum inhibitory concentration (MIC) and the second passage end-point as the minimum bactericidal concentration (MBC).

For *C. pneumoniae*, pre-clinical antibiotic susceptibility tests are often carried out in mouse models. Mice are susceptible to intranasal inoculation with *C. pneumoniae* and develop pneumonia (178). Inoculated mice are then treated with antibiotics. Antibiotic efficacy is assayed by the detection of *C. pneumoniae* from lung by isolation and PCR (179).

VIII. CONCLUSIONS

Major advances in our understanding of the immunopathology of chlamydial infections and of the development of new diagnostic methods have comprised some of the most exciting work in the field to date.

Due to the extent to which most *C. trachomatis* infections are not associated with clinical signs or symptoms, routine periodic screening of sexually active adults and adolescents continues to be an essential approach to disease control. Further, the demonstration that such routine screening effects declines in chlamydia prevalence over time (30,180,181) and prevents symptomatic pelvic inflammatory disease (182) provides hope that this strategy may evoke long-term benefits for other reproductive health outcomes in women. In fact, such favorable trends are already apparent in countries such as Sweden, where long-active *C. trachomatis* screening programs are closely linked to declines in such events as ectopic pregnancy (183). Integrating this evidence with the new diagnostic tools as described above into innovative approaches to therapy and prevention constitutes a critical challenge to public health and laboratories that are involved in the diagnosis of this common and critical sexually transmitted disease.

The emerging spectrum of diseases that are associated with *C. pneumoniae*, especially cardiovascular disease, underscore the necessity for developing rapid diagnostic methods for early identification of infection.

REFERENCES

1. Kuo C-C, Jackson LA, Campbell LA, Grayston JT. *Chlamydia pneumoniae* (TWAR). Clin Microbiol Rev 1995; 8:451-461.
2. Saikku P, Wang S-P, Kleemola M, Brander E, Rusanen E, Grayston JT. An epidemic of mild pneumonia due to an unusual strain of *Chlamydia psittaci*. J Infect Dis 1985; 151:832-839.
3. Grayston JT, Kuo C-C, Wang S-P, Altman J. A new *Chlamydia psittaci* strain, TWAR, isolated in acute respiratory tract infections. N Engl J Med 1986; 315:161-168.
4. Grayston JT, Kuo C-C, Campbell LA, Wang S-P. *Chlamydia pneumoniae* sp. nov. for *Chlamydia* strain TWAR. Int J Syst Bacteriol 1988; 39:88-90.
5. Meyer KF. Ornithosis and psittacosis. In: Biester HE, Schwarte LH, eds. Diseases of Poultry. Ames, Iowa: Iowa State College Press, 1952:569-618.
6. Stamm WE, Holmes KK. *Chlamydia trachomatis* infections of the adult. In: Holmes KK, Mårdh P-A, Sparling PF, eds. Sexually Transmitted Diseases. New York: McGraw-Hill, 1999:407-422.
7. Beatty WL, Morrison RP, Byrne GI. Persistent chlamydiae: from cell culture to a paradigm for chlamydial pathogenesis. Microbiol Rev 1994; 58:686-699.
8. Stamm WE, Wagner KF, Amsel R, Alexander ER, Turck M, Counts GW, Holmes KK. Causes of the acute urethral syndrome in women. N Engl J Med 1980; 303:409-415.
9. Paavonen J, Kiviat N, Brunham RC, Stevens CE, Kuo CC, Stamm WE, Miettinen A, Soules M, Eschenbach DA, Holmes KK. Prevalence and manifestations of endometritis among women with cervicitis. Am J Obstet Gynecol 1985; 152:280-286.
10. Stamm WE, Guinan ME, Johnson C, Starcher T, Holmes KK, McCormack WM. Effect of treatment regimens for *N. gonorrhoeae* on simultaneous infection with *C. trachomatis*. N Engl J Med 1984; 310:545-549.
11. Schachter J, Grossman M, Sweet RL, Holt J, Jordan C, Bishop E. Prospective study of perinatal transmission of *Chlamydia trachomatis*. JAMA 1986; 255:3374-3377.
12. Weiss SG, Newcomb RW, Beem MO. Pulmonary assessment of children after chlamydial pneumonia of infancy. J Pediatr 1986; 108:659-664.
13. Cates W, Joesoef MR, Goldman MB. Atypical pelvic inflammatory disease: can we identify the clinical predictors? Am J Obstet Gynecol 1993; 169:341-346.
14. Cates W, Rolfs RT, Aral SO. Sexually transmitted diseases, pelvic inflammatory disease, and infertility: an epidemiologic update. Epidemiol Rev 1990; 12:199-220.
15. Cates W, Wasserheit JN. Genital chlamydial infections: epidemiology and reproductive sequelae. Am J Obstet Gynecol 1991; 164:1771-1781.

16. Cumining DC, Honore LH, Scott JZ, Williams KE. Microscopic evidence of silent inflammation in grossly normal fallopian tubes with ectopic pregnancy. Int J Fertil 1988; 33:324-328.
17. Chow JM, Yonekura ML, Richwald GA, Greenland S, Sweet RL, Schachter J. The association between *Chlamydia trachomatis* and ectopic pregnancy. JAMA 1990; 263:3164-167.
18. Marana R, Sanna A, Lucisano A, Dell'Acqua S, Leone F, Mancuso S. High prevalence of silent chlamydia colonization of the tubal mucosa in infertile women. Fertil Steril 1990; 53:354-356.
19. Patton DL, Kuo C-C, Wang S-P, Halbert SA. Distal tubal obstruction induced by repeated *Chlamydia trachomatis* salpingeal infections in pig-tailed macaques. J Infect Dis 1987; 155:1292-1299.
20. Brunham RC, Binns B, McDowell J, Paraskevas M. *Chlamydia trachomatis* infection in women with ectopic pregnancy. Obstet Gynecol 1986; 67:722-726.
21. Hillis SD, Owens LM, Marchbanks PA, Amsterdam LE, MacKenzie WR. Recurrent chlamydial infections increase the risks of hospitalization for ectopic pregnancy and pelvic inflammatory disease. Am J Obstet Gynecol 1997; 176:103-107.
22. van der Laar MJ, van Duynhoven YT, Fennema JS, Ossewaarde JM, van den Brule AJ, van Doornum GJ, Coutinho RA, van den Hoek JA. Differences in clinical manifestations of genital chlamydial infections related to serovars. Genitourin Med 1996; 72:261-265.
23. Dean D, Schachter J, Dawson CR, Stephens RS. Comparison of the major outer membrane protein variant sequence regions of B/Ba isolates: a molecular epidemiologic approach to *Chlamydia trachomatis* infections. J Infect Dis 1992; 166:383-392.
24. Stamm WE, Hicks CB, Martin DH, Leone P, Hook EW, Cooper RH, Cohen RH, Batteiger BE, Workowski K, McCormack WM. Azithromycin for empirical treatment of the nongonococcal urethritis syndrome in men. A randomized double-blind study. JAMA 1995; 274:577-579.
25. Cohen DA, Nsuami M, Etame RB, Tropez-Sims S, Abdalian S, Farley TA, Martin DH. A school-based *Chlamydia* control program using DNA amplification technology. Pediatrics 1998; 101:E1.
26. Marrazzo JM, White CL, Lafferty WE, Krekeler B, Celum CL, Stamm WE, Handsfield HH. Community-based urine screening for *Chlamydia trachomatis* infection by ligase chain reaction. Ann Intern Med 1997; 127:796-803.
27. Beutler AM, Whittum-Hudson JA, Nanagara R, Schumacher HR, Hudson AP. Intracellular location of inapparently infecting *Chlamydia* in synovial tissue from patient with Reiter's syndrome. Immunol Res 1994; 13:163-171.
28. Sieper J, Kingsley G, Palacios-Boix A, Pitzalis C, Treharne J, Hughes R, Keat A, Panayi GS. Synovial T lymphocyte-specific immune response to *Chlamydia trachomatis* in Reiter's disease. Arthritis Rheum 1991; 34:588-598.
29. Amor B. Reiter's syndrome. Diagnosis and clinical features. Rheum Dis Clin North Am 1998; 24:677-695.
30. Centers for Disease Control and Prevention. Sexually transmitted diseases treatment guidelines. MMWR 1998; 47:RR-1.
31. Martin DH, Mroczkowski TF, Dalu ZA, McCarty J, Jones RB, Hopkins SJ, Johnson RB. A controlled trial of a single dose of azithromycin for the treatment of chlamydial urethritis and cervicitis. N Engl J Med 1992; 327:921-925.
32. Brunham RC, Peeling RW. *Chlamydia trachomatis* antigens: role in immunity and pathogenesis. Infect Agents Dis 1994; 3:218-233.
33. Jackson LA, Campbell LA, Schmidt RA, Kuo C-C, Cappuccio AL, Lee MJ, Grayston JT. Specificity of detection of *Chlamydia pneumoniae* in cardiovascular atheroma. Evaluation of the innocent bystander hypothesis. Am J Pathol 1997; 150:1785-1790.
34. Boman J, Soderberg S, Forsberg J, Birgander LS, Allard A, Persson K, Jidell E, Kumlin U, Juto P, Waldenstrom A, Wadell G. High prevalence of *Chlamydia pneumoniae* DNA in peripheral blood mononuclear cells in patients with cardiovascular disease and in middle-aged blood donors. J Infect Dis 1998; 178:274-277.
35. Moazed TC, Kuo C-C, Grayston JT, Campbell LA. Evidence of systemic dissemination of *Chlamydia pneumoniae* via macrophages in the mouse. J Infect Dis1998; 177:1322-1325.
36. Kuo C-C, Campbell LA. Detection of *Chlamydia pneumoniae* in arterial tissues. J Infect Dis 2000; Suppl. (In press)
37. Moazed TC, Kuo C-C, Grayston JT, Campbell LA. Murine models of *Chlamydia pneumoniae* infection and atherosclerosis. J Infect Dis 1997; 175:883-890.
38. Grayston JT. Infections caused by *Chlamydia pneumoniae* strain TWAR. Clin Infect Dis 1992; 15:757-763.

39. Thom DH, Grayston JT, Wang S-P, Kuo C-C, Altman J. *Chlamydia pneumoniae* strain TWAR, *Mycoplasma pneumoniae* and viral infections in acute respiratory disease in a university student health clinic population. Am J Epidemiol 1990; 132:248-256.

40. Kauppinen M, Saikku P, Kujala P, Herva E, Syrjala H. Clinical picture of community-acquired pneumonia requiring hospital treatment: a comparison between chlamydial and pneumococcal pneumonia. Thorax 1996; 51:185-189.

41. Augenbraun MH, Roblin PM, Chirgwin K, Landman D, Hammerschlag MR. Isolation of *Chlamydia pneumoniae* from the lungs of patients injected with the human immunodeficiency virus. J Clin Microbiol 1991; 29:401-402.

42. Gaydos CA, Fowler CL, Gill VJ, Eiden JJ, Quinn TC. Detection of *Chlamydia pneumoniae* by polymerase chain reaction-enzyme immunoassay in an immunocompromised population. Clin Infect Dis 1993; 17:718-723.

43. Cosentini R, Esposito S, Blasi F, Clerici Schoeller M, Pinzani R, Tarsis P, Fagetti L, Arosio C, Principi N, Allegra L. Incidence of *Chlamydia pneumoniae* infection in vertically HIV-1 infected children. Eur J Clin Microbiol Infect Dis 1998; 17:720-723.

44. Comandini UV, Maggi P Santopadre P, Monno R, Angarano G, Vullo V. *Chlamydia pneumoniae* respiratory infections among patients infected with the human immunodeficiency virus. Eur J Clin Microbiol Infect Dis 1997; 16:720-726.

45. Hashiguchi K, Ogawa H, Suzuki T, Kazuyama Y. Isolation of *Chlamydia pneumoniae* from the maxillary sinus of a patient with purulent sinusitis. Clin Infect Dis 1992; 15:570-571.

46. Ogawa H, Hashiguchi K, Kazuyama Y. Recovery of a *Chlamydia pneumoniae* in six patients with otitis media and effusion. J Laryngol Otol 1992; 106:490-492.

47. Marrie TH, Marczy M, Mann OE, Landymore RW, Raza A, Wang S-P, Grayston JT. Culture-negative endocarditis probably due to *Chlamydia pneumoniae*. J Infect Dis 1990; 161:127-129.

48. Michel D, Antoine JC, Pozetto B, Gaudin G, Lucht F. Lumbosacral mengoradiculitis associated with *Chlamydia pneumoniae* infection. J Neurol Neurosurg Psychiatr 1992; 55:511.

49. Hahn DL, Dodge RW, Golubjatnikow R. Association of *C. pneumoniae* (strain TWAR) infection with wheezing, asthmatic bronchitis, and adult-onset asthma. JAMA 1991; 266:225-230.

50. Beaty CD, Grayston JT, Wang S-P, Kuo C-C, Reto RS, Martin TR. *Chlamydia pneumoniae*, strain TWAR, infection in patients with chronic obstructive pulmonary disease. Am Rev Respir Dis 1991; 144:1408-1410.

51. Sundolof B, Gnarpe H, Gnarpe J. An unusual manifestation of *Chlamydia pneumoniae* infection: meningitis, hepatitis, iritis, and atypical erythema nodosum. Scand J Infect Dis 1993; 25:259-261.

52. Erntell M, Ljunggren K, Gadd T, Persson K. Erythema nodosum – a manifestation of *Chlamydia pneumoniae* (strain TWAR) infection. Scand J Infect Dis 1989; 21:693-696.

53. Haidl S, Ivarsson S, Bjerre I, Persson K. Guillain-Barre syndrome after *Chlamydia pneumoniae* infection. N Engl J Med 1992; 326:576-577.

54. Braun J, Laitko S, Treharne J, Eggens U, Wu P, Distler A, Sieper J. *Chlamydia pneumoniae* - a new causative agent of reactive arthritis and undifferentiated oligoarthritis. Ann Rheum Dis 1994; 53:100-105.

55. Balin BJ, G'erard HC, Arking EJ, Appelt DM, Branigan PJ, Abrams JT, Whittum-Hudson JA, Hudson AP. Identification of localization of *Chlamydia pneumoniae* in the Alzheimer's brain. Med Microbiol Immunol Berl 1998; 187:23-42.

56. Sriram S, Stratton CW, Yao SY, Tharp A, Ding L, Bannan JD, Mitchell WM. *Chlamydia pneumoniae* infection of the central nervous system in multiple sclerosis. Ann Neurol 1999; 46:6-14.

57. Grayston JT, KuoC-C, Campbell LA, Wang S-P, Jackson LA. *Chlamydia pneumoniae* and cardiovascular disease. Cardiologia 1997; 42:1145-1151.

58. Danesh J, Collins R, Peto R. Chronic infections and coronary heart disease: Is there a link? Lancet 1997; 350:430-436.

59. Campbell LA, Kuo C-C, Grayston JT. *Chlamydia pneumoniae* and cardiovascular disease. Emerg Infect Dis 1998; 4:571-579.

60. Campbell LA, Moazed TC, Kuo C-C, Grayston JT. Preclinical models for *Chlamydia pneumoniae* and cardiovascular disease: hypercholestemic mice. Clin Microbiol Infect 1998; 4:S23-S32.

61. Kuo C-C, Grayston JT. In vitro drug susceptibility of *Chlamydia* sp. strain TWAR. Antimicrob Agents Chemother 1988; 32:257-258.

62. Hammerschlag MR, Chirgwin K, Roblin PM, Gelling M, Dumornay W, Mandel L, Smith P, Schachter J. Persistent infection with *Chlamydia pneumoniae* following acute respiratory illness. Clin Infect Dis 1992; 14:178-182.

63. Welsh LE, Gaydos CA, Quinn TC. In vitro evaluation of azithromycin, erythromycin, and tetracycline against *Chlamydia trachomatis*, and *Chlamydia pneumoniae*. Antimicrob Agents Chemother 1992; 36:252-253.

64. Hammerschlag MR, Qumei KK, Roblin PM. In vitro activities of azithromycin, l-ofloxacin, and other antibiotics against *Chlamydia pneumoniae*. Antimicrob Agents Chemother 1992; 36:1573-154.

65. Jackson LA, Grayston JT. *Chlamydia pneumoniae*. In: Yu VL, Merigan TC Jr, Barriere SL, eds. Antimicrobial Therapy and Vaccines. Baltimore:Williams & Wilkins, 1999:583-586.

66. Levison DA, Guthrie W, Ward C, Green DM, Roberson PGC. Infective endocarditis as part of psittacosis. Lancet 1971; 2:844-847.

67. Jones RB, Priest JB, Kuo C-C. Subacute chlamydial endocarditis. JAMA 1982; 247:655-658.

68. Lamaury I, Sotto A, Le Quellec A, Perez C, Boussagol B, Ciurana AJ. *Chlamydia psittaci* as a cause of lethal bacterial endocarditis. Clin Infect Dis 1993; 17:821-822.

69. Jannach JR. Myocarditis in infancy with inclusion characteristic of psittacosis. Am J Dis Child 1958; 96:734-740.

70. Meyer KF. The present status of psittacosis - ornithosis. Arch Environ Health 1969; 19:461-466

71. Meyer KF. The host spectrum of psittacosis – lymphogranuloma venereum agents. Am J Ophthalmol 1967; 63:1225-1246.

72. Baker JA. A virus obtained from a pneumonia of cats and its possible relation to the cause of atypical pneumonia in man. Science 1942; 96:475-476.

73. Barwell CF. Laboratory infection of man with virus of enzootic abortion of ewes. Lancet 1955; 2:1369-1371.

74. Barnes MG, Brainered H. Pneumonitis with alveolar capillary block in a cattle rancher exposed to epizootic bovine abortion. N Engl J Med 1964; 271:981-985.

75. Schachter J, Ostler HB, Meyer KF. Human infection with the agent of feline pneumonitis. Lancet 1969; 1:1063-1065.

76. Beer RJ, Bradford WP, Hart RJC. Pregnancy complicated by psittacosis acquired from sheep. BMJ 1982; 284:1156-1157.

77. Kaiser Family Foundation. Sexually transmitted diseases in America: how many and at what cost? Report of the Kaiser Family Foundation, December, 1998.

78. Centers for Disease Control. *Chlamydia trachomatis* genital infections—United States, 1995. MMWR 1997; 46:193-198.

79. Centers for Disease Control. Ten leading nationally notifiable infectious diseases—United States, 1995. MMWR 1996; 45:883-884.

80. Suchland KL, Counts JM, Stamm WE. Laboratory methods for detection of *Chlamydia trachomatis*: survey of laboratories in Washington State. J Clin Microbiol 1997; 35:3210-3214.

81. Wills JM, Watson G, Lusher M, Mair TS, Wood D, Richmond SJ. Characterization of *Chlamydia psittaci* isolated from a horse. Vet Microbiol 1990; 24:11-19.

82. Girjes AA, Hugall A, Graham DM, McCaul TF, Lavin MF. Comparison of type I and type II *Chlamydia psittaci* strains infecting koalas (*Phascolarctos cinereus*). Vet Microbiol 1993; 37:65-83

83. Thenussen HJH, Lemmens-den Toom NA, Burggraaf A, Stolz E, Michel MF. Influence of temperature and relative humidity on the survival of *Chlamydia pneumoniae* in aerosols. Appl Environ Microbiol 1993; 59:2589-93.

84. Falsey AR, Walsh EE. Transmission of *Chlamydia pneumoniae*. J Infect Dis 1993; 168:453-6.

85. Schachter J. Biology of *Chlamydia trachomatis*. In: Holmes KK, Mårdh P-A, Sparling PF, eds. Sexually Transmitted Diseases. New York :McGraw-Hill, 1999:391-406.

86. Hatch TP, Miceli M, Sublett JE. Synthesis of disulfide-bonded membrane proteins during the developmental cycle of *Chlamydia psittaci* and *Chlamydia trachomatis*. J Bacteriol 1986; 165:379-385.

87. Schachter J, Stamm WE. *Chlamydia*. In: Murray PR, Baron EJ, Pfaller MA, Tenover FC, Tolken RH - eds. Manual of Clinical Microbiology. Washington, D.C.:American Society for Microbiology, 1999:795-806.

88. Stamm WE, Tamm MR, Koester M, Cles LD. Detection of *Chlamydia trachomatis* inclusions in McCoy cell cultures with fluorescein-conjugated monoclonal antibodies. J Clin Microbiol 1983; 17:666-668.

89. Wang S-P, Grayston JT. *Chlamydia pneumoniae* elementary body antigenic reactivity with fluorescent antibody is destroyed by methanol. J Clin Microbiol 1991; 29:1539-1541.

90. Chi EY, Kuo C-C, Grayston JT. Unique ultrastructure in the elementary body of *Chlamydia* sp. TWAR. J Bacteriol 1987; 169:3757-3763.

91. Kanamoto Y, Iikima Y, Miyashita N, Matsumoto A, Sakano T. Antigenic characterization of *Chlamydia pneumoniae* isolated in Hiroshima, Japan. Microbiol Immunol 1993; 37:495-498.

92. Perez Melgosa M, Kuo C-C, Campbell LA. Outer membrane complex proteins of *Chlamydia pneumoniae*. FEMS Microbiol Lett 1993; 112:199-204.

93. Shor A, Kuo C-C, Patton DL. Detection of *Chlamydia pneumoniae* in coronary arterial fatty streaks and atheromatous plaques. S Afr Med J 1992; 82:158-161.

94. Grayston JT, Wang S-P, Yeh LJ, Kuo C-C. Importance of reinfection in the pathogenesis of trachoma. Rev Infect Dis 1985; 7:717-725.

95. Brunham RC, MacLean IW, Binns B, Peeling RW. *Chlamydia trachomatis*: its role in tubal infertility. J Infect Dis 1985; 152:1275-1282.

96. Brunham RC, Peeling R, MacLean I, Kosseim ML, Paraskevas M. *Chlamydia trachomatis*-associated ectopic pregnancy: serologic and histologic correlation. J Infect Dis 1992; 165:1076-1081.

97. Hahn DL. *Chlamydia pneumoniae*, asthma, and COPD: what is the evidence? Ann Allergy Asthma Immunol 1999; 83:271-288.

98. Kuo C-C. Pathologic manifestation of chlamydial infection. Am Heart J 1999; 138:S496-S499.

99. Kuo C-C, Campbell LA. Is infection with *Chlamydia pneumoniae* a causative agent in atherosclerosis? Mol Med Today 1998; 4:426-430.

100. Lampe MF, Wong KG, Kuehl LM, Stamm WE. *Chlamydia trachomatis* major outer membrane protein variants escape neutralization by both monoclonal antibodies and human immune sera. Infect Immun 1997; 65:317-319.

101. Witkin SS, Jeremias J, Toth M, Ledger WJ. Cell-mediated immune response to the recombinant 57 kDa heat-shock protein of *Chlamydia trachomatis* in women with salpingitis. J Infect Dis 1993; 167:1379-1383.

102. Morrison RP, Belland RJ, Lyng K, Caldwell HD. Chlamydial disease pathogenesis. The 57 kD chlamydial hypersensitivity antigen is a stress response protein. J Exp Med 1989;170: 1271.

103. Peeling RW, Brunham RC. Chlamydiae as pathogens: new species and new issues. Emerg Infect Dis 1996; 2:307-319.

104. Persson K, Osser S, Birkelund S, Christiansen G, Brade H. Antibodies to *Chlamydia trachomatis* heat shock proteins in women with tubal factor infertility are associated with prior infection by *C. trachomatis* but not by *C. pneumoniae*. Hum Reprod 1999; 14:1969-1973.

105. Chernesky M. Can serology diagnose upper genital tract *Chlamydia trachomatis* infections? Studies on women with pelvic pain, with or without chlamydial plasmid DNA in endometrial biopsy tissue. Sex Transm Dis 1998; 25:14-19.

106. Van Voorhis WC, Barrett LK, Sweeney YT, Kuo C-C, Patton DL. Analysis of lymphocyte phenotype and cytokine activity in the inflammatory infiltrates of the upper genital tract of female macaques infected with *Chlamydia trachomatis*. J Infect Dis 1996; 174:647-650.

107. Levitt D, Berol J. The immunobiology of *Chlamydia*. Immunol Today 1987; 8:246-251.

108. Puolakkainen M, Parker J, Kuo C-C, Grayston JT, Campbell LA. Further characterization of *Chlamydia pneumoniae* specific monoclonal antibodies. Microbiol Immunol 1995; 39:551-554.

109. Campbell LA, Kuo C-C, Wang S-P, Grayston JT. Serological response to *Chlamydia pneumoniae* infection. J Clin Microbiol 1990; 28:1261-1264.

110. Carter MW, al-Mahdawi S, Giles IG, Treharne JD, Ward ME, Clarke IN. Nucleotide sequence and taxonomic value of the major outer membrane protein gene of *Chlamydia pneumoniae* IOL-207. J Gen Microbiol 1991; 137:465-475.

111. Kaltenboeck B, Kousoulas KG, Storz J. Structure of and allelic diversity and relationship among the major outer membrane protein (ompA) genes of the four chlamydial species. J Bacteriol 1993; 175:487-502.

112. Jantos CA, Heck S, Roggendorf R, Sen-Gupta M, Hegemann JH. Antigenic and molecular analyses of different *Chlamydia pneumoniae* strains. J Clin Microbiol 1997; 35:620-623.

113. Gaydos CA, Quinn TC, Bobo D, Eiden JJ. Similarity of *Chlamydia pneumoniae* strains in the variable domain IV region of the major outer membrane protein gene. Infect Immun 1992; 60:5319-5323.

114. Freidank HM, Herr AS, Jacobs E. Identification of *Chlamydia pneumoniae*-specific protein antigens in immunoblots. Eur J Clin Microbiol Infect Dis 1993; 12:947-951.

115. Iijma Y, Miyashita N, Kishimoto T, Kanamoti Y, Soejima R, Matsumoto A. Characterization of *Chlamydia pneumoniae* species-specific proteins immunodominant in humans. J Clin Microbiol 1994; 32:583-588.

116. Kol A, Sukhova GK, Lichtman AH, Libby P. Chlamydial heat shock protein 60 localizes in human atheroma and regulates macrophage tumor necrosis factor-alpha and matrix metalloproteinase expression. Circulation 1998; 98:300-307.

117. Surcel HM, Syrjala H, Leinonen M, Saikku P, Herva E. Cell-mediated immunity to *Chlamydia pneumoniae* measured as lymphocyte blast transformation in vitro. Infect Immun 1993; 61:2196-2199.

118. Brunham RC, Kuo C-C, Cles L, Holmes KK. Correlation of host immune response with quantitative recovery of *Chlamydia trachomatis* from the human endocervix. Infect Immun 1983; 39:1491-1494.
119. Heinemann M, Susa M, Simnacher U, Marre R, Essig A. Growth of *Chlamydia pneumoniae* induces cytokine production and expression of CD14 in a human monocytic cell line. Infect Immun 1996; 64:4872-4887.
120. Molestina RE, Dean D, Ramirez JA, Summersgill JT. Characterization of a strain *Chlamydia pneumoniae* isolated from a coronary atheroma by analysis of the *omp1* gene and biological activity in human endothelial cells. Infect Immun 1998; 66:1360-1376.
121. Black CM, Bullard JC, Staton GW, Jr, Hutwagner LC, Perez RL. Seroprevalence of *Chlamydia pneumoniae* antibodies in patients with pulmonary sarcoidosis in North Central Georgia. In: Mårdh P-A, La Placa M, Ward ME, eds. Proceedings of the European Society for Chlamydial Research. Stockholm:Almquist & Wicksell International, 1992 :175.
122. Grönhagen-Riska C, Saikku P, Riska H, Froseth B, Grayston JT. Antibodies to TWAR-a novel type of *Chlamydia* – in sarcoidosis. In: Grassi C, Rizzato G, Pozzi E, eds. Sarcoidosis and Other Granulomatous Disorders. Amsterdam:Excerpta Medica, 1988:297-391.
123. Moncada J, Schachter J, Shipp M, Bolan G, Wilber J. Cytobrush in collection of cervical specimens for detection of *Chlamydia trachomatis*. J Clin Microbiol 1989; 27:1863-1866.
124. Stamm WE, Tamm MR, Koester M, Cles LD. Detection of *Chlamydia trachomatis* inclusions in McCoy cell cultures with fluorescein-conjugated monoclonal antibodies. J Clin Micro 1983; 17:666-668.
125. Black CM. Current methods of laboratory diagnosis of *Chlamydia trachomatis* infections. Clin Microbiol Rev 1997; 10:160-184.
126. Marrazzo JM, Celum CL, Whittington WL, Krekeler B, Clark A, Cles L, Handsfield HH, Stamm, WE. Optimizing the use of urine ligase chain reaction assay for diagnosing *Chlamydia trachomatis* urethral infection in male STD clinic clients. 9th International Symposium on Human Chlamydial Infection. Napa, CA, June 21-26. 1998:591-594.
127. Stamm WE, Harrison HR, Alexander ER, Cles LD, Spence MR, Quinn TC. Diagnosis of *Chlamydia trachomatis* infection by direct immunofluorescence staining of genital secretions--a multicenter trial. Ann Intern Med 1984; 101:683-641.
128. Pasternack R, Vuorinen P, Kuukankorpi A, Pitkajarvi T, Miettinen A. Detection of CT infections in women by Amplicor PCR: comparison of diagnostic performance with urine and cervical specimens. J Clin Microbiol 1996; 34:995-998.
129. Schwebke JR, Clark AM, Pettinger MB, Nsubga P, Stamm WE. Use of a urine enzyme immunoassay as a diagnostic tool for *Chlamydia trachomatis* urethritis in men. J Clin Microbiol 1991; 29:2446-2449.
130. Pasternack R. Comparison of a transcription-mediated amplification assay and polymerase chain reaction for detection of *Chlamydia trachomatis* in first-void urine. Eur J Clin Microbiol Infect Dis 1999; 18:142-144.
131. Stary A. Performance of transcription-mediated amplification and ligase chain reaction assays for detection of chlamydial infection in urogenital samples obtained by invasive and noninvasive methods. J Clin Microbiol 1998; 36:2666-2670.
132. Girdner JL, Cullen AP, Salama TG, He L, Lorincz A, Quinn TC. Evaluation of the digene hybrid capture II CT-ID test for detection of *Chlamydia trachomatis* in endocervical specimens. J Clin Microbiol 1999; 37:1579-1581.
133. Stary A, Tomazic-Allen S, Choueiri B, Burczak J, Steyrer K, Lee H. Comparison of DNA amplification methods for the detection of *Chlamydia trachomatis* in first-void urine from asymptomatic military recruits. Sex Transm Dis 1996; 23:97-102.
134. Chernesky MA, Jang D, Lee H, Hu H, Sellors J, Tomazic-Allen SJ, Mahony JB. Diagnosis of *Chlamydia trachomatis* infections in men and women by testing first-void urine by ligase chain reaction. J Clin Microbiol 1994; 32:2682-2685.
135. Ridgway GL, Mumtaz G, Robinson AJ, Franchini M, Carder C, Burczak J, Lee H. Comparison of the ligase chain reaction with cell culture for the diagnosis of *Chlamydia trachomatis* infection in women. J Clin Pathol 1996; 49:116-119.
136. Schachter J, Moncada J, Whidden R, Shaw H, Bolan G, Burczak JD, Lee HH. Noninvasive tests for diagnosis of *Chlamydia trachomatis* infection: application of ligase chain reaction to first-catch urine specimens of women. J Infect Dis 1995; 172:1411-1414.
137. Lee H H, Chernesky MA, Schachter J, Burczak JD, Andrews WW, Muldoon S, Leckie G, Stamm WE. Diagnosis of *Chlamydia trachomatis* genitourinary infection in women by ligase chain reaction assay of urine. Lancet 1995; 345:213-216.

138. Rumpianesi F, Donati M, Negosanti M, D'Antuono A, LaPlaca M, Cevenini R. Detection of *Chlamydia trachomatis* by a ligase chain reaction amplification method. Sex Transm Dis 1996; 23:177-180.

139. Schachter J, Stamm WE, Quinn TC, Andrews WW, Burczak JD, Lee H. Ligase chain reaction to detect *Chlamydia trachomatis* infection of the cervix. J Clin Microbiol 1994; 32:2540-2543.

140. Domeika M, Bassiri M, Butrimiene I, Venalis A, Ranceva J, Vasjanova V. Evaluation of vaginal introital sampling as an alternative approach for the detection of genital *Chlamydia trachomatis* infection in women. Acta Obstet Gynecol Scand 1999; 78:131-136.

141. Polaneczky M. Use of self-collected vaginal specimens for detection of *Chlamydia trachomatis* infection. Obstet Gynecol 1998; 91:375-378.

142. Mahony JB, Luinstra KE, Sellors JW, Jang D, Chernesky MA. Confirmatory polymerase chain reaction testing for *Chlamydia trachomatis* in first void urine from asymptomatic and symptomatic men. J Clin Microbiol 1992; 30:2241-2245.

143. Bauwens JE, Clark AM, Loeffelholz MJ, Herman SA, Stamm WE. Diagnosis of *Chlamydia trachomatis* urethritis in men by polymerase chain reaction assay of first-catch urine. J Clin Microbiol 1993; 31:3013-3016.

144. Quinn TC, Welsh L, Lentz A, Crotchfelt K, Zenilman J, Newhall J, Gaydos C. Diagnosis by AMPLICOR PCR of *Chlamydia trachomatis* in urine samples from women and men attending sexually transmitted disease clinics. J Clin Microbiol 1996; 4:1401-1406.

145. Toye B, Peeling RW, Jessamine P, Claman P, Gemmill I. Diagnosis of *Chlamydia trachomatis* infections in asymptomatic men and women by PCR assay. J Clin Microbiol 1996; 34:1396-400.

146. Bianchi A, Scieux C, Brunat N, Vexiau D, Kermanach M, Pezin P, Janier M, Morel P, Lagrange PH. An evaluation of the polymerase chain reaction amplicor *Chlamydia trachomatis* in male urine and female urogenital specimens. Sex Transm Dis 1994; 21:196-200.

147. Bauwens JE, Clark AM, Stamm WE. Diagnosis of *Chlamydia trachomatis* endocervical infections by a commercial polymerase chain reaction assay. J Clin Microbiol 1993; 31:3023-3029.

148. Mahony J, Chong S, Jang D, Luinstra K, Faught M, Dalby D, Sellors J, Chernesky M. Urine specimens from pregnant and nonpregnant women inhibitory to amplification of *Chlamydia trachomatis* nucleic acid by PCR, ligase chain reaction, and transcription-mediated amplification: identification of urinary substances associated with inhibition and removal of inhibitory activity. J Clin Microbiol 1998; 36:3122-3126.

149. Horner PJ, Crowley T, Leece J Hughes A, Smith GD, Caul EO. *Chlamydia trachomatis* detection and the menstrual cycle. Lancet 1998; 351:341-342.

150. Jensen IP, Thorsen P, Moller BR. Sensitivity of ligase chain reaction assay of urine from pregnant women for *Chlamydia trachomatis*. Lancet 1997; 349:329-330.

151. Kluytmans JAJW, Goessens WHF, Mouton JW, van Rijsoort-Vos JH, Niesters HGM, Quint WGV, Habbema L, Stolz E, Wagenvoort JHT. Evaluation of Clearview and Magic Lite tests, polymerase chain reaction, and cell culture for detection of *Chlamydia trachomatis* in urogenital specimens. J Clin Microbiol 1994; 31:3204-3210.

152. Pate MS, Dixon PB, Hardy K, Crosby M, Hook EW 3rd. Evaluation of the Biostar Chlamydia OIA assay with specimens from women attending a sexually transmitted disease clinic. J Clin Microbiol 1998; 36:2183-2186.

153. Kacena KA, Quinn SB, Howell R, Madico GE, Quinn TC, Gaydos CA. Pooling urine samples for ligase chain reaction screening for genital *Chlamydia trachomatis* infection in asymptomatic women. J Clin Microbiol 1998; 36:481-485.

154. Peeling RW. Pooling of urine specimens for PCR testing: a cost saving strategy for *Chlamydia trachomatis* control programmes. Sex Transm Dis 1998; 74:66-70.

155. Clark AM, Marrazzo JM, Krekler B, Handsfield HH, Stamm WE. Use of pooled LCR specimens for chlamydia screening. Abstracts of the Thirteenth Meeting of the Intl Soc for STD Research, July 1999, Denver CO; p 33, #019.

156. Cles LD, Stamm WE. Use of HL cells for improved isolation and passage of *Chlamydia pneumoniae*. J Clin Microbiol 1990; 28:938-940.

157. Kuo C-C, Grayston JT. A sensitive cell line, HL cells, for isolation and propagation of *Chlamydia pneumoniae* strain TWAR. J Infect Dis 1990; 162:755-758.

158. Wong KH, Skelton SK, Chan YK. Efficient culture of *Chlamydia pneumoniae* with cell lines derived from the human respiratory tract. J Clin Microbiol 1992; 30:1625-1630.

159. Roblin PM, Dumornay W, Hammerschlag MR. Use of Hep-2 cells for improved isolation and passage of *Chlamydia pneumoniae*. J Clin Microbiol 1992; 30:1968-1971.

160. Kuo C-C, Grayston JT. Factors affecting viability and growth in HeLa 229 cells of *Chlamydia* sp. strain TWAR. J Clin Microbiol 1988; 26:812-815.

161. Kuo C-C. *Chlamydia pneumoniae*: Culture methods. In: Allegra L, Blasi F, eds. *Chlamydia pneumoniae*. Milano: Springer, 1999:9-15.

162. Maass M, Dalhoff K. Transport and storage conditions for cultural recovery of *Chlamydia pneumoniae*. J Clin Microbiol 1995; 33:1793-1796.

163. Kuo C-C. Culture and rapid methods in diagnosis of *Chlamydia pneumoniae* infections. In: Vaheri V, Tilton RC, Balows A, eds. Rapid Methods and Automation in Microbiology and Immunology. Berlin:Springer-Verlag, 1991:299-304.

164. Campbell LA, Melgosa MP, Hamilton DJ, Kuo C-C, Grayston JT. Detection of *Chlamydia pneumoniae* by polymerase chain reaction. J Clin Microbiol 1992; 30:434-439.

165. Gaydos CA, Quinn TC, Eiden JJ. Identification of the 16S rRNA gene. J Clin Microbiol 1992; 30:796-800.

166. Holland SM, Gaydos CA, Quinn TC. Detection and differentiation of *Chlamydia trachomatis*, *Chlamydia psittaci* and *Chlamydia pneumoniae* by DNA amplification. J Infect Dis 1990; 162:984-987.

167. Grayston JT, Aldous MB, Easton A, Wang S-P, Kuo C-C, Campbell LA, Altman J. Evidence that *Chlamydia pneumoniae* causes pneumonia and bronchitis. J Infect Dis 1993; 168:1231-1235.

168. Ekman MR, Grayston JT, Visakorpi R, Kleemola M, Kuo C-C, Saikku P. An epidemic of infections due to *Chlamydia pneumoniae* in military conscripts. Clin Infect Dis 1993; 17:420-425.

169. Wang S-P, Grayston JT. Immunologic relationship between genital TRIC lymphogranuloma venereum, and related organisms in a new microtiter indirect immunofluorescence test. Am J Ophthalmol 1970; 70:367-334.

170. Hukki-Immonen O, Leinonen M, Saikku P. Diagnosis of *Chlamydia pneumoniae* by microimmunofluorescence using Kajaani-6 (local epidemic) and TW-183 strains as antigens. In: Mard PA, La Placa M, Ward M, eds. Proceedings of the European Society for *Chlamydia* Research. The University of Uppsala, Uppsala, Sweden, 1992:183.

171. Black CM, Johnson JE, Farsh CE, Brown TM, Berdal BP. Antigen variation among strains of *Chlamydia pneumoniae*. J Clin Microbiol 1991; 25:1312-1316.

172. Wang S-P, Grayston JT. The similarity of *Chlamydia pneumoniae* (TWAR) isolates as antigen in the micro-immunofluroescence (MIF) test. In: Orfila J, Byrne GL, Chernesky MA, Grayston JT, Jones RP, Ridgeway GL, Saikku P, Schachter J, Stamm WE, Stephens RE, eds. Chlamydial Infections. Bologna, Italy:Societa Editrice Esculapio, 1994:549-552.

173. Verkooyen RP, Hazenberg MA, van Haasen GH, van den Bosch JM, Snijder RJ, van Helden HP, Verbrugh HA. Age-related interference with *Chlamydia pneumoniae* microimmunofluorescence serology due to circulating rheumatoid factor. J Clin Microbiol 1992; 30:1289-1290.

174. Wang SP. Serology for *Chlamydia pneumoniae*. In: Allegra L, Blasi F, eds. *Chlamydia pneumoniae*. Milan: Springer-Verlag, 1999:16-23.

175. Jones RB, Van der Pol B, Martin DH, Shepard MK. Partial characterization of *Chlamydia trachomatis* isolates resistant to multiple antibiotics. J Infect Dis 1990; 162:1309-1315.

176. Black CM, Somani J, Bhullar V, Farshy C, Workowski K. Multiple drug resistant *Chlamydia trachomatis* associated with clinical treatment failure. Thirteenth Meeting of the Intl Soc for STD Research, July 1999, Denver CO; p 56, abstract #065.

177. Kuo C-C, Wang S-P, Grayston JT. Antimicrobial activity of several antibiotics and a sulfonamide against *Chlamydia trachomatis* organisms in cell culture. Antimicrob Agents Chemother 1977; 12:80-83.

178. Yang ZP, Kuo C-C, Grayston JT. A mouse model of *Chlamydia pneumoniae*, strain TWAR pneumonitis. Infect Immun 1993; 61:2037-2040.

179. Malinverni R, Kuo C-C, Campbell LA, Lee A, Grayston JT. Experimental *Chlamydia pneumoniae* (TWAR) pneumonitis: effect of two antibiotic regimens on the cause and persistence of infection. Antimicrob Agents Chemother 1995; 39:45-49.

180. Addiss DG, Vaughn ML, Ludka D, Pfister J, Davis JP. Decreased prevalence of *Chlamydia trachomatis* infection associated with a selective screening program in family planning clinics in Wisconsin. Sex Transm Dis 1993; 20:28-35.

181. Katz BP, Blythe MJ, Van der Pol B, Jones RB. Declining prevalence of chlamydial infection among inflammatory disease by screening for cervical chlamydia infection. N Engl J Med 1996; 334:1362-1366.

182. Scholes D, Stergachis A, Heidrich FE, Andrilla H, Holmes KK, Stamm WE. Prevention of pelvic inflammatory disease by screening for cervical chlamydia infection. N Engl J Med 1996; 334:1362-1366.

183. Egger M, Low N, Smith GD, Lindblom B, Herrmann B. Screening for chlamydial infections and the risk of ectopic pregnancy in a county in Sweden: ecological analysis. BMJ 1998; 316:1776-1780.

28

Rickettsioses (with Q Fever)

Jean-Marc Rolain and Didier Raoult
Unité des Rickettsies, Faculté de Médecine, Université de la Méditerranée, Marseille, France

I. HISTORICAL BACKGROUND

Members of the family *Rickettsiaceae* are fastidious bacteria and obligate intracellular parasites. Rickettsial species are arthropod-associated bacteria which are capable of infecting vertebrates, including human beings. The order *Rickettsiales* has been divided historically into three families: *Rickettsiaceae, Bartonellaceae,* and *Anaplasmataceae.* The family *Rickettsiaceae* was divided into three tribes: *Rickettsieae, Ehrlichieae,* and *Wolbachieae,* and the tribe *Rickettsieae* has long been composed of the genera *Coxiella, Rickettsia,* and *Rochalimaea.* Phylogeny and taxonomy of rickettsiae have been studied in recent years by the introduction of new phylogenetic tools. DNA sequence analysis of 16S rRNA, citrate synthase, *rOmp*A, and *rOmp*B genes have delineated the phylogeny among rickettsial species (1-8) (Figure 1). *Coxiella burnetii,* the agent of Q fever, has been removed from the order *Rickettsiales* and replaced in the γ subgroup of *Proteobacteria,* whereas *Rickettsia* belongs to the α1 subgroup (9). Moreover, the genus *Rochalimea* has been unified to the genus *Bartonella,* removed from the order *Rickettsiales,* and replaced with *Brucella* spp. in the α2 subgroup of *Proteobacteria* (10). The *Rickettsieae* tribe now comprises only the genus *Rickettsia* which was subdivided into three subgroups: the typhus group (TG), the spotted fever group (SFG), and the scrub typhus group (STG) (Table 1). *Rickettsia tsutsugamushi,* the only member of the STG, has been recently reclassified in a new genus and is now named *Orientia tsutsugamushi* (11). The TG includes *R. prowazekii,* the agent of epidemic typhus, and *R. typhi,* the agent of murine typhus. Among the SFG, the six previously described SFG rickettsioses are Rocky Mountain Spotted Fever (RMSF) caused by *R. rickettsii,* Mediterranean Spotted Fever (MSF) caused by *R. conorii,* Siberian tick typhus caused by *R. sibirica,* Israeli spotted fever caused by *R. conorii* serotype israeli, Queensland tick typhus caused by *R. australis,* and rickettsialpox caused by *R. akari.* Since1984, six new SFG rickettsioses were described: Japanese spotted fever caused by *R. japonica* described in 1984 (12), Flinders Island spotted fever caused by *R. honei* described in 1991 (13), Astrakhan fever caused by *R. conorii* serotype astrakhan reported in 1991 (14), African tick-bite fever caused by *R. africae* described in 1992 (15), a new spotted fever due to "*Rickettsia mongolotimonae*" reported in 1996 (16,17) in France, and very recently *R. slovaca* isolated in our laboratory in a tick from a patient (18).

Until recently, species in the genus *Ehrlichia* were classified by morphological and epidemiological features. Molecular analysis of the 16S rRNA forms the basis for the current classification of the genus. The genus is now subdivided in three clades currently designated *E. canis* genogroup, *E. phago-*

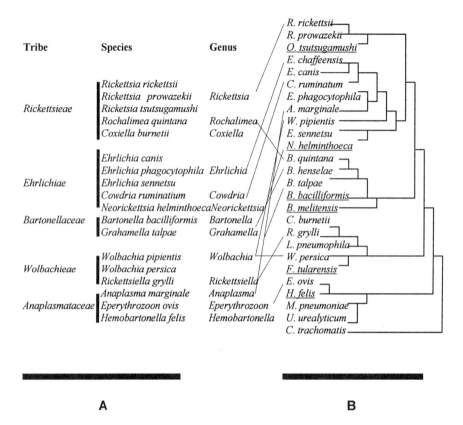

Figure 1 Classification of the *Rickettsia*. (A) The left portion illustrates a classification which is based on extractions from Bergey's Manual (100) while the right portion (B) represents a compilation of the literature for the phylogenetic tree which is based on 16S rRNA.

cytophila genogroup, and *E. sennetsu* genogroup (Figure 2). The species currently known to cause human infections include *E. chaffeensis* (19,20) in the *E. canis* genogroup, the HGE agent which is closely related to or identical with *E. equi* and *E. phagocytophila* in the *E. phagocytophila* genogroup (21), and *E. sennetsu* in the *E. sennetsu* genogroup (22).

II. CLINICAL ASPECTS

A. *Rickettsia*

The majority of human rickettsioses are diagnosed clinically with the support of a careful physical examination and epidemiological investigation. Clinically, the existence of a consistent rash often remains critical for the diagnosis, and typically the patient also presents with high fever (39 to 40°C) and headache. The symptoms and signs of rickettioses as currently recognized are summarized in Table 2.

1. Epidemic typhus

Epidemic typhus is caused by *R. prowazekii* which is transmitted by the body louse. Humans who con-

Table 1 Features of *Rickettsia* species as classified in the spotted fever group that are pathogenic for humans, the spotted fever group that are never isolated in humans, the typhus group, and the genus *Orientia*.

Species	Disease	Arthropod Vector	Distribution
Spotted fever group (human pathogens)			
R. conorii sensu stricto	Mediterranean spotted fever	*Rhipicephalus sanguineus*	Mediterrean countries, Africa, Black Sea, India
R. conorii complex	Israeli spotted fever	*Rhipicephalus sanguineus*	Israel
R. conorii complex	Astrakhan	*Rhipicephalus pumilo*	Astrakhan
R. rickettsii	RMSF	*Dermacentor variabilis* *Dermacentor andersonii* *Rhipicephalus sanguineus* *Amblyomma cajennense*	North America
R. sibirica	Siberian tick typhus	*Dermacentor nuttalli* *Dermacentor marginatus* *Haemophysalis concinna*	northern China, Pakistan, former USSR (asiatic republics, Siberia, Armenia)
R. akari	Rickettsialpox	*Allodermanyssus sanguineus*	Korea, Ukraine, United States, Slovenia
R. africae	African tick-bite fever	*Amblyomma haebraeum*	southern Africa
R. australis	Queensland tick typhus	*Ixodes holocyclus*	Australia (Queensland)
R. japonica	Japanese tick typhus	*Haemophysalis longicornis* *Dermacentor taiwanensis*	Japan (south-west)
R. honei	Flinders Island tick typhus	unknown	Flinders Island (Tasmania)
R. "mongolotimonae"	spotted fever	*Hyalomma asiaticum*	Mongolia, France
R. slovaca	spotted fever	*Dermacentor marginatus*	Slovakia, Armenia, Russia, France, Switzerland, Portugal
R. helvetica	spotted fever	*Ixodes ricinus*	Switzerland, France
Spotted fever group (not isolated from humans)			
R. massiliae		*Rhipicephalus turanicus* *Rhipicephalus sanguineus* other *Rhipicephalus* spp.	France, Greece, Spain, Portugal, central Africa
R. rhipicephali		*Rhipicephalus sanguineus*	United States, France. Portugal, central Africa
R. parkeri		*Amblyomma maculatum*	United States
R. montana		*Dermacentor variabilis*	United States
R. bellii		*Dermacentor* spp.	United States
"R. aeschlimani"		*Hyalomma marginatum*	Morocco
strain S		*Rhipicephalus sanguineus*	Armenia
"R. amblyommii"		*Amblyomma americanum*	United States
JC 880 (Pakistan) *"R. hulini"*		*Rhipicephalus sanguineus*	Pakistan
"R. heilongjiangi"		*Haemaphysalis concinna*	China
Thai tick typhus rickettsia		*Ixodes/Rhipicephalus* pool	Thailand
AB bacterium		*Adalia bipunctata* (Ladybird beetle)	England, Russia, United States

Table 1 cont'd.

	Species	Disease	Arthropod Vector	Distribution
Typhus group				
	R. prowazekii	epidemic typhus, recrudescent typhus (Brill-Zinsser disease)	*Pediculus humanus corporis*	worldwide (most in highlands of South America, Asia, Africa)
	R. typhi	murine typhus	*Xenopsylla cheopsis*	worldwide
Scrub typhus				
	O. tsutsugamushi	scrub typhus	*Leptotrombidium deliense*	east Asia, northern Australia, western Pacific Islands

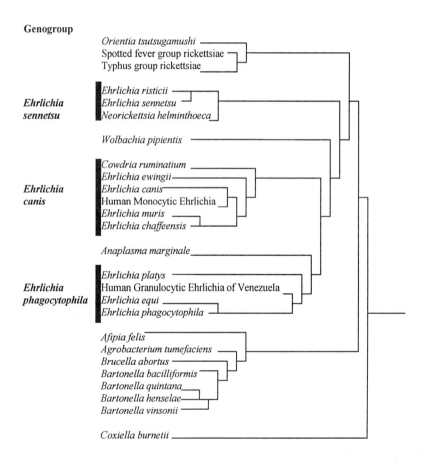

Figure 2   Classification of the genus *Ehrlichia* which is based on 16S rRNA.

Table 2   Clinical symptoms of currently recognized rickettsioses.

Disease	Agent	Rash (%)	Rash (%) specificity	Eschar (%)	Multiple eschars	Local nodes	Mortality (%)
RMSF	*R. rickettsii*	90	purpuric (45)	rare	no	no	1-5
MSF	*R. conorii*	97	purpuric (10)	72	very rare	rare	1
Astrakhan spotted fever	*R. conorii* complex	100	none	23	no	no	no
Israeli spotted fever	*R. conorii* complex	100	rarely purpuric	no	no	no	<1
Rickettsialpox	*R. akari*	100	vesicular	83	yes	yes	low
Queensland tick typhus	*R. australis*	100	vesicular	65	no	yes	low
Flinders Island spotted fever	*R. honei*	85	purpuric (8)	28	no	yes	low
Japanese spotted fever	*R. japonica*	100	none	48	no	no	low
African tick bite fever	*R. africae*	30	vesicular	100	yes	yes	very low
Siberian tick bite fever	*R. sibirica*	100	none	77	no	yes	low
Un-named spotted fevers	*R. slovaca*	?	?	yes	no	yes	no
	R. mongolotimonae	yes	?	yes	no	yes	no
	R. helvetica	?	?	?	no	no	yes
Epidemic typhus	*R. prowazekii*	40	purpuric	no	no	no	2-30
Murine typhus	*R. typhi*	50	none	no	no	no	low
Scrub typhus	*O. tsutsugamushi*	50	none	yes	no	yes	2-5

tract typhus and survive will maintain rickettsiae for the rest of their lives and become the reservoir of the disease. Under certain conditions, they may relapse and have a mild form of typhus: the Brill-Zinsser disease. Body lice may be infected by feeding on humans and subsequently initiate a new out-break of epidemic typhus. The disease is usually severe, and patients suffer from high fever, headaches, and severe myalgias. Five to ten days after the onset of symptoms, a rash appears which can become purpuric. Eschar is absent. Cough and pneumonia are often observed. Mortality rate may vary from 2 to 30% of patients if the disease is misdiagnosed. With specific antibiotic therapy, patients become afebrile within forty-eight hours, and the outcome is generally good.

2.   Murine typhus

Murine typhus is caused by *R. typhi* and is transmitted by the rat flea *Xenopsylla cheopis* (23). For this reason, the disease is probably more prevalent in tropical countries. Clinical manifestations of murine typhus are similar to those of epidemic typhus except that the disease is generally less severe (24). The rash is non- specific and is lacking in nearly 50%. The diagnosis is uncommonly made.

3.   Spotted fever group rickettsiosis

Clinical manifestations of SFG rickettsioses are summarized in Table 2. Since all organ systems are affected by rickettsial infections, patients may have common but non-specific clinical manifestations. Signs and symptoms vary and depend on the particular disease and with the respective species. Moreover, clinical presentation may vary among individual patients who are infected with the same microorganism. Patients generally suffer from fever, headache, myalgias and a rash. The quality and distribution of the rash may help to distinguish rickettsial diseases. Conjunctivitis and pharyngitis are common; malaise, anorexia, nausea, vomiting, diarrhea, or cough are noted in some patients. Pneumonia and central nervous system complications can be observed in a small percentage of patients. Thrombocytopenia and elevations in circulating liver enzymes are common.

B.   *Ehrlichia* (Table 3)

1.   Human monocytic ehrlichiosis (HME)

E. chaffeensis is the causative agent of HME and was first described in 1986. The patient had a severe febrile illness and was found to have Giemsa-stained inclusions among monocytes in a blood smear (25). Clinical manifestations of the disease may vary from asymptomatic to severe, and symptoms are similar to those of RMSF: patients typically present with high fever, headache, chills, malaise, and myalgia. Some patients may have gastrointestinal manifestations (nausea, vomiting, or diarrhea), respiratory illness (cough), or central nervous system involvement. Rash occurs in only one-third, and the lack of rash may help to distinguish ehrlichiosis from RMSF. Laboratory findings include thrombocytopenia (72%), anemia (about 50%), leukopenia (about 70%) with lymphopenia and neutropenia, and elevated serum transaminases (85%) (26). The case fatality rate is about 2-5%.

2.   Human granulocytic ehrlichiosis (HGE)

The etiological agent of HGE is closely related to the veterinary pathogens *E. phagocytophila* and *E. equi*, and has recently been described in a patient who was bitten by ticks in Wisconsin where *E. chaffeensis* and its tick vector were absent. Clinical manifestations of HGE are similar to those of ehrlichiosis due to *E. chaffeensis* but are generally more severe. Patients often present with thrombocytopenia and leukopenia. Severe opportunistic infections may occur.

3.   Sennetsu fever

Sennetsu fever is a mononucleosis-like illness due to *E. sennetsu* that has been discovered in Japan. Patients develop a self-limited febrile illness with malaise, anorexia, and lymphadenopathy. Laboratory findings include early leukopenia and atypical lymphocytes in the peripheral blood. No fatalities or severe complications have been reported.

C.   *Coxiella burnetii*

C. burnetii is the etiological agent of Q fever, a worldwide zoonosis, which may occur either in an acute or chronic form.

1.   Acute infection

The incubation period is approximately three weeks, and clinical signs are often subclinical or extremely mild, and include fever, chills, headache, fatigue, and myalgias. There is typically three distinct clinical presentations of acute Q fever: a self-limited flu-like syndrome, pneumonia, or hepatitis. The type of clinical presentation appears to vary from region to region; in Nova Scotia (Canada), Switzerland, and the Basque county (Spain), pneumonia is the main clinical presentation, whereas hepatitis

Table 3   Main clinical and epidemiological characteristics of human ehrlichiosis.

Characteristics	Sennetsu fever	Human monocytic ehrlichiosis	Human granulocytic ehrlichiosis
Etiological agent	*E. sennetsu*	*E. chaffeensis*	HGE/*E. equi*/ *E. phagocytophila*
Vector	grey mulet fish	*A. americanum*	*Ixodes* spp.
Reservoir	not known	white-tailed deer	small mammals
Geographical distribution	Japan	USA	USA, Europe
Tick bite	no	yes	yes
Fever	+++	+++	+++
Rash	--	++ (child)	?
Headaches	+	+	+++
Myalgia	+	+	++
Arthralgia	+/--	+/--	++
Sweats	+/--	+/--	++
Adenopathy	+++	++	+/--
Hepatomegaly	++	+	+/--
Splenomegaly	++	+	+/--
Meningitis	?	++	+
AST/ALT increase	+++	+++	+++
LDH increase	?	?	+++
Thrombocytopenia	+/--	++	+++
Leucopenia	+	+++	+++
Anemia	+/--	+/--	++
Positive blood smears	no	very rare	yes (80% of cases)
Target cells	monocytes/ macrophages	monocytes/ macrophages	neutrophils
Serological assay	yes	yes	yes
Doxycycline	effective	effective	effective

represents the major form in California, France, Andalusia (Spain), and Australia. Many other clinical manifestations of acute Q fever may occur but are uncommon: aseptic meningitis and/or encephalitis, hemophagocytosis, gastroenteritis, pancreatitis, lymphadenopathy mimicking lymphoma, erythema nodosum, bone marrow necrosis, hemolytic anemia, and splenic rupture.

2.   Chronic infection

Approximately 1% of patients develop chronic Q fever months to years following the initial infection. The main clinical presentation of the chronic form is represented by acute or subacute culture-negative endocarditis, but infection of vascular grafts or aneurysms, hepatitis, osteomyelitis, and prolonged fever have been described. Endocarditis occurs usually in patients with previous valvular damage or in immunocompromised patients. Symptoms are non-specific, and the diagnosis is often delayed for 12 to 24 months; this delay may contribute to increase the mortality rate.

3.   Q fever during pregnancy

Acute or chronic forms of Q fever have been reported in pregnant women. Most of the infections are asymptomatic, but complications may occur such as fetal death, placentitis, or thrombocytopenia.

III. EPIDEMIOLOGY OF INFECTION

A. *Rickettsia*

Classically, six spotted fever group rickettsiae were recognized as human pathogens and were characterized by distinct geographical distribution area: *R. rickettsii, R. conorii, R. sibirica, R. australis, R.
japonica,* and *R. akari* (27). Over recent years, several other rickettsiae have been described following
the dramatic evolution of new detection and identification techniques that have been provided by molecular biology.

 R. rickettsii is the major pathogenic strain in the New World, whereas *R. conorii* is the main
spotted fever agent in the Mediterranean area, in the Middle East, and the Far East, and is transmitted by
the brown dog tick, *Rhipicephalus sanguineus.* Another rickettsia, the agent of Israeli spotted fever is
transmitted by the same tick species in Israel and in Southern Europe (Sicilia, Portugal) (28). In the past
few years, novel rickettsial sero- and geno-types of unknown pathogenicity have been described in the
Mediterranean area, namely *R. massiliae, R. rhipicephali,* and the Mtu5 strain (29,30). Two main serotypes seemed to occupy distinct geographical regions in the centre of Europe. *R. helvetica,* isolated from
Ixodes ricinus ticks in Switzerland, is widely distributed in that country (31), and has been subsequently
found in several other European countries (France, Portugal, and the former Soviet Union) (31-33); it
has been touted as an agent of sudden death. Another pathogenic rickettsia of the Old World is *R.
sibirica,* the agent of North Asian tick typhus (or Siberian tick typhus). Its geographical distribution
spreads from the European to the Asian part of the former USSR and crosses the Chinese border (17). A
similar pathogen, isolated from *R. pumilio* ticks in the Astrakhan region, is the newly recognized agent
of Astrakhan spotted fever (34). In Asia, *R. japonica* is a human pathogen confined to the southern islands of Japan (12,35). There are at least two human pathogenic rickettsiae on the African continent, *R.
conorii* and *R. africae* (36). The vector of *R. africae* is *Amblyomma variegatum* which has a wide distribution in Africa; it has been hypothesized that *R. africae* is probably the most important rickettsial
pathogen in the world. In Australia, *R. australis* is the agent of Queensland tick typhus and is transmitted by the bite of *Ixodes holocyclus* ticks. More recently, a new rickettsial pathogen called *R. honei* has
been isolated from patients in the Flinders islands in Tasmania (13,37). The vectors of the disease are
not known. Cases of rickettsialpox have been reported from the United States and the former USSR
where the disease is transmitted by the bite of different mite vectors.

 Rickettsiae of the SFG are tick-borne organisms which infect and multiply in almost all the organs of their invertebrate hosts. When the ovaries and oocytes of an adult female are infected, rickettsiae may be infected transovarially to at least some of its offspring. Once an egg is infected, all the following life stages of the tick will be infected. Rickettsiae which infect the tick's salivary glands can be
transmitted to vertebrate hosts during feeding. Ticks represent the main reservoir for rickettsiae, but the
role of vertebrate hosts in maintaining zoonotic foci is of great importance.

 The geographic distribution of SFG rickettsiae is very wide, although reliable data on the frequency of the diseases that they cause are very fragmentary, especially in developing countries. Such
diseases are often undiagnosed because their clinical signs are usually non-specific. Moreover, the distinct epidemiological features of each SFG rickettsiosis result in different prevalences being reported
from almost each endemic area. Data may be collected in one endemic focus, or even in a small area,
and it is difficult therefore to compare these data. Moreover, serological data should be interpreted cautiously because there is extensive serological cross-reactions between rickettsial species (38). A widespread and increased incidence of spotted fever illnesses has been reported from different Mediterranean countries (40,41). The mortality of MSF in France has been estimated at 2% in patients who are
admitted to hospital (42), whereas it may be as high as 5% for RMSF in some regions of the United
States.

B. *Ehrlichia*

Sennetsu fever or glandular fever from Japan remains an enigma in terms of origin and means of transmission. Though convincing evidence is lacking, it has been suggested that the consumption of raw grey mulet fish may be the source (43).

Human monocytic ehrlichiosis is caused by *E. chaffeensis* (19). Most patients (85%) with monocytic ehrlichiosis report having been bitten by a tick within the three weeks preceding the onset of the illness (26). The tick that is responsible for transmission is *A. americanum* which is found widely across regions of the south central and southeastern United States where HME occurs (22,44). This tick has never been identified in Europe, Asia, and Africa, explaining the absence of this disease on these continents. A reservoir for *E. chaffeensis* is the white-tail deer (*Odocoileus virginianus*) (45). The rural habitat and outdoor activities in a sylvan environment are important exposure factors for the infection. Human monocytic ehrlichiosis has been diagnosed in more than 400 patients in the USA since its discovery in 1986. Most of the infections are diagnosed between May and July (46). The frequency of the disease is greater in certain states than that of RMSF (47). Geographical distribution of the disease is modelled on the geographical distribution of RMSF. No case of HME has been documented outside of the United States. Some cases, which have been reported in Europe or in Africa (48,49), were diagnosed only with serological evidence, and thus interpretation should be made cautiously due to the potential for cross-reactions. Mortality occurs in 2-3% (50,51).

The etiological agent of human granulocytic ehrlichiosis, called HGE agent, was first identified in the tick *Ixodes scapularis* (52)and has proven to be distinct from *E. chaffeensis* (21). This tick is also the main vector for *Borrelia burgdorferi*, the agent of Lyme disease. In Wisconsin and Minnesota, about 10% of the *Ixodes* spp. ticks are infected by HGE agent and some with both HGE and *B. burgdorferi* (22). The HGE agent has been detected in 2% of *Ixodes ricinus* in France (53), and we suppose that this tick would be the vector of *B. burgdorferi* and HGE in Europe. A recent report has shown that among 41 patients suffering from HGE, 61% have been in contact with animals, 90% have been exposed to ticks before the onset of the disease, and 43% were bitten by the buck tick. In North America, HGE has been reported in Wisconsin, Minnesota, Maryland (54), New York (55), Connecticut (56), Massachussets (57), and California (58). In Europe, serological evidence for the presence of HGE has been reported in Switzerland (59) (the latter where 17% of patients with antibodies that are directed against Lyme disease also have antibodies against HGE), the United Kingdom (60), Italy, Norway (61), and recently in Slovenia (62). The peak frequency of disease is bimodal with an initial prominence between May and July (68% of the diagnoses), and a second peak between October and December (22). The major reservoir for infection appears to be small mammals, especially the white-footed mouse (*Peromyscus leucopus*) in the eastern United States (63).

C. *Coxiella burnetii*

Q fever is a worldwide zoonosis. The reservoirs include mammals, birds, and arthropods (mainly ticks). The most commonly identified sources of human infection are cattle, goats, and sheep. Cats are probably a major reservoir in urban areas and may be the source of urban outbreaks (64,65). A wide variety of small animals have been suspected to be important reservoirs (66,67). Bacteria can be excreted by these mammals in urine, feces, milk, and especially birth products (68,69). Indeed, high concentrations of *C. burnetii* (of up to 10^9 bacteria per gm. of tissue) are found in the placentas of infected animals (70). Moreover, *C. burnetii* survives for long periods in the environment probably because the organism can resist physical agents and due to its capacity of sporulation (71,72).

Humans are infected by inhalation of contaminated aerosols from amniotic fluid, placenta, or contaminated wool. Moreover, Q fever is an occupational hazard, and thus, individuals who are in contact with farm animals and laboratory personnel have the greatest risk of being contaminated. Consumption of raw milk or unpasteurized dairy products could be a source of infection (73,74). Sexual transmission of Q fever has been demonstrated in mice (75) and has been suspected in humans (76).

Sporadic cases of Q fever can occur via transplacental transmission, human-to-human transmission following contact with an infected parturient woman, via intradermal inoculation, or via blood transfusion. *C. burnetii* may persist asymptomatically in humans throughout life and may be reactivated under certain circumstances, e.g., pregnancy or AIDS.

In Europe, acute Q fever is a seasonal disease which occurs mainly in spring and early summer, and is usually a benign illness. Men are more frequently infected than women. Mortality is usually low, varying from 1 to 11% of patients with chronic Q fever (77). In Southern France, 5 to 8% of endocardities are due to *C. burnetii*, and the prevalence of acute Q fever in the southeast is 50 per 100,000 inhabitants (74). Outbreaks of acute Q fever have been reported in Spain (78), Switzerland (79), Great Britain (80), Canada, Germany (81), and southern France (82).

IV. NATURE OF THE BACTERIUM AND PATHOGENESIS

A. *Rickettsia*

Bacteria of the order *Rickettsiales* were first described as short Gram negative bacillary microorganisms that retain basic fuchsin when stained by the method of Gimenez and grow in association with eukaryotic cells. They are short, rod-shaped, or coccobacillary organisms, usually 0.8 to 2 μm long and 0.3 to 0.5 μm in diameter. Rickettsiae are strict intracellular parasites, requiring host cells in which to replicate. These bacteria lie exclusively intracellularly, although not enclosed by a vacuole (83-85). SFG rickettsiae can be observed in the nuclei of host cells, perhaps because they are able to move within the cell by means of actin polymerization (83,85,86). TG rickettsiae are observed exclusively in the cytoplasm (85,86). Rickettsial genome sizes are small (1 to 1.6 Mb) and consist of a single circular chromosome (6,87,88).

Optimal temperature of growth in cell culture is 32°C for the SFG rickettsiae, and 35°C for the TG rickettsiae and *O. tsutsugamushi*. The cytopathic effects of the SFG rickettsiae occur rapidly and are prominent, leading to the formation of large plaques in culture, whereas the cytopathic effects of the TG rickettsiae are less prominent.

Antigenic properties of rickettsiae had initially been studied for taxonomic purposes and subsequently to determine antigens with protective immunity. SFG rickettsiae may be differentiated on the basis of their distinct migration patterns after polyacrylamide gel electrophoresis (89,90). Protein profiles of rickettsiae are characterized by different components: the high molecular weight species-specific proteins (rOmpA and rOmpB) and the lipopolysaccharide-like fragments (LPS) (91,92). The electrophoretic mobilities of these outer membrane proteins are different from one strain to another, whereas the LPSs have rather common features in all SFG rickettsiae. Immunological reactions of laboratory animals and humans are mainly directed against the LPS fractions (93,94), which explains the existence of cross-reacting antibodies in their sera, but mice have a specific response to the proteins which facilitates use for serotyping (95).

B. *Ehrlichia*

Ehrlichia species are obligate intracellular bacteria that infect phagocytic bone marrow-derived cells in mammalian hosts (22,44). These organisms are small (0.2-2 μ in diameter) coccobacillary Gram negative bacteria that display a variety of shapes (96). In vertebrate hosts, the ehrlichiae are found in membrane-lined vacuoles in the cytoplasm of leucocytes. Some species have a marked tropism for monocytes and others for granulocytes. This tropism is reflected in the names of the diseases that are associated with the organisms. Vacuoles which contain ehrlichieae do not fuse with lysosomes (97). The classical morula that is observed by light microscopy is an aggregate of organisms (the microcolony may comprise as few as 3 to as many as 50 or more bacteria). The inhibition of lysosomal fusion is not a generalized process in infected cells but rather is restricted to vesicles that contain *Ehrlichia* species (96,97).

C. *Coxiella burnetii*

C. burnetii is a short (0.3 to 1 μm.), pleomorphic rod that possesses a membrane similar to that of Gram negative bacteria, but it is usually not stainable by the Gram technique. The organism shares characteristics with bacteria in the genus *Rickettsia*, including a small genome (98), staining by the Gimenez method (99), strict intracellular growth in eukaryotic cells, and an association with arthropods (100). Another major characteristic of *C. burnetii* is its antigenic variation, called phase variation, which is similar to the smooth-rough variation in the family *Enterobacteriaceae*. Phase variation is related mainly to mutational variation in the lipopolysaccharide (LPS) (101-103). Phase I is the natural phase which is found in infected animals, arthropods, or humans, and is very infectious (a single bacterium may infect a human). In contrast, phase II is not very infectious and is obtained only in laboratories after serial passages in cell cultures or embryonated egg cultures. As compared to phase I, phase II displays a truncated LPS and lacks some protein cell surface determinants (104). *C. burnetii* possesses a G+C content of 43% (105). It has a sporulation-like process which confers resistance to harsh environmental conditions (106), achieves passive entry into host cells by phagocytosis, and survives in phagolysosomes where a low pH (pH 4.5) is necessary for its metabolism (107,108).

    C. burnetii expresses a low degree of genetic heterogeneity among strains. Genetic variability among different *C. burnetii* strains, however, as demonstrated by different RFLP-based genomic groups (109), specific plasmid regions (110), and LPS variation (101,111) has been reported. These variations were initially thought to be associated with virulence of these bacteria. Nevertheless, recent investigations suggest that predisposing host factors are more important than genomic strain variation in the diseases among humans (112,113). Moreover, recent data shows that genetic variation has an apparently closer connection with the geographical source of the isolate than with the clinical presentation.

V. IMMUNOLOGY OF INFECTION

C. burnetii possesses several properties that makes this bacterium unique in terms of resistance to the immune system and therefore pathogenicity. This is a strict intracellular bacterium which survives and multiplies in the phagolysosomes of host cells, which are generally mononuclear cells of the immune system. The attachment of *C. burnetii* to human monocytes occurs through a complex which is made up of LEI integrin and the IAP protein (108). The ineffectiveness of macrophages against *C. burnetii* is recognized. Immunocompromised patients develop chronic Q fever more frequently, however, which suggests that cellular immunity plays an important role for the control of infection. The hypotheses which are forwarded to explain this decrease in cellular immunity are multiple: decrease in the synthesis of Th1 lymphokines, impairment of antigenic presentation, and induction of suppressive factors. Production of interferon gamma is observed during acute Q fever but not in chronic Q fever (114). Moreover, increased production of interleukin 10 is correlated with an increased frequency of relapses (115).

    Species of the genus *Rickettsia* reach the circulation after cutaneous or conjunctival inoculation. Via blood, rickettsiae enter their host cells, the endothelial cells, through surface proteins and phospholipase activity (116-118). After penetration by induced phagocytosis, rickettsiae escape from the phagosome and multiply in the cytoplasm of the host cell. Rickettsiae of the SFG can also invade the nucleus of the cell. Patients infected with *R. conorii* have endothelial cells which contain rickettsiae (119). Increased levels of von Willebrand factor and thrombomodulin are released by damaged endothelial cells (120). Antibodies are not protective in SFG and TG rickettsiosis. TNF alpha is increased in the acute phase of MSF (121).

    Ehrlichia species are able to multiply in the phagosome of their host cells by inhibiting the phagolysosomal fusion (97,122). Histopathological studies of HME show the presence of widespread perivascular lymphohistiocytic infiltrates without true vasculitis, widespread increase in tissue infiltration with mononuclear phagocytes including non-caseating granulomas in bone marrow and liver, occasional hepatocellular apoptoses that are not associated with direct ehrlichia infection, and infrequent necrosis of spleen or lymph nodes (123). The pathology of HGE is not well-documented. It is suggested that *Ehrlichia*-induced immune dysfunction in humans is similar to that which is observed with infection of ruminants by *E. phagocytophila*; there are resulting opportunistic infections, low CD4 and CD8 lymphocyte blood counts, decreased T cell lymphoproliferative responses to mitogens, and defective neutrophil emigration and phagocytic activity (22,44).

VI. LABORATORY DIAGNOSIS (Figure 3)

Due to the non-specific clinical manifestations of rickettsial diseases, laboratory testing is necessary to confirm the diagnosis. Several techniques have been developed and evaluated, but serological testing remains the best way to diagnose rickettsial diseases because of the relative ease and simplicity. New culture methods (124), however, have led to the isolation of new strains over recent years. Laboratory methods which have been developed in recent years include immunostaining of biopsy specimens or circulating endothelial cells, isolation on shell vial cell cultures, and PCR amplification of rickettsial DNA.

A. Specimen collection

Several samples can be used for the diagnosis of rickettsiosis: blood, biopsy specimens, and arthropods. These specimens should be collected as early as possible in the course of the illness.

1. Blood

Blood can be obtained either in citrated tubes for the culture (leukocytic cell buffy coat) or in EDTA-anticoagulated tubes for PCR diagnosis. EDTA anticoagulant should be avoided for culture because it leads to detachment of the eukaryotic cell monolayer from coverslips; the best anticoagulant for an optimal yield is sodium citrate. Blood should be obtained before antimicrobial therapy. Heparinized blood can also be used for immunocytologic detection of circulating endothelial cells that contain rickettsiae (124-126). If inoculation of cell culture or the PCR assay must be delayed for more than 24 hours, plasma, buffy coat, or whole blood should be frozen at -70°C or in liquid nitrogen. Microscopic examination of Giemsa-stained blood smears provides the most rapid assessment, and it is most readily available, but it requires careful examination and experience which are important determinants for the detection of the specific inclusions (123).

  For serological diagnosis, blood samples should be collected early in the course of the disease and a second sample should be obtained after 1 or 2 weeks. If a four-fold rise in antibody titre has not occurred, a third serum sample may be useful. Serum samples can be preserved at -20°C or lower for long periods without degradation of the antibody. The use of serum samples which are dried on blotting paper is an inexpensive and convenient method for collecting, storing, and transporting blood samples for serologic studies (127).

2. Biopsy specimens

Biopsy specimens from skin lesions before antimicrobial therapy (especially a spot or the margin of an eschar) should be collected as soon as possible (128,129). Other clinical samples which are obtained at autopsy can be assessed in the same manner as skin biopsies (130,131). Cardiac valve and vascular aneurysm/graft are particularly useful for the diagnosis of endocarditis due to *C. burnetii*. Cerebrospinal fluid, bone marrow, bone biopsy, liver biopsy, milk, placenta, and post-abortal fetal specimens are also suitable for the diagnosis of rickettsiosis (132-134).

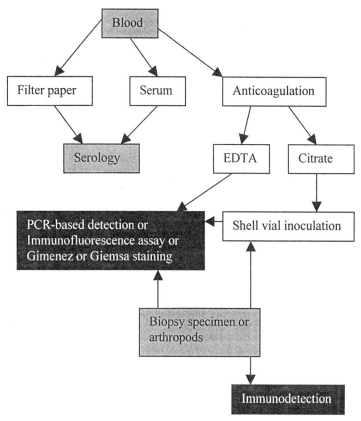

Figure 3 Practical strategies for the laboratory diagnosis of rickettsioses.

3. Arthropods

Rickettsiae can be detected and isolated in various arthropods including ticks, lice, and fleas. Ticks may be frozen (135). The hemolymph assessment should be performed while the tick remains alive (136). The distal portion of one leg is amputated to allow the collection of a hemolymph droplet which can then be spread onto a slide and then subjected to either Gimenez staining or immunodetection. The tick should then undergo surface disinfection with iodinated alcohol, crushed in medium, and inoculated onto a shell vial (135). Culture, PCR-based detection, and immunodetection methods may also be applied to ticks, fleas, and lice (31,137). Specimen collection of arthropods can be made easily (conserved dried in a box) and sent by mail to a reference laboratory for analysis.

B. Culture (Table 4)

The main characteristics of laboratory cultures for the diagnosis of rickettsiosis are summarized in Table 4. The isolation of rickettsiae must be carried out strictly in biosafety level 3 laboratories due to the high potential for infectivity. These microorganisms can be isolated by the inoculation of specimens onto conventional cell cultures (Vero, HEL, MRC5, L929, DH82, or HL60 cells) (see Table 4) or into embryonated hen yolk sacs (138,139) or laboratory animals such as mice or guinea pigs (140-142). Inoculation into animals remains helpful in situations that require isolation of the organism from postmortem tissues which are usually contaminated with other bacteria. We have also used this technique in order to remove contaminating mycoplasmas from cell cultures for rickettsia (143) and also for microsporidia (144). Cell cultures are now the most widely used method for the isolation of rickettsiae from clinical samples. *R. rickettsii* had been first isolated in vitro using a primary monocyte culture (145,147). Later, an L929 mouse fibroblast cell monolayer in tube culture was introduced for the isolation of *R. rickettsii* and *O. tsutsugamushi* from blood (125,148). More recently, the shell vial assay, developed for cytomegalovirus culture and early antigen detection, was adapted to the isolation of *R. conorii* with detection of the microorganism being possible in 48 to 72 hr. in most cases (124). The small surface area (1 cm.^{2}) of the coverslip that contains the cells enhances the ratio of the numbers of rickettsiae to the numbers of cells and allows for better recovery. Vero or L929 cells have been shown to be better than HEL or MRC5 for the isolation of rickettsiae (135). Nevertheless, HEL or MRC5 present an advantage in that once a monolayer is established, contact inhibition prevents further division, and the cells can then be used for prolonged incubation. The shell vial assay is performed routinely in triplicate in our laboratory for the isolation of rickettsiae from heparinized blood (leukocytic cell buffy coat), skin biopsy samples before antibiotic therapy, or arthropods (34,124,126,134,149). Specimens are inoculated onto human embryonic lung fibroblasts which are grown on a 1 cm.^{2} coverslip within a shell vial. The 1 hr. centrifugation step after inoculation of the shell vial is critical for the sensitivity of the technique, because it enhances rickettsial attachment and penetration of cells (124,150). For the culture of ehrlichiae, HL60 cells are used for the HGE agent, whereas DH82 cells are used for the diagnosis of HME. Detection of rickettsiae within the cells can be acccomplished by microscopic examination after Gimenez staining, immunofluorescence, or PCR. After twenty days, if immunofluorescence is negative, the culture is considered negative. If it is positive, parallel shell vials are inoculated onto confluent monolayers of HEL cells in culture flasks in an attempt to obtain isolates of *Rickettsia* spp. Isolation of rickettsiae is of greatest importance since the ultimate goal in rickettsial disease description is to isolate the bacteria from a tick or a patient. (134). In our laboratory, we systematically amplify shell vial supernatatants by PCR. Better results are obtained for the isolation of bacteria if specimens are collected prior to the initiation of antimicrobial therapy (133).

Table 4 Salient features of diagnostic laboratory culture for the rickettsioses.

Organism	Samples	Cell system	Incubation time	Growth detection	Reference
C. burnetii	blood, CSF, cardiac valve, vascular aneurysm or graft, biospsy specimens, milk, placenta, post-abortal specimens	HEL (shell vial)	5-7 days at 37°C in a 5% CO_2 atmosphere PCR	Gimenez staining IF staining	292,293
Rickettsia spp.	blood, plasma, necropsy tissue, skin biopsy, arthropods	HEL, L929, or MRC5 (shell vials)	2 wks. for SFGR (examination each week); 3 wks. for TGR (examination each 10 days)	Gimenez IF staining PCR	197,294
HGE agent *E. chaffeensis*	blood	HL60 DH82	>30 days	Diff-Quick Giemsa staining IF assay	22,44

C. Serological assays (Tables 5 and 6)

1. Microimmunofluorescence (MIF) assay

The most currently used serological test is the microimmunofluorescence assay (MIF). The test is reliable but does not always allow for differentiation of infection among SFG rickettsiae (16). The MIF is a very advantageous method because it can simultaneously detect antibodies to a number of rickettsial antigens in the same assay. Both IgM and IgG can be detected by the MIF. For the detection of IgM antibodies, the use of a rheumatoid factor absorbent before IgM determination is necessary because the assay is affected by rheumatoid factor. Non-specific fixation of antibodies can be avoided by diluting

Table 5   Serodiagnosis of rickettsial diseases: advantages and drawbacks.

Technique	Indications	Advantages	Drawbacks	Comments	References
Weil-Felix	*Rickettsia*	inexpensive	lacks sensitivity and specificity	should only be used for diagnosis of acute illnesses where resources are minimal	172,175
CF test	*Rickettsia* *C. burnetii*	highly specific	lacks sensitivity early in disease	used only for seroepidemiological studies	176
Indirect hemagglutination	*Rickettsia*	sensitive, specific, early detectable antibodies	low antibody titres in late convalescence	for the diagnosis of acute illnesses	181,182
Latex agglutination	*Rickettsia*	simple, no expensive equipment required, commercially available	kit costs	for non-equipped laboratories	183
ELISA	*Rickettsia* *C. burnetii*	specific, sensitive		for both acute cases and seroepidemiology	187-189
MIF assay	*Rickettsia* *C. burnetii* *Ehrlichia*	sensitive, specific, commercially available	need fluorescence microscopy	reference method, for both acute cases and seroepidemiology	16,153, 295,296
Line blot	*Rickettsia*	sensitive, specific, large numbers of antigens simultaneously assessed	no quantitative titres	large scale screening for seroepidemiology	166,167
Western blot	*Rickettsia* *C. burnetii* *Ehrlichia*	most sensitive and specific serological test, earliest detectable antibodies	time-consuming	probably best tool for studies of seroepidemiology	170,171, 297,298

Table 6 Cut-off proposal for the diagnosis of rickettsial diseases with the use of the microimmuno-fluorescence assay and an interpretation of serological results.

Bacteria	Antibody titres			Interpretation
Rickettsia spp.	IgG $\geq$1:128 and IgM$\geq$1:64			spotted fever group or typhus group rickettsiosis (100% predictive)
E. chaffeensis HGE agent	IgG $>$1:128 IgG $\geq$1:80			human monocytic ehrlichiosis human granulocytic ehrlichiosis
C. burnetii	phase II titre IgG $\geq$1:200	IgM $\geq$1:50	phase I titre (IgG) $>$1:800 $>$1:1600	acute Q fever (100% predictive) chronic Q fever (98% predictive) chronic Q fever (100% predictive)

sera in phosphate-buffered saline (PBS) with 3% powdered skim milk. IgM antibodies are usually detected at the end of the first week after onset of the illness, whereas IgG antibodies appear at the end of the second week (151-153).

The MIF is currently the reference method for the serodiagnosis of Q fever (154,155), human rickettsiosis, and human ehrlichiosis (156) because it is the most simple and one of the most accurate serological techniques. For the diagnosis of RMSF, sensitivity was 100% after thirty days of onset (152). A titre of $\geq$ 1:64 had a specificity of 100% and a sensitivity of 84.6%, and a titre of $\geq$ 1:32 had a specificity of 99.8% and a sensitivity of 97.4% (157). For the diagnosis of MSF, titres of $\geq$ 1:128 for IgG and 1:32 for IgM are required (158).

For the serodiagnosis of Q fever, two types of antigens are prepared for the MIF assay: phase II antigens of *C. burnetii* Nine Mile reference strain are obtained from confluent layers of L929 mouse fibroblasts, whereas phase I antigens are obtained from the spleens of mice that were infected with phase II organisms (159). In our laboratory, we use a microimmunofluorescence technique which requires very small amounts of antigens. Sera are diluted in PBS with 3% powdered skim milk to avoid the nonspecific fixation of antibody. This method can be used to determine antibodies to phase I and II in the IgG, IgM, and IgA isotypes. We use a rheumatoid factor absorbent in order to remove IgG before the determination of IgM and IgA (159). The choice of a cut-off value depends on the source and purity of the antigen and the amount of background antigen stimulation in the population to be studied. We define our cut-off value as the dilution at which less than 2% of the control population is positive. We use a 1:50 dilution as our screening dilution, achieved with anti-phase II anti-immunoglobulins. Positive sera are then serially diluted and tested for the presence of anti-phase I and II IgG, IgM, and IgA. Seroconversion is usually detected 7 to 30 days after the onset of clinical symptoms, and about 90% of infected patients will have detectable antibodies within the third week. The antigenic variation of *C. burnetii* is very useful for the differentiation of acute and chronic Q fever. In acute Q fever, antibodies to phase II antigens predominate, and their titres are higher than the phase I antibody titres. Conversely, in chronic forms of the disease such as endocarditis, elevated anti-phase I antibodies are uniformly detected. As cut-off values in the IFA, Tissot-Dupont et al. recommend titres of anti-phase II IgG of $\geq$1:200 and titres of anti-phase II IgM of $\geq$1:50 for the diagnosis of acute Q fever, and titres of anti-phase I IgG $\geq$1:800 for the diagnosis of chronic Q fever (159). We showed recently that an anti-phase I IgG titer of $\geq$1:800 was diagnostic of Q fever in a patient with endocarditis, and thus, we have modified the Duke criteria for the diagnosis of Q fever endocarditis to include one positive blood culture for *C.*

burnetii and a phase I IgG titre of ≥1:800 as a major criterion for the diagnosis of Q fever endocarditis (160). In acute Q fever, IFA titers reach their maximum levels 4 to 8 weeks after the onset of symptoms, and they decrease gradually over the following 12 months (80). IgM titres during acute Q fever declined to undetectable levels after 10 to 17 weeks (154,161).

The persistence of high levels of anti-phase I antibodies, despite appropriate therapy, or the reappearance of such antibodies, should raise suspicion of possible chronic Q fever. Patients with valvular or vascular abnormalities, those who are immunodeficient, and pregnant women should have repeated *C. burnetii* serology if they have a medical history of acute Q fever. In the case of acute Q fever, such patients should have serology assessed monthly for at least six months. For patients with chronic Q fever, serology should be done by IFA monthly for six months and every three months thereafter because the titres of antibody decline very slowly. IgM and IgA antibodies decrease during the course of the disease whereas IgG antibodies remain positive for years. Antimicrobial treatment can be stopped after 18 months to 3 years if the anti-phase I IgG titre by IFA is below 1:400 and anti-phase I IgA is undetectable (162,163).

Diagnosis of HME is most often based on the demonstration of a serological response (IgG ≥1:128) or seroconversion to *E. chaffeensis* antigens in the context of a consistent clinical illness (22,44). For HGE, diagnosis is made by using HGE agent or *E. equi* antigens (164,165). Since occasional cross-reactions with *E. chaffeensis* can occur, and clinical distinction between HME and HGE may be difficult, diagnostic tests for both agents should be performed. For HGE, diagnosis is confirmed preferably by seroconversion or by a single serological titre ≥ 1:80 in patients with a clinically compatible illness. Serological responses may persist for years in some patients and thus should be interpreted cautiously (164).

2.   *Western blot*

Western immunoblot assay with sodium dodecyl sulfate-gel electrophoresis and electroblotted antigens is a very useful assay for serological diagnosis and seroepidemiology of rickettsial infections. It allows differentiation of true-positive from false-positive results due to cross-reacting antibodies which are mainly directed against the LPS. The line blot assay is usually used for large-scale screening of sera when quantitative titers are not needed or when tests against a large number of agents are required. This assay allows an assessment of more than 45 antigens simultaneously (166) and has been adapted for the diagnosis of MSF (167). Western immunoblot was shown to be more sensitive than IFA for the detection of early antibodies in MSF (168) with the first antigen detected being the non-specific antigen LPS. Nevertheless, there is no difference in sensitivity between the Western immunoblot and the IFA technique when considering only the reaction against the specific protein antigens.

Western blotting and dot immunoblotting are both sensitive and specific methods for the diagnosis of Q fever (169-171).

3.   *Other serological techniques*

Comparison of serological tests for the diagnosis of rickettsioses are summarized in Table 5. The first technique developed for the serodiagnosis of rickettsial disease was the Weil-Felix test (172). This assay is based on the detection of antibodies to various *Proteus* species which contain LPS antigens that cross-react with antigens of the *Rickettsia* genus (173,174). By the Weil-Felix test, agglutinating antibodies are detectable within five to ten days after the onset of the symptoms (175). Patients with Brill-Zinsser disease or those infected by *R. akari* usually have no agglutinating antibodies that are detectable by the Weil-Felix test. The test lacks sensitivity and specificity, but has historically been used for laboratory diagnosis and remains useful in developing countries.

The complement fixation (CF) test used washed particulate rickettsial antigens. These antigens are species-specific for the SFG and the TG, but cross-reacting antibodies among groups have been reported (176). Various results can be obtained depending on the method of antigen production and the amount of antigen used (177). CF has also been used for the diagnosis of Q fever (155,178,179). The CF assay is less specific than IFA or ELISA (155). Seroconversion is detected later by CF than by IFA or ELISA (between ten and twenty days after the onset of symptoms) (155). A complement fixation of 1:40 is diagnostic for acute Q fever (80), whereas a 1:200 titre of antibody to phase I is diagnostic for chronic Q fever (180).

The indirect hemagglutination test detects antibodies to an antigenic erythrocyte-sensitizing substance (ESS) that is used to coat human or sheep erythrocytes (181). The ESS is specific for the rickettsial group but does not allow differentiation among RMSF, rickettsialpox, and MSF (182). This test detects both IgG and IgM antibodies but is more efficient with IgM antibodies (181).

In the latex agglutination test, ESS is used to coat latex beads (183). This test is rapid and takes only fifteen minutes and is easy to perform. The test is usually positive one week after the onset of the illness, and antibody titres disappear after two months. The antibodies which are detected belong to the IgG and IgM subclasses, but the test is more efficient when IgM is elevated. The microagglutination assay is very simple and sensitive, and can detect an early antibody response to *C. burnetii* (184,184-186). The major drawback of this technique is that it requires a relatively large quantity of antigens.

The enzyme-linked immunosorbent assay (ELISA) was first used to detect antibodies against *R. typhi* and *R. prowazekii* in contrast to other serological techniques (187). The higher sensitivity and reproducibility of this test allows for the differentiation of IgG and IgM antibodies. This technique was later adapted to the diagnosis of RMSF (188), scrub typhus (189), and Q fever (190-194). ELISA is more sensitive than IFA (169) and could also serve in the serodiagnosis of acute Q fever.

4.   Comparison among serological assays

The diagnosis of an acute rickettsial infection should be performed with a sensitive assay. For seroepidemiological studies, however, the specificity of the assay is of major concern due to the potential for false-positive results from cross-reacting antibodies. Other criteria that should be considered in selecting a serological assay include the amount of antigens needed, the cost, and the minimal material that is required.

The microagglutination assay was shown to be less sensitive than hemagglutination and IFA, but comparable in sensitivity to the CF test for both RMSF (152,157) and epidemic typhus (195). The need for a large amount of purified antigen is the major limitation of this method. The CF test is highly specific but has been reported to have poor sensitivity, especially in the early stage of the disease for the diagnosis of both RMSF (152,157,196-198) or typhus group infections (195,199). For this reason, this test is of low interest for the diagnosis of acute phases of infection but remains useful for seroepidemiological studies. The hemagglutination assay is very sensitive and detects antibodies to SFG and TG earlier than any of the other methods studied (129). This test is particularly useful for the diagnosis of acute infection; a four-fold titre rise may be detected within the first week after the onset of RMSF but not MSF (152,200). This assay should not be used for seroepidemiological studies because only very low antibody titres are observed in late convalescent-phase sera (201). The sensitivity of the latex agglutination assay is comparable to that of IFA, and this test has been proposed as an alternative to the first-line testing of sera. Its major drawback is the cost of reagents, although it does not require expensive materials.

ELISA has been shown to be as sensitive and as specific as IFA for the diagnosis of RMSF (188). The inconvenience of the ELISA technique is that it requires a complex and time-consuming antigen purification procedure (189). The Western immunoblot is therefore the most powerfool tool to determine the true prevalence of rickettsial diseases. The line blot assay has been demonstrated to be as sensitive and specific as IFA for the diagnosis of MSF (166). This assay is especially useful for the screening of many antigens that might be considered for patients who have non-specific or atypical presentations.

5. *Cross-adsorption and cross-reactions*

Cross-adsorption studies are useful as they allow for the elimination of cross-reactive antibodies with other species within the rickettsial biogroups (174,202,203). This is the case with TG because in 50% of patients, the sera had the same level of antibody against both *R. prowazekii* and *R. typhi*. Several bacteria have been reported to cross-react with *C. burnetii* including *Legionella pneumophila* (204,205), *Legionella micdadei* (206,207), *Bartonella quintana*, and *Bartonella henselae* (208).

To demonstrate that an atypical positive result is caused by cross-reacting antibodies, sera should be absorbed with the suspected cross-reacting antigens. Cross-adsorption of the serum so studied results in the disappearence of homologous and heterologous antibodies when absorption is performed with the antigen that is responsible for the disease whereas the disappearance of only homologous antibodies is observed when absorption is completed with the antigen that is responsible for the cross-reaction. Confirmation of the identity of the species responsible for the disease among a rickettsial biogroup is usually difficult. Geographical origin of the infection is a good indicator to identify the etiological agent. Moreover, homologous antibodies to a specific rickettsia are usually higher than heterologous antibodies, and differences in antibody titres between various rickettsial species are usually large enough to differentiate between biogroups. Conversely, homologous and heterologous antibodies in the same biogroup are generally identical, and thus cross-adsorption studies may help to distinguish the rickettsial species that are responsible for the disease

D. PCR-based detection from clinical specimens

1. *Diagnostic*

DNA amplification of *C. burnetii* from clinical specimens

PCR has been successfully used to detect *C. burnetii* DNA in mammalian cell cultures and clinical samples including biopsies, milk, placenta, and ticks (209). Various genes and derived primers are available for PCR amplification and detection of *C. burnetii* (Table 7) including within paraffin-embedded tissues (209,210). Moreover, PCR has proven to be more sensitive than standard culture techniques for retrospective diagnosis with and for the follow-up of patients that have been treated for chronic Q fever (209). In our experience, specimens maintained at −80°C are suitable for PCR over several years. In our laboratory, we routinely use primers derived from the *htpAB*-associated repetitive element (211,212). This element exists in at least nineteen copies in the *C. burnetii* Nine Mile I genome, and PCR-based amplification is correspondingly very sensitive (212).

DNA amplification of rickettsiae from clinical specimens

Several clinical specimens are suitable for use in PCR amplification of rickettsial DNA including blood, skin biopsy samples, and arthropods. Skin biopsy specimens are routinely used in specialized laboratories but can essentially be used in any laboratory with PCR facilities (213-215). For PCR amplification, it is necessary to used blood that is collected in EDTA or sodium citrate because heparin inhibits PCR and is difficult to neutralize. In our experience, however, we usually fail to amplify *Rickettsia* from blood. The PCR amplification must be done before antibiotic therapy. The tâche noire, when present, is the most productive clinical specimen to assess for MSF (215). Fresh tissues are preferred for PCR amplification, but paraffin-embedded tissues and even slide-fixed specimens may be useful (210). Rickettsial DNA can also be detected in ticks (216,217), fleas, and lice by PCR amplification methods (218). Detection strategies which are based on recognition of sequences within the 16S rRNA gene (1,4), and those that encode a 17-kD protein (219-221), citrate synthase (222-224), and the rOmpB (140,222) and rOmpA (for SFG rickettsiae) (8,16,225) outer membrane proteins have been described. In our laboratory, amplification of the *Omp*A and *glt*A (citrate synthase) genes are routinely used. If the former is amplified, it is further sequenced for identification. The *glt*A gene is sequenced for identification only when the *Omp*A gene fragment is not succesfully amplified.

Table 7 Genes and derived primers that are recommended for PCR amplification of *Coxiella burnetii.*

Gene	Primers (sequences)	Reference
16S rRNA	16S1 (5'-CTC CTG GCG GCG AGA GTG GC-3') 16S2N (5'-GTT AGC TTC GCT ACT AAG AAG GGA ACT TCC C-3')	299
23S rRNA	976F (5'-AGG TCC TGG TGG AAA GGA ACG-3') 1446R (5'-TCT CAT CTG CCG AAC CCA TTG C-3')	300
16S-23S	16SF (5'-TTG TAC ACA CCG CCC GTC A-3') 23SR (5'-GGG TT (CGT) CCC CAT TCG G-3') 16SS (5'-GAA GTC GTA ACA AGG TA-3') 23SS (5'-TCT CGA TGC CAA GGC ATC CAC C-3')	39
Superoxide dismutase	CB1 (5'-ACT CAA CGC ACT GGA ACG GC-3') CB2 (5'-TAG CTG AAG CCA ATT CGC C-3')	146
Plasmid QpRS	QpRS01 (5'-CTC GTA CCC AAA GAC TAT GAA TAT ATC-3') QpRS02 (5'-CAC ATT GGG TAT CGT ACT GTC CCT-3')	209
Plasmid QpH1	QpH11 (5'-TGA CAA ATA GAA TTT CTT CAT TTT GAT-3') QpH12 (5'-GCT TAT TTT CTT CCT CGA ATC TAT GAA T-3')	299
CbbE	G4131 (5'-CTG ATG TGT CAA GTA ATG TCG G-3') G4132 (5'-CTT CAT GGT TAT GAT TCT GCG-3')	299
HtpAB	Trans1 (5'-TAT GTA TCC ACC GTA GCC AGT C-3') Trans2 (5'-CCC AAC AAC ACC TCC TTA TTC-3')	299
IS 1111	Trans3 (5'-CAACTGTGTGGAATTGATGAG-3') Trans5 (5'-GCGCCATGAATCAATAACGT-3')	212

DNA amplification of *Ehrlichia* from clinical specimens

PCR was the first diagnostic tool (apart from blood smear examination) that was developed for the diagnosis of human ehrlichiosis. Indeed, the IFA method is only used when the culture of *Ehrlichia* pathogens is possible and hence the antigens are available. The most widely used target is the gene encoding the 16S rRNA. For *E. chaffeensis*, primers HE1 and HE3, which define a 389-bp product located near the 5' end of the 16S rRNA gene, are widely used for the detection of this pathogen (226-228). For the diagnosis of HGE, the initial PCR assay used the specific primer set *ge9f/ge10r*, which amplifies a 919-bp DNA sequence in the 16S rRNA gene (164). More recently, the primer set *HS43/HS45* which amplifies a 480-bp sequence of the *groESL* heat shock operon of granulocytic *Ehrlichia* has been used to confirm *E. phagocytophila* infections in European mammals (229).

3. Identification of rickettsiae

Identification of rickettsiae can be achieved either by serological or molecular methods.

Serological identification

The microimmunofluorescence method is the reference technique for the identification of rickettsiae. Recently, monoclonal antibodies have been successfully used to identify rickettsiae in place of polyclonal antibodies. Monoclonal antibodies were first raised against *R. rickettsii* (230-233) and were later raised against *R. akari* (234), *R. conorii* (235), *R. prowazekii* (236), *R. japonica* (237), and *R. afri-*

cae (238) epitopes. By using group-specific and strain-specific monoclonal antibodies, the identification of a rickettsial isolate is easily performed. Protein analysis by sodium dodecyl sulfate-polyacrylamide gel electrophoresis has also been used to differentiate rickettsial species of the SFG; the major distinctive proteins resolve in the high molecular-mass range of >90 kD (29). When studied by Western blot assay, the major antigenic protein or species-specific protein antigens are among these high molecular-mass proteins and correspond to the outer membrane proteins OmpA and OmpB (167,231,232,239-241).

Molecular biology-based identification

Molecular identification of rickettsiae should be based on the sequencing of different genes that are used for detection of these bacteria (as above).

E. Immunodetection in tissues

1.   Immunodetection of C. burnetii in tissues

The detection of *C. burnetii* in tissues is very useful among patients who are treated for chronic Q fever. Samples can be assessed whether fresh or after formalin fixation and paraffin embedding. Valvular or vascular samples are most valuable. Several techniques are available, including immunofluorescence or immunoperoxidase staining (242) using polyclonal or monoclonal antibodies (243-245). It can also be used for detection of antigen in paraffin-embedded tissues (246).

2.   Immunological detection of rickettsiae in blood and tissues

Detection of rickettsiae by the use of immunofluorescence allows for the confirmation of infection in patients prior to their seroconversion. Samples can be tested fresh (130,247-249) or after formalin fixation and paraffin embedding (130,248-251). Biopsy specimens of the skin lesion, preferably petechial lesions and tache noire specimens, are the most common samples that are used (130,248-250). Evaluations of these techniques in several cases have reported a specificity of 100% for the diagnosis of both RMSF (130) and MSF (248). Sensitivity remains low (between 53 and 75%) (130,248). We have recently described an adaptation of this technique that allows for the immunological detection of rickettsiae in circulating endothelial cells which are isolated from whole blood with immunomagnetic beads that are coated with an endothelial cell-specific monoclonal antibody (252). The sensitivity of this method is estimated to be 50% for acutely ill patients (126). Moreover, it has a prognostic use, as the number of circulating endothelial cells that are detected is proportional to the severity of the infection (119,253).

3.   Immunological detection of ehrlichiae in blood and tissues

Detection of ehrlichiae in tissue samples is very useful tool for the diagnosis of human ehrlichiosis. Samples can be used either fresh or after paraffin embedding (254). Various methods have been assessed including immunofluorescence, immunoperoxidase, or avidin-alkaline phosphatase staining (50,254) with the use of either polyclonal or monoclonal antibodies (255).

VII. ANTIBIOTIC SUSCEPTIBILITY TESTING (Table 8)

A. *Rickettsia*

1. *Methods*

Susceptibility testing of rickettsiae cannot be assessed by conventional microbiological tests. Three types of experimental models have been developed: animal models (mice and guinea pigs), the embryonated egg model, and more recently cell culture models. The animal and embryonated egg model have been abandoned because they are less practical than the in vitro systems. In vitro infected cell models allow more convenient investigation of the antibiotic susceptibility of rickettsiae, and the extracellular antibiotic concentrations which are used can be compared to antibiotic concentrations that are obtained in human sera. Three types of assay are currently used in cell culture models to assess antibiotic susceptibility: the plaque assay, the dye uptake assay, and an immunofluorescence assay.

Plaque assay

The plaque formation assay in infected cell cultures was first used for the enumeration of viable rickettsiae (256-259), and then adapted to determine their in vitro antibiotic susceptibility (256,260-263). The plaque assay is currently the recommended technique and allows for the evaluation of both the bacteriostatic and the bactericidal activities of antibiotics. Cell monolayers, usually Vero cells, are grown in tissue culture Petri dishes and are acutely infected with a rickettsial inoculum. Infected cells are then overlaid with Eagle MEM that has 2% fetal calf serum and 0.5% agar. Antibiotics are added at different concentrations at the same time, whereas no antibiotics are added in drug-free controls. Petri dishes are incubated for 7 to 10 days at 37°C in a 5% CO_2 atmosphere. Cell monolayers are then stained with crystal violet thus allowing for vizualization of the plaques. The MICs are defined as the lowest antibiotic concentration that allows for complete inhibition of plaque formation as compared to a drug-free control.

Dye uptake assay

A microplaque colorimetric assay or dye uptake assay has been described as a more convenient technique, and it allows for an accurate and more rapid determination of MICs of several strains of SFG rickettsiae (264). Vero cell cultures in 96-well microtitre plates are infected with 2000 plaque-forming units (PFU) of rickettsiae. Antibiotics are added at different concentrations in different rows. Drug-free rows infected with either 2000 PFU, 200 PFU, 20 PFU, or 0 PFU serve as controls. After four days of incubation at 37°C in 5% CO_2 atmosphere, cell monolayers are washed, and neutral red dye is introduced in to the wells. The optical density (OD) at 492 nm. of each well is determined with a spectrophotometer. The MIC corresponds to the lowest antibiotic concentration for which the mean OD at 492 nm. is lower than that of the 20 PFU controls.

IF assay

More recently, an immunofluorescence assay was described by Ives (265). Vero cells cultured in wells of chamber-culture microscope slides are infected with rickettsiae. After incubation of cultures for three hours at 37°C in a 5% CO_2 atmosphere, cell supernatants were replaced by new medium containing various concentrations of the antibiotics to be tested. Drug-free cultures served as controls. Cell culture monolayers were then fixed with methanol and stained using an immunofluorescence assay to reveal the presence of immunofluorescent foci (clusters of rickettsiae) in twenty-five random fields for each well. The minimal antibiotic concentration which allows for complete inhibition of foci formation as compared to the drug-free control was recorded as the MIC.

Table 8	Antibiotic susceptibility of rickettsiae as determined with the use of in vitro cell models.

Organism	Blm	Dox	Chm	Sxt	Rif	Ery	Cla	Amg	Qui
Rickettsia									
Spotted Fever Group									
R. conorii subgroup	R	S	S	R	S	R	S	R	S
R. massiliae subgroup[a]	R	S	S	R	R	R	S	R	S
Typhus Group[b]	R	S	S	R	S	S	S	R	S
Orientia tsutsugamushi	R	S	S	R	S	S		R	
Coxiella burnetii	R	S	R	S	S	V	S	R	S
Ehrlichia									
E. sennetsu	R	S	R	R	S	R	R	R	S
E. chaffeensis	R	S	R	R	S	R		R	R
HGE agent	R	S	R	R	S	R	R	R	S

Abbreviations: [a]Subgroup including Bar29, *R. massiliae*, *R. aeschlimanii*, *R. montana*, and *R. rhipicephali*; [b]Subgroup including *R. typhi* and *R. prowazekii*; Amg = aminoglycosides; Blm = beta-lactams; Chm = chloramphenicol; Cla = clarithromycin; Dox = doxycycline; Ery = erythromycin; Qui = quinolones; R = resistant; Rif = rifampin; S = susceptible; V = variable susceptibility among different strains

2. Results

Most experiments of antibiotic susceptibility for rickettsiae were performed using a few species, including *R. rickettsii*, *R. conorii*, *R. akari*, *R. prowazekii*, *R. typhi*, and *Orientia tsutsugamushi*. We have recently extended in vitro susceptibility data on new species or strains which have been characterized in recent years (266). Beta-lactams and aminoglycosides are not effective against rickettsiae in cell systems (256,267,268), and their ineffectiveness is probably related to poor ability of intracellular penetration (for beta-lactams) or inactivation due to local acidic pH (for aminoglycosides). Wisseman, however, has shown that penicillin G at high doses induces partial growth inhibition and spheroplast formation in *R. prowazekii* cells in vitro thus inferring that rickettsiae possess a peptidoglycan that is partially susceptible to the activity of beta-lactams compounds (269). Tetracyclines and chloramphenicol are rickettsiostatic in vitro against all rickettsial species (256,264,266-268,270). Although TG rickettsiae are susceptible to erythromycin, SFG rickettsiae were found to be more resistant (264,266,267,270). The newer macrolide compound clarithromycin possesses high rickettsiostatic activity against all SFG and TG rickettsiae that are assessed (266,271). Ives et al. reported variable susceptibility to the newer macrolides, azithromycin and clarithromycin, according to the rickettsial species considered (265). Activity of azithromycin was superior to that of clarithromycin for *R. akari*, whereas the reverse was true for *R. conorii*. MICs were comparable for both drugs among the species *R. prowazekii* and *R. rickettsii* (265). Josamycin remains the most effective compound in vitro against SFG and TG rickettsiae (266,272). All rickettsial species are highly susceptible to fluoroquinolone compounds with sparfloxacin being the most effective compound in vitro (264,266,268,273-275). Although rifampin has been demonstrated to be active in vitro against most SFG and TG rickettsiae (264,268,270), we have recently demonstrated that species or strains Bar29, *R. massiliae, R. montana*, and *R. rhipicephali*, which belong to a same phylogenetic cluster, are more resistant to this antibiotic (266,276) (Figure 4). Sulfonamides and their combination with trimethoprim are inactive in vitro against rickettsiae, and may even be used in rickettsial cultures to prevent contamination by other bacterial species (135). Moreover, we found that these antibiotics increase cytopathic effect of rickettsiae in cell cultures (unpublished data). Variability in antibiotic susceptibility among different rickettsial strains or species have been now characterized for macrolides (264,266,267,270,272) and more recently for rifampin (266) (Figure 4). All rifampin-resistant strains belong to a single phylogenetic subgroup (266), and may reflect a divergence during the evolution of this subgroup in the gene that encodes the RNA polymerase. We have recently shown that the resistance of these species to rifampin is related to mutations in the *rpo*B gene which encodes the beta subunit of the RNA polymerase (277). These mutations prevent rifampin from binding to the target enzyme and thereby inhibit its activity. Resistance to rifampin by mutation in the *rpo*B gene has been experimentally established in *R. prowazekii* (278). We may also hypothesize that the high susceptibility of the TG rickettsiae to erythromycin as compared to SFG rickettsiae may reflect a divergent strategic evolution involving macrolide antibiotic susceptibility, especially leading to different ribosomal affinity for this compound (Figure 4).

B.   *Ehrlichia*

In vitro and in vivo antibiotic susceptibility studies have been carried out on various species of *Ehrlichia*. All have been determined that doxycycline is highly effective against ehrlichiae, and this antibiotic is currently the first choice of therapy in animal and in human ehrlichiosis.

1.   Animal models

E. sennetsu was first isolated in mice (279), and subsequently infections in mice have been used as a model for Sennetsu fever. Although the growth of E. sennetsu in mice is much slower than that for other rickettsiae, treatment of mice with cyclophosphamide prior to inoculation has been found to enhance the growth of *E. sennetsu* (280), and this technique has been used for the preparation of antigen in these animals. The first report of antibiotic susceptibility in mice for *E. sennetsu* has shown that erythromy-

Non-silent rpoB sequence base positions						
aa/524	aa/640	aa/973	aa/1031	Ery	Rif	Species
Ser/AGT	Ile/ATT	Phe/ATT	Ile/ATC	R	S	*R. sibirica*
				R	S	*R. africae*
Ser/AGT	Ile/ATT	Phe/TTC	Ile/ATC	R	S	*R. conorii*
				R	S	*R. slovaca*
				R	S	*R. honei*
Ser/AGT	Ile/ATT	Phe/TTC	Thr/ACC	R	S	*R. rickettsii*
Ser/AGT	Val/GTT	Phe/TTC	Thr/ACC	R	S	*R. japonica*
Asn/AAT	Val/GTT	Leu/TAA	Thr/ACC	R	R	Bar 29
Asn/AAT	Val/GTT	Leu/TTA	Thr/ACC	R	R	*R. massiliae*
Asn/AAT	Val/GTT	Leu/TTA	Thr/ACC	R	R	*R. rhipicephali*
Ser/AGT	Val/GTT	Leu/TAA	Thr/ACC	R	R	*R. aeschlimanii*
Ser/AGT	Val/GTT	Leu/TAA	Thr/ACC	R	R	*R. montana*
				R	S	*R. helvetica*
				R	S	*R. australis*
				R	S	*R. akari*
				R	S	*R. typhi*
				R	S	*R. prowazekii*
				R	S	*R. canada*
				R	S	*R. bellii*

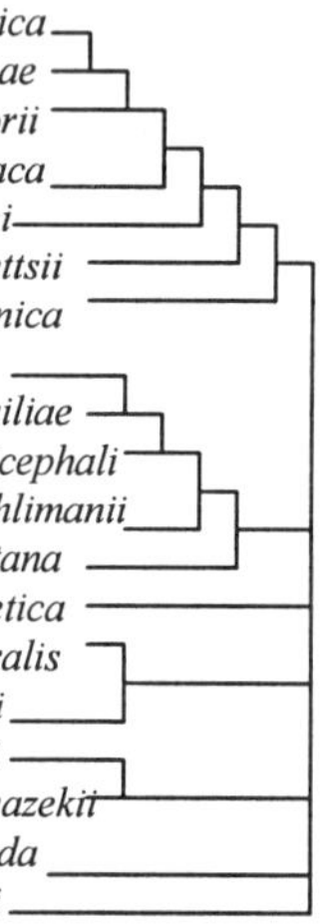

Figure 4   In vitro susceptibility of rickettsiae to erythromycin and rifampin, and *rpoB* gene alterations that are associated with rifampin resistance (266,277). Ery = erythromycin; Rif = rifampin; aa = amino acid

cin, sulfisoxazole, penicillin, streptomycin, polymyxin B, bacitracin, and chloramphenicol were ineffective even at high concentrations (281). Chlortetracycline was more effective than oxytetracycline and tetracycline. Further studies have evaluated the effect of tetracycline therapy on spleen size as a percentage of body weight, and on the splenic infectious burden in mice that are infected with *E. sennetsu* (282,283). In mice for whom tetracycline therapy was initiated at the same time as the inoculation, there were no detectable ehrlichiae in the spleen (282). Therefore, it would appear that the time for initiation of treatment may be important in controlling the course of infection with *E. sennetsu*, and that delayed therapy may allow the development of chronic infections.

2.   Cell culture model

The susceptibility of *Ehrlichia* to various antibiotics has been assessed with the use of *Ehrlichia*-infected contact-inhibition-growth cell lines that have been incubated for 48 to 72 hrs. in the antibiotic under consideration. Thereafter, the antibiotic-containing medium is removed, and *Ehrlichia*-infected cells are incubated with antibiotic-free media for at least three more days. The number of *Ehrlichia*-infected cells are counted every day, and an antibiotic was ineffective if the number of *Ehrlichia*-infected cells after exposure to the antibiotic is similar to that of control noninfected cells. If the number of *Ehrlichia*-infected cells is found to decrease during incubation with an antibiotic, the antibiotic is regarded as being bactericidal. Antibiotics are considered bacteriostatic if there is no increase or decrease in *Ehrlichia*-infected cells when the antibiotic is present, but the number of infected cells increases when antibiotic-free medium is provided. The in vitro susceptibility of *E. sennetsu* Miyayama strain to eight antibiotics was determined using Diff-Quick staining of infected P388D1 cells over a five day period (284). In this report it was also demonstrated that Diff-Quick staining was as reliable as immunofluorescence assay for detecting infected cells. It was found that *E. sennetsu* was not susceptible to penicillin, gentamicin, cotrimoxazole, erythromycin, and chloramphenicol, whereas rifampin, doxycycline, and ciprofloxacin were effective with MICs of 0.5 mg./L., 0.125 mg./L., and 0.125 mg./L., respectively.

The in vitro antibiotic suceptibility of *E. chaffeensis* has also been studied recently (285). A microplate colorimetric assay used *Ehrlichia*-infected DH82 cell culture. The percentage of infected cells was determined each day using the Diff-Quick staining which has been found to stain only viable organisms. On the third day of incubation, the antibiotic-containing medium was removed and replaced with antibiotic-free media. With these methods, it was found that *E. chaffeensis* was susceptible to 0.5 mg./L. of doxycycline and to 0.125 mg./L. of rifampin. Chloramphenicol, cotrimoxazole, erythromycin, penicillin, gentamicin, and ciprofloxacin were not effective against *E. chaffeensis*.

The HGE agent is sensitive to doxycycline, ofloxacin, ciprofloxacin, and trovafloxacin, but is resistant to clindamycin, co-trimoxazole, erythromycin, azithromycin, ampicillin, ceftriaxone, and imipenem. Chloramphenicol and aminoglycosides only display a poor bacteriostatic activity and are never bactericidal (286).

C.   *Coxiella burnetii*

Antibiotic susceptibility testing of *C. burnetii* is difficult since this organism is an obligate intracellular bacterium. Three models of infection, however, have been developed: animals, chick embryos, and cell culture. The method currently used to test antibiotic susceptibility of *C. burnetii* is based on cell culture models. Torres and Raoult (287) have developed a shell vial assay with HEL cells for assessment of the bacteriostatic effect of antibiotics. Amikacin and amoxicillin were not effective, and ceftriaxone and fusidic acid were inconsistently active (287). Co-trimoxazole, rifampin, doxycycline, clarithromycin, and the quinolones were bacteriostatic (271,273). *C. burnetii* can establish a persistent infection in several cell lines, including L929 mouse fibroblasts and J774 or P388D1 murine macrophage-like cells (288). Infected cells can be maintained in continuous cultures for months (289). Raoult et al., using

P388D1 and L929 cells, showed that pefloxacin, rifampin, and doxycycline (290) as well as clarithromycin (271) were bacteriostatic against *C. burnetii*.

An original model of the killing assay has been developed by Maurin et al. to assess the bactericidal activity of antibiotics against *C. burnetii* (Figure 5) (291). On the first day of the process, P388D1 cells were infected with *C. burnetii* that was harvested from a 150-cm.^{2} culture flask and seeded into 25-cm.^{2} flasks so that each flask received the same primary inoculum. Antibiotics were added to flasks, and flasks with or without antibiotics were incubated for 24 hrs. at 37°C. Cells were then lysed, and ten-fold serial dilutions of cell lysates were distributed into shell vials that contain uninfected HEL cells (134). After six days of incubation, *C. burnetii* on shell vials were stained by indirect immunofluorescence. It was demonstrated that doxycycline, pefloxacin, and rifampin did not show any significant bactericidal activity. The lack of bactericidal activity was probably due to the inactivation by low pH of the phagolysosomes in which *C. burnetii* survives. Maurin et al. have demonstrated that the addition of a lysosomotropic alkalinizing agent, e.g. chloroquine, to antibiotics improved the activities of doxycycline and pefloxacin, which then became bactericidal (291).

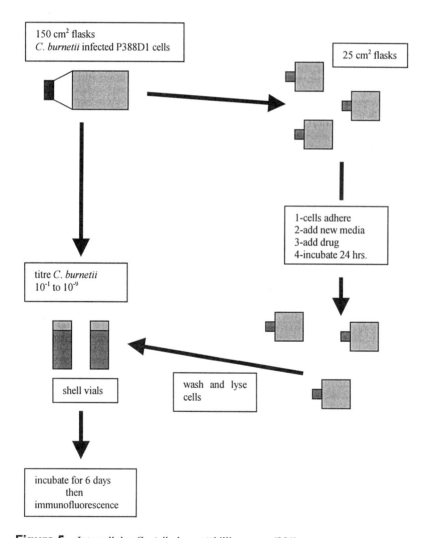

Figure 5   Intracellular *Coxiella burnetii* killing assay (291).

REFERENCES

1. Stothard DR, Fuerst PA. Evolutionary analysis of the spotted fever and typhus groups of *Rickettsia* using 16S rRNA gene sequences. Syst Appl Microbiol 1995; 18:52-61.
2. Fournier PE, Roux V, Raoult D. Phylogenetic analysis of spotted fever group rickettsiae by study of the outer surface protein rOmpA. Int J Syst Bacteriol 1998; 48:839-849.
3. Roux V, Rydkina E, Eremeeva M, Raoult D. Citrate synthase gene comparison, a new tool for phylogenetic analysis, and its application for the rickettsiae. Int J Syst Bacteriol 1997; 47:252-261.
4. Roux V, Raoult D. Phylogenetic analysis of the genus *Rickettsia* by 16S rDNA sequencing. Res Microbiol 1995; 146:385-396.
5. Roux V, Raoult D. Global genetic diversity of spotted fever group rickettsiae. In: Anderson B, Bendinelli M, Friedman H, eds. Rickettsial Infection and Immunity. New York: Plenum Press, 1997:53-64.
6. Roux V, Raoult D. Genotypic identification and phylogenetic analysis of the spotted fever group rickettsiae by pulsed-field gel electrophoresis. J Bacteriol 1993; 175:4895-4904.
7. Roux V, Fournier PE, Rydkina E. Phylogenetic study of the rickettsiae. In: Kazar J, Toman R, eds. Rickettsiae and Rickettsial Diseases. Bratislava:Veda, 1996:34-42.
8. Roux V, Fournier PE, Raoult D. Differentiation of spotted fever group rickettsiae by sequencing and analysis of restriction fragment length polymorphism of PCR amplified DNA of the gene encoding the protein rOmpA. J Clin Microbiol 1996; 34:2058-2065.
9. Weisburg WG, Dobson ME, Samuel JE, Dasch GA, Mallavia LP, Baca O, Mandelco L, Sechrest JE, Weiss E, Woese CR. Phylogenetic diversity of the rickettsiae. J Bacteriol 1989; 171:4202-4206.
10. Brenner DJ, O'Connor S, Winkler HH, Steigerwalt AG. Proposals to unify the genera *Bartonella* and *Rochalimaea*, with descriptions of *Bartonella quintana* comb. nov., *Bartonella vinsonii* comb. nov., *Bartonella henselae* comb. nov., and *Bartonella elizabethae* comb.nov., and to remove the family *Bartonellaceae* from the order *Rickettsiales*. Int J Syst Bacteriol 1993; 43:777-786.
11. Tamura A, Ohashi N, Urakami H, Miyamura S. Classification of *Rickettsia tsutsugamushi* in a new genus, *Orientia* gen nov, as *Orientia tsutsugamushi* comb. nov. Int J Syst Bacteriol 1995; 45:589-591.
12. Uchida T, Uchiyama T, Kumano K, Walker DH. *Rickettsia japonica* sp. nov., the etiological agent of spotted fever group rickettsiosis in Japan. Int J Syst Bacteriol 1992; 42:303-305.
13. Stewart RS. Flinders Island spotted fever : a newly recognised endemic focus of tick typhus in Bass Strait. Part 1. Clinical and epidemiogiocal features. Med J Aust 1991; 154:94-99.
14. Tarasevich IV, Makarova V, Fetisova NF, Stepanov A, Mistkarova E, Balayeva NM, Raoult D. Astrakhan fever: new spotted fever group rickettsiosis. Lancet 1991; 337:172-173.
15. Kelly PJ, Beati L, Mason PR, Matthewman LA, Roux V, Raoult D. *Rickettsia africae* sp nov, the etiological agent of African tick bite fever. Int J Syst Bacteriol 1996; 46:611-614.
16. Raoult D, Brouqui P, Roux V. A new spotted-fever-group rickettsiosis. Lancet 1996; 348:412.
17. Yu X, Fan M, Xu G, Liu Q, Raoult D. Genotypic and antigenic identification of two new strains of spotted fever group rickettsiae isolated from China. J Clin Microbiol 1993; 31:83-88.
18. Raoult D, Berbis P, Roux V, Xu W, Maurin M. A new tick-transmitted disease due to *Rickettsia slovaca*. Lancet 1997; 350:112-113.
19. Anderson BE, Dawson JE, Jones DC, Wilson KH. *Erhlichia chaffeensis*, a new species associated with human ehrlichiosis. J Clin Microbiol 1991; 29:2838-2842.
20. Dawson JE, Anderson BE, Fishbein DB, Sanchez JL, Goldsmith CS, Wilson KH, Duntley CW. Isolation and characterization of an *Ehrlichia* sp. from a patient diagnosed with human ehrlichiosis. J Clin Microbiol 1991; 29:2741-2745.
21. Chen S, Dumler JS, Bakken JS, Walker DH. Identification of a granulocytotropic *Ehrlichia* species as the etiologic agent of human disease. J Clin Microbiol 1994; 32:589-595.
22. Walker DH, Dumler JS. Emergence of the ehrlichioses as human health problems. Emerg Infect Dis 1996; 2:1-15.
23. Azad AF. Epidemiology of murine typhus. Ann Rev Entomol 1990; 35:553-569.
24. Weiss E. The family *Rickettsiaceae*: human pathogens. In: Starr MP, Stolp H, Trüper HG, Balows A, eds. The Prokaryotes: A Handbook on Habitats, Isolation, and Identification of Bacteria. Berlin:Springer-Verlag, 1981:2137-2160.
25. Maeda K, Markowitz N, Hawley RC, Ristic M, Cox D, McDade JE. Human infection with *Ehrlichia canis*, a leukocytic rickettsia. N Engl J Med 1987; 316:853-856.

26. Fishbein DB, Dawson JE, Robinson LE. Human ehrlichiosis in the United States, 1985 to 1990. Ann Intern Med 1994; 120:736-743.
27. Walker DH. Rickettsioses of the spotted fever group around the world. J Dermatol 1989; 16:169-177.
28. Goldwasser RA, Steiman Y, Klingberg W, Swartz TA, Klingberg MA. The isolation of strains of rickettsiae of the spotted fever group in Israel and their differentiation from other members of the group by immunofluorescence methods. Scand J Infect Dis 1974; 6:53-62.
29. Beati L, Finidori JP, Gilot B, Raoult D. Comparison of serologic typing, sodium dodecyl sulfate- polyacrylamide gel electrophoresis protein analysis, and genetic restriction fragment length polymorphism analysis for identification of rickettsiae : characterization of two new rickettsial strains. J Clin Microbiol 1992; 30:1922-1930.
30. Drancourt M, Kelly PJ, Regnery RL, Raoult D. Identification of spotted fever group rickettsiae using polymerase chain reaction and restriction-endonuclease length polymorphism analysis. Acta Virol 1992; 36:1-6.
31. Beati L, Humair PF, Aeschlimann A, Raoult D. Identification of spotted fever group rickettsiae isolated from *Dermacentor marginatus* and *Ixodes ricinus* ticks collected in Switzerland.   Am J Trop Med Hyg 1994;51:138-148.
32. Beati L, Finidori JP, Raoult D. First isolation of *Rickettsia slovaca* from *Dermacentor marginatus* in France. Am J Trop Med Hyg 1993; 48:257-268.
33. Bacellar F, Regnery RL, Nuncio MS, Filipe AR. Genotypic evaluation of rickettsial isolates recovered from various species of ticks in Portugal. Epidemiol Infect 1995; 114:169-178.
34. Eremeeva ME, Beati L, Makarova VA, Fetisova NF, Tarasevich IV, Balayeva NM, Raoult D. Astrakhan fever rickettsiae : antigenic and genotypic of isolates obtained from human and *Rhipicephalus pumilio* ticks. Am J Trop Med Hyg 1994; 51:697-706.
35. Uchida T. *Rickettsia japonica*, the etiologic agent of oriental spotted fever. Microbiol Immunol 1993; 37:91-102.
36. Kelly PJ, Beati L, Matthewman LA, Mason PR, Dasch GA, Raoult D. A new pathogenic spotted fever group rickettsia from Africa. J Trop Med Hyg 1994; 97:129-137.
37. Baird RW, Lloyd M, Stenos J, Ross BC, Stewart RS, Dwyer B. Characterization and comparison of Australian human spotted fever group rickettsiae. J Clin Microbiol 1992; 30.2896-2902.
38. Hechemy KE, Raoult D, Fox J, Han Y, Elliott LB, Rawlings J. Cross-reaction of immune sera from patients with rickettsial diseases. J Med Microbiol 1989; 29:199-202.
39. Thiele D, Willems H, Krauss H. The 16S/23S ribosomal spacer region of *Coxiella burnetii*. Eur J Epidemiol 1994; 10:421-426.
40. Raoult D, Lepeu G, de Micco P, San Marco JL, Weiller PJ, Gallais H, Casanova P. Recrudescence de la fièvre boutonneuse mediterraneenne dans le sud de la France. Méditerranée Médicale 1984; 3:102-103.
41. Mansueto S, Tringali G, Walker DH. Widespread simultaneous increase in the incidence of spotted fever group rickettsiosis. J Infect Dis 1986; 154:539-540.
42. Tissot-Dupont H, Raoult D. Epidémiologie de la fievre boutonneuse méditerraneenne en France. Med Mal Infec 1993; 23:485-490.
43. Fukuda T, Sasahara T, Kitao T. Studies on the causative agent of Hyuganetsu disease. XI. Characteristics of rickettsia-like organism isolated from metacercaria of Stellant- chasmus falcattus parasitic in grey mullet. Jpn J Assoc Infect Dis 1973; 47:474-482.
44. Dumler JS, Bakken JS. Ehrlichial diseases of humans: emerging tick-borne infections. Clin Infect Dis 1995; 20:1102-1110.
45. Lockhart JM, Davidson WR, Stallknecht DE, Dawson JE, Little SE. Natural history of *Ehrlichia chaffeensis* (rickettsiales: ehrlichieae) in the piedmont physiographic province of Georgia. J Parasitol 1997; 83:887-894.
46. Fishbein DB, Sawyer LA, Holland CJ, Hayes EB, Okoroanyanwu W, Williams D, Sikes K, Ristic M, McDade JE. Unexplained febrile illnesses after exposure to ticks. Infection with an *Ehrlichia*? JAMA 1987; 257:3100-3104.
47. Fishbein DB, Kemp A, Dawson JE, Greene NR, Redus MA, Fields DH. Human ehrlichiosis: prospective active surveillance in febrile hospitalized patients. J Infect Dis 1989; 160:803-809.
48. Brouqui P, Le Cam C, Kelly PJ, Laurens R, Tounkara A, Sawadogo S, Velo-Marcel, Gondao L, Faugere B, Delmont J, Bourgeade A, Raoult D. Serologic evidence for human ehrlichiosis in Africa. Eur J Epidemiol 1994; 10:695-698.
49. Morais JD, Dawson JE, Greene C, Filipe AR, Galhardas LC, Bacellar F. First European case of ehrlichiosis. Lancet 1991; 338:633-634.

50. Dumler JS, Brouqui P, Aronson J, Taylor JP, Walker DH. Identification of *Ehrlichia* in human tissue. N Engl J Med 1991; 325:1109-1110.

51. Dumler JS, Sutker WL, Walker DH. Persistent infection with *Ehrlichia chaffeensis*. Clin Infect Dis 1993; 17:903-905.

52. Pancholi P, Kolbert CP, Mitchell PD, Reed KD, Dumler JS, Bakken JS, Telford SR, Persing DH. *Ixodes dammini* as a potential vector of human granulocytic ehrlichiosis. J Infect 1995; 172:1007-1012.

53. Parola P, Beati L, Cambon M, Brouqui P, Raoult D. *Ehrlichia* DNA amplified from *Ixodes ricinus* (Acari : *Ixodidae)* ticks in France. J Med Entomol 1998; 35:180-183.

54. Silvers LE, Watkins S, Strickland GT, Clothier M, Grant J, Hall E, Joe L, Thompson MA, Sullivan S, Ryan J, Shanahan P, Baumann CG, Shuchel M, Burnie G, Sprouse G, Nevins JT, McQuay H. Human ehrlichiosis - Maryland, 1994. JAMA 1996; 276:1212-1213.

55. Wormser G, Mckenna D, Aguero-Rosenfeld M, Horowitz H, Munoz J, Nowakowski J, Gerina G, Welch P, Moorjani H, Rush T, Jacquette G, Stankey A, Falco R, Rapoport M, Ackamn D, Talarico J, White D, Friedlander L, Gallo R, Brady G, Mauer M, Wong S, Duncan R, Kingsley L, Taulor R, Birkhead G, Morse D, Dumler JS. Human granulocytic ehrlichiosis - New York, 1995. JAMA 1995; 274:867.

56. Hardalo CJ, Quagliarello V, Dumler JS. Human granulocytic ehrlichiosis in Connecticut: report of a fatal case. Clin Infect Dis 1995; 21:910-914.

57. Telford SR, Lepore TJ, Snow P, Warner CK, Dawson JE. Human granulocytic ehrlichiosis in Massachusetts. Ann Intern Med 1995; 123:277-279.

58. Gewirtz AS, Cornbleet PJ, Vugia DJ, Traver C, Niederhuber J, Kolbert CP, Persing DH. Human granulocytic ehrlichiosis: report of a case in Northern California. Clin Infect Dis 1996; 23:653-654.

59. Brouqui P, Dumler JS, Lienhard R, Brossard M, Raoult D. Human granulocytic ehrlichiosis in Europe. Lancet 1995; 346:782-783.

60. Sumption KJ, Wright DJM, Cutler SJ, Dale BAS. Human ehrlichiosis in the UK. Lancet 1995; 346:1487-1488.

61. Bakken JS, Krueth J, Tilden RL, Dumler JS, Kristiansen BE. Serological evidence of human granulocytic ehrlichiosis in Norway. Eur J Clin Microbiol Infect Dis 1996; 15:829-832.

62. Petrovec M, Lotric Furlan S, Avsic Zupanc T, Strle F, Brouqui P, Roux V, Dumler JS. Human disease in Europe caused by a granulocytic *Ehrlichia* species. J Clin Microbiol 1997; 35:1556-1559.

63. Telford SRI, Dawson JE, Katavalos P, Warner CK, Kolbert CP, Persing DH. Perpetuation of the agent of human granulocytic ehrlichiosis in a deer tick-rodent cycle. Proc Natl Acad Sci USA 1996; 93:6209-6214.

64. Langley JM, Marrie TJ, Covert A, Waag DM, Williams C. Poker players' pneumonia. An urban outbreak of Q fever following exposure to a parturient cat. N Engl J Med 1988; 319:354-355.

65. Marrie TJ. Q fever : clinical signs, symptoms, and pathophysiology. In: Walker DH, ed. Biology of Rickettsial Diseases. Boca Raton, Florida: CRC Press, 1988:1-16.

66. Higgins D, Marrie TJ. Seroepidemiology of Q fever among cats in New Brunswick and Prince Edward Island. Ann NY Acad Sci 1990; 590:271-274.

67. Webster JP, LLoyd G, Macdonald DW. Q fever (*Coxiella burnetii*) reservoir in wild brown rat (*Rattus norvegicus)* populations in the UK. Parasitology 1995; 110:31-35.

68. Kazar J. Q fever. In: Kazar J, Toman R - eds. Rickettsiae and Rickettsial Diseases. Bratislava: Slovak Academy of Sciences, 1996:353-362.

69. Marrie TJ, Durant H, Williams JC, Mintz E, Waag DM. Exposure to parturient cats: a risk factor for acquisition of Q fever in Maritime Canada. J Infect Dis 1988; 158:101-108.

70. Babudieri B. Q fever: A zoonosis. Adv Vet Sci 1959; 5:82-182.

71. Lang GH. Coxiellosis (Q fever) in animals. In: Marrie TJ, ed. Q Fever, The Disease. Boca Raton, FL: CRC press, 1990:23-48.

72. McCaul TF. The developmental cycle of *Coxiella burnetii*. In: Williams JC, Thompson HA, eds. Q Fever: The Biology of *Coxiella burnetii*. Boca Raton, FL: CRC Press, 1991:223-258.

73. Fishbein DB, Raoult D. A cluster of *Coxiella burnetti* infections associated with exposure to vaccinated goats and their unpasteurized dairy products. Am J Trop Med Hyg 1992; 47:35-40.

74. Tissot-Dupont H, Raoult D, Brouqui P, Janbon F, Peyramond D, Weiller PJ, Chicheportiche C, Nezri M, Poirier R. Epidemiologic features and clinical presentation of acute Q fever in hospitalized patients - 323 French cases. Am J Med 1992; 93:427-434.

75. Kruszweska D, Wirzbanowska-Tylewska S. Influence of *Coxiella burnetii* infection of male mice on their offspring. Acta Virol 1991; 35:79-82.

76. Mann JS, Douglas JG, Inglis JM, Leitch AG. Q fever: person-to-person transmission within a family. Thorax 1986; 41:974-975.

77. Raoult D. Host factors in the severity of Q fever. Ann NY Acad Sci 1990; 590:33-38.

78. Aguirre Errasti C, Montejo Baranda M, Hernandez Almaraz JL, de la Hoz Torres C, Martinez Gutierrez E, Villate Navarro JL, Sobradillo Pena V. An outbreak of Q fever in the Basque country. CMAJ 1984; 131:48-49.

79. Dupuis G, Petite J, Peter O, Vouilloz M. An important outbreak of human Q fever in a Swiss Alpine valley. Int J Epidemiol 1987; 16:282-287.

80. Guigno D, Coupland B, Smith EG, Farrell ID, Desselberger U, Caul EO. Primary humoral antibody response to *Coxiella burnetii*, the causative agent of Q Fever. J Clin Microbiol 1992; 30:1958-1967.

81. Schneider T, Jahn HU, Steinhoff D, Guschoreck HM, Liesenfeld O, Mater-Bohm H, Wesirow AL, Lode H, Ludwig WD, Dissmann T. A Q fever epidemic in Berlin. The epidemiological and clinical aspects. Dtsch Med Wochenschr 1993; 118:689-695.

82. Tissot-Dupont H, Torres S, Nezri M, Raoult D. Hyperendemic focus of Q fever related to sheep and wind. Am J Epidemiol 1999; 150:67-74.

83. Heinzen RA, Hayes SF, Peacock MG, Hackstad T. Directional actin polymerization associated with spotted fever group rickettsia infection of Vero cells. Infect Immun 1993; 61:1926-1935.

84. Teysseire N, Boudier JA, Raoult D. *Rickettsia conorii* entry into vero cells. Infect Immun 1995; 63:366-374.

85. Teysseire N, Chiche-Portiche C, Raoult D. Intracellular movements of *Rickettsia conorii* and *R. typhi* based on actin polymerization. Res Microbiol 1992; 143:821-829.

86. Burgdorfer W, Anacker RL, Bird RG, Bertram DS. Intranuclear growth of *Rickettsia rickettsii*. J Bacteriol 1968; 96:1415-1418.

87. Eremeeva ME, Roux V, Raoult D. Determination of genome size and restriction pattern polymorphism of *Rickettsia prowazekii* and *Rickettsia typhi* by pulsed field gel electrophoresis. FEMS Microbiol Lett 1993; 112:105-112.

88. Roux V, Drancourt M, Raoult D. Determination of genome sizes of *Rickettsia spp.* within the spotted fever group using pulsed-field gel electrophoresis. J Bacteriol 1992; 174:7455-7457.

89. Pedersen CE, Walters VD. Comparative electrophoresis of spotted fever group rickettsial proteins. Life Sci 1978; 22:583-587.

90. Anacker RL, McCaul TF, Burgdorfer W, Gerloff RK. Properties of selected rickettsiae of the spotted fever group. Infect Immun 1980; 27:468-474.

91. Osterman JV, Eisemann CS. Surface proteins of typhus and spotted fever group rickettsiae. Infect Immun 1978; 21:866-873.

92. Raoult D. Antibiotic susceptibility of rickettsia and treatment of rickettsioses. Eur J Epidemiol 1989; 5:432-435.

93. Philip RN, Casper EA, Ormsbee RA, Peacock MG, Burgdorfer W. Microimmunofluorescence test for the serological study of Rocky Mountain spotted fever and typhus. J Clin Microbiol 1976; 3:51-61.

94. Ormsbee RA, Peacock MG. Antigenic relationships of rickettsiae of the typhus and spotted fever groups. In: Kazar J, Ormsbee RA, Tarasevich IV, eds. Rickettsiae and Rickettsial Diseases. Proceedings of the 2nd International Symposium on Rickettsiae and Rickettsial Diseases. Smolenice, June 21-25, 1976. Bratislava:Publishing House of the Slovak Academy of Sciences, 1978:207-216.

95. Beati L, Kelly PJ, Mason PR, Raoult D. Species-specific BALB/c mouse antibodies to rickettsiae studied by Western blotting. FEMS Microbiol Lett 1994; 119:339-344.

96. Rikihisa Y. The tribe *Ehrlichieae* and ehrlichial diseases. Clin Microbiol Rev 1991; 4:286-308.

97. Wells MY, Rikihisa Y. Lack of lysosomal fusion with phagosomes containing *Ehrlichia risticii* in P388D1 cells: abrogation of inhibition with oxytetracycline. Infect Immun 1988; 56:3209-3215.

98. Heinzen RA, Stiegler GL, Whiting LL, Schmitt SA, Mallavia LP, Frazier ME. Use of pulsed field gel electrophoresis to differentiate *Coxiella burnetii* strains. Ann NY Acad Sci 1990; 590:504-513.

99. Gimenez DF. Staining rickettsiae in yolk-sac cultures. Stain Technol 1964; 39:135-140.

100. Weiss E, Moulder JW. Order I *Rickettsiales*, Gieszczkiewicz 1939. Krieg NR, Holt JG, eds. Bergey's Manual of Systematic Bacteriology. Baltimore, MD: Williams & Wilkins, 1984:687-703.

101. Hackstadt T, Peacock MG, Hitchcock PJ, Cole RL. Lipopolysaccharide variation in *Coxiella burnetti*: intrastrain heterogeneity in structure and antigenicity. Infect Immun 1985; 48:359-365.

102. Hackstadt T. Antigenic variation in the phase I lipopolysaccharide of *Coxiella burnetii* isolates. Infect Immun 1986; 52:337-340.

103. Hackstadt T. The role of lipopolysaccharides in the virulence of *Coxiella burnetii*. Ann NY Acad Sci 1990; 590:27-32.

104. Amano KI, Williams JC. Chemical and immunological characterization of lipopolysaccharides from phase I and phase II *Coxiella burnetii*. J Bacteriol 1984;160:994-1002.

105. Mallavia LP, Samuel JE, Frazier ME. The genetic of *Coxiella burnetii* etiologic agent of Q fever and chronic endocarditis. In: Williams JC, Thompson HA, eds. Q Fever : The Etiological Agent - *Coxiella burnetii*. Boca Raton, FL:CRC Press, 1991:259-284.

106. Gaburro D, Del Campo A. Considerazioni epidemiologiche e cliniche su un'infezione da *Coxiella burnetii* in tre gemelle immature. Mal Infect Parasit 1956; 8:384-390.

107. Hackstadt T, Williams JC. pH dependence of the *Coxiella burnetii* glutamate transport system. J Bacteriol 1983; 154:598-603.

108. Mege JL, Maurin M, Capo C, Raoult D. *Coxiella burnetii:* the "query" fever bacterium a model of immune subversion by a strictly intracellular microorganism. FEMS Microbiol Rev 1997; 19:209-217.

109. Hendrix LR, Samuel JE, Mallavia LP. Differentiation of *Coxiella burnetii* isolates by analysis of restriction endonuclease-digested DNA separated by SDS-PAGE. J Gen Microbiol 1991; 137:269-276.

110. Samuel JE, Frazier ME, Mallavia LP. Correlation of plasmid type and disease caused by *Coxiella burnetii*. Infect Immun 1985; 49:775-779.

111. Toman R, Kazar J. Evidence for the structural heterogeneity of the polysaccharide component of *Coxiella burnetii* strain nine mile lipopolysaccharide. Acta Virol 1991; 35:531-537.

112. La Scola B, Lepidi H, Maurin M, Raoult D. A guinea pig model for Q fever endocarditis. J Infect Dis 1998; 178:278-281.

113. Yu X, Raoult D. Serotyping *Coxiella burnetii* isolates from acute and chronic Q fever patients by using monoclonal antibodies. FEMS Microbiol Lett 1994; 117:15-20.

114. Koster FT, Williams JC, Goodwin JS. Cellular immunity in Q fever: modulation of responsiveness by a suppressor T cell-monocyte circuit. J Immunol 1985; 135:1067-1072.

115. Capo C, Zaffran Y, Zugun F, Houpikian P, Raoult D, Mege JL. Production of interleukin-10 and transforming growth factor beta by peripheral blood mononuclear cells in Q fever endocarditis. Infect Immun 1996; 64:4143-4147.

116. Li H, Walker DH. Characterization of rickettsial attachment to host cells by flow cytometry. Infect Immun 1992; 60:2030-2035.

117. Silverman DJ, Santucci LA, Meyers N, Sekeyova Z. Penetration of host cells by *Rickettsia rickettsii* appears to be mediated by a phospholipase of rickettsial origin. Infect Immun 1992; 60:2733-2740.

118. Walker DH. Pathology and pathogenesis of the vasculotropic rickettsioses. In: Walker DH - ed. Biology of Rickettsial Disease. Boca Raton, Florida: CRC Press, 1988:115-138.

119. George F, Brouqui P, Boffa MC, Mutin M, Drancourt M, Brisson C, Raoult D, Sampol J. Demonstration of *Rickettsia conorii*-induced endothelial injury in vivo by measuring circulating endothelial cells, thrombomodulin and Von Willebrand factor in patients with mediterranean spotted fever. Blood 1993; 82:2109-2116.

120. Teysseire N, Arnoux D, George F, Sampol J, Raoult D. Von Willebrand factor release, thrombomodulin and tissue factor expression in *Rickettsia conorii* infected endothelial cells. Infect Immun 1992; 60:4388-4393.

121. Oristrell J, Amengual MJ, Font-Creus B, Casanovas A, Segura-Porta F. Plasma Levels of tumor necrosis factor alpha in patients with Mediterranean spotted fever: clinical and analytical correlations. Clin Infect Dis 1994; 19:1141-1143.

122. Brouqui P, Raoult D. Effects of antibiotics on the phagolysosome fusion in *Ehrlichia sennetsu* infected P388 D1 cells. In: Kazar J, Raoult D, eds. Rickettsiae and Rickettsial Diseases. Bratislava:Publishing House of the Slovak Academy of Sciences, 1991:751-757.

123. Dumler JS, Bakken JS. Human ehrlichioses - newly recognized infections transmitted by ticks. Ann Rev Med 1998; 49:201-213.

124. Marrero M, Raoult D. Centrifugation-shell vial technique for rapid detection of Mediterranean spotted fever rickettsia in blood culture. Am J Trop Med Hyg 1989; 40:197-199.

125. Kaplowitz LG, Lange JV, Fischer JJ, Walker DH. Correlation of rickettsial titers, circulating endotoxin, and clinical features in Rocky Mountain spotted fever. Arch Intern Med 1983; 143:1149-1151.

126. La Scola B, Raoult D. Diagnosis of Mediterranean spotted fever by cultivation of *Rickettsia conorii* from blood and skin samples using the centrifugation-shell vial technique and by detection of *R. conorii* in circulating endothelial cells: a 6 year follow-up. J Clin Microbiol 1996; 34:2722-2727.

127. Fenollar F, Raoult D. Diagnosis of rickettsial diseases using samples dried on blotting paper. Clin Diagn Lab Immunol 1999; 6:483-488.

128. Montenegro MR, Mansueto S, Hegarty BC, Walker DH. The histology of "tâches noires" of boutonneuse fever and demonstration of *Rickettsia conorii* in them by immunofluorescence. Virchows Arch [A] 1983; 400:309-317.

129. Walker DH, Burday MS, Folds JD. Laboratory diagnosis of Rocky Mountain spotted fever. South Med J 1980; 73:1443-1449.

130. Walker DH, Cain BG, Olmstead PM. Laboratory diagnosis of Rocky Mountain spotted fever by immunofluorescent demonstration of *Rickettsia* in cutaneous lesions. Am J Clin Pathol 1978; 69:619-623.

131. Walker DH, Gay RM, Valdes-Dapena M. The occurrence of eschars in Rocky Mountain spotted fever. J Amer Acad Dermatol 1981; 4:571-576.

132. Gil-Grande R, Aguado JM, Pastor C, Garcia-Bravo M, Gomez-Pellico C, Soriano F, Noriega AR. Conventional viral cultures and shell vial assay for diagnosis of apparently culture-negative *Coxiella burnetii* endocarditis. Eur J Clin Microbiol Infect Dis 1995; 14:64-67.

133. Musso D, Raoult D. *Coxiella burnetii* blood cultures from acute and chronic Q-fever patients. J Clin Microbiol 1995; 33:3129-3132.

134. Raoult D, Vestris G, Enea M. Isolation of 16 strains of *Coxiella burnetii* from patients by using a sensitive centrifugation cell culture system and establishment of strains in HEL cells. J Clin Microbiol 1990; 28:2482-2484.

135. Kelly PJ, Raoult D, Mason PR. Isolation of spotted fever group rickettsias from triturated ticks using a modification of the centrifugation-shell vial technique. Trans R Soc Trop Med Hyg 1991; 85:397-398.

136. Burgdorfer W. Hemolymph test. A technique for detection of rickettsiae in ticks. Am J Trop Med Hyg 1970; 19:1010-1014.

137. Beati L, Kelly PJ, Matthewman LA, Mason P, Raoult D. Prevalence of *Rickettsia*-like organisms and spotted fever group *Rickettsiae* in ticks (Acari: *Ixodidae*) from Zimbabwe. J Med Entomol 1995; 32:787-792.

138. Cox HR. Use of yolk sac of developing chick embryo as medium for growing rickettsiae of Rocky montain spotted fever and typhus group. Public Health Rep 1938; 53:2241-2247.

139. Ormsbee RA. The growth of *Coxiella burnetii* in embryonated eggs. J Bacteriol 1952; 63:73.

140. Gilmore RD, Cieplak W, Policastro PF, Hackstadt T. The 120 kilodalton outer membrane protein (rOmpB) of *Rickettsia rickettsii* is encoded by an unusually long open reading frame. Evidence for protein processing from a large precursor. Mol Microbiol 1991; 5:2361-2370.

141. Ormsbee RA, Peacock MG, Gerloff R, Tallent G, Wike D. Limits of rickettsial infectivity. Infect Immun 1978; 19:239-245.

142. Williams JC, Thomas LA, Peacock MG. Humoral immune response to Q fever: enzyme-linked immunosorbent assay antibody response to *Coxiella burnetii* in experimentally infected guinea pigs. J Clin Microbiol 1986; 24:935-939.

143. Eremeeva ME, Balayeva NM, Raoult D. Purification of rickettsial cultures contaminated by mycoplasmas. Acta Virol 1994; 38:231-233.

144. Ridoux O, Foucault C, Drancourt M. Purification of *Encephalitozoon* cultures contaminated by mycoplasmas by murine intraperitoneal inoculation. J Clin Microbiol 1998; 36:2380-2382.

145. Buhles WC, Huxsoll DL, Ruch G, Kenyon RH, Elisberg BL. Evaluation of primary blood monocyte and bone marrow cell culture for the isolation of *Rickettsia rickettsii*. Infect Immun 1975; 12:1457-1463.

146. Stein A, Kruszewska D, Gouvernet J, Raoult D. Study of the 16S-23S ribosomal DNA internal spacer of *Coxiella burnetii*. Eur J Epidemiol 1997; 13:471-475.

147. DeShazo RD, Boyce JR, Osterman JV, Stephenson EH. Early diagnosis of Rocky Mountain spotted fever. Use of primary monocyte culture technique. JAMA 1976; 235:1353-1355.

148. Tamura A, Takahashi K, Tsuruhara T, Urakami H, Miyamura S, Sekikawa H, Kenmotsu M, Shibata M, Abe S, Nezu H. Isolation of *Rickettsia tsutsugamushi* antigenically different from Kato, Karp, and Gilliam strains from patients. Microbiol Immunol 1984; 28:873-882.

149. Espejo-Arenas E, Raoult D. First isolates of *Rickettsia conorii* in Spain using a centrifugation-shell vial assay. J Infect Dis 1989; 159:1158-1159.

150. Weiss E, Dressler HR. Centrifugation of rickettsiae and viruses into cells and its effect on infection. Proc Soc Exp Biol Med 1960; 103:691-695.

151. Bourgeois AL, Olson JG, Fang RC, Huang J, Wang CL, Chow L, Bechthold D, Dennis DT, Coolbaugh JC, Weiss E. Humoral and cellular responses in scrub typhus patients reflecting primary infection and reinfection with *Rickettsia tsutsugamushi*. Am J Trop Med Hyg 1982; 31:532-540.

152. Kleeman KT, Hicks JL, Anacker RL, Philip RL, Casper EA, Hechemy KE, Wilfert CM, MacCormack JN. Early detection of antibody to *Rickettsia rickettsii*: A comparison of four serological methods: indirect hemag-

glutination, indirect fluorescent antibody, latex agglutination, and complement fixation. In: Kazar J, ed. Rickettsiae and Rickettsial Diseases:Bratislava, 1996:171-178.

153. Raoult D, De Micco C, Gallais H. Laboratory diagnosis of Mediterranean spotted fever by immunofluorescent demonstration of *Rickettsia conorii* in cutaneous lesions. J Infect Dis 1985; 150:145-148.

154. Field PR, Hunt JG, Murphy AM. Detection and persistence of specific IgM antibody to *Coxiella burnetii* by enzyme-linked immunosorbent assay: a comparison with immunofluorescence and complement fixation tests. J Infect Dis 1983; 148:477-487.

155. Peter O, Dupuis G, Burgdorfer W, Peacock M. Evaluation of the complement fixation and indirect immunofluorescence tests in the early diagnosis of primary Q fever. Eur J Clin Microbiol Infect Dis 1985; 4:394-396.

156. Peacock MG, Philip RN, Williams JC, Faulkner RS. Serological evaluation of Q fever in humans: enhanced phase I titers of immunoglobulins G and A are diagnostic for Q fever endocarditis. Infect Immun 1983; 41:1089-1098.

157. Newhouse VF, Shepard CC, Redus MD, Tzianabos T, McDade JE. A comparison of the complement fixation, indirect fluorescent antibody, and microagglutination tests for the serological diagnosis of rickettsial diseases. Am J Trop Med Hyg 1979; 28:387-395.

158. Raoult D, Rousseau S, Toga B, Tamalet C, Gallais H, de Micco P, Casanova P. Serology diagnosis of Mediterranean Boutonneuse fever. Pathol Biol 1984; 32:791-794.

159. Tissot-Dupont H, Thirion X, Raoult D. Q fever serology: cutoff determination for microimmunofluorescence. Clin Diagn Lab Immunol 1994; 1:189-196.

160. Fournier PE, Casalta JP, Habib G, Messana T, Raoult D. Modification of the diagnostic criteria proposed by the Duke Endocarditis Service to permit improved diagnosis of Q fever endocarditis. Am J Med 1996; 100:629-633.

161. Dupuis G, Peter O, Peacock M, Burgdorfer W, Haller E. Immunoglobulin responses in acute Q fever. J Clin Microbiol 1985; 22:484-487.

162. Raoult D. Treatment of Q fever. Antimicrob Agents Chemother 1993; 37:1733-1736.

163. Raoult D, Marrie TJ. Q fever. Clin Infect Dis 1995; 20:489-496.

164. Bakken JS, Krueth J, Wilsonnordskog C, Tilden RL, Asanovich K, Dumler JS. Clinical and laboratory characteristics of human granulocytic ehrlichiosis. JAMA 1996; 275:199-205.

165. Dumler JS, Asanovich KM, Bakken JS, Richter P, Kimsey R, Madigan JE. Serologic cross-reactions among *Ehrlichia aqui*, *Ehrlichia phagocytophila*, and human granulocytic ehrlichia. J Clin Microbiol 1995; 33:1098-1103.

166. Raoult D, Dasch GA. The line blot: an immunoassay for monoclonal and other antibodies. Its application to the serotyping of gram-negative bacteria. J Immunol Meth 1989; 125:57-65.

167. Raoult D, Dasch GA. Line blot and Western blot immunoassays for diagnosis of Mediterranean spotted fever. J Clin Microbiol 1989; 27:2073-2079.

168. Teysseire N, Raoult D. Comparison of Western immunoblotting and microimmunofluoresence for diagnosis of Mediterranean spotted fever. J Clin Microbiol 1992; 30:455-460.

169. Cowley R, Fernandez F, Freemantle W, Rutter D. Enzyme immunoassay for Q Fever: comparison with complement fixation and immunofluorescence tests and dot immunoblotting. J Clin Microbiol 1992; 30:2451-2455.

170. Blondeau JM, Williams JC, Marrie TJ. The immune response to phase I and phase II *Coxiella burnetii* antigens as measured by Western immunoblotting. Ann NY Acad Sci 1990; 590:187-202.

171. Willems H, Thiele D, Glas-Adollah-Baik Kashi M, Krauss H. Immunoblot technique for Q fever. Eur J Epidemiol 1992; 8:103-107.

172. Weil E, Felix A. Zur serologischen diagnose des fleckfiebers. Wien Klin Wochenschr 1916; 29:33-35.

173. Castaneda MR, Zia S. The antigenic relationship between proteus X-19 and typhus rickettsiae. J Exp Med 1933; 58:55-62.

174. Raoult D, Dasch GA. Immunoblot cross-reactions among *Rickettsia*, *Proteus* spp. and *Legionella* spp. in patients with Mediterranean spotted fever. FEMS Immunol Med Microbiol 1995; 11:13-18.

175. Amano K, Suzuki N, Hatakeyama H, Kasahara Y, Fujii S, Fukushi K, Suto T, Mahara F. The reactivity between rickettsiae and Weil-Felix test antigens against sera of rickettsial disease patients. Acta Virol 1992; 36:67-72.

176. Shepard CC, Redus MA, Tzianabos T, Warfield DT. Recent experience with the complement fixation test in the laboratory diagnosis of rickettsial diseases in the United States. Nature 1976; 4:277-283.

177. Hersey DF, Colvin MC, Shepard CC. Studies on the serologic diagnosis of murine typhus and Rocky Mountain spotted fever. J Immunol 1957; 79:409-415.

178. Herr S, Huchzermeyer HF, Te Brugge LA, Williamson CC, Roos JA, Schiele GJ. The use of a single complement fixation test technique in bovine brucellosis, Johne's disease, dourine, equine piroplasmosis and Q fever serology. Onderstepoort J Vet 1985; 52:279-282.

179. Murphy AM, Field PR. The persistence of complement-fixing antibodies to Q-fever (*Coxiella burnetii*) after infection. Med J Aust 1970; 1:1148-1150.

180. Peter O, Flepp M, Bestetti G, Nicolet J, Luthy R, Dupuis G. Q fever endocarditis: diagnostic approaches and monitoring of therapeutic effects. Clin Invest 1992; 70:932-937.

181. Anacker RL, Philip RN, Thomas LA, Casper EA. Indirect hemagglutination test for detection of antibody to *Rickettsia rickettsii* in sera from humans and common laboratory animals. J Clin Microbiol 1979; 10:677-684.

182. Chang RS, Murray ES, Snyder JC. Erythrocyte-sensitizing substances from rickettsiae of the Rocky Mountain spotted fever group. J Immunol 1954; 73:8-15.

183. Hechemy KE, Anacker RL, Philip RN, Kleeman KT, MacCormack JN, Sasowski SJ, Michaelson EE. Detection of Rocky Mountain spotted fever antibodies by a latex agglutination test. J Clin Microbiol 1980;12:144-150.

184. Kazar J, Brezina R, Schramek S, Palanova A, Tvrda B. Suitability of the microagglutination test for detection of post- infection and post-vaccination Q fever antibodies in human sera. Acta Virol 1981; 25:235-240.

185. Fiset P, Ormsbee RA, Silberman R, Peacock M, Spielman SH. A microagglutination technique for detection and measurement of rickettsial antibodies. Acta Virol 1969; 13:60-66.

186. Nguyen SV, Otsuka H, Zhang GQ, To H, Yamaguchi T, Fukushi H, Noma A, Hirai K. Rapid method for detection of *Coxiella burnetii* antibodies using high-density particle agglutination. J Clin Microbiol 1996; 34:2947-2951.

187. Halle S, Dasch GA, Weiss E. Sensitive enzyme-linked immunosorbent assay for detection of antibodies against typhus rickettsiae, *Rickettsia prowazekii* and *Rickettsia typhi*. J Clin Microbiol 1977; 6:101-110.

188. Clements ML, Dumler JS, Fiset P, Wisseman CL, Jr., Snyder MJ, Levine MM. Serodiagnosis of Rocky Mountain spotted fever: comparison of IgM and IgG enzyme-linked immunosorbent assays and indirect fluorescent antibody test. J Infect Dis 1983; 148:876-880.

189. Dasch GA, Halle S, Bourgeois AL. Sensitive microplate enzyme-linked immunosorbent assay for detection of antibodies against the scrub typhus rickettsia, *Rickettsia tsutsugamushi*. J Clin Microbiol 1979; 9:38-48.

190. Kovacova E, Gallo J, Schramek S, Kazar J, Brezina R. *Coxiella burnetii* antigens for detection of Q fever antibodies by ELISA in human sera. Acta Virol 1987; 31:254-259.

191. Peter O, Dupuis G, Bee D, Luthy R, Nicolet J, Burgdorfer W. Enzyme-linked immunosorbent assay for diagnosis of chronic Q fever. J Clin Microbiol 1988; 26:1978-1982.

192. Uhaa I, Fishbein DB, Olson JG, Rives CC, Waag DM, Williams JC. Evaluation of specificity of indirect enzyme-linked immunosorbent assay for diagnosis of human Q fever. J Clin Microbiol 1994; 32:1560-1565.

193. Waag D, Chulay J, Marrie T, England M, Williams J. Validation of an enzyme immunoassay for serodiagnosis of acute Q fever Eur J Clin Microbiol Infect Dis 1995; 14:421-427.

194. Williams JC, Thomas LA, Peacock MG. Identification of phase-specific antigenic fractions of *Coxiella burnetti* by enzyme-linked immunosorbent assay. J Clin Microbiol 1986; 24:929-934.

195. Ormsbee R, Peacock M, Philip R, Casper E, Plorde J, Gabre-Kidan T, Wright L. Serologic diagnosis of epidemic typhus fever. Am J Epidemiol 1977; 105:261-271.

196. Kaplan JE, Schonberger LB. The sensitivity of various serologic tests in the diagnosis of Rocky Mountain spotted fever. Am J Trop Med Hyg 1986; 35:840-844.

197. La Scola B, Raoult D. Laboratory diagnosis of rickettsioses: current approaches to the diagnosis of old and new rickettsial diseases. J Clin Microbiol 1997; 35:2715-2727.

198. Philip RN, Casper EA, MacCormack JN, Sexton D, Thomas LA, Anacker RL, Burgdorfer W, Vick S. A comparison of serologic methods for diagnosis of Rocky Mountain spotted fever. Am J Epidemiol 1977; 105:56-67.

199. Shirai A, Dietel JW, Osterman JV. Indirect hemagglutination test for human antibody to typhus and spotted fever group rickettsiae. J Clin Microbiol 1975; 2:430-437.

200. Raoult D, De Micco C, Chaudet H, Tamalet J. Serological diagnosis of Mediterranean spotted fever by the immunoperoxidase reaction. Eur J Clin Microbiol Infect Dis 1985; 4:441-442.

201. Wilfert CM, Austin E, Dickinson V, Kleeman K, Hicks JL, MacCormack JN, Anacker RL, Casper EA, Philip RN. The incidence of Rocky Mountain spotted fever as described by prospective epidemiologic surveillance and the assessment of persistence of antibodies to *R. rickettsii* by indirect hemagglutination and microim-

munofluorescence tests. In: Burgdorfer W, Anacker RL, eds. Rickettsiae and Rickettsial Diseases. New York:Academic Press, 1981:179-189.

202. Sompolinsky D, Boldur I, Goldwasser RA, Kahana H, Kazak R, Keysary A, Pik A. Serological cross-reactions between *Rickettsia typhi, Proteus vulgaris* OX19, and *Legionella bozemanii* in a series of febrile patients. Isr J Med Sci 1986; 22:745-752.

203. Brouqui P, Harle JR, Delmont J, Frances C, Weiller PJ, Raoult D. African tick bite fever: an imported spotless rickettsiosis. Arch Int Med 1997; 157:119-124.

204. Dwyer DE, Gibbons VL, Brady LM, Cunningham AL. Serological reaction to *Legionella pneumophila* group 4 in a patient with Q fever. J Infect Dis 1988; 158:499-500.

205. Finidori JP, Raoult D, Bornstein N, Fleurette J. Study of cross-reaction between *Coxiella burnetii* and *Legionella pneumophila* using indirect immunofluorescence assay and immunoblotting. Acta Virol 1992; 36:459-465.

206. Dobija-Domaradzki M, Hausser JL, Gosselin F. Coexistence of Legionnaires' disease and Q fever in a single patient. CMAJ 1984; 130:1022-1023.

207. Musso D, Raoult D. Serological cross-reactions between *Coxiella burnetii* and *Legionella micdadei*. Clin Diagn Lab Immunol 1997; 4:208-212.

208. La Scola B, Raoult D. Serological cross reactions between *Bartonella quintana, Bartonella henselae*, and *Coxiella burnetii*. J Clin Microbiol 1996; 34:2270-2274.

209. Stein A, Raoult D. Detection of *Coxiella burnetii* by DNA amplification using polymerase chain reaction. J Clin Microbiol 1992; 30:2462-2466.

210. Stein A, Raoult D. A simple method for amplification of DNA from paraffin-embedded tissues. Nucleic Acids Res 1992; 20:5237-5238.

211. Hoover TA, Vodkin MH, Williams JC. A *Coxiella burnetii* repeated DNA element resembling a bacterial insertion sequence. J Bacteriol 1992; 174:5540-5548.

212. Willems H, Thiele D, Frolich-Ritter R, Krauss H. Detection of *Coxiella burnetii* in cow's milk using the polymerase chain reaction. J Vet Med B 1994; 41:580-587.

213. Horinouchi H, Murai K, Okayama A, Nagatomo Y, Tachibana N, Tsubouchi H. Genotypic identification of *Rickettsia tsutsugamushi* by restruction fragment length polymorphism analysis of DNA amplified by the polymerase chain reaction. Am J Trop Med Hyg 1996; 54:647-651.

214. Murai K, Okayama A, Horinouchi H, Oshikawa T, Tachibana N, Tsubouchi H. Eradication of *Rickettsia tsutsugamushi* from patients' blood by chemotherapy as assessed by the polymerase chain reaction. Am J Trop Med Hyg 1995; 52:325-327.

215. Williams WJ, Radulovic S, Dasch GA, Lindstrom J, Kelly DJ, Oster CN, Walker DH. Identification of *Rickettsia conorii* infection by polymerase chain reaction in a soldier returning from Somalia. Clin Infect Dis 1994; 19:93-99.

216. Gage K, Schrumpf ME, Karstens RH, Burgdorfer W, Schwan TG. DNA typing of rickettsiae in naturally infected ticks using a polymerase chain reaction/restriction fragment length polymorphism system. Am J Trop Med Hyg 1994; 50:247-260.

217. Gage KL, Gilmore RD, Karstens RH, Schwan TG. Detection of *Rickettsia rickettsii* in saliva, hemolymph and triturated tissues of infected *Dermacentor andersoni* ticks by polymerase chain reaction. Mol Cell Probes 1992; 6:333-341.

218. Higgins JA, Azad AF. Use of polymerase chain reaction to detect bacteria in arthropods: a review. J Med Entomol 1995; 32:213-222.

219. Anderson BE, Tzianabos T. Comparative sequence analysis of a genus-common rickettsial antigen gene. J Bacteriol 1989; 171:5199-5201.

220. Baird RW, Stenos J, Stewart R, Hudson B, Lloyd M, Aiuto S, Dwyer B. Genetic variation in Australian spotted fever group rickettsiae. J Clin Microbiol 1996; 34:1526-1530.

221. Balayeva NM, Eremeeva ME, Tissot-Dupont H, Zakharov IA, Raoult D. Genotype characterization of the bacterium expressing the male-killing trait in the ladybird beetle *Adalia bipunctata* with specific rickettsial molecular tools. Appl Environ Microbiol 1995; 61:1431-1437.

222. Raoult D, Roux V, Ndihokubwaho JB, Bise G, Baudon D, Martet G, Birtles RJ. Jail fever (epidemic typhus) outbreak in Burundi. Emerg Infect Dis 1997; 3:357-360.

223. Schriefer ME, Sacci JBJr, Dumler JS, Bullen MG, Azad AF. Identification of a novel rickettsial infection in a patient diagnosed with murine typhus. J Clin Microbiol 1994; 32:949-954.

224. Wood DO, Williamson LR, Winkler HH, Krause DC. Nucleotide sequence of the *Rickettsia prowazekii* citrate synthase gene. J Bacteriol 1987; 169:3564-3572.

225. Niebylski ML, Schrumpf ME, Burgdorfer W, Fischer ER, Gage KL, Schwan TG. *Rickettsia peacockii sp. nov.*, a new species infecting wood ticks, *Dermacentor andersoni*, in Western Montana. Int J Syst Bacteriol 1997;47:446-452.

226. Anderson BE, Sumner JW, Dawson JE, Tzianabos T, Greene CR, Olson JG, Fishbein DB, Olsen-Rasmussen M, Holloway BP, George EH, Azad AF. Detection of the etiologic agent of human ehrlichiosis by polymerase chain reaction. J Clin Microbiol 1992; 30:775-780.

227. Everett ED, Evans KA, Henry RB, MacDonald G. Human ehrlichiosis in adults after tick exposure. Ann Intern Med 1994; 120:730-735.

228. Standaert SM, Dawson JE, Schaffner W, Childs JE, Biggie KL, Singleton BS, Gerhardt RR, Knight ML, Hutcheson RH. Ehrlichiosis in a golf-oriented retirement community. N Engl J Med 1995; 333:420-425.

229. Sumner JW, Nicholson WL, Massung RF. PCR amplification and comparison of nucleotide sequences from the *groESL* heat shock operon of *Ehrlichia* species. J Clin Microbiol 1997; 35:2087-2092.

230. Anacker RL, List RH, Mann RE, Hayes SF, Thomas LA. Characterization of monoclonal antibodies protecting mice against *Rickettsia rickettsii*. J Infect Dis 1985; 151:1052-1060.

231. Anacker RL, List RH, Mann RE, Wiedbrauk DL. Antigenic heterogeneity in high- and low-virulence strains of *Rickettsia rickettsii* revealed by monoclonal antibodies. Infect Immun 1986; 51:653-660.

232. Anacker RL, Mann RE, Gonzales C. Reactivity of monoclonal antibodies to *Rickettsia rickettsii* with spotted fever and typhus group rickettsiae. J Clin Microbiol 1987; 25:167-171.

233. Lange JV, Walker DH. Production and characterization of monoclonal antibodies to *Rickettsia rickettsii*. Infect Immun 1984; 46:289-294.

234. McDade JE, Black CM, Roumillat LF, Redus MA, Spruill CL. Addition of monoclonal antibodies specific for *Rickettsia akari* to the rickettsial diagnostic panel. J Clin Microbiol 1988; 26:2221-2223.

235. Walker DH, Liu QH, Yu XJ, Li H, Taylor C, Feng HM. Antigenic diversity of *Rickettsia conorii*. Am J Trop Med Hyg 1992; 47:78-86.

236. Black CM, Tzianabos T, Roumillat LF, Redus MA, McDade JE, Reimer CB. Detection and characterization of mouse monoclonal antibodies to epidemic typhus rickettsiae. J Clin Microbiol 1983; 18:561-568.

237. Uchiyama T, Uchida T, Walker DH. Species-specific monoclonal antibodies to *Rickettsia japonica*, a newly identified spotted fever group rickettsia. J Clin Microbiol 1990; 28:1177-1180.

238. Xu W, Beati L, Raoult D. Characterization of and application of monoclonal antibodies against *Rickettsia africae*, a newly recognized species of spotted fever group rickettsia. J Clin Microbiol 1997; 35:64-70.

239. Dasch GA. Isolation of species-specific protein antigens of *Rickettsia typhi* and *Rickettsia prowazekii* for immunodiagnosis and immunoprophylaxis. J Clin Microbiol 1981; 14:333-341.

240. Dasch JA, Burans JP, Dobson ME, Rollwagen FM, Misiti J. Approaches to subunit vaccines against the typhus rickettsiae, *Rickettsia typhi* and *Rickettsia prowazekii*. In: Leive L, Schlessinger D, eds. Microbiology. Washington, D.C.:American Society for Microbiology, 1984:251-256.

241. Feng HM, Walker DH, Wang JG. Analysis of T-cell -dependent and -independent antigens of *Rickettsia conorii* with monoclonal antibodies. Infect Immun 1987; 55:7-15.

242. Brouqui P, Dumler JS, Raoult D. Immunohistologic demonstration of *Coxiella burnetii* in the valves of patients with Q fever endocarditis. Am J Med 1994; 97:451-458.

243. Thiele D, Karo M, Krauss H. Monoclonal antibody based capture ELISA/ELIFA for detection of *Coxiella burnetii* in clinical specimens. Eur J Epidemiol 1992; 8:568-574.

244. McCaul TF, Williams JC. Localization of DNA in *Coxiella burnetii* by post-embedding immunoelectron microscopy. Ann NY Acad Sci 1990; 590:136-147.

245. Muhlemann K, Matter L, Meyer B, Schopfer K. Isolation of *Coxiella burnetiii* from heart valves of patients treated for Q fever endocarditis. J Clin Microbiol 1995; 33:428-431.

246. Raoult D, Laurent JC, Mutillod M. Monoclonal antibodies to *Coxiella burnetii* for antigenic detection in cell cultures and in paraffin embedded tissues. Am J Clin Pathol 1994; 101:318-320.

247. Green WR, Walker DH, Cain BG. Fatal viscerotropic Rocky Mountain spotted fever. Report of a case diagnosed by immunofluorescence. Am J Med 1978; 64:523-528.

248. Raoult D, De Micco C, Gallais H, Toga M. Laboratory diagnosis of Mediterranean spotted fever by immunofluorescent demonstration of *Rickettsia conorii* in cutaneous lesions. J Infect Dis 1984; 150:145-148.

249. Woodward TE, Pedersen CE, Jr., Oster CN, Bagley LR, Romberger J, Snyder MJ. Prompt confirmation of Rocky Mountain spotted fever: identification of rickettsiae in skin tissues. J Infect Dis 1976; 134:297-301.

250. Dumler JS, Gage WR, Pettis GL, Azad AF, Kuhadja FP. Rapid immunoperoxidase demonstration of *Rickettsia rickettsii* in fixed cutaneous specimens from patients with Rocky Mountain spotted fever. Am J Clin Pathol 1990; 93:410-414.

251. Mansueto S, Tringali G, Di Leo R, Maniscalco M, Montenegro MR, Walker DH. Demonstration of spotted fever group rickettsiae in the tache noire of a healthy person in Sicily. Am J Trop Med Hyg 1984; 33:479-482.

252. George F, Brisson C, Poncelet P, Laurent JC, Massot O, Arnoux D, Ambrosi P, Klein-Soyer C, Cazenave JP, Sampol J. Rapid isolation of human endothelial cells from whole blood using S-Endo 1 monoclonal antibody coupled to immuno-magnetic beads: demonstration of endothelial injury after angioplasty. Thromb Haemost 1992; 67:147-153.

253. George F, Brouqui P, Boffa MC, Drancourt M, Raoult D, Sampol J. Demonstration of *Rickettsia conorii*-induced endothelial injury in vivo by measuring circulating endothelial cells, thrombomodulin and Von Willebrand factor in patients with Mediterranean spotted fever. Blood 1993; 82:2109-2116.

254. Dumler JS, Dawson JE, Walker DH. Human ehrlichiosis: hematopathology and immunohistologic detection of *Ehrlichia chaffeensis*. Hum Pathol 1993; 24:391-396.

255. Yu X, Brouqui P, Dumler S, Raoult D. Detection of *Ehrlichia chaffeensis* on human tissue by using species specific monoclonal antibody. J Clin Microbiol 1993; 31:3284-3288.

256. McDade JE. Determination of antibiotic susceptibility of *Rickettsia* by the plaque assay technique. Appl Microbiol 1969; 18:133-135.

257. McDade JE, Gerone PJ. Plaque assay for Q fever and scrub typhus rickettsiae. Appl Microbiol 1970; 19:963-965.

258. Weinberg EH, Stakebake JR, Gerone PJ. Plaque assay for *Rickettsia rickettsii*. J Bacteriol 1969; 98:398-402.

259. Wike DA, Tallent G, Peacock MG, Ormsbee RA. Studies of the rickettsial plaque assay technique. Infect Immun 1972; 5:715-722.

260. McDade JE, Stakebake JR, Gerone PJ. Plaque assay system for several species of *Rickettsia*. J Bacteriol 1969; 99:910-912.

261. Wisseman CL, Ordonez SV. Actions of antibiotics on *Rickettsia rickettsii*. J Infect Dis 1986; 153:626-628.

262. Wisseman CL, Waddell A. In vitro sensitivity of *Rickettsia rickettsii* to doxycycline. J Infect Dis 1982; 145:584.

263. Wisseman CL, Waddell AD, Walsh WT. In vitro studies of the action of antibiotics on *Rickettsia prowazekii* by two basic methods of cell culture. J Infect Dis 1974; 130:564-574.

264. Raoult D, Roussellier P, Vestris G, Tamalet J. In vitro antibiotic susceptibility of *Rickettsia rickettsii* and *Rickettsia conorii*: plaque assay and microplaque colorimetric assay. J Infect Dis 1987; 155:1059-1062.

265. Ives TJ, Manzewitsch P, Regnery RL, Butts JD, Kebede M. In vitro susceptibilities of *Bartonella henselae, B. quintana, B. elizabethae, Rickettsia rickettsii, R. conorii, R. akari*, and *R. prowazekii* to macrolide antibiotics as determined by immunofluorescent-antibody analysis of infected vero cell monolayers. Antimicrob Agents Chemother 1997; 41:578-582.

266. Rolain JM, Maurin M, Vestris G, Raoult D. In vitro susceptibilities of 27 rickettsiae to 13 antimicrobials. Antimicrob Agents Chemother 1998; 42:1537-1541.

267. Barker LF. Determination of antibiotic susceptibility of rickettsiae and chlamydiae in BS-C-1 cell cultures. Antimicrob Agents Chemother 1968; 8:425-428.

268. Miyamura S, Ohta T, Tamura A. Comparison of in vitro susceptibilities of *Rickettsia prowazekii, R. rickettsii, R. sibirica* and *R. tsutsugamushi* to antimicrobial agents. Nippon Saikingaku Zasshi 1989; 44:717-721.

269. Wisseman CL, Jr., Silverman DJ, Waddell A, Brown DT. Penicillin-induced unstable intracellular formation of spheroplasts by rickettsiae. J Infect Dis 1982; 146:147-158.

270. Radulovic S, Higgins JA, Jaworski DC, Azad AF. In vitro and in vivo antibiotic susceptibilities of ELB rickettsiae. Antimicrob Agents Chemother 1995; 39:2564-2566.

271. Maurin M, Raoult D. In vitro susceptibilities of spotted fever group rickettsiae and *Coxiella burnetii* to clarithromycin. Antimicrob Agents Chemother 1993; 37:2633-2637.

272. Raoult D, Roussellier P, Tamalet J. In vitro evaluation of josamycin, spiramycin, and erythromycin against *Rickettsia rickettsii* and *R. conorii*. Antimicrob Agents Chemother 1988; 32:255-256.

273. Jabarit-Aldighieri N, Torres H, Raoult D. Susceptibility of *R. conorii, R. rickettsii* and *C. burnetii* to CI- 960 (PD 127,391), PD 131,628, pefloxacin, ofloxacin and ciprofloxacin. Antimicrob Agents Chemother 1992; 36:2529-2532.

274. Maurin M, Raoult D. Bacteriostatic and bactericidal activity of levofloxacin against *Rickettsia rickettsii, Rickettsia conorii* "Israeli spotted fever group rickettsia" and *Coxiella burnetii*. J Antimicrob Chemother 1997; 39:725-730.

275. Raoult D, Bres P, Drancourt M, Vestris G. In vitro susceptibilities of *Coxiella burnetii, Rickettsia rickettsii*, and *Rickettsia conorii* to the fluoroquinolone sparfloxacin. Antimicrob Agents Chemother 1991; 35:88-91.

276. Beati L, Roux V, Ortuno A, Castella J, Segura Porta F, Raoult D. Phenotypic and genotypic characterization of spotted fever group rickettsiae isolated from Catalan *Rhipicephalus sanguineus* ticks. J Clin Microbiol 1996;34:2688-2694.

277. Drancourt M, Raoult D. Characterization of mutations in the *rpo*B gene in naturally rifampin-resistant *Rickettsia* species. Antimicrob Agent Chemother 1999; 43:2400-2403.

278. Rachek LI, Tucker AM, Winkler HH, Wood DO. Transformation of *Rickettsia prowazekii* to rifampin resistance. J Bacteriol 1998; 180:2118-2124.

279. Misao T, Kobayashi Y. Studies on infectious mononucleosis (glandular fever). Isolation of etiologic agent from blood, bone marrow, and lymph node of a patient with infectious monocleosis by using mice. Kyushu J Med Sci 1955; 6:145-152.

280. Tachibana N, Kobayashi V. Effect of cyclophosphamide on the growth of *Rickettsia sennetsu* in experimentally infected mice. Infect Immun 1975; 12:625-629.

281. Kobayashi Y, Ikeda O, Miaso T. Chemotherapy of sennetsu disease. In: Progress in Virology. Tokyo:Bainukan, 1962:130-142.

282. Kelly DJ, LaBarre DD, Lewis GEJ. Effect of tetracycline therapy on host defense in mice infected with *Ehrlichia sennetsu*. In: Winkler HH, Ristic M, eds. Microbiology. Washington, DC:American Society for Microbiology, 1986:209-212.

283. Koyama T. Immunological studies of rickettsial infection-analysis of lymphoid cell subpopulations of the spleen of mice infected with *Rickettsia sennetsu* and *Rickettsia tsutsugamushi*. Kansenshogaku Zasshi 1979; 53:243-257.

284. Brouqui P, Raoult D. In vitro susceptibility of *Ehrlichia sennetsu* to antibiotics. Antimicrob Agents Chemother 1990; 34:1593-1596.

285. Brouqui P, Raoult D. In vitro antibiotic susceptibility of the newly recognized agent of ehrhlichiosis in humans, *Ehrlichia chaffeensis*. Antimicrob Agents Chemother 1992; 36:2799-2803.

286. Klein MB, Nelson CM, Goodman JL. Antibiotic susceptibility of the newly cultivated agent of human granulocytic ehrlichiosis: promising activity of quinolones and rifamycins. Antimicrob Agents Chemother 1997; 41:76-79.

287. Torres H, Raoult D. In vitro activities of ceftriaxone and fusidic acid against 13 isolates of *Coxiella burnetii*, determined using the shell vial assay. Antimicrob Agents Chemother 1993; 37:491-494.

288. Baca OG, Akporiaye ET, Aragon AS, Martinez IL, Robles MV, Warner NL. Fate of phase I and phase II *Coxiella burnetii* in several macrophage-like tumor cell lines. Infect Immun 1981; 33:258-266.

289. Roman MJ, Coriz PD, Baca OG. A proposed model to explain persistent infection of host cells with *Coxiella burnetii*. J Gen Microbiol 1986; 132:1415-1422.

290. Raoult D, Drancourt M, Vestris G. Bactericidal effect of doxycycline associated with lysosomotropic agents on *Coxiella burnetii* in P388D1 cells. Antimicrob Agents Chemother 1990; 34:1512-1514.

291. Maurin M, Benoliel AM, Bongrand P, Raoult D. Phagolysosomal alkalinization an the bactericidal effect of antibiotics: the *Coxiella burnetii* paradigm. J Infect Dis 1992; 166:1097-1102.

292. Maurin M, Raoult D. Query fever. Clin Microbiol Rev 1999; 12:518-553.

293. Fournier PE, Marrie TJ, Raoult D. Diagnosis of Q fever. J Clin Microbiol 1998; 36:1823-1834.

294. Raoult D, Roux V. Rickettsioses as paradigms of new or emerging infectious diseases. Clin Microbiol Rev 1997;10:694-719.

295. Dawson JE, Fishbein D, Eng T, Redus M, Greene N. Diagnosis of human ehrlichiosis with the indirect fluorescent antibody test: kinetics and specificity. J Infect Dis 1990; 162:91-95.

296. Dawson JE, Rikihisa Y, Ewing SA, Fishbein DB. Serologic diagnosis of human ehrlichiosis using two *Ehrlichia canis* isolates. J Infect Dis 1991; 163:564-567.

297. Brouqui P, Lecam C, Olson J, Raoult D. Serologic diagnosis of human monocytic ehrlichiosis by immunoblot analysis. Clin Diagn Lab Immunol 1994; 1:645-649.

298. Asanovich KM, Bakken JS, Madigan JE, Aguero-Rosenfeld M, Wormser GP, Dumler JS. Antigenic diversity of granulocytic *Ehrlichia* isolates from humans in Wisconsin and New York and a horse in California. J Infect Dis 1997; 176:1029-1034.

299. Willems H, Thiele D, Krauss H. Plasmid based differentiation and detection of *Coxiella burnetii* in clinical samples. Eur J Epidemiol 1993; 9:411-417.

300. Ibrahim A, Norlander L, Macellaro A, Sjostedt A. The potential of the 23S rRNA gene for rapid detection of *Coxiella burnetii* in clinical samples. In: Kazar J, Toman R, eds. Rickettsiae and Rickettsial Diseases. Bratislava:Slovak Academy of Sciences, 1996:441-445.

29

Mycoplasmas

Nevio Cimolai
Children's and Women's Health Centre of British Columbia, Vancouver, British Columbia, Canada

I. HISTORICAL BACKGROUND

The unconventional morphology and growth characteristics of mycoplasmas have necessarily led to their historical understudy. Given the status of unusual bacteria and the ability to elude filtration processes, these microbes have disinterested the classical bacteriologist and never fully excited the virologist. Almost a century after their initial discovery, mycoplasmology continues to be seen as a difficult area by many.

The initial efforts of Nocard and Roux at the turn of the century defined what were to be the first recognized mycoplasmas. These agents were obtained from bovine pneumonia, and subsequently similar isolations were thereafter named bovine pleuropneumonia-like agents (PPLO). Whereas some work was conducted in this area, the species diversity would require major investigative efforts in the latter half of the twentieth century. Dienes and Smith demonstrated the presence of PPLO in the human genital tract by the 1940s (1). Within another decade, Morton et al. were able to document the presence of PPLO in human saliva (2). The original 'Eaton's agent' (atypical pneumonia source, filterable agent, transmissible) was so coined as a result of efforts from the mid-1940s (3), but definition of the human-associated pathogen *Mycoplasma pneumoniae* would not occur until many years later (4). It is not surprising that confusion would be had since much of this pioneering work was being performed at a time when many filterable agents of respiratory disease were becoming recognized as viruses. In addition, L forms (cell wall-less, membrane bound) of bacteria were recognized, and it was at first suspected that PPLO were but variations of the latter.

Since these pioneering efforts were published, it has become apparent that mycoplasmas are ubiquitous and may potentially serve as both pathogen and commensal for humans and other members of the animal kingdom, as well as plants. The term 'mycoplasma' continues to be used in a generic sense for these and similar cell wall-less bacteria. The name arises from a hybrid describing the microscopic morphology as "deformable like a fungus"; the class designation of Mollicutes is translated from Latin as "soft skin". Nevertheless, these designations may detract from the realization of diversity – based on metabolic and other criteria, this broad group of bacteria can be divided into mycoplasmas (proper), ureaplasmas, acholeplasmas, spiroplasmas, anaeroplasmas, and asteroleplasmas. Essentially, only mycoplasmas and ureaplasmas have been recognized as human pathogens, and then furthermore, only a small subset of these have been found in humans (Table 1). Of the human-associated mycoplasmas, again only a subset have been shown to cause disease.

The phylogeny of mycoplasmas is speculative, but it appears at this time that there may have been a degenerative evolution from some Gram positive bacteria (5). Mycoplasmas have the smallest of bacterial genomes; human mycoplasma genomes range from approximately 500 to 800 kilobase-pairs (e.g., *M. pneumoniae* ~ 816 kbp; *M. genitalium* ~ 580 kbp) (6). G+C content is in the range of 24–33 mol.%. They are generally categorized as the smallest self-replicating bacteria and are lacking of cell walls.

Table 1   Characteristics and disease-affiliations for human-associated mycoplasmas.

	Site	Characteristics	Common Disease Associations
Acholeplasma	mucosal (commensal?)	non-sterol requiring, glucose fermentation, rapid grower	none
M. buccale	oral commensal	arginine utilization	none
M. genitalium	mainly uro-genital, rarely respiratory	glucose fermentation	non-gonococcal urethritis
M. faucium	oral commensal	arginine utilization	none
M. fermentans	urogenital, oral commensal	glucose fermentation, arginine utilization	largely unknown, but found in disseminated disease among HIV+ patients
M. hominis	mainly urogenital, rarely oral commensal	arginine utilization	several uncommon or unsubstantiated associations
M. lipophilum	oral commensal	arginine utilization	none
M. orale	oral commensal	arginine utilization	none
M. penetrans	urogenital	glucose fermentation, arginine utilization, intracellular	uncertain
M. pirum	AIDS-associated (blood mononuclear cells)	glucose fermentation, arginine utilization	uncertain
M. pneumoniae	respiratory, rare genital isolation	glucose fermentation	upper and lower respiratory, numerous but uncommon extra-respiratory manifestations
M. primatum	genital	arginine utilization	none
M. salivarium	oral commensal	arginine utilization	none
M. spermatophilum	urogenital	arginine utilization	unknown
U. urealyticum	urogenital	urease activity	non-gonococcal urethritis, chorioamnionitis
Mycoplasma-Like Organisms (MLOs)	unknown	non-cultivable, morphological and clinical criteria for suspect disease	rheumatoid arthritis, uveitis, chronic fatigue (all proposed; not confirmed)

Phylogenetic positioning of human mycoplasmas into several groups has been proposed (7).

The vast majority of study in human mycoplasmology has occurred in the last forty years, and by far, this work has especially focused on *M. pneumoniae* as the respiratory pathogen and the genital mycoplasmas, specifically *M. hominis* and *U. urealyticum*, as causes of a variety of infections. *M. genitalium* has been touted as a cause of non-gonococcal urethritis within the last decade (8). *M. fermentans*, while recognized as an oral mycoplasma, has received attention as a cause of illness among HIV-infected patients among others (9). The re-discovery of the latter came about with an interesting history (10), and it was temporarily re-named *M. incognitus*. Very recently, *M. penetrans* has been discovered, and again interests have been stimulated regarding AIDS-associated mycoplasmas (11,12).

Whereas interests for *M. pneumoniae* as a common respiratory pathogen and for genital mycoplasmas as causes of a variety of urogenital and other diseases have provided a steady stream of medical literature, resurgent study has been provoked by the putative association of some mycoplasmas and HIV infection; perhaps the influences of Montagnier (13) and Lo (9) have been most appealing. In addition, mycoplasmas have occasionally been cited as possible causes of cryptic illnesses when mycoplasma-like structures have been identified by ultrastructural, especially electron microscopic, studies of diseased tissue (14). This has led to the use of 'mycoplasma-like organism' (MLO) for such elements. It is hoped that new molecular strategies (see Chapters 5 and 6) will resolve the true status of such structures. In part, the latter strategies have already been initiated and have led some to believe that detection of genetic material may implicate mycoplasmas in some illnesses where viable mycoplasmas are not actually cultivated (15,16). Mycoplasmas have also been implicated as causes of illness by extrapolation when an apparently anti-mycoplasma antibiotic has been shown to ameliorate an illness for which no conventional bacterium is found (17). Although the latter associations seem initially fallible, these and others have nevertheless led to some renewed interest in the field.

II.   CLINICAL ASPECTS

A.   *M. pneumoniae*

M. pneumoniae is a very common community-acquired cause of respiratory illness (18). The infection can occur at all levels of the respiratory tract, but there is a predominance to mid- and lower respiratory localization; perhaps recognition of the latter is better facilitated by the fact that patients with lower respiratory illness are more likely to be sufficiently ill so that they will seek medical attention. Infection may include bilateral myringitis and sinusitis, but *M. pneumoniae* is not a notable cause of illnesses that are manifest essentially as colds. Pharyngitis, when it occurs, is likely to be mild. Tracheobronchitis is a more common presentation, and less often will the disease be manifest as a focal laryngitis, or rarely as a croup or bronchiolitis of infants. Pneumonias are also a major form of illness, but clinical presentation is quite variable. Focal lobar or interstitial patterns of pneumonia are not common; rather, diffuse or multifocal bronchopneumonia patterns predominate. Nevertheless, for acute pneumonias, this bacterium essentially causes clinical presentations which are termed community-acquired atypical pneumonia. Such presentations unfortunately overlap with several other bacterial causes and with many viruses. Pleural effusions are seen in a minority of patients, either as collections which complicate an acute pneumonia or less often as a form where there may be direct bacterial infection and hence inflammation.

Bacterial infection outside of the respiratory tract has been cited on many occasions, but these ectopic sites of infection are quite uncommon. Pericardial space, central nervous system, and joint represent such sites for infection (19-21). It remains to be seen whether molecular techniques will expand our view of where *M. pneumoniae* infection occurs. An example of such insight is best exemplified by the association of *M. pneumoniae* with central nervous system disease. Narita et al. (22) have published evidence which suggests a high frequency of *M. pneumoniae* presence by molecular techniques in associated central nervous system illness. In our own experience, both culture and molecular techniques have often failed to find the bacterium in the cerebrospinal fluid (N. Cimolai, personal observations). Extra-respiratory manifestations which are not a function of documented direct bacterial invasion are evidently more common. A diverse array of such manifestations have been reported and include numerous body systems: cardiac (myocarditis, pericarditis), joint (arthritis, arthralgias), deep organ (pancreatitis, nephritis), dermatological (macular and vesicular rashes, Stevens-Johnson syndrome), hematological (hemolytic anemia), and neurological (meningitis, encephalitis, peripheral neuropathies, transverse myelitis, Guillian-Barre syndrome, cortical infarction) among others (23,24). It can only be hypothesized at this time that some form of immune dysfunction, either humoral or cell-mediated, must be responsible for this wide spectrum of disease. The frequency of extra-respiratory manifestations that accompany *M. pneumoniae* infection may as high as 5-10% (25). Associations of extra-respiratory illness with *M. pneumoniae* infection must be viewed carefully, however, for several reasons. *M. pneumoniae* infection is relatively common in the general community, and therefore infection may simply co-incide with another disease and thereby be falsely associated. Secondly, common serodiagnostic methods will have a particular frequency of false-positive indications, and the likelihood of these is greater when a fallible diagnostic that is being applied to an illness that has a low pre-test probability of true infection. It is extremely uncommon to see such an extra-respiratory manifestation unless there has been a preceding or there is an existing *M. pneumoniae* respiratory infection.

B. *U. urealyticum*

In contrast to *M. pneumoniae*, diseases that are thought to potentially be caused by *U. urealyticum* are complicated most by the fact that many of these associations have been difficult to study and hence verify. Given the localization of *U. urealyticum* to the normal genital tract, especially female, most of these disease associations relate to urogenital disease or complications of pregnancy and newborn. One of the more credible links to an illness is that of *U. urealyticum* as a cause of non-gonococcal urethritis (26). Although supported initially by treatment data, case-control studies would subsequently raise awareness of this link. Recent data, however, has challenged the relative role of *U. urealyticum* and has indicated that *M. genitalium* may actually be the more important mycoplasma in non-gonococcal urethritis (27,28). Considerable efforts in the last decade have been directed towards establishing a role for *U. urealyticum* in disease of the premature lung (29). There has been considerable controversy on the latter topic, but presently, attention is focused at a role in pneumonitis only for the very low birth-weight premature newborn. Infections of joints in hypogammaglobulinemic patients seem bonafide although rare. Central nervous system infections of premature newborns is also rare and have been the subject of some controversy mainly in respect to the frequency of illness (30,31). These bacteria have been found in amniotic fluid of pregnant females, and hence a role in chorioamnionitis seems likely (32). Other associations with disease which remain of interest, but are largely not well supported, include urinary stones, infertility, repeat spontaneous abortion and stillbirth, post-partum maternal fever, pelvic inflammatory disease of females, epididymitis, and prostatitis. Very few anecdotes of causation for wound and soft tissue infections are available. Even if *U. urealyticum* were to be a cause for some of these latter problems, the high frequency of carriage in the normal female genital tract would continue to confound.

C. *M. hominis*

Despite the high frequency of this bacterium in the female genital tract, there are fewer associations with complications of pregnancy than for *U. urealyticum*. *M. hominis* has been documented as a cause of wound infection (33). A role in Bartholin's abscesses and cysts is not clear. The bacterium has also been isolated from the joints of patients with hypogammaglobulinemia, as for *U. urealyticum*, and from amniotic fluid of pregnancy and cerebrospinal fluid of newborns. Blood culture isolates from patients with post-partum and post-abortal fever are recorded although blood culture isolation from seemingly well mothers around the time of vaginal delivery has added some confusion to the latter association. Pelvic inflammatory disease of females and bacterial vaginosis are complex conditions from a microbiological view, but there appears to be potential for *M. hominis* to exist as a co-factor in some circumstances. Challenge studies with adult volunteers have led to some suspicion that acute pharyngitis may be caused by the bacterium, but subsequent follow-through on this topic has not substantiated any such link (34,35). A role in pyelonephritis is potentially limited to very unusual circumstances. In contrast to *U. urealyticum*, *M. hominis* has not been found to be an agent of non-gonococcal urethritis or pneumonitis of the premature lung.

D. *M. genitalium*

The difficulty in cultivating this bacterium has necessarily led to the use of genetic detection methods. A proposal that *M. genitalium* might be a causative agent of non-gonococcal urethritis was made on the basis of studies in non-human primates, but a role in human disease was not substantiated (36). More recent studies, however, favour a role for *M. genitalium* in both non-gonococcal urethritis and post-gonococcal urethritis (27,28,36-38), perhaps even leading one to believe that *M. genitalium* may be a more likely and a more common urethral pathogen than *Ureaplasma urealyticum*. *M. genitalium* seems to be more commonly found in the urethrae of HIV-infected individuals. Early findings of *M. genitalium* from the respiratory tract have provided interest, but no substantiation of a role in acute respiratory disease has been clearly documented. The bacterium has not been found in amniotic fluids (39).

E. *M. fermentans*

Although recognized as a human mycoplasma for decades, a role in human disease was fortuitously discovered by Lo and others (9). Initially associated with systemic illness in HIV-infected individuals, anecdotes have emerged of an illness among non-HIV-infected patients (40,41). These findings were foreshadowed by animal studies of leukemoid reaction-associated systemic illnesses many years prior (42). *M. fermentans* is commonly found in the urine of HIV-positive individuals (43) and a role in HIV-associated nephropathy has been contemplated (44,45). Given that nephropathy may occur independently as a function of HIV infection itself, it is unclear whether *M. fermentans* has a primary, co-factor, or no role. The bacterium has been found in blood and lymph node tissue of HIV positive patients by genetic detection. There does not appear to be a role in non-gonococcal urethritis (46). Recent proposed findings of *M. fermentans* in joint fluids of arthritic patients and the blood of patients who suffer from chronic fatigue are sure to spark additional interest (15,47,48), but they must be viewed as preliminary and in need of much further substantiation.

F. *M. penetrans*

This bacterium has been isolated from the urine of HIV-infected patients (11,12), but causation of infection whether of the genitourinary system or elsewhere, is largely unexplored. A recent citation of infection in non-HIV infected patients remains of interest (73).

G. Mycoplasma-like organisms (MLOs)

MLOs have been proposed as possible etiological agents in some forms of uveitis and arthritides (14,16,49), but considerable doubt remains with respect to these findings (50,51).

H. Other

It is extremely uncommon to find any of the other commensal mycoplasmas associated with bonafide infection.

III. EPIDEMIOLOGY OF INFECTION

A. *M. pneumoniae*

M. pneumoniae is a common cause of respiratory disease in the general community throughout the world. Nosocomial infection is uncommon. The bacterium resides in the respiratory tract, but asymptomatic carriage is seemingly quite uncommon (52). It is more likely that asymptomatic excretion in the respiratory tract will follow after an active infection. There have been rare citations of *M. pneumoniae* presence in the genital tract (53). There is also the potential for *M. pneumoniae* to be present in the respiratory tract as a consequence of relatively asymptomatic infection. In essence, *M. pneumoniae* is not considered a component of normal respiratory flora.

Different sources have been consistent with the observation that periodic cycles of peak frequency seem to occur approximately every 4 to 6 years (54,55) although this pattern may be changing in modern times (56). It is unclear what impact there may be from increased use of macrolides in primary care of the general community. Infection occurs throughout the year, although for children, a higher incidence has been noted for school-aged children as might be anticipated since transmission is more likely to occur in closed populations. Indeed, outbreaks have often been documented in such settings. Infection is relatively uncommon in the first year of life, and much less common among the elderly as compared to young adults. Re-infections are known to occur, but it is unclear how often this may happen over a life-time. An incubation period of approximately 5 to 14 days is often noted, and delayed infection in a family setting at such intervals is not uncommon.

There has been little evidence to suggest that *M. pneumoniae* can be serologically heterogeneous, and therefore strain variation does not presently seem to have impact on infection and re-infection. Molecular studies have defined two genotypes of *M. pneumoniae*, but it is not clear what impact this variation has on either infection or diagnostic methods. Vaccination is not currently a feasible mode for prevention.

B. *U. urealyticum* and *M. hominis*

Although historically referred to as 'genital mycoplasmas', it is apparent that several other mycoplasmas may be preferentially acquired from the genitourinary system in addition to *U. urealyticum* and *M. hominis*. While there are parallels between the epidemiology of *U. urealyticum* and that of *M. hominis* as a consequence of their presence in genital microbial flora, there are also particular differences in the frequency of colonization. These bacteria are in general very common in the adult female genital tract; vaginal and cervical specimens have yielded frequencies of carriage in the asymptomatic state approaching 10-80% depending on the population so surveyed. Given this frequency, it is not surprising that these bacteria are likely to be present in the genital tract as a co-incidence with a variety of genitourinary problems, and then furthermore to be likely candidates for ascending infection in the pregnant and non-pregnant states. If a loose association is proposed for bacterium and disease, these bacteria will often be found when sought in the context of a genitourinary disease in a female.

Frequencies of positive genital tract culture are higher with an increasing number of sexual contacts (57), and therefore to some extent, genital mycoplasma-associated illness may be seen as a sexually transmitted disease. Nevertheless, these bacteria may still be found, albeit in lesser frequency, among those with no previous sexual encounters. As a presumed sexually transmitted disease pathogen, *U. urealyticum* has been touted as one of the more common causes (next to *Chlamydia trachomatis* and perhaps now *M. genitalium*) of non-gonococcal urethritis. There have been associations of increased genitourinary colonization with decreased socioeconomic status, but it is likely that factors which increase genital mycoplasma genitourinary colonization are multivariate. Considerable variation has been noted for different patient populations, but frequency of carriage is highest in sexually active individuals; female much more than male.

Given the reasonably high frequency of genitourinary colonization in the asymptomatic state, it is not surprising that many newborns will acquire these bacteria from their mothers. Colonization of newborn is common, and the frequency of colonization, whether of mouth, gut, or genital site, declines considerably thereafter, although pre-pubertal or non-sexually active adolescents may yet carry these bacteria. Accordingly, it is very difficult to imply that genital mycoplasma presence suggests previous sexually activity or, for that matter, sexual abuse in children. In adulthood, it is possible to find these bacteria in the oropharynx and gut, although to a much lesser frequency than the genitourinary tract.

Outside of generalizations relating to incubation for non-*Chlamydia* non-gonococcal urethritis, incubation periods for putative genital mycoplasma illnesses are difficult to define.

Both *U. urealyticum* and *M. hominis* have serotype variation (58,59). It may be possible therefore that disease variation could occur as a function of this antigenic heterogeneity (60). Such potential has been furthered for *U. urealyticum* somewhat by the recognition of two major biovars that are associated more likely each with particular serotypes (61). Separation into two biovars is supported further by genetic study (62). The role for divergent biovars or genotypes in the differential expression of disease or as etiological agents, all or none, remains a subject for study (63,64).

C. Other

M. genitalium has been found mainly in the genital tract; several studies, which have implicated this bacterium with disease, are based on genetic detection alone. *M. fermentans* has been found mainly as a genital and oral isolate (69). *M. fermentans*, *M. pirum*, and *M. penetrans* have all been in some way associated with HIV-infected patients (65,66,67). Seroprevalence studies have further suggested a link between *M. penetrans* and Kaposi's sarcoma (68), but the latter must be reassessed in light of recent findings relating to Kaposi's sarcoma and novel herpesviruses.

Given the problem with culture for the 'AIDS-associated' mycoplasmas, several studies have relied on genetic detection alone. It is unclear how accurate these methods may be (70-72). Caution must also be exercised when molecular techniques such as these alone are used to define a causal association between mycoplasmas and any other illness (15).

IV. NATURE OF THE BACTERIUM, PATHOGENESIS, AND CLINICAL MANIFESTATIONS

A. *M. pneumoniae*

The entire genome of *M. pneumoniae* is now sequenced, and it is anticipated that the resulting knowledge may further our understanding of *M. pneumoniae* infection in many ways. Like other mycoplasmas, the bacterium is devoid of a cell wall and possesses a single limiting plasma membrane. As such, the bacterium is pleomorphic. In vitro, a variety of shapes are apparent by electron microscopy (Figure 1); these are often bulbar or globular. If the bacterium has been grown on agar, colonies are pinpoint and best visualized with an inverted microscope. The bacterium can grow freely in broth media but may also be adherent to glass or plastic as a visual monolayer. The latter growth is associated with attachment to these surfaces, and structurally such attachment may be facilitated by tip-like projections from the otherwise pleomorphic bacterium. In vivo, however, electron microscopic studies demonstrate more of an elongated filamentous structure, albeit with some form of attachment tip. Complex growth requirements include a serum supplement, and in vitro, growth may require 5 days to 3 weeks of incubation; it is likely that these complex requirements are provided for in vivo. It is not surprising that mycoplasmas do have more fastidious requirements in comparison to other bacteria given their comparatively smaller genome. Utilization of glucose yields acid by-products; arginine is not converted to alkaline by-products. Colonial morphology is not sufficiently distinctive as compared to many other mycoplasmas.

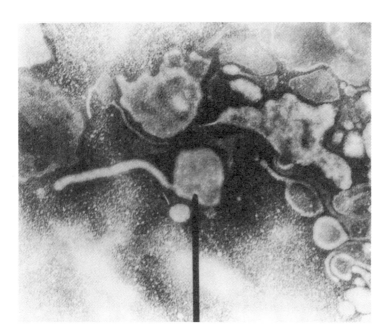

Figure 1   Electronmicrograph of *Mycoplasma pneumoniae*. Reproduced by permission from (18).

M. pneumoniae hemabsorbs red blood cells and is also able to hemolyze, albeit slowly. Attachment to eukaryotic cells is recognized. At the molecular level, these events have been researched. Cytoadherence was initially thought to occur as a function of a dominant protein adhesin, termed P1. P1 aggregates at the tip of the attachment processes. In addition to P1, however, further investigation has revealed the presence of both lower molecular weight putative adhesins and several variant weight accessory proteins. The latter presumably facilitate P1 and other protein aggregation towards the microscopically visualized attachment organelle. Attachment in vivo seems to occur preferentially to ciliated respiratory epithelial cells, and considerable work has led to the current belief that the cellular receptors are mainly sialylated oligosaccharides of the Ii type. These receptors are common on the mucosal side of ciliated respiratory epithelial cells. The pathway to host cell damage is less clear, but the most acceptable of hypotheses relates to localized effects of bacterium-generated reactive oxygen molecules. After attachment, ciliostasis occurs, and localized tissue disruption may soon follow. Local production of hydrogen peroxide and superoxides, as well as reduced host cellular catalase activity, may lead to membrane damage.

The histopathology of pulmonary infiltrates is quite unlike that which is seen for more typical pyogenic bacteria, e.g., *Streptococcus pneumoniae*. Inflammation especially occurs around the bronchi and as far as the terminal ciliated bronchioles. A perilumenal cellular infiltrate is composed mainly of lymphocytes and other mononuclear cell series. The interior of the respiratory lumen may be spared but will at times include mucous, mononuclear cells, and neutrophilic polymorphonuclear cells. These findings often mimic those that are seen with viral respiratory infections, and it is therefore evident why the clinical manifestations of pulmonary disease may be similar when caused by viruses, *M. pneumoniae*, and other atypical pneumonia agents. The pathology of the lung is based on limited human histopathological evidence since death or lung biopsy as a consequence of infection is limited. It is unclear whether recurrent infections are associated with accentuated disease in humans. Pulmonary manifestations of infection are then a result of the above events with some progression to complications of the same for individual patients. Apart from mid- to lower respiratory tract disease, there is little in the way of pathology to the upper respiratory tract.

The basis for extra-respiratory manifestations is still largely unclear although immune mechanisms are postulated. Central nervous system disease is occasionally associated with cerebrospinal fluid pleocytosis; cellular composition is variable. Some central nervous system illnesses have also been associated with an appearance that is consistent with post-infectious demyelination. Rare joint infections are accompanied by intra-articular leucocytosis.

B. *U. urealyticum*

Formerly known as T strain mycoplasmas due to the smaller colonial size in comparison to most other human-associated mycoplasmas, this genus has a number of peculiar properties. The bacterium is strong producer of urease; urea acts as an energy source with subsequent production of ammonia as a by-product. The alkaline environment which results in vitro, however, may inhibit its own growth, and thus it is apparent that *U. urealyticum* is particularly pH sensitive. It is likely that urease production in vivo is buffered. Like other mycoplasmas, more complete growth media are required in comparison to the needs of other bacteria. Glucose is not fermented, and *U. urealyticum* tends to be much more easily cultivated than *M. pneumoniae*.

There is a limited understanding of pathogenesis; this shortfall is especially complicated by the continuing uncertainty in regard to whether *U. urealyticum* is causative of varied illnesses rather than a mere associate. Phospholipases are produced as well as an IgA protease, but the role of these in disease is speculative. It must be recognized however that IgA proteases are a common feature of mucosal pathogens. Some serovars are capable of hemadsorption. Infection of fetal lung with subsequent histopathology has been detailed (74-76). In the more elaborate of these descriptions (75), histochemistry and serology were supportive of a cause and effect relationship. In the paper of Dische et al. (74), fetal lung pathology was associated with placental disease. A subsequent study has suggested an association of *U. urealyticum* with chorioamnionitis in preterm delivery (77); this study did not commonly find chorioamnionitis in early spontaneous abortions. The possibility that the particular biovar 1 may be more capable of causing disease is based on the more common finding of biovar 1 in clinical specimens (78). It is possible that phospholipase activity may vary among serovars (79). The "multiple banded antigen" is commonly recognized in the serological profile, and it has been speculated that it therefore may be more likely a candidate virulence factor (80). Progress in understanding *U. urealyticum* pathogenesis as related to human infection continues to be slow.

C. *M. hominis*

This species is a rapidly-growing mycoplasma and is capable of being visualized on agar after 2 to 4 days. Although purposely cultivated on specific mycoplasma growth media, there are many occasions when *M. hominis* is accidentally recognized on anaerobic agar media, probably due to the prolonged incubation of the latter. The large visual appearance of *M. hominis* as compared to other mycoplasma colonies is noticeable. Arginine is utilized.

Although obtained from joint and wound infections and therein associated with a pyogenic reaction, the histopathology of other disease is poorly understood, perhaps a function of the lack of common disease associations.

Putative attachment factors have been proposed. At least seven different serogroups exist, and it is apparent that clinical isolates are varied. Such variation has been documented by an examination of protein profiles, serology, and genetic restriction patterns. Monoclonal antibodies have been used to demonstrate greater variability among surface-expressed antigens in contrast to cytoplasmic antigens; antigenic variation in the host is supported by recent data (81). Restriction fragment length polymorphism types are not specific to site of isolation however. The genetic basis for such variation continues to be explored but is obviously complex.

D. *M. genitalium*

M. genitalium is seemingly more fastidious to cultivate than *M. pneumoniae* given the infrequency of isolates and given the inability to grow the bacterium despite detection by genetic amplification. It is glucose-fermenting and attaches to glassware/plastic like *M. pneumoniae*. It is also hemabsorbing.

The bacterium aggregates an attachment tip analogous to *M. pneumoniae*. Indeed, an adhesin protein of 140 kD has serological homology to the *M. pneumoniae* P1. Several other immunological epitopes are shared between these two bacteria. One would presume therefore that *M. pneumoniae* and *M. genitalium* should have tropism to identical tissue, yet *M. genitalium* is not commonly recognized in the respiratory tract, and *M. pneumoniae* is not commonly found in the urogenital tract. Although *M. genitalium* seems to be strongly associated with non-gonococcal urethritis, and therefore an inflammatory response in the urogenital lumen, there are practically no other associated diseases where pathology can be studied in the human.

E. *M. fermentans*

M. fermentans is not a common clinical isolate and the suggestion of organism presence by polymerase chain reaction amplification techniques has been used. The discordance between culture and PCR, with PCR frequency being usually more common, suggests that bacterial cultivation is more difficult than initially realized. Both glucose fermentation and arginine utilization can be documented.

In an animal model, *M. fermentans* was capable of inducing a leukemoid reaction, and the bacterium is a reasonable B and T cell mitogen. Both intracellular and extracellular replication have been proposed. Strain variation of protein expression, especially surface proteins as well as restriction fragment length polymorphism among strains, are recognized. Although it has been theorized that *M. fermentans* might activate HIV replication, perhaps even as a co-factor in AIDS, viral replication in vitro does not seem much changed in the presence of *M. fermentans*.

Much of the pathology of illness has been detailed among HIV-infected patients, but anecdotes of illness in immunocompetent patients has emerged. Host immunocompromise appears to facilitate infection. The bacterium has been found in lymph node tissue of HIV positive patients by PCR, but contamination with blood in these samples cannot be absolutely ruled out. A role in HIV nephropathy is still a subject for debate. It must be recognized that *M. fermentans* is a modestly common tissue culture contaminant.

F. *M. penetrans* and *M. pirum*

Clinical isolates and bonafide associated diseases are uncommon, and thus the pathology of illness cannot be described. Both species are capable of glucose fermentation and arginine utilization. *M. penetrans* is capable of intracellular penetration, hence the species names, and *M. pirum* may have an attachment factor with some similarity to those of *M. pneumoniae* and *M. genitalium* (82).

V. IMMUNOLOGY OF INFECTION

A. *M. pneumoniae*

A very active immune response during and after the course of respiratory infection is well-recognized. This response includes both cell-mediated and humoral responses, the latter of which are better characterized. Delayed-type hypersensitivity reactions as demonstrated by skin testing (analogous to the Mantoux test for tuberculosis) occurs after infection, but this approach has never gained favor for practical use. The high frequency of *M. pneumoniae* infection in the community may detract from such an approach especially if this delayed-type hypersensitivity persists.

The humoral immune response as indicated by conventional serodiagnostic assays and subsequently by immunoblotting has been extensively reviewed (83). Heterophil antibodies to human red blood cells have long been recognized although they do not necessarily develop on a consistent basis. The antigen which is recognized by these antibodies is the I antigen, and although not absolutely confirmed, it has been proposed that anti-I antibody evolves as a consequence of autoreactive antibodies that develop against I antigen-like receptors in the respiratory tract, the latter being bound to the *M. pneumoniae* P1 adhesin (84). A variety of other auto-antibodies have been found to arise as a consequence of *M. pneumoniae* respiratory infection including rheumatoid factor (85). Whether these antibodies arise as a function of non-specific polyclonal activation or whether they are truly cross-reactive epitopes is uncertain. Often these antibodies are IgM, and they will disappear within weeks after a respiratory infection is resolved. Cross-reactive antibodies with other mycoplasmas, and other bacteria, have been recognized (86).

As reviewed in our discussion of serodiagnosis, there are many techniques which have been used historically to detect *M. pneumoniae* antibody. These variant techniques may measure different antibodies, e.g., complement fixation by necessity detects complement fixing antibodies, e.g., hemagglutination techniques predominantly measure IgM. Neutralizing antibodies as determined by growth inhibition may not be the same as the spectrum of antibody as determined by enzyme immunoassay. Anti-*M. pneumoniae* IgG antibody is capable of crossing the maternal placenta and may last in newborn/infant circulation for 4 to 8 months. It is unclear whether anti-*M. pneumoniae* antibody in itself is protective in subsequent infection and, if so, which form of antibody, i.e., neutralizing, complement-fixing, agglutinating, etc., is protective.

IgM antibody as measured by various techniques usually first develops within 6 to 10 days after onset of infection. This timing is consistent with the timing for most other infections, whether bacterial or viral. The onset of such antibody may be delayed in states of immunocompromise, and occasionally an IgM response may not develop at all if there is re-infection; the latter is more likely to occur among adults. IgM antibody may last for many weeks to many months depending on the magnitude of the initial response. It does not appear that the severity of infection influences the maximum quantitation of *M. pneumoniae*-directed IgM. IgG antibody essentially develops concomitantly with IgM as does IgA. Both IgG and IgA, but especially the former, persist for many years. Serological surveys among varied populations throughout the world have been published (87). Mucosal antibodies to *M. pneumoniae* also arise as a consequence of infection, and secretory IgA has been found in respiratory secretions and breast milk.

Whereas most serodiagnostic techniques have detected antibody generically, immunoblotting studies have been more specific. Reducing SDS-PAGE has been used predominantly to identify anti-polypeptide responses. Immunoblotting of glycolipids has uncommonly been studied and essentially, only to confirm the nature of the reactive glycolipid antigen. The putative adhesin P1 is most commonly recognized by systemic responses, both by IgM and IgG. For the IgM response, P1 is most strongly recognized by immunoblotting, and this is also the earliest IgM response detected by this method. A number of other polypeptide antigens are consistently recognized as well, and these vary slightly depending on the publication (88-90). These antigens generally have included those with migration rates approximating 35, 45, 56, 69, 84-90, 130, 168-170 (P1), and 195 kD. Although these antigens are among those consistently found by IgG and IgM immunoblotting, there is considerable variation from person to person. In the asymptomatic state, antibody as detected by immunoblotting is common among human populations especially for IgG and especially with increasing age as the immunological experience presumably matures. Anti-P1 IgG antibody again seems to be dominant.

B. Other mycoplasmas

Apart from *M. pneumoniae*, immune responses to other mycoplasmas are considerably less well-characterized.

For *U. urealyticum*, antibody has been detected in some patients during the course of non-gonococcal urethritis, and antibody determinations in general have been used to provide some evidence for a cause and effect relationship between *U. urealyticum* and varied illnesses. Apart from conventional serological techniques, immunoblotting has also been used to demonstrate incremental and serovar-specific antibody in association with post-partum fever. The existence of 14 serotypes has the potential to complicate the appreciation of an immune response (80), although the use of a single broad reactive serovar may be sufficiently representative of the two serovars (91).

Considerable antigenic heterogeneity exists among *M. hominis* isolates (92), and this diversity complicates the ability to consistently detect an immune response, i.e., more than one serotype must be used. By immunoblotting, surface proteins that range from 102-116 kD are often recognized (93), but a 102 kD antigen is most commonly identified.

Details of the humoral response to *M. genitalium*, *M. fermentans*, and *M. penetrans* are less well-characterized, but serosurveys have been carried out especially among HIV-positive populations. There is a lack of recognized *M. genitalium* infections that are available to provide for such characterization. After *M. pneumoniae* infections, the 105 and 135 kD antigens of *M. genitalium* are especially recognized by immunoblotting. Some *M. genitalium* antibody is detected in the early ages (94). *M. penetrans* serosurveys have shown greater quantitation of antibody among HIV-seropositive than HIV-seronegative patients and further among HIV-infected patients with low CD4 counts. Among HIV-seronegative blood donors, higher antibody quantitations are found in Africa when compared to France and the United States (68,95). Indeed, a reactivation of *M. penetrans* antibody during the course of HIV infection has been demonstrated.

VI. LABORATORY DIAGNOSIS

A. General concerns

Due to the small size of mycoplasmas, routine light microscopic methods for detection are of limited value with some exceptions. The nature of mycoplasma colonies requires methods for detection that are extra-ordinary to routine bacteriology. Specialized growth media are required due to the fastidious requirements of most human-associated mycoplasmas. Due to the above dilemmae, in large part, there has been a natural progression towards the development of molecular diagnostic methods; the latter emphases have included more specific forms of serology or genetic detection.

B. *M. pneumoniae*

1.   *General*

Non-microbiological laboratory diagnostic markers of infection are essentially lacking. The systemic white blood cell count is generally of the normal range and uncommonly are there leucocytoses with polymorphonuclear cells in predominance. When neutrophil elevation does occur, it is often not overly striking (e.g., $<20x10^9$/L. among adults). Elevations much above the latter in the context of a patient with a major respiratory illness should raise the concern for other more common pyogenic bacterial causes, e.g., *Streptococcus pneumoniae*, although co-infection is possible (97). Other hematological indices, blood chemistry assessment, and urinalysis do not yield primary diagnostic information for *M. pneumoniae* infection apart from cold agglutinins which are discussed under serodiagnosis. Sputum cytological assessment, when available, may prove of some limited value, although sputum production by a patient with *M. pneumoniae* respiratory infection may be limited or relatively absent. A predominance of mononuclear cells or a modest quantitation of the same along with polymorphonuclear cells should suggest that an atypical pneumonia infectious agent is quite possible – this would then raise concern for *M. pneumoniae* as a common cause of respiratory illness. Despite the latter possibilities, some sputa from *M. pneumoniae* infections may have polymorphonuclear predominance. In the absence of other common bacterial morphotypes which are generally recognized among Gram stained sputa from patients with typical bacterial pneumonia, again *M. pneumoniae* should be considered; more so when routine cultures do not show a conventional bacterial pathogen, i.e., only usual oral flora, and especially when salivary contamination is minimal. Cellular and other compositions of diagnostic pleurocentesis are not diagnostic of *M. pneumoniae* infection. Central nervous system involvement may include meningeal inflammation which leads especially to a mononuclear predominance among the increase in cerebrospinal fluid white blood cells.

2. Microscopy

As these bacteria have a size that is at the limit of resolution for the light microscope and given their pleomorphic shape, routine light microscopy cannot be practically used to visualize *M. pneumoniae* in a respiratory specimen, even if they are stainable by a given technique. Furthermore, the presence of non-pathogenic mycoplasmas in the oropharynx would preclude identifying a mycoplasma morphology as *M. pneumoniae* specifically. Identification of *M. pneumoniae* in clinical specimens by immunofluorescnce techniques has been proposed but has not gained widespread practical use (98). The highly pleomorphic morphology and the potential for methodologically-related artifact both represent obstacles to the realization of any use. Mycoplasmas can be found by electron microscopy but only by the most experienced of electron microscopy personnel; this was more likely to occur in the era where direct electron microscopy on respiratory specimens was being used to detect respiratory viruses. Again, the specificity of such findings to indicate the presence of *M. pneumoniae* remain a concern.

3. Culture

Specimens of choice for culture will obviously include those that contain respiratory secretions such as sputa and bronchial washes. A throat swab as well as nasopharyngeal specimens are likely to yield the bacterium given the evolution of infection from upper to lower respiratory tract. The bacterium has been cultured from pleural fluid, although most pleural reactions that accompany *M. pneumoniae* infection are sterile. Isolation from pericardial fluid, cerebrospinal fluid, and joint have also been rarely detailed. During the course of an illness, antibiotic use may interrupt culture positivity, but it is not uncommon for respiratory excretion to continue after antibiotics are stopped especially if the treatment course is abbreviated. Natural growth inhibitors in clinical specimens are variable, but the quantitations of bacteria are usually so high in clinical specimens that respiratory specimens do not require dilutions prior to culture. Specimen transport media may be of value but are not absolutely required. Although a transport liquid may enhance viability, again the large numbers of bacteria per respiratory specimen usually allow for viability even if a sputum had been refrigerated at 4°C for several days without transport medium buffer. Repetitive freeze-thaw of the clinical samples will be associated with decreased yield. A suitable transport medium could simply constitute the same broth which is used for culture. Practical problems arise when similar pH color indicators are being used for viral, chlamydia, and mycoplasma culture transport, and thus, transport media must be clearly labelled for their intended use.

Selective and enrichment processes are a must due to the potential for bacterial and fungal contamination. The latter are more so likely to present a problem since mycoplasma media are maintained for up to several weeks. Enrichment is provided by the use of a broth which has essentially the same formulation as the solid medium with the exception of agar. In order to reduce contamination, antibacterial antibiotics such penicillin and polymyxin B provide for selection, and amphotericin B is more commonly used as the antifungal. Strict observation of the recommended amphotericin B concentrations is essential as it may be inhibitory at lower dilution. Use of a 0.45 micron filter to pre-treat respiratory secretions will decrease fungal contamination but may also have a minor impact on mycoplasma yield. Modified Hayflick's medium (99) or SP4 medium (100) are most commonly used. Although some believe that SP4 may be superior, a well-quality controlled Hayflick's medium may serve as an equal when all components of the culture protocol are otherwise the same. For investigative purposes, SP4 may be preferred if more fastidious mycoplasmas such as *M. genitalium* are of interest as well. Both media contain pH colour indicators which become yellow in order to indicate acid production from glucose. Colour change in this regard, though, is not absolutely diagnostic of *M. pneumoniae* presence in a broth since colour change, especially in the first 1 to 4 days, is more likely to be due to obvious or early bacterial and/or fungal overgrowth. Subculture of broth to solid medium is then essential to confirm the presence of *M. pneumoniae*. Figure 2 demonstrates an example of a *M. pneumoniae* culture protocol. In well-controlled media, growth may be apparent as early as day 5 to 7, but specimens not uncommonly will be positive over 5 days to 3 weeks. This timing will be affected by the numbers of bacteria in the initial specimen as well as inhibitors such as antibiotics. Culture plates should be placed in a humid environment since dessication of small agar plates is probable when incubated for up to and over 7 days.

Asymptomatic carriage in the oropharynx is not common in the general population, and therefore, the finding of this bacterium in a respiratory specimen in the context of an active respiratory disease has a very high predictive value for infection. It must be conceded, however, that a cause-and-effect relationship is not absolute.

Mycoplasma colonies, even when fully mature, may only reach 0.1 to 0.2 mm. in size, and therefore they are best visualized by the equivalent of an inverted microscope which is used in other circumstances to examine viral tissue culture. Colonies are clear and may or may not maintain a "fried-egg" appearance; the latter is a function of the elevation of the central colony area and an imbedding of the central colony area into the agar (Figure 3). Solid media may also begin to colour change with sufficient presence of *M. pneumoniae* colonies. Confirmation of *M. pneumoniae* can be accomplished in several ways, but the methods so chosen will depend on what degree of certainty the laboratory is willing to accept. Hemadsorption of red blood cells is probably the most commonly used of these methods on a practical basis. Although guinea pig red blood cells have been touted for this purpose, several animal

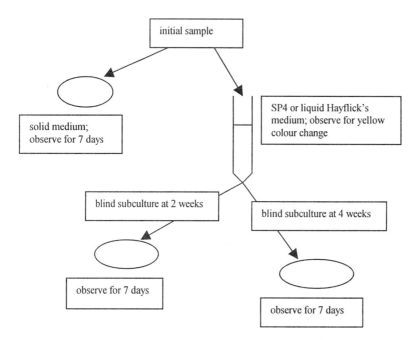

Figure 2   An example for a *M. pneumoniae* culture protocol.

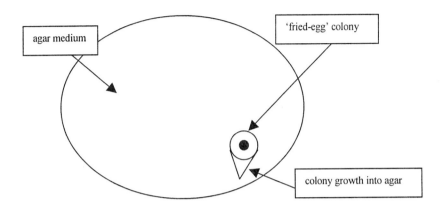

red blood cell = ○

Figure 3   Diagrammatic representation of colony appearance re: 'fried-egg' pattern.

sources can actually be used including sheep red blood cells which are more often available in laboratories where bacteriological media are produced. An overlay of suspect colonies on solid medium with a 1% suspension of red blood cells will allow for sufficient hemabsorption over 1 hr. After the suspension is washed off, suspect colonies are left with a rosette formation of adherent red blood cells (Figure 4). For respiratory specimens, the combination of acid-induced colour change along with hemadsorbing and highly suspect mycoplasma colonies gives the laboratory a very high probability for identifying *M. pneumoniae*. Most of the oral commensal mycoplasmas neither ferment glucose nor hemabsorb. *M. genitalium* is an exception, however, but true *M. genitalium* isolation from respiratory secretions is uncommon. Evidence for co-existence of both *M. pneumoniae* and *M. genitalium* in respiratory specimens has been reported. Disc diffusion inhibition of colonial growth on solid media can also be used to confirm identification, but this approach required specific antisera which are not commonly available to most laboratories. In the latter method, serum with anti-*M. pneumoniae* antibody is impregnated in paper discs and gives zones of inhibition to *M. pneumoniae* colonies, analogous to antibiotic susceptibility testing by disc diffusion. On a research basis, definitive confirmation of *M. pneumoniae* can be accomplished by immunoblotting (with or without antecedent SDS-PAGE resolution), rDNA:DNA hybridization, PCR amplification, and 16S rRNA sequencing. Many laboratories have abandoned culture due to the special medium requirements and given the emphasis on serodiagnostics. One may clearly question the ability of culture to influence the treatment of active infections given the delay of many days to weeks until culture confirmation. Nevertheless, culture may serve as a reference for quality control of molecular direct detection methods and may also be used to assess suspect tissue which is not possibly amenable to molecular diagnosis.

4.   Serology

Heterophil antibody as a consequence of infection has been exploited for diagnostic purposes. Antibodies to Streptococcus MG (expressed as agglutinins) were found historically in patients with *M. pneu-*

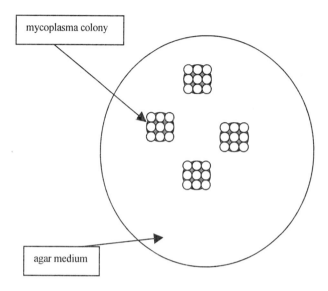

Figure 4 Diagrammatic representation of red blood cell absorption for the presumptive determination of *M. pneumoniae* colonies on agar. Each mycoplasma colony has multiple red blood cells adsorbed to it.

moniae infection, and although they emerge in a minority of those with such infection, their presence is not highly diagnostic of infection; their use has long been abandoned (96,101). Cold agglutinin heterophil antibodies have been more widely sought as diagnostic markers of acute infection (101). These antibodies are IgM, become detectable after 7 to 10 days of disease onset, peak at approximately 3 weeks, and generally disappear in 1 to 2 months. They are detected by the incubation in cold temperature of serial serum dilutions with each human adult O red blood cells and umbilical cord O red blood cells. Adult O cells possess the matured I antigen and hence agglutinate in the presence of cold agglutinin antibody while the control cord O cells (which lack mature I antigen) do not. Incubation at warm temperatures (e.g., 20 to 37°C) will not facilitate agglutination. A quantitative assessment of such agglutination is expressed as an end-point in titre of the doubling serum dilutions. Garrow's technique of qualitative assessment includes the search for agglutination when a patient's own blood agglutinates visually in a blood collection tube that has been cooled in ice; the agglutination complex will dissociate when the same tube has been warmed to approximately body temperature. In adult populations with active *M. pneumoniae* respiratory infection, approximately 30-80% will develop cold agglutinins. The frequency, however, is much lower in children. Unfortunately, low titres of cold agglutinins may be found in other illnesses including viral respiratory infections. Therefore, significant titres in adults are often indicated at the ≥1/64 level, i.e., increasing specificity by increasing the cut-off dilution that is deemed significant. This latter quantitation in an adult serum, when associated with an atypical pneumonia pattern of illness, has modest positive predictive value. Cold agglutinins should generally not be used for children. It must be recognized that although access to red blood cells may be easy, cold agglutinin determination probably adds very little to rapid diagnosis when other IgM serologies are available on an equivalent timely basis.

Immunofluorescence assays have had both historical importance and enjoy some limited current use (102). Indirect immunofluorescence studies, with *M. pneumoniae* infected tissue from embryonated eggs as substrate, proved to be critical in the historical discovery of the primary atypical pneumonia agent. For routine serological purposes, however, a more simple form of substrate was defined in the use of acetone-fixed bacterial whole cells on glass. The focus has been on using anti-*M. pneumoniae* IgM as a marker of acute infection and less so on the comparison of acute and convalescent sera for IgG titres. Immunofluorescence serology has been hindered by the technical problems which relate to consistency in end-point determination. The latter is a generic problem with immunofluorescence rather than a specific issue for *M. pneumoniae* immunofluorescence. This technical difficulty may be somewhat diminished by having the assessment performed by few and by having sufficient volume to train and maintain accuracy. Cut-off titres for clinical significance are variably defined and range from $\geq 1/4$ to $1/16$. Rheumatoid factor (IgM or IgG) may occasionally lead to false positives. IgM-IFA antibody may persist for 3 to 5 months. The IFA is a test that generally correlates well with other serological methods. The assay is commercially available, but use is not widespread.

Complement fixation (CF) serology for *M. pneumoniae* is a time-honoured method and has been of greatest use in reference centres for four decades (87). In part, the CF format in this sense has been consistent with the use of CF serology for respiratory viruses, usually in the same central laboratory. The localization of test performance has usually hindered the application of the CF test for the purposes of rapid diagnosis; until the last decade, there has been little in the way of formidable competition for this purpose. CF has often been used as a serological standard to which other diagnostics have been compared. Indeed, an incredible amount of expertise has been had in its application let alone verification (103). CF antibody is a composite of IgG and IgM especially; IgM may comprise the majority in acute infection. CF antibody peak coincides with the IgM peak and persisting CF antibody over years is especially a function of persistent IgG. Diagnostic serology will be based on either the demonstration of a four-fold change between acute and convalescent sera or by single titres above a particular cut-off (e.g., $\geq 1/64$ or $\geq 1/128$). It is possible that adults will respond to a lesser degree after infection than youth, especially when infection is recurrent and therefore the immune responses are anamnestic. The bacterial antigen for CF serology is usually a chloroform-methanol extract which much investigation has subsequently indicated is a glycolipid extract. Thin-layer chromatographic and immunoblotting analyses have proven this glycolipid antigen to be a single band, i.e., relatively homogeneous. Although this antigen is purified, it is considered to share immunological similarity to varied mammalian and plant glycolipids, and rises in CF antibody titre have been documented in non-*M. pneumoniae* associated pancreatitis and bacterial meningitis. This non-specificity raises concern, especially when the CF test is being applied to a context where the pre-test probability for *M. pneumoniae* infection is small. For example, neurological illnesses without accompanying or preceding respiratory infection are unlikely to be caused by *M. pneumoniae* even when CF antibody titres are high. Overall, there is a trend towards replacing CF serology by IgM-based assays that have better turn-around times. CF continues to be used as a comparative standard.

Measures of mycoplasma inhibitory antibody (analogous in principle to viral neutralization serology) have been assessed for diagnostic purposes by methods variably termed growth inhibition, metabolic inhibition, tetrazolium reduction inhibition, and the mycoplasmacidal assay (104). Although such inhibitory antibody includes both IgM and IgG, persistent inhibitory antibody is mainly IgG. During an acute illness, maximal inhibitory antibody titres are somewhat delayed in contrast to a simple measure of *M. pneumoniae*-specific IgM. In addition to value as a diagnostic marker, it has been suggested by some that inhibitory antibody may correlate with actual protection against subsequent disease. The latter is still the subject for debate. One major dilemma however is that these techniques are dependent on growth of the mycoplasma in vitro, and it is possible that a patient serum may contain antibiotic inhibitors, e.g., erythromycin or tetracycline. Given that patients may have already been on an antibiotic prior to specimen collection, this potential problem is real. In the current era, empiric use of new oral macrolides (e.g., clarithromycin, azithromycin) has increased significantly, and therefore, the chance of a metabolic inhibitor already being present is high. Accordingly, practical diagnostic use of such methods is limited.

Particle agglutination, with the use of a simple carrier for *M. pneumoniae* antigen, offers a technology which seemingly may be more easily implemented in a point-of-care fashion. (105). Most experience has dwelled on using the red blood cell as the antigen carrier given the potential to visually observe red blood cell agglutination (especially indirect hemagglutination [IHA]). IHA is more so a marker of IgM activity. Unfortunately, animal red blood cell antigens in themselves may be recognized by the existing specific or cross-reactive humoral response in humans, and up to 10% of sera may demonstrate such non-specific agglutination. There is also a clinical dilemma in determining cut-off values since low titres of such antibodies may exist in specimens. As an alternative, latex, gelatin, and other carrier particles, which are less likely affected by a cross-reaction, have been used as a replacement for red blood cells more recently. Although these methods have evolved in order to simplify the technology and thereby reduce time for a result as well as bring the technology closer to the clinical side, it must be recognized that there are new categories of problems which are introduced when less experienced individuals perform a test even as seemingly simple as an agglutination reaction. Both false-positive and false-negative results continue to be a concern.

The desire to increase 'signal to noise' ratios, and a context of emerging technologies in the 1970s led to the emergence of radioimmunoassay (RIA) (106) and enzyme immunoassay (EIA) (107). On a practical basis, RIA did not become widely used perhaps in large part due to the need for a radioactive label and due also to the comparable performance of EIA. EIA continues to be used, and it represents a viable alternative to other serological assays. The technology is amenable to automation although small sample numbers may also be assessed. Completion time may vary from 3 to 5 hours, and there is the potential to provide for rapid diagnosis on a same-day basis or at least within a few working days. Both IgM- and IgG- based EIAs have been detailed and indeed commercialized; the IgA format is not used. Due to the greater likelihood of pre-existing IgG and given the occasional need for acute and convalescent sera, IgM assays have been emphasized. Pioneering IgM assays were often of the indirect EIA variation whereby antigen was primarily coated onto plastic micro-titre wells. This approach led to considerable problems with false-positives due to the end-point overlap between sera from asymptomatic and infected individuals. In order to escape this dilemma, IgM-EIAs were contoured to provide for IgM capture, i.e., human IgM captured in the first step with subsequent antigen added as well as a detector layer. Although the latter does indeed represent a benefit, there continues to be concern over the definition of break-points. Break-points moved in any one direction either reduce sensitivity or increase non-specificity. The choice of a 'grey-zone' for EIA readings, which indicate an equivocal result, has been promoted for some commercial assays. Unfortunately, the physician is left with the dilemma of what an equivocal result actually implies and what impact it will have on the decision to treat. Antigen substrates for EIA have included whole cells, protein extracts, or the glycolipid (CF) antigen. There is the potential to engineer purified proteins or synthetic peptides for EIA, but a viable approach in this regard is not yet widely commercialized. Rheumatoid factor may present a problem for indirect EIA but less so for capture systems; pre-treatment with rheumatoid factor absorbent has been of value. Non-specific and generalized polyclonal IgM elevations may lead to positive IgM assays for *M. pneumoniae*. A positive IgM assay usually requires a minimum of 7 to 10 days in order to evolve, and IgM may be measured for up to many months to one year depending on the sensitivity of the assay. Immunosuppression may prevent an adequate IgM response from being measured. In general, EIAs are equal to or better than other serological assessments. IgM-EIA is not uncommonly positive in a scenario when acute sera have non-diagnostic CF titres. It is critical to remember that such assays will perform relatively well when applied to a patient population where the frequency of disease is high.

From both the perspective of *M. pneumoniae* EIA diagnostics specifically and EIA diagnostics in general, it is recognized that the signal interpretation is fundamentally an indirect one given the automated recognition of colour change. A more direct visualization that said reaction is truly bacterium-specific would be desirable, and immunoblotting provides the potential for such confirmation even when the mechanics of the test are fundamentally a form of enzyme immunoassay. Although one may conduct immunoblotting with whole bacterium or crude extract as the fixed substrate, the use of individual polypeptides, most commonly obtained by SDS-PAGE and mobilized to nitrocellulose or nylon by Western blotting, has great merit by specifically allowing for direct antibody recognition. With the latter approach in mind, it is evident why immunoblotting may be regarded as confirmatory testing while EIA, unless otherwise validated, would be most suitable to screening for possible suspect diagnoses, especially for large sample numbers. In essence, immunoblotting can be used for both screening and confirmation, and indeed this has been translated into actual value for *M. pneumoniae* diagnostics (108), including commercially available products for this end. In order to make this technology clinically relevant, IgM detection has been favoured. The major target for such serology has been the protein P1, to which early maximal and consistently common humoral responses are directed, whether IgG, IgA, or IgM. Other polypeptide targets are less reliable. Using SDS-PAGE and Western blotting to focus P1, a specific band of recognition can be visualized. Rather than an all-or-none basis, it can be anticipated that gradations of intensity will be seen which are dependent on the stage of disease. Details of how an in-house assay may be designed for anti-P1 IgM immunoblotting have been published (109,110) (Figure 5). In practice, this form of serology is as sensitive as commercial EIA and has the potential to be more specific. Once prepared, P1-containing reagent strips can be comfortably stored and the assay may be completed in several hours. A low frequency of endemic seroprevalence among controls (~2-5%) is found, and these positive assays are a testament to the fact that *M. pneumoniae* respiratory infection in general is relatively common in the community. Potential advances towards the use of synthetic peptides must be viewed with caution since P1 gene sequence divergence has been shown, albeit restricted (113), and it may be more prudent to use relatively native whole length polypeptide. Despite the possibility that anamnestic immune responses after reinfection may be associated with less IgM response, IgM anti-P1 immunoblot responses are commonly seen among sera from infected adults.

5.   Antigen detection

Direct detection of *M. pneumoniae* antigen in clinical specimens has received attention, but progress has not been considerably favourable. Whether using polyclonal or monoclonal detector antibodies and regardless of detection format, e.g., EIA, particle agglutination, or immunoblotting, the fundamental

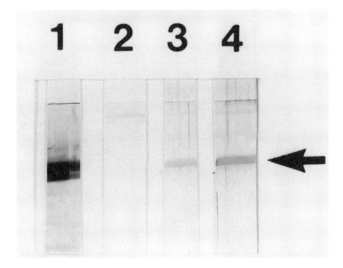

Figure 5   Anti-P1 IgM immunoblotting for *M. pneumoniae* serodiagnosis. The photograph illustrates positive (linear horizontal banding) and negative controls. Reprinted from (109) with permission.

difficulty rests with the amount of organism per specimen (111). Culture-amplified antigen detection does not seem to be a practical solution (112). Concern regarding false-positive assays is a barrier to simple agglutination assays; the mucoid nature of some clinical specimens poses a problem in this regard.

6. Genetic detection

Direct detection of *M. pneumoniae* by genetic hybridization techniques was entertained very early but, as for other diagnostic purposes, the major limiting factor was the minimal amount of genome that is required for such detection. In general, genetic detection is appealing since the bacterium does not need to be viable, and there is the potential to provide rapid diagnosis that may change management and hence clinical outcome. Various estimates claim a minimal detection limit of 10^3-10^5 genome copies. Although bacterial counts in clinical respiratory specimens may exceed this limit, many specimens do not have quantitations that approach this number. Throat swabs and nasal washes may further limit the quantity of bacterium that is available in contrast to well-collected sputa. Commercialization of a direct detection method via rDNA:DNA liquid hybridization has been achieved. Although variation for direct detection by hybridization assays has been entertained, the fundamental limitation remains the absolute number of genome copies and hence targets available.

The advent of genetic amplification technologies, especially PCR, provided the obvious opportunity to circumvent the above limitations. Numerous variations on this theme have been published (Table 2), and it is not clear that any one format is definitively superior to others. As a consequence of a restrictively small genome, few *M. pneumoniae* genes are highly repeated. The P1 gene has been a major target for PCR amplifications, perhaps as a consequence of this gene having been sequenced early. Using laboratory-cultivated bacterium as a reference, these assays have been able to detect down to 1-10 copies, but clinical application must be viewed cautiously. Many specimens have inhibitors which confer the potential to affect the amplification process. Some of this inhibition may occur on an all-or-none basis while in other circumstances there may be a gradation of inhibition, i.e., relative inhibition, which will affect the sensitivity of the test. Such inhibition must be controlled either by including a clinical sample control which has been seeded with a known threshold quantity of bacterium or by using a control for amplification of eukaryotic genes which should be present in a well-collected clinical sample. Whereas it might be projected that thick sputum samples may pose the most likely risk for inhibitors, body fluids as seemingly simplistic as cerebrospinal fluids may contain sufficient inhibitors. Preamplification treatment of specimens for the purpose of either concentrating DNA or eliminating inhibitors is often necessary, and a variety of approaches have been assessed as indicated in Table 2. There is no clear consensus as to what constitutes the best respiratory specimen, but it is evident that both throat swabs and nasopharyngeal washes often yield sufficient bacterium (126). Despite the diagnostic gain with amplification, it is unlikely that sufficient bacterial DNA will be present very late in the illness. Asymptomatic carriage of bacterium, albeit uncommon, poses another theoretical risk for interpretation. Bacterium may be detected much more early than the time it will take the immune response to emerge. Transport is less critical an issue than for culture since both living and non-viable bacteria can be detected.

7. Applications

The application of any one technology must depend on availability and then the context of the specific illness. Immunocompetent patients generally develop antibody responses within 7 to 10 days after onset of illness. Although this may seem a long interval, it must be acknowledged that patients with advanced *M. pneumoniae* respiratory illness are likely to first seek medical attention at this time, especially when this attention may relate to hospital care. Although genetic amplification is a rapid diagnostic procedure, the requisites for specimen processing as well as the timing for other components of the assay may exceed expectations, especially when a rapid serological IgM assay can be completed in a few hours. In the requisites for specimen processing as well as the timing for other components of the assay may exceed expectations, especially when a rapid serological IgM assay can be completed in a few hours. In

Table 2   A representative selection of diagnostic PCR assays for *M. pneumoniae* infection.

sample preparation	sample	primer target	cycling mode	detection method	inhibition frequency	reference
proteinase K, boiling	nasal wash	P1 gene	single	direct product visualization	2%	114
proteinase K, boiling	nasal wash	as ref. 118	nested	direct product visualization	2%	115
boiling	throat swab	as ref. 118	single	direct product visualization	ND	116
extraction	throat swab	16S rDNA	single	direct product visualization	ND	117
extraction	bronchial lavage	?	single	direct product visualization	ND	118
proteinase K, boiling	throat swab	*tuf* gene	single	colorimetric microtitre well hydridization	~15%	119
proteinase K, extraction	transthoracic aspirate	as ref. 118	single	direct product visualization	ND	120
extraction	nasal wash	as ref. 118	single	direct product visualization	~25%	121
sonication, boiling	throat swab	P1 gene	single	direct product visualization	ND	122
proteinase K, detergent, boiling	varied	16S rDNA	single	Southern blotting	5.1%	123
extraction	bronchial lavage	16S rDNA	single	colorimetric microtitre well hydridization	ND	124
freezing, boiling, extraction	nasal wash	P1 gene, 16S rDNA	single	direct product visualization	24.6%	125

ND = no data

very early disease, however, when detectable immune responses have not emerged, a PCR-based assay may have impact. For example, the early stages of a respiratory illness may trigger an asthmatic episode in an individual so predisposed. Immunocompromised patients vary in their degree of actual compromise – this may lead to a further delay in IgM development or to the absence of IgM development in its entirety. Culture may be reserved as a temporary control standard in order to assess PCR on an ongoing basis or as a technique to be applied to limited and atypical clinical specimens. Yet other circumstances will benefit from both serology and genetic amplification being available (114).

C. *U. urealyticum*

1. General

Although renowned to be relatively pH sensitive, *U. urealyticum* is somewhat less fastidious than *M. pneumoniae* and can be cultured in fewer days. Whereas the following discussion dwells heavily on culture for *U. urealyticum*, it must be emphasized that the major dilemma is not so much how and if *U. urealyticum* will be cultured but rather is centred about what such culture-positivity means in the context of a given illness. As previously detailed, many disease associations for *U. urealyticum* are tenuous at best. Given the high frequency of colonization, it is easy to find *U. urealyticum* in the genital tract of an individual, especially adult, who may suffer from an illness that has historically been of interest in mycoplasmology. For example, asymptomatic colonization in sexually active females may range from 30-80%. In this context, it is very likely that *U. urealyticum* would be found in a patient who suffers from non-gonococcal urethritis or vaginal discharge even if it has no causal relationship. Indiscriminate application of a diagnostic method for *U. urealyticum* may be problematic especially when related to the establishment of a link between the bacterium and the disease relating to the genital tract, obstetrical or not.

2. Microscopy

Again, limitation of light microscopy is a function of bacterial size. Perhaps microscopy has some value if, in a given context, it provides for exclusion of typical other microbes. Genital mycoplasmas may be found in blood culture, albeit rare, and the suspicion for such culture positivity may be highlighted when indicators (often automated) signal positive and when other conventional bacteria are not visualized or subcultured. Blind subculture for mycoplasmas in this context may be occasionally rewarding.

3. Culture

A number of specimens may be submitted purposely for *U. urealyticum* culture. These include genital specimens, operative specimens (especially gynecological), joint fluids, tracheal aspirate from low birth weight newborns, and blood. Preferably, cultures should be inoculated within hours of specimen collection although the survival of *U. urealyticum* varies considerably in different specimens, e.g., semen specimens may be relatively toxic compared to *U. urealyticum* survival on routine genital swabs. Although *U. urealyticum* can be cultured from routine swabs, maximization of culture results can occur with the use of specific transport media. If the time from collection to set-up is brief, e.g., few hours, a routine swab in conventional bacterial transport buffer may suffice. Since it is not evident that bacterial quantitation has definitive pathological correlates or etiological implications, an all-or-none assessment of *U. urealyticum* presence may suffice. Therefore, some loss of viability may be tolerable especially when an enrichment broth is part of the culture assessment. Specimens may be maintained at 4°C for several days with relatively little loss in viability if the specimen is buffered.

As for *M. pneumoniae*, both a solid medium and selective enrichment broth are used. In either medium, growth times are comparatively short and usually span 3 to 7 days. Colonial growth does not often yield the 'fried-egg' appearance that is seen with *M. pneumoniae* or *M. hominis*. Colonies are comparatively smaller and were historically termed 'T strain' mycoplasma (T for tiny) as a consequence. If it is difficult to be absolute about whether a perceived morphotype truly represents a viable colony, the agar surface may be cut, inverted, and smeared over another solid medium in order to demonstrate transferability. This approach is generally used for mycoplasmas. *U. urealyticum* will grow in various atmospheric conditions, but an anaerobic atmosphere may be preferable since yeast from genital specimens will be suppressed. Selection may include clindamycin which will inhibit *M. hominis* since the latter is commonly co-cultivated from genital specimens. Selection against other bacteria and fungi is of importance as it is for culturing other mycoplasmas. Some clinical specimens may be relatively toxic, e.g., urine or semen, either due to pH or unknown factors, and it may be prudent to dilute the specimen 1:10 with culture broth at the time of set-up.

   U. urealyticum is susceptible to pH variations, especially alkalinity, and even pH of >7.0 may prove detrimental. The sensitivity to alkalinity may vary among *U. urealyticum* isolates, and a significant reduction in numbers may occur in hours as bacterial growth and urease activity change the growth environment towards a higher pH. A variety of suitable media have been designed (variably termed U agar, A7B, A8, A5K, U9C) (127-129). In general, these media have a buffered acid pH (pH 5.5 – 6.5) when newly prepared, but *U. urealyticum* growth will lead to a pH colour indicator change as the pH approaches 7.0. Subculture is recommended shortly after this colour change occurs in order to maintain viability, and hence growth media must be inspected on a daily basis to ensure that this breakpoint is not missed. Unseeded controls should be followed as well in order to provide reference for the original colour indicator.

   Confirmation of *U. urealyticum* colonies is generally accomplished by exploiting the ubiquitous presence of urease. Solutions of $CaCl_2$ and urea or manganous sulphate, when applied directly to the colony, create a dark brown appearance. Indicators of this sort may also be incorporated into the growth medium so that colony colouration is apparent as the colony evolves.

4. Serology

Serodiagnosis is not routinely available and has been mainly used for research purposes. The definition of a serological test is somewhat complicated by the presence of 14 serotypes. A defined common antigen for *U. urealyticum* serotypes would be of potential benefit, but validation of any serological assay is a cause for concern because absolute *U. urealyticum*-caused illnesses are somewhat difficult to define in sufficient numbers.

5. Antigen detection

This prospect is experimental only.

6. Genetic detection

Direct probes again have been technically limited, and detection levels $<10^3$ are difficult to achieve. There are potential needs for PCR amplification as applied to clinical diagnosis, and indeed PCR for this purpose has been attempted (64, 130). The common presence of *U. urealyticum* in genital specimens again poses interpretive dilemmae. Differentiation between viable and non-viable bacterium may be important if contact with the bacterium is likely, i.e., PCR of endotracheal specimens from very low birth weight newborns might yield positive amplifications even when the bacterium is not viable. A precise role for this technology in laboratory diagnosis remains to be well-defined.

D. *M. hominis*

1. General

In general, interest in diagnostics for *M. hominis* are considerably less than for *U. urealyticum* and *M. pneumoniae*, even though legitimate *M. hominis*-associated infections do exist. Overall, there are few strong associations with disease.

2. Microscopy

As for *U. urealyticum*, *M. hominis* may be considered in blood culture or other specimens when conventional Gram stain/microscopy with or without culture rule out more typical bacterial pathogens.

3.   Culture

M. hominis is probably the most hardy of common human-associated mycoplasmas. Although inhibited by *U. urealyticum*-selective media, this bacterium grows well on *M. pneumoniae* media and as well on much more simple variations. The bacterium is relatively stable in clinical specimens and is not easily affected by pH. Indeed, *M. hominis* may be cultured on routine bacteriological media including blood and chocolate agars if incubation is sufficiently prolonged and care is taken to examine for suspect tiny colonies. On anaerobic media that may be incubated for 5 to 7 days, *M. hominis* may appear as small pinpoint colonies; some will initially suspect that these colonies are *Veillonella* until the Gram stain of colonies fails to identify the expected bacterial morphotype. *M. hominis* has been grown on New York City Medium (otherwise intended for the selection of *Neisseria gonorrhoeae*). Broth media will contain arginine and a pH indicator since *M. hominis* may produce an alkaline by-product which should be a signal for subculture when the initial agar medium has not yielded the organism (127). Bacterial and/or yeast contamination, if it escapes selective inhibitors, may also lead to an alkaline colour change, but broth turbidity is obvious. *M. hominis* in pure culture may lead to slight broth turbidity, but this is barely perceptable to most. Medium controls should be included again as a reference for the pH indicator. *M. hominis* is commonly referred to as a 'large colony' mycoplasma; colonies may measure up to 0.3-0.4 mm. The colonial appearance is more consistent with the classical 'fried-egg' appearance as previously detailed. Growth on agar and in broth usually takes 2 to 7 days; selection, as for *M. pneumoniae*, is generally sufficient. In positive blood cultures, direct subculture to mycoplasma or routine media will usually lead to visible colonies in1 to 2 days.

Other mycoplasmas may be arginine-positive, but this does not preclude a practical approach to *M. hominis* identification. A large colony, arginine-positive mycoplasma from genital specimens has a very high probability of being ultimately confirmed as *M. hominis*. Advanced identification may include disc inhibition whereby *M. hominis* antiserum impregnated discs create a zone of inhibition to *M. hominis*, analogous to antimicrobial disc diffusion. For research purposes, more definitive identification can be accomplished by molecular techniques.

4.   Serology

Variable proteins and multiples serotypes complicate serodiagnosis. On a practical clinical basis, serology is not available nor is there much interest in its use.

5.   Genetic detection

Such an approach, including amplification, is entirely within the realm of possibility, but practical uses are in large part lacking.

E. Other mycoplasmas

Oral commensals are easily cultivated on routine mycoplasma media for *M. pneumoniae* culture. More complicated diagnostic manoeuvres are not practically required.

Culture and confirmation of positive cultures are considerably more difficult for *M. genitalium*, *M. fermentans*, *M. penetrans*, and *M. pirum*, and so PCR-based genetic amplification has been favoured in most circumstances where these bacteria are considered whether for genital specimens, blood mononuclear cells, or other sources. In general where culture is attempted, many investigators have favoured the use of SP4 media. *M. genitalium* is inconsistently cultured, and it is not uncommon to have many more specimens as PCR-positive when cultures are negative for the same. Colonies of *M. genitalium* hemabsorb, and so there may be confusion with *M. pneumoniae*, but *M. genitalium* culture is quite uncommon. Although capable of glucose fermentation, the resulting in vitro pH colour change is apparently inconsistent. PCR methods have especially been used to determine the presence of *M. genitalium* in urethral specimens from patients with non-gonococcal urethritis. Direct DNA probes had been used for this same purpose but are now obsolete in the PCR era. In order to facilitate confirmation after culture when culture is used, PCR amplification of 16S-23S rRNA region with subsequent restriction enzyme digestion has been employed (131).

Some have expressed skepticism about the clinical value of PCR-positive assays for less cultivable mycoplasmas especially when repetitive attempts at culture are non-rewarding. Detection systems for PCR products may lead to some variability here especially if EIAs are used to assess positive product. Certainly in the case of MLOs, the presence of PCR products should be viewed with caution. As previously detailed, the association of mycoplasmas with rheumatoid arthritis and chronic fatigue are being promoted mainly on the basis of PCR products. The verification of these observations will require much more intensive study.

F. Tissue culture contamination

Tissue cultures are heavily used in diagnostic, therapeutic, and experimental endeavours. The ever-growing areas of immunology and transplantation will make the use of cell cultures for human therapy more likely. Given that critical results may be dependent on accurate assays or treatments, the need to recognize mycoplasma contamination becomes ever more so of value. When contaminated, cell culture supernatants will often have up to 10^6 mycoplasmas/ml. Apart from the supernatant burden, much of the mycoplasma contaminants will be adherent to cell lines. It has been estimated that mycoplasma DNA may comprise up to 10-25% of total DNA of a contaminated cell line. Contamination may be associated with little, if not any, appreciable effect. Conversely, presence of high numbers of mycoplasmas may also be associated with enzymatic and other biochemical aberrations, mitogenic responses with cytokine activation, alterations in antibody production for B cells, cell transformation and disarray, and ultimately cell death.

Both human and non-human (usually animal) mycoplasmas are capable of infecting cell lines. The source of cell line and the ingredients which are used to support cell line growth weigh heavily on the likelihood that a given mycoplasma is present. Animal source growth medium components such as sera are important sources for contamination. Equally though, human mycoplasmas may originate from hand or salivary contamination of the cell culture if the source is not the human tissue itself, e.g., genital tumor lines may have a higher opportunity for contamination. It must be remembered that usual antibacterial antibiotics for cell culture purposes do not inhibit mycoplasmas. Common contaminants have historically included *M. orale*, *M. hyorhinis*, *M. arginii*, *Acholeplasma*, and *M. fermentans*; it has been observed that *M. fermentans* in particular is increasing in frequency as a tissue culture contaminant.

Several methods for detection exist. Indirect indicators of enzymatic change or pH colour indicator change have a sentinel role in warning for contamination. Various direct enzymatic measurements of mycoplasma biochemical activity have been touted, but few are universal and commonly used. Culture on human infection-diagnostic mycoplasma media usually identifies the majority of contaminant mycoplasmas, and SP4 and modified Hayflick's media serve this purpose (132,133). Non-cultivable mycoplasmas do exist although on a practical basis, these are much less often a problem. Heavily colonized cell lines may also be detected by the use of DNA-binding fluorochromes (134,135) which non-specifically adhere to double-stranded DNA. The fluorochromes may be directly applied to the cell line under investigation, or a cell indicator system may be used. For the latter, supernatant from the suspect contaminated cell line is added to a mycoplasma-free cell line. Comparisons of the latter to a control by enumeration of fluorescent bodies will determine contamination. The latter approach provides a more clear substrate for fluorescence assessment since the primary cell line may have debris that can lead to interpretive artifact. Detection systems which use specific fluoresceinated antisera to contaminant mycoplasmas or dot immunobinding (antigen detection especially with monoclonal antibody) have been created, but the advent of PCR amplification (136) may render the latter obsolete. For genetic detection, it is possible to use universal amplification primers that are targeted to conserved regions of 16S rDNA. This will allow for detection of a wide range of mycoplasmas including those that may be relatively non-cultivable. There remains the possibility that PCR may detect non-viable mycoplasmas which have been inactivated and which are hence not likely to cause difficulty for cell cultures, but alternative methods may then be used as an adjunct if the circumstances require.

VII. SUSCEPTIBILITY TESTING

The susceptibility of mycoplasmas to particular antimicrobials offers the opportunity to treat infection at different body sites. Some generalizations are relevant. Macrolides and tetracyclines are commonly used to treat infections, especially *M. pneumoniae* respiratory infection. For human use, tetracyclines are avoided for children <12 yrs. and pregnant females. Beta-lactam antibiotics are not of value, and furthermore, resistance is often seen for rifampin and polymyxins. *U. urealyticum* is commonly resistant to lincomycin and often clindamycin, while *M. hominis* and *M. fermentans* are frequently erythromycin resistant. The new erythromycin analogues, clarithromycin and azithromycin, are generally as active as erythromycin. Doxycycline and other tetracycline analogues tend to be as effective in vitro as tetracycline. Most mycoplasmas are susceptible to both chloramphenicol and a wide array of new quinolone derivatives. Although isolates of both *U. urealyticum* and *M. pneumoniae* have been found to be erythromycin resistant, such citations are uncommon and therefore on a practical basis, empiric therapy of associated illnesses with erythromycin is often done without specific knowledge of susceptibility testing data. Tetracycline resistance among *U. urealyticum* and *M. hominis* is infrequent, but the presence of the *tetM* determinant among some strains and the knowledge that there is a naturally occurring presence of this factor on a mobile transposon have raised concern about emerging resistance (137). This tetracycline resistance factor is highly related to tetracycline resistance among other bacteria, especially streptococci. Therefore, antibiotic resistance among mycoplasmas can be innate, acquired by mutation, or acquired potentially by transfer.

As for other bacteria, susceptibility can be affected by a large number of variables, but the more common of these include medium composition, growth atmosphere, prolonged growth requirements, and inoculum size (138). Given the unusual growth characteristics of mycoplasmas, it is not surprising therefore that reports of antibiograms vary. A need for standardization is obvious but ultimately utility will depend on a correlation with treatment outcome. The latter requires sufficient disease to be available for study and the existence of varying degrees of resistance among bacterial isolates in order to test the in vitro-in vivo correlations.

Disc diffusion in the conventional format has not been subscribed to. Problems with diffusion for bacteria that are slow-growing has long been recognized. Nevertheless, the E test diffusion variation on this theme has been recently assessed and has been touted as a method with reasonable correlation to broth microdilution (139). More study is needed in this area.

Agar dilution minimum inhibitory concentration testing has been used. Inocula of 10^2-10^4 bacteria per spot have been recommended, and the end-point is determined by no growth of viable colonies as visualized by low power microscopy. Although amenable to standardization, this method has less appeal for routine practical use if the need specifically arises in the form of an ad hoc test. Therefore, agar dilution is likely to be chosen when reference and research studies are required.

The lack of turbidity in broths with mycoplasma growth precludes adoption of the microbroth dilution technique as it is applied to other more rapidly-growing bacteria. As a substitute, end-point determinations of growth are dependent on colour changes of pH indicators for microbroth dilution assays (140). The inoculum can be prepared by assessing the quantity of colour changing units (CCU); usually ~10^4 CCU will be used in a microtitre well. Results for dilution assays of this fashion are generally comparable to those of agar dilution.

On a practical basis, routine susceptibility testing of any mycoplasma is probably not warranted at this time. Nevertheless, there is a real and likely opportunity for resistance to emerge. Both new macrolides and quinolones are experiencing considerable use for the purposes of both community-acquired respiratory infections and varied illnesses of the genital tract. Tetracyclines continue to be used widely in veterinary practices. Selective pressure will likely become available to test susceptibility methods over the next decade.

REFERENCES

1. Dienes L, Smith WE. Relationship of pleuropneumoniae-like organisms to infections of human genital tract. Proc Soc Exp Biol Med 1942; 50:99-101.
2. Morton HE, Smith PF, Williams NB, Eickenberg CF. Isolation of pleuropneumonia-like organisms from human saliva: a newly detected member of the oral flora. J Dent Res 1951; 30:415-422.
3. Eaton MD, Meiklejohn G, Van Herick W. Studies on the etiology of primary atypical pneumonia: a filterable agent transmissible to cotton rats, hamsters, and chick embryos. J Exp Med 1944; 79:649-652.
4. Chanock RM, Hayflick L, Barile MF. Growth on artificial medium of an agent associated with atypical pneumonia and its identification as a PPLO. Proc Natl Acad Sci USA 1962: 48:41-49.
5. Woese CR, Maniloff J, Zablen LB. Phylogenetic analysis of the mycoplasmas. Proc Natl Acad Sci USA 1980; 77:494-498.
6. Fukuda Y, Washio T, Tomita M. Comparative study of overlapping genes in the genomes of *Mycoplasma genitalium* and *Mycoplasma pneumoniae*. Nucleic Acids Res 1999; 27:1847-1853.
7. Rawadi G, Dujeancourt-Henry A, Lemercier B, Roulland-Dussoix D. Phylogenetic position of rare human mycoplasmas, *Mycoplasma faucium*, *M. buccale*, *M. primatum*, and *M. spermatophilum*, based on 16S rRNA gene sequences. Int J Syst Bacteriol 1998; 48:305-309.
8. Taylor-Robinson D, Furr PM, Hanna NF. Microbiological and serological study of non-gonococcal urethritis with special reference to *Mycoplasma genitalium*. Genitourin Med 1985; 61:319-324.
9. Lo SC. Mycoplasmas and AIDS. Chapter 32. In: Maniloff J, ed. Mycoplasmas: Molecular Biology and Pathogenesis. Washington, DC:American Society for Microbiology, 1992:525-545.
10. Lo SC, Shih JW, Newton PB, Wong DM, Hayes MM, Benish JR, Wear DJ, Wang RY. Virus-like infectious agent is a novel pathogenic mycoplasma. Am J Trop Med Hyg 1989; 41:586-600.
11. Lo SC, Hayes MM, Tully JG, Wang RY, Kotani H, Pierce PF, Rose DL, Shih JW. *Mycoplasma penetrans* sp. nov. from the urogenital tract of patients with AIDS. Int J Syst Bacteriol 1992; 42:357-364.
12. Wang RY, Shih JW, Grandinetti T, Pierce PF, Hayes MM, Wear DJ, Alter HJ, Lo SC. High frequency of antibodies to *Mycoplasma penetrans* in HIV-infected patients. Lancet 1992; 340:1312-1316.
13. Tham TN, Feris S, Bahroui E, Canarelli S, Montagnier L, Blanchard A. Identification of an adhesin-like gene of *Mycoplasma pirum* isolated from AIDS patients. Ann NY Acad Sci 1994; 730:279-282.
14. Wirostko E, Johnson L, Wirostko B. Ulcerative colitis associated chronic uveitis: parasitization of intraocular leucocytes by mollicute-like organisms. J Submicrosc Cytol Pathol 1990; 22:231-239.
15. Vojdani A, Choppa PC, Tagle C, Andrin R, Samini B, Lapp CW. Detection of *Mycoplasma* genus and *Mycoplasma fermentans* by PCR in patients with chronic fatigue syndrome. FEMS Immunol Med Microbiol 1998; 22:355-365.
16. Haier J, Nasralla M, Franco AR, Nicolson GL. Detection of mycoplasmal infections in blood of patients with rheumatoid arthritis. Rheumatology 1999; 38:504-509.
17. Tilley BC, Alarcon GS, Heyse SP, Trentham DE, Neuner R, Kaplan DA, Clegg DO, Leisen JC, Buckley L, Cooper SM, Duncan H, Pillemer SR, Tuttleman M, Fowler SE, and the MIRA Trial Group. Minocycline treatment of rheumatoid arthritis. Ann Intern Med 1995; 122:81-89.
18. Cimolai N. *Mycoplasma pneumoniae* respiratory infection. Pediatr Rev 1998; 19:327-331.
19. Farraj RS, McCully RB, Oh JK, Smith TF. Mycoplasma-associated pericarditis. Mayo Clin Proc 1997; 72:33-36.
20. Abramovitz P, Schvartzman P, Harel D, Lis I, Naot Y. Direct invasion of the central nervous system by *Mycoplasma pneumoniae*: a report of two cases. J Infect Dis 1987; 155:482-487.
21. Davis CP, Cochran S. Lisse J, Buck G, DiNuzzo AR, Weber T, Reinarz JA. Isolation of *Mycoplasma pneumoniae* from synovial fluid samples in a patient with pneumonia and polyarthritis. Arch Intern Med 1988; 148:969-970.
22. Narita M, Matsuzono Y, Togashi T, Kajii N. DNA diagnosis of central nervous system infection by *Mycoplasma pneumoniae*. Pediatrics 1992; 90:250-253.

23. Murray HW, Masur H, Senterfit LB, Roberts RB. The protean manifestations of *Mycoplasma pneumoniae* infection in adults. Am J Med 1975; 58:229-242.

24. Cherry JD. Mycoplasma and ureaplasma infections. Chapter 195. In: Feigin RD, Cherry JD – eds. Textbook of Pediatric Infectious Diseases. Philadelphia, PA:WB Saunders Co., 1998:2259-2286.

25. Ponka A. The occurrence and clinical picture of serologically verified *Mycoplasma pneumoniae* infections with emphasis on central nervous system, cardiac, and joint manifestations. Ann Clin Res 1979: 24:1-25.

26. Ford DK, Henderson E. Non-gonococcal urethritis due to T-mycoplasma (*Ureaplasma urealyticum*) serotype 2 in a conjugal sexual partnership. Br J Vener Dis 1976; 52:341-342.

27. Maeda S, Tamaki M, Nakano M, Uno M, Deguchi, Kawada Y. Detection of *Mycoplasma genitalium* in patients with urethritis. J Urol 1998; 159:405-407.

28. Uno M, Deguchi T, Komeda H, Yasuda M, Tamaki M, Maeda S, Saito I, Kawada Y. Prevalence of *Mycoplasma genitalium* in men with gonococcal urethritis. Int J STD AIDS 1996; 7:443-444.

29. Wang EE, Cassell GH, Sanchez PJ, Regan JA, Payne NR, Liu PP. *Ureaplasma urealyticum* and chronic lung disease of prematurity: critical appraisal of the literature on causation. Clin Infect Dis 1993; 17 (Suppl 1):112-116.

30. Waites KB, Duffy LB, Crouse DT, Dworsky ME, Strange MJ, Nelson KG, Cassell GH. Mycoplasmal infections of cerebrospinal fluid in newborn infants from a community hospital population. Pediatr Infect Dis J 1990; 9:241-245.

31. Taylor-Robinson D, Furr PM. Update on sexually transmitted mycoplasmas. Lancet 1998; 351: (Suppl 3):12-15.

32. Yoon BH, Romero R, Park JS, Chang JW, Kim YA, Kim JC, Kim KS. Microbial invasion of the amniotic cavity with *Ureaplasma urealyticum* is associated with a robust host response in fetal, amniotic, and maternal compartments. Am J Obstet Gynecol 1998; 179:1254-1260.

33. Mossad SB, Rehm SJ, Tomford JW, Isada CM, Taylor PC, Rutherford I, Sorg S, McHenry MC. Sternotomy infection with *Mycoplasma hominis*: a cause of "culture negative" wound infection. J Cardiovasc Surg 1996; 37:505-509.

34. Mufson MA. *Mycoplasma hominis* I in respiratory tract infections. Ann NY Acad Sci 1970; 174:798-808.

35. Mufson MA. *Mycoplasma hominis*: a review of its role as a respiratory tract pathogen of humans. Sex Transm Dis 1983; 10 (Suppl 4):335-340.

36. Hooton TM, Roberts MC, Roberts PL, Holmes KK, Stamm WE, Kenny GE. Prevalence of *Mycoplasma genitalium* determined by DNA probe in men with urethritis. Lancet 1988; i:266-268.

37. Jensen JS, Orsum R, Dohn B, Uldum S, Worm AM, Lind K. *Mycoplasma genitalium*: a cause of male urethritis? Genitourin Med 1993; 69:265-269.

38. Janier M, Lassau F, Casin I, Grillot P, Scieux C, Zavaro A, Chastang C, Bianchi A, Morel P. Male urethritis with and without discharge: a clinical and microbiological study. Sex Transm Dis 1995; 22:244-252.

39. Blanchard A, Hamrick W, Duffy L, Baldus K, Cassell GH. Use of the polymerase chain reaction for detection of *Mycoplasma fermentans* and *Mycoplasma genitalium* in the urogenital tract and amniotic fluid. Clin Infect Dis 1993; 17 (Suppl 1):272-279.

40. Lo SC, Wear DJ, Green SL, Jones PG, Legier JF. Adult respiratory distress syndrome with or without systemic disease associated with infections due to *Mycoplasma fermentans*. Clin Infect Dis 1993; 17 (Suppl 1):259-263.

41. Beecham HJ, Lo SC, Lewis DE, Comer SW, Riley KJ, Oldfield EC. Recovery from fulminant infection with *Mycoplasma fermentans* (incognitus strain) in non-immunocompromised host. Lancet 1991; 338:1014-1015.

42. Plata EJ, Abell MR, Murphy WH. Induction of leukemoid disease in mice by *Mycoplasma fermentans*. J Infect Dis 1973; 128:588-597.

43. Dawson MS, Hayes MM, Wang RY, Armstrong D, Kundsin RB, Lo SC. Detection and isolation of *Mycoplasma fermentans* from urine of human immunodeficiency virus type 1-infected patients. Arch Pathol Lab Med 1993; 117:511-514.

44. Bauer FA, Wear DJ, Angritt P, Lo SC. *Mycoplasma fermentans* (incognitus strain) infection of the kidneys of patients with acquired immunodeficiency syndrome and associated nephropathy: a light microscopic, immunohistochemical, and ultrastructural study. Hum Pathol 1991; 22:63-69.

45. Ainsworth JG, Katseni V, Hourshid S, Waldron S, Ball S, Cattell V, Taylor-Robinson D. *Mycoplasma fermentans* and HIV-associated nephropathy. J Infect 1994; 29:323-326.

46. Deguchi T, Gilroy CB, Taylor-Robinson D. Failure to detect *Mycoplasma fermentans*, *Mycoplasma penetrans*, or *Mycoplasma pirum* in the urethra of patients with acute nongonococcal urethritis. Eur J Clin Microbiol Infect Dis 1996; 15:169-171.

47. Schaeverbeke T, Gilroy CB, Bebear C, Dehais J, Taylor-Robinson D. *Mycoplasma fermentans*, but not *M. penetrans*, detected by PCR assays in synovium from patients with rheumatoid arthritis and other rheumatic disorders. J Clin Pathol 1996; 49:824-828.
48. Watanabe T, Shibata K, Yoshikawa T, Dong L, Hasebe A, Domon H, Kobayashi T, Totsuka Y. Detection of *Mycoplasma salivarium* and *Mycoplasma fermentans* in synovial fluids of temporomandibular joints of patients with disorders in the joints. FEMS Immunol Med Microbiol 1998; 22:241-246.
49. Wirostko E, Johnson L, Wirostko W. Juvenile rheumatoid arthritis inflammatory eye disease: parasitization of ocular leucocytes by mollicute-like organisms. J Rheumatol 1989; 16:1446-1453.
50. Johnson L, Wirostko E, Wirostko W, Wirostko B. Mycoplasma-like organisms in Hodgkin's disease. Lancet 1996; 347:901-902.
51. Hofffman RW, O'Sullivan FX, Schafermeyeer KR, Moore TL, Rousell D, Watson-McKown R, Kim MF, Wise KS. Mycoplasma infection and rheumatoid arthritis: analysis of their relationship using immunoblotting and an ultrasensitive polymerase chain reaction detection method. Arthritis Rheum 1997; 40:1219-1228.
52. Van Kuppeveld FJ, Johansson KE, Galama JM, Kissing J, Bolske G, Hjelm E, Van Der Logt JT. 16S rRNA based polymerase chain reaction compared with culture and serological methods for diagnosis of *Mycoplasma pneumoniae* infection. Eur J Clin Microbiol Infect Dis 1994; 13:401-405.
53. Goulet M, Dular R, Tully JG, Billowes G, Kasatiya S. Isolation of *Mycoplasma pneumoniae* from the human urogenital tract. J Clin Microbiol 1995; 33:2823-2825.
54. Lind K, Bentzon MW. Epidemics of *Mycoplasma pneumoniae* infection in Denmark from 1958 to 1974. Int J Epidemiol 1976; 5:267-277.
55. Lind K, Bentzon MW. Changes in the epidemiological pattern of *Mycoplasma pneumoniae* infections in Denmark: a 30 years survey. Epidemiol Infect 1988; 101:377-386.
56. Lind K, Bentzon MW, Jensen JS, Clyde WA. A seroepidemiological study of *Mycoplasma pneumoniae* infections in Denmark over the 50-year period 1946-1995. Eur J Epidemiol 1997; 13:581-586.
57. Kovacs GT, Westcott M, Rusden J, Asche V, King H, haynes SE, Moore EK, Hall BE. Microbiological profile of the cervix in 1,000 sexually active women. Aust N Z J Obstet Gynaecol 1988; 28:216-220.
58. Zheng X, Watson HL, Waites KB, Cassell GH. Serotype diversity and antigen variation among invasive isolates of *Ureaplasma urealyticum* from neonates. Infect Immun 1992; 60:3472-3474.
59. Lin JS, Radnay K, Kendrick MI, Kass EH. Serological studies on *Mycoplasma hominis*: serotypic distribution of recent clinical isolates. Scand J Infect Dis 1976; 8:45-48.
60. Naessens A, Foulon W, Breynaert J, Lauwers S. Serotypes of *Ureaplasma urealyticum* isolated from normal pregnant women and patients with pregnancy complications. J Clin Microbiol 1988; 26:319-322.
61. Robertson JA, Vekris A, Bebear C, Stemke GW. Polymerase chain reaction using 16S rRNA gene sequences distinguishes the two biovars of *Ureaplasma urealyticum*. J Clin Microbiol 1993; 31:824-830.
62. Robertson JA, Howard LA, Zinner CL, Stemke GW. Comparison of 16S rRNA genes within the T960 and parvo biovars of ureaplasmas isolated from humans. Int J Syst Bacteriol 1994; 44:836-838.
63. Abele-Horn M, Wolff C, Dressel P, Pfaff F, Zimmerman A. Association of *Ureaplasma urealyticum* biovars with clinical outcome for neonates, obstetric patients, and gynecological patients with pelvic inflammatory disease. J Clin Microbiol 1997; 35:1199-1202.
64. Know CL, Timms P. Comparison of PCR, nested PCR, and random amplified polymorphic DNA PCR for detection and typing of *Ureaplasma urealyticum* in specimens from pregnant women. J Clin Microbiol 1998; 36:3032-3039.
65. Blanchard A, Montagnier L. AIDS-associated mycoplasmas. Annu Rev Microbiol 1994; 48:687-712.
66. Wang RY, Shih JW, Weiss SH, Grandinetti T, Pierce PF, Lange M, Alter HJ, Wear DJ, Davies CL, Mayur RK, Lo SC. *Mycoplasma penetrans* infection in male homosexuals with AIDS: high seroprevalence and association with Kaposi's sarcoma. Clin Infect Dis 1993; 17:724-729.
67. Grau O, Tuppin P, Slizewicz B, Launay V, Goujard C, Bahraoui E, Delfraissy JF, Montagnier L. A longitudinal study of seroreactivity against *Mycoplasma penetrans* in HIV-infected homosexual men: association with disease progression. AIDS Res Hum Retroviruses 1998; 14:661-667.
68. Grau O, Slizewicz B, Tuppin P, Launay V, Bourgeois E, Sagot N, Moynier M, Lafeuillade A, Bachelez H, Clauvel JP, Blanchard A, Bahraoui E, Montagnier L. Association of *Mycoplasma penetrans* with human immunodeficiency virus infection. J Infect Dis 1995; 172:672-681.
69. Chingbingyong MI, Hughes CV. Detection of *Mycoplasma fermentans* in human saliva with a polymerase chain reaction-based assay. Arch Oral Biol 1996; 41:311-314.
70. Hawkins RE, Rickman LS, Vermund SH, Carl M. Association of mycoplasma and human immunodeficiency virus infection: detection of amplified *Mycoplasma fermentans* DNA in blood. J Infect Dis 1992; 165:581-585.

71. Katseni VL, Gilroy CB, Ryait BK, Ariyoshi K, Bieniasz PD, Weber JN, Taylor-Robinson D. *Mycoplasma fermentans* in individuals seropositive and seronegative for HIV-1. Lancet 1993; 341:271-273.
72. Kovacic R, Launay V, Tuppin P, Lafeuillade A, Feullie V, Montagnier L, Grau O. Search for the presence of six *Mycoplasma* species in peripheral blood mononuclear cells of subjects seropositive and seronegative for human immunodeficiency virus. J Clin Microbiol 1996; 34:1808-1810.
73. Yanez A, Cedillo L, Neyrolles O, Alonso E, Prevost MC, Rojas J, Watson HL, Blanchard A, Cassell GH. *Mycoplasma penetrans* bacteremia and primary antiphospholipid syndrome. Emerg Infect Dis 1999; 5:164-167.
74. Dische MR, Quinn PA, Czegledy-Nagy E, Sturgess JM. Genital mycoplasma infection: intrauterine infection: pathologic study of the fetus and placenta. Am J Clin Pathol 1979; 72:167-174.
75. Quinn PA, Gillan JE, Markestad T, St. John MA, Daneman A, Lie KI, Li HCS, Czegledy-Nagy E, Klein M. Intrauterine infection with *Ureaplasma urealyticum* as a cause of fatal neonatal pneumonia. Pediatr Infect Dis J 1985; 4:538-543.
76. Waites KB, Crouse DT, Philips JB, Canupp KC, Cassell GH. Ureaplasmal pneumonia and sepsis associated with persistent pulmonary hypertension of the newborn. Pediatrics 1989; 83:79-85.
77. Joste NE, Kundsin RB, Genest DR. Histology and *Ureaplasma urealyticum* culture in 63 cases of first trimester abortion. Am J Clin Pathol 1994; 102:729-732.
78. Kong F, Zhu X, Wang W, Zhou X, Gordon S, Gilbert GL. Comparative analysis and serovar-specific identification of multiple-banded antigen genes of *Ureaplasma urealyticum* biovar 1. J Clin Microbiol 1999; 37:538-543.
79. De Silva NS, Quinn PA. Localization of endogenous activity of phospoholipases A and C in *Ureaplasma urealyticum*. J Clin Microbiol 1991; 29:1498-1503.
80. Watson HL, Blalock DK, Cassell GH. Variable antigens of *Ureaplasma urealyticum* containing both serovar-specific and serovar-cross-reactive epitopes. Infect Immun 1990; 58:3679-3688.
81. Olson LD, Renshaw CA, Shane SW, Barile MF. Successive synovial *Mycoplasma hominis* isolates exhibit apparent antigenic variation. Infect Immun 1991; 59:3327-3329.
82. Tham TN, Ferris S, Bahraoui E, Canarelli S, Montagnier L, Blanchard A. Molecular characterization of the P1-like adhesin gene from *Mycoplasma pirum*. J Bacteriol 1994; 176:781-788.
83. Cimolai N. Serodiagnosis of the Infectious Diseases: *Mycoplasma pneumoniae*. Norwell, MA, U.S.:Kluwer Academic Publishers, 1999.
84. Feizi T, Loveless RW. Carbohydrate recognition by *Mycoplasma pneumoniae* and pathlogic consequences. Am J Respir Crit Care Med 1996; 154:S133-136.
85. Cimolai N, Cheong ACH. Anti-smooth muscle antibody in clinical human and experimental animal *Mycoplasma pneumoniae* infection. J Appl Microbiol 1997; 82:389-398.
86. Cimolai N. Antigenic relationships. Chapter 4. In: Serodiagnosis of the Infectious Diseases: *Mycoplasma pneumoniae*. Norwell, MA:Kluwer Academic Publishers, 1999:25-31.
87. Cimolai N. Complement fixation. Chapter 6. In: Serodiagnosis of the Infectious Diseases: *Mycoplasma pneumoniae*. Norwell, MA:Kluwer Academic Publishers, 1999:39-52.
88. Jacobs E, Bennewitz A, Bredt W. Reaction pattern of human anti-*Mycoplasma pneumoniae* antibodies in enzyme-linked immunosorbent assays and immunoblotting. J Clin Microbiol 1986; 23:517-522.
89. Vu AC, Foy HM, Cartwright FD, Kenny GE. The principal protein antigens of isolates of *Mycoplasma pneumoniae* as measured by levels of immunoglobulain G in human serum are stable in strains collected over a 10-year period. Infect Immun 1987; 55:1830-1836.
90. Aubert G, Pozzetto B, Hafid J, Gaudin OG. Immunoblotting patterns with *Mycoplasma pneumoniae* of serum specimens from infected and non-infected subjects. J Med Microbiol 1992; 36:341-346.
91. Lee GY, Kenny GE. Humoral immune response to polypeptides of *Ureaplasma urealyticum* in women with postpartum fever. J Clin Microbiol 1987; 25:1841-1844.
92. Cassell GH, Watson HL, Blalock DK, Horowitz SA, Duffy LB. Protein antigens of genital mycoplasmas. Rev Infect Dis 1988; 10 (Suppl 2):391-398.
93. Liepmann MF, Gireaudot P, Deletrez J, De Decker L, Wattre P. Use of *Mycoplasma hominis* 102-116 kD proteins as antigen in an enzyme-linked immunosorbent assay. Microbios 1991; 65:7-13.
94. Bredt W, Kleinmann B, Jacobs E. Antibodies in the sera of *Mycoplasma pneumoniae*-infected patients against proteins of *Mycoplasma genitalium* and other mycoplasmas of man. Zentralbl Bakteriol Mikrobiol Hyg [A] 1987; 266:32-42.

95. Tuppin P, Delamare O, Launay V, Geuguen M, Samba MC, Pambou L, Montagnier L, Grau O. High preva-lence of antibodies to *Mycoplasma penetrans* in human immunodeficiency virus-seronegative and – seropositive populations in Brazzaville, Congo. Clin Diagn Lab Immunol 1997; 4:787-788.

96. Cimolai N. Historical aspects. Chapter 2. In: Serodiagnosis of the Infectious Diseases: *Mycoplasma pneumoniae*. Norwell, MA:Kluwer Academic Publishers, 1999:7-10.

97. Cimolai N, Wensley D, Seear M, Thomas ET. *Mycoplasma pneumoniae* as a co-factor in severe respiratory infections. Clin Infect Dis 1995; 21:1182-1185.

98. Hers JFP. Fluorescent antibody technique in respiratory viral diseases. Am Rev Respir Dis 1963; 88:316-333.

99. Hayflick L. Tissue cultures and mycoplasmas. Tex Rep Biol Med 1965; 23:285-303.

100. Tully JG, Rose DL, Whitcomb RF, Wenzel RP. Enhanced isolation of *Mycoplasma pneumoniae* from throat washings with a newly modified culture medium. J Infect Dis 1979; 139:478-482.

101. Cimolai N. In: Heterophil antibody. Chapter 3. In: Serodiagnosis of the Infectious Diseases: *Mycoplasma pneumoniae*. Norwell, MA:Kluwer Academic Publishers, 1999:11-24.

102. Cimolai N. Immunofluorescence. Chapter 5. In: Serodiagnosis of the infectious diseases: *Mycoplasma pneumoniae*. Norwell, MA:Kluwer Academic Publishers, 1999:33-38.

103. Kenny GE, Kaiser GG, Cooney MK, Foy HM. Diagnosis of *Mycoplasma pneumoniae* pneumonia: sensitivi-ties and specificities of serology with lipid antigen and isolation of the organism on soy peptone medium for identification of infections. J Clin Microbiol 1990; 28:2087-2093.

104. Cimolai N. Inhibitory antibody. Chapter 7. In: Serodiagnosis of the Infectious Diseases: *Mycoplasma pneumoniae*. Norwell, MA:Kluwer Academic Publishers, 1999:53-56.

105. Cimolai N. Particle agglutination. Chapter 8. In: Serodiagnosis of the Infectious Diseases: *Mycoplasma pneumoniae*. Norwell, MA:Kluwer Academic Publishers, 1999:57-63.

106. Cimolai N. Radioimmunoassay. Chapter 10. In: Serodiagnosis of the Infectious Disease: *Mycoplasma pneumoniae*. Norwell, MA:Kluwer Academic Publishers, 1999:67-68.

107. Cimolai N. Enzyme-linked immunoassay. Chapter 11. In: Serodiagnosis of the Infectious Disease: *Mycoplasma pneumoniae*. Norwell, MA:Kluwer Academic Publishers, 1999:69-76.

108. Cimolai N. Immunoblotting. Chapter 12. In: Serodiagnosis of the Infectious Diseases: *Mycoplasma pneumoniae*. Norwell, MA:Kluwer Academic Publishers, 1999:77-82.

109. Cimolai N, Mah D, Thomas E, Middleton P. Rapid immunoblot method for diagnosis of acute *Mycoplasma pneumoniae* infection. Eur J Clin Microbiol Inf Dis 1990; 9:223-226.

110. Cimolai N, Cheong ACH. IgM anti-P1 immunoblotting: a standard for the rapid serologic diagnosis of *Mycoplasma pneumoniae* infection in pediatric care. Chest 1992; 102:477-481.

111. Cimolai N, Mah D. Comparison of polyclonal antisera and anti-43 kD antigen monoclonal antibodies for the culture-amplified antigneic detection of *Mycoplasma pneumoniae* by immunoblotting. J Microbiol Meth 1991; 13:123-133.

112. Cimolai N, Bryan LE, Schryvers A, Woods DE. Culture-amplified immunological detection of *Mycoplasma pneumoniae* in clinical specimens. Diagn Micro Infect Dis 1988; 9:207-212.

113. Kenri T, Taniguchi R, Sasaki Y, Okazaki N, Narita M, Izumikawa K, Umetsu, Sasaki T. Identification of a new variable sequence in the P1 cytadhesin gene of *Mycoplasma pneumoniae*: evidence for the generation of antigenic variation by DNA recombination between repetitive sequences. Infect Immun 1999; 67:4557-4562.

114. Cimolai N, Trombley C, Mah DG. A comparison of IgM anti-P1 immunoblotting and a polymerase chain reaction assay for the diagnosis of acute *Mycoplasma pneumoniae* respiratory infection in children. Serodiagn Immunother Infect Disease 1995; 7:153-156.

115. Abele-Horn M, Busch U, Nitschko H, Jacobs E, Bax R, Pfaff F, Schaffer B, Heesemann J. Molecular ap-proaches to diagnosis of pulmonary diseases due to *Mycoplasma pneumoniae*. J Clin Microbiol 1998; 36:548-551.

116. Buck GE, Eid NS. Diagnosis of *Mycoplasma pneumoniae* pneumonia in pediatric patients by polymerase chain reaction. Pediatr Pulmonol 1995; 20:297-300.

117. Kai M, Kamiya S, Yabe H, Takakura I, Shiozawa K, Ozawa A. Rapid detection of *Mycoplasma pneumoniae* in clinical samples by the polymerase chain reaction. J Med Microbiol 1993; 38:166-170.

118. Bernet C, Garret M, DeBarbeyrac B, Bebear C, Bonnet J. Detection of *Mycoplasma pneumoniae* by using the polymerase chain reaction. J Clin Microbiol 1989; 27:2492-2496.

119. Luneberg E, Jensen JS, Frosch M. Detection of *Mycoplasma pneumoniae* by polymerase chain reaction and nonradioactive hybridization in microtiter plates. J Clin Microbiol 1993; 31:1088-1094.

120. Falguera M, Nogues A, Ruiz-Gonzalez A, Garcia M, Puig T. Detection of *Mycoplasma pneumoniae* by polymerase chain reaction in lung aspirates from patients with community-acquired pneumonia. Chest 1996; 110:972-976.

121. Skakni L, Sardet A, Just J, Landman-Parker J, Costil J, Moniot-Ville N, Bricout F, Garbarg-Chenon A. Detection of *Mycoplasma pneumoniae* in clinical samples from pediatric patients by polymerase chain reaction. J Clin Microbiol 1992; 30:2638-2643.

122. Buck GE, O'Hara LC, Summersgill JT. Rapid sensitive detection of *Mycoplasma pneumoniae* in simulated clinical specimens by DNA amplification. J Clin Microbiol 1992; 30:3280-3283.

123. Tjhie JH, van Kuppeveld FJ, Roosendaal R, Melchers WJ, Gordijn R, MacLaren DM, Walboomers JM, Meijer CJ, van den Brule AJ. Direct PCR enables detection of *Mycoplasma pneumoniae* in patients with respiratory tract infections. J Clin Microbiol 1994; 32:11-16.

124. Kessler HH, Dodge DE, Pierer K, Young KK, Liao Y, Santner BI, Eber E, Roeger MG, Stuenzner D, Sixl-Voight B, Marth E. Rapid detection of *Mycoplasma pneumoniae* by an assay based on PCR and probe hybridization in a nonradioactive microwell plate format. J Clin Microbiol 1997; 35:1592-1594.

125. Ieven M, Ursi D, Van Bever H, Quint W, Niesters HGM, Goossens H. Detection of *Mycoplasma pneumoniae* by two polymerase chain reactions and role of *M. pneumoniae* in acute respiratory tract infections in pediatric patients. J Infect Dis 1996; 173:1445-1452.

126. Dorigo-Aetsma JW, Zaat SA, Wertheim-van Dillen PM, Spanjaard L, Rijntjes J, van Waveren G, Jensen JS, Angulo AF, Dankert J. Comparison of PCR, culture, and serological tests for diangosis of *Mycoplasma pneumoniae* respiratory tract infection in children. J Clin Microbiol 1999; 37:14-17.

127. Clyde WA, Kenny GE, Schachter J. Laboratory diagnosis of chlamydial and mycoplasmal infections. Cumitech 19. Washington, D.C.:American Society for Microbiology, 1984.

128. Shepard MC. Culture media for ureaplasmas. Chapter C8. In: Razin S, Tully JG, eds. Methods in Mycoplasmology: Volume I. New York:Academic Press, Inc., 1983:137-146.

129. Taylor-Robinson D. Recovery of mycoplasmas from the genitourinary tract. Chapter A3. In: Razin S, Tully JG, eds. Methods in Mycoplasmology. Volume II. New York:Academic Press, Inc., 1983:19-26.

130. Abele-Horn M, Wolff C, Dressel P, Zimmerman A, Vahlensieck W, Pfaff F, Ruckdeschel G. Polymerase chain reaction versus culture for detection of *Ureaplasma urealyticum* and *Mycoplasma hominis* in the urogenital tract of adults and the respiratory tract of newborns. Eur J Clin Micro Infect Dis 1996; 15:595-598.

131. Hussain AI, Robson WLM, Kelley R, Reid T, Gangemi JD. *Mycoplasma penetrans* and other mycoplasmas in urine of human immunodeficiency virus-positive children. J Clin Microbiol 1999; 37:1518-1523.

132. Del Giudice RA, Tully JG. Isolation of mycoplasmas from cell cultures by axenic cultivation techniques. Chapter F2. In: Tully TG, Razin S, eds. Molecular and Diagnostic Procedures in Mycoplasmology. Volume II. San Diego, CA:Academic Press, Inc., 1996:411-418.

133. Masover GK, Becker FA. Detection of mycoplasmas in cell cultures by cultural methods. Chapter 23. In: Miles R, Nicholas R, eds. Mycoplasma Protocols. Totowa, NJ:Humana Press, Inc. 1998:207-215.

134. Masover GK, Becker FA. Detection of mycoplasmas in cell cultures by fluorescence methods. Chapter 24. In: Miles R, Nicholas R, eds. Mycoplasma Protocols. Totowa NJ:Humana Press, Inc., 1998:217-226.

135. Masover GK, Becker FA. Detection of mycoplasmas by DNA staining and fluorescent antibody methodology. Chapter F3. In: Tully JG, Razin S, eds. Molecular and Diagnostic Procedures in Mycoplasmology. Volume II. San Diego, CA:Academic Press, Inc., 1996:419-429.

136. Veilleux C, Razin S, May LH. Detection of mycoplasma infection by PCR. Chapter F4. In: Tully TG, Razin S, eds. Molecular and Diagnostic Procedures in Mycoplasmology. Volume II. San Diego,CA:Academic Press, Inc.,1996:431-438.

137. Roberts MC. Antibiotic resistance. Chapter 31. In: Maniloff J, ed. Mycoplasmas: Molecular Biology and Pathogenesis. Washington, D.C.:American Society for Microbiology, 1992:513-523.

138. Kenny GE. Problems and opportunities in susceptibility testing of mollicutes. Chapter C2. In: Tully JG, Razin S, eds. Molecular and Diagnostic Procedures in Mycoplasmology. Volume II. San Diego, CA:Academic Press, Inc., 1996:185-188.

139. Dosa E, Nagy E, Falk W, Szoke I, Ballies U. Evaluation of the E test for susceptibility testing of *Mycoplasma hominis* and *Ureaplasma urealyticum*. J Antimicrob Chemother 1999; 43:575-578.

140. Bebear C, Robertson JA. Determination of minimal inhibitory concentration. Chapter C3. In: Tully JG, Razin S, eds. Molecular and Diagnostic Procedures in Mycoplasmology. Volume II. San Diego, CA:Academic Press, Inc., 1996:189-197.

Index

AB bacterium, 825*t*
Abiotrophia,
    historical aspects, 258
    laboratory features, 307*t*, 310
Acholeplasma, 862*t*
Achromobacter,
    applied systematics, 528*t*
    clinical aspects, 534
    laboratory aspects, 537
Acidominococcus, 708*t*, 722, 729*t*
Acidovorax,
    applied systematics, 528*t*, 537
    clinical aspects, 533
Acinetobacter,
    applied systematics, 528*t*
    beta-lactamase, 174
    carbohydrate metabolism, 19
    clinical aspects, 530, 532
    epidemiology, 536
    Gram stain, 2
    intrinsic resistance, 183*t*
    KOH test, 2
    laboratory features, 540-541, 541*t*
    pathogenesis, 539
    staining, 3
    susceptibility testing, 162*t*, 180*t*, 544
    typing, 543
Acinetobacter baumannii, 532, 536, 541*t*, 544
Acinetobacter calcoaceticus, 506*f*, 541*t*, 544
Acinetobacter haemolyticus, 541*t*, 544
Acinetobacter johnsonii, 536, 541*t*
Acinetobacter junii, 532, 541*t*
Acinetobacter lwoffii, 536, 541*t*
Acquired resistance, 150
Acridine orange, 2-3
Acrodermatitis chronica atrophicans (*see*
    Borrelia)
Actinobacillus,
    clinical aspects, 560-562
    colony morphology, 5
    laboratory features, 565, 568, 569*t*, 571*t*

Actinobacillus actinomycetemcomitans, 561-
    562, 561*t*, 568
    antibiotic susceptibility, 574
Actinobacillus equuli, 558, 561*t*
Actinobacillus hominis, 558, 561*t*
Actinobacillus lignieresii, 558, 561*t*
Actinobacillus minor, 558
Actinobacillus muris, 558
Actinobacillus suis, 558, 561*t*
Actinobacillus ureae, 558, 561*t*
Actinobaculum, 343*t*
Actinomadura, 385
Actinomyces,
    antibiotic susceptibility, 737
    applied systematics, 348*f*, 708*t*
    clinical aspects, 711
    colony morphology, 5, 717
    Gram stain, 727
    immunology of infection, 724
    laboratory features, 705, 731
Actinomyces israelii,
    applied systematics, 708*t*
Actinomyces meyerii, 708*t*
Actinomyces neuii, 334*t*, 343*t*, 348*t*, 706*t*, 708*t*,
    717
Actinomyces odontolyticus, 708*t*
Actinomyces radingae, 334*t*, 343*t*, 708*t*
Actinomyces turicensis, 334*t*, 343*t*, 708*t*
Actinomyces viscosus, 708t, 717
Actinomycetes,
    clinical aspects, 384-385
    epidemiology, 387
    identification,
        restriction enzyme digests, 23
    immunology of infection, 392
    laboratory features, 402-403, 408
    microscopy, 397
    specimen collection, 394-395
    staining of, 3
    susceptibility testing, 414
    thermophilic, 385

[Actinomycetes]
    typing, 411-412
    16S rDNA digests, 23*f*
Actinomycosis (*see* Actinomyces)
Aerobes,
    atmospheric requirements, 16
Aerococcus,
    laboratory features, 311
Aeromonas,
    applied systematics, 426*f*
    clinical aspects, 438-439
    epidemiology, 443
    immunology of infection, 458
    intrinsic resistance, 183*t*
    laboratory features, 453-455, 466, 472
    serodiagnosis, 474-475
    susceptibility testing, 162*t*, 478*t*, 482
Aeromonas bestiarum, 426*f*, 455
Aeromonas caviae, 426*f*, 438, 455, 466, 472
Aeromonas hydrophila,
    clinical aspects, 438-439
    general, 426*f*, 455
Aeromonas jandaei, 426*f*, 455
Aeromonas schubertii, 426*f*, 455
Aeromonas veronii, 426*f*, 455, 472
Aerotolerance, 16
Afipia,
    applied systematics, 528*t*, 826*f*
    clinical aspects, 534
    laboratory features, 542, 544
African tick bite fever (*see* Rickettsia)
Agglutination, 63
Agrobacterium,
    applied systematics, 528*t*, 537, 589, 826*f*
    clinical aspects, 534
    KOH test, 2
Albert stain, 3
Alcaligenes,
    applied systematics, 500*f*, 528*f*, 537
    typing, 543
Allele specific oligonucleotide hybridization,
    93
Alloiococcus otitidis,
    clinical aspects, 233
    identification, 241, 309*t*
Amblyomma, 587, 754, 829*t*, 831
Aminoglycosides,
    general, 151, 153*t*, 155, 330
    modifying enzymes, 479
Amycolata, 385

Anaerobes,
    anaerobic chamber, 726
    atmospheric requirements, 16, 725-726
    Bacteroides spp., 708*t*, 720-721
    beta-lactamase, 737
    clinical aspects, 707-714
    clostridia, 708*t*, 712-714, 717-720
    definition of, 705
    epidemiology, 714-716
    fusobacteria, 708*t*, 722
    gas-liquid chromatography, 728-730
    Gram negative cocci, 722
    Gram positive cocci, 717
    Gram stain, 2, 727-728
    growth media, 726-727
    laboratory features, 724-725
    non-spore forming Gram positive
        bacilli, 717
    normal flora, 715-716
    pigmented Gram negative bacilli, 720
    pre-reduced media, 726
    selective media, 726-727, 733-734
    specimen collection, 39, 43-44, 724
    specimen processing, 725-727
    specimen transport, 43-44, 724-725
    susceptibility testing,
        broth disc elution, 736
        Etest, 736
        general, 162*t*, 173, 184*t*, 735-738
        Wilkins-Chalgren agar, 736
Anaerobiospirillum, 708t, 722, 735
Anaerorhabdus, 722
Anaerovibrio, 722
Anaplasma, 824*f*, 826*f*
Antibiotic-associated diarrhea (*see* Clostridium
    difficile)
Antibiotic classification, 152-154
Antibody,
    fetal, 77
    index, 764, 788
    maternal, 77
AntiDNAase, 56-57
Antigen,
    detection, 50-51
    for serodiagnosis, 59-60
Antihyaluronidase, 57*t*
Antistreptolysin O, 56, 58, 60, 64, 77, 291
Applied systematics,
    general, 9-30
    history of, 25-28

Approved List of Bacterial Names, 27
Arcanobacterium haemolyticum,
        applied systematics, 348*f*
        clinical aspects, 342
        epidemiology, 346
        laboratory features, 353-354
        susceptibility testing, 365
Arcanobacterium bernardiae, 334*t*, 348*t*, 365,
        361
Arcanobacterium pyogenes, 334*t*, 348*t*, 365,
        361
Arcobacter butzleri,
        applied systematics, 426*f*, 427*t*
        clinical aspects, 438
Arcobacter cryaerophilus,
        applied systematics, 426*f*
        clinical aspects, 438
Argas, 754
Arthrobacter, 334*t*, 343*t*, 346
Aspergillus fumigatus,
        molecular diagnosis, 98
Astrakhan spotted fever (*see* Rickettsia)
Atmosphere,
        growth requirements, 16, 725-726
Atopobium, 730
Auramine, 3

Bacillary angiomatosis (*see* Bartonella)
Bacillus,
        clinical aspects, 340-341
        epidemiology, 345-346
        KOH test, 2
        laboratory features, 360-361
        morphology, 15, 717
        spore formation, 351-352, 352*f*, 360
        spore selection, 360
        staining, 15
        susceptibility testing, 162*t*, 365
Bacillus anthracis,
        clinical aspects, 339-340
        epidemiology, 345
        historical background, 334-335
        immunology of infection, 355-356
        laboratory features, 359-360
        serodiagnosis, 57*t*
        susceptibility testing, 365
Bacillus cereus,
        food poisoning, 340
                epidemiology of, 345

[Bacillus cereus]
        intrinsic resistance, 183*t*
        laboratory features, 360
        selective media, 360
        susceptibility testing, 365
Bacillus thuringiensis,
        clinical aspects, 341
        laboratory features, 361
Bacterial vaginosis,
        definition of, 711-712
        microbiology, 712
        treatment, 738
Bacteriological Code, 11
Bacteroides,
        applied systematics, 708*t*
        Gram stain, 727
        immunology of infection, 724
        laboratory features, 734
        morphology, 3
        pathogenesis, 721, 734
Bacteroides capillosus, 708*t*
Bacteroides coagulans, 708*t*
Bacteroides distasonis, 708*t*, 720, 738
Bacteroides forsythus, 708*t*, 721*f*
Bacteroides fragilis,
        immunofluorescence, 3
        immunology of infection, 724
        intrinsic resistance, 184*t*
        pathogenesis, 720-721
Bacteroides fragilis group,
        antibiotic susceptibility, 738
        applied systematics, 708*t*, 721*f*
        laboratory features, 720-721, 729*f*, 734
        selective media, 734
        susceptibility testing, 738
Bacteroides gracilis, 708*t*
Bacteroides ovatus, 708*t*, 720
Bacteroides splanchnicus, 721*f*
Bacteroides thetaiotaomicron, 708*f*, 715, 720,
        721*f*
Bacteroides uniformis, 721*f*
Bacteroides ureolyticus, 708*f*, 734
Bacteroides vulgatus, 708*t*, 734
Balneatrix alpica,
        applied systematics, 528*t*
        clinical aspects, 533
        laboratory features, 542
Bannwarth's syndrome (*see* Borrelia)
Bartonella,
        applied systematics, 589, 826*t*

[Bartonella]
    bacillary angiomatosis, 96, 658
    blood culture, 672
    cat scratch disease,
        typical, 656
        atypical, 656-657
    cell culture, 673
    epidemiology, 655*t*, 659-661
    historical background, 653-654
    laboratory features, 661-665, 667-675
    microscopy, 673, 673*f*
    molecular diagnostics, 670-671, 675
    pathogenesis, 665-667
    peliosis hepatis, 658
    serodiagnosis, 55, 57*t*, 66, 667-669
    susceptibility testing, 675-677
    typing, 663-665, 666*t*
Bartonella alsatica, 655*t*
Bartonella bacilliformis,
    clinical aspects, 654-656
    epidemiology, 655*t*, 659-660
    histopathology, 666-667, 669
    historical background, 653-654
    laboratory features, 674*t*
    pathogenesis, 665-666
    serodiagnosis, 669
Bartonella clarridgeiae,
    clinical aspects, 658
    epidemiology, 655*t*, 663*t*
    laboratory features, 674*t*
Bartonella doshiae, 655*t*
Bartonella elizabethae, 654, 655*t*, 657-658
Bartonella grahamii, 655*t*
Bartonella henselae,
    16S rRNA sequencing, 120, 664
    clinical aspects, 656-659
    epidemiology, 655*t*, 660-661, 661*t*, 662*t*,
        663*t*
    histopathology, 666-667
    historical background, 653-654
    immunology of infection, 667
    laboratory features, 666*t*, 667-675
    serodiagnosis,
        EIA, 669
        IFA, 668-669
        Western blot, 669
Bartonella koelerae, 655*t*
Bartonella peromysci, 655*t*
Bartonella quintana,
    clinical aspects, 657-659

[Bartonella quintana]
    epidemiology, 660
    historical aspects, 654
    laboratory features, 667-675
    serodiagnosis, 668-669
Bartonella talpae, 655*t*
Bartonella taylorii, 655*t*
Bartonella tribocorum, 655*t*
Bartonella vinsonii, 655*t*
Bartonellosis (*see* Bartonella)
Bergey's Manual, 11, 26-27
Bergeyella zoohelcum,
    applied systematics, 528*t*
    clinical aspects, 535
Beta-lactam,
    effects on morphology, 2
    members of group, 151, 152*t*, 153*t*
    mode of action, 151
Beta-lactamase,
    anaerobes, 737
    BRO, 519
    detection of, 173-174
    extended spectrum, 173-174, 479
    general, 151
    Haemophilus, 574
    inducible, 173-174
    inhibitors, 174
    Neisseria gonorrhoeae, 518
    SHV, 478
    Staphylococcus aureus, 244
    TEM, 478, 598
Bifidobacterium,
    applied systematics, 348*f*, 708*t*
    general, 343*t*
    laboratory features, 730-731
Bilophila wadsworthia,
    antibiotic susceptibility, 738
    applied systematics, 708*t*, 722
Biotyping (*see* Typing)
Bismuth sulfite agar, 462*t*, 463*t*
Blood culture,
    acquisition of, 189-190
    BacT/Alert, 194-195, 196*t*
    BACTEC, 195-198
    Bartonella, 672
    biphasic media, 191
    Opticult, 191
    Septi-Chek, 191, 192*f*
    continuous monitoring, 194-205
    ESP, 202-205, 203*f*, 204*f*

[Blood culture]
general, 189-206
Legionella, 643
lysis centrifugation, 193*f*, 192-194, 398
miniVITAL, 198-202, 201*t*
mycobacteria, 398
Neisseria spp., 512
processing, 205-206
reporting, 206
rickettsiae, 834
sodium polyanetholsulphonate, 512
specimen collection, 37
VITAL, 198-202, 201*t*
Blue-green algae, 25
Bordetella bronchiseptica, 687
Bordetella hinzii, 687
Bordetella holmseii, 687
Bordetella parapertussis,
historical background, 687
laboratory features, 691-699
pathogenesis, 690
susceptibility testing, 700
Bordetella pertussis,
clinical aspects, 688
culture, 691-692
epidemiology, 688-689
historical background, 687
immunofluorescence, 3, 693-694
immunology of infection, 690-691
laboratory features, 691-699
molecular diagnostics, 694-697
pathogenesis, 689-693
selective media, 692-693
serodiagnosis, 57*t*, 59, 697-699
serotyping, 693
specimen collection, 34, 692
specimen preparation, 692
specimen transport, 40-41
susceptibility testing, 700
Bordetella trematum, 687
Borrelia,
clinical aspects, 749-753
epidemiology, 753-755
growth media, 760-762
historical background, 747-748
immunology of infection, 758-759
laboratory features, 755-757, 781
louse-borne, 748, 753
microscopy, 755*f*, 760
molecular diagnostics, 765-766

[Borrelia]
pathogenesis, 756-758
relapsing fever, 749-750, 756-757, 760-761
serodiagnosis, 55, 57*t*, 61, 72, 761-765
susceptibility testing, 767-768
tick-borne, 748, 754
Borrelia afzelii, 753-754, 757, 759, 764
Borrelia burgdorferi,
laboratory features, 757
Lyme disease,
clinical aspects, 750-753
clinical diagnosis, 119, 753
epidemiology, 754-755
growth media, 762
history of, 119, 748
immunology of infection, 758-759
microscopy, 761-762
molecular diagnostics, 765-766
OspA, 757, 759, 765
pathogenesis, 757-758
pathology, 757-758
sensu lato, 753
sensu strictu, 753
serodiagnosis,
enzyme immunoassay, 763-764
general, 762-764
IFA, 763
Western blot, 764
seronegative, 765
vaccination, 765
Borrelia duttonii, 749, 753-754
Borrelia garinii, 753-754, 757, 759, 764
Borrelia hermsii, 754
Borrelia japonica, 754
Borrelia parkeri, 754
Borrelia recurrentis, 749, 753, 767
Borrelia turicatae, 749
Borrelia valaisiana, 753-754, 757
Borrelia venezuelensis, 754
Botulism (*see* Clostridium botulinum)
Brachyspira aalborgii, 791
Brain-heart infusion broth, 46
Branched DNA assays, 88
Brevibacillus, 334*t*
Brevibacterium, 334*t*, 343*t*, 354
Brevundimonas, 528*t*, 532-533
Brilliant Green agar, 462*t*

Brill-Zinsser disease, 826*t*, 827
Broad range PCR, 120*f*
Bronchoalveolar lavage,
    staining, 5
Brownian movement, 1
Brucella,
    applied systematics, 590*t*, 826*t*
    blood culture, 595
    clinical aspects, 583-584, 584*t*
    epidemiology, 586
    historical background, 581-582
    immunology of infection, 594
    in blood cultures, 191
    KOH test, 2
    laboratory features, 589-590, 595-596
    laboratory safety, 223
    pathogenesis, 590-591
    serodiagnosis, 57*t*, 595
    specimen collection, 36
    susceptibility testing, 597
Brucella abortus, 581, 589, 590*t*, 594-595
Brucella canis, 581, 590*t*
Brucella melitensis, 581, 589, 590*t*, 594
Brucella neotomae, 590*t*
Brucella ovis, 589, 590*t*, 595
Brucella suis, 586, 590*t*
Budvicia, 425*f*, 436
Burkholderia cepacia complex,
    applied systematics, 500*f*, 528*t*
    clinical aspects, 530-532
    epidemiology, 536
    genomovars, 536
    intrinsic resistance, 183
    laboratory aspects, 536, 539-540
    pathogenesis, 536, 538-539
    selective media, 539-540
    susceptibility testing, 180*t*
    typing, 543
Burkholderia gladioli, 532
Burkholderia multivorans, 528*t*, 536
Burkholderia pseudomallei,
    clinical aspects, 531
    laboratory features, 540
    pathogenesis, 539
    serodiagnosis, 57*t*
Burkholderia pyrrocina, 536
Burkholderia stabilis, 528*t*
Burkholderia thailandensis, 540
Burkholderia vietnamiensis, 528*t*, 536
Buttiauxella, 425*f*, 436

Butyrovibrio, 708*t*, 722

Calymmatobacterium granulomatis,
    clinical aspects, 562
    historical background, 558
    laboratory features, 565, 570
CAMP test,
    in identification, 15, 297
Campylobacter,
    applied systematics, 426*f*, 605, 708*t*
    clinical aspects, 437-438
    DNA probes, 96
    epidemiology, 442-443
    growth requirements, 16
    historical background, 424, 427
    immunology of infection, 457-458
    in blood cultures, 205
    intrinsic resistance, 183*t*
    laboratory features, 454, 465-466, 472
    NASBA, 88
    serodiagnosis, 474
    specimen transport, 42
    susceptibility testing, 430*t*, 482
Campylobacter coli,
    applied systematics, 426*t*
    clinical aspects, 437-438
    epidemiology, 443
Campylobacter concisus, 426*f*
Campylobacter curvus, 426*f*, 427*f*, 706*t*
Campylobacter fetus,
    applied systematics, 426*t*
    clinical aspects, 438
    general, 454, 482
Campylobacter gracilis, 427*t*, 738
Campylobacter hyointestinalis, 426*f*
Campylobacter jejuni,
    antibiotic resistance, 482
    applied systematics, 426*f*
    clinical aspects, 437-438
    epidemiology, 443
    laboratory features, 454, 465-466, 472
    pathogenesis, 454
    serodiagnosis, 57*t*, 474
Campylobacter lari, 426*t*, 438
Campylobacter mucosalis, 426*t*
Campylobacter rectus, 426*f*, 427*t*, 706*t*
Campylobacter sputorum, 426*t*
Campylobacter upsaliensis,
    applied systematics, 426*f*
    clinical aspects, 438

Candida,
    DNA probes, 101
Candida albicans,
    molecular diagnostics, 101
Capnocytophaga,
    antibiotic susceptibility, 575
    clinical aspects, 561*t*, 562
    historical background, 557-558
    laboratory features, 565, 573*f*, 722
Capnocytophaga canimorsus, 558, 561*t*, 562,
        573*f*
Capnocytophaga cynodegni, 558, 561*t*, 562,
        573*f*
Capnocytophaga gingivalis, 558, 561*t*, 565,
        573*f*
Capnocytophaga granulosa, 558, 561*t*, 573*f*
Capnocytophaga haemolytica, 558, 561*t*, 573*t*
Capnocytophaga ochracea, 558, 561*t*, 565,
        573*t*, 706*t*
Capnocytophaga sputigena, 558, 561*t*, 565,
        573*t*
Capnophile, 16
Capsule,
    staining of, 2, 15
    typing, 2
Carbol fuchsin, 2
Cardiobacterium hominis,
    antibiotic susceptibility, 574
    clinical aspects, 561*t*, 562
    epidemiology, 563
    historical background, 558
    laboratory features, 565, 570*f*, 571*f*
Carrión's disease (*see* Bartonella bacilliformis)
Catalase, 17, 28
Cat scratch disease (*see* Bartonella)
Caulobacter,
    applied systematics, 528*t*, 532
    laboratory features, 542
CDC group EO-3, 528*t*, 535-536, 543
CDC group O-1, 528*t*, 535, 542
CDC group O-3, 528*t*, 535, 543
CDC group NO-1, 535, 543
CDC group WO-1, 533, 537
Cedecea,
    applied systematics, 425*f*
    clinical aspects, 436
Cellulomonas, 334*t*, 343*t*, 346, 354
Centipeda, 722
Cephalosporins, 152*t*, 153*t*
Cerebrospinal fluid,

[Cerebrospinal fluid]
    specimen transport, 41
    staining, 4
Chlamydia,
    clinical aspects, 796-799
    complement fixation, 66
    epidemiology, 799-801
    Gram stain, 2
    Giemsa stain, 2
    historical background, 795-796
    laboratory features, 801-812
    pathogenesis, 803
    serodiagnosis, 57*t*, 66
    specimen transport, 41
Chlamydia pecorum, 795
Chlamydia pneumoniae,
    antigen detection, 809-810
    antimicrobial susceptibility, 812-813
    cell culture, 808-809
    clinical aspects, 797-799
    epidemiology, 800
    historical background, 795-796
    immunology of infection, 804
    laboratory features, 801-803
    molecular diagnostics, 810
    pathogenesis, 803
    serodiagnosis, 810-811
Chlamydia psittaci,
    antimicrobial susceptibility, 813
    cell culture, 811
    clinical aspects, 799
    epidemiology, 800-801
    historical background, 796
    serodiagnostics, 812
Chlamydia trachomatis,
    antigen detection,
        DFA, 805-806
        EIA, 805-806
    antimicrobial susceptibility, 812
    cell culture, 804-805
    clinical aspects, 796-797
    epidemiology, 799-800
    historical background, 499, 795-796
    immunofluorescence, 3, 57*t*
    immunology of infection, 803-804
    molecular diagnostics,
        amplification, 806-807
        general, 99-100
        probes, 806
    pathogenesis, 803

[Chlamydia trachomatis]
    serodiagnosis, 807-808
    susceptibility testing, 812
    typing, 138
Chloramphenicol, 154*t*, 247
Chloramphenicol acetyltransferase, 248*t*, 574,
    598
Chromobacterium violaceum,
    antibiotic susceptibility, 574
    clinical aspects, 561*t*, 562
    epidemiology, 563
    laboratory features, 540, 558, 565, 570
Chryseobacterium,
    applied systematics, 528*t*
    clinical aspects, 561*t*, 562
    laboratory features, 537-538, 544
    typing, 544
Chryseobacterium gleum, 535
Chryseobacteium indologenes, 535
Chryseobacterium meningosepticum, 535
CIE (*see* Counterimmunoelectrophoresis)
CIN medium (*see* Yersinia enterocolitica)
Citrobacter,
    antibiotic resistance, 430*t*, 478*t*
    beta-lactamase, 174
    clinical aspects, 435
    intrinsic resistance, 183*t*
    pathogenesis, 452
Citrobacter amalonaticus, 425*f*
Citrobacter diversus, 425*f*
Citrobacter farmeri, 425*f*
Citrobacter freundii, 425*f*, 435
Citrobacter youngae, 425*f*
Classification (*see* Applied systematics)
Clavulanic acid, 245
Clone,
    terminology, 125
Clostridium,
    antibiotic susceptibility, 737-738
    applied systematics, 708*t*
    Gram stain, 717
    identification,
        restriction enzyme digests, 23
    immunology of infection, 723-724
    intrinsic resistance, 184
    laboratory features, 717-720, 729*f*, 730-
        734
    morphology, 15, 717-718
    staining, 15
Clostridium baratii, 718*f*

Clostridium bifermentans, 708*t*, 718
Clostridium botulinum,
    applied systematics, 718*t*
    clinical aspects, 712-713
    epidemiology, 716
    laboratory features, 731
    pathogenesis, 719
Clostridium butyricum, 718*f*
Clostridium clostridioforme, 708*t*, 715, 737
Clostridium difficile,
    antibiotic susceptibility, 738
    applied systematics, 708*t*
    clinical aspects, 713
    cytotoxin,
        agglutination, 733
        EIA, 733
        microscopy, 5
    epidemiology, 715-716
    intrinsic resistance, 184
    laboratory features, 731-734
    pathogenesis, 719
    PFGE typing, 135
    selective media, 732
    specimen collection, 37
    spore selection, 732
    toxin A, 719
    toxin B, 719
    typing, 734
Clostridium fallax, 708*t*
Clostridium histolyticum, 708*t*
Clostridium innocuum,
    applied systematics, 708*t*
    intrinsic resistance, 184
Clostridium novyi, 708*t*, 718*f*
Clostridium perfringens,
    antibiotic-associated diarrhea, 713
    applied systematics, 708*t*
    clinical aspects, 713-714
    food poisoning, 713, 731
    laboratory features, 731
    pathogenesis, 719-720
Clostridium ramosum, 708*t*, 737
Clostridium septicum, 708*t*
Clostridium sordelli, 708*t*
Clostridium sporogenes, 708*t*, 718*f*, 738
Clostridium subterminale, 718*f*, 738
Clostridium tertium, 738
Clostridium tetani,
    applied systematics, 708*t*, 718*t*
    clinical aspects, 712

[Clostridium tetani]
    laboratory features, 720
    pathogenesis, 720
    serodiagnosis, 57*t*, 60
CNA media (see colistin-nalidixic acid media)
Coagulase test, 20, 28
Coagulase-negative staphylococci,
    clinical aspects, 232
    culture, 238
    epidemiology, 234
    Gram staining of, 238
    identification, 240-241
    immunology of infection, 237
    in blood cultures, 205-206
    pathogenesis, 236
    susceptibility testing, 247-249, 162*t*
    terminology, 12, 230, 232
    typing, 242-243, 243*t*
Cold agglutinins, 62-63
Colicin (*see* Typing)
Colistin-nalidixic acid media, 46
Colonization factors, 443, 446
Comamonas,
    applied systematics, 528*t*, 537
    clinical aspects, 533
    epidemiology, 533
Complement fixation,
    anticomplementary, 55, 66
    method, 66, 67*f*
    Mycoplasma pneumoniae, 57*t*
Consensus sequence PCR, 120
Coprococcus,
    applied systematics, 708*t*
    laboratory features, 730
Corynebacterium,
    applied systematics, 348*f*, 349*f*
    clinical aspects, 335-337
    epidemiology, 344-345
    group F-1, 339*t*
    group G, 339*t*
    laboratory features, 347-350, 356-358
    morphology, 15
    susceptibility testing, 162*t*, 262-264
Corynebacterium accolens, 338*t*, 334*t*
Corynebacterium afermentans, 338*t*
Corynebacterium amycolatum, 334*t*, 338*t*
'*Corynebacterium aquaticum*',
    LANA test, 2
Corynebacterium auris, 334*t*, 338*t*
Corynebacterium bovis, 338*t*

Corynebacterium confusum, 338*t*
Corynebacterium coyleae, 338*t*
Corynebacterium diphtheriae,
    clinical aspects, 335-336
    diphtheria toxin, 347, 349
    Elek test, 357
    epidemiology, 344
    historical background, 333-334
    immunology of infection, 355
    laboratory features, 347-348
    selection, 17, 356
    serodiagnosis, 57*t*, 60
    staining, 3
    susceptibility testing, 363
Corynebacterium falsenii, 338*t*
Corynebacterium glucuronolyticum, 338*t*
Corynebacterium jeikeium,
    intrinsic resistance, 183*t*
    susceptibility testing, 364
Corynebacterium kutscheri, 338*t*
Corynebacterium macginleyi, 334*t*, 338*t*
Corynebacterium matruchotii, 338*t*
Corynebacterium minutissimum, 338*t*
Corynebacterium mucifaciens, 338*t*
Corynebacterium propinquum, 334*t*, 338*t*
Corynebacterium pseudodiphtheriticum, 338*t*
Corynebacterium pseudotuberculosis, 338*t*
Corynebacterium riegelii, 338*t*
Corynebacterium sanguinis, 338*t*
Corynebacterium simulans, 338*t*
Corynebacterium singulare, 338*t*
Corynebacterium striatum, 338*t*
Corynebacterium sundvallense, 338*t*
Corynebacterium thomssenii, 338*t*
Corynebacterium ulcerans, 338*t*
Corynebacterium urealyticum,
    applied systematics, 334*t*, 349*t*
    intrinsic resistance, 183*t*
    susceptibility testing, 364
Corynebacterium xerosis, 338*t*
Counterimmunoelectrophoresis, 64
Cowdria ruminatum, 824*t*, 826*t*
Coxiella burnetii,
    applied systematics, 824*f*, 826*f*
    clinical aspects, 828-829
    complement fixation, 66
    culture, 836*t*
    epidemiology, 831-832
    historical background, 823
    immunohistochemistry, 843

[Coxiella burnetii]
   immunology of infection, 833
   laboratory features, 833
   molecular diagnostics, 841-843
   pathogenesis, 833
   specimen collection, 834
   serodiagnosis, 57t, 837t, 837-841
   susceptibility testing, 845t, 847-848
Cultures,
   atmospheric requirements, 16, 725-726
   characterization,
      bi-state variables, 13
      continuous variables, 14
      multi-status, 13-14
      non-interpretable results, 13
   chemical requirements, 17
   differential media, 47
   enrichment culture, 45-47
   growth media, 17, 52
   macro-morphology, 15-16
   osmotic requirements, 16-17
   preservation of, 12-13
   protocols, 52
   quantitative, 48
   reference, 13
   salt requirements, 16
   selective enrichment, 17, 45-47
   temperature requirements, 16
Cytotoxicity,
   Clostridium difficile, 5
   Escherichia coli, 5

Dalfopristin, 247
Deftia acidovorans,
   applied systematics, 528t, 537
   clinical aspects, 533
Delayed-type hypersensitivity, 388
Deoxycholate-citrate agar, 462t, 463t
Dermabacter, 334t, 343t
Dermacentor, 587
Dermatophilus congolensis,
   clinical aspects, 385
   epidemiology, 387
   laboratory features, 390
   microscopy, 397
   phylogenetic positioning, 235f
Desulfomonas, 708t, 722, 735
Desulfovibrio, 708t, 722, 735
Dialister pneumosintes, 706t, 708t, 722
Differential display, 122

Diffusion assays, 63-64
Diphtheria (*see* Corynebacterium diphtheriae)
DNA arrays,
   for pathogen discovery, 164
   general, 24
DNA chips (*see also* DNA arrays), 104-105,
   106f
DNA fingerprinting (*see* Typing)
DNA hybridization,
   general 21, 27, 84-85, 126
   in situ, 85-86
   subtractive hybridization, 122
DNA probes,
   general, 22, 95-96
   GenProbe, 100
DNA sequencing,
   general, 95, 120-121
   16S rRNA gene, 107, 118-121
   23S rRNA gene, 120
Edwardsiella,
   applied systematics, 425t
   clinical aspects, 436
   epidemiology, 442
   general, 478t
   laboratory features, 452
EF-4, 562, 570, 572f, 574
Ehrlichia,
   applied systematics, 826f
   clinical aspects, 828
   culture, 836t
   epidemiology, 829t, 831
   Giemsa stain, 2
   historical background, 823-824
   immunohistochemistry, 843
   immunology of infection, 833-834
   laboratory features, 843-833
   molecular diagnostics, 842
   serodiagnosis, 57, 837t, 839
   specimen collection, 834-836
   susceptibility testing, 846-847
Ehrlichia chaffeensis,
   16S rRNA sequencing, 163
Ehrlichia canis, 823-824
Ehrlichia equi, 824
Ehrlichia phagocytophila, 823
Ehrlichia sennetsu, 824
Ehrlichiosis (*see* Ehrlichia)
Eikenella corrodens,
   antibiotic susceptibility, 574
   clinical aspects, 561t, 562

[Eikenella corrodens]
    historical background, 558
    laboratory features, 565, 570, 571*f*, 572*f*
Empedobacter breve,
    applied systematics, 528*t*
    clinical aspects, 535
Endotracheal suction,
    staining, 5
Enterobacter,
    antibiotic resistance, 430*t*, 478
    applied systematics, 425*f*
    beta-lactamase, 174
    clinical aspects, 434-435
    intrinsic resistance, 183*t*
Enterobacter aerogenes, 425*f*, 434
Enterobacter cloacae, 425*f*, 434, 478*t*
Enterobacter gergoviae, 425*f*
Enterobacter sakazakii, 425*f*
Enterobacter taylorae, 425*f*
Enterobacteriaceae,
    antimicrobial resistance, 150, 478*t*
    applied systematics, 425*f*, 500*f*
    clinical aspects, 430-436
    culture, 460-461
    differential media, 462*t*
    enrichment broths, 462*t*
    enteric screening biochemicals, 467*t*
    epidemiology, 439-442
    historical background, 423-429
    identification systems, 28, 466-467
    immunology of infection, 455-457
    intrinsic resistance, 150, 183*t*
    laboratory features, 443-452, 468-471
    lysis centrifugation, 193
    microscopy, 459-460
    morphology, 3
    ribotyping, 134
    selection, 17, 462*t*, 463*t*
    serodiagnosis, 473-474
    specimen,
        collection, 458-459
        storage, 458-459
        transport, 458-459
    staining, 3
    susceptibility testing, 160*t*, 162*t*, 477-481
    terminology, 11
    typing, 452, 475-477
Enterococcus,
    aminoglycoside resistance, 174-175

[Enterococcus]
    beta-lactamase detection, 173*t*
    clinical aspects, 269-270
    epidemiology, 275-276
    historical background, 261-262
    immunology of infection, 294
    in blood cultures, 205
    intrinsic resistance, 183*t*
    laboratory features, 305-308
    pathogenesis, 287-290
    resistance screening, 175*t*
    selection, 17
    staining, 3
    susceptibility testing, 160, 162*t*, 180*t*
    typing, 308
    vancomycin resistance, 175-176
Enterococcus casseliflavus, 306, 308*t*
Enterococcus fecalis,
    intrinsic resistance, 183*t*
Enterococcus gallinarum, 306, 308*t*
Enzyme immunoassay,
    general, 58, 62
    homogeneous assay, 71
    method, 69-71
Eosin-Methylene Blue agar, 460, 462*t*, 463*t*
Eperythozoon, 824*f*
Epidemic typhus (*see* Rickettsia)
Erwinia,
    clinical aspects, 436
Erysipelothrix rhusiopathiae,
    clinical aspects, 342
    epidemiology, 346
    intrinsic resistance, 183*t*
    laboratory features, 361
    susceptibility testing, 365
Erythema chronicum migrans (*see* Borrelia)
Escherichia coli,
    applied systematics, 425*f*
    clinical aspects, 431-432
    colonization factors, 443, 446
    cytolethal distending toxin, 447
    cytotoxic necrotizing factor, 447-448
    diffuse adherence,
        clinical aspects, 431
        general, 428
        pathogenesis, 447
    enteroaggregative,
        clinical aspects, 431
        general, 428
        laboratory features, 468

[Escherichia coli]
    pathogenesis, 447
    enterohemorrhagic,
        clinical aspects, 431
        general, 456
        laboratory features, 461, 469-470
        pathogenesis, 448
        verotoxin assay, 469
    enteroinvasive,
        clinical aspects, 431
        laboratory features, 468-469
        pathogenesis, 446
    enteropathogenic,
        historical background, 427-429
        laboratory features, 468
        pathogenesis, 445-447
    enterotoxigenic,
        clinical aspects, 431
        laboratory features, 461, 469
        pathogenesis, 446
    epidemiology, 440
    genomic structure, 127
    historic background, 423, 427-429
    immunology of infection, 456
    K1 serotype, 515
    laboratory features, 461
    localized adherence, 428
    O serotyping, 475
    pathogenesis, 446-448
    pathogenicity islands, 127
    rRNA for ribotyping, 134
    serodiagnosis, 473
    susceptibility testing, 430t, 479-480
    urinary tract infections, 431, 446
    whole genome sequencing, 103-104
Escherichia coli O157:H7,
    sorbitol MacConkey, 469
    serodiagnosis, 57t, 60
    specimen collection, 36, 458
    typing, 476-477
    verotoxin assay, 469
Escherichia fergusonii, 425f, 432
Escherichia hermanii, 425f, 432
Escherichia vulneris, 425f, 432
Etest, 168, 172, 248, 313, 575, 736
Eubacterium,
    applied systematics, 708t
    intrinsic resistance, 184t
    laboratory features, 717, 731
Eubacterium limosum, 715, 718f

Eubacterium rectale, 716
Eukaryotes, 25
Ewingella,
    clinical aspects, 436
    general, 425f
Exiguobacterium, 334t, 343t, 354

Facklamia,
    staining, 3
FIAX, 68
Fimbriae,
    electron microscopy, 15, 445f
Fingerprinting (see Typing)
Flagella,
    staining of, 2-3, 15, 445
Flavobacterium,
    applied systematics, 528t
    clinical aspects, 535
Flinders Island spotted fever (see Rickettsia)
Food poisoning (see Bacillus cereus; see
    Clostridium perfringens; see
    Staphylococcus aureus)
Francisella philomiragia, 587
Francisella tularensis,
    biovars, 587
    clinical aspects, 584-585
    epidemiology, 586-587, 587f
    historical background, 582
    immunofluorescence, 3
    immunology of infection, 594-595
    laboratory features, 591t, 596
    pathogenesis, 591-592
    serodiagnosis, 57t
    serology, 596
    susceptibility testing, 597
    Wayson stain, 2
Fusidic acid, 158, 247, 248t
Fusobacterium,
    intrinsic resistance, 184t
    laboratory features, 729f, 735
    pathogenesis, 722
Fusobacterium mortiferum, 708t
Fusobacterium necrophorum,
    applied systematics, 708t, 718t
Fusobacterium nucleatum,
    applied systematics, 708t, 718t
    laboratory features, 735
Fusobacterium prausnitzii, 716, 718
Fusobacterium varium, 706t, 708t

Gardnerella,
    bacterial vaginosis, 335, 712, 715
    clinical aspects, 342
    epidemiology, 346, 715
    laboratory features, 361-362
    LANA test, 2
    staining, 5
    susceptibility testing, 365
Gas-liquid chromatography,
    volatile esters, 21
Gastric aspirate,
    specimen collection, 36
Gastrospirillum hominis,
    historical background, 606
Gemella,
    historical aspects, 258
    laboratory features, 309*t*, 310
Genital specimens, 5
GenProbe, 100
Giemsa stain, 2, 760
GLC (*see* Gas-liquid chromatography)
Globicatella,
    laboratory features, 309*t*, 310
    staining, 3
Glomerulonephritis, 265
Glycopeptides, 154*t*, 156-157
GN broth (*see* Gram Negative broth)
Gonococcus (*see* Neisseria gonorrhoeae)
Gonorrhea (*see* Neisseria gonorhoeae)
Gordona,
    acid-fast, 3
    applied systematics, 348*f*
    clinical aspects, 385
Grahamella talpae, 654, 824*f*
Gram negative,
    cell membrane, 443, 444*f*
    cross-reactive antigens, 60
    general, 2
    identification, 26-27
    impact on processing, 51
    KOH test, 2
    LANA test, 2
    'pink cocci' (*see* Methylobacterium and
        see Roseomonas)
    staining, 15
Gram Negative broth, 46, 462*t*
Gram positive,
    cross-reactive antigens, 60
    general, 2

[Gram positive]
    identification, 20, 26-27
    KOH test, 2
    LANA test, 2
    osmotic tolerance, 16
    salt tolerance, 16
    staining, 15
Gram stain,
    for clinical specimens, 49
    for identification,
        of genital sample smears, 510
    general, 2, 15, 26, 28
Granules,
    corynebacteria, 3
    staining of, 2
Group A streptococci (*see mainly*
    Streptococcus pyogenes)
Group B streptococci (*see* Streptococcus
    agalactiae)
Group C streptococci (*see* Streptococcus
    dysgalactiae, Streptococcus equi, and
    Streptococcus zooepidemicus)
Group D streptococci (*see mainly*
    Enterococcus)
Group G streptococci (*see* Streptococcus canis)

HACEK group, 558, 571, 575
Haemophilus,
    clinical aspects, 558-560
    epidemiology, 563
    historical background, 557
    intrinsic resistance, 183*t*
    laboratory features, 564-568
    susceptibility testing, 574
    V factor, 17, 564, 567, 568*t*
    X factor, 17, 564, 567, 568*t*
Haemophilus aphrophilus,
    clinical aspects, 560
    general, 563, 568*t*, 571*t*
Haemophilus ducreyi,
    clinical aspects, 560
    enzyme immunoassay, 567
    Gram stain, 567
    immunofluorescence, 567
    probe assay, 567
    susceptibility testing, 574
Haemophilus haemolyticus, 568*t*
Haemophilus influenzae,
    antigen detection, 50-51, 566
    beta-lactamase detection, 173*t*

[Haemophilus influenzae]
    biotypes, 569*t*
    clinical aspects, 558-560
    culture,
        predictive value of, 45
    epidemiology, 563
    genomic structure, 127
    Gram stain, 566
    historical background, 557
    immunology of infection, 565-566
    in cerebrospinal fluid, 4
    laboratory features, 564, 566-567, 596
    non-typeable, 559-560
    pathogenesis, 564
    selective media, 566
    serotyping, 567
    specimen transport, 41
    susceptibility testing, 160*t*, 162*t*, 180*t*,
        574
    type b, 559, 564-566, 724
    immune response to, 60
    whole genome sequencing, 103
Haemophilus parahaemolyticus, 568*t*
Haemophilus parainfluenzae,
    biotypes, 569*t*
    clinical aspects, 560
Haemophilus paraphrophilus,
    clinical aspects, 560
    epidemiology, 563
    general, 571*f*
    laboratory features, 568*t*
Haemophilus segnis, 563
Haemophilus Test Medium, 574
Haemophysalis, 825*t*
Hafnia,
    applied systematics, 425*f*, 427*f*
    clinical aspects, 436
Haverhill fever, 585
Hayflick's medium (*see* Mycoplasma
    pneumoniae)
Hektoen enteric agar, 462*t*, 463*t*
Helcococcus,
    laboratory features, 309*t*
Helicobacter,
    clinical aspects, 438
    epidemiology, 443
    historical background, 427, 605-607
    immunology of infection, 458
    laboratory features, 455, 466, 472
Helicobacter bizzozeroni, 606*t*

Helicobacter canadensis, 606*t*
Helicobacter canis, 426*f*, 438, 455, 606*t*, 610
Helicobacter cinaedi, 426*f*, 427*t*, 438, 455,
    482, 606*t*, 617
Helicobacter felis, 606, 606*t*
Helicobacter fenelliae, 426*t*, 427*t*, 438, 455,
    606*t*
Helicobacter heilmanii, 426*f*, 606, 606*t*, 610
Helicobacter pullorum, 426*t*, 438, 606*t*, 610
Helicobacter pylori,
    antigen detection, 614, 624
    cag gene (cytotoxin-associated gene),
        102, 612
    cancer, 608
    clinical aspects, 120, 607-608
    epidemiology, 606*t*, 609-610
    fecal antigen testing, 614
    gastritis, 607
    genomic structure, 127-128
    Giemsa stain, 615
    Gram stain, 610*f*
    histopathology, 612, 614
    historical background, 605-606
    immunology of infection, 613
    in situ hybridization, 617-618
    laboratory features, 610-611, 614-621
    molecular diagnostics, 102
    non-ulcer dyspepsia, 608
    pathogenesis, 611-613
    peptic ulcer disease, 608
    PFGE typing, 135
    point-of-care testing, 624
    polymerase chain reaction, 614, 618,
        619*t*, 628
    quartz crystal microbalances, 627
    rapid urease test, 614, 617
    salivary antibody, 73
    screening tests, 625
    selective media, 616, 616*t*
    serodiagnosis,
        general, 57*t*, 71, 621, 622*t*, 623*t*
        salivary antibody, 626
        serum antibody, 621, 624
    silver stain, 615
    susceptibility testing,
        general, 162*t*, 180*t*, 628-629
        molecular methods of, 628-629
    urea breath test, 618-621
    urease gene typing, 137
    vac gene (vacuolating cytotoxin), 102,

[Helicobacter pylori]
    612
    whole genome sequencing, 104, 126-127
Helicobacter rappini, 606*t*
Helicobacter salomonis, 606*t*
Helicobacter westmeadii, 438, 455, 606*t*, 617
Hemobartonella, 824*f*
Hemolysis,
    in identification, 15
    types of, 5
Hepatitis C,
    immunoblotting, 73
Heterophil antibodies, 62-63, 596, 758, 871
Hill's criteria, 122
Histopathology,
    correlation with microbiology, 49
Human herpesvirus, 121
Human immunodeficiency virus,
    immunoblotting, 73
Human granulocytic ehrlichiosis (*see*
    Ehrlichia)
Human monocytic ehrlichiosis (*see* Ehrlichia)

Identification,
    carbohydrate metabolism, 18-19
    general, 10, 18, 22-24, 28, 30
    numerical, 28-30, 29*t*
    16S rRNA sequencing, 25-28
IgM,
    capture assay, 64, 65*f*
    cold aggutinins, 62-63
    detection, 58, 64
    enzyme immunoassay, 71
    immunofluorescence, 68
    rheumatoid factor, 62, 71
Immunoblotting,
    general, 58
    membrane assay, 71
    method, 71-72
Immunodiffusion (*see* Diffusion assays)
Immunofluorescence assay,
    general, 58-59
    method, 66-68, 67*f*
Immune response,
    antibody, 61-63
    cell-mediated immunity, 77-78
    polyclonal activation, 62
Indirect hemagglutination, 57-58, 64
Infection control, 214
Insertion sequences,

[Insertion sequences]
    mycobacterial, 22
International Committee for Systematic
    Bacteriology, 11
Intrinsic resistance, 150
Isolate,
    terminology, 12, 125
Israelii spotted fever (*see* Rickettsia)
Ixodes, 587, 654, 754, 829*t*, 831

Japanese spotted fever (*see* Rickettsia)

Ketolides, 155
Kingella,
    antibiotic susceptibility, 574
    clinical aspects, 561*t*, 562
    epidemiology, 563
    historical aspects, 558-559
    KOH test, 2
    laboratory features, 565, 570, 571*f*, 572*f*
Kingella denitrificans, 500*f*, 558, 561*t*, 562
Kingella kingae, 500*f*, 558, 561*t*, 562, 571*f*,
    572*f*
Kingella oralis, 558, 561*t*, 562, 571*t*, 572*f*
Kinyoun stain, 3, 387
Klebsiella,
    antibiotic resistance, 430*t*, 478*t*
    applied systematics, 425*f*
    clinical aspects, 435-436
    intrinsic resistance, 183*t*
    laboratory features, 461
    pathogenesis, 452
Klebsiella oxytoca, 425*f*, 435, 478*t*
Klebsiella ozaenae, 425*f*, 436
Klebsiella pneumoniae,
    applied systematics, 425*f*
    general, 435, 478*f*
    plasmid analysis, 133
Klebsiella rhinoscleromatis, 425*f*, 436, 565
Kluyvera,
    clinical aspects, 436
    general, 425*f*, 427*t*
Koch's postulates, 122
Kocuria,
    clinical aspects, 232
    phylogenetic positioning, 235*f*
    susceptibility testing, 249
KOH test, 2
Kurthia, 343*t*
Kytococcus,

[Kytococcus]
    phylogenetic positioning, 235*f*

Laboratory,
    accreditation, 219
    continuous quality improvement, 219,
        221
    informatics, 217
    infrastructure, 215-217
    management, 211-221
    proficiency testing, 219, 221
    quality assurance, 219, 221
    quality control, 219, 220*t*
    regionalization, 218
    restructuring, 218
    safety, 221-223
    standards, 218-221
    total quality management, 219, 221
Lactobacillus,
    applied systematics, 708*t*
    clinical aspects, 343*t*
    epidemiology, 346
    intrinsic resistance, 183*t*
    laboratory features, 717, 731
    susceptibility testing, 737
Lactococcus,
    historical aspects, 258
    laboratory features, 309*t*, 310
    staining, 3
Lancefield antigens, 20, 28
LANA test, 2
Latex agglutination, 64
Lautropia mirabilis, 508
Leclercia,
    clinical aspects, 436
    general, 425*f*, 427*f*
Legionnaire's disease (*see* Legionella)
Legionella,
    blood cultures, 643
    clinical aspects, 635-637
    culture, 643-644
    epidemiology, 637-638
    Gram stain, 2
    historical background, 635
    immunofluorescence, 3, 642, 644
    immunology of infection, 641
    laboratory features, 638-639, 642-645
    pathogenesis, 639-641
    polymerase chain reaction, 645
    selective media, 542

[Legionella]
    serodiagnosis, 57*t*, 644
    susceptibility testing, 645, 646*t*
Legionella anisa, 635
Legionella feelei, 635
Legionella micdadei, 635
Legionella pneumophila,
    immunofluorescence, 3, 644
    typing, 132*t*, 134
    urinary antigen test, 642
Leifsonia, 334*t*, 343*t*, 346, 354
Leminorella, 425*f*, 427*t*, 436
Leprosy (*see* Mycobacterium leprae)
Leptospira,
    clinical aspects, 778
    epidemiology, 779, 780*t*
    historical background, 777
    laboratory features, 781, 789-790
    pathogenesis, 783
    serodiagnosis, 57*t*, 790
Leptospira biflexa, 781
Leptospira icterohaemorrhagiae, 779
Leptospira interrogans, 780*t*, 791
Leptospirosis (*see* Leptospira)
Leptotrichia,
    general, 708*t*
    Gram stain, 727
    laboratory features, 729*f*, 735
Leuconostoc,
    intrinsic resistance, 183*t*
    laboratory features, 309*t*, 310
    staining, 3
Ligase chain reaction,
    for *Chlamydia trachomatis*, 100
    general, 89*f*, 90
Lincosamides, 155
Linezolid, 247
Lipopolysaccharides,
    cross-reactive antigens, 60
    Enterobacteriaceae, 445, 449
    for serology, 59
Listeria monocytogenes,
    clinical aspects, 337, 339
    enrichment culture, 46, 359
    epidemiology, 345
    historical background, 334
    immunology of infection, 355
    intrinsic resistance, 183*t*
    KOH test, 2
    laboratory features, 350-351, 358-359

[Listeria monocytogenes]
    ribotyping, 134
    selection, 17
    susceptibility testing, 162t, 364
    temperature requirements, 16
    typing, 359
Loeffler slant, 3
Lyme disease (see Borrelia)
Lymphogranuloma venereum (see Chlamydia
    trachomatis)

M type, 20, 296
MacConkey agar, 460, 462t, 463t
Macrolides, 155-156, 247, 248t
MALT lymphoma, 608
Maricaulis, 528t
Martin-Lewis medium, 511
Mass spectroscopy,
    for pathogen discovery, 122
Mediterranean spotted fever (see Rickettsia)
Megasphaera, 708t, 722, 729t
Meningococcus (see Neisseria meningitidis)
Mesophile, 16
Methicillin-resistant Staphylococcus aureus
    (MRSA) (see Staphylococcus aureus)
Methylene blue stain, 2
Methyl red test, 19
Methylobacterium,
    applied sytematics, 529t, 537
    clinical aspects, 533
    laboratory features, 537, 542
Microaerophilic,
    definition of, 16
Microbacterium, 334t, 343t, 346, 354
Micrococcus,
    clinical aspects, 232
    identification, 241
    phylogenetic positioning, 235f
    susceptibility testing, 249
Microscopy,
    clinical samples, 4-5, 26-27
    darkfield, 1
    morphological features, 3-4, 14-15
    of cell culture, 5
    of media, 5
    stains for, 1-3
MIDI system (see Sherlock Microbial
    Identification System)
Minimum bactericidal concentration (MBC),
    definition of, 177-178

Minimum inhibitory concentration (MIC),
    definition of, 148-149
    testing for, 149-150, 177
MLEE (see Multilocus enzyme
    electrophoresis)
MLO (see Mycoplasma)
Mobiluncus,
    applied systematics, 348f, 708t
    bacterial vaginosis, 712, 738
    immunology of infection, 724
    laboratory features, 717, 731
Moellerella, 425f, 426, 427f
Molecular beacons, 93-95
Molecular diagnostics,
    general, 83-108
    specimen collection, 50
Molecular epidemiology (see Typing)
Moraxella,
    applied systematics, 506f
    Gram stain, 2
    intrinsic resistance, 183t
    KOH test, 2
    LANA test, 2
    susceptibility testing, 519
Moraxella atlantae, 506f, 515f
Moraxella bovis, 506f
Moraxella catarrhalis,
    applied systematics, 500f, 506f
    beta-lactamase detection, 173t, 519
    clinical aspects, 502-503
    epidemiology of infection, 505
    historical background, 500
    immunology of infection, 509
    intrinsic resistance, 183t
    laboratory features, 505, 513t
    pathogenesis, 508
    susceptibility testing, 162t, 180t, 181,
        519
Moraxella lacunata, 503, 506f, 512, 515f
Moraxella nonliquefaciens, 506f, 575f
Moraxella osloensis, 503, 506f, 515f
Morganella,
    applied systematics, 425f, 427t, 478t
    beta-lactamase, 174
    clinical aspects, 435
    intrinsic resistance, 184t
    laboratory features, 452
Morococcus cerebrosus, 508
Morphology,
    colony, 15-16

Motility,
　　in microscopy, 1
MRSA (*see* Staphylococcus aureus)
Multilocus enzyme electrophoresis (*see*
　　Typing)
Multilocus sequence typing (*see* Typing)
Mupirocin, 330
Murine typhus (*see* Rickettsia)
Mycobacterium,
　　applied systematics, 348*f*
　　blood culture, 398, 400
　　DNA probes, 407-408
　　enrichment culture for, 46
　　Gram stain, 2
　　identification,
　　　　restriction enzyme digests, 24
　　　　in blood cultures, 205
　　Kinyoun stain, 3
　　microscopy, 395-397
　　non-tuberculous (NTM),
　　　　clinical aspects, 382-384
　　　　epidemiology, 387
　　　　historical background, 378
　　　　immunology of infection, 392
　　　　laboratory features, 404*f*
　　　　non-chromogens, 406*t*
　　　　pathogenesis, 389
　　　　photochromogens, 406*t*
　　　　rapid growers, 406*t*
　　　　scotochromogens, 406*t*
　　　　susceptibility testing, 412-413
　　probes, 22
　　specimen processing, 398
　　susceptibility testing, 412-414
　　typing, 411
　　Ziehl-Neelsen stain, 3
Mycobacterium abscessus, 3, 383*t*, 389
Mycobacterium africanum, 382
Mycobacterium asiaticum, 383*t*
Mycobacterium avium, 3, 383*t*, 389
Mycobacterium bovis, 22, 382
Mycobacterium bovis BCG, 96
Mycobacterium branderi, 383*t*
Mycobacterium celatum, 383*t*
Mycobacterium chelonae, 3, 383*t*, 389
Mycobacterium conspicuum, 383*t*
Mycobacterium flavescens, 406*t*
Mycobacterium fortuitum, 3, 383*t*, 390
Mycobacterium gastri, 383*t*
Mycobacterium genavense, 383*t*, 399

Mycobacterium gordonae, 383*t*
Mycobacterium haemophilum,
　　clinical aspects, 383*t*
　　laboratory isolation, 399
　　temperature requirements, 16
Mycobacterium heidelbergense, 383*t*
Mycobacterium interjectum, 383*t*
Mycobacterium intracellulare, 383*t*
Mycobacterium kansasii, 3, 382, 383*t*, 406*t*
Mycobacterium lentiflavum, 383*t*
Mycobacterium leprae,
　　clinical aspects, 381-382
　　epidemiology, 386-387
　　Fite stain, 388
　　immunology of infection, 391
　　laboratory features, 397
　　microscopy, 397
　　pathogenesis, 388-389
　　serodiagnosis, 57*t*
Mycobacterium malmoense, 383*t*
Mycobacterium marinum,
　　clinical aspects, 383*t*
　　laboratory isolation, 399
　　temperature requirements, 16
Mycobacterium mucogenicum, 383*t*
Mycobacterium phlei, 406*t*
Mycobacterium scrofulaceum, 383*t*
Mycobacterium shimoidei, 383*t*
Mycobacterium simiae, 383*t*
Mycobacterium smegmatis, 383*t*
Mycobacterium szulgai, 383*t*
Mycobacterium terrae, 383*t*
Mycobacterium triplex, 383*t*
Mycobacterium tuberculosis,
　　AMPLICOR MTB Assay, 410*t*
　　antigen detection, 408
　　Bactec 12B, 400*t*
　　Bactec 13A, 401*t*
　　Bactec 9000, 400
　　blood culture, 403*f*
　　clinical aspects, 379-380, 381*t*
　　cord factor, 387, 399
　　delayed-type hypersensitivity, 390
　　epidemiology, 386, 411
　　ESPII, 400, 402*t*
　　growth media, 399-400, 401*t*, 402*t*
　　historical background, 377-379
　　immunology of infection, 390-391
　　laboratory features, 387-388
　　lysis centrifugation, 192

[Mycobacterium tuberculosis]
    MB/BacT, 400, 402*t*
    MGIT, 400, 402*t*
    molecular diagnostics, 100-101, 409-
        410, 410*t*
    Mycobacterial Tuberculosis Direct Test,
        409
    NASBA, 88
    pathogenesis, 387-388
    probes, 22, 407
    Septi-Chek, 400, 402*t*
    serodiagnosis, 57*t*, 390
    specimen collection, 393-395, 394*t*
    specimen processing, 36, 398-399
    susceptibility testing, 412-414
    typing,
        binary probes, 137
        insertional sequence typing, 130,
            411
        RFLP, 136
Mycobacterium ulcerans,
    clinical aspects, 384*t*
    laboratory isolation, 399
    temperature requirements, 16
Mycobacterium vaccae, 406*t*
Mycobacterium xenopi, 384*t*
Mycoplasma,
    Gram stain, 2
    historical background, 861-863
    laboratory features, 872-885
    specimen transport, 41
    susceptibility testing, 886-887
    tissue culture contamination, 885-886
Mycoplasma arginii, 885
Mycoplasma buccale, 862*t*
Mycoplasma faucium, 862*t*
Mycoplasma fermentans,
    clinical aspects, 862*t*, 865
    epidemiology, 867
    laboratory features, 870
    pathogenesis, 870
    tissue culture contamination, 885-886
Mycoplasma genitalium,
    clinical aspects, 862*t*, 865
    epidemiology, 867
    immunology of infection, 872
    laboratory features, 870, 884
    pathogenesis, 870
    whole genome sequencing, 103, 103*f*
Mycoplasma hominis,

[Mycoplasma hominis]
    clinical aspects, 862*t*, 864-865
    culture, 884
    epidemiology, 866-867
    immunology of infection, 872
    laboratory features, 869
    microscopy, 883
    pathogenesis, 869
    serodiagnosis, 884
Mycoplasma hyorhinis, 885
Mycoplasma lipophilum, 862*t*
Mycoplasma orale, 862*t*, 885
Mycoplasma penetrans,
    clinical aspects, 862*t*, 865
    immunology of infection, 872
    laboratory features, 870, 884
Mycoplasma pirum,
    clinical aspects, 862*t*
    laboratory features, 870, 884
Mycoplasma pneumoniae,
    antigen detection, 879-880
    chloroform-methanol extract, 60
    clinical aspects, 863-864
    cold agglutinins, 62, 871
    culture, 873-875
    epidemiology, 866
    hemadsorption, 874
    heterophil antibody, 871, 875-876
    historical background, 861
    immunology of infection, 870-871
    laboratory features, 867-868
    microscopy, 873
    molecular diagnostics, 880
    mycoplasmacidal assay, 877
    pathogenesis, 867-869
    pathology, 868
    polyclonal activation, 62
    serodiagnosis,
        antibiotic effect, 106
        general, 57*t*, 58, 60, 871, 875-879
    susceptibility testing, 886
Mycoplasma primatum, 862*t*
Mycoplasma salivarium, 862*t*
Mycoplasma spermatophilum, 862*t*
Myroides,
    applied systematics, 529*t*
    clinical aspects, 535
    laboratory features, 542

NASBA (*see* Nucleic acid sequence

based amplification)
National Committee for Clinical
    Laboratory Standards (NCCLS), 159
Necrotizing fasciitis, 263
Negative predictive value,
    definition of, 74
Neisser stain, 3
Neisseria,
    applied systematics, 500*f*
    clinical aspects, 501-503
    culture, 511-512
    intrinsic resistance, 183*t*
    laboratory features, 505-508
    methylene blue stain, 2
    morphology, 15
    specimen transport, 41
    staining, 5, 505, 509-510
    susceptibility testing, 517-519
Neisseria cinerea, 503, 506*t*, 513*t*
Neisseria elongata,
    general, 513*t*
    staining, 3, 505
Neisseria flavescens, 506*f*, 513*t*
Neisseria gonorrhoeae,
    antigen detection, 514
    applied systematics, 506*f*
    beta-lactamase detection, 173*t*, 518
    clinical aspects, 501, 503
    DNA probes, 101
    epidemiology of infection, 503-504
    genomic structure, 127
    historical background, 499
    immunology of infection, 508-509
    intrinsic resistance, 184*t*
    laboratory features, 505-506, 511-517,
        513*t*, 514*f*
    ligase chain reaction, 516
    media, 511-512
    pathogenesis, 506-507
    polymerase chain reaction, 515-516
    specimen collection, 41, 45
    specimen transport, 40-41
    SPS inhibition, 190
    staining, 5, 510
    susceptibility testing, 160*t*, 162*t*, 180*t*,
        517-518
    transcription-mediated amplification,
        516
    typing,
        auxotyping, 17

[Neisseria gonorrhoeae]
    general, 137, 516
Neisseria lactamica, 503, 505, 506*f*, 511, 513*t*
Neisseria meningitidis,
    antigen detection, 50-51, 515
    applied systematics, 506*t*
    clinical aspects, 502
    epidemiology of infection, 504-505
    genetic amplification detection, 515-516
    genomic structure, 127
    historical background, 500
    immunology of infection, 509
    in cerebrospinal fluid, 4
    intrinsic resistance, 184*t*
    laboratory features, 511, 513, 515
    pathogenesis, 507
    selective media, 511-512
    serogroups, 504-505
    specimen transport, 40
    susceptibility testing, 162*t*, 180*t*, 518-
        519
    typing, 137, 516-517
Neisseria mucosa, 506*f*, 513*t*
Neisseria polysaccharea, 503, 505, 506*f*, 513*t*
Neisseria sicca, 506*f*, 513*t*
Neisseria subflava, 506*f*, 513*t*
Neisseria weaveri,
    staining, 3
Neorickettsia helminthoeca, 824*f*, 826*f*
Nesterenkonia,
    phylogenetic positioning, 235*f*
Neutralization assay, 60-64
New York City medium, 511
Nitrofurantoin, 158
Nitroimidazoles, 154*t*, 157
Nocardia,
    acid-fast, 3, 390
    agar microscopy, 5
    applied systematics, 348*f*
    clinical aspects, 384-385
    enrichment culture, 46
    intrinsic resistance, 183*t*
    serodiagnosis, 57*t*
    specimen collection, 394-395
    typing, 412
Nomenclature, 10-11
Normal flora,
    contamination with, 37-38, 724
Nucleic acid amplification, 86-92
Nucleic acid sequence based amplification, 88

Ochrobactrum,
    applied systematics, 529*t*, 537
    clinical aspects, 534
    KOH tests, 2
Oerskovia, 343*t*, 346, 354
O/F test (see Oxidation-fermentation test)
Oligella,
    clinical aspects, 503, 534
Oligella ureolytica, 515*f*
Oligella urethralis, 503, 515*f,* 544
Opacity factor, 277
Orientia tsutsugamushi, 824*f,* 826*t,* 826*f*
Ornithodoros, 754
Oroya fever (*see* Bartonella bacilliformis)
Oxidase, 17, 28
Oxidation-fermentation test, 17-18

Paenibacillus, 334*t*
Pai slant, 3
PANDAS, 265
Pandoraea,
    applied systematics, 529*t*
    clinical aspects, 530, 532
    laboratory features, 540
Pantoea,
    applied systematics, 425*f,* 427*t*
    clinical aspects, 436
Paracoccus, 529*t*
Particle agglutination, 57, 64
Pasteurella,
    clinical aspects, 561*t*, 585
    epidemiology, 588, 593*t*
    historical background, 558, 582
    immunology of infection, 595
    laboratory features, 568, 592, 596
    pathogenesis, 592
    species/subspecies, 592
    susceptibility testing, 162*t*, 597-598
Pasteurella aerogenes, 561*t*
Pasteurella bettyae, 561*t*
Pasteurella canis, 561*t*
Pasteurella dagmatis, 561*t*
Pasteurella multocida, 561*t*, 588, 597
Pasteurella pneumotropica, 561*t*
Pasteurella stomatis, 561*t*
PCR (see Polymerase chain reaction)
Pediculus humanus, 748, 826*t*
Pediococcus,
    intrinsic resistance, 183*t*

[Pediococcus]
    laboratory features, 309*t*, 310
Penicillin-binding proteins, 151, 244, 574
Peptococcus,
    applied systematics, 708*t*, 717
    laboratory features, 729*t*
Peptococcus niger, 717
Peptostreptococcus,
    applied systematics, 708*t*, 717
    intrinsic resistance, 184*t*
    laboratory features, 717, 729*f,* 730
Peptostreptococcus anaerobius, 717
Peptostreptococcus asaccharolyticus, 717
Peptostreptococcus indolicus, 717
Peptostreptococcus intermedius, 708*t*
Peptostreptococcus magnus, 717
Peptostreptococcus micros, 717
Peptostreptococcus prevotii, 717
Peptostreptococcus productus, 716, 717
Pertussis (*see* Bordetella pertussis)
Phage typing (*see* Typing)
Photorhabdus, 427*t*
Plague (*see* Yersinia pestis)
Pleisiomonas shigelloides,
    applied systematics, 426*f*
    clinical aspects, 439
    epidemiology, 443
    immunology of infection, 458
    laboratory features, 545-455, 466, 472
    susceptibility testing, 482
PPLO (*see* Mycoplasma)
Point-of-care testing, 56, 76, 218
Polymerase chain reaction,
    broad range, 121*f*
    consensus sequence, 121
    for identification, 23
    general, 88-90
    kinetic enrichment, 122
    method, 89*f*
    resistance detection, 177
Polymixins, 154*t*
Pontiac fever (*see* Legionella)
Porphyromonas,
    applied systematics, 706*t*, 708*t*, 721*f*
    intrinsic resistance, 184*t*, 738
    laboratory features, 729*t*, 734
Porphyromonas asaccharolytica, 708*t*, 721*f*
Porphyromonas gingivalis, 721*f*
Positive predictive value,
    definition of, 74

Post-mortem microbiology, 49-50
Prevotella,
        applied systematics, 706*t*, 708*t*, 721*f*
        intrinsic resistance, 184*t*, 738
        laboratory features, 729*f*, 734
Prevotella bivia, 708*t*, 721*f*
Prevotella buccae, 708*t*
Prevotella corporis, 708*t*
Prevotella dentalis, 706*t*
Prevotella denticola, 708*t*, 721*f*
Prevotella disiens, 708*t*, 721*f*
Prevotella intermedia, 708*t*
Prevotella loeschii, 708*t*, 721*f*
Prevotella melaninogenica, 708*t*, 720, 721*f*
Prevotella nigrescens, 708*t*
Prevotella oralis, 708*t*
Prevotella oris, 708*t*
Proficiency testing, 219-221
Prokaryotes, 25
Propionibacterium,
        antibiotic susceptibility, 365
        applied systematics, 348*f*, 353, 708*t*
        clinical aspects, 341
        epidemiology, 346
        laboratory features, 361, 705, 730
        susceptibility testing, 365, 737
Propionibacterium propionicus, 334*t*, 706*t*
Proteus,
        beta-lactamase, 174
        clinical aspects, 435
        laboratory features, 452, 461
Proteus mirabilis,
        applied systematics, 425*f*
        immunology of infection, 457
        intrinsic resistance, 183*t*, 478*t*
Proteus penneri,
        applied systematics, 425*f*
        intrinsic resistance, 183*t*
Proteus vulgaris,
        applied systematics, 425*f*
        intrinsic resistance, 183*t*, 478*t*
Providencia
        beta-lactamase, 174
        clinical aspects, 435
        general, 478*t*
        pathogenesis, 452
Providencia alcalifaciens, 425*f*
Providenica rettgeri, 425*f*
Providencia rustigianii, 425*f*, 427*t*
Providencia stuartii,

[*Providencia stuartii*]
        intrinsic resistance, 183*t*, 425*f*
Pseudomonads,
        Nomenclature, 528*t*, 529*t*
Pseudomonas,
        beta-lactamase, 174
        clinical aspects, 530-531
        immunofluorescence, 4
        laboratory features, 539-543
        morphology, 3
        nomenclature, 10
        staining, 3
        typing, 134, 543
Pseudomonas aeruginosa,
        clinical aspects, 530-531
        culture,
                predictive value of, 45
        epidemiology, 536
        growth requirements, 16
        immunology of infection, 538
        intrinsic resistance, 183*t*
        laboratory features, 539
        pathogenesis, 538
        PFGE analysis, 128, 129*f*
        susceptibility testing,
                general, 162*t*, 180*t*, 544
        mucoid strains, 184-185
        typing, 132*t*, 134, 543
Pseudomonas fluorescens, 542
Pseudomonas luteola, 531
Pseudomonas oryzihabitans, 531, 543
Pseudoramibacter alactolyticus, 717
Psittacosis (*see* Chlamydia psittaci)
Psychrobacter,
        clinical aspects, 535
        laboratory features, 515*t*, 542
Psychrobacter immobilis, 506*f*, 542
Psychrobacter phenylpyruvicus, 506*f*, 542
Psychrophile, 16
Pulsed field gel electrophoresis (*see* Typing)

Q fever (*see* Coxiella burnetii)
Qβ replication, 86-87, 87*f*
        for *Chlamydia trachomatis*, 99-100
        for *Mycobacterium tuberculosis*, 100-
                101
Quality control,
        for molecular diagnostics, 98-99
Queensland tick typhus (*see* Rickettsia)
Quinolones, 153*t*, 155, 247, 248*t*, 479

Quinupristin, 247

Radioimmunoassay, 58
    method, 68
Radioimmunoprecipitation, 68
Rahnella, 425*f*, 436
Ralstonia eutropha,
    applied systematics, 529*t*
    clinical aspects, 532
Ralstonia gilardii,
    applied systematics, 529*t*
    clinical aspects, 532
Ralstonia paucula,
    applied systematics, 529*t*
    clinical aspects, 530, 532
Ralstonia pickettii,
    applied systematics, 529*t*
    clinical aspects, 530, 532
    typing, 543
Ralstonia solanacearum,
    applied systematics, 529*t*
    clinical aspects, 532
Random amplification of polymorphic DNA
    (RAPD), 98, 127, 131*t*, 135-136
RAPD (*see* Random amplication of polymor-
    phic DNA)
Rat-bite fever, 791
rDNA (16S) sequencing, 126, 539
Relapsing fever (*see* Borrelia)
Rep-PCR (*see* Typing)
Representational difference analysis (RDA),
    121
Restriction enzyme digestion,
    for identification, 23-24
Restriction fragment length polymorphism
    (RFLP), 92
Rheumatic fever, 264-265
Rheumatoid factor, 62, 76-77
Rhipicephalus, 754
Rhodamine, 3
Rhodobacter, 529*t*
Rhodococcus,
    acid-fast, 3, 390
    applied systematics, 348*f*
    clinical aspects, 385
    in blood cultures, 205
    intrinsic resistance, 183*t*
Ribotyping (*see* Typing)
Rickettsia,
    applied systematics, 824*f*

[Rickettsia]
    clinical aspects, 824-828
    culture, 835-836
    epidemiology, 825*t*, 830
    Giemsa stain, 2
    Gram stain, 2
    historical background, 823-824
    identification of, 842-843
    immunohistochemistry, 843
    immunology of infection, 833
    laboratory features, 832, 834-843
    molecular diagnostics, 841
    pathogenesis, 832
    serodiagnosis, 57*t*, 837-841
    susceptibility testing,
        dye uptake assay, 844
        IF assay, 844
        plaque assay, 844
'Rickettsia aeschlimani', 825*t*
Rickettsia africae, 823
Rickettsia akari, 823
'Rickettsia amblyommii', 825*t*
Rickettsia australis, 823
Rickettsia bellii, 825*t*
Rickettsia conorii, 823
'Rickettsia heilongjiang', 825*t*
Rickettsia helvetica, 825*t*
Rickettsia honei, 823
'Rickettsia hulini', 825*t*
Rickettsia japonica, 823
Rickettsia massiliae, 825*t*
'Rickettsia mongolotimonae', 823
Rickettsia montana, 825*t*
Rickettsia parkeri, 825*t*
Rickettsia prowazekii, 823
Rickettsia rhipicephali, 825*t*
Rickettsia rickettsii, 823
Rickettsia sibirica, 823
Rickettsia slovaca, 823
Rickettsia tsutsugamushi (*see* Orientia)
Rickettsia typhi, 823
Rickettsialpox (*see* Rickettsia)
Rickettsiella, 824*f*
Rifamycins, 157
Rochalimaea (*see* Bartonella)
Rocky Mountain spotted fever (*see* Rickettsia)
Rolling circle amplification, 91*f*, 90-91
Romanowsky stain, 760
Roseomonas,
    applied systematics, 529*t*

[Roseomonas]
    clinical aspects, 533
    laboratory features, 537, 542
Rothia,
    applied systematics, 348*f*
    clinical aspects, 385
    phylogenetic positioning, 235*f*
rRNA (16S) sequencing,
    applied systematics, 22-23, 25-28, 716,
        762
Ruminococcus, 708*t*, 730

Safranin, 2
Salmonella,
    antibiotic resistance, 430*t*,
    applied systematics, 425*f*
    clinical aspects, 432-433
    culture media, 461-464
    epidemiology, 429, 441*t*, 440-441
    genomic structure, 127
    immunology of infection, 456
    laboratory features, 449, 461-464, 470
    lactose-positive, 464
    O and H typing, 28, 449, 475
    pathogenesis, 448-450
    pathogenicity islands, 127
    ribotyping, 128
    selection, 17
    serodiagnosis, 473
    specimen transport, 41
    susceptibility testing, 480
Salmonella-Shigella agar, 462*t*, 463*t*
Salmonella serotype Typhi,
    antibiotic resistance, 430*t*
    clinical aspects, 433
    epidemiology, 441
    immunology of infection, 456
    laboratory features, 470
    lactose-positive, 464
    pathogenesis, 450
    serodiagnosis, 57*t*, 473
    specimen collection, 49-50
    susceptibility testing, 480
Salmonellosis (*see* Salmonella)
Sarcina, 730
Scarlet Fever, 262-263
Schineria, 529*t*
Scrub typhus (*see* Rickettsia)
SDS-PAGE,

[SDS-PAGE]
    identification, 21
Selenite broth, 46, 462*t*
Selenomonas, 708*t*, 715, 722, 735
Sennetsu fever (*see* Ehrlichia)
Sensitivity,
    definition of, 74
Serodiagnosis,
    antibiotic effect, 77
    automation of, 75-76
    confirmatory assay, 73, 763-764
    general, 55-78
    screening assay, 73, 763
Serotyping (*see* Typing)
Serpulina hyodysenteriae, 780, 791
Serpulina pilosicoli, 791
Serratia liquefaciens, 725*f*
Serratia marcescens,
    antibiotic resistance, 430*t*, 478
    applied systematics, 425*f*
    clinical aspects, 435
    intrinsic resistance, 183*t*
    pathogenesis, 452
Serratia odifera, 425*f*
Serratia plymuthica, 425*f*
Serratia rubidea, 425*f*
Serum bactericidal titre (SBT), 178
Sherlock Microbial Identification System, 20,
        406
Shewanella,
    applied systematics, 529*t*, 533
    clinical aspects, 533
Shiga toxin (*see* Verotoxin assay)
Shiga-like toxin (*see* Verotoxin assay)
Shigella,
    applied systematics, 425*f*
    clinical aspects, 433-434
    epidemiology, 441-442
    immunology of infection, 456
    laboratory features, 450, 464, 470
    pathogenesis, 450
    serodiagnosis, 473
    specimen transport, 40-41
    susceptibility testing, 480-481
Shigella boydii, 450
Shigella dysenteriae,
    antibiotic resistance, 430*t*
    applied systematics, 425*f*
    epidemiology, 441
    laboratory features, 464

[Shigella dysenteriae]
    pathogenesis, 448, 450
Shigella flexneri, 425*f*, 450
Shigella sonnei, 425*f*, 450, 470
Shigellosis (*see* Shigella)
Siberian tick bite fever (*see* Rickettsia)
Simonsiella, 500*f*
Single strand conformation polymorphism
    (SSCP), 92-93
Southern blot (*see* DNA hybridization)
SP4 medium (*see* Mycoplasma pneumoniae)
Specificity,
    definition of, 74
Specimens,
    collection, 33-44
        post-mortem collection, 49-50
    concentration of, 47-48
    labeling, 35
    maintenance of, 45
    processing, 44-52
    record keeping, 45
    rejection, 4-5, 51
    shipping, 42-43
    transport, 33-44
Spores,
    staining of, 2-3, 15
Sphingobacterium,
    applied systematics, 529*t*
    clinical aspects, 535
Sphingomonas,
    applied systematics, 529*t*
    clinical aspects, 535
    KOH test, 2
    laboratory features, 542
Spirillum minus, 791
Sputum,
    quantitative culture, 48
    specimen collection, 34
    specimen rejection, 51
    staining, 5
Standard Precautions, 35, 39
Staphylococcus,
    general, 229-249
    glycopeptide resistance, 176-177
    intrinsic resistance, 183*t*
    morphology, 15
    penicillin resistance, 176
    resistance screening, 175*t*
    susceptibility testing, 160*t*, 180*t*
Staphylococcus aureus,

[Staphylococcus aureus]
    antibiotic-associated diarrhea, 713
    beta-lactamase,
        general, 244-245
        hyper-beta-lactamase, 245
    CAMP test, 15
    clinical aspects, 230-232
    culture, 238
    Gram stain of, 237-238
    epidemiology, 233-234
    identification, 239-240
    immunology of infection, 236-237
    in blood cultures, 198
    laboratory features, 239-240
    lysis centrifugation, 192
    *mec*A gene, 246
    MRSA, 229, 244-246
    pathogenesis, 235-236
    plasmid analysis, 133
    PFGE analysis, 128
    resistance mechanisms, 248*t*
    RFLP analysis, 92*f*
    serodiagnosis, 57*t*
    susceptibility testing, 243-249
    tolerance, 246-247
    typing, 133-134, 136, 136*f*, 242-243
    vancomycin-intermediate susceptible
        (VISA), 229, 246
Staphylococcus auricularis, 234, 240
Staphylococcus capitis, 234, 240
Staphylococcus caprae, 240
Staphylococcus cohnii, 240
Staphylococcus epidermidis,
    plasmid analysis, 133
    terminology, 234-235
    typing, 128
Staphylococcus haemolyticus, 240-241, 249
Staphylococcus hominis, 240-241
Staphylococcus hyicus, 239
Staphylococcus intermedius, 234, 239
Staphylococcus lugdunensis, 239, 240
Staphylococcus saccharolyticus, 240
Staphylococcus saprophyticus,
    identification, 241
    intrinsic resistance, 183*t*
    terminology, 12, 235
Staphylococcus schleiferi, 239-240
Staphylococcus simulans, 240
Staphylococcus warneri, 240
Staphylococcus xylosus, 240-241

Stenotrophomonas africana, 533, 536
Stenotrophomonas maltophilia,
    applied systematics, 529*t*
    clinical aspects, 530, 533
    immunofluorescence, 3
    intrinsic resistance, 183*t*
    pathogenesis, 536
    susceptibility testing, 162*t*, 180*t*, 544
    typing, 543
Stomatococcus,
    clinical aspects, 233
    identification, 241
    phylogenetic positioning, 235*f*
    susceptibility testing, 249
Strain,
    terminology, 12, 125
Streptobacillus moniliformis,
    clinical aspects, 585
    epidemiology, 588
    historical background, 582
    immunology of infection, 595
    laboratory features, 592, 596
    susceptibility testing, 598
Streptococcus,
    DNA probe identification, 96, 97*t*
    Group B,
        antigen detection, 50
    historical background, 257-262
    intrinsic resistance, 183*t*
    Lancefield grouping, 258
    morphology, 15
    staining, 3
    susceptibility testing, 160*t*, 162*t*, 180*t*
    viridans,
        clinical aspects, 267-268
        epidemiology, 273-274
        historical aspects, 259-260
        immunology of infection, 292-293
        laboratory features, 298-303
        pathogenesis, 283-284
        susceptibility testing, 312-313
Streptococcus agalactiae,
    CAMP test, 15
    clinical aspects, 266-267
    epidemiology, 272-273
    historical aspects, 258-259
    immunology of infection, 292
    intrapartum chemoprophylaxis, 259
    laboratory features, 297-298
    pathogenesis, 279-282

[*Streptococcus agalactiae*]
    rapid diagnosis, 298
    susceptibility testing, 312
Streptococcus alactolyticus,
    classification, 303
Streptococcus anginosus,
    classification, 300
    DNA probe identification, 96
    laboratory features, 299-300
Streptococcus anginosus-constellatus, 261
Streptococcus anginosus group,
    laboratory features, 299-300, 300*t*
Streptococcus bovis,
    classification, 303*t*
Streptococcus bovis group, 303
Streptococcus canis,
    laboratory features, 299*t*
    pathogenesis, 283
Streptococcus constellatus,
    classification, 300*t*
    DNA probe identification, 96
    laboratory features, 299-300
Streptococcus cricetus,
    classification, 302*t*
    laboratory features, 301
Streptococcus crista,
    classification, 301*t*
    laboratory features, 300
Streptococcus downei,
    classification, 302*t*
    laboratory features, 300
Streptococcus dysgalactiae subsp. dysgalac-
        tiae,
    laboratory features, 298, 299*t*
Streptococcus dysgalactiae subsp. equisimilis,
    clinical aspects, 267
    epidemiology, 273
    historical aspects, 259
    laboratory features, 298, 299*t*
    pathogenesis, 282-283
Streptococcus equi, 299*t*
Streptococcus equi subsp. zooepidemicus,
    clinical features, 267
    historical aspects, 259
    laboratory features, 299*t*
    pathogenesis, 273
Streptococcus equinus,
    classification, 303
Streptococcus equisimilis (*see* Streptococcus
        dysgalactiae subsp. equisimilis)

Streptococcus ferus, 302*t*
Streptococcus gordonii,
    classification, 301*t*
    laboratory features, 300-301
Streptococcus infantis,
    classification, 300
Streptococcus intermedius,
    classification, 300*t*
    laboratory features, 299-300
Streptococcus macacae,
    classification, 302*t*
    laboratory features, 301
Streptococcus MG-intermedius, 261
Streptococcus milleri,
    classification, 261*t*
    staining, 3
Streptococcus mitior, 261*t*
Streptococcus mitis,
    classification, 301*t*
    general, 261*t*
    laboratory features, 301
Streptococcus mitis group,
    general, 300-301
    laboratory features, 301*t*
Streptococcus mutans,
    classification, 302*t*
    laboratory features, 301-302
    staining, 3
Streptococcus mutans group, 301-302
Streptococcus oralis,
    classification, 301*t*
    laboratory features, 300
Streptococcus parasanguis,
    classification, 301*t*
    laboratory features, 301
Streptococcus peroris,
    classification, 261*t*
Streptococcus pneumoniae,
    antigen detection, 50
    capsule, 2
    clinical aspects, 268-269
    culture, 304
    epidemiology, 274
    historical aspects, 260-261
    immunology of infection, 293-294
    in cerebrospinal fluid, 4
    laboratory features, 303-305
    morphology, 15
    Neufeld test, 305
    pathogenesis, 284-287

[Streptococcus pneumoniae]
    penicillin resistance, 176
    Quellung reaction, 305
    resistance screening, 175*t*
    serodiagnosis, 61
    specimen collection, 33-34
    staining, 3-4
    susceptibility testing, 162*t*, 180*t*, 313-
        314
    typing, 138
Streptococcus pyogenes,
    ASOT (*see* streptolysin O)
    bacitracin susceptibility, 295
    clinical aspects, 262-265
    culture,
        predictive value of, 44
    epidemiology, 270-272
    historical aspects, 258
    immunology of infection, 290-291
    laboratory features, 295-296
    Lancefield grouping, 295
    pathogenesis, 276-279
    pyrogenic exotoxins, 278*t*
    rapid diagnosis, 295
    serodiagnosis, 57*t*, 58, 60, 64
    specimen collection, 34, 294-295
    specimen transport, 40-41
    susceptibility testing, 311-312
    typing, 296
Streptococcus rattus,
    classification, 302*t*
    laboratory features, 302
Streptococcus salivarius,
    classification, 302*t*
    DNA probe identification, 96
    laboratory features, 301
Streptococcus salivarius group, 301
Streptococcus sanguis,
    classification, 301*t*
    laboratory features, 300-301
    staining, 3
Streptococcus sobrinus,
    classification, 302*t*
    laboratory features, 302
Streptococcus thermophilus,
    DNA probe identification, 96
Streptococcus vestibularis,
    classification, 302*t*
    DNA probe identification, 96
    laboratory features, 301

Streptococcus zooepidemicus (*see* Streptococcus equi subsp. zooepidemicus)
Streptogramins, 155
Streptomyces, 385
Succinimonas, 708*t*
Succinivibrio, 708*t*
Superantigen, 291
Susceptibility testing,
     agar dilution, 166-167
     breakpoints,
          routine, 158-159
          surrogate, 180*t*
     broth macrodilution, 164-165
     broth microdilution, 165-166
     diffusion methods, 168-172
     disc diffusion, 169-171
     gradient diffusion, 172
     expert systems, 184
     general, 147-185
     intrinsic resistance, 183*t*, 184*t*
     semi-automated, 167-168
     synergy, 178
     topical antibiotics, 185
Sutterella wadworthensis, 706*t*, 708, 722, 729*t*, 735
Suttonella indologenes,
     antibiotic susceptibility, 738
     clinical aspects, 561*t*, 562
     historical background, 558
     laboratory features, 565, 570*t*, 571*f*
Systematics (*see* Applied systematics)
Syphilis (*see* Treponema pallidum)

TaqMan technology, 93-95, 108
Tatumella, 425*t*, 427*t*, 436
Taxonomy (*see* Applied systematics)
Teichoic acid antibodies, 57*t*
Teichoplanin, 249
Tetanus (*see* Clostridium tetani)
Tetracyclines,
     general, 154*t*, 156
     tetM resistance, 519
Tetrathionate broth, 462*t*
Thai tick typhus rickettsia, 825
Thayer-Martin medium, 511
Thermophile, 16
Thioglycollate broth, 46
Tissierella, 722

Tissue processing, 48
Toxic shock syndrome,
     staphylococcal, 230*f*, 231, 234
     streptococcal, 263
Trabulsiella, 425*f*, 436
Transport media,
     Amies', 41
     Cary-Blair, 41
     2-SP, 41
     Stuart's, 41
Transposons, 479
Trench fever (*see* Bartonella quintana)
Treponema carataneum, 780*t*
Treponema cuniculi, 780
Treponema denticola, 790-791
Treponema fribourg-blanc, 780
Treponema medium, 790
Treponema microdentium, 791
Treponema minutum, 791
Treponema pallidum (*see also* Syphilis),
     antimicrobial susceptibility, 791
     cardiolipin, 117
     clinical aspects, 777-778, 787*t*
     congenital syphilis, 778
     darkfield microscopy, 1, 784
     epidemiology, 779
     genomic sequencing, 117
     Gram stain, 2
     historical background, 777
     immunofluorescence, 3, 784
     immunology of infection, 781-783
     laboratory features, 783-789
     microscopy, 780, 784
     molecular diagnostics, 784
     pathogenesis, 781-783
     serodiagnosis, 55, 57*t*, 58, 63, 117, 758
          non-treponemal, 784-785
          treponemal, 785-786
     subspecies,
          endemicum, 780*t*
          pallidum, 780*t*
          pertenue, 780*t*
Treponema pectinovorum, 790
Treponema phagedenis, 783, 791
Treponema refringens, 783, 791
Treponema socranskii, 790
Treponema vincentii,
     general, 790-791
     methylene blue stain, 2
Tropheryma whippelii,

[Tropheryma whippelii]
    16S rRNA gene, 118-120
    clinical aspects, 385
    epidemiology, 387
    general, 96, 378
    molecular diagnostics, 411
    Whipple's disease, 118
Tsukamurella,
    acid-fast, 3
    applied systematics, 348*f*
    clinical aspects, 385
Tuberculosis (*see* Mycobacterium tuberculosis)
Turicella otitidis,
    antibiotic susceptibility, 366
    applied systematics, 348*f*, 349*f*
    general, 343*t*
TWAR agent (*see* Chlamydia pneumoniae)
Typhoid fever (*see* Salmonella serotype Typhi)
Typing,
    AFLP analysis, 136-137
    AP-PCR, 135, 475, 665
    bacteriocin, 475
    bacteriophage, 475
    biotyping, 133, 475
    colicin typing, 133
    definition of typeability, 130
    discriminatory power, 130
    epidemiological concordance, 131
    ERIC-PCR, 242, 243*f*, 475, 665
    general, 20-21, 125-140
    genome REA, 131*t*, 134
    mass spectrometry, 21
    multilocus enzyme electrophoresis, 127,
        135, 138, 242, 517
    multilocus sequence typing, 135, 138,
        517
    multi-state variables, 18
    nucleotide sequencing, 131*t*
    O typing, 475
    passive hemagglutination, 475
    phage typing, 133
    plasmid analysis, 133-134, 242, 475
    pneumococcal, 2
    protein electrophoresis, 133, 242
    pulsed field gel electrophoresis,
        general, 134-136, 138-139, 140*f*,
        242, 475, 665
        restriction enzymes, 132
    random amplified polymorphic DNA,
        127, 131*t*, 135-136

[Typing]
    repetitive element PCR, 136
    reproducibility, 130
    ribotyping, 134-135, 242, 475
    serotyping, 133, 475
    single locus PCR, 137
    Southern blot RFLP, 134-135
    stability, 130
    Western blotting, 133

Unitage, 212
Universal precautions, 35, 39
Ureaplasma urealyticum,
    clinical aspects, 864
    culture, 882-883
    epidemiology, 866-867
    immunology of infection, 872
    laboratory features, 869
    microscopy, 882
    molecular diagnostics, 883
    pathogenesis, 869
    serodiagnosis, 883
Urine,
    quantitative culture, 48
    specimen collection, 36
    specimen transport, 40

Vagococcus,
    historical aspects, 258
    laboratory features, 306, 307*t*
    staining, 3
Veillonella,
    antibiotic susceptibility, 738
    applied systematics, 708*t*
    Gram stain, 722, 727
    laboratory features, 722, 729*f*, 735
Verotoxin assay,
    general, 469
    toxin variants, 469
Verruga peruana (*see* Bartonella bacilliformis)
Vibrio alginolyticus, 426*f*, 436
Vibrio carchariae, 437
Vibrio cholerae,
    antibiotic resistance, 430*t*
    applied systematics, 426*t*
    classic O1, 453, 471
    clinical aspects, 436-437
    cholera toxin (choleragen), 452-453
    El Tor O1, 453, 471
    epidemiology, 442

[Vibrio cholerae]
    immunology of infection, 457
    laboratory features, 465, 471-472
    O serotypes, 453
    pathogenesis, 452-453
    selective culture, 465
    serodiagnosis, 57*t*, 474, 596
    specimen transport, 41
    string test, 471
    susceptibility testing, 162*t*, 481
    typing, 477
Vibrio cincinnatiensis, 426*f*, 436
Vibrio damsela, 426*f*, 436
Vibrio fluvialis, 426*f*, 436
Vibrio furnissii, 426*f*, 436
Vibrio harveyii, 426*f*
Vibrio hollisae, 426*f*, 436, 454
Vibrio metschnikovii, 426*f*, 453
Vibrio mimicus, 426*f*, 436, 453-454
Vibrio parahaemolyticus,
    clinical aspects, 437
    laboratory features, 454, 481
    pathogenesis, 454
    typing, 138
Vibrio vulnificus,
    clinical aspects, 436
    general, 426*f*, 453-454, 481
Viridans streptococci (*see* Streptococcus)
VISA (*see* Staphylococcus aureus)
Voges-Proskauer test, 19

Wayson stain, 2
Weeksella virosa, 529*t*
Weil-Felix test, 57*t*, 837*t*
Weil's syndrome (*see* Leptospira)
Western blotting (*see* Immunoblotting)
Whipple's disease (*see* Tropheryma whippelii)
Whooping cough (*see* Bordetella pertussis)
Widal test, 57*t*
Wolbachia, 824*f*, 826*f*
Wolinella, 708*t*, 715, 722
Workload, 212

Xenopsylla, 827
Xylose-Lysine-Deoxycholate agar, 462*t*, 463*t*

Yersinia,
    historical background, 424
    intrinsic resistance, 183*t*
    susceptibility testing, 481

Yersinia bercovieri, 424
Yersinia enterocolitica,
    applied systematics, 425*f*, 426*f*, 590
    CIN medium, 464, 470
    clinical aspects, 434
    cold enrichment, 46, 464
    epidemiology, 442
    historical background, 424
    immunology of infection, 457
    laboratory features, 464, 470-471
    pathogenesis, 450-451
    serodiagnosis, 57*t*, 473-474, 596
    specimen transport, 41
    susceptibility testing, 481
Yersinia frederiksenii, 425*f*, 426*f*
Yersinia kristensenii, 425*f*, 426*f*
Yersinia moelleretii, 425*f*, 426*f*
Yersinia pestis,
    clinical aspects, 585-586
    epidemiology, 588-589, 589*f*
    historical background, 424, 582-583
    immunology of infection, 595
    laboratory features, 592, 596-597
    pathogenesis, 592-594
    serodiagnosis, 57*t*, 597
    susceptibility testing, 598
    Wayson stain, 2
Yersinia pseudotuberculosis,
    applied systematics, 425*f*, 426*f*, 592
    clinical aspects, 434
    epidemiology, 442
    laboratory features, 464, 471
Yersiniosis (*see* Yersinia)
Yokenella,
    clinical aspects, 436
    general, 425*f*, 427*f*

Ziehl-Neelsen,
    actinomycetes, 390
    general, 15, 26, 387
    mycobacteria,
        sensitivity of, 395
        specificity of, 395-396
Zoonosis, 581

ISBN 0-8247-0589-0